国际经典内科学教科书

第10版
Cecil Essentials of Medicine
希氏内科学精要
中英双语版

原　著　**Edward J. Wing, MD, FACP, FIDSA**
Former Dean of Medicine and Biological Sciences
Professor of Medicine
Warren Alpert Medical School of Brown University, Providence, Rhode Island

Fred J. Schiffman, MD, MACP
Sigal Family Professor of Humanistic Medicine
Vice Chair, Department of Medicine
Warren Alpert Medical School of Brown University, Providence, Rhode Island

中英双语版　编辑委员会　主任委员　王　辰

—— 第10分册 ——

神经疾病·老年医学·缓和医疗·酒精和物质使用

主　译　彭　斌　王伊龙　李小鹰　宁晓红　郝　伟

北京大学医学出版社

XISHI NEIKEXUE JINGYAO（DI 10 BAN） DI 10 FENCE　SHENJING JIBING・LAONIAN YIXUE・HUANHE YILIAO・JIUJING HE WUZHI SHIYONG（ZHONGYING SHUANGYU BAN）

图书在版编目（CIP）数据

希氏内科学精要：第10版．第10分册，神经疾病・老年医学・缓和医疗・酒精和物质使用：汉、英 /（美）爱德华・温（Edward J. Wing），（美）弗雷德・谢夫曼（Fred J. Schiffman）原著；彭斌等主译．－－ 北京：北京大学医学出版社，2024．11．－－ ISBN 978-7-5659-3271-7

Ⅰ. R5

中国国家版本馆 CIP 数据核字第 20241E8E33 号

北京市版权局著作权合同登记号：图字：01-2024-4518

Elsevier (Singapore) Pte Ltd.
3 Killiney Road, #08-01 Winsland House I, Singapore 239519
Tel: (65) 6349-0200; Fax: (65) 6733-1817

Cecil Essentials of Medicine, Tenth Edition
Copyright © 2022 by Elsevier, Inc. All rights are reserved, including those for text and data mining, AI training, and similar technologies.
Publisher's note: Elsevier takes a neutral position with respect to territorial disputes or jurisdictional claims in its published content, including in maps and institutional affiliations.
Previous editions copyrighted 2016, 2010, 2007, 2004, 2001, 1997, 1993, 1990, and 1986.
ISBN-13: 978-0-323-72271-1

This translation of Cecil Essentials of Medicine, Tenth Edition by Edward J. Wing and Fred J. Schiffman was undertaken by Peking University Medical Press and is published by arrangement with Elsevier (Singapore) Pte Ltd.
Cecil Essentials of Medicine, Tenth Edition by Edward J. Wing and Fred J. Schiffman 由北京大学医学出版社进行翻译，并根据北京大学医学出版社与爱思唯尔（新加坡）私人有限公司的协议约定出版。
《希氏内科学精要（第10版）第10分册　神经疾病・老年医学・缓和医疗・酒精和物质使用（中英双语版）》（彭斌　王伊龙　李小鹰　宁晓红　郝伟　主译）
ISBN: 978-7-5659-3271-7
Copyright © 2024 by Elsevier (Singapore) Pte Ltd. and Peking University Medical Press.
All rights reserved. No part of this publication may be reproduced or transmitted in any form or by any means, electronic or mechanical, including photocopying, recording, or any information storage and retrieval system, without permission in writing from Elsevier (Singapore) Pte Ltd. and Peking University Medical Press.

注　意

本译本由北京大学医学出版社独立完成。相关从业及研究人员必须凭借其自身经验和知识对文中描述的信息数据、方法策略、搭配组合、实验操作进行评估和使用。由于医学科学发展迅速，临床诊断和给药剂量尤其需要经过独立验证。在法律允许的最大范围内，爱思唯尔、译文的原文作者、原文编辑及原文内容提供者均不对译文或因产品责任、疏忽或其他操作造成的人身及（或）财产伤害及（或）损失承担责任，亦不对由于使用文中提到的方法、产品、说明或思想而导致的人身及（或）财产伤害及（或）损失承担责任。

Published in China by Peking University Medical Press under special arrangement with Elsevier (Singapore) Pte Ltd. This edition is authorized for sale in the People's Republic of China only, excluding Hong Kong SAR, Macau SAR and Taiwan. Unauthorized export of this edition is a violation of the contract.

希氏内科学精要（第 10 版）　第 10 分册　神经疾病・老年医学・缓和医疗・酒精和物质使用（中英双语版）

主　　译：彭　斌　王伊龙　李小鹰　宁晓红　郝　伟

出版发行：北京大学医学出版社

地　　址：（100191）北京市海淀区学院路 38 号　北京大学医学部院内

电　　话：发行部 010-82802230；图书邮购 010-82802495

网　　址：http://www.pumpress.com.cn

E-mail：booksale@bjmu.edu.cn

印　　刷：北京信彩瑞禾印刷厂

经　　销：新华书店

策划编辑：高　瑾

责任编辑：畅晓燕　高　瑾　梁　洁　　责任校对：靳新强　　责任印制：李　啸

开　　本：889 mm×1194 mm　1/16　　印张：26.5　　字数：990 千字

版　　次：2024 年 11 月第 1 版　2024 年 11 月第 1 次印刷

书　　号：ISBN 978-7-5659-3271-7

定　　价：180.00 元

版权所有，违者必究

（凡属质量问题请与本社发行部联系退换）

中英双语版 编辑委员会

主任委员

王　辰

委　员（按姓氏笔画排序）

王　洁	王伊龙	王建祥	巴　一	代华平	宁　光	宁晓红	朱　兰
任景怡	刘海鹰	李小鹰	李梦涛	李雪梅	杨爱明	张福杰	郑金刚
房静远	赵　晶	赵明辉	郝　伟	姜　辉	栗占国	贾继东	夏维波
黄　慧	黄晓军	曹　彬	彭　斌	潘　慧			

第1分册　内科学概论·呼吸与危重症医学·术前和术后照护

　　　　　主译　王　辰　代华平　赵　晶　黄　慧

第2分册　心血管疾病

　　　　　主译　郑金刚　任景怡

第3分册　肾脏疾病

　　　　　主译　李雪梅　赵明辉

第4分册　胃肠疾病·肝脏与胆道系统疾病

　　　　　主译　房静远　杨爱明　贾继东

第5分册　血液疾病

　　　　　主译　黄晓军　王建祥

第6分册　肿瘤疾病

　　　　　主译　王　洁　巴　一

第7分册　内分泌疾病与代谢疾病·女性健康·男性健康·骨与骨矿物质代谢疾病

　　　　　主译　宁　光　朱　兰　姜　辉　夏维波　潘　慧

第8分册　肌肉骨骼与结缔组织疾病

　　　　　主译　栗占国　李梦涛

第9分册　感染性疾病

　　　　　主译　刘海鹰　张福杰　曹　彬

第10分册　神经疾病·老年医学·缓和医疗·酒精和物质使用

　　　　　主译　彭　斌　王伊龙　李小鹰　宁晓红　郝　伟

医学名词审定指导

任慧玲　李晓瑛　冀玉静　张燕舞　李军莲

中英双语版 序言

让我国医学生与国际医学生站在同一起跑线上的首要之事，是为其提供具有世界先进水平的标准教材。我们应争取使每一位医学生都能接触到内容经典、充分代表现代医学水平的国际权威原文教材并力求准确翻译，提供原文与中文双语对照版本，使医学生和医生在学习中形成双语医学词语、概念、概念间逻辑及由此构成的医学知识体系。在这样的思想驱动下，国际经典内科学教科书《希氏内科学精要（第10版）》中英双语版应运而生。

《希氏内科学》原著以其论述严谨准确、系统全面，被誉为"标准的内科学参考书"。自1927年首次出版以来，在内科学领域渐享世界级声誉，成为全球众多优秀医学院校，包括哈佛医学院、斯坦福大学医学院、约翰斯·霍普金斯大学医学院、牛津大学医学部、剑桥大学医学院、墨尔本大学医学院、新加坡国立大学医学院及多伦多大学医学院等普遍采用的内科学参考书。首版《希氏内科学精要》则诞生于1986年，旨在凝炼其全本的精华和要点，以最为简洁明确的方式向以医学生为主体的医学界精辟传达《希氏内科学》的核心信息，包括书中所体现出的人文精神。此后，每版精要本都力求凝炼地反映当时最新医学成果和医疗实践指南，愈来愈成为各国医学生、住院医师、专培医师及教师学习和传授内科学的主要教本，在世界医学教材体系中居引领地位。《希氏内科学》和《希氏内科学精要》两个版本不仅在英语国家被广泛使用，更被翻译为葡萄牙语、西班牙语、希腊语、意大利语、日语、简体中文版，为全球医学界广泛采用。

中国的医学生、住院医师、专培医师需要培养国际专业信息获取能力。将精要本原文引进并准确翻译，以中英文对照的形式呈现，便于读者进行双语对照阅读和学习，使之在学习理解国际标准医学内容的同时，学习好中英文医学词语，为国际医学交流打好基础。相信此举对于提高我国的医学教育水平，培养国际型医学人才至为有益。

《希氏内科学精要》精练地涵盖了内科学的所有主要领域，包括心血管疾病、呼吸疾病与危重症、消化疾病、肾脏疾病、内分泌和代谢疾病、风湿疾病、血液疾病、肿瘤、感染性疾病、神经与老年疾病等，构建了较为系统的知识体系。在翻译引进过程中，我们遵循将相关内容集中的原则，将原书按系统器官拆分为十个分册，使其更具有专科阅读的对应性，以更加灵活轻便的形式为读者提供多样化的阅读选择。

为确保译文质量，我们在译者遴选上采取了严谨的标准。从《希氏内科学（第26版）》翻译团队中择优选取责任心强、译文优质的译者，同时吸纳了临床医学专业"101"计划核心教材的编者团队。每个分册均由主译专家带领各自译者团队完成翻译、审校、交叉互审、通审四级审校工作。这些译者具备扎实的英语与专业能力，他们在翻译过程中，深入理解原文，准确阐述作者思想，并多角度审视译文的准确性、流畅性与风格一致性，确保译文的忠实性、规范性与可读性，在不同的语言和文化间架起坚实的桥梁。尤其值得称赞的是，对原著中疏漏或不够完善之处，译文中以"译者注"的形式加以适当解释和说明，使译文内容在忠实于原著的基础上更为准确。

本书读者定位于具有一定学习能力和基础的高等医学院校医学专业8年制、5年制学生以及相关医学专业人员，可作为医务人员的内科学参考书、住院医师规范化培训和专科医师规范化培训辅导教材、研究生入学考试辅导教材、内科学教师参考书、内科学各专科医师复习回顾其他专科知识的重要读本。

呼吸与危重症医学教授
中国医学科学院院长
北京协和医学院校长
2024年11月

对学习者教科书重要。
对学医者内科学重要。
世界上的内科学教科书，
首推《希氏内科学精要》。

中文是中国医生主要执业用语。
英文是国际医学交流的主要文字。
学习医学，当以双语对应阅读为好。
如此，可获纵横国际之效。

本书力求有助于此。

In Memoriam

Thomas E. Andreoli, MD

Dr. Thomas Andreoli, along with Drs. Lloyd Hollingsworth (Holly) Smith, Jr., Fred Plum, and Charles C.J. Carpenter, was one of the four founding editors of *Cecil Essentials of Medicine*. He served as editor for editions one through eight before he passed away on April 14, 2009. Dr. Andreoli was born in the Bronx, New York, in 1935, attended Catholic primary and high schools, and graduated from St. Vincent College and the Georgetown School of Medicine. He trained as a resident at Duke University under legendary Chair of Medicine Dr. Eugene Stead, who recognized him as a brilliant physician and scientist and encouraged his research career. Dr. Andreoli received his research training at the NIH and then in the laboratory of Dr. Tosteson at Duke. His research focused on the biochemical and biophysical properties of renal tubular cell membranes and their role in water and electrolyte transport. He made fundamental discoveries on the normal renal physiology, illuminating the way to subsequent work by many others on renal health and disease. His research was recognized with numerous awards and election to honorific societies both in the United States and in Europe. Dr. Andreoli also served as editor of *The American Journal of Physiology: Renal Physiology* and Editor in Chief of *Kidney International*.

Tom's national prominence and leadership qualities were recognized early in his career when he became head of Nephrology at the University of Alabama in Birmingham. There he helped faculty and trainees develop outstanding research, organized clinical services, and created a hemodialysis program to build one of the outstanding Divisions of Nephrology in the country. In 1979, Dr. Andreoli was appointed Chair of the Department of Internal Medicine at the University of Texas, Houston, where he assembled an outstanding faculty focused on research, clinical care, and teaching. In 1988, he accepted the position as Chairman of Internal Medicine at the University of Arkansas School of Medicine, a position he held until his death. There he again assembled a distinguished faculty who were outstanding researchers but also dedicated to outstanding clinical care and teaching. Morning report and clinical rounds with Dr. Andreoli were rigorous and riveting, focusing on the individual patient, not only their diagnoses and treatment but also on each patient's personal concerns and well-being. Dr. Andreoli was revered by medical students, his house staff, faculty, and colleagues, and I (EJW) personally can attest to what he regarded as his most cherished role—the mentorship and education of the next generation of physicians.

One of Dr. Andreoli's great interests was *Cecil Essentials of Medicine*, for which he was the editor/chief editor for eight of its ten editions, an interest that reflected his commitment to the education of students, house staff, and other physicians in the "essentials" of Internal Medicine.

Dr. Andreoli was devoted to his family. He was married to Elizabeth Berglund Andreoli from 1987 until his death. He was previously married to Dr. Kathleen Gainor Andreoli, mother of his three children and their ten grandchildren. Being of Italian ancestry and from Bronx, New York, it is not surprising that Dr. Andreoli was a passionate fan of the New York Yankees, Italian opera, which he could sing in Italian, and Frank Sinatra.

Dr. Andreoli's legacy lives on in his numerous previous students, house staff, colleagues, and in this book.

缅 怀

托马斯·安德里奥利博士

托马斯·安德里奥利（Thomas E. Andreoli）博士携手李奥德·霍灵斯沃斯·史密斯［Lloyd Hollingsworth（Holly）Smith］博士、弗雷德·普拉姆（Fred Plum）博士和查尔斯·卡彭特（Charles C.J. Carpenter）博士同为《希氏内科学精要》的创始编者。他在2009年4月14日去世前，曾担任该书第1至第8版的编者。安德里奥利博士于1935年出生于美国纽约布朗克斯区，就读于天主教小学和中学，后毕业于圣文森特学院和乔治城大学医学院。他在杜克大学医学院接受住院医师培训期间师从著名内科主任尤金·斯特德（Eugene Stead）博士，后者将其视为杰出的医生和科学家，并鼓励他投身科研事业。安德里奥利博士在美国国立卫生研究院接受科研训练后，前往杜克大学托斯特森（Tosteson）博士的实验室继续深造。他重点研究肾小管细胞膜的生化和生物物理特性及其在水和电解质转运中所发挥的作用。他在正常肾脏生理学方面的重要发现为后续关于肾脏健康和疾病的研究铺平了道路。安德里奥利博士的研究工作荣获多个学术奖项，并入选美国和欧洲的多个荣誉学会。他还担任《美国生理学杂志：肾脏生理学篇》（The American Journal of Physiology：Renal Physiology）的编辑以及《国际肾脏杂志》（Kidney International）的主编。

安德里奥利博士担任阿拉巴马大学伯明翰分校肾脏病学系主任后不久，即因其杰出领导力而赢得全美业内声誉。他帮助本校师生们取得科研突破，负责临床业务的组织实施，并因开创血液透析业务而使该科跻身全美顶级肾脏内科之列。1979年，安德里奥利博士被任命为得克萨斯大学休斯敦分校内科学系主任，他在该系组建了一支科研、临床诊疗和教学并重的优秀教职团队。自1988年起，他担任阿肯色大学医学院内科学系主任，直至辞世。在这里他再次组建了一支卓越的教职团队，他们不仅科研工作出色，临床诊疗和教学工作也出类拔萃。安德里奥利博士带领的晨会报告和查房非常严谨而引人入胜，不仅尽心竭力于每位患者的诊断和治疗，还关注到他们每个人的个体情况和福祉。安德里奥利博士深受医学生、住院医师、教职人员和同事的崇敬，我（EJW）可以证明，他最珍视的角色当属培养和教育下一代医生。

安德里奥利博士对《希氏内科学精要》倾注了满腔热忱，先后担任了该书10版中8版的编者/主编，践行他为医学生、住院医师和其他各科医生们传授内科学"精要"的承诺。

安德里奥利博士高度重视家庭。他与第二任妻子伊丽莎白·伯格兰德·安德里奥利（Elizabeth Berglund Andreoli）的婚姻从1987年延续到辞世。他与第一任妻子凯瑟琳·盖娜·安德里奥利（Kathleen Gainor Andreoli）博士育有三个子女和十个孙辈。作为意大利裔和纽约布朗克斯人，安德里奥利博士是纽约洋基队、意大利歌剧（他能用意大利语演唱）和美国著名歌手、演员、主持人弗兰克·辛纳屈（Frank Sinatra）的忠实拥趸。安德里奥利博士将永远被他的众多学生、住院医师和同事怀念，并因本书而流芳百世。

In Memoriam

Charles C.J. Carpenter, MD

Dr. Charles C.J. Carpenter joined Drs. Thomas Andreoli, Lloyd Hollingsworth Smith, Jr., and Fred Plum as a founder of *Cecil Essentials of Medicine.* He served as editor for seven editions and was followed in that role by Dr. Ivor Benjamin and then Dr. Edward Wing. Sadly, Chuck passed away on March 19, 2020, surrounded by his wife and children. He was Professor Emeritus of Medicine at The Warren Alpert Medical School of Brown University and Physician-in-Chief Emeritus at The Miriam Hospital.

Chuck was born in Savannah, Georgia, on January 5, 1931. He attended college at Princeton and medical school at Johns Hopkins where he also did his house staff training, including chief residency, and then joined the Johns Hopkins faculty. With his young family, he travelled to Calcutta, India, where he carried out landmark studies for the treatment of cholera.

Before coming to Brown in 1986, he was Chair of Medicine at Baltimore City Hospital and Case Western Reserve University.

His contributions to medical science and clinical care were many. While in Calcutta, using basic scientific evidence coupled with practical approaches, Dr. Carpenter developed "oral rehydration therapy" to address the cholera epidemic there. This treatment has saved millions of lives. While at Case, one of his innovations was to develop the nation's first Division of Geographic Medicine because of his strong belief that all physicians should be medical citizens of the world. In 1987, as he became deeply involved in the clinical management of persons living with HIV, he initiated a unique program in which Brown University faculty and trainees assumed responsibility for all HIV care in the Rhode Island State prison system.

Dr. Carpenter served as Chairman of the American Board of Internal Medicine and President of the Association of American Physicians. He has been a member of the NIH AIDS Executive Committee, the National Advisory Allergy and Infectious Diseases Council, and the USPHS AIDS Task Force. He was Chair of the Antiretroviral Treatment Panel of the International AIDS Society-USA and authored their recommendations on antiretroviral treatment. He also served as Chair of the Treatment Committee to evaluate the President's Emergency Plan for HIV/AIDS Relief. He became the director of the Brown University International Health Institute and the director of the Lifespan/Brown Center for AIDS Research with several Boston hospitals.

Throughout his career, Dr. Carpenter was the recipient of many international, national, and regional awards, accepting each with characteristic humility. With both small and large groups of learners, Chuck made certain that every member of his team was well educated, and each felt that they contributed to the well-being of their patients. His ability to sit calmly at the bedside, hold the patient's hand, comfort them, and listen in a genuinely focused way, influenced so many physicians. He was truly grateful for the opportunity to care for those less fortunate than he, and the feeling of being privileged to do so was clearly transmitted to all. Dr. Carpenter was a wonderful blend of profound compassion combined with the adherence to scholarship and teaching. Sir William Osler wrote that physicians should "Do the kind thing and do it first." Chuck lived by this precept. Vigor and insight characterized his approach to clinical and ethical challenges, always with younger colleagues at his side. In a recent tribute to him, many emphasized that Dr. Carpenter dedicated his life to his patients, many of whom were the most vulnerable members of society. We hope that we will have some of his strength and use his example as our compass as we are challenged to reduce suffering and improve the health of all for whom we are responsible.

He is survived by his wife of 61 years, Sally; three sons, Charles, Murray, and Andrew; and seven grandchildren.

缅 怀

查尔斯·卡彭特博士

查尔斯·卡彭特（Charles C.J. Carpenter）博士与托马斯·安德里奥利（Thomas E. Andreoli）博士、李奥德·霍灵斯沃斯·史密斯（Lloyd Hollingsworth Smith）博士和弗雷德·普拉姆（Fred Plum）博士共同开创了《希氏内科学精要》。他共担任了7版的编者，嗣后由艾弗·本杰明（Ivor Benjamin）博士和爱德华·温（Edward Wing）博士接任。查尔斯·卡彭特博士于2020年3月19日在妻子和子女们的陪伴下辞世。他曾担任布朗大学沃伦·阿尔珀特医学院的内科学系名誉教授和米里亚姆医院的名誉主任医师。

查尔斯·卡彭特博士于1931年1月5日出生于美国佐治亚州萨凡纳市。他在普林斯顿大学获得学士学位后进入约翰斯·霍普金斯大学医学院，并完成了包括住院总医师在内的住院医师培训，随后加入了约翰斯·霍普金斯大学的教职团队。他曾携妻子和年幼的孩子前往印度加尔各答，在当地对霍乱的治疗进行了具有里程碑意义的研究工作。

在1986年入职布朗大学之前，他曾担任巴尔的摩市医院和凯斯西储大学医学院的内科学主任。

他在医学科学研究和临床诊疗领域建树颇多。在加尔各答期间，基于基础科学证据及临床实践，查尔斯·卡彭特博士开创了"口服补液疗法"以遏制当地的霍乱疫情。这一疗法拯救了数百万人的生命。秉承医生无国界的世界公民理念，他在凯斯西储大学做了一项开创性工作，建立了美国首个地缘医学部（研究地理环境因素对人体健康和疾病影响的学科）。1987年，他深度参与人类免疫缺陷病毒（HIV）携带者的临床管理，并发起了一个独特的项目——由布朗大学教职团队和医学生们承担罗德岛州监狱系统内所有艾滋病相关诊疗工作。

查尔斯·卡彭特博士曾担任美国内科医师委员会主席和美国医师协会主席。他曾是美国国立卫生研究院艾滋病行政委员会、美国国家过敏与传染病咨询委员会以及公共卫生服务部艾滋病工作组的成员。他还曾担任国际艾滋病学会-美国分会抗逆转录病毒治疗组主席，并撰写了抗逆转录病毒治疗建议。他还担任过艾滋病治疗委员会主席，该委员会负责评估美国总统防治艾滋病紧急救援计划；曾担任布朗大学国际健康研究所所长，以及大学与多家波士顿当地医院合办的生命周期/布朗大学艾滋病研究中心主任。

查尔斯·卡彭特博士在职业生涯中获得过诸多国际性、全美和地区性奖项，同时展现其谦逊品格。无论学员人数多寡，查尔斯·卡彭特博士都会确保人人都能受到良好教育，并让他们感到自己也对患者的健康做出了贡献。他能够安静地坐在病床边，握住患者的手，安慰他们，并全神贯注地听取患者倾诉，这一举动深深地感染了许多医生。他十分珍视诊治不幸染病者的机会，并且能够将这种殊荣感传递给所有人。查尔斯·卡彭特博士完美地融汇了对患者的宅心仁厚与对学术和教学的坚守。威廉·奥斯勒（William Osler）爵士曾写道，医生应该"行善事，为人先"，而这正是查尔斯·卡彭特博士一生奉行的信条。他在面对临床和伦理挑战时充满活力和洞察力，始终重视提携年轻同事。许多人的悼词中都重点指出，查尔斯·卡彭特博士将毕生致力于患者福祉，其中许多人属于社会上最弱势群体。我们希望，在我们面临减少患者痛苦及改善其健康状况的挑战时，能够拥有他的力量，并以他为榜样获得指引。

查尔斯·卡彭特博士与妻子萨丽（Sally）共度了61年的婚姻时光，育有查尔斯（Charles）、穆雷（Murray）和安德鲁（Andrew）三子以及七个孙辈。

ABOUT THE EDITORS

Dr. Edward J. Wing was an editor of *Cecil Essentials of Medicine*, editions 8 and 9, and is the lead editor of edition 10. He graduated from Williams College in 1967 and from the Harvard Medical School in 1971. He was a resident in Internal Medicine at the Peter Bent Brigham and completed an Infectious Diseases Fellowship at Stanford University. Joining the faculty at the University of Pittsburgh in 1975, he focused his NIH-funded research on mechanisms of cell-mediated immunity as well as various clinical aspects of Infectious Diseases. From 1990 to 1998, the University and UPMC appointed him as Physician-in-Chief at Montefiore Hospital, then Chief of Infectious Diseases, and finally Interim Chair of Medicine.

In 1998, Dr. Wing became Chair of Medicine at Brown University (1998–2008) where he consolidated the department across hospitals, practice plans, and training programs. As Dean of Medicine and Biological Sciences at Brown University (2008–2013) he strengthened ties with affiliated hospitals (Lifespan and Care New England), increased research, and oversaw the construction of a new medical school building. International exchange programs with medical schools in Kenya, the Dominican Republic, and Haiti were established during his years as chairman and dean. Dr. Wing has cared for patients with HIV since the beginning of the epidemic in outpatient clinics. He continues to be active in research, clinical care, and teaching.

Dr. Fred J. Schiffman, who along with Dr. Edward Wing is editor of *Cecil Essentials of Medicine,* 10th edition, attended Wagner College and then the New York University School of Medicine, from which he graduated in 1973. He performed his early house staff training at Yale-New Haven Hospital and then spent two years at the National Cancer Institute. He returned to Yale as Chief Medical Resident followed by a hematology fellowship. He became Medical Director of Yale's Primary Care Center before coming to Brown University in 1983, where he has been a leader in the medical residency program as well as Associate Physician-in-Chief at The Miriam Hospital.

Dr. Schiffman holds The Sigal Family Professorship in Humanistic Medicine at The Warren Alpert Medical School of Brown University. His scholarly interests include the structure and function of the human spleen and the intersection of the arts and medical care. He has directed or championed many projects and programs, including those that encourage and reinforce wellness and resilience in patients, families, and caregivers. He began a novel program that places medical students and physicians with other nonmedical professionals as they share in the viewing of works of art in the Museum of the Rhode Island School of Design. Dr. Schiffman recently led a Brown University edX course entitled, "Artful Medicine: Art's Power to Enrich Patient Care," with worldwide participation. Dr. Schiffman has also edited texts on hematologic pathophysiology, consultative hematology, and the anemias.

原著主编

爱德华·温（Edward J. Wing）博士是《希氏内科学精要》第 8 版和第 9 版的编者，以及第 10 版的主编。他先后于 1967 年和 1971 年毕业于威廉姆斯学院和哈佛医学院。他曾在彼得·本特·布里格姆医院任内科住院医师，后在斯坦福大学完成了传染病学的专科医师（Fellowship）课程。自 1975 年加入匹兹堡大学医学院以来，他通过美国国立卫生研究院资助的研究项目，探索细胞介导免疫的机制以及传染病学各领域的临床诊疗工作。1990—1998 年期间，他先后被匹兹堡大学及其医学中心任命为蒙特菲奥里医院的主任医师、传染病科主任，后担任内科临聘主任。

1998 年起，温博士担任布朗大学医学院的内科主任（1998—2008 年）。在此期间，他在不同医院、实践计划和培训项目间对内科进行整合。在担任布朗大学医学与生物科学院院长（2008—2013 年）期间，他加强了与各附属医院（Lifespan 医院和 Care New England 医院）间的联系，提升了科研工作的水准，并为医学院建成了一座新楼。在担任主任和院长期间，他还建立了与肯尼亚、多米尼加共和国和海地的医学院的国际交流项目。温博士自艾滋病流行初期便在门诊诊治艾滋病患者，并始终工作在科研、临床和教学一线。

弗雷德·谢夫曼（Fred J. Schiffman）博士与爱德华·温（Edward Wing）博士共同担任《希氏内科学精要》第 10 版的主编。他就读于瓦格纳学院，随后进入纽约大学医学院，并于 1973 年毕业。他在耶鲁大学附属纽黑文医院接受早期住院医师培训，随后在美国国家癌症研究所工作了两年。回到耶鲁大学后，他担任住院总医师，然后完成了血液学专科医师课程，随后成为耶鲁初级保健中心医学主任。他于 1983 年入职布朗大学，领导医学住院医师项目并担任米里亚姆医院的副主任医师。

谢夫曼博士担任布朗大学沃伦·阿尔珀特医学院人文医学系的西格尔家庭医学教授。他的学术兴趣涵盖人体脾脏的结构和功能，以及艺术与医疗的交叉融合。他主持或参与了许多项目和计划，其中包括许多旨在鼓励和加强患者、家人和医护人员的福祉与康复能力的项目。他所创办的一个新项目可以让医学生和医生与其他非医学专业人士一起，共同欣赏罗德岛设计学院博物馆的艺术作品。谢夫曼博士近期还主持了布朗大学名为"艺术与医学：艺术赋能患者照护"的 edX 课程，此课程的参与者来自全球多个国家。谢夫曼博士还出版了有关血液病理生理学、血液科会诊和贫血的著作。

原著者名单

Jinnette Dawn Abbott, MD
Rajiv Agarwal, MD
Marwa Al-Badri, MD
Hyeon-Ju Ryoo Ali, MD
Jason M. Aliotta, MD
Khaldoun Almhanna, MD, MPH
Mohanad T. Al-Qaisi, MD
Zuhal Arzomand, MD
Akwi W. Asombang, MD, MPH
Su N. Aung, MD, MPH
Christopher G. Azzoli, MD
Christina Bandera, MD
Debasree Banerjee, MD
Mashal Batheja, MD
Jeffrey J. Bazarian, MD, MPH
Selim R. Benbadis, MD
Ivor J. Benjamin, MD, FAHA, FACC
Eric Benoit, MD
Marcie G. Berger, MD
Clemens Bergwitz, MD
Nancy Berliner, MD
Jeffrey S. Berns, MD
Pooja Bhadbhade, DO
Ratna Bhavaraju-Sanka, MD
Tanmayee Bichile, MD
Ariel E. Birnbaum, MD
Charles M. Bliss, Jr., MD
Andrew S. Blum, MD, PhD
Bryan J. Bonder, MD
Russell Bratman, MD
Glenn D. Braunstein, MD
Alma M. Guerrero Bready, MD
Richard Bungiro, PhD
Anna Marie Burgner, MD, MEHP
Jonathan Cahill, MD
Andrew Canakis, DO
Benedito A. Carneiro, MD, MS
Brian Casserly, MD
Abdullah Chahin, MD, MA, MSc
Philip A. Chan, MD
Kimberle Chapin, MD
William P. Cheshire, Jr., MD
Waihong Chung, MD, PhD
Emma Ciafaloni, MD

Joaquin E. Cigarroa, MD
Michael P. Cinquegrani, MD
Andreea Coca, MD, MPH
Harvey Jay Cohen, MD
Scott Cohen, MD, MPH
Beatrice P. Concepcion, MD, MS
Nathan T. Connell, MD, MPH
Maria Constantinou, MD
Roberto Cortez, MD
Timothy J. Counihan, MD, FRCPI
Anne Haney Cross, MD
Cheston B. Cunha, MD, FACP
Joanne S. Cunha, MD
Susan Cu-Uvin, MD
Noura M. Dabbouseh, MD
Kwame Dapaah-Afriyie, MD, MBA
Erin M. Denney-Koelsch, MD
Andre De Souza, MD
An S. De Vriese, MD, PhD
Neal D. Dharmadhikari, MD
Leah Dickstein, MD
Don Dizon, MD, FACP, FASCO
Robyn T. Domsic, MD, MPH
Kim A. Eagle, MD
Michael G. Earing, MD
Pamela Egan, MD
Wafik S. El-Deiry, MD, PhD, FACP
Mitchell S. V. Elkind, MD, MS
Tarra B. Evans, MD
Michael B. Fallon, MD
Dimitrios Farmakiotis, MD
Francis A. Farraye, MD
Ronan Farrell, MD
Panayotis Fasseas, MD, FACC
Mary Anne Fenton, MD
Fernando C. Fervenza, MD, PhD
Sean Fine, MD
Arkadiy Finn, MD
Timothy Flanigan, MD
Brisas M. Flores, MD
Andrew E. Foderaro, MD
Theodore C. Friedman, MD, PhD
Joseph Metmowlee Garland, MD, AAHIVM

Eric J. Gartman, MD
Abdallah Geara, MD
Raul Macias Gil, MD
Timothy Gilligan, MD, FASCO
Michael Raymond Goggins, MB BCh BAO, MRCPI
Geetha Gopalakrishnan, MD
Vidya Gopinath, MD
Susan L. Greenspan, MD, FACP
Osama Hamdy, MD, PhD
Johanna Hamel, MD
Sajeev Handa, MD, SFHM
Mitchell T. Heflin, MD, MHS
Robert G. Holloway, MD, MPH
Christopher S. Huang, MD
Zilla Hussain, MD
T. Alp Ikizler, MD
Iris Isufi, MD
Carlayne E. Jackson, MD
Paul G. Jacob, MD, MPH
Matthew D. Jankowich, MD
Niels V. Johnsen, MD, MPH
Jessica E. Johnson, MD
Rayford R. June, MD
Tareq Kheirbek, MD, ScM, FACS
Alok A. Khorana, MD, FACP, FASCO
Sena Kilic, MD
David Kim, MD
James Kleczka, MD
James R. Klinger, MD
Patrick Koo, MD, ScM
Pooja Koolwal, MD
Mary P. Kotlarczyk, PhD
Nicole M. Kuderer, MD
Awewura Kwara, MD
Jennifer M. Kwon, MD, MPH
Richard A. Lange, MD, MBA
Jerome Larkin, MD
Alfred I. Lee, MD, PhD
Daniel J. Levine, MD
David E. Lewandowski, MD
Kelly V. Liang, MD, MS
Kimberly P. Liang, MD, MS
David R. Lichtenstein, MD

扫描二维码了解更多信息

Douglas W. Lienesch, MD
Geoffrey S.F. Ling, MD, PhD
Ester Little, MD, FACP
Yi Liu, MD
Nicole L. Lohr, MD, PhD
John R. Lonks, MD, FACP, FIDSA, FSHEA
Gary H. Lyman, MD, MPH
Jeffrey M. Lyness, MD
Shane Lyons, MD, MRCPI, MRCP(UK)
Diana Maas, MD
Talha A. Malik, MD, MSPH
Sonia Manocha, MD
Susan Manzi, MD, MPH
Frederick J. Marshall, MD
F. Dennis McCool, MD
Russell J. McCulloh, MD
Kelly McGarry, MD, FACP
Eavan Mc Govern, MD, PhD
Robin L. McKinney, MD
Anthony Mega, MD
Shivang Mehta, MD
Douglas F. Milam, MD
Maria D. Mileno, MD
Abhinav Kumar Misra, MBBS, MD
Orson W. Moe, MD
Niveditha Mohan, MBBS
Larry W. Moreland, MD
Alan R. Morrison, MD, PhD
Steven F. Moss, MD
Christopher J. Mullin, MD, MHS
Sinéad M. Murphy, MB, BCh, MD, FRCPI
Sagarika Nallu, MD, FAAP, FAAN, FAASM
Javier A. Neyra, MD, MSCS
Ghaith Noaiseh, MD

Thomas A. Ollila, MD
Steven M. Opal, MD
Biff F. Palmer, MD
Jen Jung Pan, MD, PhD
Anna Papazoglou, MD
Aric Parnes, MD
Nayan M. Patel, DO, MPH
Ari Pelcovits, MD
Mark A. Perazella, MD
Michael F. Picco, MD, PhD
Kate E. Powers, DO
Laura A. Previll, MD, MPH
Nilum Rajora, MD
Adolfo Ramirez-Zamora, MD
John Reagan, MD
Rebecca Reece, MD
Harlan Rich, MD, AGAF, FACP
Jennifer H. Richman, MD
Lisa R. Rogers, DO
Ralph Rogers, MD
Michal G. Rose, MD
James A. Roth, MD
Sharon Rounds, MD
Jason C. Rubenstein, MD
Abbas Rupawala, MD
Jenna Sarvaideo, DO
Ramesh Saxena, MD, PhD
Fred J. Schiffman, MD, MACP
Ruth B. Schneider, MD
Kristin A. Seaborg, MD
Anil Seetharam, MD
Stuart Seropian, MD
Jigme Michael Sethi, MD
Sanjeev Sethi, MD, PhD
Elizabeth Shane, MD
Esseim Sharma, MD

Shani Shastri, MD, MPH
Barry S. Shea, MD
Lauren Shevell, MD, MPH
Joseph A. Smith, Jr., MD
Robert J. Smith, MD
Davendra P.S. Sohal, MD, MPH
Christopher Song, MD, FACC
Thomas Sperry, MD
Jeffrey M. Statland, MD
Emily M. Stein, MD
Jennifer L. Strande, MD, PhD
Rochelle Strenger, MD
Thomas R. Talbot, MD, MPH
Christopher G. Tarolli, MD, MSEd
Yael Tarshish, MD
Pushpak Taunk, MD
Philip Tsoukas, MD
Allan R. Tunkel, MD, PhD
Jeffrey M. Turner, MD
Zoe G.S. Vazquez, MD
Stacie A. F. Vela, MD
Paul M. Vespa, MD, FCCM, FAAN, FANA, FNCS
Wanpen Vongpatanasin, MD
Marcella D. Walker, MD
Eunice S. Wang, MD
Sharmeel K. Wasan, MD
Thomas J. Weber, MD
Brandon J. Wilcoxson, MD
Edward J. Wing, MD, FACP, FIDSA
Ellice Wong, MD
John J. Wysolmerski, MD
Rayan Yousefzai, MD
Thomas R. Ziegler, MD
Rebecca Zon, MD

ACKNOWLEDGMENTS

Dr. Schiffman and I wish to thank first of all, the authors of the 128 chapters that make up the tenth edition of *Cecil Essentials of Medicine*. They have worked diligently to compose the material for each chapter and apply their mastery as they added the newest information, in clear language, to the text. Their efforts are apparent in the excellence of the book, and we are immensely grateful for their work. We wish to also thank Marybeth Thiel, Jennifer Ehlers, and Dan Fitzgerald from Elsevier who guided and supported our work as editors and whose expertise has made this volume possible. Finally, we are always thankful to our wives, Dr. Rena Wing and Ms. Gerri Schiffman, without whose love, support, and especially humor, this book would not have happened.

致 谢

谢夫曼博士和我首先要致谢《希氏内科学精要》第 10 版全书 128 章的各位作者。感谢他们精益求精地撰写每一章节，并运用其专业知识，以简明的语言将前沿资讯呈现在书中。正是他们的辛勤努力确保了本书的卓越地位，对他们唯有由衷的感激。我们还要感谢爱思唯尔出版集团的玛丽贝丝·蒂尔（Marybeth Thiel）、詹妮弗·埃勒斯（Jennifer Ehlers）和丹·菲茨杰拉德（Dan Fitzgerald），他们对本书的编辑工作给予了指导和支持，其专业水准保障了本书的完稿。最后，要特别感谢我们的妻子——蕾娜·温（Rena Wing）博士和盖瑞·谢夫曼（Gerri Schiffman）女士，对她们的爱和支持，特别是积极乐观的心态始终心存感激，她们为本书的圆满完成发挥了不可或缺的作用。

总目录

第 1 分册

第 1 篇　内科学概论　Introduction to Medicine
第 2 篇　呼吸与危重症医学　Pulmonary and Critical Care Medicine
第 3 篇　术前和术后照护　Preoperative and Postoperative Care

第 2 分册

心血管疾病　Cardiovascular Disease

第 3 分册

肾脏疾病　Renal Disease

第 4 分册

第 1 篇　胃肠疾病　Gastrointestinal Disease
第 2 篇　肝脏与胆道系统疾病　Diseases of the Liver and Biliary System

第 5 分册

血液疾病　Hematologic Disease

第 6 分册

肿瘤疾病　Oncologic Disease

第 7 分册

第 1 篇　内分泌疾病与代谢疾病　Endocrine Disease and Metabolic Disease
第 2 篇　女性健康　Women's Health
第 3 篇　男性健康　Men's Health
第 4 篇　骨与骨矿物质代谢疾病　Diseases of Bone and Bone Mineral Metabolism

第 8 分册

肌肉骨骼与结缔组织疾病　Musculoskeletal and Connective Tissue Disease

第 9 分册

感染性疾病　Infectious Disease

第 10 分册

第 1 篇　神经疾病　Neurologic Disease
第 2 篇　老年医学　Geriatrics
第 3 篇　缓和医疗　Palliative Care
第 4 篇　酒精和物质使用　Alcohol and Substance Use

第10分册

神经疾病·老年医学·缓和医疗·酒精和物质使用

第 10 分册译者名单

主　译

彭　斌　王伊龙　李小鹰　宁晓红　郝　伟

译　者（按姓氏笔画排序）

王伊龙	首都医科大学附属北京天坛医院	陈玮琪	首都医科大学附属北京天坛医院
王婷婷	首都医科大学附属北京天坛医院	陈奕奕	首都医科大学附属北京天坛医院
牛婧雯	中国医学科学院北京协和医院	范思远	中国医学科学院北京协和医院
龙　江	上海市精神卫生中心	林　楠	中国医学科学院北京协和医院
卢　强	中国医学科学院北京协和医院	周　雁	中国医学科学院北京协和医院
付治卿	中国人民解放军总医院第二医学中心	周梦圆	首都医科大学附属北京天坛医院
付瀚辉	中国医学科学院北京协和医院	赵一龙	首都医科大学附属北京天坛医院
宁晓红	中国医学科学院北京协和医院	赵梦西	首都医科大学附属北京天坛医院
朱以诚	中国医学科学院北京协和医院	郝　伟	中南大学湘雅二医院精神卫生研究所
朱亚辉	首都医科大学附属北京天坛医院	姜　南	中国医学科学院北京协和医院
向小军	中南大学湘雅二医院精神卫生研究所	洪月慧	中国医学科学院北京协和医院
刘　韵	首都医科大学附属北京天坛医院	姚　明	中国医学科学院北京协和医院
苏　宁	中国医学科学院北京协和医院	徐　丹	中国医学科学院北京协和医院
李小鹰	中国人民解放军总医院第二医学中心	高　颖	首都医科大学附属北京天坛医院
李雨贤	首都医科大学附属北京天坛医院	曹宇泽	中国医学科学院北京协和医院
李胜德	中国医学科学院北京协和医院	阎　格	中国医学科学院北京协和医学院
杨　沫	首都医科大学附属北京天坛医院	彭　斌	中国医学科学院北京协和医院
杨洵哲	中国医学科学院北京协和医院	韩　菲	中国医学科学院北京协和医院
杨营营	首都医科大学附属北京天坛医院	鲁晓春	中国人民解放军总医院第二医学中心
沈　航	中国医学科学院北京协和医院	谭　颖	中国医学科学院北京协和医院
沈东超	中国医学科学院北京协和医院	翟菲菲	中国医学科学院北京协和医院
张梦雨	中国医学科学院北京协和医院	戴晓艳	中国医学科学院北京协和医院
张梦原	中国医学科学院北京协和医院		

第 10 分册目录

第 1 篇　神经疾病　Neurologic Disease

1. Neurologic Evaluation of the Patient, 4
   神经系统评估，5

2. Disorders of Consciousness, 14
   意识障碍，15

3. Disorders of Sleep, 26
   睡眠障碍，27

4. Cortical Syndromes, 36
   皮质综合征，37

5. Dementia and Memory Disturbances, 44
   痴呆和记忆障碍，45

6. Major Disorders of Mood, Thoughts, and Behavior, 56
   心境、思维和行为障碍，57

7. Autonomic Nervous System Disorders, 68
   自主神经系统疾病，69

8. Headache, Neck and Back Pain, and Cranial Neuralgias, 76
   头痛、颈背痛和脑神经痛，77

9. Disorders of Vision and Hearing, 92
   视觉与听觉疾病，93

10. Dizziness and Vertigo, 108
    头晕和眩晕，109

11. Disorders of the Motor System, 116
    运动系统疾病，117

12. Congenital, Developmental, and Neurocutaneous Disorders, 138
    先天性、发育性和神经皮肤疾病，139

13. Cerebrovascular Disease, 154
    脑血管疾病，155

14. Traumatic Brain Injury and Spinal Cord Injury, 180
    颅脑损伤和脊髓损伤，181

15. Epilepsy, 188
    癫痫，189

16 Central Nervous System Tumors, 216
中枢神经系统肿瘤，217

17 Demyelinating and Inflammatory Disorders, 226
脱髓鞘性和炎症性疾病，227

18 Neuromuscular Diseases: Disorders of the Motor Neuron and Plexus and Peripheral Nerve Disease, 244
神经肌肉疾病：运动神经元和神经丛疾病以及周围神经疾病，245

19 Muscle Diseases, 264
肌肉疾病，265

20 Neuromuscular Junction Disease, 286
神经肌肉接头疾病，287

第 2 篇　老年医学　Geriatrics

21 The Aging Patient, 294
老年患者，295

第 3 篇　缓和医疗　Palliative Care

22 Palliative Care, 324
缓和医疗，325

第 4 篇　酒精和物质使用　Alcohol and Substance Use

23 Alcohol and Substance Use, 344
酒精和物质使用，345

索引 Index，374

CECIL ESSENTIALS OF MEDICINE

Neurologic Disease

Geriatrics

Palliative Care

Alcohol and Substance Use

SECTION I

Neurologic Disease

1. Neurologic Evaluation of the Patient, 4
2. Disorders of Consciousness, 14
3. Disorders of Sleep, 26
4. Cortical Syndromes, 36
5. Dementia and Memory Disturbances, 44
6. Major Disorders of Mood, Thoughts, and Behavior, 56
7. Autonomic Nervous System Disorders, 68
8. Headache, Neck and Back Pain, and Cranial Neuralgias, 76
9. Disorders of Vision and Hearing, 92
10. Dizziness and Vertigo, 108
11. Disorders of the Motor System, 116
12. Congenital, Developmental, and Neurocutaneous Disorders, 138
13. Cerebrovascular Disease, 154
14. Traumatic Brain Injury and Spinal Cord Injury, 180
15. Epilepsy, 188
16. Central Nervous System Tumors, 216
17. Demyelinating and Inflammatory Disorders, 226
18. Neuromuscular Diseases: Disorders of the Motor Neuron and Plexus and Peripheral Nerve Disease, 244
19. Muscle Diseases, 264
20. Neuromuscular Junction Disease, 286

第1篇

神经疾病

1 神经系统评估，5

2 意识障碍，15

3 睡眠障碍，27

4 皮质综合征，37

5 痴呆和记忆障碍，45

6 心境、思维和行为障碍，57

7 自主神经系统疾病，69

8 头痛、颈背痛和脑神经痛，77

9 视觉与听觉疾病，93

10 头晕和眩晕，109

11 运动系统疾病，117

12 先天性、发育性和神经皮肤疾病，139

13 脑血管疾病，155

14 颅脑损伤和脊髓损伤，181

15 癫痫，189

16 中枢神经系统肿瘤，217

17 脱髓鞘性和炎症性疾病，227

18 神经肌肉疾病：运动神经元和神经丛疾病以及周围神经疾病，245

19 肌肉疾病，265

20 神经肌肉接头疾病，287

1

Neurologic Evaluation of the Patient

Frederick J. Marshall

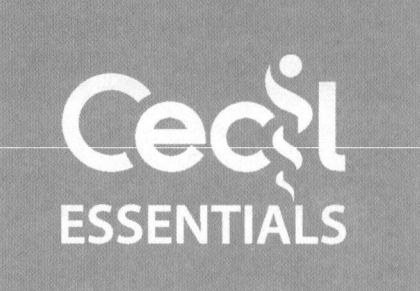

INTRODUCTION

To arrive at an accurate neurologic diagnosis, the clinician generates and tests hypotheses about the location and the mechanism of injury to the nervous system. Hypotheses are refined as the clinician progresses from the interview to the physical examination to the laboratory assessment of the patient. The focus is first placed on entities that are common, serious, and treatable. Common presentations of common diseases account for roughly 80% of cases, rare presentations of common diseases account for roughly 15%, typical presentations of rare diseases roughly 5%, and rare presentations of rare diseases less than 1% of cases. Focus your energy on common diseases but learn the rare disorders too.

TAKING A NEUROLOGIC HISTORY

The clinician should strive to determine the location, quality, and timing of symptoms. Encourage the patient to report the progression of symptoms rather than a list of diagnostic procedures and specialty evaluations. Establish when the patient last felt normal, whether the progression has been relentless or remitting, and whether it has been chronic, subacute or acute. This information substantially constrains the differential diagnosis. Ambiguous descriptors such as *dizzy* should be rejected in favor of evocative descriptors such as *light-headed* (which may implicate cardiovascular insufficiency) or *off balance* (which may implicate cerebellar or posterior column dysfunction).

Family members and other witnesses should corroborate historical information when appropriate. Historical information should include the medical and surgical histories; current medications; prior responses to efforts at treatment; allergies; family history; review of systems; and social history, including the patient's level of education, work history, possible toxin exposures, substance use, sexual history, current life circumstance, and overall function.

Clues to localization are sought during the interview. For example, pain is usually caused by a lesion of the peripheral nervous system, whereas aphasia (i.e., disordered language processing) indicates an abnormality of the central nervous system. Because sensory and motor functions are anatomically relatively distant in the cerebral cortex but progressively closer together as fibers converge in the brain stem, spinal cord, roots, and peripheral nerves, the coexistence of sensory loss and motor dysfunction in a limb implies a large lesion at the level of the cortex or a smaller lesion lower down in the neuraxis. Small lesions in areas of high traffic such as the spinal cord or brain stem can result in widespread neurologic dysfunction, whereas small lesions elsewhere may be asymptomatic.

Table 1.1 lists the potential localizing values of common neurologic symptoms to help address the issue of lesion localization. Tables 1.2 and 1.3 list symptoms that are commonly associated with lesions at specific locations in the nervous system. Some symptoms can result from a lesion at any of several levels of the nervous system. For example, double vision can result from a focal lesion in the brain stem, peripheral nerves (cranial nerve III, IV, or VI), neuromuscular junction, or extraocular muscles; or it can be nonfocal and result from an increase in intracranial pressure. Associated symptoms (or their lack) may lead the interviewer to reject certain hypotheses that at first seemed most likely. Table 1.4 lists the most important types of neuropathologic conditions and provides examples of diseases in each category.

Some neuroanatomic locations point to a specific diagnosis or a limited number of diagnoses. For example, disease of the neuromuscular junction is usually caused by an autoimmune process such as myasthenia gravis (common) or Eaton-Lambert myasthenic syndrome (uncommon). The exceptions—botulism and congenital myasthenic disorders—are rare. Alternatively, some areas of the nervous system (e.g., the cerebral hemispheres) are vulnerable to practically any of the categories of disease outlined in Table 1.4.

The pace and temporal order of symptoms are important. Degenerative diseases usually progress gradually, whereas vascular diseases (e.g., stroke, aneurysmal subarachnoid hemorrhage) progress rapidly. Certain symptoms such as double vision almost invariably develop abruptly, even if the underlying disorder has been developing gradually over days to weeks.

NEUROLOGIC EXAMINATION

Performance of the main elements of a general screening neurologic examination is imperative (Table 1.5), but the examination should be tailored to confirm or disprove the clinical hypotheses generated from the patient's history. Unexpected signs must be explained, often with a return to the history for further clarification. The goal of the exam is to determine whether the cause is diffuse, focal or multifocal.

The examination is approached as if only one of two possible injuries has occurred—the final common pathway to a structure is disrupted, or the input to that pathway is disrupted (Fig. 1.1). In the case of the motor system, the *final common pathway* is the motor unit and includes the anterior horn cells giving rise to axons in a nerve, the nerve itself, the neuromuscular junction, and the muscle. Injury to any of these structures results in dysfunction of the muscle. Conversely, if these structures are intact, observing the muscle function may be possible under the right circumstances. If all modes of engaging the final common pathway fail to elicit a response, the clinician can conclude that the lesion is located somewhere within the final common pathway.

For example, a man with paralysis of facial movement on one side that is caused by a lesion of cranial nerve VII cannot smile voluntarily, close his eye, or wrinkle his forehead on the affected side. Spontaneous laughter or smiling as an automatic response to a joke also fails to

神经系统评估

洪月慧 译　韩菲 沈航 审校　姚明 彭斌 通审

引言

在神经病学诊断中，临床医生会对神经系统损伤的部位和机制进行假设，并通过病史采集、体格检查及实验室评估对假设进行验证。诊断时优先关注常见、严重且可治疗的疾病。常见病的典型表现约占80%，常见病的罕见表现约占15%，罕见病的典型表现约占5%，而罕见病的罕见表现不到1%。临床医生应该聚焦常见病，但也要加强罕见病的学习。

采集病史

临床医生应细致采集病史，明确症状的定位、性质及演变过程。鼓励患者详细描述症状的发展过程，而非仅依赖辅助检查结果。需要明确患者最后正常状态的时间，判断病情是持续进展还是有所缓解，并区分是慢性、亚急性还是急性。这些信息有助于显著缩小鉴别诊断的范围。同时，应避免使用模糊的描述，如"头晕"，而应使用更具体的描述，如"头轻脚重"（可能提示心血管功能障碍）或"身体不稳"（可能提示小脑或脊髓后索功能障碍）。

此外，应让家属和其他目击者证实病史信息。既往史应包括患者的既往病史、手术史、用药情况、既往治疗的疗效、过敏史、家族史、系统回顾，以及个人史，包括患者的教育水平、工作史、可能的毒物暴露、物质滥用、性生活史、目前生活环境以及整体功能。

在采集病史过程中，医生应寻找有助于定位诊断的线索。例如，疼痛通常是由周围神经系统的损伤引起的，而失语（即语言障碍）则提示中枢神经系统异常。由于感觉和运动功能在大脑皮质的解剖位置相隔较远，但随着神经纤维在脑干、脊髓、神经根和周围神经汇聚，其位置逐渐接近，某个肢体的感觉和运动功能同时存在障碍提示大脑皮质较大的病变或皮质以下神经系统较小的病变。在脊髓或脑干等功能密集区域的小病变可能导致广泛的神经功能障碍，而其他部位的小病变可能无症状。

表1.1列举了常见神经系统症状的潜在定位价值。表1.2和表1.3列举了与神经系统特定部位病变相关的常见症状。某些症状可能由神经系统不同部位的病变引起。例如，复视可能由脑干、周围神经（第Ⅲ、Ⅳ或Ⅵ脑神经）、神经-肌肉接头或眼外肌的局灶病变引起；它也可能并非神经系统局灶病变导致，而是由颅内压升高引起。医生可能会根据伴随症状（或阴性症状）推翻某些最初看似最有可能的假设。表1.4列出了神经系统疾病的最重要类别，并在每个类别下提供了疾病示例。

某些神经解剖部位的病变，往往指向特定的诊断或少数几个可能的诊断。例如，神经肌肉接头疾病通常由自身免疫机制导致，如重症肌无力（常见）或兰伯特-伊顿肌无力综合征（少见）。肉毒中毒症和先天性肌无力症则是更为罕见的情况。此外，神经系统的某些部位（如大脑半球）容易在多种疾病（表1.4）中受损。

症状的进展速度和时间顺序对诊断至关重要。退行性疾病通常缓慢进展，而血管性疾病（如卒中、动脉瘤性蛛网膜下腔出血）则迅速发作。某些症状，如复视，可能突然出现，即使潜在的疾病在数天至数周内也已经逐渐发展。

神经系统检查

进行全面的神经系统检查至关重要（表1.5），但应根据患者病史调整，来验证或推翻临床假设。意外发现的体征通常需要通过回顾病史来进一步确证。查体的目的是明确病变是弥漫性的、局灶性的还是多灶性的。

神经系统检查通常基于两种可能的损伤机制来进行：一是最终共同通路的某一结构被破坏，二是通往该通路的传入途径被阻断（图1.1）。以运动系统为例，最终共同通路是运动单位，包括形成神经轴突的前角细胞、神经本身、神经肌肉接头及肌肉。这些结构中任何一个损伤都会导致肌肉功能障碍。相反，如果这些结构是完整的，通过检查方法就能观察到这些肌肉的正常功能反应。如果所有尝试激活最终共同通路的方式都未能引起反应，临床医生可以得出结论，病变位于最终共同通路内的某个位置。

例如，面神经（第Ⅶ脑神经）损伤导致面肌瘫痪患者的受损侧不能主动地微笑、闭眼或皱眉。当听到笑话时本应自然出现的不自主大笑或微笑也不能让瘫痪侧的面肌运动。然而，如果病变位于中枢神经系统，

move the paretic side. If the problem is central, however, facial movement with involuntary (spontaneous) smiling may be preserved or increased. This observation is common in patients with facial weakness caused by a stroke.

Central input to a final common pathway in the nervous system is usually tonically inhibitory. Damage to this input typically results in overactivity of the involved muscle group. Signs of damage to central inhibitory systems include spasticity and hyperreflexia (i.e., motor cortex, subcortical white matter, or corticospinal pathways in the brain stem and spinal cord); dystonia, rigidity, tremor, and tic (i.e., basal ganglia or extrapyramidal systems); and ataxia and dysmetria (i.e., cerebellum). An exception is hypotonia, which may be seen in cerebellar disease.

TECHNOLOGIC ASSESSMENT

Laboratory investigations and special testing should be used to confirm a clinical suggestion and to finalize the diagnosis. Testing should be selectively performed because of expense, risk, and discomfort to the patient. Frequently helpful tests are discussed in subsequent sections. Diagnostic tests should never be ordered without a specific differential diagnosis firmly in mind. Many neurodiagnostic tests disclose incidental abnormalities unrelated to a patient's symptomatic disease process.

Lumbar Puncture

Investigation of the cerebrospinal fluid (CSF) is indicated in a small number of specific circumstances, usually infections, malignancy, or inflammatory/immune mediated conditions (Table 1.6). When taken, a CSF specimen should be routinely sent for laboratory testing to determine cell and differential counts, protein and glucose levels, and bacterial cultures. The CSF should also be examined for its color and clarity. Cloudy or discolored CSF should be centrifuged and examined for xanthochromia in comparison with water. Additional, special studies may be obtained as appropriate, including Gram stain; fungal, viral, and tuberculous cultures; cryptococcal and other antigens; tests for syphilis; Lyme titers; malignant cytologic patterns; paraneoplastic and other specific protein antibodies; and oligoclonal bands. Polymerase chain reaction for specific viruses may also be appropriate. Assessment of specific CSF proteins such as tau, phosphorylated tau, and amyloid-β in selected patients at risk for dementia may be considered. The 14-3-3 protein, found in Creutzfeldt-Jakob disease, may be found in patients with rapid-onset dementia.

Recording the opening and closing pressures is important. Tissue infection in the region of the puncture site is an absolute contraindication to lumbar puncture. Relative contraindications include known or probable intracranial or spinal mass lesion, increased intracranial pressure as a result of mass lesions, coagulopathy caused by thrombocytopenia (usually correctable), anticoagulant therapy, and bleeding disorders.

Rare but severe complications of lumbar puncture include transtentorial or foramen magnum herniation, spinal epidural hematoma, spinal abscess, herniated or infected disk, meningitis, and adverse reaction to a local anesthetic agent. More common and relatively benign complications include headache and backache.

Tissue Biopsies

In selected specialty centers, a diagnostic biopsy is performed on various tissues, including brain, peripheral nerve (see Chapter 18),

TABLE 1.1 Potential Localizing Value of Common Neurologic Symptoms

Potential Localizing Value	Sign or Symptom
High	Focal weakness, sensory loss, or pain
	Focal visual loss
	Language disturbance
	Neglect or anosognosia
Medium	Vertigo
	Dysarthria
	Clumsiness
Low	Fatigue
	Headache
	Insomnia
	Dizziness
	Anxiety, confusion, or psychosis

TABLE 1.2 Symptom Localization in the Central Nervous System

Sign or Symptom	Location
Cerebral Hemispheres	
Unilateral weakness or sensory complaints	Contralateral cerebral hemisphere
Language dysfunction	Left hemisphere (frontal and temporal)
Spatial disorientation	Right hemisphere (parietal and occipital)
Anosognosia (lack of insight into deficit)	Right hemisphere (parietal)
Hemivisual loss	Contralateral hemisphere (occipital, temporal, and parietal)
Flattening of affect or social disinhibition	Bihemispheric (frontal and limbic)
Alteration of consciousness	Bihemispheric (diffuse)
Alteration of memory	Bihemispheric (hippocampus, fornix, amygdala, and mammillary bodies)
Cerebellum	
Limb clumsiness	Ipsilateral cerebellar hemisphere
Unsteadiness of gait or posture	Midline cerebellar structures
Basal Ganglia	
Slowness of voluntary movement	Substantia nigra and striatum
Involuntary movement	Striatum, thalamus, and subthalamus
Brain Stem	
Contralateral weakness or sensory complaints in the body with ipsilateral weakness or sensory complaints in the face	Midbrain, pons, and medulla
Double vision	Midbrain and pons
Vertigo	Pons and medulla
Alteration of consciousness	Midbrain, pons, medulla (reticular formation)
Spinal Cord	
Weakness and spasticity (ipsilateral) and anesthesia (contralateral) below a specified level	Corticospinal and spinothalamic tracts
Unsteadiness of gait	Posterior columns
Bilateral (can be asymmetrical) weakness and sensory complaints in multiple contiguous radicular distributions	Central cord

面部不自主（自发）微笑动作可能保留或增加。这种情况常见于因卒中导致的面瘫患者。

神经系统中最终共同通路的中枢传入通常是抑制性的。中枢传入损伤通常会导致相应肌群的过度活动。中枢抑制系统损伤的体征包括痉挛性瘫痪和反射亢进（如运动皮质、皮质下白质、脑干和脊髓中的皮质脊髓束）、肌张力障碍、强直、震颤和抽动（如基底节或锥体外系）、共济失调和辨距不良（如小脑）。小脑疾病中出现的肌张力低下则是一个例外。

辅助检查

实验室检查和特殊检查用于确证临床推测并得到最终诊断。然而，由于成本、风险和检查可能给患者带来的不适，应选择性安排辅助检查。在后续章节中，我们将讨论一些常用且有用的检查。诊断性检查绝不应该在没有鉴别诊断思路的情况下进行。许多神经系统诊断性检查可能会偶然发现与患者疾病过程无关的异常结果。

腰椎穿刺

少数特定情况下，需行脑脊液（CSF）检查，主要包括感染、恶性肿瘤或炎症/免疫介导疾病（表1.6）。常规检查应包括脑脊液细胞计数和分类、蛋白质和葡萄糖水平，以及细菌培养。应检查脑脊液的颜色和透明度。浑浊或变色的脑脊液应离心，以评估是否存在黄变（xanthochromia）。此外，可能还需要根据具体情况进行特殊检查，包括：革兰染色，真菌、病毒和结核培养，隐球菌和其他抗原检测，梅毒检测，莱姆病滴度，恶性细胞学改变，副肿瘤和其他特定蛋白抗体，以及寡克隆带检测。针对特定病毒的聚合酶链反应可能是合适的。对于某些有痴呆风险的患者，可考虑检测特定的脑脊液蛋白，如tau蛋白、磷酸化tau蛋白和β淀粉样物质。对于快速进展性痴呆患者，可能会发现与克-雅病相关的14-3-3蛋白。

记录脑脊液的初压和末压非常重要。穿刺部位组织感染是腰椎穿刺的绝对禁忌证。相对禁忌证包括已知或很可能的颅内或脊髓占位、占位病变引起的颅内压增高、血小板减少（通常可纠正）导致的凝血障碍、抗凝治疗和出血性疾病。

腰椎穿刺的罕见但严重的并发症包括小脑幕切迹疝或枕骨大孔疝、脊髓硬膜外血肿、脊柱脓肿、椎间盘突出或感染、脑膜炎和对局部麻醉剂的不良反应。更常见且相对良性的并发症包括头痛和背痛。

组织活检

在某些专业医疗中心，会对各种组织进行诊断性活检，包括大脑、周围神经（见第18章）、肌肉（见

表1.2　中枢神经系统的症状定位

体征或症状	定位
大脑半球	
一侧无力或感觉障碍	对侧大脑半球
言语障碍	左侧大脑半球（额叶和颞叶）
空间定向障碍	右侧大脑半球（顶叶和枕叶）
病感失认症（对疾病缺乏感知）	右侧大脑半球（顶叶）
偏盲	对侧大脑半球（枕叶、颞叶和顶叶）
情感淡漠或社交抑制减弱	双侧大脑半球（额叶和边缘叶）
意识改变	双侧大脑半球（弥漫）
记忆障碍	双侧大脑半球（海马、穹窿、杏仁核、乳头体）
小脑	
肢体笨拙	同侧小脑半球
步态或姿势不稳	小脑中线结构
基底节	
运动迟缓	黑质和纹状体
不自主运动	纹状体、丘脑和底丘脑
脑干	
对侧无力或感觉障碍及同侧面部无力或感觉障碍	中脑、脑桥和延髓
复视	中脑和脑桥
眩晕	脑桥和延髓
意识改变	中脑、脑桥、延髓（网状结构）
脊髓	
损伤平面以下无力和痉挛（同侧）、感觉障碍（对侧）	皮质脊髓束和脊髓丘脑束
步态不稳	后索
多个连续节段根性分布的双侧无力（可不对称）、感觉障碍	中央管

表1.1　常见神经系统症状的潜在定位价值

潜在定位价值	体征或症状
高	局灶无力、感觉丧失或疼痛 局灶视力下降 言语障碍 忽视或病感失认症
中	眩晕 构音障碍 笨拙
低	乏力 头痛 失眠 头晕 焦虑、意识模糊或精神异常

TABLE 1.3 Symptom Localization in the Motor Unit[a]

Sign or Symptom	Location
Anterior Horn Cell	
Weakness and wasting with muscle twitching (fasciculation) but no sensory complaints	Anterior horn of spinal cord (diffuse or segmental)
Spinal Root	
Weakness and sensory loss confined to a known radicular distribution (pain, a common feature, may spread)	Cervical, thoracic, lumbar, and sacral
Plexus	
Pain, weakness, and sensory loss in a limb; not limited to a single radicular or peripheral nerve distribution	Brachial and lumbosacral (may also be caused by polyradiculopathy)
Nerve	
Pain, distal weakness, and/or sensory changes confined to a single peripheral nerve distribution	Peripheral nerves (mononeuropathy)
Pain, distal weakness, and/or sensory changes affecting both sides symmetrically (usually starting in feet)	Peripheral nerves (polyneuropathy)
Pain, distal weakness, and/or sensory changes affecting scattered single peripheral nerve distributions	Peripheral nerves (mononeuropathy multiplex)
Unilateral special sensory loss	Cranial nerves I, II, V, VII, VIII, and IX
Unilateral facial weakness involving entire one half of face	Cranial nerve VII (ipsilateral)
Neuromuscular Junction	
Progressive weakness with repeated use of a muscle; no sensory complaints	Ocular, pharyngeal, and skeletal
Muscle	
Proximal weakness; no sensory complaints	Diffuse and various patterns

[a]Anterior horn cell and the peripheral nervous system.

TABLE 1.4 Categories of Neurologic Disease

Disease Category	Example
Genetic	
Autosomal dominant	Huntington's disease
Autosomal recessive	Friedreich's ataxia
X-linked recessive	Duchenne muscular dystrophy
Mitochondrial	Progressive external ophthalmoplegia
Sporadic	Down syndrome
Neoplastic	
Intrinsic	Glioblastoma
Extrinsic	Metastatic melanoma
Paraneoplastic	Cerebellar degeneration
Vascular	
Stroke	Thrombotic, embolic, lacunar, hemorrhagic
Structural	Arteriovenous malformation
Inflammatory	Cranial arteritis
Infectious	
Bacterial	Meningococcal meningitis
Viral	Herpes encephalitis
Protozoal	Toxoplasmosis
Fungal	Cryptococcal meningitis
Helminthic	Cysticercosis
Prion	Creutzfeldt-Jakob disease
Degenerative	
Central	Parkinson's disease
Central and peripheral	Amyotrophic lateral sclerosis
Autoimmune	
Central demyelinating	Multiple sclerosis
Peripheral demyelinating	Guillain-Barré syndrome
Neuromuscular junction	Myasthenia gravis
Toxic and Metabolic	
Endogenous	Uremic encephalopathy
Exogenous	Alcoholic neuropathy
Other Structural	
Trauma	Spinal cord injury
Hydrodynamic	Normal pressure hydrocephalus
Psychogenic	Hysterical paraparesis

muscle (see Chapter 19), and skin. Occasionally, biopsy provides the only means of arriving at a definitive diagnosis.

Electrophysiologic Studies

Electrophysiologic studies include electroencephalography, electromyography, nerve conduction studies, and evoked potentials. These studies are helpful in situations in which the patient cannot be examined or interviewed adequately.

Electroencephalography is most often used to investigate seizures (see Chapter 15). It can document encephalopathy, in which case the background electrical activity of the brain is slowed, and it is also used in the evaluation of brain death.

Electromyography is useful in the differential diagnosis of muscle disease, neuromuscular junction disease, peripheral nerve disease, and anterior horn cell disease. Nerve conduction studies (see Chapters 18 and 19) may show decreased amplitude (characteristic of axonal neuropathy) or decreased velocity (characteristic of demyelinating neuropathy).

Visual-evoked potential studies are commonly used in the evaluation of possible multiple sclerosis (see Chapter 17). Asymmetrical slowing of the cortical response to visual pattern stimulation suggests demyelination in the optic nerve or central optic pathways. Brain stem auditory-evoked potential studies are useful in the diagnosis of diseases affecting cranial nerve VIII or its central projections. Lesions at the cerebellopontine angle and the brain stem cause abnormal delay in conduction. Brain stem auditory-evoked potentials are helpful in the diagnosis of deafness in infants. Somatosensory-evoked potentials are used to identify a slowing of central sensory conduction that results from demyelinating disease, compression, or metabolic derangements. They are also used to evaluate spinal cord–mediated sensory abnormalities.

Imaging Studies

Magnetic resonance imaging (MRI) and computed tomography (CT) are high-resolution imaging techniques that provide extraordinary

表1.3 运动单位的症状定位 a	
体征或症状	定位
前角细胞	
肢体无力、萎缩伴肌肉颤搐（肌束震颤），但无感觉障碍	脊髓前角（弥漫或节段性）
脊髓神经根	
根性分布的肢体无力、感觉障碍（疼痛为常见特征，可能扩散）	颈、胸、腰、骶髓
神经丛	
单肢疼痛、无力、感觉障碍，不局限于一个神经根或周围神经分布区	臂丛、腰骶丛（可能由多神经根病导致）
神经	
局限于单神经分布区的疼痛、远端无力和（或）感觉障碍	周围神经（单神经病）
两侧对称性疼痛、远端无力和（或）感觉障碍	周围神经（多发性神经病）
多个单神经分布区的疼痛、远端无力和（或）感觉障碍	周围神经（多发性单神经病）
一侧特殊感觉障碍	脑神经 I、II、V、VII、VIII或IX
一侧面部肌肉无力，累及整个半侧面部	脑神经VII（同侧）
神经肌肉接头	
肌肉反复用力后进展性无力（疲劳现象），无感觉障碍	眼肌、咽肌、骨骼肌
肌肉	
近端无力，无感觉障碍	弥漫或多种受累模式

a 前角细胞和周围神经系统。

表1.4 神经系统疾病分类	
疾病分类	举例
遗传性	
常染色体显性遗传	亨廷顿病
常染色体隐性遗传	费里德赖希共济失调
X连锁隐性遗传	进行性假肥大性肌营养不良
线粒体	进行性眼外肌麻痹
散发	唐氏综合征
肿瘤性	
原发	胶质母细胞瘤
转移	转移性黑色素瘤
副肿瘤	小脑变性
血管性	
卒中	血栓、栓塞、腔隙性、出血性
结构	动静脉畸形
炎症	脑动脉炎
感染性	
细菌性	脑膜炎球菌性脑膜炎
病毒性	疱疹性脑炎
原虫	弓形虫病
真菌性	隐球菌脑膜炎
蠕虫	囊尾蚴病
朊病毒	克-雅病
退行性	
中枢神经	帕金森病
中枢和周围神经	肌萎缩侧索硬化
自身免疫性	
中枢神经炎性脱髓鞘	多发性硬化
周围神经炎性脱髓鞘	吉兰-巴雷综合征
神经肌肉接头	重症肌无力
中毒和代谢性	
内源性	尿毒症脑病
外源性	酒精性神经病
其他结构性	
外伤	脊髓损伤
液体动力学	正常颅压脑积水
心因性	癔症性截瘫

第19章）和皮肤。在少数情况下，活检是明确诊断的唯一手段。

电生理检查

电生理检查包括脑电图、肌电图、神经传导检查和诱发电位。这些检查在患者无法配合或交流受限时非常有用。

脑电图通常用于评估癫痫发作（见第15章）。它可提示脑功能障碍，如在脑病情况下大脑的背景电活动会减慢。此外，脑电图也用于评估脑死亡。

肌电图在肌肉疾病、神经肌肉接头疾病、周围神经疾病以及前角细胞疾病的鉴别诊断中具有重要作用。神经传导检查（见第18章和第19章）可显示波幅降低（轴索性神经病的特征）或传导速度下降（脱髓鞘性神经病的特征）。

视觉诱发电位检查通常用于评估可能的多发性硬化患者（见第17章）。对视觉刺激的皮质反应不对称性减慢提示视神经或视通路中枢部分发生了脱髓鞘。脑干听觉诱发电位检查对于诊断累及第VIII脑神经或其中枢投射的疾病非常有帮助，桥小脑角和脑干的病变会导致其传导异常延迟，脑干听觉诱发电位有助于诊断婴儿耳聋。体感诱发电位用于识别由脱髓鞘疾病、压迫或代谢紊乱引起的中枢感觉传导减慢。它们也用于评估脊髓病变导致的感觉异常。

影像检查

磁共振成像（MRI）和计算机断层成像（CT）是高分辨率成像技术，为中枢神经系统病变的精准诊断

TABLE 1.5 Elements of a General Screening Neurologic Examination

Systemic Physical Examination
Head (trauma, dysmorphism, and bruits)
Neck (tone, bruits, and thyromegaly)
Cardiovascular (heart rate, rhythm, and murmurs; peripheral pulses and jugular venous distention)
Pulmonary (breathing pattern, cough and cyanosis)
Abdomen (hepatosplenomegaly)
Back and extremities (skeletal abnormalities, peripheral edema, and straight-leg raising)
Skin (neurocutaneous stigmata and hepatic stigmata)

Mental Status
Level of consciousness (awake, drowsy, and comatose)
Attention (coherent stream of thought, serial 7s)
Orientation (temporal and spatial)
Memory (short and long term)
Language (naming, repetition, comprehension, fluency, reading, and writing)
Visuospatial skills (clock drawing and figure copying)
Judgment, insight, thought content (psychotic)
Mood (depressed, manic, and anxious)

Cranial Nerves
Olfactory (smell in each nostril)
Optic (afferent pupillary function, funduscopic examination, visual acuity, visual fields, and structural eye findings)
Oculomotor, trochlear, and abducens (smooth pursuit and saccadic eye movements, nystagmus, efferent pupillary function, and eyelid opening)
Trigeminal (jaw jerk, facial sensation, afferent corneal reflex, and muscles of mastication)
Facial (efferent corneal reflex, facial expression, eyelid closure, nasolabial folds, and power and bulk)
Vestibulocochlear (nystagmus, speech discrimination, Weber test, and Rinne test)
Glossopharyngeal and vagus (afferent and efferent gag reflex and uvula position)
Spinal accessory (power and bulk of sternocleidomastoid and trapezii muscles)
Hypoglossal (position, bulk, and fasciculations of tongue)

Motor Examination
Pronator drift (subtle corticospinal lesion)
Tone and bulk of muscles (basal ganglia lesion yields rigidity, cerebellar lesion yields hypotonia, corticospinal lesion yields spasticity, nonspecific bihemispheric disease yields paratonia [inability to relax muscles], hypertrophy indicates dystonia, pseudohypertrophy indicates muscle disease, and atrophy indicates lower motor neuron disease)
Adventitious movements (tremor, tic, dystonia, and chorea indicate disease of the basal ganglia; asterixis and myoclonus may indicate toxic metabolic process)
Power of major muscle groups (scale 0-5)
Upper extremities: deltoids, biceps, triceps, wrist extension and flexion, finger extension and flexion, and interossei
Lower extremities: hip flexion, extension, abduction, and adduction; knee extension and flexion; ankle dorsiflexion, plantar flexion, inversion, and eversion; toe extension and flexion

Sensory Examination
Light touch (posterior columns)
Pinprick (spinothalamic tract)
Temperature (spinothalamic tract)
Joint position sense (posterior columns)
Vibration (posterior columns)
Graphesthesia (cortical sensory)
Double simultaneous stimulation (cortical sensory)
Two-point discrimination (posterior columns and cortical sensory)

Reflex Examination
Standard reflexes (grades 0-4)
Biceps
Triceps
Brachioradialis
Knee jerk
Ankle jerk
Pathologic reflexes
Babinski sign (if present)
Myerson sign (glabellar sign) (if present)
Snout (if present)
Jaw jerk (if brisk)
Palmomental (twitch of chin muscles when palm is stroked) (if present)
Hoffmann sign (thumb or index finger flexion when nail of middle finger is flicked) (if brisk)

Coordination and Gait
Finger-nose-finger (action tremor suggesting cerebellar disease)
Rapid alternating movements (dysdiadochokinesia suggesting cerebellar disease)
Fine motor movements (slowness and small amplitude suggesting basal ganglia or corticospinal tract abnormalities)
Heel-to-shin (ataxia suggesting cerebellar disease)
Arising from chair with arms folded across chest (inability in advanced basal ganglia, cerebellar, corticospinal, or muscle disease)
Walking naturally (look for decreased arm swing, spasticity, broad base, festination (quickening and shortening of normal gait), waddle, footdrop, start hesitation, and dystonia)
Tandem gait (look for ataxia)
Walking with feet everted or inverted (look for latent dystonia)
Hopping on each foot separately (look for latent dystonia)
Stand with feet together and eyes open, eyes closed (sensory ataxia and cerebellar disease)
Response to retropulsive stress (loss of postural righting mechanisms)

---

diagnostic precision for central nervous system lesions. Most neurologic diseases, however, can have normal CT and MRI findings. Moreover, many abnormal findings on CT and MRI bear no relation to the diagnosis responsible for the patient's symptoms.

Table 1.7 compares CT with MRI. MRI is used for most purposes, although CT has the advantage of wider accessibility, greater speed of acquisition, and better tolerability by the patient. CT detects acute hemorrhage and is preferred for emergencies. MRI provides more detail and simultaneously obtains images in the horizontal, vertical, and coronal planes. Contrast media for CT or MRI are useful in the diagnosis of tumors, abscesses, and other processes that derange the blood-brain barrier. MRI can be used for functional imaging and spectroscopy; both techniques have great promise for the evaluation of cognitive and metabolic disorders, epilepsy, multiple sclerosis, and many other conditions.

MR- and CT-angiography allow noninvasive visualization of the major vessels of the head and neck. Conventional angiography with an intra-arterial injection of contrast agent is used for evaluation of

表 1.5　全面神经系统检查的组成

系统体格检查
头（外伤、畸形、杂音）
颈（肌张力、杂音、甲状腺肿大）
心血管（心率、心律、心脏杂音、脉搏、颈静脉扩张）
肺（呼吸节律、咳嗽、发绀）
腹部（肝脾大）
背及四肢（骨骼异常、肢体水肿、直腿抬高）
皮肤（神经皮肤征、肝病的皮肤征象）

意识状态
意识水平（清醒、嗜睡、昏迷）
注意力（思维连贯性、连续减 7 测试）
定向力（时间、空间）
记忆（近、远）
语言（命名、复述、理解、流利性、读、写）
视空间（画钟、模仿画图）
判断力、洞察力、思维内容（精神病性）
情绪（抑郁、躁狂、焦虑）

脑神经
嗅觉（每侧鼻的嗅觉）
视神经（瞳孔传入神经、眼底检查、视力、视野、眼结构改变）
动眼神经、滑车神经、展神经（平滑追踪、扫视、眼震、瞳孔传出神经、睁眼）
三叉神经（下颌反射、面部感觉、角膜反射传入神经、咀嚼肌）
面神经（角膜反射传出神经、面部表情、闭眼、鼻唇沟、面部肌肉的力量和容积）
前庭蜗神经（眼震、言语辨别、韦伯试验、林纳试验）
舌咽、迷走神经（咽反射的传入和传出神经、悬雍垂位置）
副神经（胸锁乳突肌和斜方肌的肌力和容积）
舌下神经（舌的位置、肌力、纤颤）

运动系统
旋前肌轻瘫（轻微皮质脊髓束损害）
肌张力、肌容积［基底节病灶导致僵硬，小脑病灶导致肌张力低下，皮质脊髓束病灶导致痉挛，非特异性双侧半球疾病导致肌张力异常（肌肉无法放松），肥大提示肌张力障碍，假性肥大提示肌肉疾病，肌萎缩提示下运动神经元疾病］
附加运动（震颤、抽动、肌张力障碍，舞蹈动作提示基底节病变，扑翼样震颤和肌阵挛提示中毒代谢性过程）
主要肌群的肌力（0～5 级）
上肢：三角肌、肱二头肌、肱三头肌、屈腕和伸腕、屈指和伸指、骨间肌
下肢：髋的屈、伸、外展和内收，伸膝和屈膝，踝的背屈、跖屈、内翻和外翻，足趾的屈、伸

感觉系统
轻触觉（后索）
针刺觉（脊髓丘脑束）
温度觉（脊髓丘脑束）
关节位置觉（后索）
振动觉（后索）
图形觉（皮质感觉）
双侧同时刺激（皮质感觉）
两点辨别觉（后索、皮质感觉）

反射
标准反射（0～4 级）
肱二头肌
肱三头肌
肱桡肌
膝反射
踝反射

病理反射
巴宾斯基征（是否存在）
迈尔森征（眉间征）（是否存在）
撅嘴反射（是否存在）
下颌反射（是否活跃）
掌颏反射（划手掌时颏肌收缩）（是否存在）
霍夫曼征（弹拨中指指甲时，拇指或示指屈曲）（是否活跃）

共济与步态
指鼻试验（动作性震颤提示小脑病变）
快速轮替动作（轮替障碍提示小脑病变）
精细运动（动作慢、幅度小提示基底节或皮质脊髓束异常）
跟膝胫试验（共济失调提示小脑病变）
双臂交叉抱在胸前从椅子上起身（无法完成则提示严重的基底节、小脑、皮质脊髓束或肌肉病变）
自然行走［观察是否存在摆臂幅度减小、痉挛、步基增宽、慌张步态（步速快、步幅小）、蹒跚步态、足下垂、启动困难、肌张力障碍］
串联行走（观察是否存在共济失调）
行走时足外翻或内翻（观察是否存在潜在的肌张力障碍）
分别单脚跳（观察是否存在潜在肌张力障碍）
睁眼、闭眼并足站立（感觉性共济失调、小脑病变）
后拉试验（观察姿势矫正能力是否下降）

提供了重要的价值。然而，值得注意的是，许多神经系统疾病可能在 CT 和 MRI 扫描中呈现为正常表现。同样，CT 和 MRI 扫描有时会发现与患者当前症状无关的异常结果。

表 1.7 对 CT 与 MRI 进行了比较。尽管 CT 可及性更高、采集速度更快、患者耐受性更好，但大多数情况下，MRI 仍是首选的检查方法。CT 扫描可显示急性出血，是急诊的首选检查。MRI 可提供更多信息，可同时获得轴位、矢状位和冠状位图像。CT 或 MRI 增强扫描在诊断肿瘤、脓肿和其他破坏血脑屏障的疾病时非常有用。MRI 还可用于功能成像和波谱成像，这两种影像技术在认知障碍、代谢紊乱、癫痫、多发性硬化等疾病的评估中显示出巨大潜力。

MR 和 CT 血管成像可对头颈部主要血管进行无创可视化评估。传统脑血管造影，即在动脉内注入造影

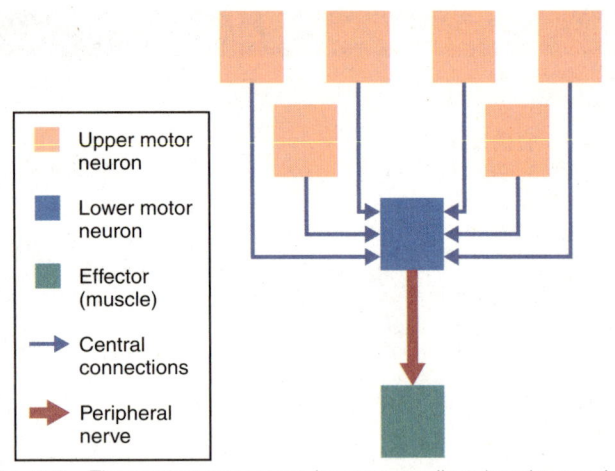

Fig. 1.1 The nervous system can be conceptually reduced to a series of higher-order inputs that converge on final common pathways. For example, upper motor neurons converge on lower motor neurons, whose axons form the final common pathway to an effector muscle.

TABLE 1.6	Indications for Lumbar Puncture
Urgent (Do Not Wait for Brain Imaging)	
Acute central nervous system infection in the absence of focal neurologic signs	
Less Urgent (Wait for Brain Imaging)	
Vasculitis, subarachnoid hemorrhage, or cryptic process	
Increased intracranial pressure in the absence of mass lesion on magnetic resonance imaging or computed tomography	
Intrathecal therapy for fungal or carcinomatous meningitis	
Symptomatic treatment for headache from idiopathic intracranial hypertension or subarachnoid hemorrhage	

TABLE 1.7	Magnetic Resonance Imaging Versus Computed Tomography
Magnetic Resonance Imaging (MRI)	
Resolution 1-2 mm (higher with newer 3-Tesla magnets)	
Gadolinium contrast relatively safe, except in severe renal insufficiency	
Unaffected by bone; multiple planes of imaging available; functional (physiologic) imaging capacity	
Computed Tomography	
Resolution >5 mm	
Iodine contrast associated with anaphylaxis and rash	
Faster acquisition than MRI	
Metallic objects such as pacemaker or aneurysm clip preclude MRI	
Acute hemorrhage well visualized	
Better tolerated by patients who are severely ill or claustrophobic	

TABLE 1.8	Some Neurologic Conditions for Which Genetic Tests Are Commercially Available
• Neuromuscular diseases: *n*erve (Charcot-Marie-Tooth disease); *m*uscle (myotonic dystrophy, Duchenne-Becker muscular dystrophy); *s*pinal muscular atrophy, familial amyotrophic lateral sclerosis	
• Movement disorders: ataxia (spinal cerebellar ataxias, Friedreich ataxia); dystonia, parkinsonism, chorea	
• Dementias: Alzheimer's disease, frontotemporal dementia, hereditary prion disease	
• Mental retardation (fragile X syndrome)	
• Mitochondrial diseases: *m*itochondrial *e*ncephalomyelopathy, *l*actic *a*cidosis, and *s*troke-like symptoms (MELAS syndrome); *m*yoclonus *e*pilepsy with *r*agged *r*ed *f*ibers (MERRF syndrome)	

many intracranial vascular abnormalities, including small aneurysms and arteriovenous malformations, and inflammation of small blood vessels.

Noninvasive ultrasonography of the carotid and vertebral arteries can define stenotic vessels. It has been supplemented by transcranial Doppler technology, which allows characterization of blood flow in intracranial arteries.

Single-photon emission CT (SPECT) is useful for the evaluation of intracranial blood flow. The development of iodine-123 ioflupane injection (DaTscan) makes it possible to visualize the dopamine transporter to follow cell loss in patients with Parkinson's disease.

Positron-emission tomography (PET) is a functional imaging technology that can demonstrate specific metabolic derangements. It is useful for evaluating local abnormalities of glucose and oxygen metabolism. PET is of particular value in defining the site of origin of focal seizures. Customized ligands can be used to identify specific pathologic processes. Examples include three FDA-approved agents for estimating β-amyloid neuritic plaque density in Alzheimer's disease and fluorodopa F18 in Parkinson's disease.

Genetic and Molecular Testing

There are more neurologic diseases than diseases of all other systems combined. Discoveries have revolutionized the diagnostic approach to many of these diseases, and new genetic tests are discovered every year. Table 1.8 outlines the tests that are commercially available.

Genetic testing for a disorder requires the clinician to perform a thoughtful and caring evaluation of the patient, usually with input from and evaluation of the patient's family. Important ethical issues surround the use of genetic tests, including the ability to ensure privacy, to ensure adequate psychological and social support for patients who may be given devastating news, and to address adequately the appropriateness of prenatal screening or presymptomatic testing when no treatment is available.

PROSPECTS FOR THE FUTURE

Novel imaging techniques and molecular diagnostic studies are beginning to shed light on the pathogenesis of neurologic conditions that have been identifiable only by clinical phenomenology. Studies of previously untreatable neurodegenerative disorders are now targeting presymptomatic individuals in the hope that earlier intervention can modify disease outcomes. Despite these and foreseeable future advances, the clinical aspects of neurologic disease remain fundamentally important in understanding the impact of disease on patients and their families.

SUGGESTED READINGS

Biller J, editor: Practical neurology, ed 4, Philadelphia, 2012, Lippincott Williams & Wilkins.

DeLuca GC, Griggs RC: Approach to the patient with neurologic disease. In Goldman L, Schafer AI, editors: Goldman-Cecil medicine, ed 26, 2020, pp 2298–2304, Philadelphia.

Ropper, AH, Samuels MA, Leine JP, Prasad S, editors: Adams and victor's principles of neurology, ed 11, New York, McGraw Hill.

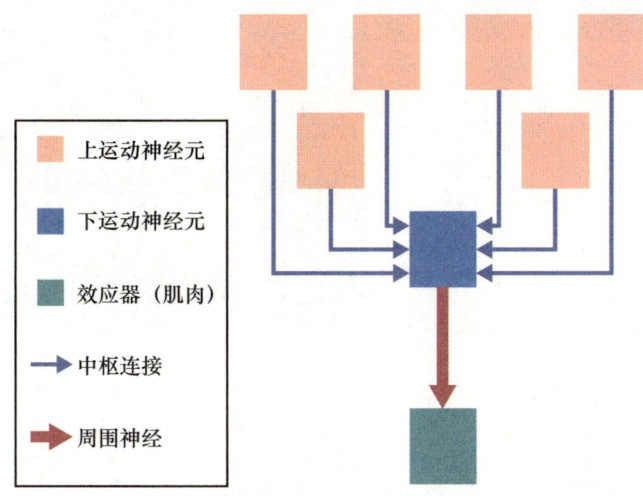

图1.1 简单来说，神经系统可以看作一系列汇聚在最终共同通路上的高阶传入系统。例如，上运动神经元汇聚于下运动神经元，其轴突经最终共同通路将信号传至效应肌

表 1.6　腰椎穿刺的适应证
紧急（不需要等待头部影像）
急性中枢神经系统感染，无局灶神经功能异常体征
不紧急（需要等待头部影像）
血管炎、蛛网膜下腔出血，或其他不明原因
颅内压升高，头 MRI 或 CT 无占位病灶
真菌性脑膜炎或脑膜癌病需鞘内治疗
特发性颅内高压或蛛网膜下腔出血相关头痛的对症治疗

表 1.7　MRI vs. CT
MRI
分辨率 1～2 mm（使用更新的 3-特斯拉磁场时更高）
钆造影剂相对安全，但严重肾功能不全者除外
不受骨骼影响，可多平面成像，可完成功能成像
CT
分辨率＞5 mm
碘造影剂可能引起过敏、皮疹
成像速度比 MRI 更快
有金属物质（如起搏器、动脉瘤夹）不能行 MRI 检查，可行 CT 检查
对急性出血显示清晰
病情危重或幽闭恐惧症患者可耐受

表 1.8　一些可商业化基因检测的神经系统疾病
• 神经肌肉疾病：周围神经疾病[夏科-马里-图思病（CMT）]；肌肉疾病（强直性肌营养不良、杜氏-贝克肌营养不良）；脊髓性肌萎缩，家族性肌萎缩侧索硬化症
• 运动障碍：共济失调（脊髓小脑共济失调、弗里德赖希共济失调）；肌张力障碍，帕金森综合征，舞蹈病
• 痴呆：阿尔茨海默病、额颞叶痴呆、遗传性朊病毒病
• 智力发育迟滞（脆性 X 综合征）
• 线粒体疾病：线粒体脑肌病伴乳酸中毒和卒中样发作（MELAS 综合征），肌阵挛性癫痫伴破碎红纤维（MERRF 综合征）

剂，可以评估多种颅内血管异常，包括小动脉瘤、动静脉畸形和小血管炎症。

无创的颈动脉、椎动脉超声检查可用于评估血管狭窄。经颅多普勒超声进一步补充了对血管功能的评估，能够描述颅内动脉的血流特征。

单光子发射计算机断层成像（SPECT）可用于评估脑血流。碘[^{123}I]氟潘可显示多巴胺转运体，从而评估帕金森病患者脑内的多巴胺能神经元丢失情况。

正电子发射断层成像（PET）是一种功能成像技术，可显示特定的代谢异常，它有助于评估局部葡萄糖和氧代谢异常。PET 在确定局灶性癫痫发作的起源部位方面具有特殊价值。此外，使用定制的配体可用于识别特定的病理过程。例如，美国食品和药物管理局（FDA）批准的 3 种示踪剂，可用于评估阿尔茨海默病中的 β 淀粉样物质神经炎斑块密度和帕金森病中的氟多巴 F18。

基因和分子检测

神经系统疾病的数量超过了所有其他系统疾病的总和。一些研究进展已经彻底改变了许多疾病的诊断方法，并且每年都会有新的基因检测方法被发现。表 1.8 概述了市面上可用的检测方法。

对某种疾病的基因检测要求临床医生对患者进行周到细致的评估，通常还需要患者的家庭成员提供信息并参与评估。基因检测的应用伴随着重要的伦理问题，包括能否保证患者隐私，能否为可能收到坏消息的患者提供足够的心理和社会支持，以及在没有治疗方法的情况下，能否妥善解决产前筛查或症状前检测的合理性问题。

未来展望

新型成像技术和分子诊断检测开始揭示那些从前只能通过临床表现来识别的神经系统疾病的发病机制。对于以前无法治疗的神经退行性疾病，正在开展针对症状前患者的研究，希望通过早期干预改变疾病结局。尽管上述进展突飞猛进，但临床评估对于理解神经系统疾病对患者及其家庭的影响仍然至关重要。

推荐阅读

Biller J, editor: Practical neurology, ed 4, Philadelphia, 2012, Lippincott Williams & Wilkins.

DeLuca GC, Griggs RC: Approach to the patient with neurologic disease. In Goldman L, Schafer AI, editors: Goldman-Cecil medicine, ed 26, 2020, pp 2298–2304, Philadelphia.

Ropper, AH, Samuels MA, Leine JP, Prasad S, editors: Adams and victor's principles of neurology, ed 11, New York, McGraw Hill.

Disorders of Consciousness

Leah Dickstein, Paul M. Vespa

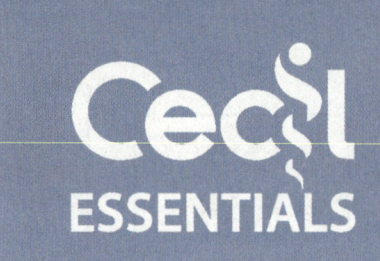

INTRODUCTION

Coma is a state in which the patient is unresponsive and the eyes remain closed even with vigorous stimulation. A poorly responsive state in which the eyes are spontaneously open, or an agitated and confused state, or delirium is not coma but may represent early stages of the same disease processes and should be investigated in the same manner.

Consciousness requires that the brain stem reticular activating system and its cortical projections be intact and functioning. The reticular formation begins in the mid pons and ascends through the dorsal midbrain to synapse in the thalamus; it then innervates higher centers through thalamocortical connections. Knowledge of this anatomic substrate provides the short list of regions to be investigated in the search for a structural cause of coma: Brain stem or bihemispheric dysfunction, be it medication or lesion-related, is typically needed to impede consciousness, whereas structural lesions elsewhere are not the cause of the patient's unconsciousness. In addition to structural lesions, meningeal inflammation, metabolic encephalopathy, sedation, and seizures diffusely affect the brain and complete the differential diagnosis for the patient in coma.

PATHOPHYSIOLOGIC FACTORS

Meningeal irritation caused by infection or blood in the subarachnoid space is an essential early consideration in coma evaluation because its cause requires immediate attention (especially with purulent meningitis) and may not be diagnosed by computed tomography (CT).

Hemispheric mass lesions result in coma either by expanding across the midline laterally to compromise both cerebral hemispheres or by impinging on the brain stem to compress the rostral reticular formation. These processes—*lateral herniation* (lateral movement of the brain) and *transtentorial herniation* (vertical movement of the brain)—most commonly occur together. At the bedside, clinical signs of an expanding hemispheric mass evolve in a level-by-level, rostral-caudal manner (Fig. 2.1). Hemispheric lesions of adequate size to produce coma are readily seen on CT.

Brain stem mass lesions produce coma by directly affecting the reticular formation. Because the pathways for lateral eye movements—the pontine gaze center, medial longitudinal fasciculus, and oculomotor (third nerve) nucleus—traverse the reticular activating system, impairment of reflex eye movements is often the critical element of diagnosis of a brain stem lesion. A comatose patient without impaired reflex lateral eye movements does not have a mass lesion compromising brain stem structures in the posterior fossa. CT is not able to show some lesions in this region. Posterior fossa lesions may block the flow of cerebrospinal fluid from the lateral ventricles, resulting in the dangerous situation of *noncommunicating hydrocephalus*.

Metabolic abnormalities are caused by deficiency states (e.g., thiamine, glucose), by derangements of metabolism (e.g., hyponatremia), or by the presence of *exogenous toxins* (e.g., drugs) or *endogenous toxins* (e.g., organ system failure). Metabolic abnormalities result in diffuse dysfunction of the nervous system; therefore, with rare exceptions, they produce no localized signs such as hemiparesis or unilateral papillary dilation. The diagnosis of *metabolic encephalopathy* means that the examiner has found no focal anatomic features on examination or neuroimaging studies to explain coma but that a specific metabolic cause has not been established. Drugs have a predilection for affecting the reticular formation in the brain stem and for producing paralysis of reflex eye movement on examination. *Multifocal structural disorders* may simulate metabolic coma (Table 2.1).

In the late stages of status epilepticus, motor movements may be subtle even though *seizure activity* is continuing throughout the brain (nonconvulsive status epilepticus). Once seizures stop, the so-called *postictal state* can also cause unexplained coma.

DIAGNOSTIC APPROACH

The history and examination are essential in the diagnosis and are not replaced by brain imaging (Table 2.2). A history of a premonitory headache supports a diagnosis of meningitis, encephalitis, or intracerebral or subarachnoid hemorrhage. A preceding period of intoxication, confusion, or delirium points to a diffuse process such as meningitis or endogenous or exogenous toxins. The sudden apoplectic onset of coma is particularly suggestive of ischemic or hemorrhagic stroke affecting the brain stem or of subarachnoid hemorrhage or intracerebral hemorrhage with intraventricular rupture. Lateralized symptoms of hemiparesis or aphasia before coma occur in patients with hemispheric masses or infarctions.

The physical examination is critical, quickly accomplished, and diagnostic. The issues are three: (1) Does the patient have meningitis? (2) Are signs of a mass lesion present? and (3) Is this condition a diffuse syndrome of exogenous or endogenous metabolic etiology? Emergency management should then be instituted accordingly (Table 2.3).

Identification of Meningitis

Signs of meningeal irritation are not invariably present and have differing sensitivities depending on the cause: They are extremely common with acute pyogenic meningitis and subarachnoid hemorrhage and less common with indolent, fungal meningitis. Nevertheless, the presence of these signs on examination is the central clue to the diagnosis. Missing these signs results in time-consuming additional tests such as brain imaging and the potential loss of a narrow window of opportunity for directed therapy.

意识障碍

李胜德 译 谭颖 周雁 审校 姚明 彭斌 通审

引言

昏迷是指患者无法对外界产生应答，即使受到强烈刺激仍然闭眼的状态。反应不良状态不是昏迷，患者存在自发睁眼、烦躁伴意识模糊或谵妄，但可能提示是疾病加重的早期征象，需要进一步寻找病因。

意识由脑干网状激活系统及完整正常的皮质投射功能维持。网状结构始于脑桥中部，沿中脑背侧上升至丘脑，然后经丘脑-皮质上行纤维投射到皮质进而支配高级中枢。对该解剖的了解令我们在判断昏迷病因时得以重点关注关键的脑结构：脑干或大脑半球，无论是药物性或结构性损害，这些部位病变都可以导致意识障碍，而其他部位脑损害不能导致昏迷。除结构性病变外，脑膜炎、代谢性脑病、镇静和癫痫也会造成弥漫性脑损害导致昏迷，需要纳入鉴别诊断。

病理生理因素

评估昏迷患者时，感染或蛛网膜下腔出血导致的脑膜刺激征是需要尽早关注的体征。这是因为其潜在病因可能无法通过计算机断层成像（CT）识别，但是需要及时识别和干预（特别是化脓性脑膜炎）。

幕上占位性病变可导致昏迷，原因是病变扩大跨越中线而损害双侧大脑半球，或压迫脑干喙侧网状结构。侧型脑疝（译者注：大脑镰下疝）（脑横向移动）和小脑幕切迹疝（脑纵向移动）的过程经常同时发生。床旁观察，可见幕上占位扩大的临床体征按照"从上到下"逐级演变（图2.1）。造成昏迷的幕上占位一般较大，在CT上很容易看到。

脑干占位性病变造成昏迷的原因是直接压迫网状结构。由于控制眼球水平活动的通路——脑桥侧视中枢、内侧纵束和动眼神经核——贯穿网状激活系统，眼球反射活动异常通常提示脑干损伤。若一名昏迷患者没有眼球反射性活动异常，提示不存在损伤脑干的颅后窝占位。CT可能无法显示某些颅后窝病变。颅后窝病变可能造成侧脑室的脑脊液流出道下游梗阻，导致严重的非交通性脑积水。

代谢异常是由营养缺乏（如维生素B_1、葡萄糖）、代谢紊乱（如低钠血症）、外源性毒素（如药物）或内源性毒素（如器官衰竭）引起的。代谢异常造成广泛的神经系统功能障碍。因此，除个别罕见情况，代谢异常不会出现偏瘫或单侧瞳孔扩大等定位体征。代谢性脑病在诊断时，检查者通过查体和影像找不到可以解释昏迷的明确病变，也尚未找到明确的代谢诱因。药物更容易影响脑干网状结构，查体时可见反射性眼球运动消失。多灶性脑组织病变的表现可类似代谢性昏迷（表2.1）。

在癫痫持续状态的末期，肢体抽搐逐渐缓解，但整个大脑的癫痫放电仍在继续（非惊厥性癫痫持续状态）。一旦癫痫中止，所谓的"癫痫发作后状态"也可导致不明原因的昏迷。

诊断方法

病史和体格检查在诊断中至关重要，不能被脑影像检查取代（表2.2）。有前驱性头痛病史支持脑膜炎、脑炎、颅内或蛛网膜下腔出血。中毒史、意识模糊或谵妄等症状提示广泛损害，应考虑脑膜炎、内源或外源性中毒。突发昏迷高度提示脑干缺血或出血性卒中、蛛网膜下腔出血或颅内出血破入侧脑室。昏迷前出现偏瘫或失语提示幕上占位或梗死。

体格检查非常重要且便捷，具有诊断价值。此过程围绕三个问题展开：①是否提示脑膜炎？②是否提示占位性病变？③是否提示广泛损害，有无外源性或内源性的代谢性病因？据此采取相应的急诊管理措施（表2.3）。

脑膜炎的诊断

脑膜刺激征不是必需的，取决于具体病因：在急性化脓性脑膜炎和蛛网膜下腔出血中脑膜刺激征极为常见，而在慢性真菌性脑膜炎中则较少出现。然而，检查时发现脑膜刺激征是诊断的重要线索。忽略了这些体征，临床医生会消耗不必要的时间去进行头部影像检查，并有可能错失治疗的最佳时机。

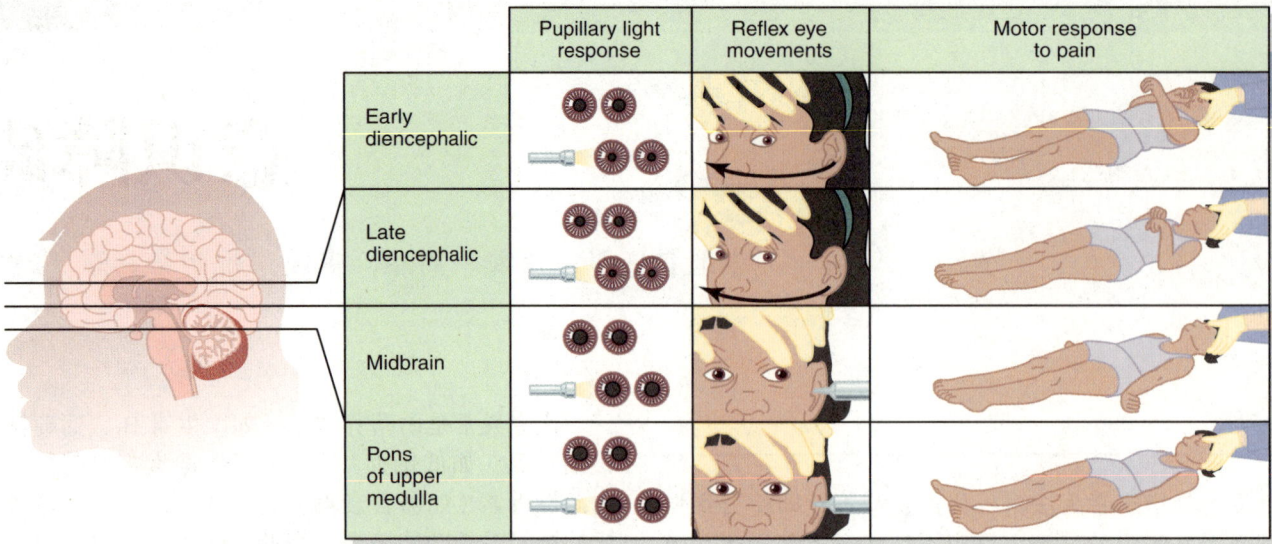

Fig. 2.1 The evolution of neurologic signs in coma from a hemispheric mass lesion as the brain becomes functionally impaired in a rostral-caudal manner. The terms *early diencephalic* and *late diencephalic* refer to levels of dysfunction just above and just below the thalamus, respectively. (From Aminoff MJ, Greenberg DA, Simon RP: Clinical neurology, Stamford, Conn., 1996, Appleton and Lange.)

TABLE 2.1 Multifocal Disorders Indicating Metabolic Coma
Disseminated intravascular coagulopathy
Sepsis
Pancreatitis
Vasculitis
Thrombotic thrombocytopenic purpura
Fat emboli
Hypertensive encephalopathy
Diffuse micrometastases

Passive neck flexion should be tested (Fig. 2.2) in all comatose patients unless a history of head trauma exists. When the neck is passively flexed by attempting to bring the chin within a few fingerbreadths of the chest, patients with irritated meninges reflexively flex one or both knees. This sign, called the *Brudzinski reflex*, is usually asymmetrical and not dramatic, but any evidence of knee flexion during passive neck flexion mandates that the cerebrospinal fluid be examined.

Is CT required before lumbar puncture in this setting? In the absence of lateralized signs (e.g., hemiparesis) supporting a superimposed mass lesion, a spinal puncture should be performed immediately. Although rare cases of herniation after lumbar puncture have been reported in children with bacterial meningitis, the urgency of diagnosis and treatment at the point of coma is paramount. The time required for CT may result in a fatal therapeutic delay. An alternative approach involves obtaining blood cultures and immediately initiating antibiotic therapy with subsequent lumbar puncture. With this approach, the cerebrospinal fluid cell count, glucose determination, and protein content are unchanged, and Gram stain and culture often remain positive despite a short period of antibiotic treatment. Bacterial antigens in the cerebrospinal fluid or blood can also be detected.

Separation of Structural From Metabolic Causes of Coma

The goal of this differential diagnosis is achieved by neurologic examination. Because the evaluation and potential treatments for structural and metabolic coma are widely divergent and the disease processes in both categories are often rapidly progressive, initiating prompt medical and surgical evaluation may be life-saving. Identification of a structural versus a metabolic cause is accomplished by focusing on three features of the neurologic examination: the *motor response* to a painful stimulus, *pupillary function,* and *reflex eye movements*.

Motor Response

Asymmetrical or reflex function of the motor system provides the clearest indication of a mass lesion. Elicitation of a *motor response* requires that a painful stimulus be applied, to which the patient will react. The patient's arms should be placed in a semiflexed posture, and a painful stimulus should be applied to the head or trunk. Strong pressure on the supraorbital ridge or pinching of the skin on the anterior chest or inner arm is the most useful method; finger nail bed pressure is also used, but it makes the interpretation of upper limb movement difficult.

The neurologic examination of a patient with an expanding hemispheric mass lesion is shown in Fig. 2.1. Hemispheric masses in their *early diencephalic* stage (i.e., compromising the brain above the thalamus) produce appropriate movement of one upper extremity—that is, movement toward the painful stimulus. The attenuated contralateral arm movement reflects a hemiparesis. This lateralized motor response in a comatose patient establishes the working diagnosis of a hemispheric mass. As the mass expands to involve the thalamus (*late diencephalic* stage), the response to pain becomes reflex arm flexion associated with extension and internal rotation of the legs (*decorticate posturing*); asymmetry of the response in the upper extremities is seen. With further brain compromise at the midbrain level, the reflex posturing in the arms changes such that both arms and legs respond by extension (*decerebrate posturing*); at that level, the asymmetry tends to

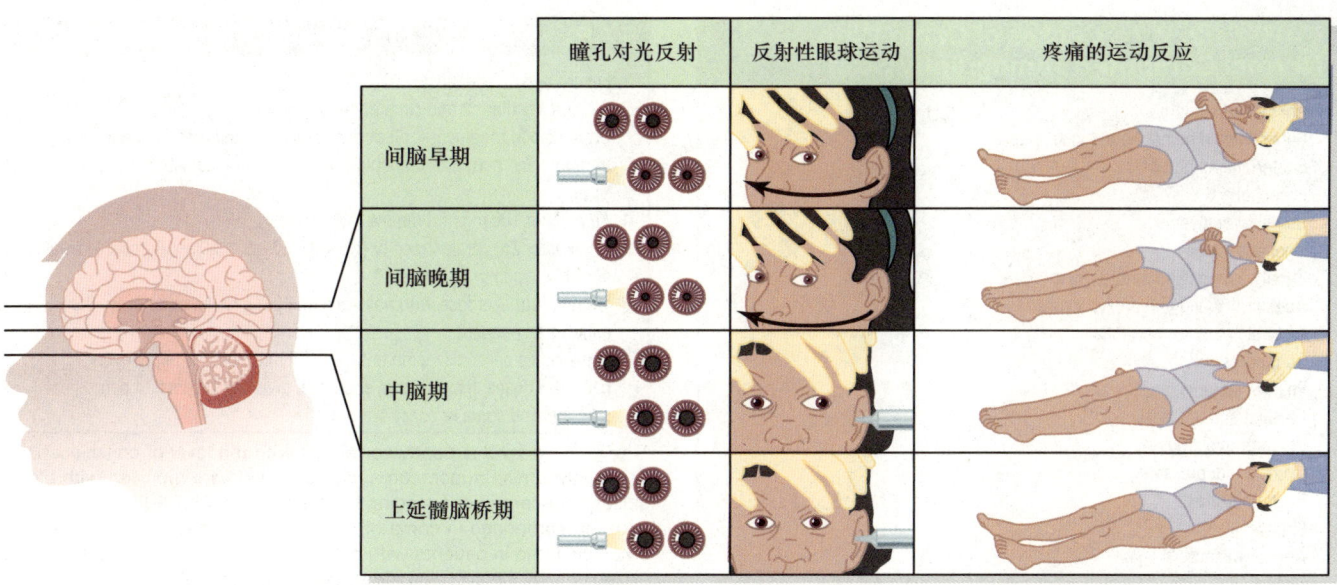

图 2.1 幕上占位性病变导致昏迷的患者神经系统体征演变，损害以"从上到下"的模式呈现。间脑早期和间脑晚期分别指丘脑上方和下方的功能障碍水平。（引自 Aminoff MJ，Greenberg DA，Simon RP：Clinical neurology，Stamford，Conn.，1996，Appleton and Lange.）

表 2.1 代谢性昏迷相关的多灶性疾病
弥散性血管内凝血
感染中毒症
胰腺炎
血管炎
血栓性血小板减少性紫癜
脂肪栓塞
高血压脑病
弥漫性微转移灶

除头部外伤外，昏迷患者都应做被动屈颈检查（图 2.2）。具有脑膜刺激征的患者被动屈颈时会反射性地屈曲一侧或双侧膝关节，这个体征被称为布鲁津斯基反射，此反射通常双侧不对称且不明显。在被动屈颈查体中一旦发现屈膝现象则必须完善脑脊液检查。

在这种情况下腰椎穿刺前是否需要完善 CT？如果没有偏侧体征（如偏瘫）提示占位，应立即进行腰椎穿刺。极少数情况下，细菌性脑膜炎患儿在腰椎穿刺后发生脑疝，但患者昏迷时的紧急诊疗更加重要。CT 检查可能会延误治疗，造成致命的严重后果。另一替代方案为完善血培养后即刻予抗生素治疗，随后进行腰椎穿刺。脑脊液细胞数、葡萄糖和蛋白质含量都不会因此改变，短期抗生素治疗也不会改变革兰染色和病原培养的阳性结果。脑脊液或血液中的细菌抗原也可被测出。

结构性原因和代谢性原因所致昏迷的鉴别

神经系统查体有助于鉴别诊断。由于结构性和代谢性昏迷的评估和治疗方法差异很大，且这两种疾病进展通常迅速，及时的药物和手术治疗可能挽救患者的生命。可以从神经系统查体的三个方面进行结构性昏迷与代谢性昏迷的鉴别：疼痛刺激的运动反应、瞳孔对光反射及反射性眼球运动。

运动反应

运动系统反射的不对称性是占位性病变的最明显征象。给予患者疼痛刺激，可诱发运动反应。令患者的双臂置于半屈曲位，向其头部或躯干施以疼痛刺激。压眶或者掐前胸或手臂内侧的皮肤是最有效的方法。也可压甲床，但可能掩盖真实的上肢运动。

图 2.1 显示了一位幕上占位性病变患者的神经系统检查。幕上占位在间脑早期（丘脑以上水平损害）出现一侧上肢对疼痛刺激的运动反应正常，对侧上肢运动减弱则提示偏瘫。昏迷患者的这种不对称运动反应提示幕上占位。随着占位扩大并累及丘脑水平（间脑晚期），患者对疼痛的反应变成手臂屈曲伴双腿伸直和内旋（去皮质强直），可观察到上肢反应不对称。随着占位累及中脑水平，反射姿势变为手臂和双腿伸直（去大脑强直），在这一水平上不对称现象会消失。此

TABLE 2.2 Causes of Coma With Normal Computed Tomography Scan

Meningeal disorders
   Subarachnoid hemorrhage (uncommon)
   Bacterial meningitis
   Encephalitis
   Subdural empyema
Exogenous toxins
   Sedative drugs and barbiturates
   Anesthetics and γ-hydroxybutyrate[a]
   Alcohol
   Stimulants
   Phencyclidine[b]
   Cocaine and amphetamine[c]
   Psychotropic drugs
   Cyclic antidepressants
   Phenothiazines
   Lithium
   Anticonvulsants
   Opioids
   Clonidine[d]
   Penicillins
   Salicylates
   Anticholinergics
   Carbon monoxide, cyanide, and methemoglobinemia
Endogenous toxins, deficiencies, derangements
   Hypoxia and ischemia
   Hypoglycemia
   Hypercalcemia
Osmolar causes
   Hyperglycemia
   Hyponatremia
   Hypernatremia
Organ system failure
   Hepatic encephalopathy
   Uremic encephalopathy
   Pulmonary insufficiency (carbon dioxide narcosis)
Seizures
   Prolonged postictal state
   Spike-wave stupor
Hypothermia or hyperthermia
Brain stem ischemia
Basilar artery stroke
Pituitary apoplexy
Conversion or malingering

[a]General anesthetic, similar to γ-aminobutyric acid; used as a recreational drug and body building aid. It has a rapid onset and rapid recovery, often with myoclonic jerking and confusion. It causes deep coma lasting 2 to 3 hours (Glasgow Coma Scale score = 3) with maintenance of vital signs.
[b]Coma associated with cholinergic signs: lacrimation, salivation, bronchorrhea, and hyperthermia.
[c]Coma after seizures or status epilepticus (i.e., a prolonged postictal state).
[d]An antihypertensive agent that is active through the opiate receptor system; overdose is frequent when used to treat narcotic withdrawal.

be lost. At this point, the pupils become mid-position in size, and the light reflex is lost, first unilaterally and then bilaterally. With further progression to the level of the pons, the most frequent finding is no response to painful stimulation, although spinal-mediated movements of leg flexion may occur.

TABLE 2.3 Emergency Management

1. Ensure airway adequacy.
2. Support ventilation and circulation.
3. Obtain blood for glucose, electrolytes, hepatic and renal function, prothrombin and partial thromboplastin times, complete blood count, and drug screen.
4. Administer 100 mg of thiamine intravenously (IV).
5. Administer 25 g of dextrose IV (typically 50 mL of 50% dextrose) to treat possible hypoglycemic coma.[a]
6. Treat opiate overdose with naloxone (0.4-2 mg IV repeated every 2-3 minutes as needed).
7. The specific benzodiazepine antagonist flumazenil (0.2 mg IV every 1 min, ×1-5 doses; max is 1 mg) should be given for reversal of benzodiazepine-induced coma or conscious sedation.[b]

[a]The glucose level is poorly correlated with the level of consciousness in hypoglycemia; stupor, coma, and confusion are reported with blood glucose concentrations ranging from 2 to 60 mg/dL.
[b]Not recommended in coma of unknown origin because seizures may be precipitated in patients with polydrug overdoses that include benzodiazepines with tricyclic antidepressants or cocaine.

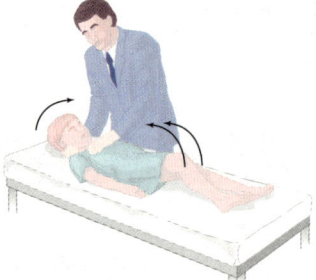

Fig. 2.2 Elicitation of Brudzinski sign of meningeal irritation, as seen in infectious meningitis or subarachnoid hemorrhage. (From Aminoff MJ, Greenberg DA, Simon RP: Clinical neurology, Stamford, Conn., 1996, Appleton and Lange.)

The classic postures illustrated in Fig. 2.1, and particularly their asymmetry, strongly support the presence of a mass lesion. However, these motor movements, especially early in coma, are most frequently seen as fragments of the fully developed, asymmetrical flexion or extension of the arms (illustrated as decorticate and decerebrate postures in Fig. 2.1). A small amount of asymmetrical flexion or extension of the arms in response to a painful stimulus carries the same implications as the full-blown postures of decortication or decerebration.

Metabolic lesions do not compromise the brain in a progressive, level-by-level manner as do hemispheric masses, and they rarely produce the asymmetrical motor signs typical of masses. Reflex posturing may be seen, but it lacks the asymmetry of decortication seen with a hemispheric mass, and it is not associated with the loss of pupillary reactivity at the stage of decerebration.

Pupillary Reactivity

In metabolic coma, one feature is central to the examination: Pupillary reactivity is present. This reactivity is seen both early in metabolic coma, when an appropriate motor response to pain may be retained, and late in coma, when no motor responses can be elicited. The pupillary reaction in metabolic coma is lost only when coma is so deep that the patient requires ventilatory and blood pressure support.

表 2.2　计算机断层成像正常的昏迷原因
脑膜疾病
蛛网膜下腔出血（不常见）
细菌性脑膜炎
脑炎
硬膜下积脓
外源性毒素
镇静药和巴比妥酸盐
麻醉剂和 γ- 羟基丁酸盐[a]
乙醇
兴奋剂
苯环利定[b]
可卡因和苯丙胺[c]
精神类药物
环类抗抑郁剂
吩噻嗪类药物
锂
抗惊厥药
阿片类药物
可乐定[d]
青霉素类
水杨酸盐
抗胆碱能药
一氧化碳、氰化物和高铁血红蛋白血症
内源性毒素、营养缺乏、代谢紊乱
缺氧和缺血
低血糖症
高钙血症
渗透性病因
高血糖症
低钠血症
高钠血症
器官衰竭
肝性脑病
尿毒症脑病
肺功能不全（二氧化碳中毒）
癫痫发作
长时间的发作后状态
棘波昏睡
低体温或高体温
脑干缺血
基底动脉卒中
垂体卒中
癔症或诈病

[a] 全身麻醉剂，类似于 γ- 氨基丁酸；可用作娱乐药物和健美辅助药物。它起效快，恢复也快，通常伴有肌阵挛样抽搐和意识模糊。它会导致持续 2～3 h 的深度昏迷（格拉斯哥昏迷量表评分＝3），但生命体征仍可维持。
[b] 昏迷伴有胆碱能样表现：流泪、流涎、支气管溢液和高热。
[c] 癫痫发作或癫痫持续状态后昏迷（即长时间的发作后状态）。
[d] 一种通过阿片受体系统发挥活性的降压药；用于治疗麻醉药戒断时，经常出现用药过量的情况。

表 2.3　急诊管理
1. 保持气道通畅。
2. 呼吸循环支持。
3. 采血检测葡萄糖、电解质、肝肾功能、凝血酶原和部分凝血活酶时间、全血细胞计数和药物筛查。
4. 静脉注射（IV）100 mg 维生素 B_1（硫胺素）。
5. 静脉注射 25 g 葡萄糖（通常是 50 ml 50% 葡萄糖）来治疗可能的低血糖昏迷[a]。
6. 使用纳洛酮（0.4～2 mg 静脉注射，根据需要每 2～3 min 重复一次）来治疗阿片类药物过量。
7. 为逆转苯二氮䓬类药物引起的昏迷或意识镇静状态，应使用特定的苯二氮䓬类药物拮抗剂氟马西尼（0.2 mg，静脉注射，每分钟一次，1～5 次剂量；最大剂量为 1 mg）[b]。

[a] 血糖水平与低血糖患者的意识水平关系不大；据报道，血糖浓度为 2～60 mg/dl 时都可出现昏睡、昏迷和意识模糊。
[b] 不推荐在原因不明的昏迷患者中使用，因为在过量服用多种药物（包括苯二氮䓬类药物和三环类抗抑郁药或可卡因）的患者中使用可能会诱发癫痫发作。

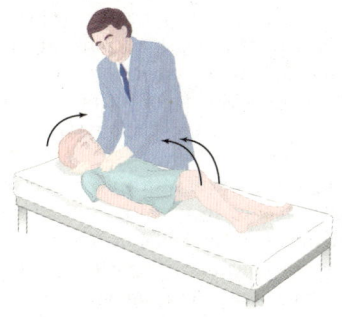

图 2.2　脑膜刺激的布鲁津斯基征，可见于感染性脑膜炎或蛛网膜下腔出血。（引自 Aminoff MJ, Greenberg DA, Simon RP: Clinical neurology, Stamford, Conn., 1996, Appleton and Lange.）

图 2.1 所示的典型姿势，特别是不对称性，强烈提示幕上占位性病变。然而，这些肢体运动，尤其在昏迷早期，常被视作上肢完全的、不对称的屈曲或伸直的不完全表现（如图 2.1 中的"去皮质"和"去大脑"强直所示）。疼痛刺激后上肢小幅度的不对称屈曲或伸直动作提示的意义与完全的去皮质和去大脑强直相同。

代谢性因素对大脑的损害不会像占位那样逐级递进，也很少出现占位那样典型的不对称运动症状。反射性姿势可能会出现，但不会出现幕上占位那样不对称性去皮质强直，在去大脑强直状态下也不会出现瞳孔反射消失。

瞳孔对光反射

瞳孔对光反射存在是代谢性昏迷患者的一个核心体征。在代谢性昏迷的早期（疼痛刺激可诱发运动反应）和晚期（疼痛刺激不能诱发运动反应），这种瞳孔对光反射始终存在。在代谢性昏迷中，只有当深度昏迷需要呼吸和血压支持时，瞳孔反射才会消失。

时，瞳孔变为中等大小，对光反射消失，从一侧进展到双侧。病情进一步进展至脑桥水平，最常见的症状是对疼痛刺激无反应，但可能会出现脊髓介导的腿部屈曲运动。

Reflex Eye Movements

The presence of inducible lateral eye movements reflects the integrity of the pons and midbrain. These reflex eye movements (see Fig. 2.1) are brought about with the use of passive head rotation to stimulate the semicircular canal input to the vestibular system (so-called *doll's eyes maneuver*) or by inhibiting the function of one semicircular canal by infusing ice water against the tympanic membrane (caloric testing).

In metabolic coma, reflex eye movements may be lost or retained. Lack of inducible eye movements with the doll's eyes maneuver, in the setting of preserved pupillary reactivity, is virtually diagnostic of drug toxicity. With metabolic coma of non–drug-induced origin, such as organ system failure, electrolyte disorders, or osmolar disorders, reflex eye movements are preserved.

Brain stem mass lesions are most commonly caused by hemorrhage or infarction. Reflex lateral eye movements, the pathways for which traverse the pons and midbrain, are particularly affected, and the reflex postures of decortication and decerebration typical of brain stem injury are common. Lesions restricted to the midbrain (e.g., embolization from the heart to the top of the basilar artery) cause sluggish pupillary reflexes or their absence, with or without impaired medial eye movements; both are controlled by the third cranial nerve. With lesions restricted to the pons (e.g., intrapontine hypertensive hemorrhage), pupils are reactive but very small (pinpoint or pontine pupils), reflecting focal impairment of sympathetic innervations; pinpoint pupils are rare. Ocular bobbing (spontaneous symmetrical or asymmetrical rhythmic vertical ocular oscillations) is most often a manifestation of a pontine lesion.

Seizures occurring in a patient with acute brain injury (such as that resulting from encephalitis, hypertensive encephalopathy, hyponatremia, hypernatremia, hypoglycemia, or hyperglycemia) or chronic brain injury (such as dementia or mental retardation) often result in prolonged postictal coma. The examination shows reactive pupils and inducible eye movements (in the absence of overtreatment with anticonvulsants), and often up-going toes or focal signs are observed (Todd paresis).

Nonconvulsive status epilepticus should be considered as a diagnosis even if there are no obvious seizure movements. Nonconvulsive seizures can cause coma and also can complicate other etiologies of coma, including infectious and metabolic disorders. Nonconvulsive seizures should be suspected in patients with (1) a seemingly prolonged "postictal state" after generalized convulsive seizures or prolonged alteration of alertness after an operative procedure or neurologic insult; (2) acute onset of impaired consciousness or fluctuating mentation interspersed with episodes of normal awareness; (3) altered mental status or consciousness associated with facial myoclonus or nystagmoid eye movements; or (4) episodic blank staring, aphasia, automatisms (e.g., lip-smacking, fumbling with fingers), or acute-onset aphasia without an acute structural lesion. The diagnosis is made by electroencephalography (EEG) (see Chapter 15). EEG provides information about brain electrical activity even when brain function is depressed and cannot be evaluated otherwise, as in comatose patients. EEG is essential to detect electrical seizures and document their duration as well as the response to therapy and to improve coma prognostication.

Current evidence suggests that the presence of nonconvulsive seizures or periodic discharges, delay to diagnosis, and duration of nonconvulsive status in patients with or without acute brain injury are independent predictors of worse outcome.

PROGNOSIS IN COMA AFTER CARDIAC ARREST

Historically, prognostication after cardiac arrest was solely based on neurologic examination. Pupillary, corneal, and motor responses are

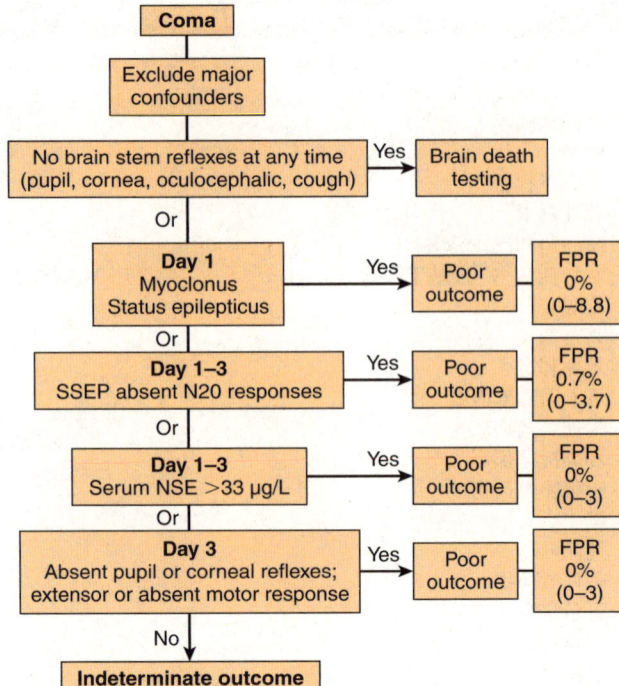

Fig. 2.3 Decision algorithm for use in prognostication of comatose survivors after cardiopulmonary resuscitation (CPR). The numbers in parentheses show the exact 95% confidence intervals. *FPR*, False-positive rate; *N20*, a negative peak at 20 ms on SSEP; *NSE*, neuron-specific enolase; *SSEP*, somatosensory evoked potential. (Data from Wijdicks EFM, Hijdra A, Young GB, et al: Practice parameter: prediction of outcome in comatose survivors after CPR [an evidence-based review]: report of the Quality Standards Subcommittee of the American Academy of Neurology, Neurology 67:203-210, 2006.)

the best clinical indicators of prognosis that can be assessed at bedside. Such responses reflect the functionality of the brain stem, which is the most resilient portion of central nervous system (Fig. 2.3).

Although the neurologic exam is still the cornerstone of prognostication, there has been extensive work using other modalities to better predict prognosis. Current guidelines endorse using EEG to guide prognostication in comatose survivors of cardiac arrest. The absence of normal background activity or reactivity predicts a poor prognosis. Conversely, continuous background activity and the presence of reactivity are among the few reliable predictors of good neurologic recovery. Somatosensory evoked potentials (SSEPs), another electrophysiologic marker of cortical responsiveness, are most helpful for predicting which patients will remain in a persistent coma. By 24 hours after cardiac arrest, bilateral absence of the N20 cortical response (a negative peak at 20 ms) to median nerve stimulation predicts a grave outcome. The early onset of generalized myoclonic status is an ominous sign. Neuron-specific enolase (NSE) is the most promising of several serum biomarkers that have been evaluated. NSE level greater than 30 ng/mL predicts persistent coma. Despite tremendous potential, the role of neuroimaging as a prognostic tool after hypoxic-ischemic injury from cardiac arrest has yet to be clearly defined. Severe reductions in the apparent diffusion coefficient (ADC), as well as bilateral hippocampal hyperintensities on magnetic resonance imaging (MRI), suggest severe global damage and extensive ischemic injury and are predictive of poor neurologic recovery.

Therapeutic hypothermia has been demonstrated to improve neurologic outcomes in patients who have return of spontaneous circulation

反射性眼球运动

可诱发的单侧反射性水平眼球运动的存在，提示脑桥和中脑的功能完整。通过被动旋转头部刺激半规管及前庭系统（所谓的玩偶眼试验）来诱发反射性眼球运动，或通过向鼓膜注入冰水来抑制单个半规管的功能（冷热水试验）来诱发（见图2.1）。

在代谢性昏迷时，反射性眼球运动可能消失或保留。在瞳孔对光反射保留的情况下，玩偶眼试验中反射性眼球运动消失，基本可诊断为药物中毒。非药物中毒如器官衰竭、电解质紊乱或渗透压引起的代谢性昏迷，反射性眼球运动正常。

脑干占位性病变最常见于出血或梗死。反射性眼球运动通路贯穿脑桥和中脑，容易受到影响，脑干病变经常导致典型的去皮质强直和去大脑强直。局限于中脑的病变（如心脏到基底动脉尖的栓塞）会导致瞳孔反射迟钝或消失，伴或不伴眼球内收障碍；瞳孔对光反射和眼球内收都受第Ⅲ对脑神经控制。如果病变局限于脑桥（如高血压性脑桥出血），瞳孔对光反射存在但直径缩小（针尖样瞳孔或脑桥瞳孔），反映出交感神经的局灶性损害；针尖样瞳孔很少见。眼球浮动（自发性对称或非对称性节律性垂直眼球摆动）是脑桥病变的一种最常见表现。

急性脑损伤（如脑炎、高血压脑病、低钠血症、高钠血症、低血糖或高血糖所致）或慢性脑损伤（如痴呆或精神发育迟滞）继发的癫痫发作通常会导致发作后长时间的昏迷。神经系统查体可见瞳孔对光反射正常和诱导的眼球运动（在没有过度使用抗惊厥药的情况下），通常还会见到足趾上翘或局灶性体征（Todd瘫痪）。

即使没有明显的癫痫发作，也应该鉴别非惊厥性癫痫持续状态。非惊厥性癫痫发作可导致昏迷，也可合并昏迷的其他诱因，包括感染性和代谢性疾病。当患者出现以下情况时，应怀疑非惊厥性癫痫发作：①全面性惊厥发作后出现一个看似长时间的"发作后状态"，或在手术或神经系统损伤后出现长时间的警觉性改变；②急性发作的意识障碍或波动性精神异常，伴间断性意识正常；③伴有面肌痉挛或眼震样运动的精神或意识改变；④发作性愣神、失语、自动症（如咂嘴或摸索动作），或不伴急性结构性病变的突发失语症。诊断主要依靠脑电图（EEG）（见第15章）。即使是脑功能受损，无法用其他方法评估的昏迷患者，脑电图依然可以提供脑电活动的信息。脑电图对于监测癫痫电活动、记录其持续时间和对治疗的反应以及改善昏迷预后至关重要。

现有证据表明，无论急性脑损伤是否存在，非惊厥性癫痫发作或周期性放电、延迟诊断以及非惊厥状态持续时间，都是患者病情恶化的独立预测因素。

心脏停搏后昏迷患者的预后

长期以来，心脏停搏的预后仅以神经系统检查作为判断基础。瞳孔对光反射、角膜反射以及运动反应是床边评估预

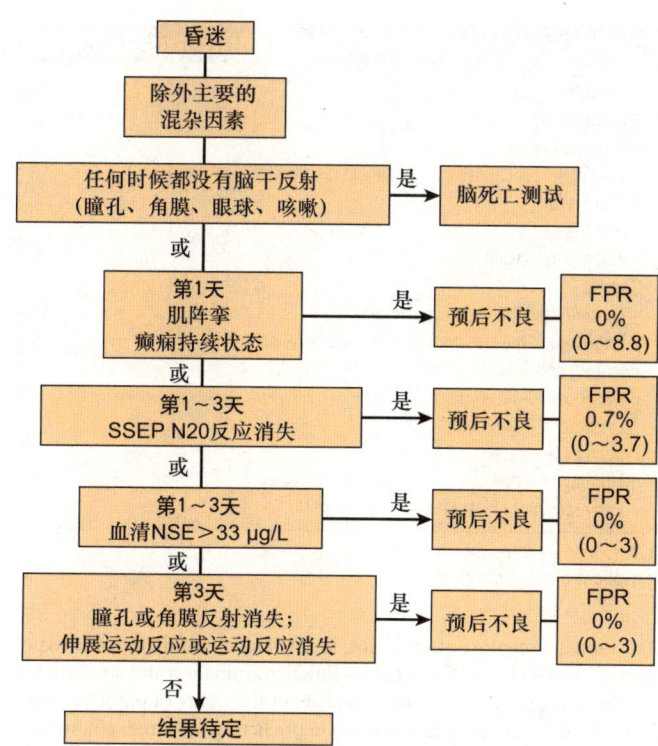

图2.3 心肺复苏术（CPR）后昏迷幸存者预后预测的决策图。括号中的数字表示精确的95%置信区间。FPR，假阳性率；N20，SSEP 20 ms处的负峰值；NSE，神经元特异性烯醇化酶；SSEP，体感诱发电位。[数据引自 Wijdicks EFM, Hijdra A, Young GB, et al: Practice parameter: prediction of outcome in comatose survivors after CPR (an evidence-based review): report of the Quality Standards Subcommittee of the American Academy of Neurology, Neurology 67: 203-210, 2006.]

后的最佳临床指标。这些反应体现了脑干的功能，而脑干是中枢神经系统中功能修复能力最强的部分（图2.3）。

虽然神经系统检查仍是判断预后的基石，现已有大量研究采用其他方法以更好地预测患者预后。现有指南推荐使用脑电图来评估心脏停搏后昏迷患者的预后。正常的背景活动或反应的消失提示预后不良。相反，作为少数可靠的预测指标之一，持续正常的背景活动和反应性存在则预示神经功能恢复良好。作为大脑皮质反应性的另一种电生理标志，体感诱发电位（SSEP）最有助于预测哪些患者会长时间昏迷。心脏停搏24 h后，正中神经刺激诱发的双侧N20反应（20 ms处的负峰）消失，提示预后严重不良。早期出现全身性肌阵挛状态也提示预后不良。在诸多被研究评估过的血清生物标志物中，神经元特异性烯醇化酶（NSE）被认为是最有前景的标志物，NSE水平超过30 ng/ml提示有可能出现持续性昏迷。神经影像学在预测心脏停搏缺氧缺血性损伤的预后方面的作用尚待研究，未来潜力巨大。双侧海马的磁共振成像（MRI）高信号以及表观弥散系数（ADC）显著减低则提示严重的全脑损伤和广泛的缺血性损害，这预示神经功能预后不良。

对于心脏停搏后自主循环恢复但仍处于昏迷状态的患者，治疗性低温已被证实可改善其神经功能预后。

TABLE 2.4	Locked-In Syndrome
Clinical features	
Eye opening	
Reactive pupils	
Volitional vertical eye movements in response to command	
Muteness	
Quadriparesis	
Sleep-wake cycles	
Causes	
Pontine vascular lesions (common)	
Head injury, brain stem tumor, pontine myelinolysis (rare)	
Recovery possible	
Onset over 1-12 wk (vascular)[a] *or*	
Onset over 4-6 mo (nonvascular)[a]	
Prognosis favorable	
Normal CT scan[a]	
Early recovery of lateral eye movements[a]	

CT, Computed tomography.
[a]Implications for care.

but remain comatose after cardiac arrest. The use of therapeutic hypothermia quite likely influences the clinical examination and ancillary test findings. There are a scarcity of data about the utility of physical examination, EEG, and evoked potentials in predicting outcomes among cardiac arrest patients with induced hypothermia. It is well accepted that one should consider observation for longer than 72 hours before prognosticating outcome in patients treated with hypothermia.

COMA-LIKE STATES

Patients with *locked-in syndrome* have a lesion (usually a hemorrhage or an infarct) that transects the brain stem at a point below the reticular formation (thereby sparing consciousness) but above the ventilatory nuclei of the medulla (thereby maintaining cardiopulmonary function) (Table 2.4). Such patients are awake, with eye opening and sleep-wake cycles, but the descending pathways through the brain stem that are necessary for volitional vocalization or limb movement have been transected. Voluntary eye movement, especially vertically, is preserved, and patients can open and close their eyes or produce appropriate numbers of blinking movements in answer to questions. The EEG is usually normal, reflecting normal cortical function.

Psychogenic unresponsiveness is a diagnosis of exclusion. The neurologic examination shows reactive pupils and no reflex posturing in response to pain. Eye movements during the doll's eyes maneuver show volitional override rather than the smooth, uninhibited reflex lateral eye movements of coma. Ice water caloric testing either arouses the patient because of the discomfort produced or induces cortically mediated nystagmus rather than the tonic deviation typical of coma. The slow, conjugate roving eye movements of metabolic coma cannot be imitated and therefore rule out psychogenic unresponsiveness. Likewise, the slow, often asymmetrical, and incomplete eye closure seen after passive eye opening in a comatose patient cannot be feigned. In contrast, conscious patients usually exhibit some voluntary muscle tone in the eyelids during passive eye opening. The EEG in psychogenic unresponsiveness is that of normal wakefulness, with reactive posterior rhythms on eye opening and eye closing. In patients with catatonic stupor, lorazepam administration may produce awakening.

Unresponsive wakefulness syndrome, previously called vegetative state (VS), is exhibited by patients with eye opening and sleep-wake cycles. The reticular activating system of the brain stem is intact to produce wakefulness, but the connections to the cortical mantle are interrupted, precluding awareness.

A VS is termed *persistent* after 3 months if the brain injury was ischemic in nature or after 12 months if the brain injury was traumatic in nature. The determination as to when *persistent* equals *permanent* cannot be stated absolutely. Prediction early in VS of which patients will remain persistently vegetative is particularly difficult in cases of trauma. Lesions of the corpus callosum and dorsolateral brain stem seen on MRI 6 to 8 weeks after trauma correlated with persistence of VS at 1 year. A combined analysis of morphologic MRI studies and post-traumatic brain stem spectroscopy can be a predictor of persistent vegetative states (PVS) and minimally conscious states (MVS). In rare cases, patients show late improvement, but they do not return to normal. Bilateral absence of SSEPs in the first week predicts death or VS.

Patients in a PVS open their eyes diurnally and in response to loud sounds; blinking occurs with bright lights. Pupils react and eye movements occur both spontaneously and with the doll's eyes maneuver. Yawning, chewing, swallowing, and, uncommonly, guttural vocalizations and lacrimation may be preserved. Spontaneous roving eye movements (very slow, with constant velocity) are particularly characteristic and distressing to the patient's visitors because the patient appears to be looking about the room. The brain stem origin of the eye movements is documented by their being readily redirected by the oculocephalic (doll's eyes) reflex. The limbs may move, but motor responses are only primitive; pain usually produces decorticate or decerebrate postures or fragments of these movements.

Minimally conscious state (MCS) is a newly described entity in which patients do not meet criteria for PVS. Both patients in PVS and those in MCS demonstrate severe alteration in consciousness. In contrast to PVS, subjects with MCS exhibit evidence of limited interaction with the environment by visually tracking, following simple commands, answering yes or no (not necessarily reliably), or having intelligible verbalization or restricted purposeful behavior. It is estimated that the rate of misdiagnosis between the VS and MCS is about 40%.

Novel applications of functional neuroimaging in patients with disorders of consciousness may aid in differential diagnosis, prognostic assessment, and identification of pathophysiologic mechanisms. In one study, authors prospectively evaluated cortical activation in response to a familiar voice in seven patients in VS and four subjects in MCS. All four of the MCS patients and only two of the VS patients showed activation that extended beyond the primary auditory cortex to hierarchically higher-order associative temporal areas. Over the course of 3 months, these two VS patients improved clinically to MCS.

Brain death characterizes the *irreversible cessation* of brain function. Therefore, death of the organism can be determined based on death of the brain. Although local laws may dictate some details, the standard definition permits a diagnosis of brain death based on documentation of irreversible cessation of all brain function, including function of the brain stem (Table 2.5). Documentation of *irreversibility* requires that the cause of the coma is known, that the cause is adequate to explain the clinical findings of brain death, and that exclusionary criteria are absent (Table 2.6). Confirmatory tests are sometimes used but are not required for diagnosis (Table 2.7). Brain death results in asystole, usually within days (mean, 4 days), even if ventilatory support is continued. Recovery after appropriate documentation of brain death has never been reported. Removal of the ventilator results in terminal rhythms (most often complete heart block without ventricular response), junctional rhythms, or ventricular tachycardia. Purely spinal motor movements may occur in the moments of terminal apnea (or during apnea testing in the absence of passive administration of oxygen); these may include arching of the back, neck turning, stiffening of the legs, and upper extremity flexion.

表 2.4 闭锁综合征
临床特征
睁眼
瞳孔对光反射存在
遵嘱自主完成眼球垂直运动
缄默
四肢瘫
睡眠-觉醒周期
病因
脑桥血管病变（常见）
头部外伤、脑干肿瘤、脑桥髓鞘溶解（罕见）
可能恢复的时间
起病 1～2 周（血管性）[a] 或
起病 4～6 个月（非血管性）[a]
支持良好预后
正常的 CT 扫描结果[a]
水平眼球运动早期恢复[a]

CT，计算机断层成像。
[a] 对临床照护的意义。

采用治疗性低温很可能会影响临床检查和辅助检查的结果。目前缺乏证据指导临床医师如何使用体格检查、脑电图和诱发电位在心脏停搏患者中预测诱导性低温治疗的预后。普遍认为，对接受低温治疗的患者在进行预后评估前，需观察 72 h 以上。

类昏迷状态

闭锁综合征患者的病变（通常是出血或梗死）是一种横贯性损伤，损伤部位是脑干网状结构以下（保存了意识）、延髓呼吸运动核团以上（维持了心肺功能）（表2.4）。这类患者是清醒的，存在睁眼和睡眠-觉醒周期，但支配自主发声或肢体运动的脑干下行通路已受到横贯性损害。患者的眼球活动自如，尤其是垂直方向的运动不受影响，可以通过睁闭眼，或通过对应次数的眨眼动作来回答问题。他们的脑电图通常是正常的，提示大脑皮质功能正常。

心因性反应迟钝是排除性诊断。神经系统检查显示瞳孔对光反射存在，但对疼痛刺激没有反应。玩偶眼试验显示的眼球活动提示受意识控制，而非昏迷患者那样平滑、无抑制的反射性眼球水平运动。冷热水试验要么会因不适而唤醒患者，要么会诱发大脑皮质介导的眼球震颤，而非昏迷患者那样典型的强直性眼球偏转。代谢性昏迷患者的缓慢、共轭徘徊样眼球运动，是难以模仿的，可用于除外心因性无反应的可能性。同样，在被动睁眼后，昏迷患者的缓慢、不对称和不完全的闭眼动作也无法假装。与此相反，清醒患者在被动睁眼时眼睑的肌肉张力常表现出一定程度的主动违抗。心因性反应迟钝患者的脑电图提示正常清醒状态，并存在睁闭眼的反应性后节律。对于紧张性木僵患者，给予劳拉西泮可能会使其苏醒。

无反应觉醒综合征以前被称为植物状态（VS），患者表现出睁眼和睡眠-觉醒周期。脑干的网状激活系统保持完整，所以可产生觉醒，但其与大脑皮质的连接中断，导致缺乏意识。

持续植物状态的定义是缺血性脑损伤超过 3 个月或创伤性脑损伤超过 12 个月。持续植物状态保持多长时间后称为永久性植物状态，并没有绝对的定论。在外伤患者中，更加难以在早期预测哪些患者会一直处于植物状态。磁共振成像显示，外伤后 6～8 周出现的胼胝体和脑干背外侧的损伤与植物状态持续 1 年相关。磁共振成像形态和创伤后脑干光谱的联合分析可以预测持续植物状态（PVS）和最小意识状态（MCS）。极少数情况下，患者在很长时间后会出现好转，但不会恢复正常。双侧体感诱发电位（SSEP）在第 1 周消失预示死亡或植物状态（VS）。

持续植物状态的患者每日都会睁眼，对响亮的声音有反应，在强光下会眨眼。瞳孔有对光反射，眼球也会自发转动或在做玩偶眼试验时运动。患者可以打哈欠、咀嚼、吞咽，偶尔发出咕噜声和流泪。眼球自发来回运动（非常缓慢，速度恒定）是一种特征性表现，像在环顾房间，这会令探视者感到伤感。眼球运动反射（玩偶眼征）直接证明了眼动的支配源于脑干。患者肢体可运动，但只保留了本能运动；疼痛刺激通常产生完全或不完全的去皮质或去大脑强直。

最小意识状态（MCS）是一个新的疾病名词，用来描述不符合持续植物状态的昏迷患者。持续植物状态和最小意识状态的患者都存在严重的意识障碍。与持续植物状态相反，最小意识状态患者可通过视觉跟踪、执行简单指令、回答是或否（不一定可靠）、可被理解的语言或有限制的目的性行为与周围环境进行有限的互动。据估计，持续植物状态和最小意识状态间的误诊率约为 40%。

功能神经影像技术的创新和应用可能有助于意识障碍的鉴别诊断、预后评估以及病理生理机制的推断。一项研究前瞻性地评估了 7 名植物状态患者和 4 名最小意识状态患者对熟悉声音的皮质激活反应。4 名最小意识状态患者和 2 名植物状态患者的皮质激活范围从初级听觉皮质延伸至高级听觉皮质相关的颞叶。此后 3 个月，这 2 名植物状态患者改善至最小意识状态。

脑死亡是指大脑功能不可逆转地停止。因此，生物体的死亡可以依据大脑死亡来判定。尽管各地法律在细节上有些不同，但标准的定义允许根据所有脑功能（包括脑干功能在内）不可逆转的停止来诊断脑死亡（表 2.5）。若记录为不可逆转，则要求昏迷的原因是明确的，并足以解释脑死亡的临床表现，且不存在其他排除性标准（表 2.6）。有时会采用确证检查，但这并非诊断的必要条件（表 2.7）。即使存在呼吸支持，脑死亡通常在数天内（平均 4 天）导致心搏停止。从未有脑死亡患者恢复的案例。撤除呼吸机会导致终末心律（最常见的是无室性反应的完全性心脏传导阻滞）、交界性节律或室性心动过速。在呼吸停止的最后时刻（窒息测试没有被动给氧的情况下）可能会出现纯脊髓反射运动，这些运动可能包括角弓反张、转颈、下肢强直及上肢屈曲。

TABLE 2.5 Criteria for Cessation of Brain Function[a]

Anatomic Region Tested	Confirmatory Sign
Hemispheres	Unresponsive and unreceptive to sensory stimuli including pain[b]
Midbrain	Unreactive pupils[c]
Pons	Absent reflex eye movements[d]
Medulla	Apnea[e]

CO_2, Carbon dioxide; PCO_2, partial pressure of carbon dioxide.

[a]Sequential testing is necessary for a clinical diagnosis of brain death; it should be done at least every 6 hours in all cases and at least every 24 hours in the setting of anoxic-ischemic brain injury.

[b]The patient does not rouse, groan, grimace, or withdraw limbs. Purely spinal reflexes (deep tendon reflexes, plantar flexion reflex, plantar withdrawal, and tonic neck reflexes) may be maintained.

[c]Most easily assessed by the bright light of an ophthalmoscope viewed through its magnifying lens when focused on the iris. Unreactive pupils may be either midposition, as they will be in death, or dilated, as they often are in the setting of a dopamine infusion.

[d]No eye movement toward the side of irrigation of the tympanic membrane with 50 mL of ice water. The oculocephalic response (doll's eyes maneuver) is always absent in the setting of absent oculovestibular testing.

[e]No ventilatory movements in the setting of maximum CO_2 stimulation (≥60 mm Hg); with apnea, PCO_2 passively rises 2 to 3 mm Hg/min). Disconnect the ventilator from the endotracheal tube and insert a cannula with 6 L of oxygen per minute.

TABLE 2.6 Exclusionary Criteria for Brain Death

Seizures
Decorticate or decerebrate posturing
Sedative drugs
Hypothermia (<32.2° C)
Neuromuscular blockade
Shock

TABLE 2.7 Confirmatory Tests for Brain Death

EEG isoelectricity	Deep coma from sedative drugs or hypothermia (temperature <20° C) can produce EEG flattening.
Nuclear medicine	The most common radionuclide modality for brain imaging uses the tracer HMPAO. Absence of isotope uptake ("hollow skull phenomenon") indicates no brain perfusion and supports the diagnosis of brain death.
Transcranial Doppler	Findings of small systolic peaks without diastolic flow or a reverberating flow pattern suggest high vascular resistance and support the diagnosis of brain death. No cerebral blood flow is the most definitive confirmatory test.
CT angiography	Nonopacification of the cortical segments of MCAs and ICVs appears to be highly sensitive for confirming brain death, with a specificity of 100%. Lack of opacification of the ICVs is the most sensitive sign.

CT, Computed tomographic; EEG, electroencephalogram; HMPAO, ^{99m}Tc-labeled hexamethylpropyleneamine oxime; ICV, internal cerebral vein; MCA, middle cerebral artery.

SUGGESTED READINGS

Bernard SA, Gray TW, Buist MD, et al: Treatment of comatose survivors of out-of-hospital cardiac arrest with induced hypothermia, N Engl J Med 346:557–563, 2002.

Bernat JL: Chronic disorders of consciousness, Lancet 367:1181–1192, 2006.

Fins JJ, Master MG, Gerber LM, et al: The minimally conscious state: a diagnosis in search of an epidemiology, Arch Neurol 64:1400–1405, 2007.

Greer DM, Scripko PD, Wu O, et al: Hippocampal magnetic resonance imaging abnormalities in cardiac arrest are associated with poor outcome, J Stroke Cerebrovasc Dis 22:899–905, 2013.

Laureys S, Celesia GG, Cohadon F, et al: Unresponsive wakefulness syndrome: a new name for the vegetative state or apallic syndrome, BMC Med 8:68, 2010.

Laureys S, Schiff ND: Coma and consciousness: paradigms (re)framed by neuroimaging, Neuroimage 61(2):478–491, 2012.

Meaney PA, Bobrow BJ, Mancini ME: Cardiopulmonary resuscitation quality: improving cardiac resuscitation outcomes both inside and outside the hospital–a consensus statement from the American Heart Association, Circulation 124:417–435, 2013.

Peberdy MA, Callaway CW, Neumar RW, et al: Cardiac arrest care: 2010 American Heart Association guidelines for cardiopulmonary resuscitation and emergency cardiovascular care, Circulation 122(18 Suppl 3):S768–S786, 2010. [Errata in Circulation 123:e237, 2011, and Circulation 124:e403, 2011.].

Plum F, Posner JB: The diagnosis of stupor and coma. Contemporary Neurology Series, vol. 71, ed 3, New York, 2007, Oxford University Press.

Rodriguez RA, Nair S, Bussiere M, et al: Long-lasting functional disabilities in patients who recover from coma after cardiac operations, Ann Thorac Surg 95:884–891, 2013.

Rossetti AO, Rabinstein AA, Oddo ML: Neurological prognostication of outcome in patients in coma after cardiac arrest, Lancet Neurol 15(6):597–609, 2016.

Wijdicks EFM: The diagnosis of brain death, N Engl J Med 344:1215–1221, 2001.

Wijdicks EFM, Hijdra A, Young GB, et al: Practice parameter: prediction of outcome in comatose survivors after cardiopulmonary resuscitation (an evidence-based review), Neurology 67:203–210, 2006.

Wu O, Soresnen AG, Benner T, et al: Comatose patients with cardiac arrest: predicting clinical outcome with diffusion-weighted MR imaging, Radiology 252:173–181, 2009.

Young GB: Neurologic prognosis after cardiac arrest, N Engl J Med 361:605–611, 2009.

Zandbergen EGJ, Hijdra A, Koelman JH, et al: Prediction of poor outcome within the first 3 days of postanoxic coma, Neurology 66:62–68, 2006.

表 2.5 脑功能丧失的标准[a]

受检解剖区域	确证体征
大脑半球	对包括疼痛在内的感觉刺激反应迟钝或无反应[b]
中脑	瞳孔对光反射消失[c]
脑桥	反射性眼球运动消失[d]
延髓	呼吸暂停[e]

CO_2，二氧化碳；PCO_2，二氧化碳分压。

[a] 连续检测是临床诊断脑死亡所必需的。在所有情况下至少每 6 h 进行一次，在缺氧缺血性脑损伤的情况下至少每 24 h 进行一次。

[b] 患者不会唤醒、呻吟、龇牙或回缩肢体。纯脊髓反射（深反射、跖屈反射、足底退缩反射和颈部强直反射）可能会保留。

[c] 通过放大镜观察眼底镜的强光，聚焦在虹膜上时最容易进行评估。无反应的瞳孔可以是中等大小（如死亡时），也可以是散大（如输注多巴胺时）。

[d] 用 50 ml 冰水冲洗鼓膜时，眼球不向冲洗侧移动。在眼前庭测试缺失的情况下，眼球反应（玩偶眼动作）总是消失。

[e] 在最大 CO_2 浓度（≥ 60 mmHg）刺激下无呼吸运动；呼吸暂停时，PCO_2 以 2 ~ 3 mmHg/min 速度被动上升。断开呼吸机与气管导管的连接，予插管，供氧速度 6 L/min。

表 2.6 脑死亡的排除标准

癫痫发作
去皮质或去大脑强直
镇静药物
体温过低（< 32.2℃）
神经肌肉阻滞
休克

表 2.7 脑死亡确证检查

等电位 EEG	镇静药物或低体温（体温 < 20℃）引起的深度昏迷会导致脑电图变平。
核医学	最常见的放射性核素脑成像方法使用示踪剂 HMPAO。无同位素摄取（"空颅现象"）表明没有脑灌注，支持脑死亡诊断。
经颅多普勒	收缩期峰值减低且无舒张期血流，或存在混杂血流模式，则表明血管阻力大，支持脑死亡诊断。无脑血流是最确切的确诊检查。
CT 血管成像	在确认脑死亡方面，MCA 和颅内静脉皮质段不显影似乎具有高度敏感性，特异性高达 100%。

EEG，脑电图；HMPAO，锝 -99m 标记的六甲基丙烯胺肟；MCA，大脑中动脉。

推荐阅读

Bernard SA, Gray TW, Buist MD, et al: Treatment of comatose survivors of out-of-hospital cardiac arrest with induced hypothermia, N Engl J Med 346:557–563, 2002.

Bernat JL: Chronic disorders of consciousness, Lancet 367:1181–1192, 2006.

Fins JJ, Master MG, Gerber LM, et al: The minimally conscious state: a diagnosis in search of an epidemiology, Arch Neurol 64:1400–1405, 2007.

Greer DM, Scripko PD, Wu O, et al: Hippocampal magnetic resonance imaging abnormalities in cardiac arrest are associated with poor outcome, J Stroke Cerebrovasc Dis 22:899–905, 2013.

Laureys S, Celesia GG, Cohadon F, et al: Unresponsive wakefulness syndrome: a new name for the vegetative state or apallic syndrome, BMC Med 8:68, 2010.

Laureys S, Schiff ND: Coma and consciousness: paradigms (re)framed by neuroimaging, Neuroimage 61(2):478–491, 2012.

Meaney PA, Bobrow BJ, Mancini ME: Cardiopulmonary resuscitation quality: improving cardiac resuscitation outcomes both inside and outside the hospital–a consensus statement from the American Heart Association, Circulation 124:417–435, 2013.

Peberdy MA, Callaway CW, Neumar RW, et al: Cardiac arrest care: 2010 American Heart Association guidelines for cardiopulmonary resuscitation and emergency cardiovascular care, Circulation 122(18 Suppl 3):S768–S786, 2010. [Errata in Circulation 123:e237, 2011, and Circulation 124:e403, 2011.].

Plum F, Posner JB: The diagnosis of stupor and coma. Contemporary Neurology Series, vol. 71, ed 3, New York, 2007, Oxford University Press.

Rodriguez RA, Nair S, Bussiere M, et al: Long-lasting functional disabilities in patients who recover from coma after cardiac operations, Ann Thorac Surg 95:884–891, 2013.

Rossetti AO, Rabinstein AA, Oddo ML: Neurological prognostication of outcome in patients in coma after cardiac arrest, Lancet Neurol 15(6):597–609, 2016.

Wijdicks EFM: The diagnosis of brain death, N Engl J Med 344:1215–1221, 2001.

Wijdicks EFM, Hijdra A, Young GB, et al: Practice parameter: prediction of outcome in comatose survivors after cardiopulmonary resuscitation (an evidence-based review), Neurology 67:203–210, 2006.

Wu O, Soresnen AG, Benner T, et al: Comatose patients with cardiac arrest: predicting clinical outcome with diffusion-weighted MR imaging, Radiology 252:173–181, 2009.

Young GB: Neurologic prognosis after cardiac arrest, N Engl J Med 361:605 611, 2009.

Zandbergen EGJ, Hijdra A, Koelman JH, et al: Prediction of poor outcome within the first 3 days of postanoxic coma, Neurology 66:62–68, 2006.

3

Disorders of Sleep

Sagarika Nallu, Selim R. Benbadis

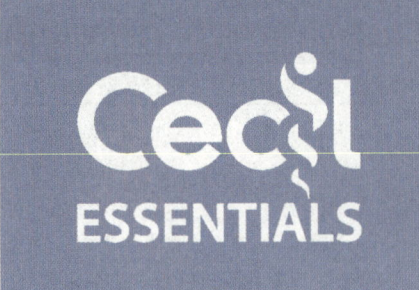

INTRODUCTION

The *International Classification of Sleep Disorders* (ICSD-3) groups disorders with sleep into six major categories: insomnia, sleep-related breathing disorders, central disorders of hypersomnolence, circadian rhythm sleep-wake disorders, parasomnias, and sleep-related movement disorders. From a practical point of view, sleep disorders are better classified by their clinical presentation, which is the approach taken here. This chapter focuses on primary sleep disorders rather than sleep disturbances that result from self-evident medical or psychiatric diseases.

DISORDERS OF EXCESSIVE DAYTIME SLEEPINESS

History and Examination

Evaluating patients with sleep disorders should include a thorough sleep history and physical examination that includes the respiratory, cardiovascular, and neurologic symptoms. The majority of the patients with sleep disorders present with excessive daytime somnolence (EDS) as their chief symptom. A careful history is the starting point and often uncovers the likely causes (e.g., insufficient sleep time with sleep deprivation, lifestyles, circadian rhythm disorders, medications, systemic illnesses). Most of these causes do not require any diagnostic interventions. To subjectively quantify EDS, various scales have been developed. The most validated and useful in the clinical practice is the Epworth Sleepiness Scale (ESS). The ESS consists of a brief questionnaire on the likelihood of dozing off in eight situations. This yields a score between 0 and 24 (Table 3.1). Scores of 10 or above warrant investigation.

Sleep Studies

Polysomnography (PSG) is an all-night sleep study that measures multiple parameters such as sleep staging, respiration, leg movements, and electrocardiographic patterns. The limited channel sleep monitoring version is also called portable home sleep testing (HST) and is used in patients with high probability of obstructive sleep apnea (OSA). The multiple sleep latency test (MSLT) and the maintenance of wakefulness test (MWT) are used to measure and quantify EDS. They consist of a series of daytime naps during which sleep latency is measured and sleep stages are determined. MSLT must be performed with a prior night PSG.

SLEEP-DISORDERED BREATHING

Definition and Epidemiology

Sleep-disordered breathing encompasses a spectrum of chronic conditions in which partial or complete cessation of breathing occurs multiple times throughout sleep. This group includes the most common disorders: OSA, central sleep apnea, and sleep-related hypoventilation. Respiratory events are classified as apneas and hypopneas; apneas are further subdivided into obstructive, central or mixed. Obstructive apneas are episodes of complete upper airway collapse, defined as a greater than 90% drop in the airflow/thermal sensor in the presence of continued respiratory effort lasting at least 10 seconds. Hypopnea is defined as a 30% or more drop in the nasal pressure signal lasting for at least 10 seconds, associated with a 3% or more oxygen desaturation or an arousal. In contrast, central apnea is defined as a greater than 90% drop in the airflow/thermal sensor accompanied by absent respiratory effort that lasts for at least 10 seconds. The severity of sleep apnea is based on the polysomnographic scoring and is defined by the apnea-hypopnea index (AHI), a ratio of the sum of all respiratory events to the total hours of sleep on the PSG or HST.

The estimated prevalence rates of obstructive sleep apnea have increased substantially over the last two decades, most likely due to the obesity epidemic. It is now estimated that 26% of adults between the ages of 30 and 70 years have sleep apnea.

Pathophysiology

The pathophysiology of OSA is recurrent upper airway closure/collapse with resulting oxygen desaturation leading to arousals. The sleep fragmentation caused by arousal is responsible for sleep deprivation and EDS.

Clinical Manifestation

OSA patients typically present with at least one of these symptoms: snoring, waking up with gasping/choking or witnessed apneas in sleep by their bed partners. EDS, nonrestorative sleep, fatigue, and insomnia also have comorbid conditions such as hypertension, coronary artery disease (CAD), mood disorders, cognitive dysfunction or type 2 diabetes. Risk factors for OSA are both modifiable and nonmodifiable. Modifiable risk factors include sedative medication, alcohol, tobacco use, obesity, endocrine disorders (e.g., hypothyroidism, polycystic ovary syndrome, acromegaly) and nasal obstruction/congestion. Nonmodifiable factors include genetic predisposition, craniofacial anomalies and congenital syndromes (e.g., Down, Pierre Robin, and Treacher Collins syndromes).

Treatment and Prognosis

Depending on the severity, treatment modalities of OSA include positive airway pressure therapy (PAP), oral appliance therapy, surgical modifications of upper airway, weight loss, and positional measures to prevent sleeping supine (positional therapy). Initial treatment of OSA requires close monitoring and early identification of difficulties with PAP use (including troubleshooting and monitoring of objective efficacy and usage data to ensure adequate treatment and adherence). Success over the first few days to weeks has been shown to predict long-term adherence.

睡眠障碍

林楠 译　韩菲 沈航 审校　姚明 彭斌 通审

引言

《国际睡眠障碍分类》(ICSD-3)将睡眠障碍分为六大类别：失眠、睡眠呼吸障碍、中枢性过度睡眠、昼夜节律睡眠-觉醒障碍、异态睡眠以及睡眠相关运动障碍。本章将从实用性角度出发，依据临床症状对睡眠障碍进行分类，重点介绍原发性睡眠障碍，明确的器质性或精神性疾病继发的睡眠障碍不在此处讨论。

白天过度嗜睡障碍

病史和查体

睡眠障碍患者的评估应包括详尽的睡眠病史和全面的体格检查，包括对呼吸、心血管及神经系统的检查。白天过度嗜睡(EDS)是睡眠障碍患者最常见的主诉。通过详细的病史询问，医生通常可以发现可能的病因(例如，睡眠时间不足导致的睡眠剥夺、生活方式、昼夜节律障碍、药物、系统性疾病等)。这些病因中的大多数不需要进一步的诊断性干预。为了量化EDS的严重程度，多种量表被开发应用。在临床实践中，Epworth嗜睡量表(ESS)被证实为有效工具。ESS是一个简短的问卷，评价8种不同情境下的嗜睡情况。量表得分范围为0~24分(表3.1)。得分10分或以上通常提示需要进一步检查。

睡眠检查

多导睡眠监测(PSG)是一项全夜睡眠检查，可记录睡眠分期、呼吸、腿部运动、心电等多种参数。有限导联睡眠监测，也称为便携式家庭睡眠监测(HST)，可用于高度怀疑阻塞性睡眠呼吸暂停(OSA)的患者。多次小睡睡眠潜伏时间试验(MSLT)和清醒维持测验(MWT)是用于EDS检测和量化的工具。它们包括一系列日间小睡，并检测其睡眠潜伏期和睡眠分期。进行MSLT前一晚需要先进行PSG检查。

睡眠呼吸障碍

定义和流行病学

睡眠呼吸障碍是一组慢性疾病，睡眠过程中多次出现部分或完全性呼吸停止是其特征。这组谱系疾病包括最常见的睡眠障碍类型：阻塞性睡眠呼吸暂停(OSA)、中枢性睡眠呼吸暂停以及睡眠相关低通气。

呼吸事件分为呼吸暂停和低通气，呼吸暂停进一步分为阻塞性、中枢性及混合性。阻塞性呼吸暂停是指上呼吸道完全塌陷，定义为在持续呼吸努力的情况下，气流/热传感器下降90%以上，持续时间至少10 s。低通气定义为鼻压信号下降30%或以上，持续至少10 s，伴有3%或以上的氧饱和度下降或觉醒。相反，中枢性呼吸暂停是指气流/热传感器下降90%以上，伴呼吸努力消失，持续至少10 s。基于多导睡眠监测评分，睡眠呼吸暂停的严重程度通过呼吸暂停-低通气指数(AHI)来评定，即所有呼吸事件的总和与PSG或HST上睡眠总时长的比率。

阻塞性睡眠呼吸暂停患病率在过去20年明显升高，这主要与肥胖症的流行相关。目前估计，30~70岁成年人中有26%患有睡眠呼吸暂停。

病理生理机制

OSA的病理生理机制是反复上呼吸道闭塞或塌陷，导致氧饱和度降低和觉醒。因觉醒导致的睡眠碎片化是造成睡眠剥夺和白天过度嗜睡(EDS)的原因。

临床表现

OSA患者会出现至少一项以下症状：打鼾，窒息或呛咳引起觉醒，或其床伴观察到睡眠中有呼吸暂停。EDS、非恢复性睡眠、疲劳、失眠，以及高血压、冠状动脉疾病、情绪障碍、认知障碍或2型糖尿病等都是常见并发症。OSA的风险因素包括可干预的和不可干预的因素。可干预的风险因素包括镇静药物、酒精、烟草使用、肥胖、内分泌障碍(如甲状腺功能减退、多囊卵巢综合征、肢端肥大症)和鼻塞/鼻充血。不可干预的风险因素包括遗传易感性、颅面异常和先天性综合征(如唐氏综合征、Pierre Robin综合征和Treacher Collins综合征)。

治疗和预后

根据严重程度，OSA的治疗方法包括正压通气(PAP)治疗、口腔矫治器治疗、上呼吸道手术修正、减重，以及体位措施以防止仰卧睡眠(体位治疗)。OSA的初始治疗需要密切监测和早期识别PAP使用中的困难(包括故障排除、客观效果和使用数据的监测，以确保治疗的充分性和依从性)。已证实治疗初期的良好疗效有助于长期的治疗依从性。

TABLE 3.1 Epworth Sleepiness Scale

How likely are you to doze off or fall asleep in the following situations in contrast to just feeling tired? The situations refer to your usual way of life. Even if you have not done some of these things recently, try to work out how they would have affected you. Use the following scale to choose the most appropriate number for each situation.

0 = would never doze
1 = slight chance of dozing
2 = moderate chance of dozing
3 = high chance of dozing

What is your chance of dozing in the following situations?

Situation	
Sitting and reading	_____
Watching TV	_____
Sitting and inactive in a public place (theater or meeting)	_____
As a passenger in a car for an hour without a break	_____
Lying down to rest in the afternoon when possible	_____
Sitting and talking to someone	_____
Sitting quietly after lunch (without alcohol)	_____
In a car while stopped for a few minutes in traffic	_____
Total	_____

Modified from Johns MW: A new method for measuring daytime sleepiness: the Epworth Sleepiness Scale, Sleep 14:540-545, 1991.

TABLE 3.2 Agents Promoting Wakefulness

Drug	Dose Range (mg)
Amphetamine (Dexedrine, Desoxyn, Adderall, Adderall XR)	5-60
Methylphenidate (Ritalin, Metadate, Methylin, Concerta)	10-60
Modafinil (Provigil)	200-400
Armodafinil	150-250

Central sleep apnea (CSA) is seen in a variety of settings, including periodic breathing in infancy, healthy adults at altitude, and Cheyne-Stokes respirations in heart failure. In most cases of CSA, the cyclic absence of effort is a paradoxical consequence of hypersensitive ventilatory chemo reflex responses that oppose changes in airflow, producing elevated loop gain and leading to overshoot/undershoot ventilatory oscillations. Therapies for CSA affect loop gain by improving lung volumes (PAP therapy), reducing the alveolar-inspired Pco_2 difference (stimulants) and lowering chemosensitivity (supplemental oxygen). CSA is further differentiated by a hypercapnic (e.g., brain stem lesions, opioids, obesity hypoventilation syndrome, congenital central alveolar hypoventilation syndrome, neuromuscular disorders, chest wall deformities) or hypocapnic response (e.g., Cheyne-Stokes respiration).

NARCOLEPSY

Narcolepsy is a complex sleep disorder that can manifest in childhood or adolescence. It is the most common cause of excessive daytime sleepiness and can occur in isolation or in combination with other symptoms such as cataplexy, hypnogogic/hypnopompic hallucinations, disturbed nocturnal sleep, and sleep paralysis. Cataplexy distinguishes type 1 (narcolepsy with cataplexy) from type 2 narcolepsy (narcolepsy without cataplexy). Cataplexy is reported by 60% to 75% of patients with narcolepsy and is defined as a transient, sudden-onset loss of skeletal muscle tone with retained consciousness. It is often in seen in response to a strong emotion (e.g., laughter, startle, anger). Hypnagogic or hypnopompic hallucinations are vivid, dreamlike sensations that an individual feels, hears or sees and that occur near the onset of sleep (hypnogogic) or upon waking up from sleep (hypnopompic). Sleep paralysis is defined as temporary inability to move or speak while being conscious and that occurs when a person is falling asleep or waking up from sleep.

Pathophysiology

Genetic and environmental factors reportedly play a role in the etiology of narcolepsy. Evidence suggests that the loss of hypocretin is highly associated with its development. Hypocretin, a neuropeptide found in the lateral and posterior hypothalamus, targets monoaminergic and cholinergic areas. The loss of hypocretin neurons results in characteristic symptoms of narcolepsy including the inability to sustain long periods of wakefulness and frequent lapses into sleep. Evidence suggests a link between HLA DQB1*06:02 and narcolepsy, indicating an autoimmune basis for narcolepsy that is mediated by hypocretin neurons.

Diagnosis and Differential Diagnosis

Diagnosis of narcolepsy requires a detailed clinical history and diagnostic studies such as an overnight PSG followed by an MSLT. An MSLT with sleep latency of 8 minutes or less and two or more sleep-onset REM periods and the exclusion of other sleep disorders on PSG provide a definitive diagnosis of narcolepsy. The PSG performed the night prior to MSLT is important for excluding other primary sleep disorders such as sleep apnea and periodic limb movement disorder. Abnormal MSLT findings are not specific for narcolepsy and may be produced by other sleep disorders such as sleep apnea, circadian misalignment, other mental or medical conditions, medications or substance use or sleep deprivation. An alternative criterion for diagnosis is a CSF hypocretin level 110 pg/mL or less.

Treatment

Narcolepsy treatment includes a multimodal approach with both nonpharmacologic and pharmacologic components. Pharmacologic therapy includes stimulant therapy, which aims to improve alertness and functioning (Table 3.2). Wake-promoting medications such as modafinil and armodafinil are considered first-line therapy for excessive daytime sleepiness. Sodium oxybate (Xyrem), a precursor for GABA, is the only treatment for cataplexy that has been approved by the FDA. Tricyclic antidepressants (e.g., clomipramine), selective serotonin reuptake inhibitors (e.g., fluoxetine), and serotonin and norepinephrine reuptake inhibitors (e.g., venlafaxine) have all been used to treat cataplexy. Nonpharmacologic treatments include scheduled brief naps, practicing good sleep hygiene, and regular exercise during the day to improve alertness.

IDIOPATHIC HYPERSOMNIA

Definition and Epidemiology

Idiopathic hypersomnia (IH) is a chronic neurologic disorder that manifests as pathologic daytime sleepiness with or without prolonged sleep durations. Etiology of IH is presently unknown, although a genetic predisposition is suggested by the strong family history of similar symptoms. Patients report unrefreshed (i.e., sleep inertia) nocturnal sleep and long daytime naps, and they can have prolonged states of fogginess despite long sleep hours (i.e., sleep drunkenness).

表 3.1　Epworth 嗜睡量表
下列情况下你打瞌睡（不仅仅是感到疲倦）的程度如何？这是指你平常的生活情况。假如你最近没有做过其中的某些事情，请试着填上它们可能给你带来的影响。运用下列指标给每种情况选出最适当的数字。
0 = 从不打瞌睡；1 = 很少打瞌睡；2 = 有时打瞌睡；3 = 经常打瞌睡
在下列情况中你打瞌睡的程度是什么？
坐着阅读时 _____
看电视时 _____
在公共场所坐着不动时（如剧院或会议）_____
乘车 1 h 期间无休息时 _____
下午有条件静卧休息时 _____
坐着与人谈话时 _____
午饭后安静坐着时（无饮酒）_____
开车等红绿灯时 _____
总分 _____

改编自 Johns MW：A new method for measuring daytime sleepiness：the Epworth Sleepiness Scale，Sleep 14：540-545，1991.

中枢性睡眠呼吸暂停（CSA）可见于多种情况，包括婴儿期周期性呼吸、高海拔区健康成人的生理性呼吸变化，以及心力衰竭时的 Cheyne-Stokes 呼吸。在大多数 CSA 病例中，通气化学反射反应高度敏感，与气流改变相反，导致呼吸周期性努力消失，这种矛盾的结果会引起环路增益升高，并导致过度/不足的通气振荡。CSA 治疗方法通过改善肺容积（PAP 治疗）、减少肺泡吸入 PCO_2 差（呼吸刺激药）和降低化学敏感性（氧疗）来影响环路增益。CSA 进一步可分为高碳酸血症型（如脑干病变、阿片类药物、肥胖低通气综合征、先天性中枢性肺泡低通气综合征、神经肌肉疾病、胸壁畸形相关）和低碳酸血症型（如 Cheyne-Stokes 呼吸）。

发作性睡病

发作性睡病是一种复杂的睡眠障碍，可见于儿童或青少年期。这是引起白天过度嗜睡的最常见病因，伴或不伴猝倒、睡前或醒后幻觉、夜间睡眠障碍以及睡眠麻痹等症状。根据是否存在猝倒，分为发作性睡病 1 型（伴猝倒的发作性睡病）与 2 型（不伴猝倒的发作性睡病）。猝倒是指清醒时短暂突发的骨骼肌张力消失，可见于 60%～75% 的发作性睡病患者。通常由强烈情绪触发（例如，大笑、惊吓、愤怒）。睡前或醒后幻觉是患者感受到、听见或看到生动、梦境般的感觉，发生于刚入睡时（睡前）或从睡眠中醒来时（醒后）。睡眠麻痹定义为意识清醒但暂时无法活动或言语，出现在患者刚入睡或从睡眠中将醒来时。

病理生理机制

发作性睡病的病理生理机制涉及遗传和环境因素。研究显示，下丘脑分泌素的缺失与疾病的发生发展密切相关。下丘脑分泌素是一种存在于下丘脑外侧和后侧的神经肽，作用于单胺能和胆碱能区。下丘脑分泌素神经元的缺失导致无法保持长时间清醒和频繁入睡等发作性睡病的临床症状。此外，HLA DQB1*06：02 与发作性睡病有关，提示下丘脑分泌素神经元介导的自身免疫性机制参与其发病。

表 3.2　促觉醒药物	
药物	有效剂量范围（mg）
苯丙胺（Dexedrine、Desoxyn、Adderall、Adderall XR）	5～60
哌甲酯（利他林、Metadate、Methylin、专注达）	10～60
莫达非尼（Provigil）	200～400
阿莫非尼	150～250

诊断和鉴别诊断

发作性睡病诊断需要详细的临床病史和诊断性检查，如全夜 PSG 及次日 MSLT。MSLT 显示睡眠潜伏期少于或等于 8 min，2 次或以上睡眠起始快速眼动（REM）期，以及 PSG 除外其他睡眠障碍，可以确诊发作性睡病。在 MSLT 前一晚进行 PSG 检查对于排除其他睡眠障碍（如睡眠呼吸暂停和周期性肢体运动障碍）非常重要。异常 MSLT 结果并不是发作性睡病特有的，也可能由其他睡眠障碍（如睡眠呼吸暂停、昼夜节律错位、其他精神或器质性情况、药物治疗或滥用、睡眠剥夺）引起。脑脊液下丘脑分泌素水平低于 110 pg/ml 是诊断的另一替代标准。

治疗

发作性睡病的治疗包括非药物和药物联合治疗。药物治疗包括神经兴奋治疗，旨在改善警觉性和功能（表 3.2）。促觉醒药物如莫达非尼和阿莫非尼被认为是白天过度嗜睡的一线治疗。GABA 前体羟丁酸钠（Xyrem）是 FDA 批准的唯一治疗猝倒药物。三环类抗抑郁药（如氯米帕明）、选择性 5-羟色胺再摄取抑制剂（如氟西汀）和 5-羟色胺、去甲肾上腺素再摄取双重抑制剂（如文拉法辛）都已用于治疗猝倒。非药物治疗包括规律短时间小睡、良好的睡眠卫生习惯以及日间规律锻炼来提高警觉性。

特发性嗜睡症

定义和流行病学

特发性嗜睡症（IH）是一种慢性神经系统疾病，表现为病理性白天嗜睡，伴或不伴睡眠时间延长。尽管存在家族史可能提示具有遗传倾向，但 IH 的确切病因目前仍未知。患者无法从夜间睡眠和长时间日间小睡中恢复精神（即睡眠惰性），并在睡眠数小时后长时间持续迷离状态（即醉梦状态）。

Diagnosis and Differential Diagnosis

Diagnosis of IH involves a careful history, with particular attention to the possibility of other disorders with similar symptomatology, and objective testing with sleep studies. Other causes of EDS must be excluded, and the PSG should be normal with no sleep-disordered breathing. MSLT confirms sleep latency of less than 8 minutes but without sleep-onset REM.

Treatment and Prognosis

There are no FDA-approved treatments for IH symptoms, which are typically treated with off-label use of medications approved for narcolepsy.

KLEINE-LEVIN SYNDROME

Kleine-Levin syndrome is a rare, recurrent or cyclic hypersomnia with a prevalence of 1 case per 1 million people. Its cause is unknown. Its onset is usually in the second decade of life.

These episodes of hypersomnia are also associated with other symptoms including hyperphagia, hypersexuality, confusion and hallucinations. Episodes can last days to weeks and reoccur every few months, and at least once a year. Lithium is the choice of medication along with other stimulants and wake-promoting agents (see Table 3.2).

Other symptomatic causes of EDS must be excluded. With time, episodes tend to become less severe, less prolonged, and less frequent.

RESTLESS LEGS SYNDROME, PERIODIC LIMB MOVEMENTS IN SLEEP, AND PERIODIC LIMB MOVEMENT DISORDER

Restless legs syndrome (RLS), also known as Willis-Ekbom disease, is a common neurologic sensorimotor disorder that manifests as an irresistible urge to move the body to relieve the uncomfortable sensations. These sensations always occur during resting, sitting or sleeping. Symptoms commonly worsen at night, causing difficulties with initiating sleep. It is more prevalent in females, and a family history of RLS was detected in 90.9% of the patients with RLS, indicating high heritability.

Periodic limb movements in sleep (PLMS) are polysomnographic findings and are characterized by stereotypical jerks lasting between 0.5 to 10 seconds and occurring at 15- to 40-second intervals. PLMS are present in approximately 80% of patients with RLS. A periodic limb movement index of 15 or greater, when associated with a sleep complaint not accountable by any other sleep disorder, may suggest a periodic limb movement disorder (PLMD).

Clinical Manifestations

Leg movements may be reported by the bed partner, and the patient may report EDS, insomnia, or symptoms of RLS (i.e., urge to move legs or walk due to unpleasant "creepy-crawly" sensations at rest). Most patients with RLS have PLMD, but the reverse is not true.

Treatment and Prognosis

The management of RLS and PLMD involves both nonpharmacologic and pharmacologic approaches. Secondary causes that can aggravate both RLS and PLMD symptoms should be investigated, which includes polyneuropathy, spinal cord disease, pregnancy, iron and B_{12} deficiencies, uremia, sleep deprivation, irregular sleep schedules, caffeine, nicotine, alcohol, and certain medications (e.g., antihistamines, serotonergic antidepressants, neuroleptics).

Dopamine agonists and alpha2delta calcium-channel ligands are considered first-line treatments, but these treatments have very different side effect profiles that should be taken into consideration. Doses of dopamine agonists used for RLS treatment are much lower than typical doses in patients with Parkinson's disease and are timed to be taken approximately 2 hours before typical symptom onset. The starting dose of ropinirole is 0.25 mg/d, then is titrated as follows: 0.25 mg for 2 days, then 0.5 mg for 5 days, then may increase by 0.5-mg increments every week until an effective or maximum dose is achieved, whichever comes first. Doses above 4 mg/d should be avoided in patients with RLS whenever possible. The pramipexole starting dose is 0.125 mg/d, and it may be increased by 0.125-mg increments every 4 to 7 days until symptom control or maximum dose is reached. The maximum recommended RLS dose of pramipexole is 0.75 mg/d (although this is an expert consensus recommendation that differs from the FDA labeling of 0.5 mg/d). Rotigotine is the only dopamine agonist that is dosed via daily transdermal patch, which is initiated at 1 mg/d, and may be escalated to 2 mg/d or 3 mg/d in increments of 1 mg/d every week (Table 3.3).

For a deeper discussion of these topics, please see Chapter 382, "Other Movement Disorders," in *Goldman-Cecil Medicine*, 26th Edition.

TABLE 3.3 Treatments for Restless Legs Syndrome

Drug	Dose Range (mg)
Levodopa or carbidopa (Sinemet)	50-200
Ropinirole (Requip)	0.25-4.0
Pramipexole (Mirapex)	0.125-0.5
Rotigotine (Neupro) transdermal patch	1-3

INSOMNIA

Definition and Epidemiology

Insomnia is the most common sleep complaint in the United States, affecting as many as 30 million people in the general population. A diagnosis of insomnia can be present either with or without a comorbid mental or physical disorder. Insomnia is defined as persistent difficulty with sleep initiation, duration, and consolidation, or sleep quality that occurs despite adequate opportunity and circumstances for sleep, and results in some form of daytime impairment. Individuals who report these sleep-related symptoms in the absence of daytime impairment are not regarded as having insomnia disorder that warrants clinical attention other than education and reassurance. The three diagnostic categories for insomnia include chronic insomnia, short-term insomnia, and other insomnia disorder.

Pathophysiology

Acute or short-term insomnia is caused by identifiable factors and can become a chronic, persistent problem. Chronic insomnia results from predisposing (genetic), precipitating (environmental), and perpetuating (behaviors) factors. With the exception of rare conditions such as the prion disease of fatal familial insomnia, insomnia alone is almost never the symptom of a neurologic disease.

Clinical Manifestations

Insomnia may manifest as the inability to fall asleep (i.e., onset insomnia) or to stay asleep (i.e., maintenance insomnia). In addition to nighttime symptoms, the diagnosis demands daytime symptoms considered to be the consequence of insomnia (e.g., fatigue, EDS, poor concentration, altered mood, headache).

诊断和鉴别诊断

IH 的诊断需要详尽的病史记录，特别需要注意排除其他可引起类似症状的疾病，并使用客观的睡眠检查协助诊断。必须排除其他可能导致 EDS 的病因，同时 PSG 结果应该是正常的，且没有睡眠呼吸障碍。此外，MSLT 确认睡眠潜伏期少于 8 min，但没有睡眠起始 REM 期。

治疗和预后

目前尚没有 FDA 批准的专门用于 IH 治疗的药物，IH 症状通常采用治疗发作性睡病的药物进行超说明书治疗。

克莱恩-莱文综合征

克莱恩-莱文综合征是一种罕见的复发或周期性嗜睡症，患病率为 1/100 万。其病因未明。通常十几岁发病。

嗜睡发作期间，还可能伴随其他症状，包括过度进食、性欲亢进、意识模糊及幻觉。发作可以持续数天至数周，每隔数月复发，每年至少发作一次。锂剂以及其他神经兴奋和促觉醒药物是可选治疗方案（见表 3.2）。

在诊断克莱恩-莱文综合征时，须排除其他可引起白天过度嗜睡（EDS）的器质性病因。随着时间推移，部分患者发作程度会逐渐减轻，持续时间缩短，复发频率降低。

不宁腿综合征、睡眠周期性肢体运动和周期性肢体运动障碍

不宁腿综合征（RLS），也被称为 Willis-Ekbom 病，是一种常见的神经感觉运动障碍，患者会感到不可抗拒的冲动，通过活动身体以缓解不适感。这些感觉多在休息、坐位或睡眠时出现。症状常在晚上加重，导致入睡困难。RLS 在女性中更为常见，且具有明显的家族遗传倾向，RLS 家族史见于 90.9% 的 RLS 患者。

睡眠周期性肢体运动（PLMS）由多导睡眠监测发现，表现为持续 0.5～10 s、间隔 15～40 s 的刻板性抽动。约 80% RLS 患者表现有 PLMS。当周期性肢体运动指数达到 15 及以上，且合并睡眠障碍且无法由任何其他睡眠障碍解释时，可能提示周期性肢体运动障碍（PLMD）。

临床表现

腿部运动可能由床伴发现，患者则可能主诉 EDS、失眠或 RLS 症状（即休息时因不舒服的"虫爬样"感觉而有活动腿部或行走的冲动）。大多数 RLS 患者合并 PLMD，但反之则不然。

治疗和预后

RLS 和 PLMD 的治疗包括非药物和药物治疗。须排除可能加重 RLS 和 PLMD 症状的继发性病因，包括多发性周围神经病、脊髓病、怀孕、缺铁和维生素 B_{12} 缺乏症、尿毒症、睡眠剥夺、不规律睡眠作息、咖啡因、尼古丁、酒精以及药物（例如，抗组胺药、5-羟色胺抗抑郁药、神经阻滞剂）。

表 3.3　不宁腿综合征治疗方案	
药物	有效剂量范围（mg）
左旋多巴或卡比多巴（息宁）	50～200
罗匹尼罗（Requip）	0.25～4.0
普拉克索（Mirapex）	0.125～0.5
罗替戈汀（Neupro）经皮贴剂	1～3

多巴胺受体激动剂和 alpha-2-delta 钙离子通道拮抗剂是一线治疗，但需综合考虑这些药物的不良反应。用于 RLS 治疗的多巴胺受体激动剂的剂量明显低于帕金森病患者的常规剂量，并应在典型症状出现前约 2 h 服用。罗匹尼罗起始剂量为 0.25 mg/d，然后按照以下方案调整：0.25 mg/d 用 2 天，0.5 mg/d 用 5 天，之后可每周增加 0.5 mg 直到达到有效剂量或最大剂量，尽可能避免超过 4 mg/d。普拉克索起始剂量是 0.125 mg/d，可以每 4～7 天增加 0.125 mg，直到症状控制或最大剂量。普拉克索用于 RLS 治疗的推荐最大剂量为 0.75 mg/d（此为专家共识推荐剂量，不同于 FDA 说明书标注的 0.5 mg/d）。罗替戈汀是唯一每日经皮贴剂给药的多巴胺受体激动剂，起始剂量为 1 mg/d，可以每周以 1 mg/d 增量至 2 mg/d 或 3 mg/d（表 3.3）。

有关此专题的深入讨论，请参阅 *Goldman-Cecil Medicine* 第 26 版第 382 章"其他运动障碍"。

失眠

定义和流行病学

失眠是睡眠障碍最常见的主诉，在美国，高达 3000 万人受失眠影响。失眠可以单独出现，也可以与其他精神或器质性疾病共病。失眠被定义为持续的睡眠启动、维持和巩固困难，或在充足睡眠条件和环境中发生的睡眠质量问题，并导致日间功能障碍。如果有睡眠相关症状，但日间没有功能障碍，通常不被视为是需要临床关注的失眠，而是可能只需要教育和安抚。失眠的诊断分为三个类别：慢性失眠、短期失眠和其他失眠障碍。

病理生理机制

由已知诱因引起的急性或短期失眠，可能发展为长期的慢性失眠。慢性失眠的发展可能与易感性（遗传）、诱发性（环境）和维持性（行为）因素有关。除了一些罕见病因，如致死性家族性失眠症等朊病毒病，失眠一般不会是神经系统疾病的唯一症状。

临床表现

失眠可能表现为难以入睡（即入睡困难）或难以维持睡眠（即维持睡眠困难）。除了夜间症状，诊断还需有因失眠引起的日间功能受损（例如，疲劳、EDS、注意力不集中、情绪改变、头痛）。

TABLE 3.4 Sleep Hygiene

1. Maintain a regular schedule each day.
2. Wake at the same time each morning.
3. Exposure to natural light entrains the circadian rhythm.
4. Exercise in the morning or early afternoon; avoid vigorous exercise in the evening.
5. Avoid napping during the day, especially after 3 PM.
6. Avoid stimulants such as caffeine and nicotine and avoid alcohol close to bedtime.
7. Avoid large meals close to bedtime.
8. Maintain regular and relaxing routines at bedtime.
9. Maintain a comfortable sleep environment.
10. Reserve the bed for sleep; avoid other activities (e.g., TV, radio, reading).
11. Sleep only when sleepy.
12. Try to resolve worries (or list for future thought) before sleeping.
13. Get out of bed if not sleeping in 20 minutes.

Adjustment insomnia is an acute reaction to some type of stress. When the trigger combines with a propensity for poor or fragile sleep, the condition can become chronic (>1 month) and lead to maladaptive behaviors and a conditioned arousal associated with sleep. This is known as *psychophysiologic insomnia,* and it is by far the most common insomnia syndrome. A vicious cycle is created by poor sleep habits that worsen the insomnia. Because of its chronicity, it is typically associated with poor sleep habits, multiple treatment trials, and anxiety about sleep. If there was no trigger at onset, there may be a lifelong history of poor sleep (i.e., idiopathic insomnia) with the same end result of psychophysiologic insomnia.

Paradoxical insomnia and *sleep-state misperception* are terms applied to patients who claim to not sleep. However, when studied objectively, they have normal sleep amounts and architecture.

Diagnosis and Differential Diagnosis

The diagnosis is based on the history, which should include a sleep diary. Identifiable medical, psychiatric, or drug-related disease and other sleep disorders (e.g., OSA) require exclusion. Sleep studies (PSG and MSLT) are occasionally helpful.

Treatment and Prognosis

Nondrug treatments include commonsense sleep hygiene recommendations (e.g., avoiding caffeine, exercising late in the day) (Table 3.4) and behavior modifications to avoid the conditioned arousal responses associated with sleep (e.g., using the bedroom only for sleep and sex). Other strategies include cognitive behavior therapy specifically for insomnia (CBT-I), relaxation techniques, biofeedback, and behavioral changes such as sleep restriction therapy and stimulus control therapy.

The principles of the pharmacologic treatment of insomnia include using the lowest effective dose, intermittent (not daily) use, using the appropriate (i.e., short or intermediate half-life) drug based on the type of insomnia (i.e., onset or maintenance), and limiting the duration of treatment. Treatment should be tapered to avoid rebound. Medications should be used only in combination with nondrug (i.e., behavioral) treatments. Behavioral treatment has been effective.

Over-the-counter sleep aids (usually antihistamines) are typically safe, but use is limited by anticholinergic and hangover effects. Melatonin may promote sleep and be used for circadian rhythm disorders, including jet lag. The selective melatonin agonist ramelteon is helpful for sleep-onset insomnia.

Prognosis is usually good with the combination of drug and nondrug treatments. Behavior modification may be limited by the willingness of patients to participate.

PARASOMNIAS

Parasomnias are undesirable phenomena that occur in sleep or during transition to or from sleep. They may occur in REM or NREM sleep. They usually consist of complex and seemingly purposeful behaviors, sometimes dramatic, of which the patient is not aware. They are often classified by the sleep stage in which they arise.

NREM Parasomnias

NREM-related parasomnias include confusional arousals, sleep walking (somnambulism), and sleep terrors (pavor nocturnus), and arise as a result of incomplete arousals from deep sleep. They tend to begin in childhood and a family history of similar symptoms is common. The events usually occur during the first third of sleep when delta sleep predominates. Episodes are often triggered by precipitants such as intercurrent illness, sleep deprivation, alcohol use, and stress. Sleep walking episodes typically begin as confusional arousals. These patients often start with sitting up in bed and looking about in a confused manner. Sleep terrors differ from sleep walking in that episodes are more dramatic, with abrupt arousal, a scream or cry and autonomic hyperactivity (e.g., mydriasis, diaphoresis, flushing, piloerection, tachycardia). The child appears terrified and is inconsolable.

Diagnosis and Differential Diagnosis

The main differential diagnosis is nocturnal seizures, which requires video-monitored electroencephalogram (EEG) for diagnosis. Nocturnal seizures tend to be more stereotyped than parasomnias, and they often include tonic or clonic motor activity. Treatment consists of reassurances and measures to avoid injuries during these episodes. Other sleep disorders such as OSA can precipitate these episodes and should be ruled out as part of the treatment. For severe episodes with injurious behaviors, low-dose benzodiazepines such as clonazepam are often recommended.

Treatment and Prognosis

Reassurance and measures to avoid injuries usually are sufficient. For episodes with injurious behaviors, low-dose benzodiazepines (clonazepam, 0.5 to 1 mg) are often effective. Prognosis is good, and most patients do not require treatment.

Rapid Eye Movement Behavior Disorder
Definition and Epidemiology

REM behavior disorder (RBD) is a disorder of REM sleep regulation in which there is a dissociation of REM features with loss of the muscle atonia, leading to patients acting out their dreams. RBD typically affects patients after the age of 50 (usually older) and the male-to-female ratio is 10:1.

Pathophysiology

REM inhibition is lost due to bilateral degeneration of REM atonic neurons in the pons. RBD occurs with α-synucleinopathies (i.e., Parkinson's disease, multiple system atrophy, and dementia with Lewy bodies), and RBD typically heralds these neurodegenerative diseases, sometimes by 10 to 15 years.

Clinical Manifestations

Typically, the episodes are reported by the bed partner and consist of high-amplitude, flailing, injurious behaviors during sleep. When awakened, the patient typically recalls the dream. As is typical of REM arousals, the patient is alert and coherent immediately (unlike slow-wave sleep arousal). Medications, especially psychotropics, can exacerbate RBD.

表 3.4	睡眠卫生
1. 每天保持规律的生活作息。
2. 每天早晨在同一时间醒来。
3. 接触自然光有益于昼夜节律。
4. 早晨或下午早些时候进行锻炼,避免夜间剧烈运动。
5. 避免在白天小睡,尤其是在下午 3 点之后。
6. 避免使用兴奋剂,如咖啡因和尼古丁,避免睡前饮酒。
7. 避免睡前大量进食。
8. 保持睡前规律且放松的日常活动。
9. 保持舒适的睡眠环境。
10. 床只用于睡眠,避免进行其他活动(例如,看电视、听收音机、读书)。
11. 只有在困倦时睡觉。
12. 尝试在睡前解决担忧(或列出以后考虑)。
13. 如果 20 min 内没有入睡就起床。

适应性失眠是对某种压力的急性反应。当个体存在较差的睡眠质量倾向时,可能发展成慢性(>1个月)状态,并导致不良睡眠行为以及睡眠相关的条件性觉醒。这种称为心理生理性失眠,是目前最常见的失眠综合征。不良睡眠习惯进一步加重失眠,形成恶性循环。由于其慢性特性,通常伴有不良睡眠习惯,采用多种治疗方案,并对睡眠产生焦虑。如果没有诱因,则可能存在长期睡眠障碍的病史(如特发性失眠),预后类似心理生理性失眠。

矛盾性失眠和失眠状态错觉是指患者声称自己没有睡眠,但客观检查显示他们实际上有正常的睡眠时长和结构。

诊断和鉴别诊断

失眠的诊断依赖于病史,包括睡眠日记的记录。需要排除器质性、精神性或药物相关疾病以及其他睡眠障碍(如 OSA)。睡眠检查(PSG 和 MSLT)在某些情况下可能会有所帮助。

治疗和预后

非药物治疗包括常识性的睡眠卫生建议(例如,避免咖啡因和晚间锻炼)(表 3.4),行为改变以避免与睡眠相关的条件性觉醒反应(例如,只在卧室睡觉和性行为)。其他治疗方案包括针对失眠的认知行为疗法(CBT-I)、放松训练、生物反馈治疗以及行为改变(如睡眠限制和刺激控制疗法)。

失眠药物治疗的原则包括使用最低有效剂量,间断性(非每日)给药,根据失眠类型(即入睡或维持)使用适当(即短效或中效半衰期)药物,并限制疗程。治疗应逐渐减药以避免病情反弹。且药物通常需要与非药物(如行为疗法)治疗同时使用。行为疗法已被证实有效。

非处方睡眠药(多为抗组胺药)通常是安全的,但由于抗胆碱和宿醉效应,应用受到限制。褪黑素可能促进睡眠,并用于治疗昼夜节律障碍(包括时差反应)。选择性褪黑素激动剂雷美替安有助于治疗入睡困难的失眠。

药物和非药物的联合治疗通常有良好预后。行为疗法的效果可能会受限于患者参与的意愿。

异态睡眠

异态睡眠是一组在睡眠中或睡眠转换期间发生的复杂睡眠行为障碍。可出现于快速眼动(REM)或非快速眼动(NREM)睡眠。症状多为复杂且看似有目的的行为,甚至可能很激烈,而患者在这些行为发生时并不清醒。通常根据症状出现的睡眠时期进行分类。

NREM 异态睡眠

NREM 相关异态睡眠包括意识模糊性觉醒、睡行症(梦游)和睡惊症(夜惊),因深度睡眠阶段不完全唤醒而引起。多于儿童期起病,常合并家族史。事件通常发生于第 1 个三期睡眠(慢波睡眠)。发作可由多种因素诱发,包括疾病、睡眠剥夺、酒精摄入和压力。睡行发作常继发于意识模糊性觉醒。这些患者通常表现为在床上坐起并意识模糊地四处张望。睡惊症与睡行症不同,发作更为剧烈,伴有突然觉醒、尖叫或哭喊以及自主神经功能亢进(例如,瞳孔扩大、多汗、面色发红、皮肤鸡皮疙瘩、心动过速)。患儿看起来非常害怕且无法安抚。

诊断和鉴别诊断

主要与夜间癫痫发作相鉴别,后者需要视频脑电图(EEG)监测来诊断。夜间癫痫发作相比异态睡眠更为刻板,常有强直或阵挛性运动活动。治疗包括安抚和发作期避免受伤措施。可以引发这些发作的其他睡眠障碍(如 OSA)应被除外,该过程应作为治疗的一部分。对于有伤害行为的严重发作,通常推荐使用低剂量苯二氮䓬类药物(如氯硝西泮)。

治疗和预后

安抚和避免受伤的措施常常是足够的。对于伴有伤害行为的发作,低剂量苯二氮䓬类药物(氯硝西泮,0.5~1 mg)通常是有效的。预后良好,大多数患者不需要治疗。

快速眼动行为障碍

定义和流行病学

REM 行为障碍(RBD)是一种 REM 期睡眠调节障碍,因 REM 期失去了正常的肌张力弛缓状态,导致患者演绎梦境。RBD 通常影响 50 岁以上人群,男/女比例为 10:1。

病理生理机制

由于脑桥两侧 REM 弛缓神经元退化,导致 REM 抑制消失。RBD 可合并 α 突触核蛋白病(如帕金森病、多系统萎缩和路易体痴呆),RBD 常是这些神经退行性疾病的早期症状,有时甚至在确诊前 10~15 年出现。

临床表现

发作事件多由床伴发现,包括睡眠中大幅的挥舞、伤害动作。当被叫醒时,患者常可回忆梦境。正如 REM 觉醒一样,患者可立即清醒并正常表达(与慢波睡眠觉醒不同)。药物(特别是精神类药物)可加重 RBD。

Diagnosis and Differential Diagnosis

The diagnosis can usually be made by the history alone, and PSG is not needed. When performed, PSG shows a lack of REM atonia or increased phasic and tonic REM. Like slow-wave parasomnias, the main differential diagnosis is nocturnal seizure, and this occasionally requires epilepsy monitoring. Home video (cell phone) recordings can be useful.

Treatment and Prognosis

Low-dose clonazepam (0.5 to 2 mg) is usually effective. Symptoms initially respond to treatment, but a neurodegenerative disease is likely to become evident.

For a deeper discussion of these topics, please see Chapter 377, "Sleep Disorders," in *Goldman-Cecil Medicine*, 26th Edition.

SUGGESTED READINGS

Berry RB, Wagner MH: Sleep medicine pearls, ed 3, 2014, Elsevier/Saunders.

Ebisawa T: Analysis of the molecular pathophysiology of sleep disorders relevant to a disturbed biological clock, Mol Genet Genomics 288:185–193, 2013.

Handbook of sleep disorders. In Thorpy MJ, editor: Neurological disease and therapy, New York, 1990, Taylor & Francis.

International Classification of Sleep Disorders: ed 3, Darien, IL USA, 2014, American Academy of Sleep Medicine.

Kryger MH, Rosenberg R, Kirsch D: Kryger's sleep medicine review E-Book: a problem-oriented approach, ed 3, 2019, Elsevier.

诊断和鉴别诊断

一般通过病史即可进行诊断，无需 PSG 检查。PSG 可显示 REM 期肌张力弛缓消失或 REM 期时相性持续性肌电活动增加。与慢波期异态睡眠一样，RBD 主要与夜间癫痫发作鉴别，后者可能需视频脑电图监测来诊断。居家视频（手机）记录可有助于诊断。

治疗和预后

低剂量氯硝西泮（0.5～2 mg）通常有效。症状初期对治疗反应好，但神经退行性疾病可能会更明显和难以控制。

❖ 有关此专题的深入讨论，请参阅 *Goldman-Cecil Medicine* 第 26 版第 377 章 "睡眠障碍"。

推荐阅读

Berry RB, Wagner MH: Sleep medicine pearls, ed 3, 2014, Elsevier/Saunders.

Ebisawa T: Analysis of the molecular pathophysiology of sleep disorders relevant to a disturbed biological clock, Mol Genet Genomics 288:185–193, 2013.

Handbook of sleep disorders. In Thorpy MJ, editor: Neurological disease and therapy, New York, 1990, Taylor & Francis.

International Classification of Sleep Disorders: ed 3, Darien, IL USA, 2014, American Academy of Sleep Medicine.

Kryger MH, Rosenberg R, Kirsch D: Kryger's sleep medicine review E-Book: a problem-oriented approach, ed 3, 2019, Elsevier.

4

Cortical Syndromes

Sinéad M. Murphy, Timothy J. Counihan

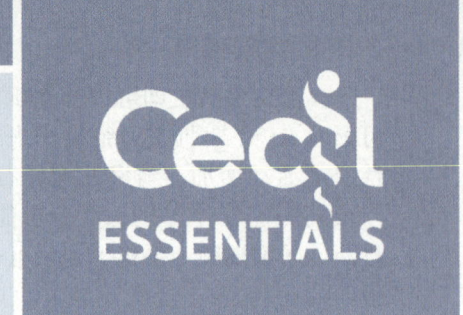

FUNCTIONAL ANATOMY

The cerebral cortex consists of two hemispheres connected by a large band of white matter fibers, the *corpus callosum*. Each hemisphere consists of four anatomically and functionally distinct regions: the frontal, temporal, parietal, and occipital lobes (Fig. 4.1). It is worth considering in some detail the regional functionality of specific brain regions, as they can provide valuable localizing information in assessing patients with cerebral dysfunction syndromes.
- Frontal Lobe: Motor control of the opposite side of the body, attention, executive function, social cognition, language production
- Temporal Lobe: Memory, emotion, speech comprehension
- Parietal Lobe: Sensation for the opposite side of the body, spatial perception
- Occipital Lobe: Vision

Although the two cerebral hemispheres share a number of behavioral and sensorimotor tasks, certain functions, particularly language, manual dexterity, and visuospatial perception are strongly lateralized to one hemisphere. Language function is lateralized to the left hemisphere in 95% of the population; although 15% of people are left-handed, the right hemisphere is dominant for language in only about 10%. Visuospatial perception is largely a function of the right (nondominant) hemisphere. On either side of the central sulcus lie the pre- and post-central gyri; in these regions, cortical representations of the different parts of the body are arranged as the motor (frontal lobe) and sensory (parietal lobe) homunculi (Fig. 4.2). It is worth noting that the juxtaposition of facial and hand representation in the homunculus accounts for the facio-brachial predominant pattern of weakness in syndromes affecting the cerebral lateral convexity such as is seen in many patients with ischemic stroke. Similarly, motor or sensory signs confined to the lower extremities may suggest a parasagittal lesion.

CLINICAL ASSESSMENT

Although lesions in specific regions of the cerebral cortex can result in well-defined syndromes, it is important to be aware of potential pitfalls in interpreting symptoms and signs of cortical origin.
- Patients with lesions of the nondominant hemisphere are often unaware of the extent of their deficit.
- Symptoms and signs caused by cortical lesions may be less consistent than deficits caused by lesions of the spinal cord or more peripheral nerves.

REGIONAL SYNDROMES

Table 4.1 summarizes some of the more common syndromes associated with damage to individual cerebral lobes.

Aphasia

Aphasia or *dysphasia* refers to a loss or impairment of language function as a result of damage to the specific language centers of the dominant hemisphere. It is distinct from dysarthria, which is a disturbance in the articulation of speech. The principal types of aphasia are summarized in Table 4.2.

Clinical assessment for aphasia requires testing of fluency, comprehension, repetition, naming, reading, calculation, and writing. *Anomia* refers to difficulty in the naming of objects. Patients may

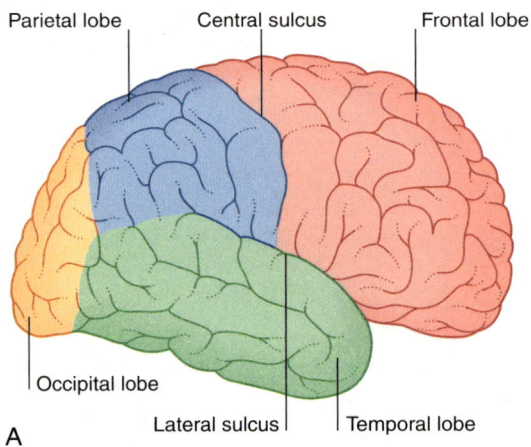

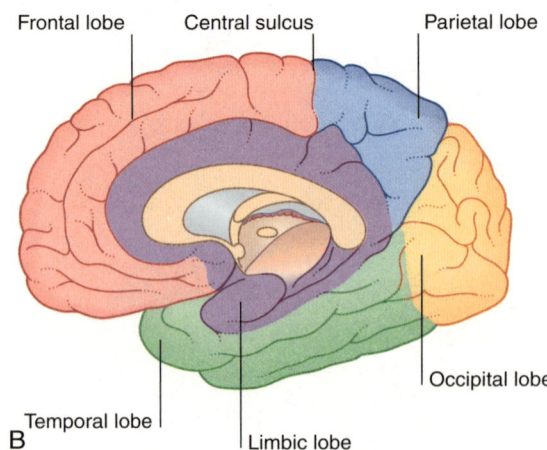

Fig. 4.1 Lateral (A) and medial (B) views of the cerebral hemispheres. (From FitzGerald MJT, editor: Clinical neuroanatomy and neuroscience, ed 6, Philadelphia, 2011, Saunders, Fig. 2-1.)

皮质综合征

徐丹 译 谭颖 周雁 审校 姚明 彭斌 通审

功能解剖学

两侧大脑半球由一条大的白质纤维带，即胼胝体相连。每个半球包含四个解剖和功能截然不同的区域：额叶、颞叶、顶叶和枕叶（图4.1）。在评估脑功能障碍的患者时，应尤其注意询问和检查可提供定位诊断信息的细节。具体脑区对应功能如下：

- 额叶：控制对侧运动、注意力、执行功能、社会认知、语言产生。
- 颞叶：记忆、情感、言语理解。
- 顶叶：对侧感觉、空间感知。
- 枕叶：视觉。

两侧大脑半球协同完成许多行为和感觉运动任务，但某些功能却以单侧半球支配为主，尤其是语言、动手能力、视空间感知。95%的人语言功能由左半球控制；尽管15%的人是左利手，但仅约10%的人语言功能主要由右半球控制。与之相反，视空间功能主要由右半球（非优势半球）控制。以中央沟为界，分为中央前回（运动皮质）和中央后回（感觉皮质），身体各部位的皮质代表区在运动（额叶）和感觉（顶叶）排列呈"倒人状"分布（图4.2）。值得注意的是，由面部和手部代表区的分布可见，若面部和上肢联合受累，提示病变位于皮质外侧凸面，多见于缺血性卒中患者。同样，当运动和感觉症状局限于下肢，提示为矢状窦旁区域病变。

临床评估

尽管大脑皮质局灶性损害可导致明确的综合征，但在理解某些皮质损害的症状和体征时，要注意以下一些误区。

- 非优势半球病变的患者往往意识不到自己存在神经功能缺损。
- 与脊髓或周围神经病变相比，皮质病变引起的症状和体征一致性略差。

局灶综合征

表4.1总结了一些常见的脑叶损害综合征。

失语症

失语症或语言障碍是指由于优势半球的特定语言中枢受损而导致的语言功能丧失或受损。它有别于构音障碍，后者是言语发音紊乱。失语症的主要类型总结于表4.2。

失语症的临床评估包括流畅度、理解、复述、命名、阅读、计算及书写。命名性失语指的是对物体的命名困难。患者可能叫不出常用物体的准确名称，例

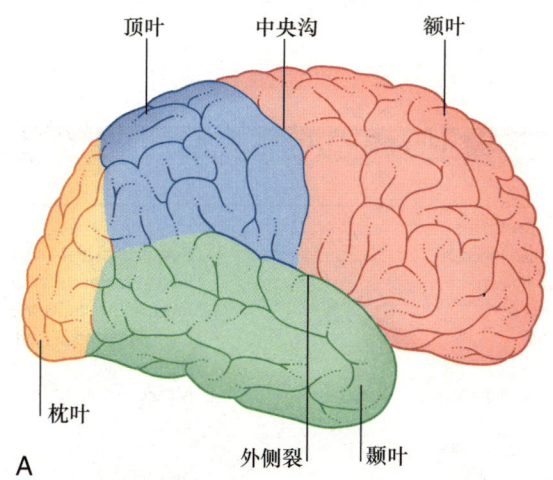

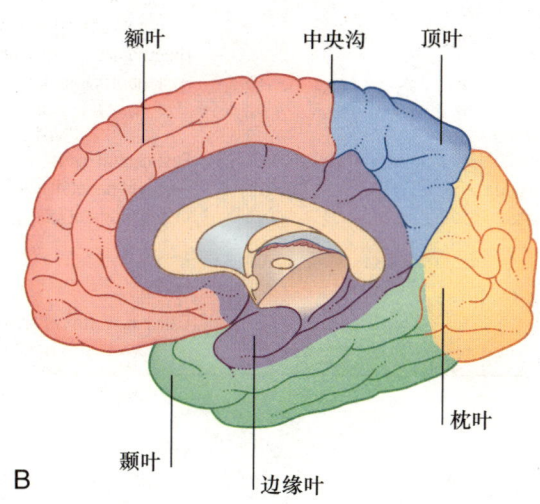

图4.1 大脑半球的外侧视图（A）和内侧视图（B）。（引自 FitzGerald MJT, editor: Clinical neuroanatomy and neuroscience, ed 6, Philadelphia, 2011, Saunders, Fig. 2-1.）

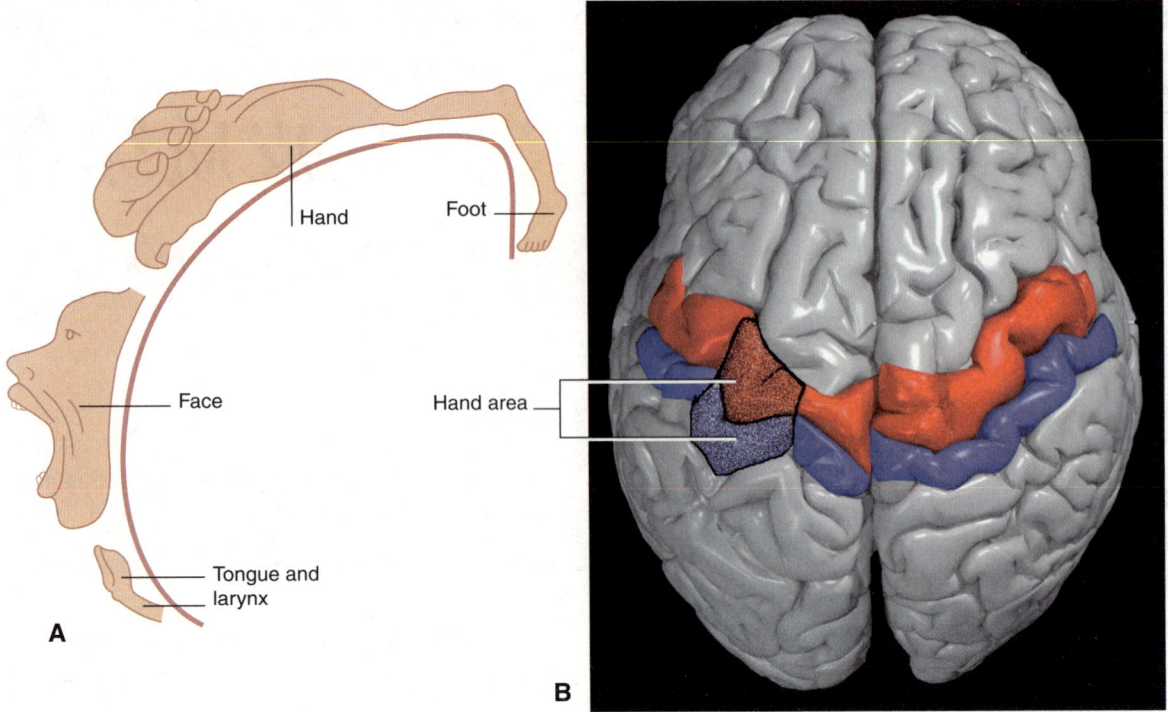

Fig. 4.2 (A) Homuncular arrangement shows the correlations with the primary motor cortex lying anterior to the central sulcus and the somatosensory cortex posteriorly (B). (Modified from Kretschmann HJ, Weinrich W: Neurofunctional systems: 3D reconstructions with correlated neuroimaging: text and CD-ROM, New York, 1998, Thieme.)

TABLE 4.1 Cortical Syndromes and Their Localization

Function	Location	Clinical Signs
Frontal Lobe		
Executive function	Dorsolateral prefrontal cortex	Motor sequencing
Motor function	Primary motor cortex (prefrontal gyrus)	Contralateral weakness
Language	Broca area (inferior frontal cortex)	Expressive aphasia
Behavior	Cingulate (medial frontal lobe)	Obsessive-compulsive traits
	Orbitofrontal	Disinhibition apathy
Oculomotor (frontal eye fields)	Middle frontal gyrus	Forced contralateral eye deviation
Temporal Lobe		
Hearing	Superior temporal gyrus	Auditory hallucinations
Smell	Uncus of temporal lobe	Olfactory hallucinations
Emotion	Amygdala of temporal lobe	Irrational fear
Memory	Hippocampus (medial temporal lobe)	Amnesia; déjà vu
Language	Posterior superior temporal lobe	Wernicke aphasia
Parietal Lobe		
Sensation	Post-central gyrus	Contralateral sensory loss
Visuo-spatial	Posterior parietal lobe	Constructional apraxia
Language	Inferior parietal lobe	Gerstmann syndrome (acalculia, finger agnosia, agraphia, left-right disorientation)
Occipital Lobe		
Vision	Calcarine cortex of occipital lobe	Cortical blindness; visual hallucinations; contralateral homonymous hemianopia

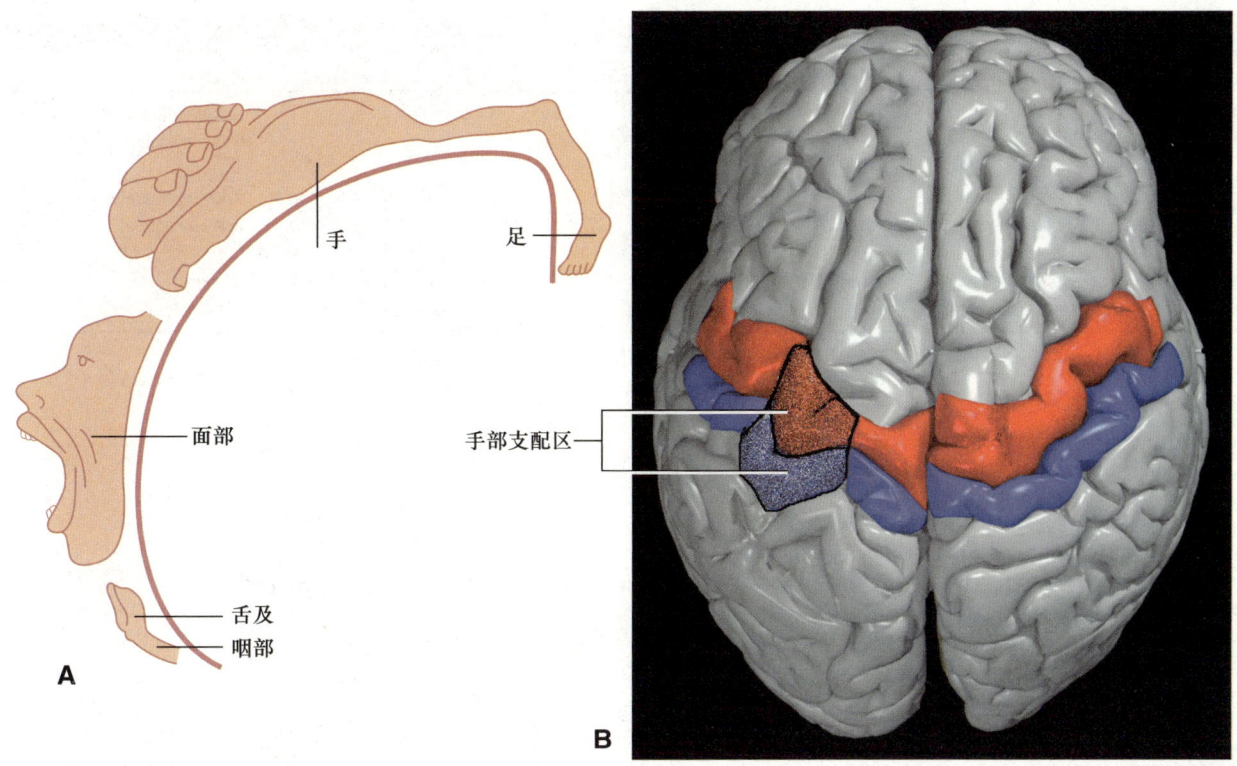

图 4.2 "倒人状"排列（A）显示了皮质支配区与位于中央沟前后的初级运动皮质及躯体感觉皮质间的位置关系（B）。（改编自 Kretschmann HJ，Weinrich W：Neurofunctional systems：3D reconstructions with correlated neuroimaging：text and CD-ROM，New York，1998，Thieme.）

表 4.1 皮质综合征及其定位

功能	定位	临床症状或体征
额叶		
执行功能	前额叶皮质背外侧	运动序列障碍
运动功能	初级运动皮质（中央前回）	对侧无力
语言	Broca 区（额下回皮质）	运动性失语
行为	扣带回（额叶内侧）	强迫症状
	额叶眶回	失抑制、淡漠
眼球运动（前额眼动区）	额中回	眼球向对侧凝视
颞叶		
听觉	颞上回	幻听
嗅觉	颞叶钩回	幻嗅
情感	颞叶杏仁核	无端恐惧
记忆	海马体（颞叶内侧）	失忆，似曾相识感
语言	颞上回后部	Wernicke 失语
顶叶		
感觉	中央后回	对侧感觉缺失
视空间	后顶叶	结构性失用
语言	顶下小叶	格斯特曼（Gerstmann）综合征：计算不能、手指失认、失写、左右失认
枕叶		
视觉	枕叶距状裂	皮质盲、幻视、对侧同向性偏盲

TABLE 4.2 Principal Types of Aphasia

Type	Lesion Site	Fluency	Comprehension	Repetition	Naming	Other Signs
Broca (expressive)	Inferior frontal lobe	↓	Good	↓	↓	Contralateral weakness
Wernicke (receptive)	Posterior superior temporal lobe	Good	↓	↓	↓	Homonymous hemianopia
Transcortical motor	Inferior frontal gyrus	↓	Good	Good	May be normal	May be contralateral weakness
Transcortical sensory	Middle temporal gyrus, thalamus	Good	↓	Good	Usually normal	May be normal
Conduction	Supramarginal gyrus	Good	Good	↓	↓	None
Global	Frontal lobe (large)	↓	↓	↓	↓	Hemiplegia

↓, Reduced.

have difficulty with the correct identification of common items such as a watch, often using a word that either sounds like the intended word ("a spotch"—a literal paraphasic error) or a word with a broadly similar meaning ("a clock"—a semantic paraphasic error). There are two broad types of aphasia depending on the anatomic site of the lesion: anterior (Broca) aphasia and posterior (Wernicke) aphasia.

Broca aphasia is characterized by a severe disruption in the fluency of speech, with profound impairments of expression in both speech and writing. Comprehension may be mildly affected. The language disturbance is almost invariably accompanied by contralateral face and arm weakness as a result of the proximity of the motor homunculus to the Broca speech area in the inferior frontal lobe.

Wernicke aphasia is characterized by an inability to comprehend spoken or written language. Affected patients speak fluently, but the content is meaningless. The lesion is located in the posterior superior temporal area and may be associated with a homonymous hemianopic visual field deficit.

Conduction aphasia is characterized by normal comprehension and fluent speech but a striking inability to repeat a phrase. The responsible lesion lies in the arcuate fasciculus connecting the Broca and Wernicke areas. *Global aphasia* results from large lesions of the frontal lobe; all aspects of language are affected. Lesions of the language areas of the nondominant hemisphere result in *dysprosody*. For instance, patients with lesions in the inferior frontal lobe of the nondominant hemisphere, analogous to the Broca area, speak with a monotonous voice, losing the ability to add emotional cadence to their speech. Similarly, lesions affecting the nondominant Wernicke area result in patients failing to pick up on the emotional inflexions (such as anger) of what is said to them.

Writing is almost invariably affected in patients with disturbances of language (Fig. 4.3). An exception to this occurs in the syndrome of *alexia without agraphia*, which results from a lesion in the dominant occipital lobe and splenium of the corpus callosum (usually caused by infarction in the territory of the posterior cerebral artery). The patient's language center is "disconnected" from the contralateral (unaffected) visual cortex. Such patients can write a sentence but are unable to read what they have written.

Agnosia and Apraxia

Agnosia is the inability to recognize a specific sensory stimulus despite preserved sensory function. For instance, visual agnosia is the inability to recognize a visual stimulus despite normal visual acuity. Other agnosia syndromes include the inability to recognize sounds (auditory agnosia), color (color agnosia), or familiar faces (prosopagnosia). Usually, the responsible lesions are located in the occipitotemporal region.

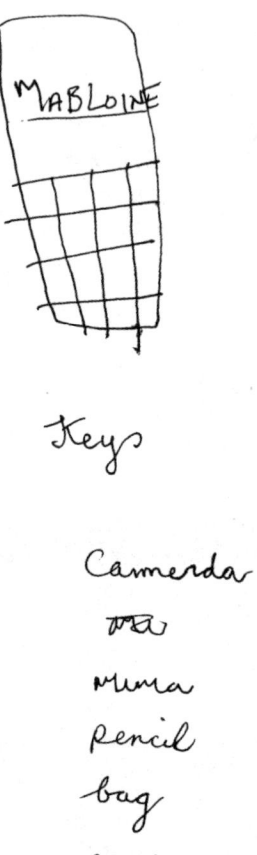

Fig. 4.3 Neologisms written by a patient with aphasia who was attempting to name cell phone, keys, camera, watch, pen, bag, and boots.

Apraxia refers to an inability to perform learned motor tasks despite sufficient sensorimotor function to physically execute the movement; it is a disorder of motor planning (Fig. 4.4). The responsible lesions are usually in the dominant inferior parietal lobe. A simple test of apraxia is to ask the patient to perform a pantomime (e.g., combing the hair, blowing out a candle). Lesions of the nondominant parietal lobe often result in *hemispatial neglect:* the patient does not attend to stimuli in the contralateral (usually the left) visual field or on the contralateral side of the body. In a milder form of neglect, called *extinction*, patients can attend to stimuli contralateral to the side of the brain with the lesion (typically the right hemisphere), but

表 4.2 失语症的主要类型

类型	病变部位	流畅性	理解能力	复述	命名	其他体征
运动性（Broca）	额叶下部	↓	正常	↓	↓	对侧力弱
感觉性（Wernicke）	颞上回后部	正常	↓	↓	↓	同向性偏盲
经皮质运动性	额下回	↓	正常	正常	可能正常	可能有对侧力弱
经皮质感觉性	颞中回、丘脑	正常	↓	正常	通常正常	可能正常
传导性	缘上回	正常	正常	↓	↓	无
全面性	额叶（大面积）	↓	↓	↓	↓	偏瘫

↓，下降。

如"手表"，他们使用的词语在语音或者语义上与目标词汇相近。根据病变的解剖部位，失语症可分为两大类：前部（Broca）失语症和后部（Wernicke）失语症。

Broca 失语症（运动性失语症）的特点是言语流畅性严重受损，伴有突出的言语和书写表达障碍。理解力可能轻微受损。Broca 失语症通常伴有对侧面部及上肢无力，因为相应的运动区与 Broca 区在额下回后部相邻。

Wernicke 失语症（感觉性失语症）的特点是无法理解口头或书面语言。患者说话流利，但内容毫无意义。病变位于颞上回后部，可能伴有同向性偏盲。

传导性失语症的特点是理解力正常、语言流畅，但却无法复述。病灶位于连接 Broca 区和 Wernicke 区的弓状纤维。全面性失语症由额叶大面积病变造成，语言的各个方面都受累。非优势半球语言区的病变会导致言语声律障碍。例如，非优势半球额下回（类似于 Broca 区）病变的患者说话声音单调，失去自然语调的抑扬顿挫性。同样，病变累及非优势半球 Wernicke 区时，患者无法理解别人对他们说话时言语中所表达的情绪（如愤怒等）。

语言障碍的患者书写通常受累（图 4.3）。但不伴有失写症的失读症是个例外，其与优势半球枕叶和胼胝体压部病变相关（通常由大脑后动脉区域的梗死引起）。患者的语言中枢与对侧（无病变侧）视觉皮质"失联络"，他们可以写出一个句子，却无法读出其内容。

失认症和失用症

失认症是指感觉功能保持正常却无法识别特定的感觉刺激。例如，视觉失认症就是在视力正常的情况下无法识别视觉刺激。其他失认症还包括无法识别声音（听觉失认）、颜色（颜色失认）或熟悉的面孔（面孔失认）。责任病灶通常位于枕颞部。

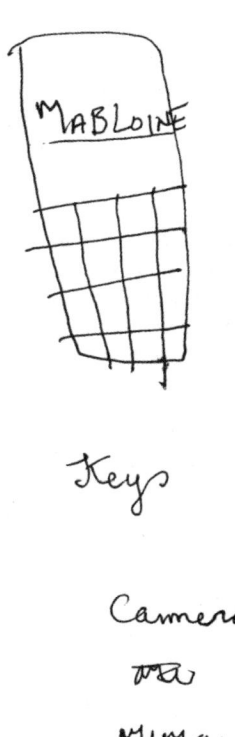

图 4.3 失语症患者被要求命名手机、钥匙、照相机、手表、笔、包和靴子，图示因功能障碍所写出的新词

失用症是指尽管感觉运动功能足以执行动作，但仍无法完成所习得的运动任务；这是一种运动规划障碍（图 4.4）。病变通常位于优势半球顶下小叶。一个简单的失用症检查就是让患者做个动作（如梳头、吹蜡烛）。非优势半球顶叶病变通常会导致偏侧忽视：患者注意不到对侧（通常是左侧）视野范围内或对侧身体的刺激。一种较轻的忽视被称为对侧消退：患者可以注意到大脑病变对侧（通常是右半球病变）的刺

Copy this cube:

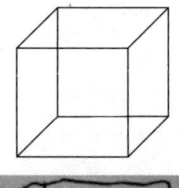

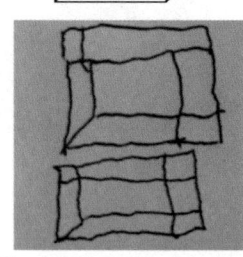

Draw a clock, fill in the numbers and put the time at ten after 2:

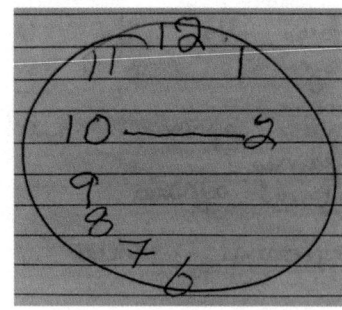

Fig. 4.4 Attempts to copy a cube and draw a clock by patients with neurodegenerative disorders demonstrate constructional apraxia and right-sided neglect.

when presented with bilateral stimuli simultaneously, they respond to stimuli only on the right hemibody side. *Anosognosia,* or the lack of awareness of one's deficit, frequently accompanies hemispatial neglect. In severe cases, patients may even deny that the affected limb belongs to them. Patients with anosognosia may present a challenge to rehabilitation therapists.

PROSPECTUS FOR THE FUTURE

Recent advances in neuroimaging technology have added to our understanding not only of the structural and functional anatomy of the brain but also its metabolic activity. Functional magnetic resonance imaging (fMRI) permits mapping of the metabolic anatomy of subcortical gray and white matter structures, such as the basal ganglia, and their roles in conditions such as dystonia. Furthermore, a modality known as diffusion tensor imaging allows for the mapping of white matter tracts (tractography) in great detail.

Several new strategies are emerging in an attempt to reverse the deficit in self-awareness in patients with neglect or anosognosia resulting from degenerative or ischemic lesions of the nondominant hemisphere. The development of virtual reality computer interface programs has opened the possibility to generate a variety of computer-based simulation environments to provide patients with detailed feedback options to improve self-awareness as part of a rehabilitation program.

SUGGESTED READINGS

Brazis PW, Masdeu JC, Biller J: Localization in clinical neurology, ed 7, Philadelphia, 2016, Wolters Kluwer.

Fitzgerald MJT, Gruener G, Estomih M: Clinical neuroanatomy and neuroscience, ed 6, Saunders, 2011.

Muratore M, Tuena C, Pedroli E, Cipresso P, Riva G: Virtual reality as a possible tool for the assessment of self-awareness, Front Behav Neurosci 13:62, 2019. https://doi.org/10.3389/fnbeh.2019.00062.

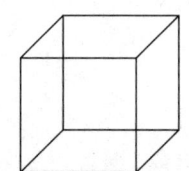
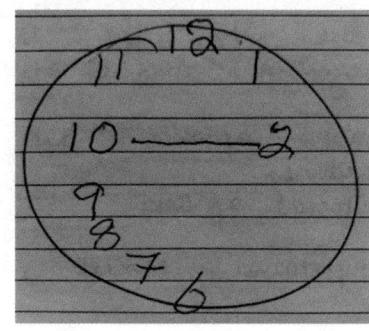
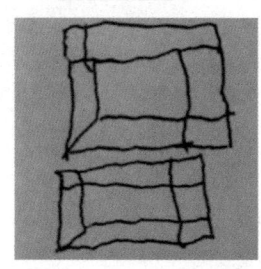

图 4.4　神经退行性疾病患者尝试临摹立方体和绘制时钟时，表现出结构性失用和右侧忽视

激，但当受到双侧同时刺激时，他们只能对右侧肢体受到的刺激有反应。病感失认症，即无法意识到自己的缺陷，常伴偏侧忽视。严重的患者甚至会否认患肢属于自己。对病感失认症患者进行康复治疗可能会是一项挑战。

未来展望

神经影像技术的最新进展增加了我们对脑结构和功能解剖、脑代谢活动的认识。功能磁共振成像（fMRI）可以绘制皮质下灰白质结构（如基底节）的代谢解剖图，以及它们在某些疾病（如肌张力障碍）中的作用图。此外，一种被称为"弥散张量成像（DTI）"的方法可以详细绘制白质束（纤维束成像）。

对于非优势半球的退行性病变或缺血性病变导致的忽视或病感失认症患者，一些新的治疗策略有助于改变其自我意识缺陷。计算机虚拟现实接口提供了广泛的基于计算机的刺激环境，为患者提供具体化的反馈选项，可作为提高患者自我意识的康复手段。

推荐阅读

Brazis PW, Masdeu JC, Biller J: Localization in clinical neurology, ed 7, Philadelphia, 2016, Wolters Kluwer.

Fitzgerald MJT, Gruener G, Estomih M: Clinical neuroanatomy and neuroscience, ed 6, Saunders, 2011.

Muratore M, Tuena C, Pedroli E, Cipresso P, Riva G: Virtual reality as a possible tool for the assessment of self-awareness, Front Behav Neurosci 13:62, 2019. https://doi.org/10.3389/fnbeh.2019.00062.

5

Dementia and Memory Disturbances

Frederick J. Marshall

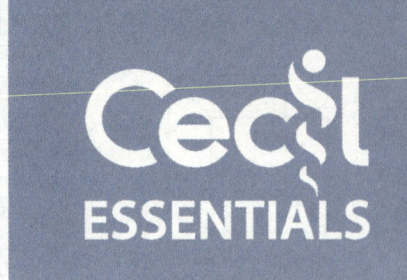

MAJOR DEMENTIA SYNDROMES

Dementia places an enormous burden on the patient, family, and society. A third of older adults in the United States die of Alzheimer disease (AD) or other form of dementia, but only one in six older adults receives routine cognitive screening. The annual direct and indirect expenditure for AD and other dementias in the United States was $290 billion in 2019.

The term *dementia* refers to a syndrome of progressive cognitive decline leading to the loss of fully independent function in daily life. Memory loss is the most common central feature, and specific dementia syndromes characteristically cause particular forms of memory impairment. Different dementias produce specific abnormalities of cognition in language, spatial processing, praxis (the ability to execute learned motor behaviors), and executive function (the ability to plan and sequence thoughts and activities), and many have associated non-cognitive features. *Cortical dementia* and *subcortical dementia*, although older terms, remain helpful for subdividing the dementias (Table 5.1).

Neurodegeneration is the most common underlying cause of dementia. Table 5.2 provides the differential diagnosis of neurodegenerative causes of dementia. Table 5.3 outlines other causes of dementia.

Most causes of dementia are currently untreatable. Potentially correctable causes account for less than 5% of dementia cases. Structural processes or infections must be considered, along with metabolic and nutritional diseases. Every patient with dementia should have tests of serum electrolytes and vitamin B_{12} and assessments of liver, renal, and thyroid function. Serologic studies for syphilis, human immunodeficiency virus (HIV), and Lyme exposure should be done if risk factors are identified. Chronic infections, normal-pressure hydrocephalus (NPH), and autoimmune encephalopathies should be considered. Brain imaging should be performed.

Neuropsychological testing characterizes the pattern of cognitive and memory impairments and is helpful in the differential diagnosis. The Montreal Cognitive Assessment (MoCA) (Table 5.4) is a standard test that can be used as a bedside or office screening tool for identifying patients with dementia. It typically takes about 10 minutes to administer. This examination is superior to the Mini-Mental Status Examination (MMSE) in that it is more sensitive to abnormalities in a wider array of cognitive domains, including visual-spatial or executive function, naming, attention, fluency; abstract reasoning, short-term memory encoding and retrieval, and orientation.

In addition to the MoCA, patients with dementia should have tests of praxis (e.g., show how you would comb your hair; show how you would blow out a match) and neglect (e.g., testing of double-simultaneous extinction to visual, tactile, and auditory stimuli). Depending on the results of these screening procedures, more detailed neuropsychological studies can be pursued.

Alzheimer Disease

AD accounts for approximately 70% of dementia cases among older adults. There is widespread confusion among the lay population about the relationship between the terms *Alzheimer disease, senility,* and *dementia*. Patients and their family members often need clarification. Alzheimer *disease* (a specific diagnosis) is only one possible cause (albeit by far the most common cause) of *dementia* (a syndrome). Nearly six million persons in the United States are affected, and this number is estimated to approach 14 million by 2050 as the population ages. The disease occurs in 32% to 47% of persons older than 80 years of age. Incidence at age 65 is one in 200 people per year. Incidence at age 80 is one case per 10 people per year. More than 50% of caregivers develop depression or a major medical illness. Deaths from heart disease decreased 9% between 2000 and 2017, while deaths from AD increased 145%.

AD has many causes, but none is fully defined. All causes produce similar clinical and pathologic findings. The disease is characterized by the progressive loss of cortical neurons and the formation of amyloid plaques and intraneuronal neurofibrillary tangles. β-Amyloid (Aβ) is the major component of the plaques, while hyperphosphorylated tau protein is the major constituent of the neurofibrillary tangles. The process starts in the hippocampus and entorhinal cortex and spreads to involve diffuse areas of association cortex in the temporal, parietal, and frontal lobes. The relative deficiency of cortical acetylcholine (resulting from the loss of neurons in the nucleus basalis) provides the rationale for symptomatic treatment of the disease with centrally acting acetylcholinesterase inhibitors.

Pathogenesis

AD is often categorized as a young-onset hereditary or familial form, which is rare (≈5% overall) and for which three specific genetic abnormalities have been determined, or as a common (≈95% overall), sporadic form that typically occurs in persons older than 65 years of age (Table 5.5).

The autosomal dominant early-onset forms of AD have in common abnormalities of Aβ production and processing that have provided clues to the molecular pathogenesis of sporadic AD. Abnormal processing of amyloid precursor protein into the amyloidogenic peptide Aβ (1-42) is thought to be important in the pathogenesis of AD. It is thought to provoke downstream abnormalities of tau protein processing, with hyperphosphorylation of tau yielding intraneuronal tangles.

The apolipoprotein E (Apo E) gene *(APOE)* is a susceptibility locus for sporadic AD in late-onset familial AD pedigrees. The gene is

痴呆和记忆障碍

翟菲菲 译 周雁 卢强 审校 姚明 彭斌 通审

痴呆综合征

痴呆给患者、家庭和社会带来了巨大负担。在美国，约有 1/3 的老年人死于阿尔茨海默病（Alzheimer disease，AD）或其他类型的痴呆，但只有 1/6 的老年人接受常规认知筛查。2019 年，美国在阿尔茨海默病和其他类型痴呆的年度直接和间接支出合计 2900 亿美元。

痴呆（dementia）是指进行性认知功能下降、导致日常生活能力丧失的一种临床综合征。记忆减退是最常见的核心特征，特定类型的痴呆综合征会导致特定形式的记忆障碍。不同类型的痴呆会在语言、空间处理、实践能力（执行已学会的运动行为的能力）和执行功能（计划和顺序思维及活动的能力）方面产生特定的认知异常，许多痴呆患者还伴有非认知症状。虽然"皮质性痴呆"和"皮质下痴呆"是较老的术语，但仍有助于痴呆分类（表 5.1）。

神经退行性变是痴呆最常见的潜在病因。表 5.2 列出了导致痴呆的神经退行性疾病的鉴别诊断，表 5.3 概述了痴呆的其他病因。

大多数痴呆的病因目前无法治愈，潜在的可纠正病因小于 5%。在可纠正的病因里需要考虑结构性异常、感染、代谢和营养障碍相关疾病。每位痴呆患者都应进行血清电解质和维生素 B_{12} 检测，并评估肝功能、肾功能以及甲状腺功能。如果存在暴露风险，还应行梅毒、人类免疫缺陷病毒（HIV）及莱姆病的血清学检查。此外，还应考虑慢性感染、正常压力脑积水（NPH）和自身免疫性脑病。应进行脑影像学评估。

神经心理学测试可以评估认知和记忆障碍的模式，有助于鉴别诊断。蒙特利尔认知评估量表（MoCA）（表 5.4）是一个标准测试，可以用作床旁或诊室筛查工具来识别痴呆患者。该测试通常需要 10 min 左右完成。MoCA 优于简易精神状态检查量表（MMSE）是因为它在检测更广泛认知领域的异常时更加敏感，这些认知领域包括视空间或执行功能、命名、注意力、流畅性、抽象推理、短期记忆编码和提取以及定向力。

除了 MoCA，痴呆患者还应接受失用（例如，展示如何梳头、如何吹灭火柴）和忽视（例如，双侧同时给予视觉、触觉或听觉刺激，病灶侧不能感知）测试。根据这些筛查的结果，可以进行更详细的神经心理学测试。

阿尔茨海默病

AD 约占老年人痴呆病例的 70%。非专业人士对"阿尔茨海默病""老年痴呆（senility）"和"痴呆（dementia）"这几个术语之间的关系存在混淆，通常需要对患者及其家属进行澄清。AD 是一个具体疾病诊断，它只是痴呆（一个综合征）的一种可能病因（尽管是迄今为止最常见的病因）。美国有近 600 万人患有 AD，随着人口老龄化的加剧，预计到 2050 年，这个数字将接近 1400 万。该病在 80 岁以上人群中的患病率为 32%～47%。65 岁人群 AD 的年发病率为 1/200，80 岁人群 AD 的年发病率为 1/10。超过 50% 的照料者会患上抑郁症或重大疾病。2000—2017 年间，死于心脏病的人数减少了 9%，而死于 AD 的人数增加了 145%。

AD 有多种病因，但目前尚未被完全明确，所有病因都导致相似的临床和病理学表现。该病的病理特点是大脑皮质神经元的进行性丢失和淀粉样斑块及神经元内神经纤维缠结的形成。β 淀粉样蛋白（Aβ）是淀粉样斑块的主要成分，而过度磷酸化 tau 蛋白是神经纤维缠结的主要成分。该过程始于海马和内嗅皮质，并逐渐累及颞叶、顶叶和额叶的广泛联络皮质区域。大脑皮质乙酰胆碱的相对缺乏（由于基底核神经元丢失导致）为使用中枢作用的胆碱酯酶抑制剂进行对症治疗提供了理论依据。

发病机制

阿尔茨海默病（AD）通常分为两种类型：一种是年轻起病的遗传性或家族性 AD，较为罕见（约占 5%），目前已确定了 3 种特定的基因异常；另一种是常见的散发类型（约占 95%），通常见于 65 岁以上的人群（表 5.5）。

常染色体显性遗传早发型 AD 的共同特征是 Aβ 生成和加工异常，这为散发性 AD 发病的分子机制提供了线索。淀粉样前体蛋白异常加工生成淀粉样肽 Aβ（1-42）被认为在 AD 的发病机制中起重要作用。这种异常加工会引发下游的 tau 蛋白加工异常，导致 tau 蛋白的过度磷酸化，进而形成神经元内的神经纤维缠结。

载脂蛋白 E（Apo E）基因（APOE）是晚发型家

TABLE 5.1 Distinguishing Characteristics of Cortical and Subcortical Dementias

Cortical Dementia
Symptoms: major changes in memory, language deficits, perceptual deficits, praxis disturbances
Affected brain regions: temporal cortex (medial), parietal cortex, and frontal lobe cortex
Examples: Alzheimer disease, diffuse Lewy body disease, vascular dementia, frontotemporal dementias

Subcortical Dementia
Symptoms: behavioral changes, impaired affect and mood, motor slowing, executive dysfunction, less severe changes in memory early on in the course
Affected brain regions: thalamus, striatum, midbrain, striatofrontal projections, subcortical white matter
Examples: Parkinson's disease, progressive supranuclear palsy, normal-pressure hydrocephalus, Huntington's disease

TABLE 5.2 Etiologic Diagnosis of Neurodegenerative Dementia in Adults

Alzheimer disease[a] (AD)
Parkinson's disease[a] (PD)
Diffuse Lewy body disease[a] (DLBD)
Progressive supranuclear palsy (PSP)
Corticobasal ganglionic degeneration (CBGD)
Striatonigral degeneration
Huntington's disease[a]
Frontotemporal dementias (FTD)
Frontotemporal dementia without characteristic neuropathology
Frontotemporal dementia with motor neuron disease
Neurodegeneration with brain iron accumulation
Dentatorubral-pallidoluysian atrophy (DRPLA)
Spinal-cerebellar ataxias (SCAs)

[a]Denotes conditions for which symptomatic pharmacologic treatment is available.

TABLE 5.3 Other Causes of Progressive Dementia in Adults

Structural Disease or Trauma
Normal-pressure hydrocephalus (NPH)[a]
Neoplasms[a]
Dementia pugilistica (multiple concussions in boxers)
Chronic traumatic encephalopathy (CTE)

Vascular Disease
Vascular dementia[b] (also called multi-infarct dementia)
Vasculitis[a]

Heredometabolic Disease
Wilson's disease[a]
Neuronal ceroid lipofuscinosis (Kufs disease)
Other late-onset lysosomal storage diseases

Demyelinating or Dysmyelinating Disease
Multiple sclerosis[b]
Metachromatic leukodystrophy

Infectious Disease
Human immunodeficiency virus type 1[a]
Tertiary syphilis[a]
Creutzfeldt-Jakob disease
Progressive multifocal leukoencephalopathy
Whipple disease[a]
Chronic meningitis[a]
Cryptococcal meningitis[a]
Others

Metabolic or Nutritional Disease
Vitamin B_{12} deficiency[a]
Thyroid hormone deficiency or excess[a]
Thiamine deficiency[a] (Korsakoff syndrome)
Alcoholism[b]

Psychiatric Disease
Pseudodementia from depression[a]

[a]Denotes conditions for which preventive or corrective treatment is available.
[b]Denotes conditions for which symptomatic treatment is available.

polymorphic (ε2, ε3, ε4), and first-degree relatives of AD patients who inherit both ε4 alleles have a greater than 60% lifetime risk of developing AD. Apo E-ε4 interacts selectively with Aβ and with tau protein, but how Apo E-ε4 increases the risk of AD remains unknown.

Clinical Features

AD begins gradually and affects memory, orientation, language, visuospatial processing, praxis, judgment, and insight. Depression is common early in AD, and psychosis with agitation and behavioral disinhibition often occur in advanced stages. Patients become dependent on others for all activities of daily living. The rate of progression of AD varies but usually takes 5 to 15 years to progress from presentation to advanced illness.

Diagnostic criteria are outlined in Table 5.6. Although a definitive diagnosis of AD requires biopsy (rarely done) or autopsy confirmation, these diagnostic criteria establish the diagnosis with more than 85% specificity in moderately demented patients.

There are now three different positron emission tomography (PET) ligands that bind to Aβ plaques approved by the US Food and Drug Administration (FDA) for use in the clinical diagnosis of AD. These compounds are costly, however, and not universally approved by insurances, limiting their utility in clinical practice. Cerebral amyloid accumulation is largely completed at a relatively early stage of AD when patients may be asymptomatic or have only isolated impairment of memory but no overt loss of independent function in daily life (a stage known as *mild neurocognitive disorder*). Research efforts are underway to find disease modifying approaches that ameliorate plaque and possibly prolong the time to patients' loss of independence.

Another protein, known as *tau*, plays an important role in the stabilization of microtubules involved in the transport of nutrients and other substances within the neuron. In AD, tau becomes hyperphosphorylated and forms intraneuronal neurofibrillary tangles that cannot be effectively disposed of by the cell. Smaller forms of tau (oligomers) are known to circulate among neurons and interfere with their function and can be found in AD brains more than a decade prior to symptom onset. Because tau continues to accumulate throughout the course of AD, it is a potentially useful marker of disease progression. The FDA has recently approved a PET ligand that binds to tau.

表 5.1　皮质性痴呆和皮质下痴呆的区别

皮质性痴呆
症状：记忆力显著下降、语言障碍、感知障碍、实践能力障碍
受影响的脑区：颞叶皮质（内侧）、顶叶皮质、额叶皮质
例如：阿尔茨海默病、弥漫性路易体病、血管性痴呆、额颞叶痴呆

皮质下痴呆
症状：行为改变、情感和情绪受损、运动迟缓、执行功能障碍，病程早期记忆力变化较轻
受影响的脑区：丘脑、纹状体、中脑、纹状体额叶投射、皮质下白质
例如：帕金森病、进行性核上性麻痹、正常压力脑积水、亨廷顿病

表 5.2　成人神经退行性痴呆的病因诊断

阿尔茨海默病[a]（AD）
帕金森病[a]（PD）
弥漫性路易体病[a]（DLBD）
进行性核上性麻痹（PSP）
皮质基底节变性（CBGD）
纹状体黑质变性
亨廷顿病[a]（HD）
额颞叶痴呆（FTD）
无特征性神经病理的额颞叶痴呆
伴运动神经元病的额颞叶痴呆
伴脑铁沉积的神经退行性疾病
齿状核红核苍白球路易体萎缩症（DRPLA）
脊髓小脑性共济失调（SCA）

[a] 表示有可用的药物对症治疗。

表 5.3　成人进行性痴呆的其他病因

结构性异常或外伤
正常压力脑积水（NPH）[a]
肿瘤[a]
拳击手痴呆（拳击运动员多次脑震荡）
慢性创伤性脑病（CTE）

血管疾病
血管性痴呆[b]（也称多发梗死性痴呆）
血管炎[a]

遗传代谢性疾病
肝豆状核变性[a]
神经元蜡样脂褐质沉积症（Kufs 病）
其他晚发型溶酶体贮积病

脱髓鞘或髓鞘发育不良性疾病
多发性硬化[b]
异染性脑白质营养不良

感染性疾病
人类免疫缺陷病毒 1 型[a]
三期梅毒[a]
克-雅病
进行性多灶性白质脑病
惠普尔病
慢性脑膜炎
隐球菌性脑膜炎[a]
其他

代谢或营养性疾病
维生素 B_{12} 缺乏[a]
甲状腺功能减退或亢进[a]
维生素 B_1 缺乏（科萨科夫综合征）[a]
酗酒[b]

精神疾病
抑郁症引起的假性痴呆[a]

[a] 表示可以进行预防或矫正治疗。
[b] 表示有可用的药物对症治疗。

族性 AD 谱系中散发性 AD 的易感基因。该基因具有多态性，有 ε2、ε3、ε4 几种形式。AD 患者的一级亲属若遗传了 2 个 ε4 等位基因，其终生罹患 AD 的风险超过 60%。Apo E-ε4 选择性地与 Aβ 和 tau 蛋白相互作用，但 Apo E-ε4 是如何增加 AD 风险尚不清楚。

临床特征

AD 通常隐匿起病、逐渐加重，影响记忆力、定向力、语言、视空间处理、实践能力、判断力以及洞察力。抑郁在 AD 早期常见，在晚期常有易激惹、行为失抑制等精神症状，患者的所有日常生活活动都需要依赖他人。AD 的进展速度各不相同，通常在发病后 5～15 年进展到疾病晚期。

表 5.6 列出了 AD 的诊断标准。虽然 AD 的确诊需要活检（很少进行）或尸检，但这些诊断标准在中度痴呆患者中的特异性超过 85%。

目前美国食品和药物管理局（FDA）已批准了三种与 Aβ 斑块结合的不同正电子发射断层成像（PET）配体，用于 AD 的临床诊断。然而，这些化合物价格昂贵，而且医保通常不覆盖，限制了它们在临床实践中的应用。大脑中淀粉样蛋白的沉积在 AD 早期就已大部分完成，此时患者可能无症状或仅有孤立的记忆障碍，但无明显的日常生活能力丧失（这一阶段被称为轻度认知障碍）。研究人员正在努力寻找能够减少淀粉样斑块、延长患者独立生活时间的疾病修饰疗法。

另一种被称为 tau 的蛋白质在微管稳定中发挥重要作用，微管参与神经元内营养物质和其他物质的运输。在 AD 中，tau 蛋白过度磷酸化，形成神经元内的神经纤维缠结，这些缠结无法被细胞有效清除。已知较小形式的 tau 蛋白（寡聚体）可以在神经元之间循环并干扰神经元功能，并且在症状出现前十多年就可以见于 AD 患者的大脑中。由于 tau 蛋白在 AD 的整个病程中不断积累，因此它是一个潜在有用的疾病进展标志物。FDA 最近批准了一种与 tau 结合的 PET 配体。

TABLE 5.4 Elements of the Montreal Cognitive Assessment

Cognitive Domain	Items	Score
Visual-spatial or executive	Complete a trail-making task, copy a cube, draw a clock	5
Naming	Name three depicted animals	3
Attention	Recall five digits forward, three digits backward, maintain letter vigilance, subtract 7s serially	6
Language	Repeat two phrases, generate a list of words starting with a specific letter	3
Abstraction	Identify the similarity between nouns (train/bicycle; watch/ruler)	2
Delayed recall	Recall five words rehearsed twice previously (face, velvet, church, daisy, red)	5
Orientation	Identify the date, month, year, day, place, and city	6
Total possible score		30

A score of 26 or greater is considered normal.
From Nasreddine ZS, Phillips NA, Bedirian V, et al: The Montreal Cognitive Assessment, MoCA: a brief screening tool for mild cognitive impairment, J Am Geriatr Soc 53:695-699, 2005.

TABLE 5.5 Familial Versus Sporadic Alzheimer Disease

Chromosome and Gene	Age at Onset (Yr)	% of All FAD Cases	% of All SAD Cases
Familial Alzheimer Disease[a]			
Chromosome 1, *PSEN2* (presenilin 2)	40-80	5-10	<0.5
Chromosome 14, *PSEN1* (presenilin 1)	30-60	70	<1
Chromosome 21, *APP* (amyloid-β precursor protein)	35-65	5	<0.5
Sporadic Alzheimer Disease[b]			
No single determinant gene[c]	Usually >60	—	98

[a]Familial Alzheimer disease (FAD) has early onset and is autosomal dominant.
[b]Sporadic Alzheimer disease (SAD) has late onset and may be polygenetic and/or environmental.
[c]Apolipoprotein E-ε4 allele on chromosome 19 increases the risk compared with the ε2 or ε3 allele.

TABLE 5.6 Diagnostic Criteria for Probable Alzheimer Disease

Progressive functional decline and dementia established by clinical examination and mental status testing and confirmed by neuropsychological assessment
Insidious onset
Clear-cut history of worsening cognition by report or observation
Initial and most prominent cognitive deficits evident on history and examination in one of the following categories:
    Amnestic presentation (plus at least one other domain)
    Nonamnestic presentations (plus deficits in other domains): language, visuospatial, executive dysfunction
No evidence of vascular dementia, dementia with Lewy bodies, frontotemporal dementias, or other concurrent active neurologic or non-neurologic medical comorbidity or use of medication that could have a substantial effect on cognition

---

Tau has been implicated in several other neurodegenerative diseases, but the abnormal tau in these diseases is not identical. Along with AD, these diseases are sometimes referred to as *tauopathies*. These include: chronic traumatic encephalopathy (CTE), corticobasal-ganglionic degeneration (CBGD), frontotemporal dementia with parkinsonism-17 (FTDP-17), Pick disease, and progressive supranuclear palsy (PSP) (see later for further discussion).

Analysis of cerebrospinal fluid (CSF) for Aβ, total-tau, and phosphorylated-tau protein levels has been commercialized as an aid to diagnosis. Because amyloid plaques accumulate extraneuronally and sequester soluble Aβ, the level of Aβ found in CSF samples from patients with AD is lower than normal. Alternatively, tau is intraneuronal and is released into the CSF when neurons die, thereby increasing the level of tau in CSF from patients with AD and a variety of other diseases that involve neuronal cell death. In AD, the ratio of CSF tau to CSF Aβ goes up. Because of the invasive nature of the testing (involving a spinal tap) and the relatively high pretest probability of AD in older individuals with dementia who meet diagnostic criteria, CSF analysis is more commonly performed in young-onset patients.

Treatment

Although their benefits are modest, the cholinesterase-inhibiting drugs donepezil (Aricept), rivastigmine (Exelon), and galantamine (Razadyne) represent important advances. These drugs may be given in once-daily formulations. Rivastigmine is also available as a transdermal patch.

In clinical trials, cholinesterase inhibitors benefited less than 50% of patients. They have not been shown to prevent AD in patients with mild cognitive impairment (MCI), a condition in which the memory or another domain of cognition is impaired in the absence of meaningful

表 5.4 蒙特利尔认知评估的要素

认知域	项目	分数
视空间或执行功能	完成一项路径绘制任务，临摹一个立方体，画一个钟表	5
命名	命名图片上的 3 种动物	3
注意力	数字顺背（5 个数字）、数字倒背（3 个数字）、保持字母警觉性，连续减 7	6
语言	重复两句话，说出以特定字母开头的单词列表	3
抽象思维	说出词语之间的相似性（火车/自行车，手表/尺子）	2
延迟回忆	回忆之前练习过两次的 5 个词语（面孔、天鹅绒、教堂、雏菊、红色）	5
定向力	确定日期、月份、年份、星期几、地点、城市	6
总分		30

得分 ≥ 26 分视为正常。

引自 Nasreddine ZS, Phillips NA, Bedirian V, et al: The Montreal Cognitive Assessment, MoCA: a brief screening tool for mild cognitive impairment, J Am Geriatr Soc 53: 695-699, 2005.

表 5.5 家族性与散发性阿尔茨海默病比较

染色体和基因	发病年龄（岁）	占所有 FAD 病例的百分比（%）	占所有 SAD 病例的百分比（%）
家族性阿尔茨海默病[a]			
1 号染色体，*PSEN2*（早老蛋白 2 基因）	40～80	5～10	< 0.5
14 号染色体，*PSEN1*（早老蛋白 1 基因）	30～60	70	< 1
21 号染色体，*APP*（β 淀粉样前体蛋白基因）	35～65	5	< 0.5
散发性阿尔茨海默病[b]			
无单一致病基因[c]	通常 > 60	—	98

[a] 家族性阿尔茨海默病（FAD）早发，为常染色体显性遗传。
[b] 散发性阿尔茨海默病（SAD）晚发，可能与多基因遗传和（或）环境因素有关。
[c] 与 ε2 或 ε3 等位基因相比，19 号染色体上的载脂蛋白 E-ε4 等位基因增加患病风险。

表 5.6 可能的阿尔茨海默病诊断标准

通过临床检查和精神状态测试确定进行性功能下降和痴呆，并通过神经心理评估加以确认
隐匿起病
报告或观察到明确的认知恶化病史
根据病史和检查发现的最初和最突出的认知障碍属于以下类别之一：
　　遗忘症状（+至少一个其他认知域）
　　非遗忘症状（+其他认知域损害）：语言、视空间、执行功能障碍
无血管性痴呆、路易体痴呆、额颞叶痴呆或其他同时存在的活动性神经系统或非神经系统合并症的证据，没有使用可能对认知产生重大影响的药物的证据

Tau 蛋白也与其他几种神经退行性疾病有关，但这些疾病中的异常 tau 蛋白并不相同，这些疾病有时与 AD 一起被称为 tau 蛋白病。这些疾病包括：慢性创伤性脑病（CTE）、皮质基底节变性（CBGD）、17 号染色体相关的额颞叶痴呆合并帕金森综合征（FTDP-17）、皮克病和进行性核上性麻痹（PSP）（见后续讨论）。

脑脊液（CSF）中 Aβ、总 tau 蛋白及磷酸化 tau 蛋白水平的分析已经商业化，可以作为辅助诊断手段。由于淀粉样斑块在神经元外积聚并隔离可溶性 Aβ，所以 AD 患者 CSF 标本中的 Aβ 水平低于正常。另一种情况是，tau 蛋白存在于神经元内，当神经元死亡时会释放到 CSF 中，因此 AD 患者和其他多种涉及神经元细胞死亡的疾病患者 CSF 中 tau 蛋白水平升高。在 AD 患者中，CSF 中 tau 蛋白与 Aβ 的比值升高。由于脑脊液检测具有侵入性（需要腰椎穿刺），并且符合诊断标准的老年痴呆患者在脑脊液检测之前已经有较高的可能性被诊断为 AD，因此 CSF 分析更多用于年轻起病的患者。

治疗

尽管胆碱酯酶抑制剂多奈哌齐（安理申）、卡巴拉汀（艾斯能）及加兰他敏（Razadyne）获益有限，但它们代表了痴呆治疗领域的重要进步。这些药物可以每日一次给药。卡巴拉汀还有透皮贴剂可供使用。

在临床试验中，不到 50% 的患者从胆碱酯酶抑制剂中获益。对于记忆或其他认知域受损、但日常生活功能尚未受到明显影响的轻度认知障碍（MCI）患者，这些药物尚未被证明能预防 AD。每年大约 12% 的

dysfunction in daily life. Approximately 12% of patients with MCI go on to develop AD per year, with roughly two thirds of patients with MCI developing clinical AD within 5 years of symptom onset.

The glutamate antagonist memantine (Namenda) has been shown to prolong daily function in patients with moderate to advanced AD.

Treatment strategies in clinical trials over the past decade have included decreasing Aβ peptide production by blocking α-secretase or β-secretase or upregulating cleavage of the amyloid precursor protein at the α-secretase site. Studies of active and passive immunization have been designed to lower brain Aβ levels. However, these approaches have failed to deliver on the promise of disease modification, necessitating a wide-reaching reassessment of current theories of disease pathogenesis.

Nursing services provide oversight of hygiene, nutrition, and medication compliance. Antipsychotics, antidepressants, and anxiolytics are useful for patients with behavioral disturbances, which are the most common cause of nursing home placement. Patients and families can be referred to a local Alzheimer's Association chapter for further information on available community support.

Prevention

There is relatively strong epidemiologic evidence, but no well controlled prospective randomized clinical trial evidence, that the following five things lower the lifetime incidence of dementia in populations: (1) alcohol in moderation (no more than one drink per day), (2) cardiovascular risk-factor mitigation, (3) regular socialization, (4) Mediterranean diet, and (5) regular exercise (three times weekly to the point of sweating). There is some epidemiologic evidence that statin medications and fish oil lower the risk of AD in populations (though there are individuals for whom statins may provoke encephalopathy). There is randomized clinical trial evidence that *gingko biloba* does not have benefit in AD. There is a moderate level of scientific evidence that conjugated equine estrogen with methyl-progesterone increases the risk of AD. There is a low level of scientific evidence that some nonsteroidal anti-inflammatory drugs, depressive disorder, diabetes mellitus, hyperlipidemia in midlife, current tobacco use, traumatic brain injury, pesticide exposure, and relative social isolation increase the risk of AD.

Diffuse Lewy Body Disease

Lewy bodies are pathologic intraneuronal alpha-synuclein inclusions that are the hallmark of Parkinson's disease when they are restricted to the brain stem (see Chapter 11). Patients with diffuse Lewy body disease have clinical parkinsonism (i.e., slow movement, rigidity, and balance problems) combined with early and prominent dementia. Pathologically, Lewy bodies are found in the brain stem, limbic system, and cortex. Visual hallucinations and cognitive fluctuations are common, and patients are unusually sensitive to the adverse effects of neuroleptic medication.

Diffuse Lewy body disease may represent the second most common cause of dementia after AD. However, the common concurrence of the pathologic features of diffuse Lewy body disease with the classic neuritic plaques and neurofibrillary tangles of AD complicates the identification of the cause of dementia in a given patient.

Vascular Dementia

Approximately 10% to 20% of older patients with dementia have radiographic evidence of focal stroke on magnetic resonance imaging (MRI) or computed tomography (CT), combined with focal signs on the neurologic examination. When the dementia syndrome begins with a stroke and progression of the illness is stepwise (suggesting recurrent vascular events), the diagnosis of vascular dementia is likely.

Patients typically develop early incontinence, gait disturbances, and flattening of affect. A subcortical dementing process attributed to small vessel disease in the periventricular white matter has been referred to as *Binswanger disease,* but it may be a radiographic finding rather than a true disease. Appropriate treatment of risk factors for vascular disease—blood pressure control, smoking cessation, diet modification, and anticoagulation (in select settings such as atrial fibrillation)—is mandatory and may be of benefit.

Frontotemporal Dementias

Patients with the behavioral variant of frontotemporal dementia (FTD) are frequently socially disinhibited, but they may also be lethargic and lack motivation and spontaneity. Patients with the progressive nonfluent aphasia variant of FTD have loss of speech fluency with poor articulation and syntactic errors but relative preservation of comprehension. Those with the semantic dementia variant of FTD remain fluent with normal phonation but have progressive difficulty with naming and word comprehension. Memory and spatial skills and praxis are relatively preserved early on in all of these forms, whereas executive function, emotional regulation, and conduct are relatively impaired.

There are several frontotemporal lobar degenerations (FTLDs), including Pick disease (now referred to as FTLD-tau). In some families, a mutation in the microtubule-associated protein tau gene *(MAPT)* on chromosome 17 causes tau-positive frontotemporal dementia with parkinsonism (FTDP-17). Transactive response DNA-binding protein (TDP-43) pathology accounts for 40% of FTD with or without motor neuron disease. Although mutations in the fused sarcoma gene *(FUS)* had previously been identified as a cause of familial amyotrophic lateral sclerosis (ALS), some also give rise to 5% to 10% of clinically diagnosed FTD (typically the behavioral variant). Hexanucleotide repeat expansions in *C9orf72* cause neurodegeneration in FTD and ALS. RNA processing is abnormal in both conditions.

As in AD, all forms of FTD progress over years. No intervention slows the inevitable decline of these patients. Approximately 50% of patients have a family history of the disease.

Parkinson's Disease

The majority of patients with Parkinson's disease (see Chapter 11) become demented in the later stages of illness. The dementia of Parkinson's disease affects executive function out of proportion to its impact on language. Thought processes appear to slow down *(bradyphrenia),* analogous to the slowing of movement *(bradykinesia).*

Because dementia occurs relatively late in the progression of Parkinson's disease, most patients are taking drugs to improve their movement disorder by enhancing dopaminergic neurotransmission. These drugs can induce psychosis. Dose reductions should be attempted before the diagnosis of underlying dementia is made for these patients. Acetylcholinesterase inhibition has been helpful for patients with dementia caused by Parkinson's disease, and the FDA has specifically approved rivastigmine for this indication.

Normal-Pressure Hydrocephalus

The triad of dementia (typically subcortical), gait instability, and urinary incontinence suggests the possibility of normal-pressure hydrocephalus. These patients appear to walk with their feet stuck to the floor, without lifting up the knees and with a broad base. Symptoms evolve over the course of weeks to months, and brain imaging reveals ventricular enlargement out of proportion to the degree of cortical atrophy.

Numerous diagnostic tests have been described, including radionuclide cisternography and MRI flow studies. The most important test remains the clinical response to removal of large volumes of CSF

MCI 患者发展为 AD，约 2/3 的 MCI 患者在症状出现 5 年内发展为临床 AD。

谷氨酸拮抗剂美金刚（Namenda）已被证明可以改善中-晚期 AD 患者的日常生活能力。

临床试验过去 10 年的治疗策略包括通过阻断 α 分泌酶或 β 分泌酶，或上调淀粉样前体蛋白在 α 分泌酶位点的裂解来减少 Aβ 的产生。主动和被动免疫研究旨在降低大脑中的 Aβ 水平。然而，这些方法未能达到预期的疾病修饰效果，因此需要对当前的疾病发病理论进行全面的重新评估。

护理服务提供对卫生、营养及药物依从性的监督。抗精神病药、抗抑郁药及抗焦虑药对有行为异常的患者有帮助，而这些行为异常是患者被安置在疗养院的最常见原因。患者和家属可以向当地的阿尔茨海默病协会分会咨询有关社区支持的更多信息。

预防

尽管缺乏严格的前瞻性随机临床试验证据，但相对有力的流行病学证据显示以下 5 种方式可以降低人群中痴呆的终生发病率：①适量饮酒（每天不超过 1 标准杯）；②控制心血管危险因素；③定期社交；④地中海饮食；⑤定期锻炼（每周 3 次，达到出汗的程度）。一些流行病学证据表明，他汀类药物和鱼油可以降低人群罹患 AD 的风险（尽管某些人服用他汀类药物可能会引起脑病）。有随机临床试验证据表明，银杏叶提取物对 AD 没有益处。有中等水平的科学证据表明，含有甲羟孕酮的马结合雌激素会增加 AD 的风险。有低水平的科学证据表明，某些非甾体抗炎药、抑郁症、糖尿病、中年高脂血症、吸烟、创伤性脑损伤、杀虫剂暴露及相对的社交孤立增加 AD 的风险。

弥漫性路易体病

路易体是病理性的神经元内 α 突触核蛋白包涵体，当它们局限于脑干时，是帕金森病的标志性特征（见第 11 章）。弥漫性路易体病患者表现为帕金森综合征（即动作迟缓、肌强直和平衡障碍）以及早发且显著的痴呆。病理学上，路易体存在于脑干、边缘系统及皮质。在弥漫性路易体病患者中，视幻觉和认知波动很常见，而且患者对抗精神病药物的不良反应异常敏感。

弥漫性路易体病可能是继 AD 之后第二常见的痴呆原因。然而，弥漫性路易体病的病理特征与 AD 典型的淀粉样斑块和神经纤维缠结经常共存，这增加了鉴别痴呆患者病因的难度。

血管性痴呆

10%～20% 的老年痴呆患者在磁共振成像（MRI）或计算机断层成像（CT）上有局灶性卒中的影像学证据，并且神经系统查体存在局灶体征。当痴呆综合征发生在卒中后，并且病情呈阶梯样进展（提示反复的血管事件），则提示诊断可能是血管性痴呆。

血管性痴呆患者通常早期出现尿失禁、步态障碍及淡漠。脑小血管病导致侧脑室旁白质受累所引起的皮质下痴呆被称为 Binswanger 病，但这可能只是一个影像学表现，而非真正的疾病。对于血管病危险因素的适当治疗——血压控制、戒烟、饮食调整及抗凝（在某些情况下如心房颤动）——是必要且可能获益的。

额颞叶痴呆

行为变异型额颞叶痴呆（FTD）的患者常表现出社交脱抑制，但他们也可能表现出懒散、缺乏动力和主动性。进行性非流利性失语变异型 FTD 患者的语言流利性下降，发音不清晰并且语法错误多，但理解能力相对保留。语义性痴呆变异型 FTD 患者的语言流利性和发音正常，但存在进行性加重的命名和词汇理解障碍。在所有这些类型中，记忆、空间技能及实践能力在早期相对保留，而执行功能、情绪调节及行为控制则相对受损。

额颞叶变性（FTLD）包括多种类型，例如皮克病（现称为 FTLD-tau）。在一些家族中，17 号染色体上的微管相关蛋白 tau 基因（*MAPT*）突变导致 tau 阳性额颞叶痴呆伴帕金森综合征（FTDP-17）。转录激活响应 DNA 结合蛋白（TDP-43）病理改变见于 40% 伴或不伴运动神经元病的 FTD。尽管融合肉瘤基因（*FUS*）突变之前被确定为家族性肌萎缩侧索硬化（ALS）的病因，但其中一些突变也导致了 5%～10% 临床诊断的 FTD（通常是行为变异型）。*C9orf72* 基因的六核苷酸重复扩增会导致 FTD 和 ALS 的神经退行性变，这两种情况下 RNA 处理均存在异常。

与 AD 一样，所有类型的 FTD 都会在数年内进展。没有任何干预措施可以减缓这些患者的进展。大约 50% 的 FTD 患者有家族史。

帕金森病

大多数帕金森病患者（见第 11 章）在病程晚期会出现痴呆。帕金森病痴呆对执行功能的影响大于对语言功能的影响。类似于动作缓慢［动作迟缓（bradykinesia）］，思维过程似乎也逐渐减慢［思维迟钝（bradyphrenia）］。

由于痴呆通常在帕金森病的较晚阶段出现，大多数患者正在服用增强多巴胺能神经传递的药物以改善其运动障碍，这些药物可能引起精神症状。这些患者诊断潜在的痴呆之前，应尝试减少药物剂量。胆碱酯酶抑制剂对帕金森病引起的痴呆有效，FDA 已专门批准卡巴拉汀用于该适应证。

正常压力脑积水

正常压力脑积水的三联征包括痴呆（通常为皮质下痴呆）、步态不稳和尿失禁。这些患者行走时双脚贴地，抬不起膝盖并且步基宽。症状在数周到数月内逐渐发展，影像学显示脑室扩大与皮质萎缩程度不成比例。

目前有多种诊断方法，包括放射性核素脑池显像和 MRI 流量研究，最重要的方法仍然是通过腰椎穿刺或临时放置腰椎引流管放出大量 CSF 后观察临床反应，

through serial lumbar punctures or the temporary placement of a lumbar drain, followed by examination of the patient's gait and cognitive function. Neurosurgical placement of a permanent ventriculoperitoneal shunt may correct the problem. Patients likely to benefit from shunt placement have a clear response to the removal of 30 to 40 mL of spinal fluid, with improved gait and alertness within minutes to hours of the procedure. The cause of normal-pressure hydrocephalus is a derangement of the CSF hydrodynamics. Shunt placement is most likely to be effective if normal-pressure hydrocephalus occurs after severe head trauma or subarachnoid hemorrhage.

Prion Infection, Chronic Meningitis, and Dementia Related to Acquired Immunodeficiency Syndrome

Creutzfeldt-Jakob disease (CJD) is a subacute, dementing, transmissible illness with typical onset between 40 and 75 years of age and an incidence of one case per 1 million people. The disease causes spongiform degeneration and gliosis in widespread areas of the cortex. Clinical variants of the disorder are differentiated by the relative predominance of cerebellar symptoms, extrapyramidal hyperkinesias, or visual agnosia and cortical blindness (*Heidenhain variant*).

Ninety percent of patients with CJD have myoclonus, compared with 10% of patients with AD. Patients with all forms of the disease share a relentlessly progressive dementia and disruption of personality over weeks to months. The electroencephalogram shows characteristic abnormalities, including diffuse slowing and periodic sharp waves or spikes.

The transmissible agent, a prion protein, is invulnerable to routine modes of antisepsis. CSF can be tested for the 14-3-3 protein, although this test is not as sensitive or specific for CJD as once hoped. Real-time quaking-induced conversion (RT-QuIC) assays are currently considered more sensitive and specific but can be adversely effected if the protein, red or white cell count in the CSF sample studied is elevated.

Certain infectious agents can cause the subacute or chronic development of subcortical dementia. These chronic meningitides are discussed in Section "Infectious Disease" Chapter 5.

Human immunodeficiency virus accesses the central nervous system through monocytes and the microglial system and causes associated neuronal cell loss, vacuolization, and lymphocytic infiltration. The dementia associated with this infection is characterized by bradyphrenia and bradykinesia. Patients have executive dysfunction, impaired memory, poor concentration, and apathy. Treatment of the underlying viral infection with effective antiretroviral therapy may slow the progression of the dementia.

There is increasing recognition of the potential for abnormal production of antibodies misdirected against brain epitopes to cause encephalopathy that can sometimes mimic classical dementia. Waxing and waning mental status rather than insidious progression of cognitive decline should prompt consideration of this category of illness as should cancer comorbidity, a history of autoimmune disease, or seizures in a patient presenting with cognitive changes. CSF should be sent for analysis to centers specializing in this emerging area of neuroimmunology.

OTHER MEMORY DISTURBANCES

Structure of Memory

Memory function is divided into introspective processes (i.e., declarative, explicit, aware memories) and processes that are not accessible to introspection (i.e., nondeclarative, implicit, procedural memories). Short-term memory (e.g., words on a list) is a form of declarative memory. Other forms include the conscious recall of episodes from personal experience (i.e., episodic memory) and factual knowledge (i.e., semantic memory) that can be consciously recalled and stated (i.e., declared). Declarative memory involves consciously *knowing that*… Patients with amnesia resulting from lesions of the medial temporal lobes or midline diencephalic structures have deficits of declarative memory.

Nondeclarative memory encompasses several distinct and neuroanatomically less clearly localized functions related to the performance of specific learned motor, cognitive, or perceptual tasks. Nondeclarative (procedural) memories involve unconsciously *knowing how*… Deficits in nondeclarative memory may involve various areas of association neocortex, depending on the nature of the task (e.g., parietal-temporal-occipital junction cortex for visual perceptual tasks, frontal association cortex for motor tasks). Patients with amnesia resulting from lesions of the medial temporal lobes tend to perform normally on tests of nondeclarative memory.

Anterograde amnesia is the inability to learn new information. It commonly occurs after brain injury or in association with dementia. The inability to recollect prior information is retrograde amnesia. Both types of amnesia usually occur together in brain injury syndromes, although the extent of one type or the other may vary. The degree of anterograde amnesia after head injury correlates with the severity of the injury.

Isolated Disorders of Memory Function

Memory can be impaired in relative isolation as a consequence of head injury, thiamine deficiency (i.e., Korsakoff syndrome), benign forgetfulness of aging, transient global amnesia, or psychogenic disease.

Head injury typically results in retrograde amnesia in excess of anterograde amnesia, with both forms stretching out over time from the discrete event. As time passes, these disrupted memories gradually return, although rarely to the point at which the events immediately surrounding the trauma are recalled.

Korsakoff syndrome is characterized by the near-total inability to establish new memory. Patients often confabulate responses when they are asked to convey the details of their current circumstance or to relay the content of a recently presented story. Deficiency of thiamine and other nutritional deficiencies in the context of chronic alcoholism are the most common underlying causes. Thiamine is a necessary cofactor in the metabolism of glucose, and thiamine must be replenished at the same time glucose is administered whenever a comatose patient is seen in the emergency department.

Aging is associated with mild loss of memory, exhibited by difficulty in recalling names and by forgetfulness for dates. Population-based assessments of neuropsychological function have demonstrated that poor performance on delayed-recall tasks is the most sensitive indicator of cognitive change with advancing age. Verbal fluency, in contrast, remains intact with advancing age, and vocabulary may increase with time, even into old age.

Transient global amnesia is a dramatic memory disturbance that affects older patients (>50 years). Patients usually have only one episode; occasionally, episodes recur over the course of several years. Patients have complete temporal and spatial disorientation; orientation for person is preserved. Near-total retrograde and anterograde amnesia persists for various periods, typically 6 to 12 hours. Patients are often anxious and may repeat the same question over and over again. Transient global amnesia may be confused with psychogenic amnesia, fugue state, or partial complex status epilepticus. Transient global amnesia is thought to reflect underlying vascular insufficiency to the hippocampus or midline thalamic projections.

Unlike patients with organic memory disturbances, patients with psychogenic amnesia typically have inconsistent loss of recent and remote memory, relatively more loss of emotionally charged memory

评估患者的步态和认知功能。通过神经外科手术置入永久性脑室腹腔分流管可以治疗该病症。那些在放出30～40 ml脑脊液后步态和警觉性在几分钟到数小时内显著改善的患者，很可能从分流术中获益。正常压力脑积水的原因是CSF动力学紊乱。如果在严重头部创伤或蛛网膜下腔出血后出现正常压力脑积水，分流术最有可能奏效。

朊病毒感染、慢性脑膜炎和获得性免疫缺陷综合征相关痴呆

克-雅病（CJD）是一种亚急性、痴呆性、可传染的疾病，典型发病年龄为40～75岁，发病率为1/100万。该疾病导致大脑皮质广泛区域海绵状变性和胶质增生。其临床变异型根据小脑症状、锥体外系多动症状或视觉失认和皮质盲（Heidenhain变异型）等症状进行鉴别。

90%的CJD患者有肌阵挛，而AD患者中只有10%有此症状。所有类型的CJD患者都会在数周到数月内出现持续进展的痴呆和人格分裂。脑电图显示特征性异常，包括弥漫性慢波和周期性尖波或棘波。

常规的消毒剂对这种可传染性朊病毒蛋白无效。可以检测CSF中的14-3-3蛋白，但14-3-3蛋白对CJD诊断的敏感性和特异性并不尽如人意。目前认为实时震荡诱导转化（RT-QuIC）检测法对CJD的诊断更敏感、更特异，但如果CSF样本中的蛋白质、红细胞或白细胞计数升高，检测结果会受到影响。

某些传染性病原体可以导致亚急性或慢性皮质下痴呆，这些慢性脑膜炎在《感染性疾病分册》第5章中有讨论。

人类免疫缺陷病毒（HIV）通过单核细胞和小胶质细胞系统进入中枢神经系统，导致神经元细胞丢失、空泡化和淋巴细胞浸润。与该感染相关的痴呆特征是思维迟钝和动作迟缓。患者会出现执行功能障碍、记忆力减退、注意力不集中和淡漠。有效的抗逆转录病毒治疗可能会减缓痴呆的进展。

越来越多的证据表明，异常产生的针对大脑表位的抗体可能导致脑病，有时会类似经典的痴呆。如果患者的精神状态时好时坏，而不是缓慢进展的认知功能减退，同时合并肿瘤、自身免疫性疾病病史，或出现癫痫，需要考虑到这种抗体介导的脑病。应将CSF送往专门从事这一新兴神经免疫学领域的中心进行分析。

其他记忆障碍
记忆的结构

记忆功能分为内省过程（即陈述性记忆、显性记忆、知觉记忆）和无法进入内省的过程（即非陈述性记忆、隐性记忆、程序性记忆）。短期记忆（例如单词表上的单词）是陈述性记忆的一种形式。其他形式的陈述性记忆包括有意识地回忆个人经历中的情节（即情景记忆）和可以有意识回忆和陈述的事实知识（即语义记忆）。陈述性记忆涉及"有意识地知道……"，因内侧颞叶或中线间脑结构病变而导致失忆的患者，其陈述性记忆功能会受损。

非陈述性记忆包括几种不同的功能，这些功能在神经解剖学上定位不太清晰，主要与特定的已学到的运动、认知或感知任务的执行有关。非陈述性（程序性）记忆涉及"无意识地知道如何做……"。非陈述性记忆的缺陷可能涉及不同的新皮质联合区域，具体取决于任务的性质（例如，视觉感知任务涉及顶叶-颞叶-枕叶交界区皮质，运动任务涉及额叶联合皮质）。因内侧颞叶损伤导致失忆的患者在非陈述性记忆测试中通常表现正常。

顺行性遗忘是无法学习新信息，它通常发生在脑损伤后或与痴呆并发。逆行性遗忘是无法回忆以前的信息。在脑损伤综合征中，这两种类型的遗忘通常同时出现，但在程度上可能会有所不同。头部外伤后顺行性遗忘的程度与受伤的严重程度相关。

孤立性记忆功能障碍

头部外伤、维生素B_1缺乏症（即科萨科夫综合征）、老年良性健忘、短暂性全面性遗忘或精神性疾病可导致相对孤立的记忆受损。

头部外伤通常导致逆行性遗忘比顺行性遗忘更严重，这两种形式的遗忘都是从离散事件开始随着时间逐渐延伸。随着时间的推移，这些被打乱的记忆会逐渐恢复，但很少恢复到能够回忆起外伤前后事件的程度。

科萨科夫综合征的特征是几乎完全无法建立新的记忆。患者在被问及当前情况的细节或转述故事内容时经常编造答案。慢性酗酒导致的维生素B_1（硫胺素）和其他营养缺乏是最常见的根本原因。维生素B_1是葡萄糖代谢过程中必需的辅酶，在急诊科接诊昏迷患者时，在补充葡萄糖的同时必须同时补充维生素B_1。

随着年龄增长，记忆力可能会轻度减退，表现为回忆名字困难和忘记日期。基于人群的神经心理学功能评估表明，延迟回忆任务表现变差是随着年龄增长最敏感的认知变化指标。相对而言，语言流畅性随着年龄增长变化不大，词汇量甚至可能在老年时增加。

短暂性全面性遗忘是一种影响老年患者（50岁以上）的严重记忆障碍。患者通常只有一次发作，偶尔会在数年内反复发作。患者会出现完全的时间和空间定向障碍，但人物定向力保留。近乎完全的逆行性和顺行性遗忘持续不同的时间，通常为6～12 h。患者常常焦虑不安，可能反复问同一个问题。短暂性全面性遗忘可与心因性遗忘症、漫游状态或复杂部分性癫痫持续状态相混淆。短暂性全面性遗忘被认为反映了海马或中线丘脑投射区的供血不足。

与器质性记忆障碍患者不同，心因性遗忘症患者的近期和远期记忆丧失表现通常不一致，情感性记忆

(rather than relatively less loss of such memory in organic disease), and an apparent indifference to their own plight; they ask few questions. Most characteristically, patients with psychogenic amnesia tend to express disorientation to person (asking, *Who am I?*), a phenomenon seldom seen in organic memory disturbance.

Patients with severe depression may exhibit pseudodementia. Vegetative signs, including changes in appetite, weight, and sleep pattern, are common, whereas signs of cortical impairment, such as aphasia, agnosia, and apraxia, are rare. Memory and bradyphrenia improve with antidepressant therapy. Depression often coexists with other causes of dementia, such as AD, Parkinson's disease, and vascular dementia.

❖ For a deeper discussion on this topic, please see Chapter 374, "Cognitive Impairment and Dementia," in *Goldman-Cecil Medicine*, 26th Edition.

SUGGESTED READINGS

Femminella GD, Thayanandan T, Calsolaro V, Komici K, Rengo G, Corbi G, Ferrara N: Imaging and molecular mechanisms of Alzheimer's disease: a review, Int J Mol Sci 19(12):3702, 2018.

Gomperts SN: Lewy body dementias: dementia with lewy bodies and Parkinson disease dementia, Continuum 22:435–463, 2016.

Hane FT, Robinson M, Lee BY, Bai O, Leonenko Z, Albert MS: Recent progress in Alzheimer's disease research, Part 3: diagnosis and treatment, J Alzheimers Dis 57:645–665, 2017.

Jack Jr CR, Bennett DA, Blennow K, Carrillo MC, Dunn B, Elliott C, et al: NIA-AA research framework: towards a biological definition of Alzheimer's disease, Alzheimer Dement 14:535–562, 2018.

O'Brien JT, Thomas A: Vascular dementia, Lancet 386:1698–1706, 2015.

Sivasathiaseelan H, Marshall CR, Agustus JL, Benhamou E, Bond RL, van Leeuwen JEP, Hardy CJD, Rohrer JD, Warren JD. Frontotemporal dementia: a clinical review. Semin Neurol 2019;266:2075-2086.

Villain N, Dubois B: Alzheimer's disease including focal presentations, Semin Neurol 39:213–226, 2019.

丧失较多（而此在器质性疾病中相对丧失较少），并且对自己的困境表现出明显的冷漠，他们很少提问。最具特征的是，心因性遗忘症患者往往表现出人物定向障碍（问"我是谁？"），这种现象在器质性记忆障碍中很少见。

重度抑郁患者可能表现出假性痴呆。自主神经症状，包括食欲、体重和睡眠模式的变化很常见，而大脑皮质受损的症状如失语、失认和失用则很少见。记忆力和思维迟钝在抗抑郁治疗后会得到改善。抑郁症常与其他病因导致的痴呆并存，如阿尔茨海默病、帕金森病和血管性痴呆。

❖ 有关此专题的深入讨论，请参阅 *Goldman-Cecil Medicine* 第 26 版第 374 章"认知障碍和痴呆"。

推荐阅读

Femminella GD, Thayanandan T, Calsolaro V, Komici K, Rengo G, Corbi G, Ferrara N: Imaging and molecular mechanisms of Alzheimer's disease: a review, Int J Mol Sci 19(12):3702, 2018.

Gomperts SN: Lewy body dementias: dementia with lewy bodies and Parkinson disease dementia, Continuum 22:435–463, 2016.

Hane FT, Robinson M, Lee BY, Bai O, Leonenko Z, Albert MS: Recent progress in Alzheimer's disease research, Part 3: diagnosis and treatment, J Alzheimers Dis 57:645–665, 2017.

Jack Jr CR, Bennett DA, Blennow K, Carrillo MC, Dunn B, Elliott C, et al: NIA-AA research framework: towards a biological definition of Alzheimer's disease, Alzheimer Dement 14:535–562, 2018.

O'Brien JT, Thomas A: Vascular dementia, Lancet 386:1698–1706, 2015.

Sivasathiaseelan H, Marshall CR, Agustus JL, Benhamou E, Bond RL, van Leeuwen JEP, Hardy CJD, Rohrer JD, Warren JD. Frontotemporal dementia: a clinical review. Semin Neurol 2019;266:2075-2086.

Villain N, Dubois B: Alzheimer's disease including focal presentations, Semin Neurol 39:213–226, 2019.

6

Major Disorders of Mood, Thoughts, and Behavior

Jeffrey M. Lyness, Jennifer H. Richman

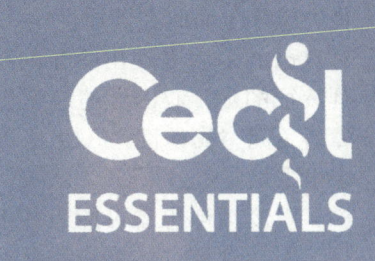

CLASSIFICATION OF MENTAL DISORDERS

Mental (psychiatric) disorders are alterations in thoughts, feelings, or behaviors that produce substantive subjective distress or affect the patient's functional status. Many mental disorders are caused by the direct effects of drugs, systemic disease, or neurologic disease on brain physiology. They may be broadly considered as secondary psychiatric disorders, as opposed to the primary or idiopathic psychiatric disorders. The distinguishing feature of neurocognitive disorders is impairment in intellectual functions such as level of consciousness, orientation, attention, or memory; however, these disorders also often include disruption of mood, thoughts, and behaviors similar to that seen in other psychiatric syndromes. Neurocognitive disorders are the focus of Chapter 21.

The noncognitive secondary syndromes by definition cause psychiatric phenomena similar to their idiopathic counterparts. During the evaluation of any patient with new or worsened psychiatric symptoms, it is essential to conduct a thorough evaluation for other medical causes, including a careful history and physical examination (with a screening neurologic examination) that often are supplemented by laboratory evaluations. Table 6.1 outlines important causes of psychiatric syndromes. Although some conditions are likely to produce certain psychiatric syndromes, many manifest as any of several psychiatric syndromes. Conversely, a psychiatric syndrome may be caused by a wide range of conditions.

Because the cause of primary psychiatric disorders is unknown, approaches to classification depend on reliable empirical observations of phenomena clustered into recognizable syndromes. Table 6.2 shows the most important psychiatric syndromes and the disorders in which they may manifest. Table 6.3 shows the major idiopathic disorders, excluding addictive disorders (see Chapter 23). Many psychiatric disorders manifest with multiple syndromes. For example, major depression with psychotic features manifests with a depressive syndrome and a psychotic syndrome. In evaluating a patient with new or worsened psychiatric symptoms, the clinician must construct a differential diagnosis based on syndromes alongside the differential diagnosis based on potential secondary causes.

DEPRESSIVE AND BIPOLAR DISORDERS

Depressive and bipolar disorders are characterized by idiopathic episodes of depression alone (i.e., unipolar) or mania and depression (i.e., bipolar). The core symptoms of depressive episodes include emotional symptoms (e.g., dysphoria, irritability, anhedonia, loss of interests), ideational symptoms (e.g., thoughts with hopeless, worthless, guilty, or suicidal themes), and neurovegetative symptoms and signs (e.g., anergia; psychomotor slowing or agitation; decreased concentration; altered sleep, appetite, and weight).

Major depressive disorder is defined by episodes of a least five symptoms, including depressed mood, anhedonia, or loss of interests, that occur almost every day for at least 2 consecutive weeks, sufficient to cause significant distress and affect functional status. Other prominent symptoms may include associated anxiety, somatic worry, or new somatic symptoms, and in the most severe cases, psychotic symptoms, including nihilistic or self-deprecatory (i.e., mood-congruent) delusions.

Major depression is common, with a 12-month prevalence of approximately 7% and a lifetime prevalence of up to 10% among men and 20% to 25% in women. New depressive episodes have an annual incidence of approximately 3%. First onset may occur at any age but is most common in the third through fifth decades of life. Whereas most episodes of major depression fully remit spontaneously or with treatment, the lifetime risk of recurrence is at least 50% to 70%, and up to 20% of patients may experience chronic symptoms over many years. Major depression is a leading correlate of disability worldwide, is an important determinant of death by suicide, and is associated with increased risk of death from comorbid physical illnesses. Major depression also causes significant economic burden, costing approximately 210.5 billion inflation-adjusted dollars in the United States alone in 2010. Persistent depressive disorder (i.e., dysthymia) is a condition defined by chronic depressive symptoms, often of insufficient severity to meet criteria for major depression.

Depressive disorders are heterogeneous, with many potential pathogenic mechanisms. Genetic factors, such as polymorphisms of the serotonin transporter protein, affect vulnerability to depressive episodes in the face of psychosocial stressors. Depression is polygenic and multifactorial, with genetic factors accounting for about 40% of the risk. Alterations in the functioning of brain serotonergic and noradrenergic systems and of the hypothalamic-pituitary-adrenal axis are found in depression. Neuroimaging studies show smaller hippocampal volumes and altered metabolic activity in several regions, including the anterior cingulate cortex. However, the information in these studies is not sufficient for making the clinical diagnosis, which depends on identification of the clinical syndrome. Dysfunctional, negativistic patterns of thinking, impaired social relationships, and stressful life events also contribute to depression.

Mild to moderate forms of major depression respond to focused psychotherapies or antidepressant medications (Table 6.4). More severe forms of depression do not respond to psychosocial interventions alone. Severe or refractory depression may be treated safely and effectively with electroconvulsive therapy. Other evidence-based somatic therapies include light therapy (for depression with a seasonal component) and vagal nerve stimulation. Data suggest that the dissociative anesthetic ketamine, an N-methyl-D-aspartate (NMDA)

心境、思维和行为障碍

曹宇泽 译 周雁 卢强 审校 姚明 彭斌 通审

精神障碍的分类

精神（精神病性）障碍是指思维、情感或行为的改变，导致显著的主观痛苦或影响患者的功能状态。许多精神障碍是由药物、全身性疾病或神经系统疾病对大脑生理的直接影响引起的。这些可以被广泛地视为继发性精神障碍，与原发性或特发性精神障碍相对应。神经认知障碍的显著特征是存在智能的损害，如意识水平、定向力、注意力或记忆力；然而，这些障碍通常还包括心境、思维以及行为的紊乱，与其他精神病综合征相似。神经认知障碍是第 21 章的重点内容。

根据定义，非认知性继发性综合征导致的精神现象与特发性综合征类似。在评估任何出现新的或恶化的精神症状患者时，必须对其他医学原因进行全面评估，包括详细的病史采集和体格检查（包括神经系统筛查），通常还需辅以实验室评估。表 6.1 列出了精神病综合征的重要病因。尽管某些疾病可能会导致特定的精神病综合征，但许多疾病可表现为几种精神病综合征中的任意一种。反之，一种精神病综合征也可能由多种疾病引起。

由于原发性精神障碍的病因尚不清楚，其分类方法依赖于对现象进行可靠的经验观察，并将其归类为可识别的综合征。表 6.2 展示了最重要的精神病综合征及其可能表现的障碍。表 6.3 列出了主要的特发性障碍，不包括成瘾性障碍（见第 23 章）。许多精神障碍表现为多种综合征。例如，伴有精神病特征的重度抑郁表现为抑郁综合征和精神病综合征。对新发精神症状患者或原有精神症状恶化的患者进行评估时，临床医生必须基于综合征进行鉴别诊断，同时鉴别潜在的继发性原因。

抑郁和双相障碍

抑郁和双相障碍的特征是特发性的单独抑郁发作（即单相）或躁狂和抑郁发作（即双相）。抑郁发作的核心症状包括情感症状（如烦躁不安、易怒、快感缺失、兴趣丧失）、观念症状（如绝望、无价值感、内疚或自杀的想法）和自主神经系统症状和体征（如无力、精神运动迟缓或激越、注意力下降，以及睡眠、食欲和体重变化）。

重度抑郁障碍的定义为至少包含 5 种症状的发作，包括抑郁心境、快感缺失或兴趣丧失，这些症状几乎每天发生，且持续至少 2 周，足以引起显著的痛苦并影响功能状态。其他突出的症状可能包括伴随的焦虑、躯体担忧或新的躯体症状，在最严重的情况下，还可能出现包括虚无主义或自我贬低（即心境一致性）妄想在内的精神病性症状。

重度抑郁很常见，12 个月患病率约为 7%，男性终生患病率为 10%，女性终生患病率高达 20%～25%。新发抑郁的年发病率约为 3%。首次发病可发生在任何年龄，但最常见于 30～50 岁。尽管大多数重度抑郁发作会自发或通过治疗完全缓解，但终生复发风险至少为 50%～70%，多达 20% 的患者可能经历多年的慢性症状。重度抑郁是全球残疾的主要相关因素，是自杀死亡的重要决定因素，并与合并身体疾病的死亡风险增加相关。重度抑郁还带来巨大的经济负担，仅在美国，2010 年就造成约 2105 亿美元（通货膨胀调整后）的经济损失。持续性抑郁障碍（即心境恶劣障碍）是一种以慢性抑郁症状为特征的状态，其严重程度通常不足以达到重度抑郁的标准。

抑郁障碍是异质性的，具有多种潜在的致病机制。遗传因素，例如 5-羟色胺转运蛋白的多态性，会影响面对社会心理压力时对抑郁发作的易感性。抑郁是一种多基因和多因素疾病，遗传因素约占患病风险的 40%。已发现抑郁患者的大脑 5-羟色胺和去甲肾上腺素系统以及下丘脑-垂体-肾上腺轴的功能发生了改变。神经影像学研究显示，海马体积缩小，包括前扣带回皮质在内的多个区域的代谢活动发生改变。然而，这些研究的信息不足以做出临床诊断，临床诊断依赖于临床综合征的识别。功能失调、消极的思维模式、社交关系受损以及应激性生活事件也会导致抑郁。

轻中度的重度抑郁对于针对性心理治疗或抗抑郁药物治疗有反应（表 6.4）。单纯的社会心理干预对更严重的抑郁无效。重度或难治性抑郁可通过电休克疗法进行安全有效的治疗。其他基于循证的躯体疗法包括光疗（用于季节性抑郁）和迷走神经刺激。数据表明，解离性麻醉药物氯胺酮，一种 N-甲基-D-天冬氨酸

TABLE 6.1 Important Causes of Psychiatric Syndromes

Central Nervous System Conditions
Tumor
Toxins
Vascular disorders
Seizure
Infection
Genetic disorders
Congenital malformation
Demyelinating conditions
Degenerative conditions
Hydrocephalus

Systemic Diseases
Cardiovascular diseases
Pulmonary diseases
Cancer
Infection
Nutritional disorders
Endocrine disorders
Metabolic disorders
Autoimmune disorders

Drugs
Drug intoxication
Drug withdrawal

receptor antagonist, may rapidly improve patients with treatment-resistant depression, although the general clinical applicability of ketamine remains to be determined.

Bipolar disorder (i.e., bipolar I) is characterized by recurrent episodes of mania, usually with episodes of major depression. Manic episodes include elevated (euphoric) or irritable mood, goal-directed hyperactivity (often for pleasurable activities with poor judgment leading to substantial adverse consequences such as sexual, spending, or gambling sprees), pressured speech, increased energy level with a decreased need for sleep, and distractibility.

Compared with unipolar depression, bipolar disorder has a lower 12-month prevalence (approximately 0.6%) and a younger average age of onset (typically late teens to 20s). Unlike unipolar depression, bipolar disorder is slightly more common among males. Most patients return to baseline functioning between acute mood episodes, but some have a deteriorating course, and others have frequent debilitating episodes (i.e., rapid cycling of four episodes per year).

Genetic factors play a greater role in the pathogenesis of bipolar disorder than in major depressive disorder, accounting for approximately 50% of the risk and representing a greater than 50-fold increase over the population base rate. Bipolar disorder is polygenic and has been linked in individual families to different loci. The pathogenesis is unclear but likely involves dysregulation of frontostriatal systems. Structural neuroimaging studies show increased ventricular-to-brain ratios, suggesting parenchymal atrophy. Psychosocial stressors often play a role in precipitating episodes of mania and depression.

The mainstay of treatment for bipolar disorder is mood stabilizer medications (e.g., lithium, anticonvulsants such as valproic acid and

TABLE 6.2 Important Psychiatric Syndromes

Syndrome	Main Symptoms and Signs	Disorders
Neurocognitive	Impairment in intellectual functions (e.g., level of consciousness, orientation, attention, memory, language, praxis, visuospatial, executive functions)	Neurocognitive disorders Intellectual disability (if onset in childhood)
Mood	Depressive: lowered mood, anhedonia, negativistic thoughts, neurovegetative symptoms Manic: elevated or irritable mood; grandiosity; goal-directed hyperactivity with increased energy; pressured speech; decreased sleep need	Neurocognitive disorders Mood disorders (bipolar or depressive) (primary or secondary) Trauma- and stressor-related disorders Psychotic disorders (schizoaffective disorder)
Anxiety	All include anxious mood and associated physiologic signs and symptoms (e.g., palpitations, tremors, diaphoresis) May include various types of dysfunctional thoughts (e.g., catastrophic fears, obsessions, flashbacks) and behaviors (e.g., compulsions, avoidance behaviors)	Neurocognitive disorders Mood disorders (bipolar or depressive) (primary or secondary) Psychotic disorders (primary or secondary) Anxiety disorders (primary or secondary) Obsessive-compulsive and related disorders Trauma- and stressor-related disorders
Psychotic	Impairments in reality testing: hallucinations, thought process derailments	Neurocognitive disorders Mood disorders (bipolar or depressive) (primary or secondary) Psychotic disorders
Somatic symptom syndromes	Somatic symptoms with associated distressing thoughts, feelings, or behaviors	Mood disorders (bipolar or depressive) (primary or secondary) Anxiety disorders (primary or secondary) Obsessive-compulsive and related disorders Trauma- and stressor-related disorders Somatic symptom disorders
Personality pathology	Dysfunctional enduring patterns of emotional regulation, thought patterns, interpersonal behaviors, impulse regulation	Neurocognitive disorders Personality change due to another medical condition Personality disorders

Data from American Psychiatric Association: Diagnostic and statistical manual of mental disorders, ed 5, Washington, D.C., 2013, American Psychiatric Association.

表 6.1　精神病综合征的重要病因
中枢神经系统疾病
肿瘤
毒素
血管疾病
癫痫发作
感染
遗传性疾病
先天畸形
脱髓鞘疾病
退行性疾病
脑积水
全身性疾病
心血管疾病
肺部疾病
癌症
感染
营养障碍
内分泌障碍
代谢障碍
自身免疫性疾病
药物
药物中毒
药物戒断

（NMDA）受体拮抗剂，可快速改善难治性抑郁患者的病情，但氯胺酮在临床上的普遍适用性仍有待确定。

双相障碍（即双相Ⅰ型）以反复躁狂发作为特征，通常伴有重度抑郁发作。躁狂发作包括心境高涨（欣快）或易怒、目标导向性过度活跃（通常为了愉悦的活动，但判断力差，导致严重不良后果，如性冲动、挥霍或赌博等）、言语急促、精力旺盛且睡眠需求减少，以及注意力分散。

与单相抑郁相比，双相障碍的 12 个月患病率较低（约 0.6%），且平均发病年龄较小（通常在青春期后期至 20 多岁）。与单相抑郁不同，双相障碍在男性中略多见。大多数患者在急性心境发作间期可恢复到基线水平，但部分患者病情会恶化，另一部分患者会频繁经历令人痛苦的发作（即每年 4 次发作的快速循环）。

与重度抑郁障碍相比，遗传因素在双相障碍的发病机制中起着更重要的作用，约占发病风险的 50%，且比一般人群的基础发病率增加了 50 倍以上。双相障碍是多基因遗传，并且已在个别家族中发现与不同的基因位点有关。其发病机制尚不明确，但可能涉及额叶-纹状体系统的功能失调。结构性神经影像研究显示脑室与脑实质的比率增加，提示存在脑实质萎缩。社会心理压力往往在躁狂和抑郁发作中发挥作用。

双相障碍的主要治疗方法是使用心境稳定剂（例如锂、抗惊厥药物如丙戊酸和卡马西平）治疗急性发

表 6.2　重要的精神病综合征

综合征	主要症状和体征	障碍
神经认知	智力障碍（例如，意识水平、定向力、注意力、记忆力、语言、实践能力、视空间能力、执行功能）	神经认知障碍 智力残疾（如果在儿童期发病）
心境	抑郁：心境低落、快感缺失、消极思维、自主神经系统症状 躁狂：心境高涨或易怒，自大，目标导向性的过度活跃且精力充沛，言语急促，睡眠需求减少	神经认知障碍 心境障碍（双相或抑郁）（原发或继发） 创伤和应激相关障碍 精神病性障碍（分裂情感障碍）
焦虑	所有类型均包括焦虑心境及相关的生理体征和症状（例如，心悸、震颤、出汗） 可能包括各种类型的功能失调性思维（例如，灾难性恐惧、强迫观念、闪回）和行为（例如，强迫行为、回避行为）	神经认知障碍 心境障碍（双相或抑郁）（原发或继发） 精神病性障碍（原发或继发） 焦虑障碍（原发或继发） 强迫症及相关障碍 创伤和应激相关障碍
精神病性	现实测试障碍：幻觉、思维过程脱轨	神经认知障碍 心境障碍（双相或抑郁）（原发或继发） 精神病性障碍
躯体症状综合征	伴有相关痛苦思维、感受或行为的躯体症状	心境障碍（双相或抑郁）（原发或继发） 焦虑障碍（原发或继发） 强迫症及相关障碍 创伤和应激相关障碍 躯体症状障碍
人格病理	情绪调节、思维模式、人际交往行为、冲动调节的功能失调持久模式	神经认知障碍 由其他疾病引起的人格改变 人格障碍

引自 American Psychiatric Association：Diagnostic and statistical manual of mental disorders, ed 5, Washington, D.C., 2013, American Psychiatric Association.

TABLE 6.3 Major Idiopathic (Primary) Disorders of Mood, Thoughts, and Behavior

Mood Disorders
Depressive (Unipolar)
Major depressive disorder
Persistent depressive disorder (dysthymia)

Bipolar
Bipolar disorder
Cyclothymic disorder
Bipolar II disorder (bipolar disorder not otherwise specified)

Anxiety Disorders
Panic disorder (without or with agoraphobia)
Generalized anxiety disorder
Social phobia
Specific phobia

Other Conditions With Anxiety as a Prominent Feature
Obsessive-compulsive disorder
Acute stress disorder, post-traumatic stress disorder

Psychotic (Schizophrenia and Related) Disorders
Schizophrenia
Schizophreniform disorder
Brief psychotic disorder
Schizoaffective disorder
Delusional disorder

Somatic Symptom Disorders
Somatic symptom disorder
Illness anxiety disorder
Conversion (functional neurologic symptom) disorder
Psychological factors affecting physical condition
Factitious disorder (i.e., Munchausen syndrome)

Personality Disorders
Cluster A: Odd Eccentric
Schizoid personality disorder (detachment from social relationships, restricted emotional expression)
Schizotypal personality disorder (social and emotional deficits, cognitive or perceptual distortions, eccentric behavior)
Paranoid personality disorder (pervasive distrust and suspiciousness)

Cluster B: Dramatic or Emotional
Borderline personality disorder (instability of interpersonal relationships, self-image, and affects, and impulsivity)
Narcissistic personality disorder (grandiosity, need for admiration, lack of empathy)
Antisocial personality disorder (disregard for and violation of the rights of others)
Histrionic personality disorder

Cluster C: Anxious or Fearful
Avoidant personality disorder (social inhibition, feelings of inadequacy, hypersensitivity to criticism)
Dependent personality disorder (pervasive and excessive need to be taken care of, leading to submissive and clinging behavior and fears of separation)
Obsessive-compulsive personality disorder (preoccupation with orderliness, perfectionism, and mental and interpersonal control, at the expense of flexibility, openness, and efficiency)

Data from American Psychiatric Association: Diagnostic and statistical manual of mental disorders, ed 5, Washington, D.C., 2013, American Psychiatric Association.

---

carbamazepine) for acute episodes and maintenance therapy. The anticonvulsant lamotrigine may be particularly useful for bipolar depression. Antipsychotic medications are useful for acute manic episodes and may have a role in maintenance therapy. Benzodiazepines may be used to treat acute agitation and aggression while waiting for more definitive antimanic therapies to take effect. Antidepressants have long been used for depressive episodes, although they may precipitate manic episodes.

Electroconvulsive therapy is effective for refractory mania and depression. Psychosocial treatments alone do not effectively treat mania and may be less effective for bipolar depression, but psychoeducation and support to manage psychosocial stressors and encourage medication compliance improve longer-term outcomes.

A spectrum of less severe bipolar disorders includes conditions marked by episodes of hypomania (i.e., low-level manic symptoms without psychosis or significant impairment in functioning). They include bipolar II disorder, characterized by episodes of hypomania and major depression, and cyclothymic disorder, characterized by hypomania and low-level depression not meeting criteria for major depression. Because patients with bipolar II disorder are most likely to seek care during depressive episodes, it is important to inquire about a history of manic symptoms to avoid precipitating mania with the use of antidepressant medications. The pathogeneses of these less severe mood disorders is unclear.

DISORDERS WITH ANXIETY AS A PROMINENT FEATURE

The idiopathic anxiety disorders manifest with troublesome thoughts and somatic symptoms (Table 6.5) along with the emotional sensation of anxiety. A panic attack is a transient episode of crescendo anxiety, catastrophic thoughts (e.g., fears of dying, going insane, losing self-control), and somatic symptoms. If panic attacks or other clinically significant anxiety symptoms occur only in predictable response to environmental stimuli, the anxiety disorder is known as a *phobia*, which may further be classified as agoraphobia (i.e., anxiety about being in places from which escape may be difficult or embarrassing such as being alone, in crowds, in tunnels, or on bridges), social phobia (i.e., anxiety in interpersonal situations), and specific phobia (i.e., anxiety provoked by other situations or objects such as blood, animals, or heights). *Panic disorder* manifests with recurrent panic attacks, some of which are unexpected and unpredictable, along with anticipatory anxiety (i.e., fear of having another attack) and avoidance behaviors (i.e., avoiding situations that may provoke a panic attack or in which having an attack is perceived to be embarrassing or dangerous). Other disorders may not cause discrete panic attacks. Enduring anxiety in various domains that the individual finds difficult to control is classified as *generalized anxiety disorder*. Those with generalized anxiety disorder may also experience physical symptoms such as feeling keyed up, muscle tension or fatigue; however, they are not in discrete episodes.

Obsessive-compulsive disorder is characterized by recurrent obsessions (i.e., thoughts, impulses, or mental images that are anxiety-producing, perceived as intrusive and inappropriate, and resistant to attempts to suppress or neutralize them) and compulsions (i.e., repetitive behaviors or mental acts performed in response to obsessions or other rigid rules). Recognizing its distinct pathogenesis involving striatofrontal function and central serotonergic systems, it has been classified separately from the anxiety disorders.

Individuals exposed to severely stressful events (typically involving the actual or threatened loss of life or limb) may experience any of a wide variety of psychiatric sequelae. If the sequelae include symptoms of intrusion (e.g., intrusive memories, dreams, flashbacks,

表 6.3 主要特发性（原发性）心境、思维和行为障碍
心境障碍
抑郁（单相）
重度抑郁障碍
持续性抑郁障碍（心境恶劣障碍）
双相
双相障碍
周期性情感障碍
双相Ⅱ型障碍（未特定的双相障碍）
焦虑障碍
惊恐障碍（伴或不伴广场恐惧症）
广泛性焦虑障碍
社交恐惧症
特定恐惧症
以焦虑为显著特征的其他疾病
强迫症
急性应激障碍、创伤后应激障碍
精神病性（精神分裂症及相关）障碍
精神分裂症
精神分裂样障碍
短暂精神病性障碍
分裂情感障碍
妄想性障碍
躯体症状障碍
躯体症状障碍
疾病焦虑障碍
转换（功能性神经症状）障碍
影响躯体状况的心理因素
做作性障碍（即 Munchausen 综合征）
人格障碍
A组：奇怪、古怪
类分裂型人格障碍（脱离社会关系，情感表达受限）
分裂型人格障碍（社交和情感障碍，认知或感知扭曲，行为古怪）
偏执型人格障碍（广泛的不信任和猜疑）
B组：戏剧化或情绪化
边缘型人格障碍（人际关系、自我形象和情感不稳定，易冲动）
自恋型人格障碍（自大、需要赞美、缺乏同情心）
反社会型人格障碍（漠视和侵犯他人权利）
表演型人格障碍
C组：焦虑或恐惧
回避型人格障碍（社交抑制、自卑感、对批评过度敏感）
依赖型人格障碍（广泛和过度需要被照顾，导致顺从和依附行为，分离恐惧）
强迫型人格障碍（对秩序、完美主义、心理和人际控制过度关注，以牺牲灵活性、开放性和效率为代价）

引自 American Psychiatric Association: Diagnostic and statistical manual of mental disorders, ed 5, Washington, D.C., 2013, American Psychiatric Association.

作和维持治疗。抗惊厥药物拉莫三嗪可能特别适用于双相抑郁。抗精神病药物可用于急性躁狂发作，并可在维持治疗中起作用。在等待特异性抗躁狂治疗起效时，可以使用苯二氮䓬类药物治疗急性激越和攻击性行为。长期以来，抗抑郁药物被用于治疗抑郁发作，尽管它们可能会诱发躁狂发作。

电休克疗法对难治性躁狂和抑郁有效。单纯的心理社会治疗对躁狂的治疗效果不佳，对双相抑郁可能效果较差，但通过心理教育和支持以管理社会心理压力，并鼓励服药依从性，可改善长期预后。

轻度双相障碍谱系包括表现为轻躁狂发作为特征的疾病（即没有精神病或功能严重受损的低水平躁狂症状）。它们包括以轻躁狂发作和重度抑郁发作为特征的双相Ⅱ型障碍，以及以轻躁狂发作和未达到重度抑郁标准的低水平抑郁为特征的周期性情感障碍。由于双相Ⅱ型障碍患者最有可能在抑郁发作期间寻求治疗，因此询问躁狂症状病史很重要，以避免使用抗抑郁药物诱发躁狂。这些不太严重的心境障碍的发病机制尚不清楚。

以焦虑障碍为突出特征的疾病

特发性焦虑障碍表现为令人困扰的想法和躯体症状（表6.5），同时伴有焦虑的情感体验。惊恐发作是一种短暂发作的渐增性焦虑、灾难性想法（例如，害怕死亡、精神错乱、失去自控力）和躯体症状。如果惊恐发作或其他临床上显著的焦虑症状仅在对环境刺激做出可预测反应时发生，则这种焦虑障碍称为恐惧症，可进一步分类为广场恐惧症（即对身处难以逃脱或令人尴尬的地方感到焦虑，例如独处、人群中、隧道中或桥上）、社交恐惧症（即在人际交往中的焦虑）和特定恐惧症（即其他情境或物体引发的焦虑，例如血液、动物或高度）。惊恐障碍表现为反复的惊恐发作，其中一些是意外和不可预测的，并伴有预期焦虑（即害怕再次发作）和回避行为（即回避可能引发惊恐发作的情境，或回避认为发作时会令人尴尬或危险的情境）。其他障碍可能不会引起明显的惊恐发作。个体难以控制的、在各种领域中的持久焦虑被归类为广泛性焦虑障碍。广泛性焦虑障碍患者还可能会经历诸如紧张感、肌肉紧张或疲劳等躯体症状。然而，这些症状并不是断断续续的。

强迫症的特征是反复出现的强迫观念（即引起焦虑、被认为是侵入性的和不适当的想法、冲动或心理图像，并对试图压制或消除它们的努力产生抵触）和强迫行为（即基于强迫观念或其他硬性规则做出的重复行为或心理活动）。由于其独特的发病机制涉及纹状体-额叶功能和中枢5-羟色胺系统，因此已将其从焦虑障碍中单独分类出来。

遭受严重应激事件（通常涉及实际或可能丧失生命或肢体）的个体可能会经历各种各样的精神后遗症。如果这些后遗症包括侵入症状（如侵入性记忆、梦境、

TABLE 6.4 Psychotherapies for Depression and Antidepressant Medications

Name	Approach or Mechanism of Action
Psychotherapy	
Cognitive psychotherapy	Identify and correct negativistic patterns of thinking
Interpersonal psychotherapy	Identify and work through role transitions or interpersonal losses, conflicts, or deficits
Problem-solving therapy	Identify and prioritize situational problems; plan and implement strategies to deal with top-priority problems
Commonly Used Antidepressants	
Selective serotonin reuptake inhibitors (SSRIs)	Inhibit presynaptic reuptake of serotonin
Citalopram and escitalopram	
Fluoxetine	
Fluvoxamine	
Paroxetine	
Sertraline	
Serotonin and norepinephrine reuptake inhibitors (SNRIs)	Inhibit presynaptic reuptake of serotonin and norepinephrine
Duloxetine	
Venlafaxine and desvenlafaxine	
Milnacipran and levomilnacipran	
Tricyclic antidepressants (TCAs)	Inhibit presynaptic reuptake of serotonin and norepinephrine (in various proportions depending on the specific TCA)
Amitriptyline	
Desipramine	
Doxepin	
Imipramine	
Nortriptyline	
Monoamine oxidase inhibitors (MAOIs)	Inhibit monoamine oxidase, the enzyme that catalyzes oxidative metabolism of monoamine neurotransmitters
Isocarboxazid	
Phenelzine	
Selegiline	Selective MAO-B inhibitor
Tranylcypromine	
Other drugs	
Bupropion	Unknown, although it is weak inhibitor of presynaptic reuptake of norepinephrine and dopamine
Mirtazapine	Serotonin (5-hydroxytryptamine [5-HT]) antagonist at α_2 and 5-HT2 receptors
Trazodone	Inhibits presynaptic reuptake of serotonin; antagonist at 5-HT2 and 5-HT3 receptors
Vilazodone	Inhibits presynaptic reuptake of serotonin; agonist at 5-HT1A receptors
Vortioxetine	Inhibits the reuptake of serotonin (5-HT); antagonist at 5-HT3, 5-HT1D, and 5-HT7 receptors; agonist at 5-HT1A receptors; 5-HT1B receptor partial agonist

intense distressing responses to reminders of the trauma), avoidance of distressing memories or external reminders, negative cognitions and mood (e.g., amnesia for aspects of the event, negativistic thoughts about oneself in general or self-blame for the event, diminished interests or activities, feelings of detachment), and alterations in arousal and reactivity, the disorder is called *acute stress disorder* (duration up to 1 month) or *post-traumatic stress disorder* (duration is more than 1 month). These disorders also have been classified separately, as in addition to anxiety symptoms, they can present with prominent dysphoric symptoms, externalizing aggressive symptoms, or dissociative symptoms.

These disorders are common, with point prevalence of 1% to 2% each for panic disorder and obsessive-compulsive disorder and up to 10% for phobias. Although there are fewer data on long-term outcome than for mood disorders, many of these disorders tend to have a chronic waxing and waning course. Most of these disorders have a first onset in the teens, 20s, and 30s. Although new-onset anxiety is common in later life, the cause is rarely a late-onset primary anxiety disorder (see Table 6.2).

The pathogeneses of most anxiety disorders may be understood as inappropriate activation of the stress response system involving a variety of neuroendocrine and autonomic outputs and coordinated by the central nucleus of the amygdala and other brain structures. The amygdala receives excitatory glutamatergic inputs from cortical sensory areas and the thalamus and has outputs to the major monoaminergic centers (e.g., noradrenergic neurons of the locus coeruleus, dopaminergic neurons of the ventral tegmental area, and serotonergic neurons of the raphe nuclei), which project to the many brain regions subserving the symptoms of anxiety.

The identification and correction of dysfunctional patterns of thinking (i.e., cognitive therapy) and the extinction of pathologic behaviors and positive reinforcement of more functional behaviors (i.e., behavior therapy) are evidence-based psychotherapies useful in most anxiety disorders. They are the sole therapies for specific phobias and may be the sole or primary therapy for most other anxiety disorders or combined with pharmacotherapy.

Antidepressant, anxiolytic, and other drug therapies are used in treatment. Increasingly, antidepressant medications have replaced anxiolytics as the mainstay of pharmacotherapy for panic disorder, post-traumatic stress disorder, generalized social phobia, and generalized anxiety disorder. For obsessive-compulsive disorder, only antidepressant agents with pronounced activity on the serotonergic system (i.e., clomipramine and selective serotonin reuptake inhibitors [SSRIs]; see Table 6.4) are efficacious.

表 6.4　抑郁的心理治疗和抗抑郁药物治疗

名称	方法或作用机制
心理治疗	
认知心理治疗	识别并纠正消极思维模式
人际关系心理治疗	识别并处理角色转变或人际关系中的失落、冲突或缺陷
问题解决疗法	识别并优先处理情境问题，计划并实施应对首要问题的策略
常用抗抑郁药物	
选择性 5- 羟色胺再摄取抑制剂（SSRI）	抑制突触前 5- 羟色胺的再摄取
西酞普兰和艾司西酞普兰	
氟西汀	
氟伏沙明	
帕罗西汀	
舍曲林	
5- 羟色胺和去甲肾上腺素再摄取抑制剂（SNRI）	抑制突触前 5- 羟色胺和去甲肾上腺素的再摄取
度洛西汀	
文拉法辛和去甲文拉法辛	
米那普仑和左米那普仑	
三环类抗抑郁药（TCA）	抑制突触前 5- 羟色胺和去甲肾上腺素的再摄取（比例取决于具体的 TCA）
阿米替林	
地昔帕明	
多塞平	
丙米嗪	
去甲替林	
单胺氧化酶抑制剂（MAOI）	抑制单胺氧化酶（MAO），一种催化单胺类神经递质氧化代谢的酶
异卡波肼	
苯乙肼	
司来吉兰	选择性 MAO-B 抑制剂
反苯环丙胺	
其他药物	
安非他酮	未知，尽管它是去甲肾上腺素和多巴胺突触前再摄取的弱抑制剂
米氮平	5- 羟色胺（5-HT）α_2 受体和 5-HT2 受体拮抗剂
曲唑酮	抑制突触前 5-HT 再摄取，5-HT2 和 5-HT3 受体拮抗剂
维拉唑酮	抑制突触前 5-HT 再摄取，5-HT1A 受体激动剂
沃替西汀	抑制 5-HT 的再摄取；5-HT3、5-HT1D 和 5-HT7 受体拮抗剂，5-HT1A 受体激动剂，5-HT1B 受体部分激动剂

闪回、对创伤提醒的强烈痛苦反应）、回避痛苦记忆或外部提醒、负面认知和心境（如对事件某些方面的失忆、自我否定或自责、兴趣或活动的减少、疏离感）以及觉醒和反应性的改变，则这种疾病被称为急性应激障碍（持续时间不超过 1 个月）或创伤后应激障碍（持续时间超过 1 个月）。这些疾病也被单独分类，因为除了焦虑症状外，它们还可能表现为突出的烦躁症状、外化攻击症状或分离症状。

这些疾病很常见，惊恐障碍和强迫症的时点患病率（point prevalence）为 1% ～ 2%，恐惧症的时点患病率则高达 10%。尽管与心境障碍相比，这些障碍的长期预后数据较少，但许多此类障碍往往表现为慢性波动性病程。这些疾病大多在青少年时期、20 多岁或 30 多岁时首次发病。尽管晚年新发焦虑很常见，但其原因很少是晚发性原发性焦虑障碍（见表 6.2）。

大多数焦虑障碍的发病机制可理解为应激反应系统的不适当激活，涉及多种神经内分泌和自主神经输出，并由杏仁核的中央核和其他脑结构协调。杏仁核接收来自大脑皮质感觉区和丘脑的兴奋性谷氨酸能输入，并输出到主要的单胺能中枢（如蓝斑的去甲肾上腺素能神经元、腹侧被盖区的多巴胺能神经元和中缝核的 5- 羟色胺能神经元），这些神经元投射到推动焦虑症状的许多脑区。

识别和纠正功能失调的思维模式（即认知疗法）以及消除病态行为并积极强化更具功能性的行为（即行为疗法）是对大多数焦虑障碍有效的循证心理疗法。它们是特定恐惧症的唯一疗法，也可能是其他大多数焦虑障碍的唯一或主要疗法，亦可与药物治疗相结合。

抗抑郁药、抗焦虑药和其他药物疗法被用于治疗该类疾病。抗抑郁药越来越多地取代了抗焦虑药，成为惊恐障碍、创伤后应激障碍、广泛性社交恐惧症和广泛性焦虑障碍的主要治疗药物。对于强迫症，只有对 5- 羟色胺通路具有显著活性的抗抑郁药［如氯米帕明和选择性 5- 羟色胺再摄取抑制剂（SSRI）］是有效的（见表 6.4）。

PSYCHOTIC DISORDERS

Psychosis is a loss of reality testing, manifested as hallucinations (i.e., false sensory perceptions), delusions (i.e., fixed false beliefs), and thought process derailments. Schizophrenia is the prototypic psychotic disorder; it includes acute episodes of psychosis (i.e., positive symptoms) and often declining overall functioning over time related to the negative symptoms such as affective flattening, abulia, apathy, and social withdrawal.

The lifetime prevalence of schizophrenia is slightly less than 1%, and its chronic, debilitating course takes a considerable toll on patients, families, and society. Peak onset is in late adolescence to young adulthood, with slightly younger ages for males than females. The annual incidence is approximately 15 cases per 100,000 people, but with marked variability across study samples and populations. The condition is slightly more common in males than females.

The pathogenesis of schizophrenia remains unknown, but it is clearly multifactorial. Genetic factors account for up to 50% of the risk, with multiple loci implicated. Studies of postmortem brains indicate a nongliotic neuropathologic process with subtle disruptions of cortical cytoarchitecture. It is likely that psychosocial factors and neurodevelopment interact with a nonlocalizable brain lesion present at birth or acquired early in life. Dopaminergic mesocortical and mesolimbic pathways are important in the production of psychotic symptoms.

Antipsychotic medications, often with adjunctive benzodiazepines, are used to treat acute psychotic episodes (Table 6.6). Although maintenance antipsychotic medications help reduce the severity and frequency of acute psychotic episodes, comprehensive psychosocial rehabilitation programs are required to help patients manage interpersonal and other stressors and to improve overall clinical outcomes. Adjunctive cognitive-behavioral therapy also may improve outcomes for some patients. Second-generation (atypical) antipsychotic medications have replaced first-generation antipsychotics in common US practice because of their lower rates of extrapyramidal side effects, including tardive dyskinesia. However, second-generation drugs contribute to an increase in obesity and metabolic syndrome.

Schizoaffective disorder is a chronic, recurrent disorder with a prevalence slightly lower than that of schizophrenia. It is characterized by episodes of non-mood psychosis and mood episodes (i.e., manic or depressed) with psychotic features. Its diagnosis therefore cannot be based on the patient's clinical findings at any one point in time but requires knowledge of the overall course. The outcomes of schizoaffective disorder are heterogeneous but on average are intermediate between schizophrenia and mood disorders. Treatment is symptomatic, using antipsychotic, mood stabilizing, and antidepressant medications to target specific psychotic and mood symptoms.

Delusional disorder is characterized by delusions in the absence of thought process disorder, prominent hallucinations, or the negative symptoms of schizophrenia. The delusions may be potentially

TABLE 6.5 Common Somatic Symptoms of Anxiety

Cardiorespiratory
- Palpitations
- Chest pain
- Dyspnea or sensation of being smothered

Gastrointestinal
- Sensation of choking
- Dyspepsia
- Nausea
- Diarrhea
- Abdominal bloating or pain

Genitourinary
- Urinary frequency or urgency

Neurologic or Autonomic
- Diaphoresis
- Warm flushes
- Dizziness or presyncope
- Paresthesia
- Tremor
- Headache

TABLE 6.6 Commonly Used Antipsychotic Medications

Name	Mechanism of Action/Side Effect Profile
First Generation ("Typical")	Blocks D2 receptors in addition to some level of muscarinic, histaminic and alpha-adrenergic blockade; tend to have higher rates of neurologic side effects
Chlorpromazine	High blockade of histaminic, alpha adrenergic receptors, higher likelihood of sedation and anticholinergic effects, "low potency"
Fluphenazine	
Haloperidol	Higher blockade of D2 receptors with little blockade of others, higher likelihood of extrapyramidal side effects, "high potency"
Perphenazine	
Thioridazine	
Thiothixene	
Trifluorophenazine	
Second Generation ("Atypical")	Blocks D2 receptors and 5-HT2A receptors; higher rates of metabolic side effects
Aripiprazole	Partial D2 agonist
Asenapine	
Brexipiprazole	
Cariprazine	
Clozapine	
Iloperidone	
Lurasidone	

精神病性障碍

精神病是一种现实感的丧失，表现为幻觉（即错误的感官知觉）、妄想（即固定的错误信念）和思维过程脱轨。精神分裂症是典型的精神病性障碍，它包括急性精神病发作（即阳性症状），以及随着时间的推移，往往呈现与情感平淡、意志缺乏、淡漠和社交退缩等负面症状有关的整体功能下降。

精神分裂症的终生患病率略低于1%，其慢性、致残性的病程给患者、家庭和社会带来了重大负担。发病高峰在青少年晚期至成年早期，男性发病年龄略早于女性。年发病率约为15/10万，但在不同的研究样本和人群之间存在显著差异。该病男性患病率略高于女性。

精神分裂症的发病机制尚不清楚，但显然是多因素作用的结果。遗传因素占患病风险的50%，涉及多个基因位点。对尸检脑组织的研究表明，这是一种非胶质细胞性神经病理过程，伴有皮质细胞结构的微小破坏。推测该病很可能是社会心理因素和神经发育与出生时就存在或生命早期获得的非定位性脑损伤相互作用所致。多巴胺能中脑皮质和中脑边缘系统通路在精神病症状的产生中起着重要作用。

抗精神病药物通常与苯二氮䓬类药物联合使用来治疗精神病急性发作（表6.6）。尽管维持性抗精神病药物有助于降低急性精神病发作的严重程度和频率，但需要全面的社会心理康复计划来帮助患者管理人际和其他压力，以此改善整体临床预后。辅助认知行为疗法也可能改善部分患者的预后。第二代（非典型）抗精神病药物由于锥体外系副作用（包括迟发性运动障碍）发生率较低，已取代第一代抗精神病药物，成为美国的常用药物。然而，第二代药物会增加肥胖和代谢综合征的风险。

分裂情感障碍是一种慢性、复发性疾病，患病率略低于精神分裂症。其特征是出现非心境性精神病发作和伴有精神病特征的心境发作（即躁狂或抑郁）。因此，其诊断不能仅基于患者在某一时间点的临床表现，而需要了解其整体病程。分裂情感障碍的预后差异很大，但平均来说介于精神分裂症和心境障碍之间。分裂情感障碍的治疗主要针对特定的精神症状和心境症状使用抗精神病药物、心境稳定剂及抗抑郁药物。

妄想性障碍的特征是在没有思维过程障碍、显著幻觉或精神分裂症阴性症状的情况下出现妄想。这些

表 6.5 焦虑的常见躯体症状

心血管和呼吸系统
心悸
胸痛
呼吸困难或窒息感

消化系统
哽噎感
消化不良
恶心
腹泻
腹胀或腹痛

泌尿生殖系统
尿频或尿急

神经系统或自主神经系统
出汗
潮热
头晕或晕厥前状态
感觉异常
震颤
头痛

表 6.6 常用的抗精神病药物

名称	作用机制 / 副作用
第一代（"典型"）	除了在一定程度上阻断毒蕈碱、组胺和 α 肾上腺素能之外，还能阻断 D_2 受体；神经系统副作用发生率较高
氯丙嗪	高度阻断组胺能和 α 肾上腺素能受体；较高的镇静和抗胆碱能副作用，"低效力"
氟奋乃静	
氟哌啶醇	高度阻断 D_2 受体，对其他受体阻断较少；锥体外系副作用发生率高，"高效力"
奋乃静	
硫利达嗪	
氨砜噻吨	
三氟奋乃静	
第二代（"非典型"）	阻断 D_2 受体和 5-HT2A 受体；代谢副作用发生率较高
阿立哌唑	部分 D_2 受体激动剂
阿塞那平	
依匹哌唑	
卡利拉嗪	
氯氮平	
伊洛哌酮	
鲁拉西酮	

plausible (i.e., not bizarre). Delusional disorder has a lifetime prevalence of approximately 0.2%. It often is only partially responsive to antipsychotic medications, but patients' functioning may be largely unimpaired if they are able with the aid of antipsychotics and psychotherapy to avoid acting on their delusions. The pathogeneses of the non-schizophrenic primary psychotic disorders remain largely unknown.

SOMATIC SYMPTOM DISORDER AND RELATED DISORDERS

Formerly called *somatoform disorders*, these conditions include somatic symptoms and associated thoughts, feelings, or behaviors that are distressing and disabling. Prominent types include somatic symptom disorder (i.e., excessive thoughts, feelings, or behaviors associated with one or more somatic symptoms), illness anxiety disorder (i.e., illness preoccupation and health-related behaviors disproportionate to somatic symptoms), conversion (i.e., functional neurologic symptom) disorder (i.e., neurologic somatoform symptoms incompatible with recognized neurologic or general medical conditions), and psychological factors affecting physical conditions. Factitious disorder (i.e., Munchausen syndrome) is a mental disorder in which patients consciously produce stigmata of disease (e.g., simulated or artificially induced fever or hypoglycemia) for the unconscious gain of assuming the sick role.

Although identifiable physical disease is insufficient to fully explain the patient's presentation, in all these conditions other than factitious disorder, the patient's distress and dysfunction are *not* consciously produced and are just as distressing to patients as would be similar symptoms produced by other medical conditions. Malingering is the conscious feigning of illness for conscious gain and therefore is not a mental disorder.

PERSONALITY DISORDERS

Personality is defined as the repertoire of enduring patterns of inner mental experience and behavior, including affect and impulse regulation, defense and coping mechanisms, and interpersonal relatedness. Personality traits must be distinguished from time-limited states. For example, a patient who exhibits dependent features solely while acutely depressed does not have a dependent personality.

A personality disorder is diagnosed when personality traits lead to pervasive (if variable) subjective distress or dysfunction in a broad range of situations. The major personality disorders are listed in Table 6.3. Personality and personality disorders are the result of complex interactions among genetic, environmental, and developmental factors. Approaches to patients with personality disorders depend on the specific type, but in most clinical circumstances other than long-term psychotherapy, the realistic goal is not to alter fundamental personality structure but to help the patient maximize use of personality strengths (e.g., optimal defense mechanisms) while minimizing the harmful effects of emotional dysregulation, unhelpful defenses, and destructive behaviors.

Although not the mainstay of most treatments for personality disorders, pharmacotherapy can be useful in selected patients (e.g., antipsychotics to target escalating paranoia in paranoid personality disorder, mood stabilizers or antidepressants to target emotional dysregulation in borderline personality disorder). Patients with personality disorders are also prone to mood, anxiety, eating, addictive, and other treatable psychiatric disorders.

PROSPECTUS FOR THE FUTURE

Advances in neuroscience will lead to not only better pharmacologic and other somatic therapies, but may hold the key to more accurate diagnosis of psychiatric illness. In the future, precision medicine in psychiatry will allow us to use information such as genomics and brain imaging to more accurately define, diagnose, and treat illness. Although not ready to be used clinically, the National Institute of Mental Health (NIMH) has initiated the Research Domains Criteria in order to test a framework of mental illness that goes beyond the traditional syndrome-based diagnosis by aligning more closely with underlying neural systems. The recent approval of two drugs with different mechanisms of action from previous antidepressants, intranasal esketamine and brexanolone, exemplifies the potential to discover new ways to treat mood and other psychiatric disorders. What is particularly exciting regarding these new medications is that they appear to work more quickly than other antidepressants. It remains to be seen how they will be optimally deployed among other therapeutic choices. Prevention remains an important area of growth in psychiatry, albeit an area that historically had lagged behind many other medical specialties. Promising data showing that early intervention teams for patients suffering from first onset psychosis improve long-term outcomes is a step in the right direction. Evidence is also growing that late-life depression can be prevented by cost-effective preventive interventions in at-risk patients in primary care and several specialty settings. Advances in prevention, diagnosis, and treatment will contribute to a new understanding of mental illness and lead to a future in which the global burden of mental illness can be decreased.

SUGGESTED READINGS

American Psychiatric Association: Diagnostic and statistical manual of mental disorders, ed 5, Arlington, VA, 2013, American Psychiatric Association.

Batelaan NM, Bosman RC, Muntingh A, et al: Risk of relapse after antidepressant discontinuation in anxiety disorders, obsessive compulsive disorder and post-traumatic stress disorder: systematic review and meta-analysis of relapse prevention trials, BMJ 358:j3927, 2017.

Bateman AW, Gunderson J, Mulder R: Treatment of personality disorder, Lancet 385:735–743, 2015.

Cipriani A, Furukawa TA, Salanti G, et al: Comparative efficacy and acceptability of 21 antidepressant drugs for the acute treatment of adults with major depressive disorder: a systematic review and network meta-analysis, Lancet 391:1357–1366, 2018.

Grande I, Berk M, Birmaher B, Vieta E: Bipolar disorder, Lancet 387:1561–1572, 2016.

Leucht S, Cipriani A, Spineli L, et al: Comparative efficacy and tolerability of 15 antipsychotic drugs in schizophrenia: a multiple-treatments meta-analysis, Lancet 382:951–962, 2013.

Lieberman JA, First MB: Psychosis, N Engl J Med 379:270–280, 2018.

Malhi GS, Mann JJ: Depression, Lancet 392:2299–2312, 2018.

O'Neal MA, Baslet G: Treatment for patients with a functional neurologic disorder (conversion disorder): an integrated approach, Am J Psychiatry 175:307–314, 2018.

Sanacors G, Frye MA, McDonald W, et al: A consensus statement on the use of ketamine in the treatment of mood disorders, JAMA Psychiatry 74:399–405, 2017.

Slee A, Nazareth I, Bondarek P, et al: Pharmacological treatments for generalized anxiety disorder: a systematic review and network meta-analysis, Lancet 393:768–777, 2019.

Stroup TS, Gerhard T, Crystal S, et al: Comparative effectiveness of clozapine and standard antipsychotic treatment in adults with schizophrenia, Am J Psychiatry 173:166–172, 2016.

妄想可能是看似合理的（即不是离奇的）。妄想性障碍的终生患病率约为0.2%。虽然抗精神病药物仅部分有效，但如果患者在抗精神病药物和心理治疗的帮助下能够避免对妄想采取行动，他们的功能可能在很大程度上不受影响。非精神分裂症的原发性精神障碍的发病机制仍不甚明了。

躯体症状障碍及相关疾病

这些疾病以前被称为躯体形式障碍，包括躯体症状和相关的令人痛苦和致残的想法、感受或行为。主要类型包括躯体症状障碍（即与一种或多种躯体症状相关的过度想法、感受或行为）、疾病焦虑障碍（即与躯体症状不相称的疾病担忧和健康相关行为）、转换障碍（即功能性神经症状；例如，与已知的神经或全身疾病不相符的神经性躯体形式症状），以及影响身体状况的心理因素。做作性障碍（即Munchausen综合征）是一种精神障碍，患者有意识地制造疾病的假象（例如，模拟或人为诱发发热或低血糖），以达到无意识地扮演患者角色的目的。

尽管可识别的躯体疾病无法完全解释患者的表现，但除了做作性障碍之外，在所有这些病症中，患者的痛苦和功能障碍并不是有意识制造的，对患者来说，这些症状与由其他疾病引起的类似症状一样令人痛苦。诈病是为了谋取利益而有意装病，因此不属于精神障碍。

人格障碍

人格被定义为内在心理体验和行为的持久模式的集合，包括情感和冲动调节、防御和应对机制以及人际关系。人格特质必须与时限性状态区分开来。例如，仅在急性抑郁时表现出依赖特征的患者并不具有依赖型人格。

当人格特质导致在各种情况下普遍存在的（如果可变的）主观痛苦或功能障碍时，则可诊断为人格障碍。主要的人格障碍列于表6.3。人格和人格障碍是遗传、环境和发育因素复杂相互作用的结果。对人格障碍患者的治疗方法取决于其具体类型，但除长期心理治疗外，在大多数临床情况下，现实目标不是改变基本的人格结构，而是帮助患者最大限度地利用人格优势（例如最佳防御机制），同时最大限度地减少情绪调节障碍、不利防御和破坏性行为的有害影响。

尽管药物治疗并非大多数人格障碍治疗的主要手段，但在特定患者中可能是有用的（例如，使用抗精神病药物治疗偏执型人格障碍患者不断升级的偏执，使用心境稳定剂或抗抑郁药物治疗边缘型人格障碍中的情绪失调）。人格障碍患者也容易患上心境障碍、焦虑障碍、进食障碍、成瘾以及其他可治疗的精神障碍。

未来展望

神经科学的进步不仅将带来更好的药物治疗和其他躯体治疗方法，而且可能成为更准确诊断精神疾病的关键。未来，精神病学中的精准医学将允许我们利用基因组学和脑成像等信息，更准确地定义、诊断和治疗疾病。尽管尚未准备好在临床中使用，美国国立精神卫生研究所（NIMH）已经启动了研究领域标准（Research Domains Criteria），以测试一种超越传统基于综合征诊断框架的精神疾病模型，以此与潜在的神经系统更加紧密地贴近。最近，2种具有不同于以往抗抑郁药作用机制的新药——鼻喷艾司氯胺酮（esketamine）和别孕烯醇酮（brexanolone）获得了批准，这充分体现了探索治疗心境障碍和其他精神障碍新方法的潜力。尤其令人兴奋的是，这些新药物似乎比其他抗抑郁药物起效更快。至于如何在其他治疗选择中优化配置这些药物，仍有待观察。预防仍然是精神病学发展中的一个重要领域，尽管这一领域在历史上落后于许多其他医学专业。令人鼓舞的数据表明，针对首次发病的精神病患者进行早期团队干预能够改善长期预后，这是朝着正确方向迈出的一步。越来越多的证据表明，在初级保健和一些专科医疗机构中，对高危患者采取具有成本-效益的预防性干预措施，可有效预防老年抑郁。预防、诊断和治疗的进步将有助于人们对精神疾病有一个新的认识，并在未来减轻全球精神疾病的负担。

推荐阅读

American Psychiatric Association: Diagnostic and statistical manual of mental disorders, ed 5, Arlington, VA, 2013, American Psychiatric Association.

Batelaan NM, Bosman RC, Muntingh A, et al: Risk of relapse after antidepressant discontinuation in anxiety disorders, obsessive compulsive disorder and post-traumatic stress disorder: systematic review and meta-analysis of relapse prevention trials, BMJ 358:j3927, 2017.

Bateman AW, Gunderson J, Mulder R: Treatment of personality disorder, Lancet 385:735–743, 2015.

Cipriani A, Furukawa TA, Salanti G, et al: Comparative efficacy and acceptability of 21 antidepressant drugs for the acute treatment of adults with major depressive disorder: a systematic review and network meta-analysis, Lancet 391:1357–1366, 2018.

Grande I, Berk M, Birmaher B, Vieta E: Bipolar disorder, Lancet 387:1561–1572, 2016.

Leucht S, Cipriani A, Spineli L, et al: Comparative efficacy and tolerability of 15 antipsychotic drugs in schizophrenia: a multiple-treatments meta-analysis, Lancet 382:951–962, 2013.

Lieberman JA, First MB: Psychosis, N Engl J Med 379:270–280, 2018.

Malhi GS, Mann JJ: Depression, Lancet 392:2299–2312, 2018.

O'Neal MA, Baslet G: Treatment for patients with a functional neurologic disorder (conversion disorder): an integrated approach, Am J Psychiatry 175:307–314, 2018.

Sanacors G, Frye MA, McDonald W, et al: A consensus statement on the use of ketamine in the treatment of mood disorders, JAMA Psychiatry 74:399–405, 2017.

Slee A, Nazareth I, Bondarek P, et al: Pharmacological treatments for generalized anxiety disorder: a systematic review and network meta-analysis, Lancet 393:768–777, 2019.

Stroup TS, Gerhard T, Crystal S, et al: Comparative effectiveness of clozapine and standard antipsychotic treatment in adults with schizophrenia, Am J Psychiatry 173:166–172, 2016.

Autonomic Nervous System Disorders

William P. Cheshire, Jr.

DEFINITION AND EPIDEMIOLOGY

The autonomic nervous system reaches throughout the body and governs all visceral activity. Its central network and peripheral sympathetic and parasympathetic divisions integrate complex organ functions, maintain internal homeostasis in response to environmental change, modulate the flight-or-fight physiologic response to stress, and enable circulation, digestion, and procreation.

Benign dysautonomias are common. Neurally mediated syncope and situational reflex syncope in response to emotional distress, carotid sinus stimulation, micturition, defecation, coughing, straining, or other factors occur in about 20% of people during a lifetime and account for 1% to 3% of all emergency room visits. Hyperhidrosis of the palms and soles affects about 1% of the population. Anhidrosis can contribute to increased mortality rates during severe heat stress.

One of the most disabling manifestations of autonomic failure is orthostatic hypotension, the prevalence of which increases with age, physical inactivity, and in diseases that impair sympathetic adrenergic nerves. Orthostatic hypotension affects about 5% to 20% of the elderly.

Diabetes mellitus is the most common cause of autonomic neuropathy in industrialized nations. About 30% of diabetics develop autonomic neuropathy, and symptomatic orthostatic hypotension occurs in 5% of patients. Other features of autonomic neuropathy include constipation in 40% to 60% of diabetics, gastroparesis in 20% to 40%, bladder dysfunction in 30% to 80%, and erectile impotence in more than 30% of men.

For a deeper discussion of these topics, please see Chapter 22, "Common Clinical Sequelae of Aging," and Chapter 216, "Diabetes Mellitus," in *Goldman-Cecil Medicine*, 26th Edition.

PATHOLOGY

Many brain, spinal cord, peripheral nerve, and systemic disorders that impair autonomic nerves can cause autonomic dysfunction or failure. They include a wide range of degenerative, traumatic, cerebrovascular, autoimmune, genetic, metabolic, toxic, and pharmacologic conditions.

Small-caliber peripheral autonomic nerves are unmyelinated or thinly myelinated, and small-fiber peripheral neuropathies that cause distal sensory loss may also involve sympathetic or parasympathetic nerves. Diabetic autonomic neuropathy results from microvascular damage to autonomic nerves. Several hereditary, infectious, metabolic, toxic, and drug-induced sensory and autonomic neuropathies are recognized causes.

Accumulation of abnormal proteins distinguishes some of the degenerative dysautonomias. Oligodendroglial cytoplasmic inclusions composed of aggregates of misfolded α-synuclein are pathognomonic of multiple system atrophy. Abnormally folded sympathetic neuronal accumulation of α-synuclein occurs in Lewy body disorders such as Parkinson's disease. Peripheral autonomic nerve deposition of β-pleated sheet amyloid protein causes a severe autonomic neuropathy, which is frequently seen in primary amyloidosis, immunoglobulin light chain–associated disease, and hereditary amyloidosis, although rarely in reactive amyloidosis.

Other dysautonomias have an autoimmune basis. Autonomic instability has long been recognized in Guillain-Barré syndrome, which is an acute inflammatory, demyelinating polyradiculoneuropathy associated with antiganglioside antibodies (e.g., anti-GM_1, anti-GM_3). The list of autoimmune autonomic neuropathies includes acute autonomic ganglionopathy; patients with acute pandysautonomia have antibodies against the nicotinic acetylcholine receptor in autonomic ganglia, which is sometimes associated with lung cancer or thymoma. Additional paraneoplastic autonomic neuropathies include those associated with antineuronal nuclear antibody type 1 (i.e., ANNA-1 or anti-Hu) and antibodies against collapsing response mediator proteins (i.e., CRMP-5 or anti-CV2). Lambert-Eaton myasthenic syndrome is associated with antibodies to voltage-gated calcium channels. Antibodies to voltage-gated potassium channels cause autoimmune neuromyotonia and dysautonomia with hyperhidrosis and orthostatic intolerance.

Pharmacologic agents frequently alter autonomic function. Diuretics, sympatholytic drugs, α-adrenoreceptor blockers, and vasodilators can cause or contribute to orthostatic hypotension. Anticholinergics and carbonic anhydrase inhibitors decrease sweating, whereas opioids and selective serotonin reuptake inhibitors increase sweating. Opioids slow intestinal transit. Anticholinergics, tricyclic antidepressants, and antihistamines may cause urinary retention.

Functional dysautonomias are medical conditions in which autonomic function is impaired in the absence of a known structural neurologic deficit. Some psychological disorders may manifest with autonomic symptoms because emotional and autonomic centers are closely linked in the limbic system.

For a deeper discussion of these topics, please see Chapter 392, "Peripheral Neuropathies," Chapter 179, "Amyloidosis," and Chapter 41, "Mechanisms of Immune-Mediated Tissue Injury," in *Goldman-Cecil Medicine*, 26th Edition.

CLINICAL PRESENTATION

Clinical manifestations of autonomic disorders vary according to which nerves are involved and how severely. Autonomic signs and symptoms may be benign or serious, paroxysmal or continuous, or localized or generalized, and they may represent hypofunction or hyperfunction.

Afferent autonomic lesions that separate central autonomic nuclei from incoming information needed to gauge an appropriate response may cause excessive or erratic autonomic outflow. An example of afferent dysautonomia is the volatile hypertension in carotid arterial baroreceptor failure after irradiation to treat laryngeal carcinoma. Spinal cord injuries above the level of sympathetic outflow at T5 can cause autonomic dysreflexia, a condition of paroxysmal sympathetic surges

自主神经系统疾病

范思远 译 卢强 韩菲 审校 姚明 朱以诚 通审

定义和流行病学

自主神经系统遍布全身,支配所有内脏活动。其中枢网络与外周的交感和副交感神经分支整合复杂的器官功能,维持应对环境变化的内环境稳态,调节针对应激的"逃跑或战斗"生理反应,并使循环、消化和生殖得以进行。

良性的自主神经功能障碍很常见。大约20%的人在一生中会因情绪困扰、颈动脉窦刺激、排尿、排便、咳嗽、用力或其他因素而发生神经性晕厥和情景反射性晕厥,这类情况占急诊就诊总量的1%~3%。手掌和足底的多汗症影响大约1%的人口。无汗症可能导致严重热应激期间的死亡率增加。

体位性低血压是自主神经功能衰竭最具致残性的表现之一,其患病率随年龄增长、缺乏运动以及损害交感肾上腺素能神经的疾病而增加。5%~20%的老年人受体位性低血压的影响。

在工业化国家中,糖尿病是自主神经病变的最常见原因。大约30%的糖尿病患者出现自主神经病变,5%的患者出现症状性体位性低血压。自主神经病变的其他特点包括40%~60%糖尿病患者出现便秘,20%~40%有胃轻瘫,30%~80%出现膀胱功能障碍,以及超过30%的男性有勃起功能障碍。

❖ 有关此专题的深入讨论,请参阅 Goldman-Cecil Medicine 第26版第22章"衰老的常见临床后遗症"和第216章"糖尿病"。

病理学

多种损伤自主神经的脑、脊髓、周围神经和系统性疾病都可能导致自主神经功能障碍或衰竭。这类疾病包括一系列退行性、创伤性、脑血管性、自身免疫性、遗传性、代谢性、中毒性和药物性疾病。

小直径的周围自主神经是无髓或薄髓的,导致远端感觉缺失的小纤维周围神经病也可能累及交感或副交感神经。糖尿病自主神经病变是由于自主神经的微血管损伤引起的。一些遗传性、感染性、代谢性、中毒性和药物诱导的感觉和自主神经病变是已知的原因。

异常蛋白质的沉积是一些退行性自主神经功能障碍的特征。由错误折叠的α突触核蛋白聚集构成的少突胶质细胞胞质内包涵体是多系统萎缩的病理特征。在帕金森病等路易体疾病中,存在异常折叠的交感神经元α突触核蛋白沉积。周围自主神经的β折叠片状淀粉样蛋白沉积会引起严重的自主神经病变,这种情况在原发性淀粉样变性、免疫球蛋白轻链相关疾病和遗传性淀粉样变性中常见,但在反应性淀粉样变性中少见。

其他自主神经功能障碍存在自身免疫基础。自主神经功能失衡在吉兰-巴雷综合征中早已被认识,这是一种与抗神经节苷脂抗体(如抗GM_1和抗GM_3抗体)相关的急性炎症性脱髓鞘性多发性神经根神经病。自身免疫性自主神经病变包括急性自主神经节病,急性泛自主神经功能障碍的患者存在针对自主神经节中的烟碱型乙酰胆碱受体抗体,有时与肺癌或胸腺瘤相关。其他的副肿瘤性自主神经病变包括与抗神经元核抗体1型(即ANNA-1或抗-Hu)和抗坍塌反应调节蛋白抗体(即CRMP-5或抗CV2抗体)相关的疾病。兰伯特-伊顿肌无力综合征与电压门控钙通道抗体相关。电压门控钾通道抗体会引起自身免疫性神经性肌强直和自主神经功能障碍,伴有多汗和直立不耐受。

药物常改变自主神经功能。利尿剂、交感神经抑制剂、α肾上腺素能受体阻滞剂和血管扩张剂可导致或加剧体位性低血压。抗胆碱能药物和碳酸酐酶抑制剂减少出汗,而阿片类药物和选择性5-羟色胺再摄取抑制剂增加出汗。阿片类药物会减慢肠道转运。抗胆碱能药物、三环类抗抑郁药和抗组胺药物可能导致尿潴留。

功能性自主神经功能障碍是指在没有已知结构性神经系统缺陷的情况下,出现自主神经功能障碍的一种医学状况。一些心理疾病可能表现出自主神经症状,因为情感中枢和自主神经中枢在边缘系统中紧密相连。

有关此专题的深入讨论,请参阅 Goldman-Cecil ❖ Medicine 第26版第392章"周围神经病"、第179章"淀粉样变性"和第41章"免疫介导的组织损伤机制"。

临床表现

自主神经疾病的临床表现因受累神经和严重程度而异。自主神经的体征和症状可能是良性的,也可能是严重的;可能是阵发性的,也可能是持续性的;可能是局部性,也可能是全身性的;并且可能表现为功能低下,也可能表现为功能亢进。

传入性自主神经病变,将中枢自主神经核与判断适当反应所需的传入信息分离开来,可能导致自主神经输出过度或不稳定。传入性自主神经功能障碍的一个例子是喉癌放疗后,颈动脉压力感受器功能衰竭导致不稳定性高血

with hypertension, diaphoresis, flushing, and headache. Catastrophic brain disorders such as subarachnoid hemorrhage, trauma, or hydrocephalus may also cause autonomic storms if hypothalamic circuits are released from cortical inhibition.

More common are efferent autonomic lesions, which cause failure of outflow to neuroeffector junctions, resulting in inadequate excitatory or inhibitory autonomic responses. An example of efferent dysautonomias is autonomic peripheral neuropathy, which may accompany distal sensory loss and decreased Achilles tendon jerks.

Cardiovascular adrenergic failure impairs the cardiac and peripheral vascular response needed to maintain blood pressure during orthostatic stress. Patients present with orthostatic hypotension and may report lightheadedness or fatigue on standing that is relieved by sitting.

Vagal failure impairs cardiac parasympathetic tone that may protect against arrhythmogenic sympathetic activity. Patients have a fixed heart rate that does not vary with respiration.

Sudomotor failure (failure to stimulate the sweat glands) with extensive anhidrosis may coexist with tonic pupils (sluggish response to light) and areflexia (i.e., Ross syndrome), and it can increase the risk of heat exhaustion or heat stroke. A dramatic example of regional sudomotor failure is harlequin syndrome, in which hemifacial cutaneous sympathetic denervation divides the pale and dry denervated half of the face from the intact half that flushes red in response to heat stress. Horner syndrome (i.e., unilateral ptosis, miosis, and anhidrosis) may be identified.

The clinical hallmark of generalized autonomic failure is severe orthostatic hypotension without pulse acceleration. In at least one half of patients, it is accompanied by supine and nocturnal hypertension, a reversal of the normal diurnal decrease in blood pressure during sleep. In addition to vagal and sudomotor failure, patients with generalized autonomic failure may have constipation, gastroparesis, bladder dysfunction, male erectile dysfunction, dry mouth, or dry eyes. Some have postprandial hypotension, in which a large meal high in carbohydrate content causes a reduction in blood pressure.

One of the most severe autonomic disorders is multiple system atrophy, which is a sporadic, progressive, ultimately fatal neurodegenerative disorder in which autonomic failure occurs in combination with parkinsonism or cerebellar ataxia. Bladder hypotonia with overflow incontinence and nocturnal respiratory stridor may occur. The parkinsonian phenotype (i.e., Shy-Drager syndrome) tends to respond poorly to levodopa. Orthostatic hypotension is also common in Lewy body disorders such as Parkinson's disease. Pure autonomic failure consists of widespread autonomic failure without other neurologic features.

In contrast to autonomic failure, neurally mediated syncope occurs in patients with a functioning autonomic nervous system in which there is a reversal of normal autonomic outflow. Prodromal features typically include pallor, sweating, nausea, abdominal discomfort, mydriasis, increased respiratory rate, and cognitive slowing, which may progress to transient loss of consciousness if the patient continues in an upright posture. Withdrawal of peripheral sympathetic vasomotor tone (i.e., vasodepressor syncope) or an increase in parasympathetic tone (i.e., vasovagal syncope) causes a fall in blood pressure, heart rate, and cerebral perfusion.

Orthostatic intolerance refers to a heterogeneous group of conditions in which patients have difficulty sustaining the autonomic outflow needed to maintain blood pressure during the gravitational stress of prolonged standing. Some patients experience a gradual decline in blood pressure, but others experience an abnormal increase in heart rate without a drop in blood pressure.

❖ For a deeper discussion of these topics, please see Chapter 56, "Approach to the Patient with Suspected Arrhythmia," Chapter 70, "Arterial Hypertension," Chapter 127, "Disorders of Gastrointestinal Motility," and Chapter 381, "Parkinsonism," in *Goldman-Cecil Medicine*, 26th Edition.

DIAGNOSIS AND DIFFERENTIAL DIAGNOSIS

A careful history and discerning physical examination are essential for reaching a diagnosis. The astute clinician inquires about the time course of symptoms and the circumstances that provoke or modify them. How long have they been present? Are they stable, improving, or worsening? Do they occur consistently or episodically? Orthostatic disorders are typically worse in the early morning, in heat, and after physical exercise or a large meal. How well the patient tolerates standing in line or taking a warm shower are helpful clues to identifying orthostatic intolerance.

Physical signs of autonomic dysfunction may include pupillary asymmetry or sluggishness, ptosis, or mucosal dryness. An acutely distended bladder may be suspected by percussion. Asymmetrical sweating may be visible or palpable.

The most important part of the examination, but one that is frequently omitted, is measurement of orthostatic blood pressure (Fig. 7.1). Blood pressure and heart rate should be assessed when the patient is resting supine and again after standing for 1 to 3 minutes. Correlation with symptoms is key. Patients with orthostatic

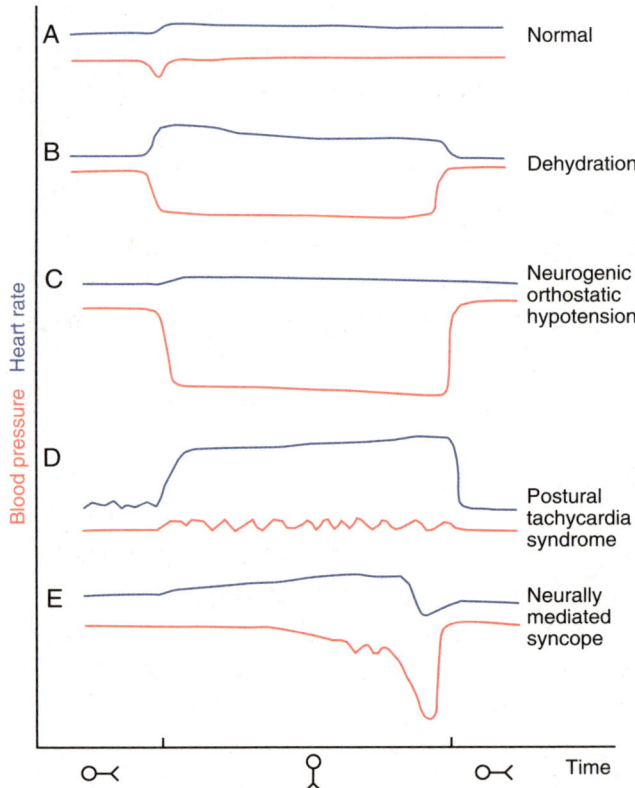

Fig. 7.1 Orthostatic blood pressure profiles. (A) The normal response to standing or head-up tilt is no change or a small decrease in blood pressure that recovers within half a minute and a small increase in heart rate. (B) Dehydration causing intravascular hypovolemia may cause a fall in blood pressure accompanied by reflex tachycardia. (C) Neurogenic orthostatic hypotension may cause a more profound drop in blood pressure. Hypotension occurs immediately and is sustained without recovery during standing and often without adequate compensatory tachycardia. (D) Postural tachycardia syndrome is characterized by an abnormal increase in heart rate without orthostatic hypotension. (E) Neurally mediated syncope develops after standing for some time, may be preceded by oscillations in blood pressure, and may be accompanied by bradycardia with loss of consciousness in about 7 seconds if cerebral perfusion is not restored.

压。T5 水平（交感输出）以上的脊髓损伤可导致自主神经反射异常，这是一种阵发性交感神经功能亢进状态，伴有高血压、大汗、潮红和头痛等症状。蛛网膜下腔出血、外伤或脑积水这类灾难性脑部疾病中，若下丘脑环路从大脑皮质抑制中得以释放，也可能导致自主神经风暴。

更常见的是传出性自主神经病变，这导致神经-效应器接头的输出失败，从而引起自主神经的兴奋性或抑制性反应不足。传出性自主神经功能障碍的一个例子是自主神经周围神经病，它可能伴随远端感觉缺失和跟腱反射减弱。

心血管肾上腺素能衰竭可损害直立应激下维持血压所需的心脏和外周血管反应。患者表现为体位性低血压，并可出现站立时头晕或疲劳，坐下后症状会有所缓解。

迷走神经功能衰竭可损害心脏副交感神经张力，这种张力可防止交感神经活动导致心律失常。患者的心率固定不变，不随呼吸而变化。

汗腺功能衰竭（无法刺激汗腺）伴广泛无汗症，可能与强直瞳孔（对光反射迟钝）和反射消失［即罗斯综合征（Ross syndrome）］共存，这种情况可能增加热衰竭或热射病的风险。区域性汗腺功能衰竭的一个显著例子是丑角综合征（harlequin syndrome），其中半侧面部皮肤的交感神经去神经支配，导致苍白、干燥的去神经支配半侧面部与对热应激反应而潮红的正常半侧面部形成对比。可能会出现霍纳综合征（即单侧眼睑下垂、瞳孔缩小和无汗症）。

严重的体位性低血压而不伴脉搏加速是全身性自主神经功能衰竭的临床特点。至少一半的患者伴有仰卧位和夜间高血压，这是睡眠期间正常日间血压下降的逆转。除了迷走神经和汗腺功能衰竭外，全身性自主神经功能衰竭的患者还可出现便秘、胃轻瘫、膀胱功能障碍、男性勃起功能障碍、口干或眼干。有些患者存在餐后低血压，碳水化合物含量高的一顿大餐可导致血压降低。

最严重的自主神经疾病之一是多系统萎缩，这是一种散发性、进行性、最终致命的神经系统退行性疾病，其中自主神经功能衰竭与帕金森综合征或小脑性共济失调同时发生。可能出现膀胱张力降低伴充盈性尿失禁和夜间呼吸喘鸣。帕金森病表型［即夏-德综合征（Shy-Drager syndrome）］往往对左旋多巴反应不佳。体位性低血压也常见于帕金森病等路易体疾病。纯自主神经功能衰竭出现广泛的自主神经功能衰竭，不伴其他神经系统表现。

与自主神经功能衰竭不同，神经性晕厥发生在自主神经系统功能正常的患者中，其中正常的自主神经输出发生逆转。前驱表现通常包括面色苍白、出汗、恶心、腹部不适、瞳孔散大、呼吸频率加快和认知减慢，如果患者继续保持直立姿势，可能会发展为一过性意识丧失。外周交感神经血管运动张力减弱（即血管减压性晕厥）或副交感神经张力增加（即血管迷走性晕厥）导致血压、心率和脑灌注下降。

直立不耐受是一组异质性疾病，患者在长时间站立的重力应激下，维持血压所需的自主神经输出难以维持。一些患者血压逐渐下降，另一些患者则出现心率异常加快，但不伴血压下降。

有关此专题的深入讨论，请参阅 Goldman-Cecil Medicine 第 26 版第 56 章"疑似心律失常患者的处理方案"、第 70 章"动脉性高血压"、第 127 章"胃肠动力疾病"和第 381 章"帕金森综合征"。

诊断和鉴别诊断

仔细询问病史并进行鉴别性的体格检查对于确诊至关重要。敏锐的临床医生会询问症状出现的时间过程，以及诱发或改变症状的因素。症状存在多久了？症状是稳定、好转还是恶化？症状是持续性的还是间歇性的？直立性疾病通常在早晨、炎热天气、体育锻炼或大餐后加重。患者对站立排队或洗热水澡的耐受性如何，是识别直立不耐受的有用线索。

自主神经功能障碍的体征可能包括瞳孔不对称或反射迟钝、眼睑下垂或黏膜干燥。叩诊可能发现膀胱的急性扩张。不对称的出汗可以通过观察和触诊来识别。

在检查中，最重要但常被忽略的部分，是测量直立位血压（图 7.1）。在患者静卧时测量血压和心率，并在站起 1～3 min 后再次测量。与症状之间的相关性

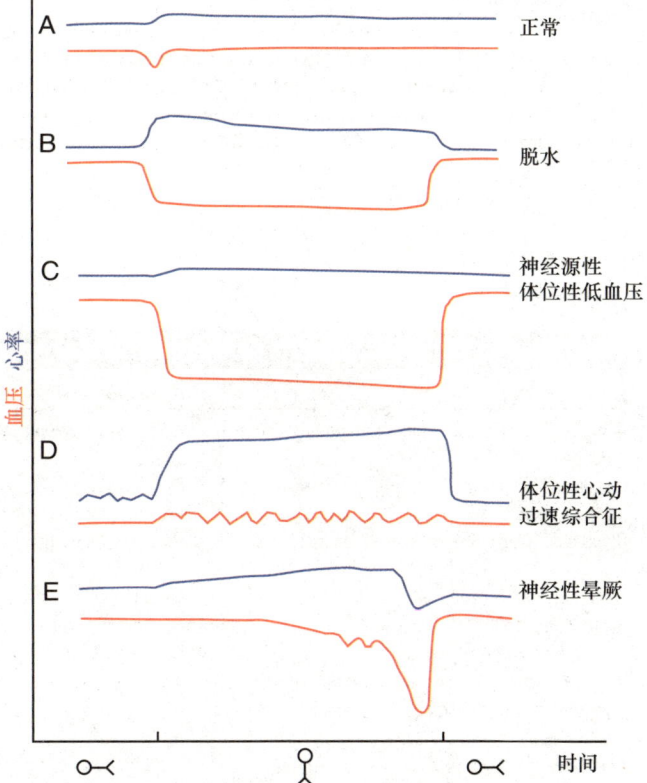

图 7.1 直立位血压曲线图。（A）站立或仰头时的正常反应是血压无变化或轻度下降，但在半分钟内恢复，伴心率轻度增加。（B）脱水导致血管内低血容量可引起血压下降，伴有反射性心动过速。（C）神经源性体位性低血压可引起更大幅度的血压下降。低血压在站起时立即发生，在站立期间持续不恢复，且通常缺乏足够的代偿性心动过速。（D）体位性心动过速综合征的特点是心率异常增快，但没有体位性低血压。（E）神经性晕厥在站立一段时间后发生，可能先有血压波动，若脑灌注未恢复，可能在 7 s 内出现心动过缓伴意识丧失

hypotension may appear less alert, or they may shift weight from one leg to the other to improve venous return, lower the head to bring the cerebral circulation closer to the level of the heart, or exhibit lower extremity rubor if cutaneous vasomotor function is impaired.

Orthostatic hypotension is a reduction in systolic blood pressure of at least 20 mm Hg or a reduction in diastolic blood pressure of at least 10 mm Hg, with or without symptoms, within 1 to 3 minutes of assuming an erect posture. Neurogenic orthostatic hypotension, a cardinal manifestation of sympathetic adrenergic failure, is typically sustained with continued standing and may lack the reflex tachycardia seen when hypotension is caused by blood loss, dehydration, or excessive venous pooling.

Orthostatic intolerance is difficulty tolerating the upright posture because of symptoms that resolve when supine. These patients do not have orthostatic hypotension but may have a sustained increase in postural heart rate (postural tachycardia syndrome) of more than 30 beats per minute in adults (40 in adolescents).

Laboratory testing of autonomic responses under controlled conditions is useful to determine the presence, severity, and distribution of autonomic failure and to distinguish neurogenic from other causes of orthostatic hypotension. Clinical autonomic testing typically evaluates beat-to-beat blood pressure and heart rate responses to the Valsalva maneuver, upright tilt, and periodic deep breathing, along with quantitative assessment of axons that produce sweating responses. Ambulatory blood pressure testing is useful for the assessment of episodic or postprandial hypotension, nocturnal hypertension, and the volatile hypertension of autonomic storms.

TREATMENT

Treatment options for orthostatic hypotension are outlined in Table 7.1. The goal is to enable the patient to stand long enough to engage in daily activities without symptoms. Medication is not always needed and can potentially exacerbate recumbent hypertension. Orthostatic intolerance was shown in a randomized controlled trial to improve after endurance exercise training.

Generalized hyperhidrosis may be reduced by oral anticholinergic agents such as 1 to 2 mg of glycopyrrolate taken one to three times daily. Topical glycopyrrolate reduces regional gustatory sweating. Subdermal botulinum toxin injections are helpful for some forms of focal hyperhidrosis, and palmar hyperhidrosis may respond to tap water iontophoresis or, in severe cases, to endoscopic thoracic sympathotomy.

For a deeper discussion of these topics, please see Chapter 390, "Autonomic Disorders and Their Management," in *Goldman-Cecil Medicine*, 26th Edition.

PROGNOSIS

Orthostatic intolerance and neurally mediated syncope are frequently benign, manageable, and improve or recover with time. Autonomic failure, in contrast, can signify a more serious prognosis, depending on the nature and extent of its pathophysiology. Persistent or severe orthostatic hypotension carries a worse prognosis.

Diabetic cardiovascular autonomic neuropathy doubles the risk for silent myocardial ischemia and overall mortality. Amyloid autonomic neuropathy is especially grave, with a median survival of less than 1 year if the patient has orthostatic hypotension. Pure autonomic failure may remain stable for many years, although some patients with this phenotype eventually develop signs of multiple system atrophy, which denotes a life expectancy of 7 to 9 years after diagnosis.

Regular physical exercise can reverse the autonomic deconditioning that comes from inactivity. In the elderly, it may compensate for some age-associated decline in autonomic function.

For a deeper discussion of these topics, please see Chapter 390, "Autonomic Disorders and Their Management," in *Goldman-Cecil Medicine*, 26th Edition.

TABLE 7.1 Treatment of Orthostatic Hypotension

Intervention	Rationale	Dosage
Avoid prolonged bed rest and increase time spent upright	Reverses physiologic deconditioning	
Liberalize fluid intake	Expands plasma volume	2-2.5 L/day
Increase sodium intake	Expands plasma volume	Salt 10-20 g/day
Compressive leg garments and abdominal binder	Reduces venous pooling	20-40 mm Hg (10 mm Hg for abdominal binder)
Physical counter-maneuvers	Tensing limb muscles augments venous return	Isometric contractions for 30 sec
Water bolus treatment	Sympathetic reflex increases blood pressure for 1-2 hr	16 oz. plain water
Elevate head of bed 4 inches	Decreases nocturnal natriuresis and nocturnal hypertension	
Avoid large meals high in carbohydrate content	If patient is subject to postprandial hypotension	
Discontinue or decrease dose of blood pressure–lowering drugs		
Midodrine	α-Adrenergic agonist, constricts capacitance vessels	5-10 mg tid
Droxidopa	Norepinephrine prodrug, stimulates sympathetic nerves	100-600 mg tid
Fludrocortisone	Retains sodium and sensitizes peripheral vascular α-adrenergic receptors	0.1-0.4 mg/day
Pyridostigmine	Stimulates sympathetic ganglionic transmission	30-60 mg bid or tid

是至关重要的。体位性低血压的患者可能表现出较低的警觉性，或者他们可能会将重心从一条腿转移至另一条腿以改善静脉回流，低头以使脑循环更接近心脏水平，或者在皮肤血管运动功能受损时出现下肢发红。

体位性低血压是指在保持直立姿势 1～3 min 内，收缩压降低至少 20 mmHg 或舒张压降低至少 10 mmHg，伴或不伴症状。神经源性体位性低血压是交感肾上腺素能衰竭的主要表现，通常在持续站立时血压持续降低，并且在失血、脱水或静脉过度淤滞引起的低血压时缺乏相应的反射性心动过速。

直立不耐受是指由于症状在仰卧时缓解而难以忍受直立姿势。这些患者没有体位性低血压，但可能存在持续的体位性心率增加（体位性心动过速综合征），在成人中每分钟超出 30 次（青少年每分钟超出 40 次）。

在控制条件下对自主神经反应进行实验室检查，有助于确定自主神经功能衰竭的存在、严重程度和分布，并区分神经源性和其他原因引起的体位性低血压。临床自主神经检查通常包括评估患者对瓦尔萨尔瓦动作（Valsalva maneuver）、直立倾斜和周期性深呼吸的逐搏（beat-to-beat）血压和心率反应，以及对出汗反应相关轴突的定量评估。动态血压监测有助于评估间歇性或餐后低血压、夜间高血压以及自主神经风暴引起的波动性高血压。

治疗

表 7.1 列出了治疗体位性低血压的各种方案。目标是让患者能够站立足够长的时间来从事日常活动而不出现症状。并非总是需要药物治疗，而且药物治疗可能会加重卧位高血压。一项随机对照试验表明，经过耐力运动训练后，直立不耐受得到改善。

口服抗胆碱能药物，如格隆溴铵 1～2 mg，每天 1～3 次，可减轻全身性多汗症。外用格隆溴铵可以减轻区域性味觉性出汗。皮下注射肉毒素对某些形式的局部多汗症有效，而手掌多汗症可能对自来水离子电渗疗法有反应，严重的病例还可能对胸腔镜下交感神经切断术有反应。

有关此专题的深入讨论，请参阅 *Goldman-Cecil Medicine* 第 26 版第 390 章"自主神经疾病及其治疗"。

预后

直立不耐受和神经性晕厥通常是良性的、可治的，并且会随时间推移而改善或恢复。相比之下，自主神经功能衰竭可能意味着预后更差，这取决于其病理生理学的性质和程度。持续或严重的体位性低血压预后较差。

糖尿病心血管自主神经病变导致无症状性心肌缺血和总体死亡率的风险加倍。淀粉样变性自主神经病变尤其严重，若患者出现体位性低血压，中位生存期不到 1 年。纯自主神经功能衰竭可能在多年内保持稳定，但一些具有这种表型的患者最终会出现多系统萎缩的症状，这意味着诊断后的预期寿命为 7～9 年。

规律的体育锻炼可以逆转因缺乏运动而导致的自主神经功能失调。在老年人中，它可以代偿一些与年龄相关的自主神经功能衰退。

有关此专题的深入讨论，请参阅 *Goldman-Cecil Medicine* 第 26 版第 390 章"自主神经疾病及其治疗"。

表 7.1 体位性低血压的治疗

干预措施	原理	剂量
避免长时间卧床，增加直立时间	逆转生理性功能失调	
增加液体摄入量	扩大血浆容量	每天 2～2.5 L
增加钠摄入量	扩大血浆容量	每天 10～20 g 盐
使用弹力袜和腹带	减少静脉淤滞	20～40 mmHg（腹带为 10 mmHg）
身体对抗动作	肢体肌肉紧张增加静脉回流	等长收缩 30 s
水负荷治疗	交感神经反射性升高血压 1～2 h	16 oz（译者注：473 ml）纯净水
抬高床头 4 in（译者注：10 cm）	减少夜间尿钠排泄和减轻夜间高血压	
避免碳水化合物含量高的大餐	如果患者存在餐后低血压	
停用或减少降压药的剂量		
米多君	α 肾上腺素能激动剂，收缩容量血管	5～10 mg，3 次/日
屈昔多巴	去甲肾上腺素前体药，刺激交感神经	100～600 mg，3 次/日
氟氢可的松	保钠并使外周血管 α 肾上腺素能受体致敏	0.1～0.4 mg/d
溴吡斯的明	刺激交感神经节传输	30～60 mg，2～3 次/日

SUGGESTED READINGS

Cheshire WP: Syncope, Continuum 23:335–358, 2017.

Cheshire WP, Goldstein DS: Autonomic uprising: the tilt table test in autonomic medicine, Clin Auton Res 29:215–230, 2019.

Cheshire WP, Goldstein DS: The physical examination as a window into autonomic disorders, Clin Auton Res 28:23–33, 2018.

Eschlböck S, Wenning G, Fanciulli A: Evidence-based treatment of neurogenic orthostatic hypotension and related symptoms, J Neural Transm 124:1567–1605, 2017.

Feldstein C, Weder AB: Orthostatic hypotension: a common, serious and under-recognized problem in hospitalized patients, J Am Soc Hypertens 6:27–39, 2013.

Figueroa JJ, Basford JR, Low PA: Preventing and treating orthostatic hypotension: as easy as A, B, C, Cleve, Clin J Med 77:298–306, 2010.

Goldstein DS, Cheshire WP: The autonomic medical history, Clin Auton Res 27:223–233, 2017.

Guzman JC, Armaganijan LV, Morillo CA: Treatment of neurally mediated reflex syncope, Cardiol Clin 31:123–129, 2013.

Karayannis G, Giamouzis G, Cokkinos DV, et al: Diabetic cardiovascular autonomic neuropathy: clinical implications, Expert Rev Cardiovasc Ther 10:747–765, 2012.

Koike H, Watanabe H, Sobue G: The spectrum of immune-mediated autonomic neuropathies: insights from the clinicopathological features, J Neurol Neurosurg Psychiatry 84:98–106, 2013.

Spallone V, Ziegler D, Freeman R, et al: Cardiovascular autonomic neuropathy in diabetes: clinical impact, assessment, diagnosis, and management, Diabetes Metab Res Rev 27:639–653, 2011.

Stewart JM: Common syndromes of orthostatic intolerance, Pediatrics 131:968–980, 2013.

Wenning GK, Geser F, Krismer F, et al: The natural history of multiple system atrophy: a prospective European cohort study, Lancet Neurol 12:264–274, 2013.

推荐阅读

Cheshire WP: Syncope, Continuum 23:335–358, 2017.

Cheshire WP, Goldstein DS: Autonomic uprising: the tilt table test in autonomic medicine, Clin Auton Res 29:215–230, 2019.

Cheshire WP, Goldstein DS: The physical examination as a window into autonomic disorders, Clin Auton Res 28:23–33, 2018.

Eschlböck S, Wenning G, Fanciulli A: Evidence-based treatment of neurogenic orthostatic hypotension and related symptoms, J Neural Transm 124:1567–1605, 2017.

Feldstein C, Weder AB: Orthostatic hypotension: a common, serious and under-recognized problem in hospitalized patients, J Am Soc Hypertens 6:27–39, 2013.

Figueroa JJ, Basford JR, Low PA: Preventing and treating orthostatic hypotension: as easy as A, B, C, Cleve, Clin J Med 77:298–306, 2010.

Goldstein DS, Cheshire WP: The autonomic medical history, Clin Auton Res 27:223–233, 2017.

Guzman JC, Armaganijan LV, Morillo CA: Treatment of neurally mediated reflex syncope, Cardiol Clin 31:123–129, 2013.

Karayannis G, Giamouzis G, Cokkinos DV, et al: Diabetic cardiovascular autonomic neuropathy: clinical implications, Expert Rev Cardiovasc Ther 10:747–765, 2012.

Koike H, Watanabe H, Sobue G: The spectrum of immune-mediated autonomic neuropathies: insights from the clinicopathological features, J Neurol Neurosurg Psychiatry 84:98–106, 2013.

Spallone V, Ziegler D, Freeman R, et al: Cardiovascular autonomic neuropathy in diabetes: clinical impact, assessment, diagnosis, and management, Diabetes Metab Res Rev 27:639–653, 2011.

Stewart JM: Common syndromes of orthostatic intolerance, Pediatrics 131:968–980, 2013.

Wenning GK, Geser F, Krismer F, et al: The natural history of multiple system atrophy: a prospective European cohort study, Lancet Neurol 12:264–274, 2013.

8

Headache, Neck and Back Pain, and Cranial Neuralgias

Shane Lyons, Timothy J. Counihan

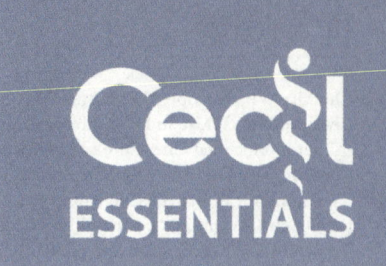

HEADACHE

Definition and Epidemiology

Headache is caused by irritation of pain-sensitive intracranial structures, including the dural sinuses; the intracranial portions of the trigeminal, glossopharyngeal, vagus, and upper cervical nerves; the large arteries; and the venous sinuses. Many structures are insensitive to pain, including the brain parenchyma, the ependymal lining of the ventricles, and the choroid plexuses. The insensitivity of the brain parenchyma to pain accounts for the common clinical observation of patients who, despite having large intracerebral lesions (such as a hematoma or a brain tumor), complain of little or no headache. The term "cervicogenic" headache is sometimes used to indicate that the source of headache (usually occipital in location) arises from an abnormality in the cervical spine.

Classification of Headache

Headache is generally classified into primary, secondary, and cranial neuralgia syndromes (Table 8.1, Table 8.2, Table 8.3). It is essential that the clinician make every effort to make an accurate clinical diagnosis of the presenting headache syndrome; Table 8.4 provides some key questions in the assessment of the patient with headache.

Migraine

Definition. Migraine is a common episodic neurologic disorder characterized by disabling headache and reversible neurologic and systemic symptoms. Migraine may be heralded by a premonitory phase of fatigue and neck stiffness, which precedes attacks by hours or days. One third of patients with migraine experience various combinations of neurologic, gastrointestinal, and autonomic phenomena (termed the "aura"). The diagnosis is based on the headache's characteristics and associated symptoms. Results of the physical examination as well as the laboratory studies are usually normal.

Every year, up to 18% of women and 6% of men experience a migraine attack. It is estimated that 28 million Americans have disabling migraine headaches. All varieties of migraine may begin at any age from early childhood on, although peak ages at onset are adolescence and early adulthood.

Several subtypes of migraine are described (Table 8.5). The two most common are migraine without aura and migraine with aura; migraine without aura accounts for 70% of patients. Migraine auras are focal neurologic symptoms that precede, accompany, or, rarely, follow an attack. The aura usually develops over 5 to 20 minutes, lasts less than 60 minutes, and can involve visual, sensorimotor, language, or brain stem disturbances. The most common aura is typified by positive visual phenomena (such as scintillating scotomata [zig zag, shimmering or colored lines] or fortification spectra [more complex images sometimes resembling a fortress]) that often precede the headache. Auras may also occur in the absence of headache (acephalgic migraine), particularly later in life. Migraine auras are stereotyped and a sudden change in a previously predictable aura pattern should prompt evaluation for an aura mimic.

The differential diagnosis of an aura includes a focal epileptic seizure arising from the visual cortex of the occipital lobe, a transient ischemic attack (TIA), or "amyloid spells" occurring in the context of cerebral amyloid angiopathy. In the latter, there is no evolution of symptoms, and the symptoms themselves are typically "negative" (such as a hemianopia) rather than the "positive" visual phenomenon of phosphenes that is characteristic of the migrainous aura. Amyloid spells are associated with evolving and "positive" symptoms and may be difficult to accurately distinguish clinically from migraine aura. The pain of migraine is often pulsating, unilateral, frontotemporal in distribution, exacerbated by movement, and usually accompanied by anorexia, nausea, and, occasionally, vomiting. In characteristic attacks, patients are markedly intolerant of light (photophobia) and seek rest in a dark room. There may also be intolerance to sound (phonophobia) and occasionally to odors (osmophobia). The diagnosis of migraine requires the presence of at least one of these features, particularly in the absence of gastrointestinal symptoms. The presence of these symptoms results in a syndrome that is invariably disabling for the patient, to the extent that for the duration of the attack he or she is unable to function normally. Following resolution of headache, a postdromal phase characterized by asthenia, fatigue, poor concentration, and nausea may persist for hours. In children, migraine is often associated with episodic abdominal pain, motion sickness, vertigo, and sleep disturbances. Onset of typical migraine late in life (older than age 50) is rare, although recurrence of migraine that had been in remission is not uncommon. Recurrent migraine headache associated with transient hemiparesis or hemiplegia occurs rarely as a clearly genetically determined (mendelian) disease, most commonly due to mutations of the *CACNA1A* gene *(familial hemiplegic migraine).*

Migraine with basilar aura is unusual and occurs primarily in childhood. Severe episodic headache is preceded, or accompanied by, signs of bilateral occipital lobe, brain stem, or cerebellar dysfunction (e.g., diplopia, bilateral visual field abnormalities, ataxia, dysarthria, bilateral sensory disturbances, other cranial nerve signs, and occasionally coma). *Vestibular migraine* is characterized by symptoms of vertigo with or without the other typical migraine symptoms. A number of episodic syndromes have been identified that bear similarities to migraine; these include cyclical vomiting, abdominal migraine, benign paroxysmal vertigo, and benign paroxysmal torticollis.

Complications of migraine. Status migrainosus refers to a severe migraine lasting greater than 72 hours. *Migrainous infarction* is a rare complication of migraine with aura. The term *migralepsy* has been suggested for patients in whom an aura triggers a seizure.

头痛、颈背痛和脑神经痛

姜南 译 沈航 韩菲 审校 姚明 朱以诚 通审

头痛

定义和流行病学

头痛由颅内痛敏结构受到刺激引起。颅内痛敏结构包括：硬膜窦，三叉神经、舌咽神经、迷走神经和上颈段神经的颅内部分，大动脉和静脉窦。脑实质、脑室的室管膜层和脉络丛等结构对疼痛不敏感。脑实质对疼痛不敏感解释了临床上的常见现象，即尽管存在大的颅内病变（如血肿或脑肿瘤），但患者头痛轻微或没有头痛主诉。"颈源性"头痛有时用来表示头痛（通常位于枕部）来源于颈椎异常。

头痛分类

头痛通常分为原发性头痛、继发性头痛以及脑神经痛综合征（表8.1、表8.2和表8.3）。临床医生必须尽最大努力对头痛综合征做出准确的临床诊断。表8.4提供了评估头痛患者时的一些关键问题。

偏头痛

定义 偏头痛是一种常见的发作性神经系统疾病，以致残性头痛、可逆的神经和系统性症状为特征。偏头痛发作前数小时或数天可出现前驱期症状，表现为疲劳、颈僵。1/3的偏头痛患者会经历神经、胃肠道和自主神经症状的各种组合（称为"先兆"）。诊断基于头痛的特点和伴随症状。体格检查和实验室检查结果通常正常。

每年，多达18%的女性和6%的男性会经历偏头痛发作。据估计，有2800万美国人患有致残性偏头痛。各种类型的偏头痛虽然可在儿童早期任何年龄发病，但好发于青春期和成年早期。

几种偏头痛亚型已被描述（表8.5）。最常见的两种亚型是无先兆偏头痛和有先兆偏头痛，前者占偏头痛患者的70%。偏头痛先兆是局灶神经系统症状，可在头痛前或头痛期出现，罕见情况下也可在头痛后出现。先兆通常逐渐发展超过5～20 min，持续时间小于60 min，可表现为视觉、感觉运动、语言或脑干功能障碍。最常见的先兆表现为阳性视觉症状［如闪烁暗点（锯齿状、闪光或彩色的线条）或堡垒幻影（有时类似于城堡的复杂图案）］，通常发生在头痛之前。先兆也可能在没有头痛的情况下出现（无头痛性偏头痛），尤其是在晚年时。偏头痛的先兆是刻板的，如果先前规律的先兆模式突然改变，应该对表现类似先兆的疾病进行评估。

先兆的鉴别诊断包括起源于枕叶视觉皮质的局灶性癫痫发作、短暂性脑缺血发作（TIA）或脑淀粉样血管病的"淀粉样发作"。TIA的症状缺乏演变，症状本身通常是"阴性"症状（如偏盲）而不是偏头痛先兆特有的"阳性"光幻视等视觉现象。淀粉样发作症状表现为逐渐发展的"阳性"症状，在临床上可能难以与偏头痛先兆准确区分。偏头痛的疼痛通常是搏动性的、单侧的，位于额颞部，运动可加重疼痛，通常伴有厌食、恶心，有时伴呕吐。在典型的偏头痛发作中，患者明显对光不耐受（畏光），会寻求在黑暗的房间中休息。还可能出现对声音不耐受（畏声），偶有对气味不耐受（畏嗅）。偏头痛的诊断需要具备上述特征中的至少一项，特别是在没有胃肠道症状的情况下。这些症状不可避免地使患者失能，以至于在发作期无法正常工作或生活。头痛缓解后，可能会出现持续数小时的恢复期症状，如虚弱、疲劳、注意力不集中和恶心。儿童偏头痛常伴随发作性腹痛、晕动病、眩晕和睡眠紊乱。虽然先前已缓解的偏头痛在年龄大时复发并不少见，但是晚发（年龄大于50岁）的典型偏头痛罕见。伴有短暂性轻瘫或偏瘫的复发性偏头痛是一种罕见（孟德尔）遗传病，最常由于 *CACNA1A* 基因突变导致（家族性偏瘫型偏头痛）。

基底先兆性偏头痛不常见，主要见于儿童。在重度发作性头痛之前，或发作过程中，出现双侧枕叶、脑干或小脑功能障碍的体征（例如，复视、双侧视野异常、共济失调、构音障碍、双侧感觉障碍、其他脑神经体征，偶见昏迷）。前庭性偏头痛表现为眩晕症状，伴或不伴其他典型偏头痛症状。已经确定了一些类似偏头痛的发作性综合征，包括周期性呕吐、腹型偏头痛、良性阵发性眩晕和良性阵发性斜颈。

偏头痛并发症 偏头痛持续状态是指持续时间大于72 h的严重偏头痛。偏头痛性梗死是有先兆偏头痛的罕见并发症。"偏头痛癫痫"被建议用于偏头痛先兆诱发的痫性发作患者。

TABLE 8.1 Primary Headache Syndromes

Migraine
Tension-type headache
Trigeminal autonomic cephalgias
- Cluster
- Paroxysmal hemicrania
- SUNCT

Other primary headache syndromes
- Primary stabbing headache
- Exertional/sex headache
- Primary thunderclap headache
- Hemicrania continua

SUNCT, Sudden-onset unilateral neuralgiform (headache with) conjunctival tearing.

TABLE 8.2 Secondary Headache Syndromes

Post-traumatic
Vascular
- Subarachnoid hemorrhage
- Vasculitis
- Arterial Dissection (carotid or vertebral)

Nonvascular
- Idiopathic intracranial hypertension (pseudotumor cerebri)
- Low CSF pressure (e.g., post lumbar puncture or CSF leak)
- Tumor
- Chiari malformation

Infection
- Meningitis
- Abscess
- Sinusitis

Disordered Homeostasis
- Hypoxia or hypercapnia (e.g., obstructive sleep apnea)
- Dialysis-associated headache
- Hypoglycemia

Medication
- Side effects (e.g., dipyridamole, nitrates, cyclosporine)
- Withdrawal

Syndrome of Transient Headache and Neurological Deficits With CSF Lymphocytosis (HANDL)
Cervicogenic

CSF, Cerebrospinal fluid.

TABLE 8.3 Common Cranial Neuralgias and Related Disorders

Trigeminal neuralgia
Glossopharyngeal neuralgia
Occipital neuralgia
Other cranial branch neuralgias (e.g., superior orbital neuralgia)
Central facial pain syndromes (e.g., cold-stimulus headache)

TABLE 8.4 Key Questions in the Assessment of Headache

1. For how long have you been having headaches?
2. What were they like when they first began? Were they intermittent, daily persistent, or progressive from the beginning?
3. What is the length of time from the start of the headache until its peak intensity?
4. Are there any warning symptoms (e.g., aura)?
5. Does the headache interfere significantly with normal activity (e.g., work, school)?
6. What aggravates the headache (e.g., light, noise, odors)?
7. What do you do for relief from the headache (e.g., rest, move around, take medication)?
8. What time of day are the headaches most likely to occur? Do they regularly awaken you from sleep?
9. Are you aware of any specific triggers (e.g., foods, stress, lack of sleep, menstrual cycle)?
10. Does anyone else in the family have headaches?

TABLE 8.5 Classification of Migraine

Migraine without aura
Migraine with aura
Migraine variants
- Hemiplegic migraine
- Migraine with basilar aura
- Vestibular migraine
- Retinal migraine

Pathophysiology of migraine. A migraine attack is the end result of the interaction of a number of factors of varying importance in different individuals. These factors include a genetic predisposition, a susceptibility of the central nervous system to certain stimuli, hormonal factors, and a sequence of neurovascular events. A positive family history is reported in 65% to 91% of cases. Three distinct ion channel gene mutations have been identified in patients with familial hemiplegic migraine (FHM), including a mutation in the *P/Q* type calcium channel on chromosome 19 (FHM 1) and a gene encoding a Na/K− ion pump on chromosome 1 (FHM 2). These findings lend support to the theory that migraine may be a true channelopathy in which mutations of diverse channels result in a common phenotype. The etiology of migraine in the majority of patients remains unknown.

The migrainous aura is likely caused by a "cortical spreading depression," corresponding to a wave of neuronal depolarization spreading over the cortex from posterior to anterior. One of the key structures in the mechanism of pain in migraine is the trigeminal vascular system. Stimulation of the trigeminal nucleus caudalis can activate serotonin receptors and nerve endings on small dural arteries and result in a state of neurogenic inflammation. Activation of the trigeminal ganglion nociceptive (pain) neurons results in the release of calcitonin gene-related peptide (CGRP), a vasoactive peptide that is strongly implicated in the generation of migraine. The critical role of CGRP in migraine has been demonstrated through the induction of migraine by infusing CGRP, while treatment with potent CGRP inhibitors can abort an acute migraine attack. It is postulated that these processes, in turn, stimulate perivascular nerve endings, with resultant orthodromic (normal direction) stimulation of trigeminal nerve and pain referred to its territory. Furthermore, positron emission tomographic (PET) studies have demonstrated activation of brain stem neuromodulatory structures, including the periaqueductal gray matter, locus coeruleus, and raphe nuclei during a migraine attack.

Treatment of migraine. The goals of treatment are (1) making an accurate and confident diagnosis of migraine to reassure the patient that there is no more sinister cause for the headache; (2) relieving acute attacks; and (3) preventing pain and associated symptoms

表 8.1 原发性头痛综合征

偏头痛
紧张型头痛
三叉神经自主神经性头痛
- 丛集性头痛
- 阵发性偏侧头痛
- SUNCT

其他原发性头痛综合征
- 原发性针刺样头痛
- 劳力性/性交头痛
- 原发性霹雳性头痛
- 持续性偏侧头痛

SUNCT，伴结膜充血和流泪的短暂性单侧神经痛样头痛。

表 8.2 继发性头痛综合征

外伤后
血管性
- 蛛网膜下腔出血
- 血管炎
- 动脉夹层（颈动脉或椎动脉）

非血管性
- 特发性颅内高压（假脑瘤）
- 脑脊液低压（例如，腰椎穿刺后或脑脊液漏）
- 肿瘤
- Chiari 畸形

感染
- 脑膜炎
- 脓肿
- 鼻窦炎

内环境紊乱
- 缺氧或高碳酸血症（例如，阻塞性睡眠呼吸暂停）
- 透析相关头痛
- 低血糖

药物
- 副作用（例如，双嘧达莫、硝酸盐、环孢素）
- 戒断

短暂性头痛和神经功能缺损伴脑脊液淋巴细胞增多（HANDL）综合征
颈源性

表 8.3 常见的脑神经痛和相关疾病

三叉神经痛
舌咽神经痛
枕神经痛
其他脑神经分支神经痛（如眶上神经痛）
中枢性面痛综合征（如冷刺激性头痛）

表 8.4 头痛评估中的关键问题

1. 您头痛多久了？
2. 头痛刚开始的时候是什么样的？是间歇性的，每日持续性的，还是从一开始就进行性加重？
3. 头痛从开始到最严重用了多长时间？
4. 是否有任何预警症状（如先兆）？
5. 头痛是否显著干扰正常活动（如工作、上学）？
6. 什么会加重头痛（如光、声、气味）？
7. 做什么可缓解头痛（如休息、走动、服药）？
8. 一天中什么时候最容易头痛？你会在睡眠中被痛醒吗？
9. 你是否知道特定的诱因（如食物、压力、睡眠不足、月经周期）？
10. 家里还有其他人头痛吗？

表 8.5 偏头痛的分类

无先兆偏头痛
有先兆偏头痛
偏头痛变异型
- 偏瘫型偏头痛
- 基底先兆性偏头痛
- 前庭性偏头痛
- 视网膜型偏头痛

65%～91% 的病例有阳性家族史。在家族性偏瘫型偏头痛（FHM）患者中已确定三种不同的离子通道基因突变，包括 19 号染色体上的 P/Q 型钙通道基因突变（FHM 1）和 1 号染色体上编码 Na/K 离子泵的基因突变（FHM 2）。这些发现支持偏头痛可能是一种真正的通道病的理论，不同的通道突变导致共同的表型。大多数偏头痛患者的病因仍然未知。

偏头痛先兆可能是由"皮质扩散性抑制"引起的，对应了沿皮质从后向前的神经元去极化波。偏头痛的疼痛机制中，一个关键结构是三叉神经血管系统。刺激三叉神经尾核可以激活 5-羟色胺受体和硬膜小动脉上的神经末梢，导致神经源性炎症状态。激活三叉神经节伤害性（疼痛）神经元会释放降钙素基因相关肽（CGRP），CGRP 是一种与偏头痛的发生密切相关的血管活性肽。注射 CGRP 可诱发偏头痛，使用强效 CGRP 抑制剂治疗可终止急性偏头痛发作，这证明 CGRP 在偏头痛中起关键作用。据推测，这些过程反过来刺激血管周围神经末梢，导致三叉神经的顺向（正向）刺激，产生其支配区的疼痛。此外，正电子发射断层成像（PET）研究表明，在偏头痛发作时，导水管周围灰质、蓝斑和中缝核等脑干神经调节结构均被激活。

偏头痛的治疗 治疗的目标包括：①准确且自信地诊断偏头痛以使患者安心，使患者确信头痛没有其他不祥的原因；②缓解急性发作；③预防复发性头痛

偏头痛的病理生理学 偏头痛发作是多种因素相互作用的结果，这些因素在不同个体中有不同的重要性。这些因素包括遗传易感性、中枢神经系统对特定刺激的敏感性、激素因素以及一系列神经血管事件。

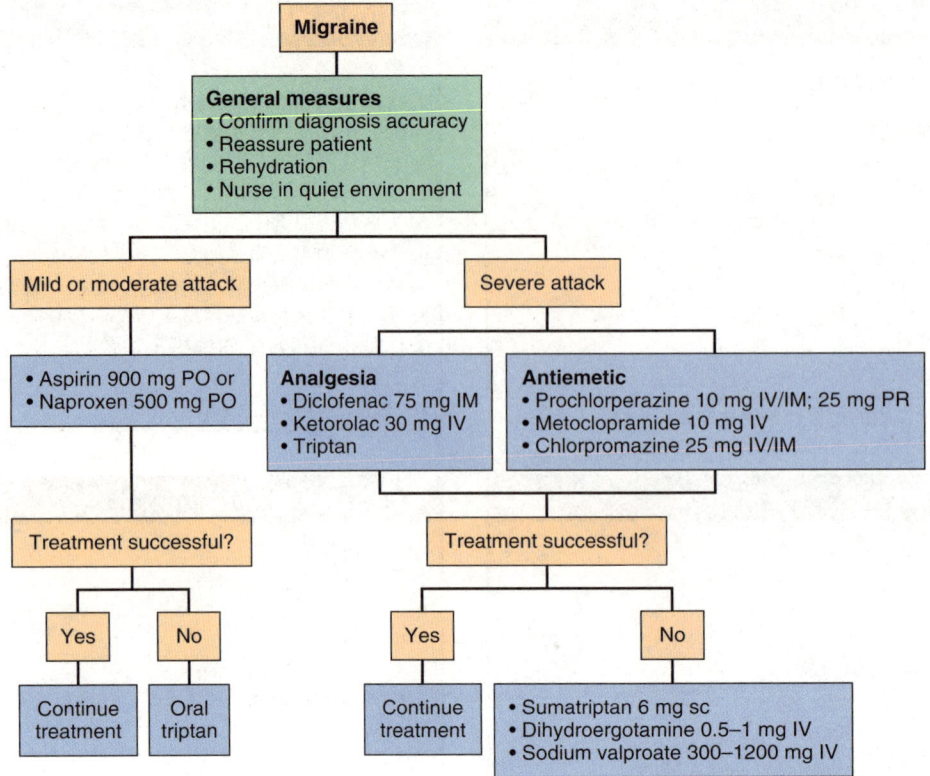

Fig. 8.1 Algorithm for the treatment of migraine. *DHE*, Dihydroergotamine; *IM*, intramuscular; *IV*, intravenous; *NS*, normal saline; *NSAIDs*, nonsteroidal anti-inflammatory drugs; *SC*, subcutaneous.

of recurrent headaches. The first step is to inform the patient that he or she has a migraine. The benign nature of the disorder and the patient's central role in the treatment plan should be emphasized. It is important that the patient keep a headache diary, which serves to help identify covert headache triggers, assists in monitoring headache frequency and response to treatment, and actively involves the patient in the management of the condition. A sustained pain-free therapeutic response should aim to have the patient pain-free at 2 hours with no recurrence and no need for subsequent rescue medication.

Acute migraine attack. Acute attacks are best alleviated using a stratified, rather than stepped care approach, using single agents or varying combinations of drugs as well as with behavioral modification therapy. Many attacks of migraine respond to simple analgesics, such as acetaminophen, aspirin, or nonsteroidal anti-inflammatory agents (NSAIDs). Opioid drugs and butalbital should not be used in the routine management of patients with migraine. Overuse of analgesics is particularly frequent in headache patients; therefore, one of the most important aspects of therapy is the monitoring of amounts of analgesic used to avoid both side effects and the emergence of medication-associated headache. In patients who are nauseated, it is often helpful to prescribe an antiemetic agent early in an attack. Phenothiazine drugs have antiemetic, prokinetic, and sedative properties, but they can produce involuntary movements as an acute adverse effect (acute dystonic reaction) or with prolonged use (tardive dyskinesias).

A number of *migraine-specific* serotonin agonist drugs have become available. These agents, commonly referred to as "triptans," are useful in the acute treatment of migraine, having a rapid onset of action. The increasing availability of non-oral (parenteral, inhaled, and transdermal) preparations has largely circumvented the problem of emesis and gastroparesis in migraine patients resulting in greater efficacy. For instance, sumatriptan, available as a subcutaneous preparation, results in a headache response rate of close to 70% (Fig. 8.1). Although triptans are highly effective in alleviating migraine, patients must be carefully instructed in their appropriate use. Moreover, a response to these medications does not confirm a diagnosis of migraine.

Treating acute migraine in the emergency room. Migraine is one of the most common reasons for emergency room visits and presents some treatment challenges; typically migraine is more difficult to treat once it is fully established. It is essential to confirm that the diagnosis is accurate, even in patients with an established history of migraine. Patients will usually be aware that the headache will have started as their typical migraine, although it may be more severe than usual. In patients who state that the new headache is different than their usual headache, consideration should be given to exclude a more sinister cause. Thereafter the core principles of treatment include reassurance that the headache can be treated effectively, hydration, pain control, and relief of accompanying symptoms such as nausea and photophobia. The majority of patients presenting with acute migraine as an emergency will have already tried some form of abortive therapy, and they are likely to be dehydrated. In this setting parenteral therapy with an NSAID, a triptan, and an antiemetic is often effective. 5-HT1F receptor agonists (ditans), such as lamiditan, may offer similar benefits to triptans without the vasoconstrictive effect of triptans.

Migraine prevention. Several agents have a strong evidence base for efficacy in the prevention of migraine (Table 8.6). The use of these agents should be restricted to patients who have frequent attacks (usually more than four per month) and who are willing to take daily medication. With any of the medications, an adequate trial period should be given, using adequate doses, before it is declared ineffective. Combination therapy is occasionally required but is not routinely prescribed. For a preventative drug to be considered successful, it should reduce the headache frequency rate by at least

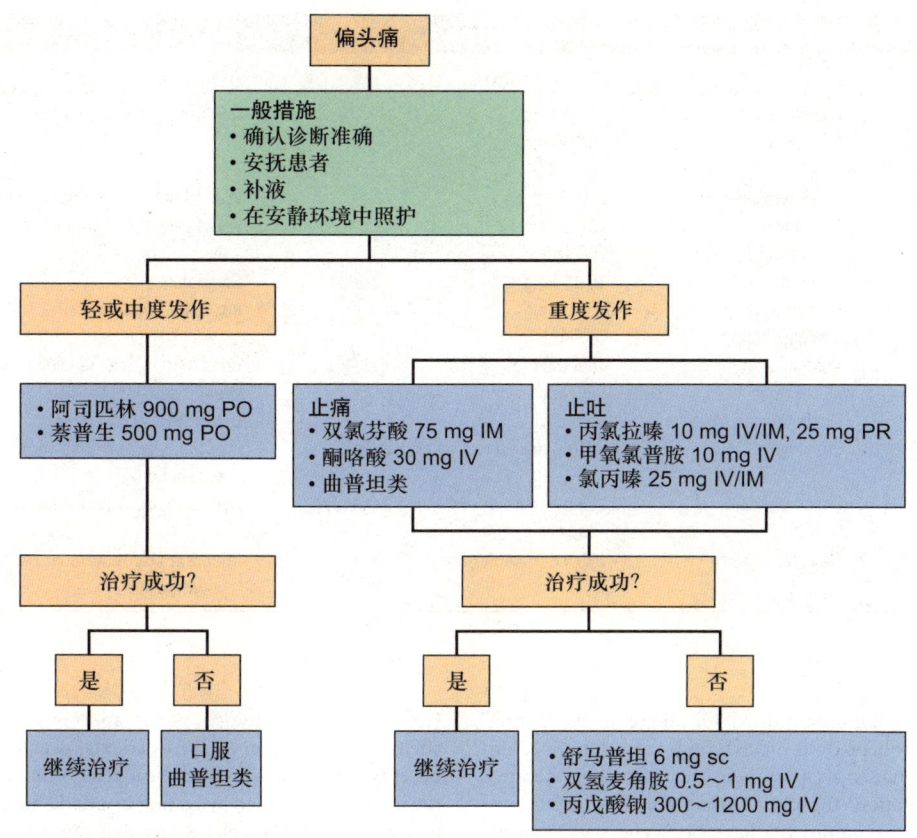

图 8.1 偏头痛的治疗流程图。IM，肌内注射；IV，静脉注射；PO，口服；PR，灌肠；SC，皮下

的疼痛和伴随症状。第一步是告知患者患有偏头痛。应强调这种疾病的良性本质以及患者在治疗计划中的核心作用。患者坚持记录头痛日记非常重要，这有助于识别隐匿的头痛诱发因素，帮助监测头痛频率和对治疗的反应，并让患者积极参与疾病管理。持续无痛的治疗反应旨在使患者在 2 h 内达到无痛状态，且无复发、无需后续的补救药物。

急性偏头痛发作 急性发作的最佳缓解方式是分层治疗，而不是阶梯治疗，可以使用单一药物或不同药物的组合，还可以结合行为矫正疗法。对乙酰氨基酚、阿司匹林或非甾体抗炎药（NSAID）等简单的镇痛药对许多偏头痛发作有效。阿片类药物和布他比妥不应常规用于治疗偏头痛。头痛患者过度使用镇痛药的情况特别常见；因此，治疗中重要的一点是监测镇痛药的用量，以避免副作用和药物相关性头痛的出现。对于伴有恶心的患者，在发作早期开具止吐药通常会有帮助。吩噻嗪类药物具有止吐、促胃动力和镇静作用，但它们可能会产生不自主运动，可为急性不良反应（急性肌张力障碍反应）或在长期使用后出现（迟发性运动障碍）。

一些偏头痛特异性 5-羟色胺激动剂药物已经问世。这些药物通常被称为"曲普坦类"，用于偏头痛的急性治疗，它们有效且起效快。非口服（胃肠外、吸入和透皮）制剂的日益普及大大规避了偏头痛患者的呕吐和胃轻瘫问题，从而提高了疗效。例如，舒马普坦皮下给药，头痛缓解率接近 70%（图 8.1）。虽然曲普坦类药物在缓解偏头痛方面非常有效，但是必须仔细指导患者正确使用。此外，对这些药物有反应并不能证实偏头痛的诊断。

在急诊室治疗急性偏头痛 偏头痛是急诊室就诊的最常见原因之一，治疗具有挑战性；典型的偏头痛一旦完全发作就更难治疗。准确诊断至关重要，即使是对有偏头痛病史的患者也应再确认。患者通常会意识到头痛开始时是典型的偏头痛，尽管它可能比平时更严重。对于声称新发头痛与既往不同的患者，应考虑排除更严重的病因。此后，治疗的核心原则包括保证头痛可得到有效治疗、水化、控制疼痛以及缓解伴随症状如恶心和畏光。就诊于急诊室的大多数急性偏头痛患者已尝试过某种中止头痛的急性治疗，并可能出现脱水。在这种情况下，胃肠外给予非甾体抗炎药（NSAID）、曲普坦类和止吐药通常有效。5-HT1F 受体激动剂（地坦类），如拉米地坦，可能具有与曲普坦类相似的益处，但没有曲普坦类的缩血管作用。

偏头痛的预防 一些药物在预防偏头痛方面有很强的疗效证据（表 8.6）。用药应仅限于偏头痛频繁发作（通常每月 4 次以上）和愿意每天服药的患者。对于任何一种药物，在判定无效之前，应给予充足的用药观察期，并使用足够的剂量。偶尔需要联合用药但不建议常规使用。有效的预防药物应该将头痛发作频率降低至少

TABLE 8.6 Preventive Therapies for Migraine

Drug Class	Agent	Dose Range	Adverse Effects
β-Adrenoceptor blockers	Propranolol	80-240 mg	Contraindicated in asthma, syncope
	Metoprolol	50-150 mg	
	Timolol	10-20 mg	
Antiepileptic drugs	Divalproex sodium	200-1500 mg	Weight gain, thrombocytopenia, tremor
	Topiramate	25-150 mg	Renal calculi, weight loss, amnesia, glaucoma, dysequilibrium
	Gabapentin	300-1800 mg	
Antidepressants	Amitriptyline	10-150 mg	Somnolence
	Nortriptyline	25-100 mg	Insomnia, hypertension
	Venlafaxine	37.5-150 mg	
Calcium-channel blockers	Verapamil	180-480 mg	Constipation, hypotension, edema
	Flunarizine[a]	5-10 mg	Weight gain, depression
Other	Onabotulinum toxin A	Variable	Discomfort, ecchymosis
CGRP monoclonal antibodies	Erenumab	70-140 mg every 4 week, subcut	Injection site reactions, muscle spasm, hypersensitivity reaction.
	Fremanezumab	225 mg monthly or 675 mg 3-monthly, subcut	Hypersensitivity and injection site reactions
	Galcanezumab	120 mg monthly subcut	Injection site reactions, vertigo, pruritus, constipation

[a]Not available in the United States.

50%. Other medications commonly used for migraine prevention include gabapentin, cyproheptadine, methysergide, and clonidine, but these have limited evidence to support their use as first-line therapy. Magnesium supplementation, the plant extract feverfew, butterbur, and high-dose riboflavin (vitamin B_2) have been effective in some patients.

Recent years have seen the emergence of the first medications specifically designed to treat migraine based on pathophysiologic understanding of migraine; monoclonal antibodies directed against CGRP. A number of medications targeting the CGRP cascade in migraine have been developed, including small molecule CGRP antagonists (gepants) and monoclonal antibodies directed against both the CGRP receptor and the CGRP molecule itself. Three CGRP monoclonal antibodies have been approved for the prevention of migraine (erenumab, fremanezumab, and galcanezumab). They are administered by infusion or subcutaneous injection and in trials improved headache by 75% in one third of patients.

A variety of interventional procedures including greater occipital nerve blockade, botulinum toxin injection to the scalp and cervical musculature, and sphenopalatine ganglion (SPG) blockade are deployed in the management of severe and chronic migraine. Neuromodulation, by means of noninvasive vagal nerve stimulation, external trigeminal nerve stimulation, and transcranial magnetic stimulation represents a novel, nonpharmacologic method of migraine management.

Cluster Headache

Clinical features. Cluster headache is the prototypic trigeminal autonomic cephalgia, entirely distinct from migraine, although there may be some clinical overlap. It is uncommon, occurring in less than 10% of all patients with headache. Unlike migraine, it is much more common in men than in women, and the mean age at onset is later in life. Also, unlike migraine, cluster headache rarely begins in childhood, and there is less often a family history. The pain in cluster headache is extremely intense, is strictly unilateral, and is associated with congestion of the nasal mucosa and injection of the conjunctiva on the side of the pain. Increased sweating of the ipsilateral side of the forehead and face may occur. There may be associated ocular signs of Horner syndrome: miosis, ptosis, and the additional feature of eyelid edema. Attacks often awaken patients, usually 2 to 3 hours after the onset of sleep ("alarm-clock headache"). In contrast to migraineurs, the pain is not relieved by resting in a dark, quiet area; on the contrary, patients sometimes seek activity that can distract them. The duration of headache is usually around 1 hour, although it may recur several times in a day, paroxysmally (in *clusters*) for several weeks.

These periods of frequent headaches are separated by headache-free periods of varying duration, often several months or years. Attacks have a striking tendency to be precipitated by even small amounts of alcohol. There are rare variants of cluster headache: a "chronic variety" in which remissions are brief (less than 14 days); *chronic paroxysmal hemicrania,* in which attacks are shorter and strikingly more prevalent in women; and *hemicrania continua,* in which there is continuous, moderately severe, unilateral headache. The cause of all these syndromes is unknown, although the distribution of the pain suggests dysfunction of the trigeminal nerve.

Treatment. Therapy for cluster headache may be abortive for acute headache or prophylactic to prevent headache. Acute headache may respond to oxygen by mask (7 to 10 L/min for 15 minutes), which is effective within several minutes in 70% of patients. Sumatriptan and dihydroergotamine are also effective. Preventive medications include lithium, divalproex sodium, verapamil, methysergide, melatonin, and corticosteroids. Noninvasive vagal nerve stimulation is now licensed for the acute treatment of episode cluster headache and has evidence to support its use in prevention. Emerging treatments include galcanezumab and SPG stimulation. Paroxysmal hemicrania and related syndromes are often strikingly responsive to indomethacin.

Tension-Type Headache

In contrast to migraine, tension-type headache is featureless. The pain is usually not throbbing, but rather steady and often described as a "pressure feeling" or a "viselike" sensation. It is usually not unilateral and may be frontal, occipital, or generalized. There is frequently pain in the neck area, unlike in migraine. Pain commonly lasts for long periods of time (days) and does not rapidly appear and disappear in attacks. There is no "aura." Photophobia and phonophobia are not

表 8.6 偏头痛的预防性治疗

药物分类	药剂	剂量范围	不良反应
β 肾上腺素受体阻滞剂	普萘洛尔	80~240 mg	哮喘、晕厥禁用
	美托洛尔	50~150 mg	
	噻吗洛尔	10~20 mg	
抗癫痫药	双丙戊酸钠	200~1500 mg	体重增加、血小板减少、震颤
	托吡酯	25~150 mg	肾结石、体重下降、记忆下降、青光眼、平衡障碍
	加巴喷丁	300~1800 mg	
抗抑郁药	阿米替林	10~150 mg	嗜睡
	去甲替林	25~100 mg	失眠、高血压
	文拉法辛	37.5~150 mg	
钙通道阻滞剂	维拉帕米	180~480 mg	便秘、低血压、水肿
	氟桂利嗪[a]	5~10 mg	体重增加、抑郁
其他	A 型肉毒毒素	可变	不适、瘀斑
CGRP 单克隆抗体	依瑞奈尤单抗（Erenumab）	每 4 周 70~140 mg，皮下注射	注射部位反应、肌肉痉挛、过敏反应
	瑞玛奈珠单抗（Fremanezumab）	每月 225 mg 或每 3 个月 675 mg，皮下注射	过敏和注射部位反应
	加卡奈珠单抗（Galcanezumab）	每月 120 mg，皮下注射	注射部位反应、眩晕、瘙痒、便秘

[a] 在美国无法获得。

50%。其他常用于预防偏头痛的药物包括加巴喷丁、赛庚啶、美西麦角和可乐定，但这些药物作为一线治疗的支持证据有限。补充镁、植物提取物小白菊、蜂斗菜和大剂量核黄素（维生素 B_2）对一些患者有效。

近年来，首次出现了基于对偏头痛病理生理机制的理解而设计的偏头痛治疗药物，这些药物是抗 CGRP 的单克隆抗体。已经开发出了治疗偏头痛的靶向 CGRP 通路的药物，包括小分子 CGRP 拮抗剂（吉泮类）以及抗 CGRP 受体和抗 CGRP 分子本身的单克隆抗体。已经有三种 CGRP 单克隆抗体获批用于偏头痛的预防性治疗［依瑞奈尤单抗（erenumab）、瑞玛奈珠单抗（fremanezumab）和加卡奈珠单抗（galcanezumab）］。它们通过静脉输注或皮下注射的方式给药，在试验中使 1/3 的患者头痛改善 75%。

多种介入操作已被用于治疗重度和慢性偏头痛，包括枕大神经阻滞、肉毒毒素头皮和颈部肌内注射、蝶腭神经节（SPG）阻滞。神经调控是一种新的非药物疗法，包括非侵入性迷走神经刺激、外周三叉神经刺激和经颅磁刺激。

丛集性头痛

临床特征 丛集性头痛是典型的三叉神经自主神经性头痛，虽然与偏头痛可能存在一些临床重叠，但两者完全不同。它并不常见，只出现在不到 10% 的头痛患者中。与偏头痛不同的是，丛集性头痛在男性中要远比女性更多见，平均发病年龄较晚。同样，与偏头痛不同的是，丛集性头痛很少在儿童期开始发病，家族史也少见。丛集性头痛的疼痛极其剧烈，严格单侧疼痛，并伴有疼痛同侧的鼻塞和结膜充血，可能出现同侧额面部出汗增加，可能伴有霍纳综合征的眼征：瞳孔缩小、上睑下垂，以及眼睑水肿的额外特征。头痛发作通常在入睡后 2~3 h 发作（"闹钟性头痛"），常使患者痛醒。与偏头痛患者不同，丛集性头痛患者在黑暗、安静的地方休息并不能缓解疼痛；相反，患者有时会寻求能分散注意力的活动。头痛持续时间通常约为 1 h，可能在一天内多次发作，反复阵发发作（成簇）持续数周。

头痛频发期与无头痛期交替出现，无头痛期通常持续几个月或几年。少量的饮酒往往就能促发头痛发作。丛集性头痛有一些罕见的变异型："慢性型"的缓解期很短（小于 14 天）；慢性阵发性偏侧头痛，发作持续时间更短，女性患者更多见；持续性偏侧头痛，表现为持续中重度的单侧疼痛。虽然疼痛的分布提示三叉神经功能障碍，但是所有这些综合征的病因都是未知的。

治疗 丛集性头痛的治疗包括终止头痛发作的急性治疗和防止头痛再发的预防性治疗。对于急性治疗，面罩吸氧（7~10 L/min，持续 15 min）可能有效，70% 的患者可在数分钟内见效；舒马普坦和双氢麦角胺也可能有效。预防性治疗药物包括锂剂、双丙戊酸钠、维拉帕米、美西麦角、褪黑素和皮质类固醇。非侵入性迷走神经刺激现已获批用于发作性丛集性头痛的急性治疗，并有证据支持其用于预防性治疗。新的治疗方法包括加卡奈珠单抗和蝶腭神经节刺激。对于阵发性偏侧头痛和相关综合征，吲哚美辛治疗常有显著效果。

紧张型头痛

与偏头痛相比，紧张型头痛缺乏特征。疼痛通常不是搏动性痛而是稳定的痛，常被描述为"压迫感"或"紧箍感"。疼痛通常不是单侧的，可能位于额部、枕部或整个头部。与偏头痛不同，紧张型头痛经常会有颈部疼痛。每次发作，疼痛通常持续很长时间（数天），疼

prominent. Although tension-type headache may be related by the patient to occur or be exacerbated at times of particular emotional stress, the pathophysiology may relate to sustained craniocervical muscle contraction; hence, a more useful term for this syndrome is *muscle-contraction headache.*

A careful evaluation should be made of the patient's psychosocial milieu and the presence of anxiety or depression. The tricyclic antidepressant drugs in low doses have proven the most useful for prevention of tension-type headache. Although the best documented is amitriptyline, newer agents with fewer side effects may be equally effective. Nonpharmacologic therapies such as relaxation therapy, massage, physiotherapy, or acupuncture may be useful in refractory cases. Intramuscular botulinum toxin injections have been used both in migraine and tension-type headache but are of established benefit only in patients with chronic migraine.

Other Defined Primary Headache Syndromes

Other acute short-lasting headache syndromes need to be differentiated from migraine, cluster, or tension headache. These include primary "thunderclap" headache, *primary stabbing headache, primary exertional headache,* and coital headache. The latter may be indistinguishable from the headache of intracranial aneurysm rupture and requires computed tomography (CT) and lumbar puncture to exclude subarachnoid hemorrhage (SAH). All of these headache syndromes are more common in migraineurs. Two additional rare, short-lasting headache syndromes deserve mention: short-lasting unilateral neuralgiform headache with conjunctival tearing (SUNCT) and *hypnic* headache. The latter refers to multiple episodes of very brief headache that awaken the patient (typically an older woman) from sleep. The syndrome of SUNCT causes multiple very brief (seconds to minutes) episodes of cluster-like headache and autonomic disturbance.

Chronic daily headache is defined arbitrarily as headache lasting for more than 4 hours on more than 15 days in the month for more than 3 months. In clinical practice this means that the patient has a headache more often than not. In these cases it is important to establish whether the headache syndrome began as an episodic disorder (as in migraine or tension-type headache) or whether it consists of new daily persistent headaches.

New daily persistent headache. New daily persistent headache needs to be distinguished from tension-type or migraine headaches that have transformed into chronic daily headache and necessitates investigation to exclude a secondary cause.

Headache may be a manifestation of underlying structural brain disease (see Table 8.2). Headache can be seen in all forms of cerebrovascular disease, including infarction, intracerebral hemorrhage, and SAH, although headache is rarely prominent in cerebral infarction. In contrast, the headache in SAH is usually extremely severe and often described by the patient as "the worst headache of my life." Nuchal rigidity, third nerve palsy (usually involving the pupil), and retinal, preretinal, or subconjunctival hemorrhages may be found. CT of the head usually shows subarachnoid, intraventricular, or other intracranial blood.

Certain symptoms raise suspicion for a structural brain lesion (Tables 8.7 and 8.8).

The patient with headache and fever presents a common diagnostic problem in the emergency department. Neck stiffness is a common symptom. Meningismus is confirmed by eliciting Brudzinski and Kernig signs. Vomiting occurs in about 50% of patients. Suspicion for meningitis should prompt immediate investigation, including a lumbar puncture. If the patient shows focal signs, papilledema, or profound alteration in level of consciousness, CT of the head before lumbar puncture is required to rule out focal disease such as an abscess or subdural empyema. These lesions, however, are rare.

Acute sinusitis. Head and face pain is the most prominent feature of sinusitis. Malaise and low-grade fever are usually present. The pain is dull, aching, and nonpulsatile; is exacerbated by movement, coughing, or straining; and is improved with nasal decongestants. The pain is most pronounced on awakening or after any prolonged recumbency and is diminished with maintenance of an upright posture.

The location of the pain depends on the sinus involved. Maxillary sinusitis provokes ipsilateral malar, ear, and dental pain with significant overlying facial tenderness. Frontal sinusitis produces frontal headache that may radiate behind the eyes and to the vertex of the skull. Tenderness to frontal palpation may be present with point tenderness on the undersurface of the medial aspect of the superior orbital rim. In ethmoidal sinusitis, the pain is between or behind the eyes with radiation to the temporal area. The eyes and orbit are often tender to palpation, and, in fact, eye movements themselves may accentuate the pain. Sphenoidal sinusitis causes pain in the orbit and at the vertex of the skull and occasionally in the frontal or occipital regions. Given that the trigeminal nerve mediates pain perception from the sinuses, many patients who complain of "sinus headaches" are probably suffering from the trigeminovascular disturbance of migraine, rather than sinusitis. Chronic sinusitis is seldom a cause of headache.

Brain tumors. Posterior fossa tumors (particularly of the cerebellum) frequently produce headache, especially if hydrocephalus

---

TABLE 8.7 Differential Diagnosis of Acute Headache: Major Causes

Migraine
Cluster headache
Stroke
- Subarachnoid hemorrhage
- Intracerebral hemorrhage
- Cerebral infarction
- Arterial dissection (carotid or vertebral)

Acute hydrocephalus
Meningitis or encephalitis
Giant cell arteritis (often chronic)
Tumor (usually chronic)
Trauma

TABLE 8.8 Clinical Features of Headaches Suggesting a Structural Brain Lesion

Symptoms
Worst of the patient's life
Progressive
Onset >50 years
Worse in early morning—awakens patient
Marked exacerbation with straining
Focal neurologic dysfunction

Signs
Nuchal rigidity
Fever
Papilledema
Pathologic reflexes or reflex asymmetry
Altered state of consciousness

痛的出现和消失不是很迅速。没有"先兆"。无明显畏光和畏声。虽然情绪紧张与紧张型头痛的发生或加重有关，但是其病理生理机制可能与持续的头颈肌肉收缩有关。因此，对该综合征更有用的术语是肌收缩性头痛。

应仔细评估患者的心理社会环境和是否存在焦虑或抑郁。已证实小剂量三环类抗抑郁药对预防紧张型头痛最有用。虽然阿米替林被认为最有效，但副作用更少的新型药物可能同样有效。非药物疗法，如放松疗法、按摩、理疗或针灸，对难治性病例可能有效。肉毒毒素肌内注射已经用于偏头痛和紧张型头痛，但只对慢性偏头痛患者有效。

其他已定义的原发性头痛综合征

其他急性短暂性头痛综合征需要与偏头痛、丛集性头痛或紧张型头痛鉴别，这些综合征包括原发性霹雳性头痛、原发性针刺样头痛、原发性劳力性头痛和性交头痛。性交头痛可能与颅内动脉瘤破裂的头痛难以区分，需要计算机断层成像（CT）和腰椎穿刺以排除蛛网膜下腔出血（SAH）。所有这些头痛综合征在偏头痛患者中更常见。值得一提的还有另外两种罕见的短暂性头痛综合征：伴结膜充血和流泪的短暂性单侧神经痛样头痛（SUNCT）和睡眠性头痛。睡眠性头痛是指很短的头痛多次发作并且使患者（通常是老年女性）从睡眠中醒来。SUNCT综合征引起多次非常短的（数秒至数分钟）丛集样头痛发作和自主神经障碍。

慢性每日头痛被定义为每次头痛超过4 h，每月头痛大于15天，并且持续3个月以上。在临床实践中，这意味着患者头痛日多于无痛日。这种情况下，重要的是确定这种头痛综合征是否以发作性疾病（如偏头痛或紧张型头痛）开始，还是它包含了新发每日持续性头痛。

新发每日持续性头痛 新发每日持续性头痛需要与转变为慢性每日头痛的紧张型头痛或偏头痛相鉴别，并需要检查以排除继发性头痛。

头痛可能是潜在结构性脑部疾病的表现（见表8.2）。头痛可见于所有形式的脑血管病，包括脑梗死、脑出血和蛛网膜下腔出血（SAH），尽管头痛很少是脑梗死的突出表现。相反，SAH的头痛通常极为严重，常被患者描述为"一生中最严重的头痛"。可能发现颈强直、第Ⅲ脑神经麻痹（通常累及瞳孔），以及视网膜、视网膜前或结膜下出血。头部CT通常显示蛛网膜下腔、脑室内或其他颅内出血。

某些症状需要怀疑结构性脑损伤（表8.7和表8.8）。

发热伴头痛的患者是急诊室中常见的诊断问题。颈部僵硬是常见症状。引出布鲁津斯基征和克尼格征可以确认存在脑膜刺激征。约50%的患者发生呕吐。怀疑脑膜炎应立即检查，包括腰椎穿刺。如果患者有局灶性体征、视盘水肿或意识水平显著改变等表现，则应在腰椎穿刺前进行头部CT检查以排除脓肿或硬膜下积脓等局灶性疾病。然而，这些病变很少见。

急性鼻窦炎 头面部痛是鼻窦炎的主要特征，通常伴有不适和低热。疼痛性质为钝痛、酸痛和非搏动性痛，运动、咳嗽或用力时加重，鼻腔减充血剂可缓解。疼痛在醒后或任何原因长时间卧床后最为明显，保持直立姿势则可减轻。

疼痛部位取决于受累的鼻窦。上颌窦炎引起同侧颧部、耳部痛和牙痛，并有明显的面部压痛。额窦炎引起额部头痛，可能放射到眼后和头顶。额部可能存在触痛，压痛点位于上眶缘内侧的下表面。筛窦炎的疼痛位于两眼之间或眼球后方，并放射到颞部。眼球和眼眶常有触诊压痛，眼球运动也可能加重疼痛。蝶窦炎引起眼眶和头顶痛，偶尔也有额部或枕部疼痛。由于来自鼻窦的疼痛感知是由三叉神经传导的，因此许多主诉"窦性头痛"的患者很可能是偏头痛引起的三叉神经血管紊乱，而不是鼻窦炎。慢性鼻窦炎很少引起头痛。

脑肿瘤 颅后窝肿瘤（尤其是小脑肿瘤）常引起

表 8.7　急性头痛的鉴别诊断：主要病因

偏头痛
丛集性头痛
卒中
- 蛛网膜下腔出血
- 脑出血
- 脑梗死
- 动脉夹层（颈动脉或椎动脉）

急性脑积水
脑膜炎或脑炎
巨细胞动脉炎（常为慢性）
肿瘤（通常为慢性）
外伤

表 8.8　提示结构性脑损伤的头痛的临床特征

症状
患者一生中最严重的头痛
进行性加重
起病 > 50 岁
晨起时加重——患者痛醒
用力时明显加重
局灶性神经功能障碍

体征
颈强直
发热
视盘水肿
病理反射或反射不对称
意识状态改变

occurs because cerebrospinal fluid (CSF) flow is partially obstructed. Supratentorial tumors, however, are less likely to cause headache and are more frequently heralded by altered mental status, focal deficits, or seizures. Although increased intracranial pressure is often associated with headache, it is usually not the primary mechanism because uniform pressure elevations do not usually produce distortions of pain-sensitive structures.

Idiopathic intracranial hypertension. Idiopathic intracranial hypertension (IIH), also called *benign intracranial hypertension*, is defined as a syndrome of elevated intracranial pressure without evidence of focal lesions, hydrocephalus, or frank brain edema. It usually occurs between the ages of 15 and 45 years and is more frequent in obese women. The disorder is characterized by headache with features of raised intracranial pressure. The headache is usually insidious in onset, is typically generalized, is relatively mild in severity, and is often worse in the morning or after exertion (e.g., straining or coughing).

At times, patients have visual disturbances, such as restricted peripheral visual fields, enlarged blind spots, visual blurring (*obscurations*), or diplopia secondary to abducens nerve palsies. Funduscopic examination shows papilledema, which is often more impressive than the clinical picture. IIH is usually a benign and self-limited disorder, but it may lead to visual loss, including blindness. IIH often coexists with other disorders, including polycystic ovary syndrome, sleep apnea, anxiety, and cognitive dysfunction.

The condition has been associated with drugs—vitamin A intoxication, nalidixic acid, danazol (Danocrine), and isotretinoin (Accutane)—as well as corticosteroid withdrawal and systemic disorders such as hypoparathyroidism and lupus.

CT scans are usually normal but can show small ventricles and an "empty sella"; in some cases flattening of the posterior aspect of the ocular globe, tortuosity of the optic nerve, and distension of the perioptic subarachnoid space may be seen. CSF opening pressure is elevated, usually in the range of 250 to 450 mm of water, with the pressure fluctuating markedly when monitoring occurs over a prolonged period. Some cases of IIH are caused by cerebral venous sinus occlusion. These cases can occur in hypercoagulable states, including peripartum, in association with the combined oral contraceptive pill, and in association with antiphospholipid antibody syndrome. After secondary causes of IIH have been eliminated, the patient should have dietary counseling for weight loss; up to 15% weight loss is required to put IIH into remission. Carbonic anhydrase inhibitors (acetazolamide) and corticosteroids have proved useful in headache control. As a second-line agent, furosemide also acts to lower CSF production. In cases where the headache has migrainous features (68%), acute and preventative treatments for migraine may be useful. Topiramate can prevent headache and may facilitate weight loss. Serial lumbar punctures are understandably unpopular with patients even though transient headache relief is obtained. CSF shunting procedures (ventriculoperitoneal shunt) are occasionally necessary. For patients with progressive visual loss, optic nerve sheath fenestration preserves or restores vision in 80% to 90% of cases and provides headache relief in a majority. Patients should be followed for visual acuity, pupil examination, formal visual field assessment, dilated fundal examination to grade papilledema, and BMI monitoring.

Idiopathic intracranial hypotension. Also known as *low pressure headache*, idiopathic intracranial hypotension is commonly encountered as a sequela of lumbar puncture, resulting from leakage of CSF through the dural sac. Low pressure headaches may also occur spontaneously as a result of rupture of subarachnoid cysts. The headache is initially characteristically positional, being severe on standing but relieved rapidly on lying down. Occasionally the headache is associated with focal or "false localizing" signs, especially abducens nerve palsies.

Post-traumatic headache. Headache following trauma has no specific quality and is associated with irritability, concentration impairment, insomnia, memory disturbance, and lightheadedness. Anxiety and depression are present to variable degrees. Multiple treatment options are available, and amitriptyline and nonsteroidal anti-inflammatory agents are useful. Occasionally, muscle relaxants and anxiolytics are beneficial. Training is occasionally associated with the onset of typical migraine.

Medication-associated headache. Medication overuse of "rebound" headache accounts for a significant portion of the headache burden in the population and in headache clinics. The term describes a chronic (≥15 days/month) headache that occurs in patients with a preexisting headache syndrome (most commonly migraine or tension-type headache) who use analgesic medication. Opioids, such as codeine, are particularly apt to give rise to this syndrome, but triptans, NSAIDs, and even paracetamol may have the same effect. Treatment involves the reduction or cessation of analgesic medication with a "washout" period of several weeks, during which time the headaches may worsen. Nonpharmacologic methods of pain management play a crucial role in this period. A range of other medications and substances, such as nitrous oxide, carbon monoxide, cocaine, alcohol, and phosphodiesterase inhibitors have also been reported to induce headache.

Giant cell arteritis. Headache occurs in 60% of patients with giant cell arteritis, a granulomatous vasculitis of medium and large arteries. Over 95% of patients are 50 years of age or older. Malaise, fever, weight loss, and jaw claudication occur early, in addition to headache. Polymyalgia rheumatica, a syndrome of painful stiffness of the neck, shoulders, and pelvis, is found in half the patients. Visual impairment secondary to ischemic optic neuritis may occur. The headache is usually described as aching and is exacerbated at night and after exposure to cold. The superficial temporal artery is frequently swollen, tender, and may be pulseless. The erythrocyte sedimentation rate is usually elevated; the mean is 100 mm/hr. Anemia is frequently present. Doppler ultrasound of the temporal arteries demonstrates a hypoechoic "halo sign" around the lumen of affected arteries. Temporal artery biopsy usually confirms the diagnosis, but, because the arteritis is segmental, large or multiple sections may be required. Prednisone therapy is often dramatically effective and must be given promptly to preserve vision on the affected side. Tocilizumab, a monoclonal antibody directed against the interleukin-6 receptor, is now available for the treatment of GCA, particularly in refractory or relapsing disease.

Evaluation of the Patient With Acute Headache

It is important to distinguish benign from ominous causes of headache. A detailed history (the quality, location, duration, and time course of the headache) helps in determination of which patients have a symptomatic structural intracranial lesion (see Table 8.7, Table 8.8, Table 8.4). Pain intensity is not of much diagnostic value, except for the patient who complains of the acute onset of the worst headache of his or her life. The quality of pain ("throbbing," "pressure," "jabbing") and the location may also be helpful, especially if the pain is of extracranial origin, such as temporal in temporal arteritis. Posterior fossa lesions cause occipitocervical pain, occasionally associated with unilateral retro-orbital pain. In general, multifocal pain usually implies a benign cause. It is most important to clarify the acuity of onset of the headache; patients who describe the onset of pain as "like being hit on the head with a bat" should be suspected of having the sentinel headache of subarachnoid headache. Equally important is to establish the time course of the headache. Is this paroxysmal, nonprogressive

头痛，尤其是当脑脊液（CSF）流动部分受阻引起脑积水时。幕上肿瘤不太可能引起头痛，而更常表现为精神状态改变、局灶神经功能缺损或癫痫发作。虽然颅内压增高常与头痛相关，但通常不是头痛的主要机制，因为均匀的压力升高通常不会使痛敏结构受压变形。

特发性颅内高压 特发性颅内高压（IIH），也称为良性颅内高压，定义为无局灶性病变、脑积水或明显脑水肿证据的颅内压升高综合征。通常发生在 15～45 岁，更常见于肥胖女性。本病的特征是伴有颅内压增高的头痛。头痛通常起病隐袭、范围弥漫、严重程度相对较轻，常在早晨或劳力（如用力或咳嗽）后加重。

有时患者出现视觉障碍，如周边视野缩小、盲点扩大、视物模糊（昏暗）或继发于展神经麻痹的复视。眼底检查显示的视盘水肿通常比临床表象更令人印象深刻。IIH 通常是良性、自限性疾病，但可能导致视力丧失，包括失明。IIH 常与其他疾病共存，包括多囊卵巢综合征、睡眠呼吸暂停、焦虑和认知功能障碍。

该病与药物有关——维生素 A 中毒、萘啶酸、达那唑（Danocrine）和异维 A 酸（Accutane），也与皮质类固醇撤药和系统性疾病如甲状旁腺功能减退和狼疮有关。

CT 扫描通常正常，但可显示脑室变小和"空蝶鞍"；有时可见眼球后部扁平、视神经扭曲和视神经周围蛛网膜下腔扩张。脑脊液开放压升高，通常在 250～450 mmH$_2$O 范围内，长时间监测可观察到压力显著波动。一些 IIH 病例由脑静脉窦堵塞引起。这些病例可发生于包括围生期在内的高凝状态，部分与复方口服避孕药或抗磷脂抗体综合征相关。在排除 IIH 的继发性原因后，患者应进行饮食咨询以减重；需要减轻多达 15% 的体重才能使 IIH 缓解。碳酸酐酶抑制剂（乙酰唑胺）和皮质类固醇已被证明在控制头痛中有用。呋塞米作为二线药物也能减少 CSF 产生。在头痛有偏头痛特征的情况下（68%），采用对偏头痛的急性和预防性治疗可能有用。托吡酯可预防头痛，并可能有助于减重。虽然连续腰椎穿刺能够短暂缓解头痛，但可想而知患者难以接受。脑脊液分流手术（脑室腹腔分流术）有时是必要的。对于进行性视力丧失的患者，视神经鞘开窗术可保护或恢复 80%～90% 患者的视力，并可缓解大多数患者的头痛。应随访患者，进行视力、瞳孔检查、正式的视野评估、散瞳眼底检查以评估视盘水肿，并监测体重指数（BMI）。

特发性颅内低压 特发性颅内低压也称为低颅压头痛，通常作为腰椎穿刺的后遗症，因脑脊液通过硬膜囊漏出所致。低颅压头痛也可能因蛛网膜下腔囊肿破裂而自发产生。头痛最初的特征是体位性头痛，站立时严重，平躺后迅速缓解。头痛偶尔伴随局灶性或"假定位"体征，尤其是展神经麻痹。

外伤后头痛 外伤后的头痛没有特定的性质，常伴有易怒、注意力不集中、失眠、记忆障碍和头晕。患者存在不同程度的焦虑和抑郁。有多种治疗选择，阿米替林和非甾体抗炎药有用。偶尔，肌松剂和抗焦虑药有益。本病偶尔与典型偏头痛的起病有关。

药物相关性头痛 在人群和头痛门诊中，很大一部分头痛是"反跳性"的药物过度使用性头痛。该术语描述了在使用镇痛药的患者中发生的慢性（每月 ≥ 15 天）头痛，这些患者先前已存在一种头痛综合征（最常见的是偏头痛或紧张型头痛）。阿片类药物，如可待因，特别容易引起该综合征，但曲普坦类、非甾体抗炎药甚至对乙酰氨基酚也可能有同样的作用。治疗包括在数周的"洗脱"期内减少或停用镇痛药，在此期间头痛可能加重。非药物疼痛管理方法在此期间发挥至关重要的作用。据报道，其他药物和物质，如一氧化氮、一氧化碳、可卡因、酒精和磷酸二酯酶抑制剂，也可引起头痛。

巨细胞动脉炎 巨细胞动脉炎是一种累及大到中等动脉的肉芽肿性血管炎，60% 的巨细胞动脉炎患者发生头痛。95% 以上的患者年龄在 50 岁或以上。除头痛外，早期还可出现全身不适、发热、体重减轻和下颌跛行。风湿性多肌痛是颈、肩和骨盆的疼痛僵硬综合征，见于半数巨细胞动脉炎患者。可能出现继发于缺血性视神经炎的视力障碍。头痛通常描述为隐痛，夜间和暴露于寒冷后加重。颞浅动脉常有肿胀、压痛，可能无脉。红细胞沉降率通常升高，平均为 100 mm/h。贫血常见。颞动脉多普勒超声显示受累动脉腔周围的低回声"晕轮征"。颞动脉活检通常可确诊，但由于动脉炎是节段性的，可能需要大切片或多段切片。泼尼松治疗通常效果显著，必须及时给药以保护病变侧的视力。托珠单抗是针对白细胞介素-6 受体的单克隆抗体，如今也可用于治疗巨细胞动脉炎，尤其是难治性或复发性病例。

急性头痛患者的评估

重要的是区分有特定病因的头痛和良性头痛。详细的病史（头痛的性质、部位、持续时间和病程经过）有助于确定哪些患者是症状性的，存在颅内结构性病变（见表 8.7、表 8.8、表 8.4）。疼痛程度对诊断价值不大，除非患者主诉为一生中急性起病的最严重头痛。疼痛性质（"搏动样痛""压迫样痛""刺痛"）和疼痛部位也可能对诊断有帮助，尤其是如果疼痛起源于颅外，如颞动脉炎的颞部疼痛。颅后窝病变引起枕颈部疼痛，偶尔伴有单侧眼眶后疼痛。一般来讲，多灶性疼痛通常提示良性病因。最重要的是明确头痛起病时的急性程度；将疼痛起病描述为"像被球棒击中头部"的患者，应怀疑蛛网膜下腔出血（SAH）的前哨头痛。同样重要的是确定头痛的病程经过。头痛是阵发性的、

headache (typical of migraine or tension-type headache)? Or is the headache daily persistent (such as in temporal arteritis) or progressive (suggesting the presence of a structural brain lesion)? Patients should be asked about any known triggers for the headache, such as menses, particular foods, caffeine, alcohol, or stress. Positional headache (headache that is maximal in the upright position and disappears rapidly on lying down) is characteristic of intracranial hypotension (low pressure headache). Diurnal variation in headache severity may give a clue to cause; morning headache or headache that awakens a patient from sleep may indicate raised intracranial pressure or sleep apnea as a cause. The presence of associated symptoms such as visual disturbances, nausea, or vomiting should be noted. The history should include inquiries about medications, especially use of analgesics and over-the-counter remedies. Information regarding the patient's past medical history as well as family history should also be taken into consideration. In the majority of patients with headache, the physical and neurologic examination findings are normal, although special attention may be directed toward examination of the eyes for papilledema, as well as the temporal arteries for a palpable nonpulsatile artery. Assessment of the patient with acute nontraumatic headache in the emergency room can be challenging; it is essential to establish how the headache evolved. Acute-onset severe headache should prompt investigation to exclude SAH, intracranial hemorrhage, acute obstructive hydrocephalus, and meningitis (see Table 8.7). Appropriate initial investigations should include brain imaging with CT or magnetic resonance imaging (MRI). Patients with suspected meningitis without focal neurologic signs or impaired consciousness should not have their lumbar puncture delayed unnecessarily before imaging. All patients should have standard blood tests, including blood cultures if bacterial meningitis is suspected.

A wide variety of systemic diseases have headache as a prominent symptom; some of the more prevalent disorders are summarized in Table 8.2.

CRANIAL NEURALGIAS

Neuralgias are differentiated from other head pains by the brevity of the attacks (usually 1 to 2 seconds or less) and by the distribution of the pain (see Table 8.3).

Trigeminal Neuralgia

In trigeminal neuralgia (tic douloureux), stabbing, spasmodic pain occurs unilaterally in one of the divisions of the trigeminal nerve. It lasts seconds, but it may occur many times a day for weeks at a time. It is characteristically induced by even the lightest touch to particular areas of the face, such as the lips or gums. Trigeminal neuralgia is the most frequent neuralgia of the elderly and is thought to be caused by compression of the trigeminal nerve root in the pons by an aberrant arterial loop. A small minority of cases are caused by multiple sclerosis, cerebellopontine angle tumors, aneurysms, or arteriovenous malformations, although in these cases (unlike "true" trigeminal neuralgia) there are usually objective signs of neurologic deficit, such as areas of diminished sensation. In these cases of "symptomatic" neuralgia, the pain is often atypical. MRI is indicated in patients who have sensory loss, those who are under 40, and those with bilateral or atypical symptoms. Trigeminal neuralgia may be life threatening when it interferes with eating. Neuralgic pain is often responsive to treatment with standard doses of an anticonvulsant such as phenytoin, carbamazepine, gabapentin, pregabalin, and, occasionally, baclofen. Antidepressant drugs such as amitriptyline and, more recently, duloxetine may also be useful in this setting. Combination therapy, including an antidepressant, anticonvulsant, and opiate analgesic, has been shown to have synergistic effects.

If medical treatments are unsuccessful, surgical treatment may be indicated: microvascular decompression or radiofrequency lesioning of the sensory portion of the trigeminal nerve. The latter occasionally gives rise to the complication of anaesthesia dolorosa, in which the loss of sensation resulting from the procedure is experienced as being extremely unpleasant.

Glossopharyngeal Neuralgia

Glossopharyngeal neuralgia is less common than trigeminal neuralgia. Brief paroxysms of severe, stabbing, unilateral pain radiate from the throat to the ear or vice versa and are frequently initiated by stimulation of specific "trigger zones" (e.g., tonsillar fossa or pharyngeal wall). Swallowing often provokes an attack; yawning, talking, and coughing are other potential triggers. Microvascular decompression is necessary if medical treatment is ineffective.

Postherpetic Neuralgia

Herpes zoster produces head pain by cranial nerve involvement in one third of cases. In some cases a persistent intense burning pain follows the initial acute illness. The discomfort may subside after several weeks or persist (particularly in the elderly) for months or years. The pain is localized over the distribution of the affected nerve and associated with exquisite tenderness to even the lightest touch. The first division of the trigeminal nerve is the most frequent cranial nerve involved (ophthalmic herpes) and is occasionally associated with keratoconjunctivitis. When the seventh nerve is affected ("geniculate herpes"), the pain involves the external auditory meatus and pinna. Occasionally, concomitant facial paralysis may occur (Ramsay Hunt syndrome).

Occipital Neuralgia

Occipital neuralgia is a syndrome that includes occipital pain starting at the base of the skull and often provoked by neck extension. Physical examination shows tenderness in the region of the occipital nerves and altered sensation in the C2 dermatome. Treatment includes the use of a soft collar, muscle relaxants, physical therapy, and local injections of analgesics and anti-inflammatory agents. The term *cervicogenic headache* is often used to describe headache associated with myofascial trigger points in the neck. Importantly, cervical spondylosis (discussed next) is not usually typically associated with headache.

CERVICAL SPONDYLOSIS

Cervical spondylosis is a degenerative disorder of the cervical intervertebral disks leading to osteophyte formation and hypertrophy of adjacent facet joints and ligaments. In contrast to the lumbar spine, herniation of cervical intervertebral disks (nucleus pulposus) accounts for only 20% to 25% of cervical root irritation. Cervical spondylosis is one of the most common pathologies seen in office practice and is present radiographically in over 90% of the population older than 60 years. For unknown reasons, the degree of anatomic abnormality is not directly correlated with the clinical signs and symptoms. Clinical disease may represent a combination of normal, age-related, degenerative changes in the cervical spine and a congenital or developmental stenosis of the cervical canal; the process may be aggravated by trauma. Cervical spinal myelopathy results from a combination of degenerative disc disease, spondylosis aggravated by biomechanical instability, as well as stiffening and buckling of the ligamentum flavum. It may manifest as a painful stiff neck, with or without symptoms or signs of cervical root irritation or spinal cord compression. Patients with root irritation (cervical radiculopathy) complain of pain and paresthesias radiating down the arm roughly in the dermatomal distribution of the affected nerve root. More typically, the pain radiates in a myotomal

非进行性加重的头痛（典型的偏头痛或紧张型头痛）？还是每日持续性头痛（如颞动脉炎）或进行性加重的头痛（提示存在脑内结构性病变）？应询问患者已知的头痛诱因，如月经、特定的食物、咖啡因、酒精或压力。体位性头痛（站立时最严重、平躺后迅速消失的疼痛）是颅内低压（低颅压头痛）的特征。头痛严重程度的昼夜变化可能为病因提供线索，清晨头痛或将患者从睡眠中唤醒的头痛可能提示病因为颅内压升高或睡眠呼吸暂停。应注意伴随症状，如视觉障碍、恶心或呕吐。病史采集应包括药物的使用，特别是镇痛药和非处方药的使用。应采集患者的既往史和家族史。大多数头痛患者的体格检查和神经系统检查结果正常，但应特别注意眼部检查是否存在视盘水肿以及颞动脉触诊是否无脉。急诊室中评估急性非外伤性头痛患者可能具有挑战性，确定头痛如何演变至关重要。急性起病的重度头痛应立即检查以排除 SAH、颅内出血、急性梗阻性脑积水和脑膜炎（见表 8.7）。适当的初步检查应包括头 CT 或头磁共振成像（MRI）。疑似脑膜炎且无局灶性神经系统体征或无意识受损的患者不应在影像学检查前不必要地延迟腰椎穿刺。所有患者应进行标准血液检查，如果怀疑细菌性脑膜炎则应进行血培养。

很多系统性疾病都以头痛为突出症状，表 8.2 总结了一些较常见的疾病。

脑神经痛

神经痛与其他头痛的区别在于发作时间短暂（通常 1～2 s 或更短）和疼痛的分布（见表 8.3）。

三叉神经痛

三叉神经痛（痛性抽搐）表现为一侧三叉神经分支的针刺样、痉挛性疼痛。它持续数秒，但可能一天多次发作并持续数周。即使轻触面部的特定区域（如嘴唇或牙龈）也能诱发发作。三叉神经痛是老年人最常见的神经痛，被认为是由异常动脉袢压迫脑桥的三叉神经根引起。少数病例由多发性硬化、小脑脑桥角肿瘤、动脉瘤或动静脉畸形引起，尽管在这些病例中（不像"真正的"三叉神经痛）通常有神经缺损的客观体征，例如存在感觉减退区。在这些"症状性"神经痛病例中，疼痛常不典型。对伴有感觉丧失、40 岁以下和双侧症状或不典型症状的患者应进行 MRI 检查。当三叉神经痛影响进食时可能威胁生命。神经痛通常用标准剂量的抗癫痫药治疗有效，如苯妥英钠、卡马西平、加巴喷丁、普瑞巴林，以及偶尔巴氯芬有效。抗抑郁药如阿米替林和更新的度洛西汀，在这种情况下也可能有用。包括抗抑郁药、抗癫痫药和阿片类镇痛药在内的联合治疗已显示具有协同作用。

如果药物治疗不成功，可能需要手术治疗：三叉神经感觉部分的微血管减压或射频损毁术。后者偶尔会引起痛性感觉缺失的并发症，即手术所致的感觉丧失导致极不愉快的感受。

舌咽神经痛

舌咽神经痛比三叉神经痛少见。重度、针刺样、单侧疼痛反复短暂发作，从喉咙放射到耳部或者相反，发作通常由特定"触发区"（如扁桃体窝或咽壁）的刺激引发。吞咽常诱发发作，打哈欠、说话和咳嗽是其他潜在的诱因。如果药物治疗无效，可能需要微血管减压术。

带状疱疹后神经痛

1/3 的带状疱疹患者因累及脑神经引起头部疼痛。在一些病例中，早期急性病程后会出现持续的强烈灼痛。疼痛可能在几周后消退或持续数月乃至数年（尤其在老年人中）。疼痛位于受累神经的分布区，伴随着对最轻的触碰也会出现严重的疼痛。三叉神经第一支是最常受累的脑神经（眼带状疱疹），偶尔伴有角结膜炎。当第Ⅶ脑神经受累时（"膝状神经节疱疹"），疼痛累及外耳道和耳廓。偶尔并发面瘫（拉姆齐·亨特综合征）。

枕神经痛

枕神经痛是一种起自颅底的枕部疼痛综合征，通常由伸颈引起。体格检查显示枕神经区压痛和 C2 皮节感觉异常。治疗包括穿软领衣服、使用肌松剂、理疗以及局部注射镇痛药和抗炎药。颈源性头痛，常用于描述伴有颈部肌筋膜触发点的头痛。重要的是，颈椎病（接下来将讨论）通常不伴有头痛。

颈椎病

颈椎病是颈椎间盘退行性疾病，导致邻近的关节突关节和韧带骨赘形成和肥大。与腰椎不同，仅有 20%～25% 的颈神经根刺激由颈椎间盘（髓核）突出导致。颈椎病是临床最常见的疾病之一，在 60 岁以上人群中，超过 90% 的人存在颈椎病影像学表现。由于未知的原因，解剖异常的程度与临床症状和体征无直接相关性。临床上可能表现为正常的与年龄相关的颈椎退行性变和先天性或发育性颈椎管狭窄的组合，这一过程可能因外伤而加剧。脊髓型颈椎病是椎间盘退行性疾病、因生物力学不稳定而加重的颈椎病，以及黄韧带僵硬和扭曲的综合结果。它可表现为颈部疼痛性僵硬，伴或不伴颈神经根刺激或脊髓压迫的症状或体征。伴颈神经根刺激（颈神经根病）症状的患者诉手臂疼痛和感觉异常，症状沿受累神经根的皮节分布

TABLE 8.9	Common Cervical Root Syndromes				
Disk Space	Root Affected	Muscles Affected	Distribution of Pain	Distribution of Sensory Symptoms	Reflex Affected
C4-5	C5	Deltoid; biceps	Medial scapula; shoulder	Shoulder	Biceps
C5-6	C6	Wrist extensors	Lateral forearm	Thumb; index finger	Triceps
C6-7	C7	Triceps	Medial scapula	Middle finger	Brachioradialis
C7-T1	C8	Hand intrinsics	Medial forearm	Fourth and fifth fingers	Finger flexion

pattern, whereas numbness and paresthesias follow a dermatomal distribution. Discrete sensory loss is uncommon and less prominent than symptoms (Table 8.9). For relief, patients often adopt a position with the arm elevated and flexed behind the head. Pain is exacerbated by turning the head, ear down, to the side of the pain (Spurling maneuver). Objective neurologic findings may be limited to reflex asymmetry because weakness may be obscured by pain. Patients who have some degree of spinal cord compression demonstrate gait and bladder disturbances and evidence of spasticity on examination of the lower extremities. These patients require investigation with MRI. Plain radiographs of the cervical spine add little information except in patients with rheumatoid arthritis in whom basilar invagination or atlantoaxial subluxation is suspected.

Cervical spondylosis is so common in the general population that it may be present coincidentally in a patient with another disease of the spinal cord. Among other diseases that may mimic cervical spondylosis are multiple sclerosis, amyotrophic lateral sclerosis, and, less commonly, subacute combined system disease (vitamin B_{12} deficiency). Conservative treatment includes the use of anti-inflammatory medication, cervical immobilization, and physical therapy for isometric strengthening of neck muscles once pain has subsided. Surgery should be considered if there is progression of the neurologic deficit, especially the emergence of signs of cervical cord compression. There is some evidence to suggest that cervical spondylosis is an active degenerative disease rather than simply the process. Furthermore, early studies with the glutamate antagonist riluzole suggest a potential role in reducing disease progression.

ACUTE LOW BACK PAIN

Low back pain without sciatica (radiating radicular pain) is common, with a reported point prevalence of up to 33%. Acute low back pain lasting several weeks is usually self-limiting, with a low risk for serious permanent disability. Risk factors for prolonged disability include psychological distress, compensation conflict over work-related injury, and other coexistent pain syndromes. The evaluation of patients with acute low back pain should focus on distinguishing pain of mechanical origin from neurogenic pain caused by nerve root irritation. The same pathologic changes that affect the cervical spine may also affect the lumbar spine. Because the spinal cord ends at the level of the first lumbar vertebra, lumbar canal stenosis from intervertebral disk disease and degenerative spondylosis will affect the roots of the cauda equina. The most common levels for lumbar degenerative disk disease are at L4 to L5 and L5 to S1, resulting in the common complaint of sciatica caused by irritation of the lower lumbar roots. Pain tends to improve with sitting or lying down, in contrast to the pain from spinal or vertebral tumors, which is aggravated by prolonged recumbency. Examination shows loss of the normal lumbar lordosis, paraspinal muscle spasm, and exacerbation of pain with straight leg rising, owing to stretching of the lower lumbar roots. About 10% of disk herniations occur lateral to the spinal canal, in which case the more rostral root is compressed. Percussion of the spine may elicit focal tenderness of one of the vertebrae, suggesting bony infiltration by infection or tumor.

Spinal stenosis of the lumbar region may manifest as "neurogenic claudication," which is usually described as unilateral or bilateral buttock pain that is worse on standing or walking and relieved by rest or flexion at the waist. Patients may have pain that is worse when walking downhill, in contrast to patients with vascular claudication, whose pain is maximal when walking up an incline.

MRI in many patients with isolated low back pain shows nonspecific findings; MRI assessment early in the course of an episode of low back pain does not improve clinical outcome. MRI should be limited to patients with back pain who have associated neurologic symptoms or signs, especially new-onset disturbances of bladder or bowel continence or perineal sensory symptoms suggestive of a *cauda equina syndrome*. Patients with risk factors for malignancy, infection, or osteoporosis, as well as those with pain maximal at rest (or nocturnal pain) require imaging. Patients with primary and metastatic tumor can present with acute back pain. Moreover, developmental anomalies are often associated with pain (see Chapter 12).

Treatment strategies for lumbar pain are similar to those for cervical pain, with surgery reserved for patients with neurologic signs and clear pathologic processes seen on imaging studies. Most cases of acute low back pain, even with rupture of an intervertebral disk, can be treated conservatively with a short period of rest, muscle relaxants, and analgesics. Prolonged bed rest is recommended only for patients in severe pain. Patient education regarding proper posture and appropriate back exercises is helpful, as is a formal physical therapy program. Chiropractic manipulation should not be performed for patients who have evidence of neurologic injury or spine instability.

For a deeper discussion on this topic, please see Chapter 370, "Headaches and Other Head Pain," in *Goldman-Cecil Medicine*, 26th Edition.

SUGGESTED READINGS

Bronfort G, Evans R, Anderson AV, et al: Spinal manipulation, medication, or home exercise with advice for acute and subacute neck pain: a randomized trial, Ann Intern Med 156:1–10, 2012.

Cherkin DC, Sherman KJ, Kahn J, et al: A comparison of the effects of 2 types of massage and usual care on chronic low back pain: a randomized, controlled trial, Ann Intern Med 155:1–9, 2011.

El Barzouhi A, Vleggeert-Lankamp CL, Lycklama à Nijeholt GJ, et al: Magnetic resonance imaging in follow up assessment of sciatica, N Engl J Med 368:999–1007, 2013.

Fehlings MG, Tetreault LA, Wilson JR, et al: Cervical spondylitic myelopathy. Current state of the art and future directions, Spine 38:S1–S8, 2013.

Gelfand AA, Goadsby PJ: A neurologist's guide to acute migraine treatment in the emergency room, Neurohospitalist 2:51–59, 2012.

Headache Classification Subcommittee of the International Headache Society: The international classification of headache disorders: 3rd edition, Cephalalgia 33:629-808, 2013. Available at: http://ihs.classification.org/en/.

Rana MV: Managing and treating headache of cervicogenic origin, Med Clin North Am 97:267–280, 2013.

Rizzoli PB: Acute and preventive treatment of migraine, Continuum 18:764–782, 2012.

表 8.9 常见颈神经根综合征

椎间隙	受累神经根	受累肌肉	疼痛分布	感觉症状分布	受累的反射
C4-5	C5	三角肌、肱二头肌	肩胛内侧、肩部	肩部	肱二头肌
C5-6	C6	腕伸肌	前臂外侧	拇指、示指	肱三头肌
C6-7	C7	肱三头肌	肩胛内侧	中指	肱桡肌
C7-T1	C8	手内在肌	前臂内侧	第四和第五指	屈指

区向远端放射。更典型的情况是，疼痛沿肌节放射，而麻木和感觉异常沿皮节分布。离散性感觉丧失不常见且不明显（表 8.9）。为缓解症状，患者常采取手臂抬高并在头后屈曲的姿势。头、耳向疼痛侧下转可加重疼痛（Spurling 手法）。因为疼痛可能掩盖无力，客观神经系统检查可能只发现反射不对称。脊髓一定程度受压的患者表现出步态异常和膀胱功能障碍，下肢检查显示痉挛体征。这些患者需要 MRI 检查。除了类风湿关节炎患者怀疑颅底凹陷或寰枢椎半脱位，颈椎 X 线平片几乎不能提供任何信息。

颈椎病在人群中如此常见，以至于它可能碰巧出现在患有另一种脊髓病的患者身上。其他可能类似颈椎病的疾病包括多发性硬化、肌萎缩侧索硬化和较少见的亚急性联合系统疾病（维生素 B_{12} 缺乏）。保守治疗包括使用抗炎药物、颈椎制动和疼痛消退后的颈部肌肉等长强化理疗。如果神经功能缺损进展，特别是出现脊髓压迫体征时，应考虑手术。一些证据表明，颈椎病是一种活动性的退行性疾病，而不仅仅是个过程。此外，谷氨酸拮抗剂利鲁唑的早期研究提示其可能在减轻疾病进展方面具有潜在作用。

急性腰痛

不伴坐骨神经痛（放射性根性疼痛）的腰痛很常见，报告的时点患病率高达 33%。急性腰痛持续数周，通常有自限性，严重永久性残疾的风险低。长期残疾的危险因素包括心理困扰、工伤赔偿冲突和其他共存的疼痛综合征。评估急性腰痛患者应重点区分机械源性疼痛和由神经根刺激引起的神经源性疼痛。影响颈椎的病理性变化也可能影响腰椎。由于脊髓的末端在第一腰椎水平，椎间盘疾病和退行性脊椎病导致的腰椎管狭窄将影响马尾神经根。最常见的退行性腰椎间盘疾病位于 L4 至 L5 和 L5 至 S1 水平，导致常见的坐骨神经痛，这是因下腰神经根受刺激引起。坐位或卧位疼痛往往会改善，这与脊柱或椎体肿瘤的疼痛不同，后者因长时间卧床而加重。检查显示正常的腰椎前凸消失、脊旁肌痉挛和直腿抬高动作牵拉下腰神经根引起疼痛加重。约 10% 的椎间盘突出发生在椎管外侧，导致更多的神经根受压。脊柱叩诊引起椎骨的局部疼痛提示感染或肿瘤浸润。

腰椎管狭窄可能表现为"神经源性跛行"，通常被描述为单侧或双侧臀部疼痛，站立或行走时加重，休息或弯腰时缓解。患者下坡行走时疼痛可能更严重，这与血管性跛行患者相反，后者上坡时疼痛最严重。

许多孤立性腰痛患者的 MRI 表现无特异性，在腰痛发作的早期进行 MRI 评估不会改善临床结局。MRI 应仅限于伴有相关神经症状或体征的腰痛患者，尤其是提示马尾综合征的新发膀胱障碍或大便失禁或会阴感觉症状。有恶性肿瘤、感染或骨质疏松危险因素的患者，以及静息时疼痛（或夜间疼痛）最重的患者需要影像学检查。原发和转移性肿瘤患者可能出现急性腰背痛。此外，发育异常经常伴有疼痛（见第 12 章）。

腰痛的治疗策略与颈痛相似，手术仅限于有神经系统体征和影像学检查显示明确病理性过程的患者。大多数急性腰痛病例，即使椎间盘破裂，也可通过短期休息、肌松剂和镇痛药进行保守治疗。仅建议重度疼痛患者长期卧床休息。与正式的物理治疗计划一样，关于正确姿势和适当背部锻炼的患者教育也有帮助。有神经损伤或脊柱不稳定证据的患者，不应进行整脊手法。

有关此专题的深入讨论，请参阅 *Goldman-Cecil Medicine* 第 26 版第 370 章"头痛和其他头部疼痛"。

推荐阅读

Bronfort G, Evans R, Anderson AV, et al: Spinal manipulation, medication, or home exercise with advice for acute and subacute neck pain: a randomized trial, Ann Intern Med 156:1–10, 2012.

Cherkin DC, Sherman KJ, Kahn J, et al: A comparison of the effects of 2 types of massage and usual care on chronic low back pain: a randomized, controlled trial, Ann Intern Med 155:1–9, 2011.

El Barzouhi A, Vleggeert-Lankamp CL, Lycklama à Nijeholt GJ, et al: Magnetic resonance imaging in follow up assessment of sciatica, N Engl J Med 368:999–1007, 2013.

Fehlings MG, Tetreault LA, Wilson JR, et al: Cervical spondylitic myelopathy. Current state of the art and future directions, Spine 38:S1–S8, 2013.

Gelfand AA, Goadsby PJ: A neurologist's guide to acute migraine treatment in the emergency room, Neurohospitalist 2:51–59, 2012.

Headache Classification Subcommittee of the International Headache Society: The international classification of headache disorders: 3rd edition, Cephalalgia 33:629-808, 2013. Available at: http://ihs.classification.org/en/.

Rana MV: Managing and treating headache of cervicogenic origin, Med Clin North Am 97:267–280, 2013.

Rizzoli PB: Acute and preventive treatment of migraine, Continuum 18:764–782, 2012.

9
Disorders of Vision and Hearing

Eavan Mc Govern, Timothy J. Counihan

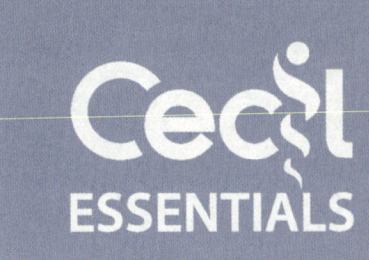

DISORDERS OF VISION AND EYE MOVEMENTS

Examination of the Visual System

Visual Acuity
The clinical examination of visual function begins with testing visual acuity.

Examination technique.
- Use a Snellen chart at a distance of 20 feet (Fig. 9.1).
- If applicable, test visual acuity with a patient's corrective lenses.
- Examine each eye separately.
- Record the smallest line the patient can read. This is the visual acuity for the eye tested; for instance, acuity of 20/40 refers to letters that the patient sees maximally at 20 feet, which a normal individual can see at 40 feet.
- If a patient is unable to read the largest letter, visual acuity is recorded using finger counting or light perception.

Clinical clues. When errors of refraction are responsible for decreased visual acuity, vision may be improved by having the patient look through a pinhole. Corrected vision in one eye of less than 20/40 suggests damage to the lens (cataract) or retina or a disorder of the anterior visual (prechiasmal) pathway. Color vision should be tested using Ishihara color plates to detect an acquired unilateral or bilateral cause of color loss. Patients with optic nerve lesions with normal visual acuity can report that colors appear "washed out" in the affected eye (color desaturation).

Visual Fields
Confrontational examination of visual fields is helpful when localizing lesions interrupting the afferent visual system (Fig. 9.2).

Examination technique.
- The examiner's head should be level with the patient's head.
- Test each eye separately, by initially asking the patient to cover the other eye.
- Visual fields should be tested in all four quadrants using finger counting by comparing the patient's field with that of the examiner.
- Use a white pin to map peripheral visual fields and a red pin to assess for the presence of a central area of visual field loss (referred to as a scotoma).

Examination tips. Finger counting is more sensitive than presenting moving objects in detecting visual field deficits. The field should be tested first unilaterally and then bilaterally. A defect (particularly in the left hemifield) with bilateral testing only (extinction) suggests visual neglect and a lesion in the contralateral parietal lobe.

Clinical clues. The following questions are helpful to help localize the lesion within the visual afferent system.
- Is the defect monocular or binocular? Monocular lesions localize the defect to the retina or to the optic nerve. A binocular lesion localizes posterior to and including the optic chiasm.
- Is the defect central or peripheral? *Scotomas* are areas of partial or complete visual loss and may be central or peripheral. Central scotomas result from damage to the macula. A scotoma affecting one half of a visual field is known as a *hemianopia.* Field defects are said to be *homonymous* if the same part of the visual field is affected in both eyes; a homonymous hemianopia implies a postchiasmal lesion.
- Is the defect congruous or incongruous? A homonymous defect may be *congruous* (the visual defect is identical in each hemifield) or *incongruous* (the visual defect is not identical in each hemifield). The closer the visual field defect to the occipital lobe the more congruous the defect.
- Does the defect involve the superior, inferior or bitemporal visual fields? Quadrantanopsias are smaller defects in the visual field and may be superior (which suggests a temporal lobe lesion) or inferior (which suggests a parietal lobe lesion). Bitemporal hemianopia implies a lesion at the chiasm, such as a pituitary tumor. An altitudinal hemianopia occurs with vascular damage to the retina.
- Is the visual defect associated with positive symptoms? Scintillating scotomas are hallucinations of flashing lights. If they are monocular, they may be caused by retinal detachment; binocular scintillations suggest occipital oligemia (as in migraine) or seizure.

Any suspicious findings on bedside confrontation testing warrant formal visual field testing using perimetry (Fig. 9.3).

Pupils
Pupil constriction is mediated by the parasympathetic system of the oculomotor (third cranial) nerve, whereas dilation is mediated by the sympathetic system. If the balance of these systems is disrupted, *anisocoria* (unequal pupil size) results.

Examination technique.
- Observe the pupillary size and shape at rest.
- Examine the pupils in both dim and bright light.
- Note the direct and consensual light responses for each eye. This is best tested using the "swinging light test," in which the light is moved quickly from one eye to the other.
- Test for accommodation by asking the patient to first look at a distant object and then at the examiner's fingers, held 12 inches away.

Clinical clues. If the degree of anisocoria increases going from dim to bright light, this suggests that the larger lesion is failing to constrict due to a lesion of the parasympathetic system. Similarly, if the degree of pupillary asymmetry is maximal in a dimly lit environment, this suggests that the smaller pupil fails to dilate appropriately due to a lesion of the sympathetic nervous system. *Physiologic anisocoria* is characterized by pupillary asymmetry that is unchanged irrespective of the ambient light intensity; this occurs in approximately 20% of the population. When light is shone into one eye, both eyes should

视觉与听觉疾病

张梦雨 译 卢强 牛婧雯 审校 姚明 朱以诚 通审

视觉与眼动疾病

视觉系统检查

视力

视觉功能的临床检查首先是测试视力。

检查技术
- 使用斯内伦视力表（Snellen chart），距离为 20 英尺（约 6 m）（图 9.1）。
- 如适用，患者佩戴矫正镜片测试视力。
- 分别检查每只眼睛。
- 记录患者能够阅读的最小行，即是所测眼睛的视力。例如，视力为 20/40 意味着患者最远在 20 英尺（约 6 m）处能看到的字母，而一个正常人可以在 40 英尺（约 12 m）处看到。
- 如果患者无法阅读最大的字母，视力记录使用手指计数或光感来表示。

临床线索 当视力下降是由于屈光不正所致时，让患者通过小孔视物有可能改善视力。单眼的矫正视力低于 20/40 提示晶状体损伤（白内障）或视网膜损伤或前视觉（视交叉前）通路疾病。应使用石原色盲板（Ishihara color plates）测试色觉，以检测单侧或双侧色觉丧失的后天获得性原因。视神经病变的患者即使视力正常，也可能主诉患眼的颜色看起来"褪色"（颜色不饱和）。

视野

视野检查对于定位累及视觉传入系统的病变有帮助（图 9.2）。

检查技术
- 检查者的头部应与患者的头部在同一水平线上。
- 分别测试每只眼睛，让患者遮住另一只眼睛。
- 视野应在四个象限内使用手指计数进行测试，将患者的视野与检查者的视野进行比较。
- 使用白色针绘制周边视野，使用红色针评估是否存在中心视野缺失区域（称为暗点）。

检查提示 在检测视野缺损时，数手指比展示移动物体更灵敏。应首先测试单侧视野，然后双侧同时测试。如果仅在双侧测试时出现缺损（特别是在左侧视野），即视觉消失现象，则提示视觉忽视及对侧顶叶病变。

临床线索 以下问题有助于定位视觉传入系统中的病变位置。

- 缺损是单眼还是双眼？单眼病变定位于视网膜或视神经。双眼病变定位于视交叉后，包括视交叉。
- 缺损是中心还是周边？暗点是视力部分或完全丧失的区域，可能是中心或周边的。中心暗点是由黄斑损伤所致。影响半侧视野的暗点称为偏盲。如果双眼的同一部分视野受到影响，则称为同向偏盲，同向偏盲提示视交叉后病变。
- 缺损是对称的还是不对称的？同向偏盲可能是对称的（每侧视野的缺损相同）或不对称的（每侧视野的缺损不同）。病变越靠近枕叶，缺损越对称。
- 缺损涉及上、下还是双颞侧视野？象限偏盲是视野中的较小缺损，可能是上象限（提示颞叶病变）或下象限（提示顶叶病变）。双颞侧偏盲提示视交叉处的病变，如垂体瘤。视网膜血管受损时会出现上下性偏盲。
- 视觉缺陷是否与阳性症状有关？闪光暗点是闪光的幻觉。单眼闪光暗点，可能是由视网膜脱离引起的；双眼闪光暗点提示枕叶缺血（如偏头痛）或癫痫发作。

床旁视野测试中发现的任何可疑结果都需要使用视野计进行正式的视野测试（图 9.3）。

瞳孔

瞳孔缩小是由动眼神经（第Ⅲ脑神经）的副交感神经系统控制的，而瞳孔扩张是由交感神经系统控制的。如果这些系统的平衡被打破，就会导致瞳孔不等（瞳孔大小不等）。

检查技术
- 观察瞳孔在静止时的大小和形状。
- 在昏暗和明亮的光线下检查瞳孔。
- 注意每只眼睛的直接和间接对光反射。最好的测试方法是使用"摆动光测试"，即快速地将光从一只眼睛移动到另一只眼睛。
- 通过让患者先看一个远处的物体，然后看距离 12 英寸（约 30 cm）的检查者的手指，以测试调节反应。

临床线索 如果从昏暗到明亮的光线下，瞳孔不等的程度增加，这表明副交感神经系统的病变更重，导致瞳孔无法缩小。同样，如果瞳孔不等在昏暗的环境中最明显，这表明由于交感神经系统病变，较小的瞳孔无法

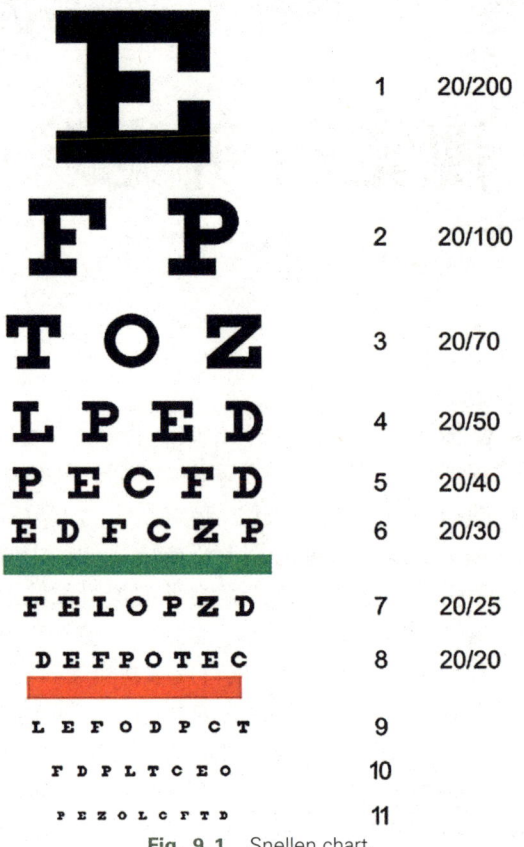

Fig. 9.1 Snellen chart.

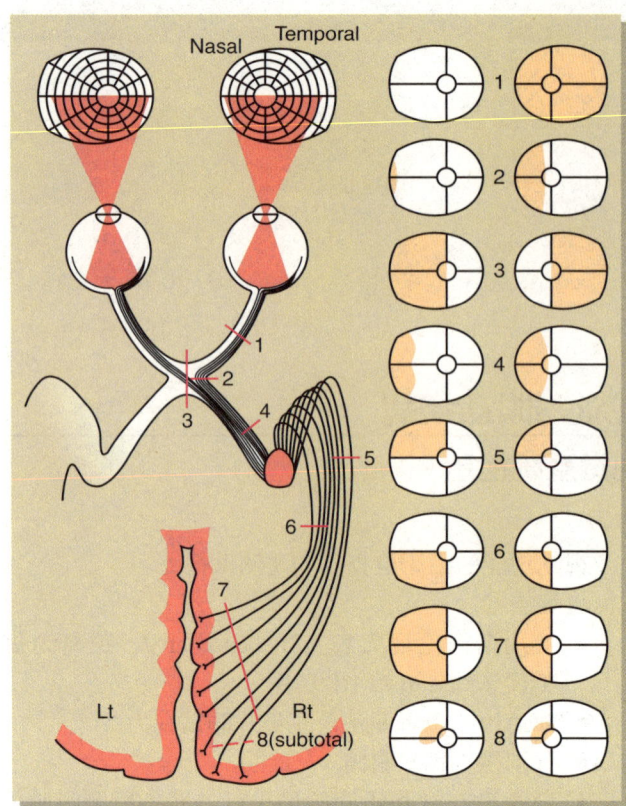

Fig. 9.2 Visual fields that accompany damage to the visual pathways. *1*, Optic nerve: unilateral amaurosis. *2*, Lateral optic chiasm: grossly incongruous, incomplete (contralateral) homonymous hemianopia. *3*, Central optic chiasm: bitemporal hemianopia. *4*, Optic tract: incongruous, incomplete homonymous hemianopia. *5*, Temporal (Meyer) loop of optic radiation: congruous partial or complete (contralateral) homonymous superior quadrantanopia. *6*, Parietal (superior) projection of the optic radiation: congruous partial or complete homonymous inferior quadrantanopia. *7*, Complete parieto-occipital interruption of optic radiation: complete congruous homonymous hemianopia with psychophysical shift of foveal point often sparing central vision, giving "macular sparing." *8*, Incomplete damage to visual cortex: congruous homonymous scotomas, usually encroaching at least acutely on central vision. (From Baloh RW: Neuro-ophthalmology. In Goldman L, Bennett JC, editors: Cecil textbook of medicine, ed 21, Philadelphia, 1998, WB Saunders, p 2236.)

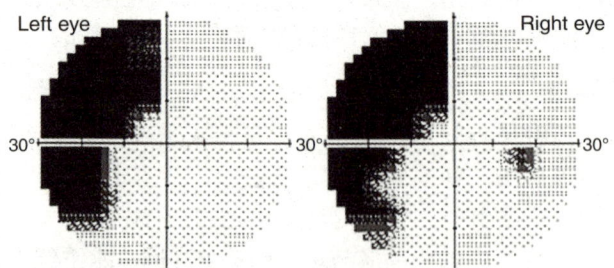

Fig. 9.3 Humphrey visual fields demonstrating an incongruent homonymous hemianopia.

constrict simultaneously. When the light source is shone from a normal eye to an affected, relative dilatation of both pupils is observed. This abnormality is referred to as an *afferent pupillary defect* and indicates severe retinal disease or an optic neuropathy. *Argyll-Robertson pupils* are small, irregular pupils that constrict to near vision (accommodation reflex) but not in response to light. They are associated with neurosyphilis, diabetes, and other disorders. This so-called *light-near dissociation* may also occur in rostral dorsal midbrain lesions, in which there may be associated abnormalities of vertical gaze, eyelid retraction, and convergence retraction nystagmus (Parinaud syndrome). This constellation of clinical findings is occasionally found in patients with lesions of the pineal gland.

The presence of drooping of the eyelid (ptosis) should be noted. A large, unreactive pupil with complete ptosis indicates a lesion of the oculomotor nerve *(third cranial nerve palsy)* interrupting the parasympathetic nerve supply to the pupil. The associated paralysis of the medial and inferior rectus and inferior oblique muscles (see later discussion) results in distortion of the eye (inferolaterally, "*down and out*") and a subjective complaint of diplopia by the patient. Common causes of a third nerve palsy include compression by an aneurysm of the posterior communicating artery, by transtentorial herniation, or from ischemia, usually in the setting of diabetes or vasculitis. A third cranial nerve palsy caused by ischemia often spares the pupil but results in complete paralysis of the oculomotor and eyelid levator muscles. Acute painful third nerve palsy should be treated as an emergency, with the need to investigate for an intracranial aneurysm.

A small, poorly reactive pupil with associated partial ptosis is known as *Horner syndrome* and results from damage to the sympathetic fibers to the pupil, which may occur anywhere along their course from the hypothalamus, brain stem, and ascending sympathetic chain from the superior cervical ganglion to the orbit. There may be associated unilateral anhidrosis resulting from damage to sympathetic fibers. Horner syndrome may be the first sign of an apical lung tumor (Pancoast) or may occur in diseases affecting the carotid artery such as dissection.

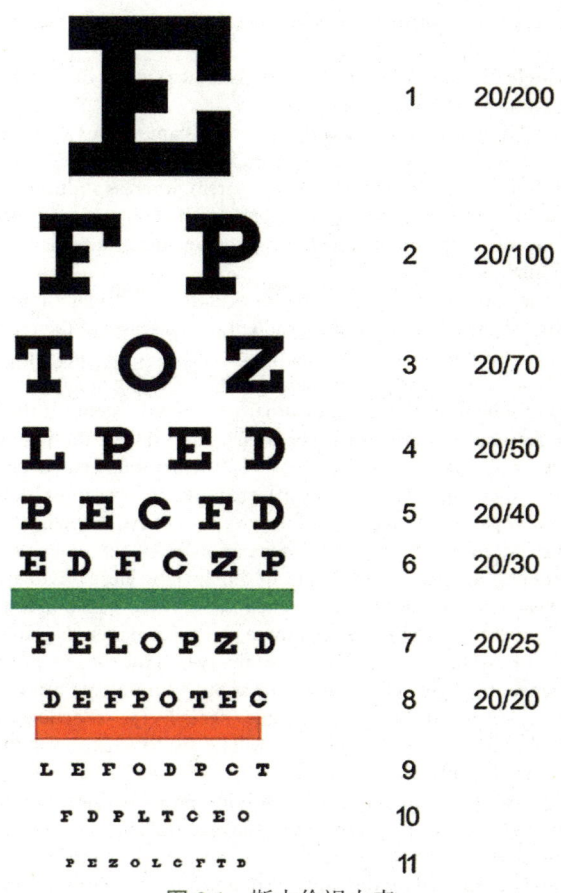

图9.1 斯内伦视力表

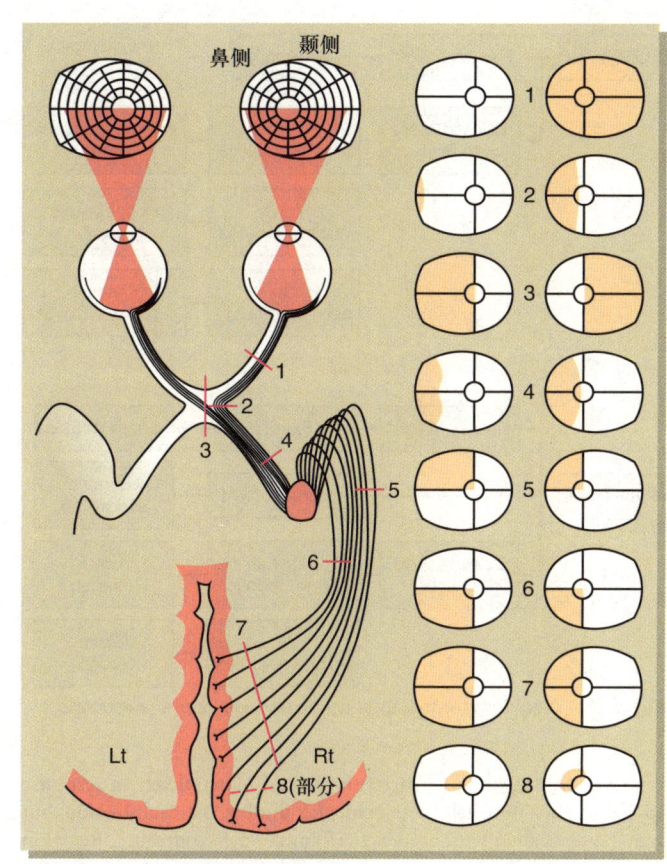

图9.2 视觉通路损伤伴随的视野变化。1. 视神经：单侧黑矇。2. 外侧视交叉：严重不对称、不完全（对侧）同向偏盲。3. 中央视交叉：双颞侧偏盲。4. 视束：不对称、不完全（对侧）同向偏盲。5. 视放射颞（Meyer）袢：对称的部分或完全（对侧）同向上象限盲。6. 顶叶（上部）视放射投射：对称的部分或完全（对侧）同向下象限盲。7. 顶枕部视放射完全中断：完全的对侧同向偏盲，通常保留中央视力，形成"黄斑回避"。8. 视皮质不完全损伤：对称的同向暗点，通常至少会严重影响中央视力。（引自 Baloh RW: Neuro-ophthalmology. In Goldman L, Bennett JC, editors: Cecil textbook of medicine, ed 21, Philadelphia, 1998, WB Saunders, p 2236.）

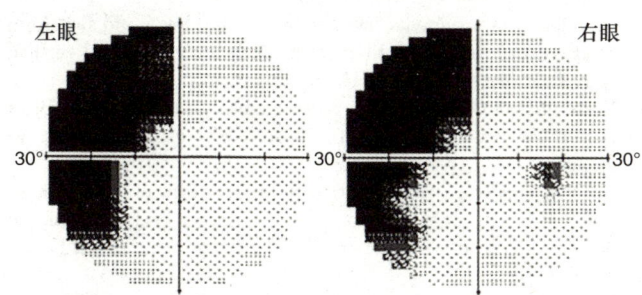

图9.3 Humphrey 视野图显示不一致的同向偏盲

适当地扩张。生理性瞳孔不等的特征为瞳孔的不对称性在不同光线强度下保持不变，大约20%的正常人群会出现这种情况。当光线照射到一只眼睛时，双眼瞳孔应同时缩小。当光源从正常眼照射到患眼时，可观察到双侧瞳孔相对扩张。这种异常称为传入性瞳孔障碍，表明存在严重的视网膜疾病或视神经病变。阿-罗瞳孔（Argyll-Robertson pupil）是小而不规则的瞳孔，视近物时会收缩（调节反射），但对光反射无反应。这与神经梅毒、糖尿病及其他疾病有关。这种所谓的光-近分离现象也可能出现在中脑背侧上部病变中，此时可能伴有垂直凝视异常、眼睑回缩和辐辏回缩性眼球震颤（帕里诺综合征）。松果体病变患者偶尔也会出现这一系列临床表现。

应注意眼睑是否下垂（上睑下垂）。瞳孔大而无反应伴完全的上睑下垂表明动眼神经病变（第Ⅲ脑神经麻痹），导致副交感神经对瞳孔失支配。与此相关的内直肌、下直肌和下斜肌麻痹（见后续讨论）导致眼球向下和向外斜视，患者主诉复视。引起动眼神经麻痹的常见原因包括后交通动脉瘤压迫、小脑幕切迹疝或常由糖尿病或血管炎导致的缺血。由缺血引起的动眼神经麻痹通常会避开瞳孔，但会导致眼外肌和上睑提肌完全麻痹。急性痛性动眼神经麻痹应作为急症处理，需要检查是否有颅内动脉瘤。

瞳孔小、反应迟钝并伴有部分性上睑下垂称为霍纳综合征，其原因是瞳孔的交感神经纤维受损，这种损伤可能发生在从下丘脑、脑干到上行性交感神经链（从颈上神经节至眼眶）的全程中。可能伴有单侧无汗症，这是由于交感神经纤维损伤引起的。霍纳综合征可能是肺尖肿瘤（Pancoast）的首发症状，也可能发生在颈动脉疾病（如颈动脉夹层）中。

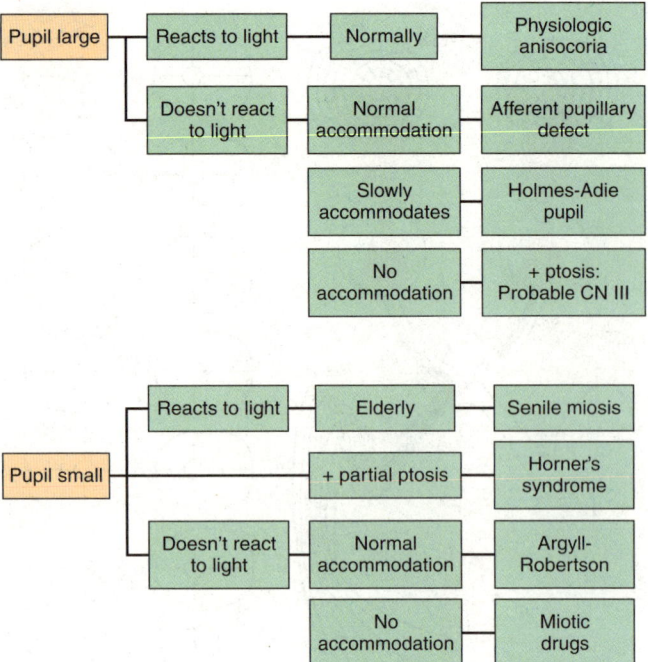

Fig. 9.4 Algorithm for the approach to unequal pupils (anisocoria).

Tonic (Adie) pupils constrict slowly and incompletely in response to light. This is usually an incidental finding on examination but may be associated with areflexia (Holmes-Adie syndrome). Reaction to accommodation is preserved, and it has been suggested that the disorder is a result of parasympathetic denervation. *Hippus* refers to pupillary unrest with synchronous oscillation of the pupil size; it is considered a normal phenomenon. Fig. 9.4 summarizes common pupillary abnormalities and their associated features.

Eye Movements

Abnormalities in ocular motility may arise from lesions of the cerebral hemisphere, brain stem, cranial nerves and ocular muscles. The ability to localize lesions disrupting binocular vision can provide valuable diagnostic information for the clinician.

Examination technique. First note the position of the head and eyes with the eyes in primary gaze. Next, the four components of oculomotor function should be tested:

1. Pursuit eye movements: Smooth pursuit eye movements allow fixation on a moving object. Ask the patient to follow a moving target such as a pin in all directions of gaze.
2. Saccadic eye movements: These movements allow rapid switching of gaze from one target to another. Both horizontal and vertical saccadic movements should be checked.
3. Vestibulo-ocular reflex: This reflex enables fixation on an object even if the head is moving. It is assessed by using the *doll's eye maneuver*.
4. Convergence response: This tests the ability of the eyes to track an object as it is brought close to the limit of accommodation. Ask the patient to look into the distance and then at your finger held close to their eyes.

Both smooth pursuit and (voluntary) saccadic eye movements in horizontal and vertical directions are checked to determine whether the movements are conjugate or dysconjugate.

Clinical clues from history. The following questions from the clinical history can be helpful in evaluating the patient with diplopia.

- Is the diplopia primarily horizontal or vertical, or is it greater looking to the right or to the left?
- Is there diurnal variation? Double vision that varies during the day suggests myasthenia gravis.
- Is the diplopia maximal with near or distant vision? Greater difficulty with near vision suggests impairment of the medial rectus, oculomotor nerve, or convergence system, whereas abducens nerve weakness results in horizontal diplopia when objects are viewed at a distance. Diplopia that worsens on going down stairs may suggest a fourth nerve lesion.
- Is the diplopia monocular or binocular? Monocular diplopia is usually caused by an optical problem (i.e., diseases of the retina or lens). It is corrected by having the patient look through a pinhole, unless the cause is psychogenic. Binocular diplopia suggests ocular misalignment that is a disorder of the brain stem (at the level of the ocular motor nuclei or their connections), the peripheral nerves (cranial nerves III, IV, or VI), the neuromuscular junction (myasthenia gravis or botulism) or individual eye muscles (ocular myopathy). A large deficit in the range of eye movements may provide sufficient diagnostic information. However, in many cases, although the patient complains of diplopia, no clear misalignment is visible on testing eye movements. The corneal reflection test may help identify misalignment in these cases. The patient is instructed to look at a light shining directly at the eyes. If the eyes are normally aligned, the light reflection will be about 1 mm nasal to the center of the cornea. If one eye is deviated medially, the reflection will be displaced outward; the reflection will be displaced inward if the eye is deviated outward.

When assessing eye movements, it is important to know the cranial nerves and muscles involved in eye movement. The abducens (sixth cranial) nerve supplies the lateral rectus muscle. The trochlear (fourth cranial) nerve subserves the superior oblique muscle, which intorts the eye as well as depresses the eye in adduction (such as when a patient tries to look downstairs). All other muscles are supplied by the oculomotor nerve (Fig. 9.5). Abnormalities of the cranial nerves in the brain stem are usually accompanied by other signs, such as weakness, ataxia, or dysarthria. The abducens nerve has a long ascending course through the posterior fossa, where it is prone to compression at multiple sites and as a result of raised intracranial pressure; hence, a sixth nerve palsy may be a false localizing sign. Conjugate eye movement is regulated by supranuclear pathways from the cerebral hemisphere to the medial longitudinal fasciculus in the brain stem. A lesion in the cerebral hemisphere resulting from hemorrhage, infarction, or tumor disrupts conjugate gaze to the contralateral side, so that the eyes "look away" from the hemiplegia. Lesions of the brain stem cause conjugate paralysis to the ipsilateral side (eyes looking toward the side of the hemiplegia). Lesions of the medial longitudinal fasciculus, which connects the nuclei of the oculomotor and abducens nerves, lead to *internuclear ophthalmoplegia*. In this case, horizontal gaze results in failure of adduction in one eye and nystagmus in the abducting eye. The lesion is on the side of failed adduction; bilateral lesions are frequently seen in multiple sclerosis. Table 9.1 lists the major causes of acute ophthalmoplegia.

Funduscopy

The retina should be carefully examined in each patient by direct ophthalmoscopy, which provides a magnified view of the fundus without the necessity for dilation of the pupil (Fig. 9.6).

Examination technique.
- The examiner's head should be level with the patient's head.
- The examiner's right eye should be used to examine the patient's right eye.

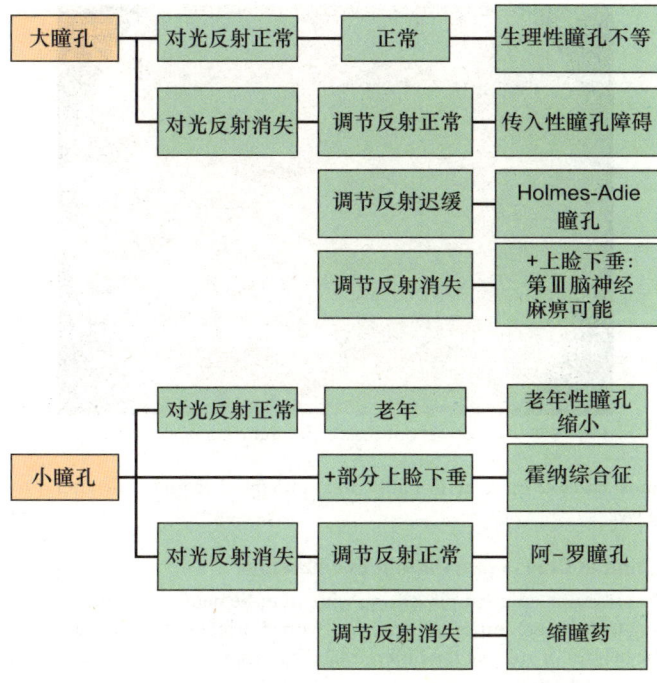

图9.4 瞳孔不等的鉴别流程

强直性瞳孔（阿迪瞳孔）对光反射缓慢且不完全。通常是在检查中偶然发现，但可能与反射消失（Holmes-Adie综合征）有关。调节反应保留，目前认为这种疾病是由副交感神经失神经支配造成的。虹膜震颤指的是瞳孔大小同步振荡的不稳定现象，是一种正常现象。图9.4总结了常见的瞳孔异常及其相关特征。

眼球运动

眼球运动异常可能源于大脑半球、脑干、脑神经和眼肌的病变。对破坏双眼视觉的病变进行定位的能力可为临床医生提供宝贵的诊断信息。

检查技术 首先要注意头部和眼睛在初始注视时的位置。接下来，应测试眼球运动功能的四个组成部分：

1. 追踪眼球运动：平滑的追踪眼球运动能够使视线固定在移动的物体上。让患者从各个注视方向追踪一个移动目标（如大头针）。

2. 眼扫视运动：这种运动可使视线从一个目标快速切换到另一个目标。应检查水平和垂直方向的眼扫视运动。

3. 前庭-眼反射：即使头部移动，这种反射也能使视线固定在一个物体上。可通过玩偶眼动作进行评估。

4. 辐辏反射：在物体靠近调节极限时，测试眼睛跟踪物体的能力。让患者先看远处，然后看你靠近他们眼睛的手指。

应检查水平和垂直方向上的平滑追踪运动和（自主的）眼扫视运动，以确定这些运动是否协调。

从病史中获得的临床线索 以下临床病史有助于评估患者的复视情况。

- 复视主要是水平的还是垂直的，或者在向右看或向左看时更明显？
- 是否存在昼夜变化？日间波动性的复视提示重症肌无力。
- 复视在近距离视物还是远距离视物时最明显？近距离视物困难较大提示内直肌、动眼神经或会聚系统受损，而展神经受损在远距离视物时导致水平复视。下楼梯时复视加重可能提示第Ⅳ脑神经病变。
- 复视是单眼还是双眼？单眼复视通常由光学问题引起（如视网膜或晶状体疾病）。除非是心因性的，否则可以让患者通过小孔视物来纠正复视。双眼复视提示眼位不正，病变位置可能是脑干（在眼动神经核团或其连接处）、周围神经（第Ⅲ、Ⅳ、Ⅵ脑神经）、神经肌肉接头（重症肌无力或肉毒毒素中毒）或个别眼肌（眼肌病）。眼动范围的明显缺陷可能提供足够的诊断信息。然而，在许多病例中，尽管患者主诉复视，但测试眼动时却没有明显的眼位不正。在这种情况下，角膜映光测试可能有助于识别眼位不正。请患者注视直射眼睛的光线，如果眼位正常，将在角膜中心偏鼻侧约1 mm处看到映光点。如果一只眼睛向内侧偏斜，映光点将向外移位；如果眼睛向外偏斜，映光点将向内移位。

在评估眼动时，了解参与眼动的脑神经和肌肉非常重要。展神经（第Ⅵ脑神经）支配外直肌。滑车神经（第Ⅳ脑神经）支配上斜肌，上斜肌内旋眼球并在眼球内收时将眼球向下旋转（类似于患者下楼梯时向下看的状态）。其他眼外肌由动眼神经支配（图9.5）。脑干中的脑神经受损通常伴有其他体征，如无力、共济失调或构音障碍。展神经在颅后窝的上升路线较长，容易受到多个部位的压迫以及颅内压升高的影响；因此，第Ⅵ脑神经麻痹可能是一个假定位体征。从大脑半球到脑干内侧纵束的核上性神经通路调节眼球的共轭运动。由于脑出血、脑梗死或肿瘤导致的大脑半球病变会破坏眼球向对侧凝视的共轭运动，使眼睛"不看"偏瘫肢体。脑干病变导致同侧凝视麻痹（眼睛看向偏瘫肢体）。连接动眼神经核和展神经核的内侧纵束病变会导致核间性眼肌麻痹。在这种情况下，水平凝视会出现一侧眼球内收不能而另一侧眼球外展出现眼震。病变在内收不能的一侧。双侧病变常见于多发性硬化。表9.1列出了急性眼肌麻痹的主要原因。

眼底镜检查

应通过直接眼底镜检查仔细检查每位患者的视网膜，眼底镜检查可提供放大后的眼底视图而不需散瞳（图9.6）。

检查技术

- 检查者的头部应与患者的头部保持同一水平。
- 用检查者的右眼检查患者的右眼。

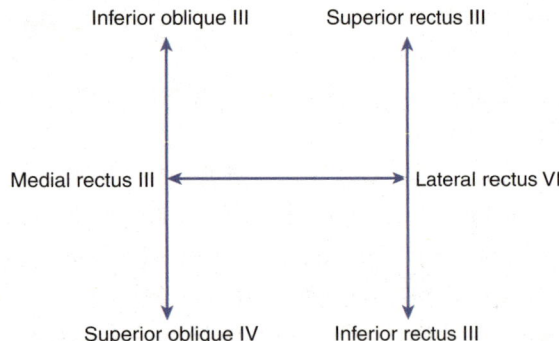

Fig. 9.5 Movements of eye muscles and their innervation.

TABLE 9.1 Major Causes of Acute Ophthalmoplegia

Condition	Diagnostic Features
Bilateral	
Botulism	Contaminated food; high-altitude cooking; pupils involved
Myasthenia gravis	Fluctuating degree of paralysis; responds to edrophonium chloride (Tensilon) IV
Wernicke encephalopathy	Nutritional deficiency; responds to thiamine IV
Acute cranial polyneuropathy	Antecedent respiratory infection; elevated CSF protein level
Brain stem stroke	Other brain stem signs
Unilateral	
P Comm aneurysm	Third cranial nerve, pupil involved
Diabetic-idiopathic	Third or sixth cranial nerve, pupil spared
Myasthenia gravis	As above
Brain stem stroke	As above

CSF, Cerebrospinal fluid; *IV*, intravenous; *P Comm*, posterior communicating artery.

- Locate the red reflex in both eyes. While focusing on one eye, move closer until the retina comes into view.
- While focusing on the retina, follow the vessels toward the patient's nose to locate the optic disc.
- To view the macula, ask the patient to look directly at the light.

Clinical clues from patient history. In eliciting the history the most important thing to establish is whether the visual loss is monocular or binocular.

Monocular Visual Loss

Loss of vision in one eye localizes to the prechiasmatic visual pathway (i.e., the eye itself or the optic nerve). Causes include lesions of the cornea, lens, vitreous, retina, or optic nerve. Loss of the red reflex suggests a lesion of the anterior chamber. Careful funduscopic examination will usually reveal ocular and retinal lesions, but acute lesions of the optic nerve (optic neuritis) may not be associated with abnormalities of the optic nerve head.

Optic neuritis is characterized by inflammation of the optic nerve accompanied by non-homonymous visual defects. Optic neuropathies acutely associated with a normal appearing optic disk on funduscopic examination are posterior or *retrobulbar optic neuritis* ("the doctor sees nothing and the patient sees nothing"). Those with a swollen disk on funduscopic examination are anterior optic neuropathies. In most cases of optic neuropathy, the optic disc becomes pale after 4 to 6 weeks.

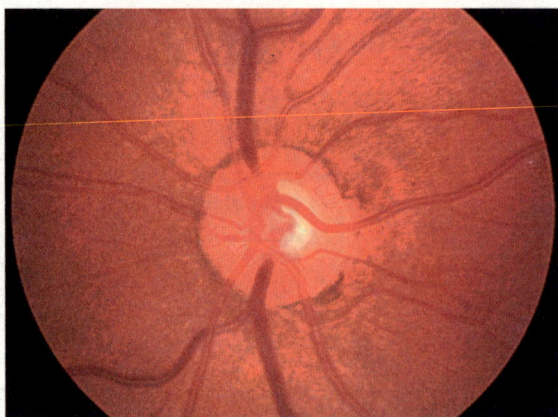

Fig. 9.6 A normal optic disk on funduscopic examination.

Clinical Clues From Patient Examination

In assessing a patient presenting with an optic neuropathy the following features are important to identify on clinical examination and can be helpful in guiding the differential diagnosis:
- Visual acuity
- Color vision
- Visual field
- The presence or absence of a relative afferent pupillary defect (RAPD)
- Optic nerve head appearance on funduscopic examination

The patient with optic neuritis complains of difficulty with vision in the affected eye. Loss of vision may be insidious and recognized only when the unaffected eye is accidentally occluded. Patients often complain of periorbital pain on eye movement on presentation. The evolution of visual loss is highly variable, progressing over a period ranging from less than a day to several weeks, although most patients will have reached their maximal visual deficit in 3 to 7 days.

At the time the patient is first examined, visual acuity may range from almost 20/20 to the extreme of total blindness. Patients may describe their vision as blurred or dim, and colors may appear less bright than usual or "gray." Red desaturation may occur with optic neuritis and may be detected using Ishihara color plates. Examination of the visual field shows defects within the central 25 degrees, with central and paracentral scotomas being the most common types. An afferent pupillary defect is frequently present. The funduscopic examination is abnormal in only about one half of the cases. The disc may appear hyperemic with blurred margins, and hemorrhages, when present, are few and found only on the disc or in the area immediately surrounding the disc.

There are many causes of optic neuropathy. Broadly speaking, the causes may be divided into inflammatory, vascular, or compressive/infiltrative. Treatment is directed at the underlying cause. Inflammatory causes usually result in subacute painful loss of central vision. In this instance, high-dose intravenous corticosteroids should be used to shorten time to recovery. The most common cause of inflammatory optic neuritis is multiple sclerosis. Bilateral optic neuritis is much less common and may coincide with longitudinally extensive transverse myelitis, known as *neuromyelitis optica* (NMO) or *Devic disease*. The recent discovery of antibodies directed toward aquaporin 4 (a water channel present on astrocytes and vascular endothelial cells), associated with NMO, has identified this as a separate disease entity, with a different treatment regimen emerging for it. The NMO antibody

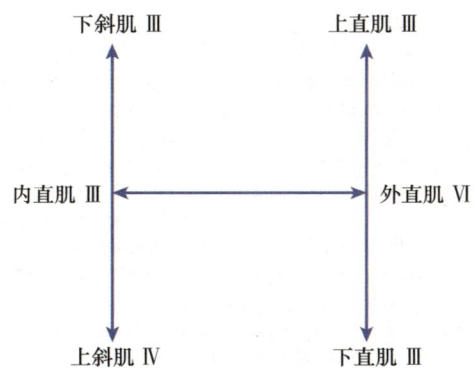

图 9.5 眼外肌的运动及其神经支配

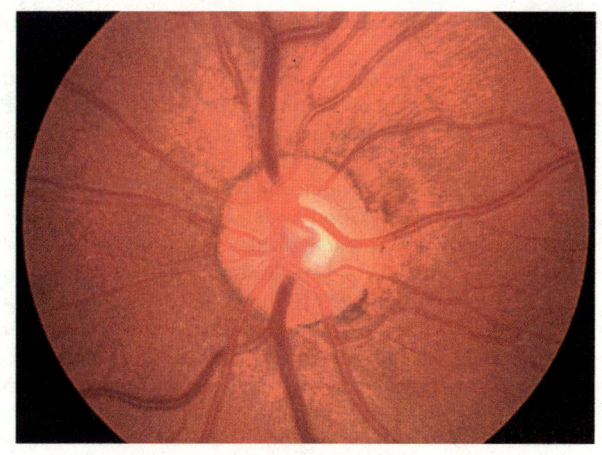

图 9.6 眼底镜检查中正常的视盘

表 9.1 急性眼肌麻痹的主要病因	
病因	诊断特点
双侧	
肉毒毒素中毒	食物中毒，高海拔烹饪，累及瞳孔
重症肌无力	眼肌麻痹程度有波动性，对静注依酚氯铵（腾喜龙）有效
韦尼克脑病	营养缺乏，对静注维生素 B_1 有效
急性多发性脑神经病	前驱呼吸系统感染史，脑脊液蛋白质水平升高
脑干梗死	其他脑干体征
单侧	
后交通动脉瘤	第Ⅲ脑神经麻痹，瞳孔受累
糖尿病（特发性）	第Ⅲ或第Ⅵ脑神经麻痹，瞳孔不受累
重症肌无力	如前所述
脑干梗死	如前所述

- 找到双眼的红光反射。聚焦于一只眼睛靠近，直到视网膜进入视野。
- 当聚焦于视网膜时，沿着血管向患者鼻子的方向寻找视盘。
- 让患者直视光源以查看黄斑。

从病史中获得的临床线索　在病史采集过程中，最重要的是确定视力丧失是单眼还是双眼。

单眼视力丧失

单眼视力丧失定位于视交叉前的视觉通路（即眼本身或视神经）。其原因包括角膜、晶状体、玻璃体、视网膜或视神经的病变。红光反射消失提示前房病变。仔细的眼底镜检查通常会发现眼部和视网膜的病变，但急性视神经病变（视神经炎）可能不伴随视盘异常。

视神经炎的特征是视神经的炎症，伴有非同向视力缺损。在眼底镜检查中视盘外观正常的急性视神经病变为后部视神经病或称为球后视神经炎（"医生看不到任何异常，患者什么也看不见"）。眼底镜检查发现视盘肿胀的为前部视神经病。在大多数视神经病变的病例中，视盘在 4～6 周后会变得苍白。

体格检查中的临床线索

在对视神经病变患者进行评估时，临床体格检查中识别以下特征非常重要，这些特征有助于指导鉴别诊断：

- 视力
- 色觉
- 视野
- 是否存在相对性传入性瞳孔障碍（RAPD）
- 眼底镜检查中视盘外观

视神经炎患者主诉为患侧眼视物困难。视力下降可能是隐匿性的，只有在健侧眼被偶然遮住时才被发现。患者通常在就诊时主诉眼球活动时眼眶周围疼痛。视力下降的进展速度非常不一致，从不到 1 天到数周不等，大多数患者会在 3～7 天内达到最大视力缺损。

在患者初次检查时，视力可能从接近 20/20 到完全失明不等。患者可能描述视物模糊或暗淡，颜色看起来不如平时那么鲜艳或"灰暗"。视神经炎可能出现红色饱和度下降现象，可使用石原色盲板检测。视野检查显示中央 25°范围内的缺损，中央和旁中央暗点是最常见的类型。常见传入性瞳孔障碍。仅在大约一半的病例眼底镜检查异常。视盘可能出现充血，边界模糊，较少有出血，且仅出现在视盘或其周围区域。

视神经病的病因有很多。大致上，病因可分为炎症性、血管性或压迫/浸润性。治疗应针对根本病因。炎症性疾病通常导致亚急性疼痛性中央视力丧失。在这种情况下，应使用大剂量静脉皮质类固醇以缩短恢复时间。最常见的炎症性视神经病是多发性硬化。双侧视神经炎较少见，可能伴有长节段横贯性脊髓炎，称为视神经脊髓炎（NMO）或 Devic 病。最近发现与 NMO 相关的水通道蛋白 4（存在于星形胶质细胞和血管内皮细胞上）抗体，已将其确定为一种独立的疾病实体，并且针对该病制订了不同的治疗方案。NMO 抗

is the first sensitive and specific biomarker associated with a central demyelinating disorder.

The optic nerve may be compressed by tumors that originate in the nerve itself or in the region of the optic chiasm. Compressive/infiltrative causes typically cause progressive visual loss, color desaturation, and no pain on eye movement. Headache may result in the presence of raised intracranial pressure. Proptosis and diplopia occurs with orbital lesions. Cranial nerve palsies result with lesions involving the cavernous sinus. Causes may be broadly divided into neoplastic and nonneoplastic causes such as thyroid eye disease.

Ischemic optic neuropathy (ION) is the most common cause of acute optic neuropathy in patients over 50 years. The posterior ciliary artery, a branch of the ophthalmic artery, supplies the optic nerve. Due to its anatomic arrangement, optic nerve ischemia results in superior or inferior segmental optic nerve atrophy and clinically manifests as altitudinal defects. ION occurs in two forms. The *atherosclerotic* variety occurs mostly between the ages of 50 and 70 years, and typically no evidence of systemic disease is present. The *arteritic* form is usually a manifestation of giant cell arteritis. There may be systemic manifestations of the disease, including headache, scalp tenderness, and generalized myalgias. Laboratory evaluation shows anemia and elevated erythrocyte sedimentation rate in almost every case. Patients with arteritis should be treated with high doses of corticosteroids to prevent permanent loss of vision.

Acute transient monocular blindness is usually the result of embolization to the central retinal artery from an atheromatous plaque in the carotid artery *(amaurosis fugax)*. Any complaint of transient visual loss constitutes an emergency, and steps must be taken to prevent permanent loss of vision by making a prompt diagnosis and initiating appropriate therapy. Examples of sight-saving procedures include corticosteroid therapy for cranial arteritis, reduction of intraocular pressure for acute glaucoma, and carotid surgery, anticoagulation, or antiplatelet therapy for embolic cerebrovascular disease.

Binocular Visual Loss

Binocular visual loss usually suggests retro-chiasmatic pathology. Gradual bilateral visual loss caused by optic nerve lesions is rare. Causes include Leber hereditary optic neuropathy and a toxic nutritional–deficiency state. Acute transient bilateral visual loss (visual obscuration) may be a symptom of raised intracranial pressure caused by a brain tumor or idiopathic intracranial hypertension (IIH); papilledema is often severe. IIH, formerly known as *pseudotumor cerebri*, requires prompt investigation and treatment to prevent potential bilateral visual failure. It is often associated with a high body mass index (BMI) and is more common in young females. Vitamin A and tetracycline ingestion have been associated with the condition. Unilateral or bilateral lateral rectus palsy may be present. It is one of the few situations in which, after imaging, performance of a lumbar puncture is safe in the setting of marked bilateral papilledema. Cerebral venous sinus thrombosis may mimic IIH and should be screened for with neuroimaging.

Bilateral damage to the optic radiations or visual cortex results in cortical blindness. The pupillary light reflex is normal, as are the funduscopic examination findings, and the patient may occasionally be unaware that he or she is blind *(Anton syndrome)*. Patients are often misdiagnosed as having a conversion reaction. Transient cortical blindness occurs most often in basilar artery insufficiency but is also seen in hypertensive encephalopathy. Positive visual phenomena (e.g., phosphenes, scintillating scotomas) are characteristic of migrainous aura and probably reflect oligemia to the occipital lobes from vasoconstriction. Arteriovenous malformations, tumors, and seizures may produce similar symptoms and should be distinguished from migraine with aura by a careful history and examination as well as by imaging in appropriate cases.

Visual hallucinations are visual sensations independent of external light stimulation; they may be either simple or complex, may be localized or generalized, and may occur in patients with a clear or clouded sensorium. Visual illusions are alterations of a perceived external stimulus in which some features are distorted. The simplest visual phenomena consist of flashes of light (photopsias), blue lights (phosphenes), or scintillating zigzag lines, which last a fraction of a second and recur frequently or which appear to be in constant motion. These can arise from dysfunction within the optic pathways at any point from the eye to the cortex. Glaucoma, incipient retinal detachment, retinal ischemia, or macular degeneration can cause simple visual hallucinations. Lesions of the occipital lobe are often associated with simple hallucinations; classic migraine is by far the most common condition of this type. Complex visual hallucinations such as seeing objects as people, animals, landscapes, or various indescribable scenes occur most frequently with temporal lobe lesions or parieto-occipital association areas. Visual hallucinations of epileptogenic origin are typically stereotyped.

HEARING AND ITS IMPAIRMENTS

Symptoms of Auditory Dysfunction

The two main symptoms of lesions affecting the auditory system are hearing loss and tinnitus. Hearing loss can be classified as conductive, sensorineural, mixed, or central, based on the anatomic site of pathology (Figs. 9.7 and 9.8). Tinnitus can be either subjective or objective. Conductive hearing loss results when there is difficulty transferring sound waves from the external to the middle ear. Any lesion along this pathway can cause conductive hearing loss. Patients with conductive loss have particular difficulty hearing low-frequency sounds and hear better in noisy backgrounds than in quiet environments. Patients often report frequently ear fullness as if their ear is blocked.

Sensorineural hearing loss usually results from lesions of the cochlea or the auditory division of the vestibulocochlear (eighth cranial) nerve. The cochlea analyzes the frequency of sounds and activates appropriate sensory cells depending on the frequency. Patients with sensorineural hearing loss often have difficulty hearing speech that is mixed with background noise and may be annoyed by loud speech. Low tones are better heard than high-frequency ones. Distortion of sounds is common with sensorineural hearing loss. Central (retrocochlear) hearing disorders are rare and result from bilateral lesions of the central auditory pathways, including the cochlear and dorsal olivary nuclear complexes, inferior colliculi, medial geniculate bodies, and auditory cortex in the temporal lobes. Damage to both auditory cortices may result in pure word deafness, in which patients are selectively unable to discriminate language but may be able to hear nonverbal sounds.

Tinnitus is the perception of a noise or ringing in the ear that is usually audible only to the patient (subjective), although, rarely, an examiner can hear the sound as well. The latter, so-called *objective tinnitus*, can be heard when the examining physician places a stethoscope against the patient's external auditory canal. Tinnitus that is pulsatory and synchronous with the heartbeat suggests a vascular abnormality within the head or neck. Aneurysms, arteriovenous malformations, and vascular tumors can produce this type of tinnitus.

Subjective tinnitus, heard only by the patient, can result from lesions involving the external ear canal, tympanic membrane, ossicles, cochlea, auditory nerve, brain stem, and cortex. The character of the tinnitus does not usually aid in determining the site of the disturbance. For this, one must rely on associated symptoms and signs. When tinnitus results from a lesion of the external or middle ear, it is usually accompanied by a

体是首个与中枢神经系统脱髓鞘疾病相关的敏感且特异的生物标志物。

起源于神经本身或视交叉区域的肿瘤可能会压迫视神经。压迫/浸润性原因通常导致进行性视力减退、色觉饱和度下降，且眼球运动时无疼痛感。颅内压升高可能导致头痛。眼眶病变导致眼球突出和复视。涉及海绵窦的病变可导致脑神经麻痹。病因可大致分为肿瘤性和非肿瘤性原因，如甲状腺眼病。

缺血性视神经病变（ION）是50岁以上患者急性视神经病变的最常见原因。睫状后动脉是眼动脉的分支，为视神经供血。由于其解剖结构，视神经缺血导致上部或下部节段性视神经萎缩，临床表现为视野垂直缺损。ION有两种类型。动脉粥样硬化型多发病于50～70岁，通常没有全身性疾病证据。动脉炎型通常是巨细胞动脉炎的一种表现，可能有疾病的全身表现，包括头痛、头皮触痛和全身肌痛。实验室检查显示，几乎每例都会出现贫血和红细胞沉降率升高。动脉炎患者应使用大剂量皮质类固醇治疗，以防止永久性视力丧失。

急性短暂性单眼失明（一过性黑矇）通常是由于颈动脉粥样斑块导致视网膜中央动脉栓塞所致。任何短暂性视力丧失的主诉都属于急症，必须及时诊断并采取适当的治疗措施，以防止永久性视力丧失。挽救视力的措施包括脑动脉炎的皮质类固醇疗法、急性青光眼的降低眼内压，以及栓塞性脑血管疾病的颈动脉手术、抗凝或抗血小板治疗。

双眼视力丧失

双眼视力丧失通常提示视交叉后病变。由视神经病变引起的渐进性双侧视力丧失较为罕见，原因包括莱伯（Leber）遗传性视神经病和营养缺乏引起的毒性状态。急性短暂性双侧视力丧失（视觉模糊）可能是由于脑肿瘤或特发性颅内高压（IIH）引起的颅内压升高症状，视盘水肿通常很严重。IIH，曾被称为假性脑瘤，需要及时检查和治疗以防止潜在的双眼视力丧失。它通常与高体重指数（BMI）相关，在年轻女性中更为常见。维生素A和四环素摄入与该病有关。可出现单侧或双侧外直肌麻痹。IIH是少数在双侧视盘水肿明显的情况下，影像学检查后进行腰椎穿刺仍是安全的情况之一。脑静脉窦血栓形成可能与IIH相似，应通过神经影像学进行筛查。

双侧视辐射或视觉皮质损伤会导致皮质盲。瞳孔对光反射正常，眼底检查结果也正常，患者有时可能意识不到自己失明（安东综合征）。患者常被误诊为转换障碍。短暂性皮质盲最常发生于基底动脉供血不足，但也见于高血压脑病。阳性视觉现象（如光幻视、闪光暗点）是偏头痛先兆的特征，可能反映了由血管收缩导致的枕叶供血不足。动静脉畸形、肿瘤和癫痫发作可能会产生类似症状，应通过仔细询问病史和体格检查，并在适当情况下通过影像学检查将其与伴有先兆的偏头痛区分开来。

幻视是不依赖于外部光刺激的视觉感觉，可能是单纯的或复杂的，可能是局灶的或全面的，可能发生在清醒或神志不清的患者中。视错觉是对外部刺激的感知改变，其中某些特征被扭曲。最简单的视觉现象包括光的闪烁（闪光感）、蓝光（光幻视）或闪烁的锯齿状线条，持续时间极短（仅几分之一秒），且经常复发，或者看起来在不断运动。这些现象可以从眼睛到大脑皮质的任何视觉通路位置发生功能障碍时出现。青光眼、初期视网膜脱离、视网膜缺血或黄斑变性可导致单纯的幻视。枕叶病变通常与单纯幻视有关，经典的偏头痛是这种类型中最常见的情况。复杂的幻视，如将物体看作人、动物、风景或各种难以描述的场景，最常见于颞叶病变或顶枕联合区病变。癫痫发作的幻视通常是刻板的。

听力及其障碍

听觉功能障碍的症状

听觉系统病变的两个主要症状是听力损失和耳鸣。根据病变解剖部位，听力损失可分为传导性、感音神经性、混合性或中枢性（图9.7和图9.8）。耳鸣可以是主观的，也可以是客观的。传导性听力损失是指声波难以从外耳传递到中耳。该路径上的任何病变都可能导致传导性听力损失。传导性听力损失的患者尤其难以听到低频声音，在嘈杂的环境中比在安静的环境中听得更清楚。患者常主诉耳朵有满胀感，仿佛被堵住。

感音神经性听力损失通常是由耳蜗或前庭蜗神经（第Ⅷ脑神经）听觉部分的病变引起的。耳蜗对声音频率进行分析，并根据频率激活相应的感觉细胞。患有感音神经性听力损失的患者通常难以在背景噪声中听清讲话，并可能对大声讲话感到厌烦。低频声音比高频声音更容易听到。感音神经性听力损失常伴有声音失真。中枢性（耳蜗后）听力障碍较为罕见，是由双侧中枢听觉传导通路病变引起的，包括耳蜗、背侧橄榄核复合体、下丘、内侧膝状体和颞叶听觉皮质。双侧听觉皮质损伤可能导致纯词聋，即患者选择性无法辨别语言，但可以听到非语言声音。

耳鸣是指耳中感知到噪声或鸣响，通常只有患者自己能听到（主观性），尽管在极少数情况下，检查者也能听到这种声音。这种情况下的耳鸣被称为客观性耳鸣，当检查医生将听诊器放在患者的外耳道时就能听到。与心跳同步的搏动性耳鸣提示头颈部血管异常。动脉瘤、动静脉畸形和血管肿瘤都可能产生这种类型的耳鸣。

只有患者能听到的主观性耳鸣可能是外耳道、鼓膜、听小骨、耳蜗、听神经、脑干或大脑皮质病变所致。耳鸣的特征通常不能帮助确定病变部位，为此需要依靠伴随的症状和体征。当耳鸣由外耳或中耳病变

conductive hearing loss. The patient may complain that his or her voice sounds hollow and that other sounds are muffled. Because the masking effect of ambient noise is lost, the patient may be disturbed by normal muscular sounds such as chewing, tight closure of the eyes, or clenching of the jaws. The characteristic tinnitus associated with Meniere's syndrome is low pitched and continuous, although fluctuating in intensity. Often the tinnitus becomes very loud immediately preceding an acute attack of vertigo and then may disappear after the attack. Tinnitus resulting from lesions within the central nervous system is usually not associated with hearing loss but is nearly always associated with other neurologic symptoms and signs. High-dose salicylates frequently result in tinnitus.

Examination of the Auditory System
Examination Technique
Hearing is first tested in the speech range to observe the response to spoken commands at different intensities (whisper, conversation, and shouting). The examiner must be careful to prevent the patient from reading his or her lip movement. A high-frequency stimulus such as a watch tick should also be used because sensorineural disorders often involve only the higher frequencies. Tuning fork tests permit a rough assessment of the hearing level for pure tones of known frequency. The Rinne test compares a patient's hearing by air and by bone conduction. A 512-cps tuning fork is first held against the mastoid process until the sound fades. It is then placed 1 inch from the ear. Normal subjects can hear the fork about twice as long by air conduction as compared with bone conduction. If hearing by bone conduction is longer than by air conduction, a conductive hearing loss is suggested. The Weber test compares the patient's hearing by bone conduction in the two ears. The fork is placed at the center of the forehead, and the patient is asked where he or she hears the tone. Normal subjects hear it in the center of the head, patients with unilateral conductive loss hear it on the affected side, and patients with unilateral sensorineural loss hear it on the side opposite the loss. Otoscopic examination may reveal impacted cerumen as a cause of conductive hearing loss.

Causes of Hearing Loss
Presbycusis is bilateral hearing loss associated with advancing age. It is not a distinct disease entity. It represents multiple effects of aging on

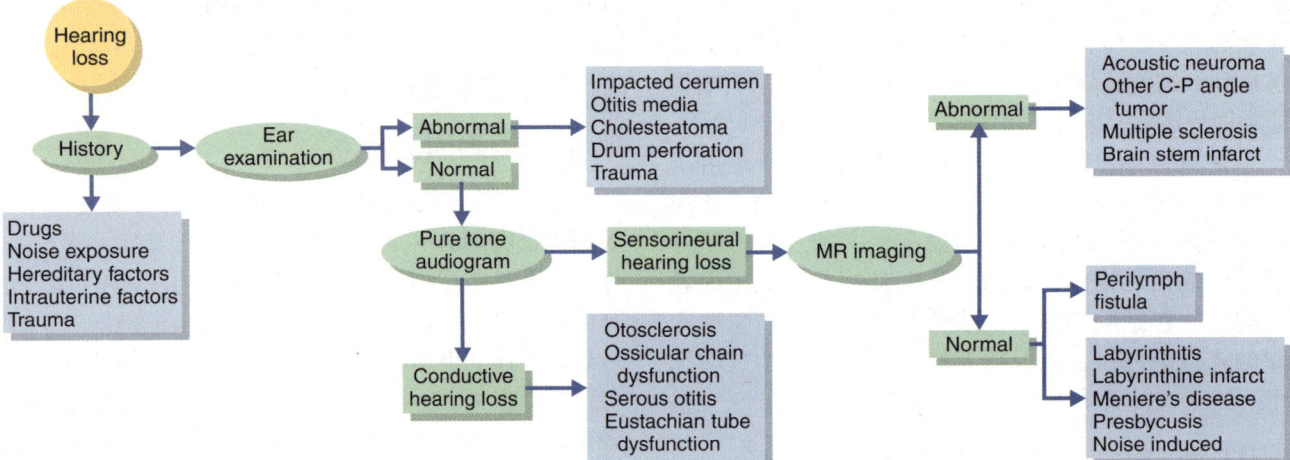

Fig. 9.7 Evaluation of deafness (unilateral and bilateral). *C-P,* Cerebellopontine; *MR,* magnetic resonance. (Modified from Baloh RW: Hearing and equilibrium. In Goldman L, Bennett JC, editors: Cecil textbook of medicine, ed 21, Philadelphia, 1998, WB Saunders, p 2250.)

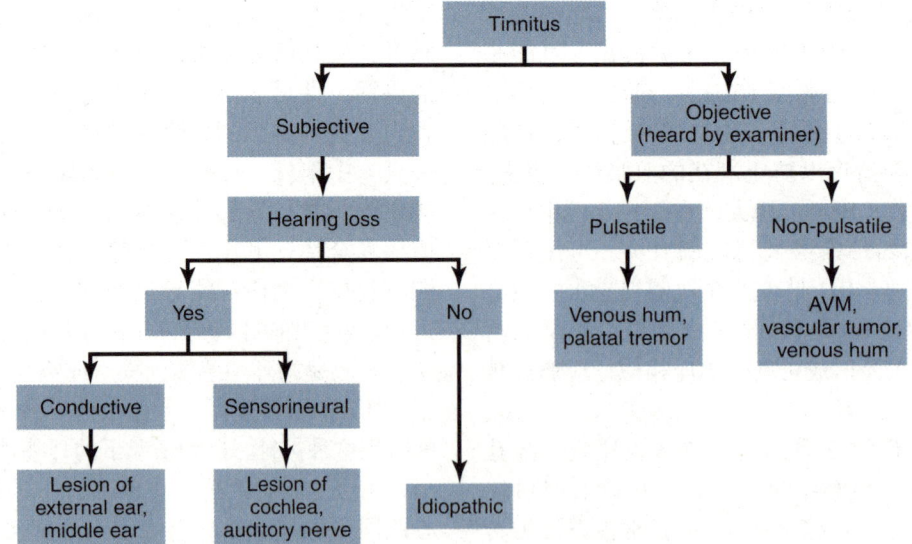

Fig. 9.8 Algorithm for the approach to the patient with tinnitus. *AVM,* Arteriovenous malformation.

引起时，通常伴有传导性听力损失。患者可能主诉自己的声音听起来空洞，听不清其他声音。由于失去了环境噪声的掩蔽效应，患者可能会受到正常肌肉声音的干扰，如咀嚼、紧闭眼睛或咬紧下颌等声音。梅尼埃综合征的特征性耳鸣音调低且持续，但强度有波动。通常在急性眩晕发作前，耳鸣变得非常响亮，发作后可能会消失。由中枢神经系统病变引起的耳鸣通常不伴有听力损失，但几乎总是伴有其他神经系统症状和体征。大剂量水杨酸盐常导致耳鸣。

听觉系统检查

检查技术

首先在整个音量范围内测试听力，观察患者对不同强度的口头指令（耳语、对话及大声呼喊）的反应。检查者必须注意防止患者看出自己的唇部动作。还应使用高频刺激（如手表滴答声），因为感音神经性疾病常常仅影响高频声音。音叉测试可以粗略评估已知频率纯音的听力水平。林纳试验（Rinne试验）比较患者的气导和骨导听力。首先将一个512 Hz的音叉放在乳突上，直到声音消失。然后将音叉放置在距离耳朵1英寸（约2.5 cm）处。正常人通过气导听到声音的时间约为骨导的2倍。如果通过骨导听到的时间比气导长，则提示传导性耳聋。韦伯试验（Weber试验）比较患者双耳的骨导听力。将音叉放在前额中央，询问患者听到声音的位置。正常人听到的声音在头部中央，单侧传导性耳聋患者听到的声音在患侧，而单侧感音神经性耳聋患者听到的声音在健侧。耳镜检查可能会发现耵聍阻塞，这是导致传导性听力损失的原因之一。

听力损失的病因

老年性耳聋是与年龄增长相关的双侧听力损失。它不是一个独立的疾病实体，而是代表了衰老对听觉

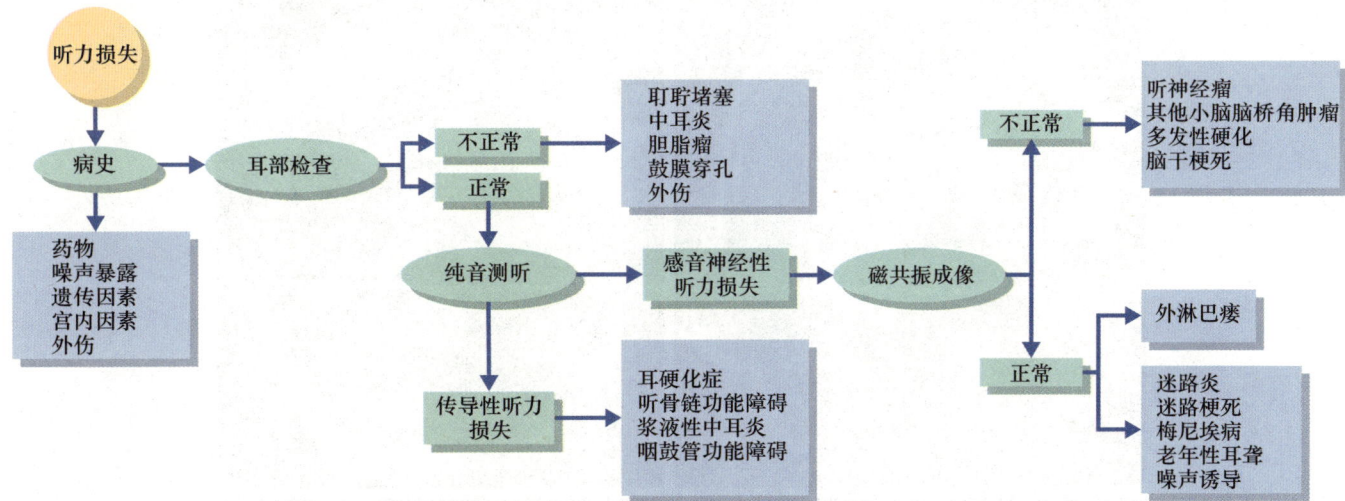

图9.7 单侧和双侧耳聋的评估。（改编自 Baloh RW：Hearing and equilibrium. In Goldman L，Bennett JC，editors：Cecil textbook of medicine，ed 21，Philadelphia，1998，WB Saunders，p 2250.）

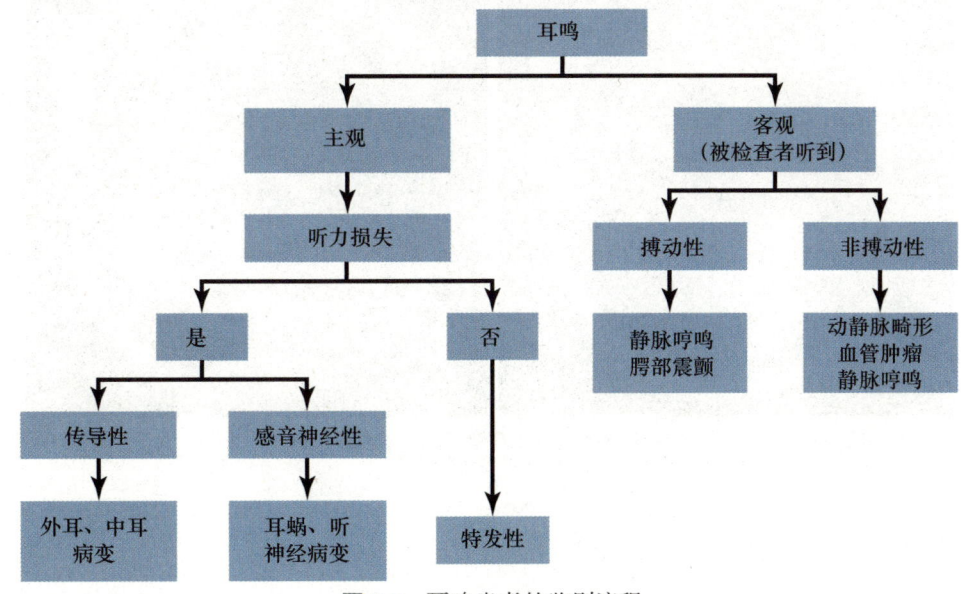

图9.8 耳鸣患者的鉴别流程

the auditory system. Presbycusis may include conductive and central dysfunction, although the most consistent effect of aging is on the sensory cells and neurons of the cochlea; as a result, higher tones are lost early.

TABLE 9.2 Cause of Acute Unilateral Sensorineural Deafness

Cochlear
Idiopathic (85%)
Trauma
Meniere's disease
Lyme disease
Syphilis
Autoimmune disease
Retrocochlear
Demyelination
Vestibular schwannoma (usually gradual onset)
Stroke

Otosclerosis is a disease of the bony labyrinth that usually manifests itself by immobilizing the stapes, thereby producing a conductive hearing loss. Seventy percent of patients with clinical otosclerosis notice hearing loss between the ages of 11 and 30. A family history of otosclerosis is observed in approximately 50% of cases. *Stapedectomy,* a procedure in which the stapes is replaced with a prosthesis, is effective in correcting the conductive component of hearing loss.

A lesion of the cerebellopontine angle, such as a vestibular schwannoma, causes slowly progressive unilateral hearing loss (Table 9.2). Symptoms are caused by compression of the nerve in the narrow confines of the canal (Fig. 9.9). The most common symptoms associated with vestibular schwannomas are slowly progressive hearing loss and tinnitus from compression of the cochlear nerve. Vertigo occurs in fewer than 20% of patients, but approximately 50% complain of imbalance or disequilibrium. Next to the auditory nerve, the cranial nerves most commonly involved by compression are the seventh (facial weakness) and fifth (sensory loss). Loss of the corneal reflex on the affected side is often the first clinical sign. Diagnosis is confirmed with gadolinium-enhanced MRI brain imaging. Treatment in most cases is surgical removal.

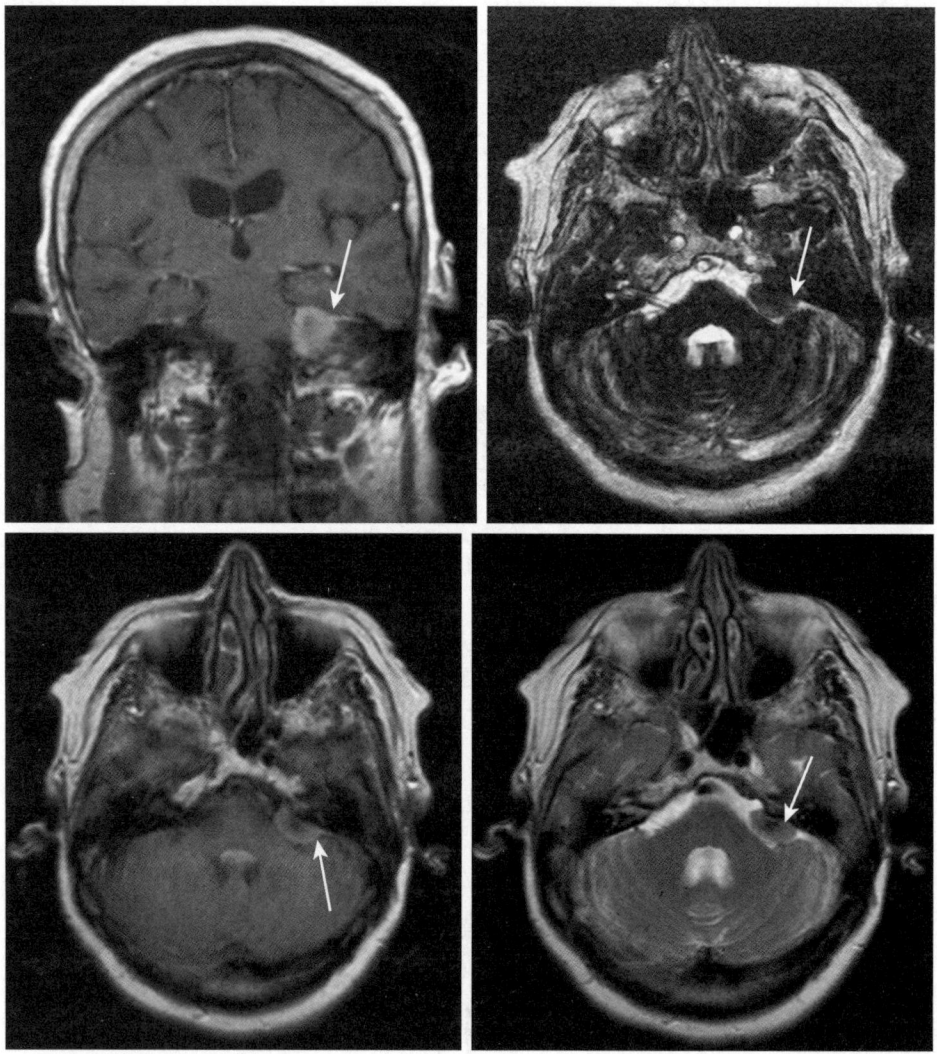

Fig. 9.9 Magnetic resonance imaging scan of the brain showing coronal and axial views of a tumor of the left cerebellopontine angle, consistent with a schwannoma.

系统的多重影响。老年性耳聋可能包括传导性和中枢性功能障碍，但老化对耳蜗感觉细胞和神经元的影响最为一致；因此，高频声音较早损失。

表 9.2　急性单侧感音神经性耳聋的病因
耳蜗
特发性（85%）
外伤
梅尼埃病
莱姆病
梅毒
自身免疫性疾病
耳蜗后结构
脱髓鞘疾病
前庭神经鞘瘤（通常逐渐进展）
脑卒中

耳硬化症是一种骨迷路疾病，通常表现为镫骨固定，从而导致传导性听力损失。临床上，70% 的耳硬化症患者在 11～30 岁出现听力损失。大约 50% 的病例有耳硬化症的家族史。镫骨足板切除术，即用假体替换镫骨的手术，可有效纠正传导性听力损失。

小脑脑桥角病变，例如前庭神经鞘瘤，会导致缓慢进展的单侧听力损失（表 9.2）。症状是由于神经在狭窄的管腔内受压所致（图 9.9）。前庭神经鞘瘤最常见的症状是耳蜗神经受压引起的缓慢进展的听力损失和耳鸣。不到 20% 的患者会出现眩晕，但约 50% 的患者会主诉行走不稳或失衡。除了听神经外，最常受压的脑神经是第Ⅶ脑神经（面瘫）和第Ⅴ脑神经（感觉缺失）。患侧角膜反射消失往往是第一个临床征象。通过钆增强头 MRI 可以确诊。大多数病例的治疗方法是手术切除。

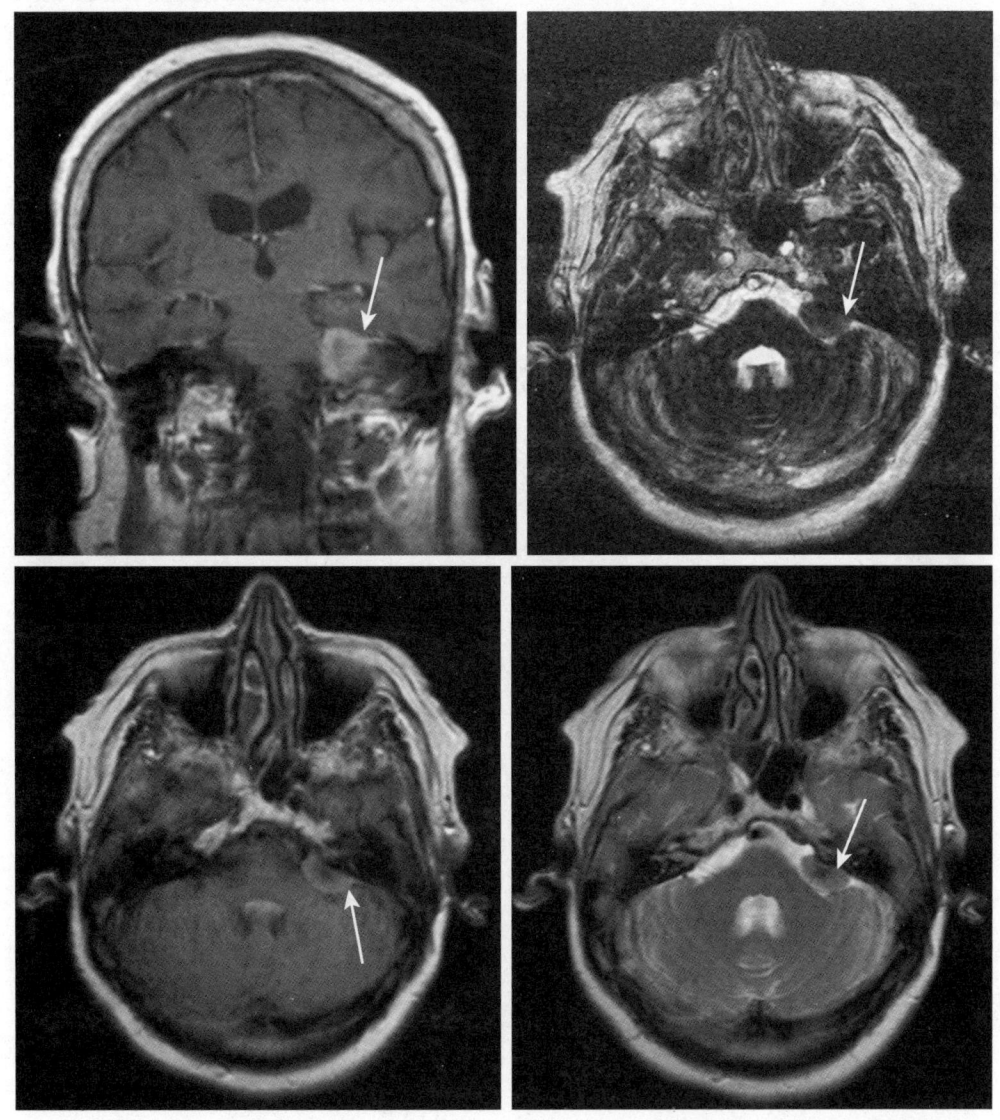

图 9.9　头 MRI 扫描冠状位和轴位，显示左侧小脑脑桥角肿瘤，符合神经鞘瘤

Meniere's syndrome presents with a clinical triad of fluctuating hearing loss, tinnitus, and episodic vertigo. It is thought to be caused by endolymphatic hydrops in the lymphatic system of the inner ear. Typically the patient develops a sensation of fullness and pressure, along with decreased hearing and tinnitus in one ear. Vertigo rapidly follows, reaching a maximum intensity within minutes and then slowly subsiding over the next several hours. The patient is usually left with a sense of unsteadiness and dizziness for days after the acute vertiginous episode. In the early stages the hearing loss is completely reversible, but in later stages a residual hearing loss remains. Up to 50% of patients with idiopathic Meniere's syndrome have a positive family history, suggesting genetic predisposing factors. The key to the diagnosis of Meniere's syndrome is to document fluctuating hearing levels in a patient with the characteristic clinical history. Medical therapy for endolymphatic hydrops includes dietary sodium restriction and oral diuretics.

Acute unilateral deafness usually results from damage to the cochlea and may be caused by viral or bacterial labyrinthitis or vascular occlusion in the territory of the anterior inferior cerebellar artery. Perilymphatic fistulas may also cause abrupt unilateral deafness, usually in association with tinnitus and vertigo.

Drugs that cause acute irreversible bilateral hearing loss include aminoglycosides, cisplatin, and furosemide. Salicylates may cause reversible hearing loss and tinnitus.

Treatment of Hearing Loss

The best treatment is prevention, particularly by the appropriate use of earplugs for those working in a noisy environment. Hearing aids help patients with conductive hearing loss, and developments with cochlear implants may help patients with sensorineural hearing loss.

Prospectus for the Future

Ophthalmology has experienced significant advances in imaging modalities that evaluate the retina. Optical coherence tomography (OCT) is one such technique that provides high-resolution images of retina and optic nerve. Cross section images of the retina, optic nerve, and peripapillary areas are produced. It is helpful at detecting macular disease that is not readily detected on funduscopic examination. In addition, OCT is helpful for monitoring disease activity in various optic neuropathies. OCT angiography is a noninvasive imaging technique that uses OCT technology to visualize retinal and choroidal vasculature. This technique assists with diagnosis and provides insight into the vascular contribution of various retinal diseases.

For a deeper discussion on this topic, please see Chapter 395, "Diseases of the Visual System," and Chapter 396, "Neuro-Ophthalmology," in *Goldman-Cecil Medicine*, 26th Edition.

SUGGESTED READINGS

Margolin E: The swollen optic nerve; an approach to diagnosis and management, Practical Neurol 19(4):302–309, 2019.

Toosy AT, Mason DF, Miller DH: Optic neuritis, Lancet Neurol 13:83–99, 2014.

梅尼埃综合征表现为波动性听力损失、耳鸣和阵发性眩晕的临床三联征。其病因被认为是内耳淋巴系统中的内淋巴积液。典型表现为患者一侧耳朵内感到满胀感，伴随听力下降和耳鸣。随后迅速出现眩晕，在几分钟内达到最大强度，然后在接下来的几小时内逐渐减轻。急性眩晕发作后的数天内，患者通常会感到站立不稳和头晕。在早期阶段，听力损失是完全可逆的，但在后期阶段会残留听力损失。多达50%的特发性梅尼埃综合征患者有阳性家族史，这表明该病存在遗传易感因素。诊断梅尼埃综合征的关键是在具有典型临床病史的患者中记录到听力水平波动情况。内淋巴积液的内科治疗包括饮食限盐和口服利尿剂。

急性单侧耳聋通常是由于耳蜗损伤引起的，可能由病毒性或细菌性迷路炎或小脑前下动脉血管闭塞引起。外淋巴瘘也可能导致突发性单侧耳聋，通常伴有耳鸣和眩晕。

导致急性不可逆双侧听力损失的药物包括氨基糖苷类药物、顺铂和呋塞米。水杨酸盐可能导致可逆性听力损失和耳鸣。

听力损失的治疗

最好的治疗方法是预防，尤其是在嘈杂环境中工作的人应适当使用耳塞。助听器对传导性听力损失的患者有帮助，人工耳蜗的开发则可以帮助感音神经性听力损失患者。

未来展望

眼科学在评估视网膜的成像技术方面取得了显著进展。光学相干断层成像（OCT）就是这样一种可提供视网膜和视神经高分辨率图像的技术。它可以生成视网膜、视神经和视盘周围区域的横截面图像，有助于检测到眼底镜检查不易发现的黄斑病变。此外，OCT还有助于监测各种视神经病变的疾病活动情况。OCT血管造影是一种无创成像技术，利用OCT技术有助于可视化视网膜和脉络膜血管系统。这项技术有助于诊断并深入了解各种视网膜疾病的血管因素。

有关此专题的深入讨论，请参阅 *Goldman-Cecil Medicine* 第26版第395章"视觉系统疾病"和第396章"神经眼科学"。

推荐阅读

Margolin E: The swollen optic nerve; an approach to diagnosis and management, Practical Neurol 19(4):302–309, 2019.

Toosy AT, Mason DF, Miller DH: Optic neuritis, Lancet Neurol 13:83–99, 2014.

10

Dizziness and Vertigo

Jonathan Cahill

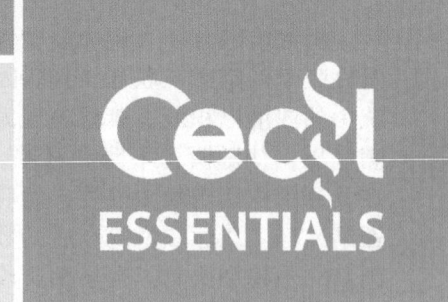

DEFINITIONS AND EPIDEMIOLOGY

Vertigo is defined as the sensation of self-motion in the absence of motion or the sensation of distorted self-motion during normal movement. Traditionally, vertigo is described as a spinning sensation, though other descriptions such as a rising, sinking, or floating sensation may also be vertiginous. Dizziness has a less specific definition and has often been further categorized into sensations of vertigo, disequilibrium, lightheadedness, or presyncope. Patients with dizziness frequently describe multiple different and simultaneous symptoms, and their descriptions of symptoms are frequently inconsistent, which makes accurate diagnosis challenging. Throughout this chapter, the terms *vertigo* and *dizziness* will be used almost interchangeably.

Dizziness is a very commonly reported symptom. As a chief complaint, dizziness accounts for 3% of adult primary care clinic visits and 4% of adult emergency department visits. Approximately 30% of the general population reports having had some type of bothersome dizziness.

THE VESTIBULAR SYSTEM AND BRAIN STEM CIRCUITRY

The sense of balance is maintained by a complicated network of afferent (vestibular, visual, and proprioceptive) and efferent (motor, cerebellar, and oculomotor) systems. The vestibular system consists of the vestibular labyrinth in the temporal bone of the inner ear and its projections to the vestibular portion of the eighth cranial nerve. The eighth cranial nerve projects to the vestibular nuclear complex in the brain stem, which in turn projects widely to the cerebellum, other brain stem nuclei, thalamus, and cerebral cortex.

The paired vestibular systems (left and right) maintain balanced tonic input to the brain. Perturbation of any portion of the circuit by focal lesions or aberrant stimulation can lead to dizziness. The connection of the vestibular system to the oculomotor system, demonstrated by the vestibulo-ocular reflex (VOR), is vital in maintaining clear vision during movement. In many cases, vestibular system abnormalities can be detected by examination of eye movements and the VOR. Nystagmus, alternating fast and slow rhythmic eye movements, is a characteristic sign of vestibular system dysfunction. The type and pattern of nystagmus can assist in more accurately localizing the vestibular disorder. Table 10.1 summarizes common patterns of nystagmus observed in patients with vestibular disorders.

DIFFERENTIATING CENTRAL FROM PERIPHERAL

Most causes of dizziness and vertigo are benign. But it is important to consider the rare more serious causes, such as brain stem infarct or a posterior fossa mass, and to understand the strengths and limitations of available diagnostic testing. The goal of most diagnostic tests is to differentiate causes of vertigo localized to the peripheral (e.g., vestibule, labyrinth, or vestibular nerve) or central (e.g., vestibular nuclear complex, other brain stem connections, cerebellum) vestibular systems.

Computed tomography (CT) scan of the brain is sensitive to rule out acute intracerebral hemorrhage but has limited sensitivity for other etiologies of vertigo. The contents of the posterior fossa (brain stem, cerebellum, and supporting structures) are not well imaged with CT. Furthermore, acute intracerebral hemorrhage commonly presents with additional symptoms and signs and is rarely confused for the other etiologies considered here. Magnetic resonance imaging (MRI) of the brain has better sensitivity for acute ischemic stroke, but in the posterior fossa MRI can miss 15% to 20% of acute ischemic strokes, especially in cases of small (<1 cm) infarctions and when MRI imaging is performed within 24 to 48 hours of symptom onset.

In cases of acute onset dizziness and vertigo, the acute vestibular syndrome, a three-step bedside oculomotor examination is more sensitive than MRI for acute ischemic stroke. The Head-Impulse—Nystagmus—Test-of-Skew (HINTS) examination can be performed in less than 1 minute and can lead to accurate diagnosis in many cases. Table 10.2 summarizes the possible findings of the HINTS examination. It is important to recognize that the HINTS examination findings can only be interpreted when the examination is performed in symptomatic patients.

CLINICAL PRESENTATION PATTERNS

For patients presenting with dizziness, the traditional approach had been to specify the nature or quality of the dizziness as vertigo, imbalance, lightheadedness, or presyncope. The differential diagnosis would then be informed by the specific symptom type. This approach, however, does not lead to accurate diagnosis in many cases and has been replaced by a focus on the timing and triggers of symptoms, rather than the quality of dizziness.

There are four patterns of dizziness presentation: (1) acute persistent, (2) episodic-spontaneous, (3) episodic-triggered, and less commonly, (4) chronic/progressive. It is important to note that no pattern is definitively associated with a particular diagnosis but that the examination and additional testing can be used to home in on a specific disorder and rule out others.

The three most common peripheral vestibular disorders can be thought of as prototypes for most pathology involving the peripheral vestibular system. Each of these three disorders (vestibular neuronitis, Meniere's disease, and benign-paroxysmal positional vertigo [BPPV]) can be diagnosed using the tests described previously and after consideration of possible red flag symptoms. The timing of symptom onset and the triggers of symptoms are the most important features to consider. Table 10.3 summarizes the symptom onset, triggers, and

头晕和眩晕

苏宁 译 牛婧雯 杨洵哲 审校 姚明 朱以诚 通审

定义和流行病学

眩晕（vertigo）是指在没有运动的情况下出现自我运动的感觉，或在正常运动时出现自我异常运动的感觉。通常眩晕被描述为一种旋转的感觉，其他的描述如上升、下沉或漂浮的感觉也可能是眩晕。头晕（dizziness）的定义不太明确，通常被进一步分为眩晕、不平衡感、头昏或晕厥前期。头晕患者经常描述多种不同的且同时出现的症状，而且他们对症状的描述往往不一致，这给准确诊断带来了挑战。在本章中，眩晕和头晕这两个术语几乎可以互换使用。

头晕是一种非常常见的症状。以头晕为主诉的患者占成人初级诊所就诊人数的3%，占成人急诊就诊人数的4%。约30%的普通人都曾有过某种令人烦恼的头晕。

前庭系统和脑干回路

平衡感是通过复杂的神经网络来维持的，包含传入神经系统（前庭系统、视觉系统和本体感觉系统）和传出神经系统（运动系统、小脑系统和眼动系统）。前庭系统包括内耳颞骨部的前庭迷路及其对第Ⅷ脑神经前庭部分的投射纤维。第Ⅷ脑神经投射至脑干的前庭核复合体，而前庭核复合体又广泛地投射至小脑、其他脑干核团、丘脑和大脑皮质。

成对的前庭系统（左侧和右侧）共同维持大脑的平衡性张力信号输入。局部病变或异常刺激对该神经环路任何部位的干扰都可导致头晕。前庭系统与眼动系统的神经纤维连接可通过前庭-眼反射（VOR）来体现，这两部分的神经纤维连接对运动过程中保持清晰的视觉至关重要。在许多情况下，前庭系统的异常可通过眼球运动和前庭-眼反射来检测。眼球震颤，即快速和缓慢交替的眼球节律性运动，是前庭系统功能障碍的特征性表现。眼球震颤的类型和模式有助于更准确地定位前庭功能障碍。表10.1总结了前庭疾病患者眼球震颤的常见模式。

中枢性头晕及周围性头晕的鉴别

大多数引起头晕和眩晕的病因是良性的。但重要的是要考虑到罕见的更严重的病因，例如脑干梗死或颅后窝肿物，并了解目前诊断辅助工具的优势及局限性。大多数诊断性试验的目的是区分眩晕的病因定位于周围（如前庭、迷路或前庭神经）或中枢（如前庭核复合物、其他脑干连接、小脑）前庭系统。

颅脑计算机断层成像（CT）在排除急性颅内出血方面是敏感的，但对其他病因造成的眩晕敏感性有限。颅后窝的内容物（脑干、小脑及其关联结构）在CT上成像不佳。此外，急性脑出血通常合并其他症状和体征，很少与其他病因混淆。颅脑磁共振成像（MRI）对急性缺血性卒中具有更好的敏感性，但可能会遗漏15%～20%的后循环急性缺血性卒中，尤其当梗死病灶小（＜1 cm）以及在症状出现后24～48 h内进行头颅MRI扫描的情况下。

对于急性起病的头晕、眩晕和急性前庭综合征，床旁三步眼动检查对急性缺血性卒中的识别比头颅MRI更敏感。头部脉冲-眼球震颤-眼偏斜测试（HINTS）检查可在不到1 min内完成，并可在许多情况下准确诊断。表10.2总结了HINTS检查的可能结果。需要注意，只有在有症状的患者中进行HINTS检查时才能解释相应的检查结果。

临床表现模式

对于表现为头晕的患者，传统的诊断思路是明确头晕的本质或性质，包括眩晕、不平衡感、头昏或晕厥前期。然后根据具体的症状类型进行鉴别诊断。然而，在许多情况下这种方法并不能帮助明确诊断，因此取而代之的方法是，关注症状的持续时间和诱发因素，而不是头晕的性质。

头晕的表现有四种类型：①急性持续性；②发作性-自发性；③较少见的发作性-诱发性；④慢性/进行性。值得注意的是，没有一种发作形式与特定的诊断有明确的联系，但检查和额外的测试可以用来确定特定的疾病，并排除其他疾病。

三种最常见的前庭周围性病变可以被认为是累及周围前庭系统的大多数病变的原型。这三种疾病[前庭神经炎、梅尼埃病及良性阵发性位置性眩晕（BPPV）]均可通过前面描述的检查并考虑相关的警示征象后进行诊断。症状发作的时间和症状的诱发因素是需要考虑的最重要的特征。表10.3总结了急性前庭

TABLE 10.1 Nystagmus Patterns

	Pattern	Localization	Principal Causes
Spontaneous	Unidirectional, horizontal > torsional	Vestibular nerve, less commonly brain stem	Vestibular neuronitis, less commonly stroke
	Downbeat, upbeat, or pure torsional	Brain	Stroke, brain stem mass, brain stem demyelination
Gaze-evoked	Unidirectional	Vestibular nerve	Vestibular neuronitis
	Bidirectional	Brain	Stroke, cerebellar syndrome, medication side effect
Positional	Burst of upbeat torsional with Dix-Halpike maneuver	Semicircular canal of labyrinth	Benign-paroxysmal-positional vertigo (BPPV)
	Horizontal with supine positional testing	Semicircular canal of labyrinth, less commonly brain stem	BPPV, brain stem lesion
	Persistent downbeat	Brain	Chiari malformation, cerebellar degeneration

TABLE 10.2 HINTS Examination

	Technique	Findings Suggestive of Central Etiology	Findings Suggestive of Peripheral Etiology
Head-Impulse	Patient attempts to maintain visual fixation while the examiner quickly turns the patient's head 5-10 degrees horizontally	Normal fixation, no corrective saccade (rapid eye movements that change the point of fixation)	Abnormal corrective horizontal saccade when the head is turned toward the affected ear
Nystagmus	Extraocular movements examined for nystagmus	Direction changing nystagmus, pure vertical nystagmus	Unidirectional horizontal nystagmus, with some rotary component, worst with gaze in the direction of the fast phase nystagmus
Test-of-Skew	Alternate eye cover testing while patient maintains fixation	Vertical skew with corrective saccade upon uncovering of the eye	Normal, no skew or corrective saccade

TABLE 10.3 Acute Persistent, Episodic-Spontaneous, and Episodic-Triggered Acute Vestibular Syndromes

	Acute Persistent	Episodic-Spontaneous	Episodic-Triggered
Primary consideration	Vestibular neuronitis	Meniere's disease	BPPV
Key features	Constant vertigo, unidirectional horizontal nystagmus, HINTS suggestive of peripheral etiology	Vertigo lasting hours, no specific triggers, unilateral auditory symptoms	Positionally triggered, brief (<1 min) attacks, upbeat torsional nystagmus
Other considerations	Stroke, metabolic disorder, brain stem lesion (mass, demyelination)	TIA, vestibular migraine, panic/anxiety	Orthostatic hypotension
Red flags	Abnormal neurologic examination, HINTS suggestive of central etiology	HINTS (during symptoms) suggestive of central etiology	Prolonged duration of symptoms. Neurologic symptoms other than vertigo.

examination findings for these three common presentations of the acute vestibular syndrome (AVS).

DIFFERENTIAL DIAGNOSIS

For vestibular syndromes, the determination of a peripheral or central etiology and the pattern of presenting symptoms serve as the framework for generating the differential diagnosis. In addition to the peripheral and central causes of vertigo and dizziness considered here, there are several other general medical conditions that can present with symptoms mimicking a vestibular syndrome. And despite careful history, examination, and diagnostic testing selection, many cases of dizziness and vertigo remain idiopathic.

The three common causes of a peripheral vestibular disorder (see Table 10.3) are vestibular neuronitis, Meniere's disease, and BPPV. Vestibular neuronitis, caused by a viral infection of the vestibular nerve, typically presents with abrupt onset vertigo (acute-persistent pattern) and nausea, most commonly lasting for several days. The vertigo attacks of Meniere's disease are shorter in duration, typically hours, and accompanied by nausea and prominent auditory symptoms of hearing loss, ear fullness, and tinnitus. The auditory symptoms of Meniere's disease become more prominent as the disease progresses and can occur outside of specific vertigo attacks. Meniere's disease attacks occur without provocation (episodic-spontaneous), unlike the attacks of BPPV (episodic-triggered). BPPV is caused by otoliths entering the semicircular canals of the inner ear and causing aberrant stimulation of the vestibule and vestibular nerve. In BPPV, sudden movement of the head, such as rolling over in bed or turning one's head to the side, can provoke severe vertigo and nausea, which lasts typically for less than 1 minute if the head is held still. Despite the short duration of vertigo in BPPV, the symptoms can be severe and disabling.

表 10.1 眼球震颤（眼震）类型

	类型	定位	主要病因
自发性眼震	单向的，水平的>扭转的	前庭神经，少见于脑干	前庭神经炎，少见于卒中
	下跳性、上跳性、或单纯扭转性	脑	卒中、脑干肿物、脑干脱髓鞘
凝视诱发性眼震	单向的	前庭神经	前庭神经炎
	双向的	脑	卒中、小脑综合征、药物不良反应
位置性眼震	Dix-Halpike 试验出现上跳伴扭转性眼震	迷路半规管	良性阵发性位置性眩晕（BPPV）
	仰卧翻滚试验出现水平性眼震	迷路半规管，少见于脑干	BPPV、脑干病变
	持续下跳性眼震	脑	Chiari 畸形、小脑退行性变

表 10.2 HINTS 检查

	操作	检查结果提示中枢性病因	检查结果提示周围性病因
头部脉冲试验	患者尝试保持视觉固定，检查者快速将患者头部水平转动 5°~10°	正常注视，没有矫正性扫视（快速眼球运动来改变眼球注视点）	当往患侧耳转头时出现异常的矫正性水平扫视
眼震检查	眼球运动检查眼震	改变方向的眼震，单纯垂直性眼震	单一方向水平眼震，合并部分旋转性成分，当往快速眼震方向注视时会加重
眼偏斜试验	当患者双眼注视时交替遮盖患者眼球	去除遮盖时眼睛出现垂直斜视及矫正性扫视	正常，没有斜视或矫正性扫视

表 10.3 急性持续性、发作性-自发性和发作性-诱发性的急性前庭综合征

	急性持续性	发作性-自发性	发作性-诱发性
主要考虑	前庭神经炎	梅尼埃病	BPPV
主要特点	持续眩晕，单一方向水平眼震，HINTS 提示周围性病变	眩晕持续数小时，无特殊诱因，单侧听觉症状	体位变化诱发，短暂发作（<1 min），向上的旋转性眼震
其他考虑	卒中、代谢性疾病、脑干病变（肿物、脱髓鞘）	短暂性脑缺血发作，前庭性偏头痛，惊恐、焦虑	体位性低血压
警示征象	异常神经系统查体，HINTS 提示中枢性病变	HINTS（症状存在时）提示中枢性病变	症状持续，合并眩晕之外的神经系统症状

综合征（AVS）这三种常见表现的发病症状、诱发因素和检查结果。

鉴别诊断

对于前庭综合征，确定周围或中枢性病因以及症状的表现模式可作为鉴别诊断的框架。除了本文所讨论的引起眩晕和头晕的周围性和中枢性原因外，还有其他的一些医学情况表现为类前庭综合征。尽管进行了仔细的病史询问、查体和诊断性检查选择，许多头晕和眩晕病例仍然原因未明。

周围前庭神经病变的三个常见原因（见表 10.3）是前庭神经炎、梅尼埃病及 BPPV。前庭神经炎由前庭神经的病毒感染引起，典型表现为突然起病的眩晕（急性持续性）和恶心，症状常持续数天。梅尼埃病的眩晕发作持续时间较短，通常为数小时，并伴有恶心和明显的听觉症状，如听力减退、耳胀和耳鸣。梅尼埃病的听觉症状随着疾病的进展而更加突出，并且可以在眩晕不发作时出现。与 BPPV 的发作（发作性-诱发性）不同，梅尼埃病发作无特定诱发因素（发作性-自发性）。BPPV 是由耳石进入内耳半规管，引起前庭和前庭神经异常刺激导致的。对 BPPV 患者，头部的突然运动，如在床上翻身或把头转向一侧，可诱发严重的眩晕和恶心，如果头部保持不动，症状通常持续不到 1 min。尽管 BPPV 的眩晕持续时间很短，但症状可能很严重，甚至致残。

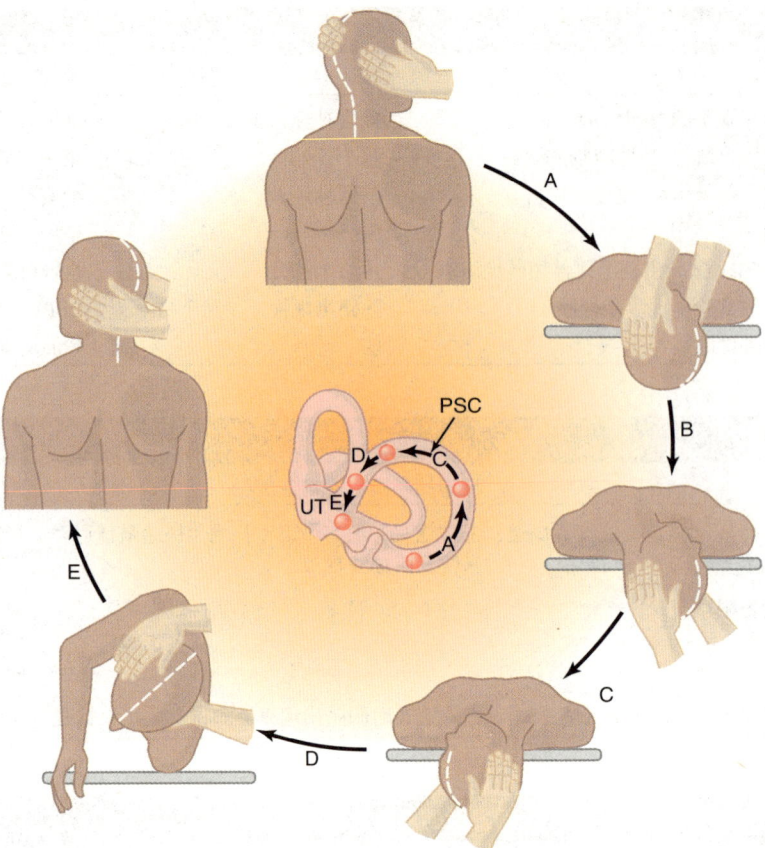

Fig. 10.1 Repositioning treatment for benign paroxysmal positional vertigo designed to move endolymphatic debris out of the posterior semicircular canal (PSC) of the right ear and into the utricle (UT). The patient is seated, and the patient's head is turned 45 degrees to the right (A). The head is then lowered rapidly to below the horizontal (B). The examiner shifts hand positions (C), and the patient's head is rotated rapidly 90 degrees in the opposite direction, so it now points 45 degrees to the left, where it remains for 30 seconds (D). The patient then rolls onto the left side without turning the head in relation to the body and maintains this position for another 30 seconds (E) before sitting up. The treatment is repeated until nystagmus is abolished. The procedure is reversed for treating the left ear. (Modified from Foster CA, Baloh RW: Episodic vertigo. In Rakel RE, editor: Conn's Current Therapy, Philadelphia, 1995, WB Saunders.)

Central causes of vertigo include numerous pathologies that cause structural or functional disturbance of the brain stem and cerebellum. For acute vestibular syndromes, ischemic stroke and/or transient ischemic attack (TIA) should be considered, especially in cases where the HINTS examination is concerning or there are other neurologic symptoms or signs in addition to vertigo and dizziness. Migraine may be one of the most common central causes of vertigo, with up to 40% of migraine patients reporting some accompanying vertigo with their migraine attacks. Both vestibular migraine and migraine with brain stem aura can have vertigo as a prominent symptom, though it is usually not the lone symptom. Space occupying lesions in the brain stem or cerebellum (neoplasm, abscess) should be considered in patients with risk factors. And unlike acute ischemic stroke, which can be missed by MRI up to 20% of the time, mass lesions of the brain stem or cerebellum will typically be seen on MRI. Hydrocephalus, which can be readily diagnosed on CT or MRI imaging, may cause symptoms of dizziness, but more typically it would present with a gait ataxia in the absence of dizziness. Degenerative disorders of the cerebellum can cause vertigo, but the pattern of symptoms would not be confused with that of stroke or other AVS.

A wide array of other general medical conditions can cause dizziness or vertigo as well. Dizziness as a side effect of medications is probably the most common. Dizziness can also be a prominent symptom of panic and anxiety. Symptomatic anemia can cause lightheadedness and dizziness. And following significant head trauma, a post-traumatic dizziness can last for several weeks.

TARGETED TREATMENT

Because most causes of vertigo are benign and the symptoms typically resolve spontaneously in hours to days, conservative treatments are most often appropriate. Symptomatic relief of vertigo can be achieved with antihistamines, benzodiazepines, or antiemetics, but their side effects in the long term and in older patients limit their use. More specific, targeted treatment to the underlying cause of vertigo is preferable.

Vestibular rehabilitation as directed by a physical therapist is the most helpful treatment for prolonged vertigo, such as with vestibular neuronitis. Meniere's disease is commonly treated with a low salt diet or diuretics to reduce the frequency of attacks. The Epley maneuver (Fig. 10.1) for repositioning semicircular canal otoliths is highly effective for BPPV, especially in the most common circumstance where the posterior semicircular canal is affected. For

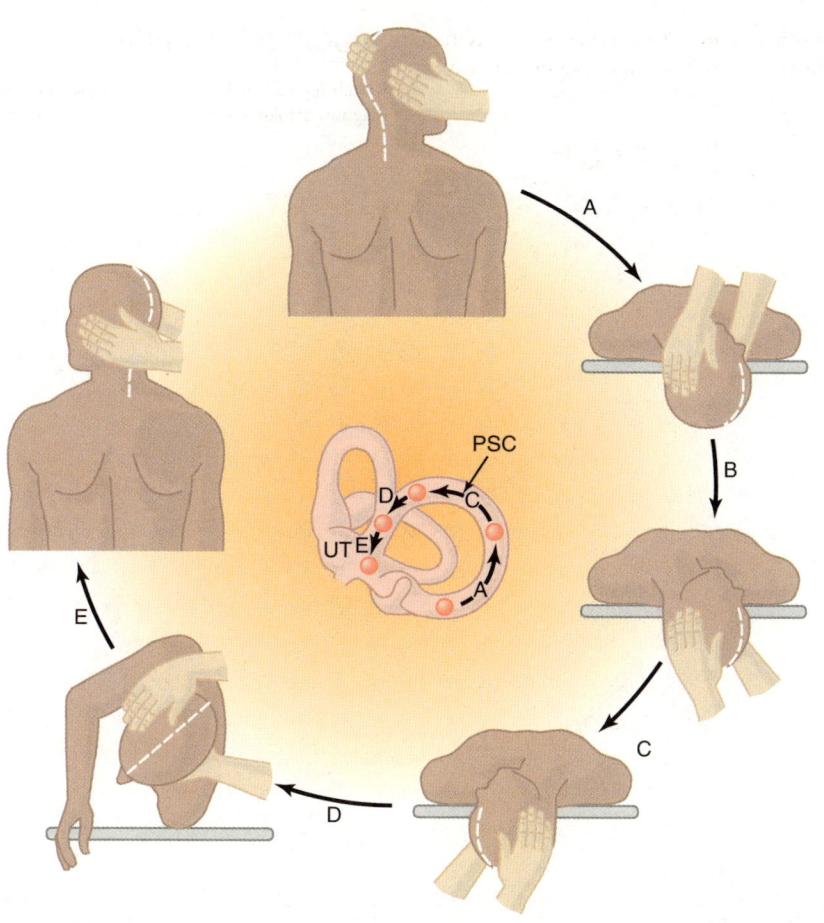

图 10.1　良性阵发性位置性眩晕的复位治疗，旨在将内淋巴的耳石移出右耳后半规管，并转移至椭圆囊。患者坐位，检查者将患者头部向右转动 45°（**A**）。然后检查者将患者头部迅速下降到水平位以下（**B**）。检查者移动手的位置（**C**），将患者的头部向相反方向快速旋转 90°，因此头部现在是向左 45°，保持该姿势 30 s（**D**）。患者随后向左侧转身，头部相对于身体不转动，并保持该姿势 30 s（**E**），然后坐起来。重复治疗直到眼球震颤完全消失。治疗左耳则相反。PSC，后半规管；UT，椭圆囊。（改编自 Foster CA, Baloh RW: Episodic vertigo. In Rakel RE, editor: Conn's Current Therapy, Philadelphia, 1995, WB Saunders.）

眩晕的中枢性病因包括一系列能引起脑干和小脑结构或功能紊乱的病变。对于急性前庭综合征，应考虑缺血性卒中和（或）短暂性脑缺血发作（TIA），尤其是当 HINTS 检查提示合并眩晕和头晕之外的神经系统症状及体征表现时。偏头痛可能是中枢性眩晕最常见的原因之一，高达 40% 的偏头痛患者报告偏头痛发作时伴有眩晕。前庭偏头痛和脑干先兆偏头痛都可以眩晕为突出症状之一，尽管眩晕通常不是唯一的症状。对于有危险因素的患者，需要考虑脑干或小脑占位性病变（肿瘤、脓肿）。MRI 检查可能遗漏 20% 的急性缺血性卒中，而脑干或小脑的占位病变通常能通过 MRI 被发现。脑积水患者也可能会出现头晕症状，通过 CT 或 MRI 即可诊断脑积水，但脑积水更典型的症状是不伴头晕的共济失调步态。小脑退行性疾病可引起眩晕，但其症状模式很容易与卒中或其他 AVS 相区别。

其他许多临床状况也会导致头晕或眩晕。其中药物副作用引起的头晕可能是最常见的。头晕也可能是恐慌和焦虑的一个突出症状。症状性贫血会引起头昏和头晕。严重的头部外伤后，创伤性头晕可持续数周。

针对性治疗

由于大部分眩晕的病因是良性的，症状通常在几小时到几天内自行好转，保守治疗通常是最合适的。抗组胺药、苯二氮䓬类药物或止吐药可以缓解眩晕症状，但药物的长期副作用和对老年患者的副作用限制了这些药物的使用。针对眩晕的潜在病因进行治疗更有效。

理疗师指导下的前庭神经康复是治疗长时间眩晕（如前庭神经炎）最有效的方法。梅尼埃病通常通过低盐饮食或利尿剂来减少发作的频率。Epley 手法（图 10.1）对 BPPV 的半规管耳石复位非常有效，特别是针

central causes of vertigo, both stroke and migraine have specific treatments proven to be effective as both abortive and preventative therapies.

SUGGESTED READING

Kattah JC, Talkad AV, Wang DZ, Hsieh YH, Newman-Toker DE: HINTS to diagnose stroke in the acute vestibular syndrome, Stroke 40:3504–3510, 2009.

对最常见的后半规管受累情况。对于中枢性眩晕如卒中和偏头痛，都有特定的有效的治疗方法，包括终止发作和预防性的治疗。

推荐阅读

Kattah JC, Talkad AV, Wang DZ, Hsieh YH, Newman-Toker DE: HINTS to diagnose stroke in the acute vestibular syndrome, Stroke 40:3504–3510, 2009.

11

Disorders of the Motor System

Ruth B. Schneider, Adolfo Ramirez-Zamora, Christopher G. Tarolli

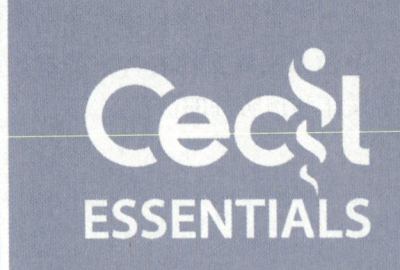

INTRODUCTION

The motor system is broadly divided into the pyramidal and extrapyramidal systems. The pyramidal system functions to execute motor activity, while the extrapyramidal system provides feedback to the pyramidal system, allowing selection of wanted patterns of movement and suppression of unwanted patterns. The pyramidal system is a two-neuron system, which originates in the primary motor cortex of the frontal lobes and, with white matter projections, coalesces to form the internal capsule; it then traverses the brain stem (as the cerebral peduncles in the midbrain, the basis pontis in the pons, and the pyramids in the medulla where the majority of neurons decussate to form the corticospinal tracts) and ultimately synapses on the lower motor neurons in the anterior horn of the spinal cord. The extrapyramidal system consists primarily of the basal ganglia and the cerebellum and provides coordinating and integrating information to the pyramidal tract system under the influence of various afferent feedback loops. The components and pathways of the basal ganglia (Fig. 11.1) and cerebellum (Fig. 11.2) influence and modulate voluntary motor activity of the motor cortex.

Disorders of the motor system affect the components of the pyramidal and extrapyramidal systems. The approach to the patient with motor dysfunction depends on the ability to accurately localize the neuroanatomic region affected through a careful history and focused examination. Disorders of the pyramidal system (central and peripheral) will be described in other chapters of this text (Chapters 4, 14, 18, and 20). Here, we will focus on disorders of the extrapyramidal system, which present with a variety of disorders of movement.

INTRODUCTION TO MOVEMENT DISORDERS

Movement disorders are a heterogeneous group of disorders associated with basal ganglia dysfunction. Movement disorders refer to a broad group of conditions leading to involuntary or abnormal movement as a prominent feature. In contrast to most seizures, the involuntary movements occur when the patient is conscious but are absent during sleep (with very few exceptions).

Movement disorders can be classified as either hyperkinetic or hypokinetic. Hyperkinetic phenomena include tremor, chorea, dystonia, tics, myoclonus, and other involuntary movements (Table 11.1). Hypokinetic disorders encompass the parkinsonian disorders characterized by a paucity of spontaneous movement (akinesia), slow movements (bradykinesia), and low amplitude movements (hypokinesia). The term bradykinesia is commonly used to encompass all three of these phenomena. While this classification strategy is a valuable means for approaching the patient with abnormal movements, many movement disorders display a combination of both hyperkinetic and hypokinetic phenomena. Idiopathic Parkinson's disease is the prototypical hypokinetic movement disorder, but it is associated with the hyperkinetic phenomenon of tremor in over 60% of patients. Similarly, Huntington's disease, a traditionally hyperkinetic disorder, is associated with bradykinesia.

Parkinsonism

Parkinsonism is characterized by bradykinesia, rigidity, tremor, and postural instability. It can be caused by a wide variety of degenerative disorders, medications, toxins, and systemic diseases. Table 11.2 summarizes the differential diagnosis of parkinsonism.

Idiopathic Parkinson's Disease

Idiopathic Parkinson's disease (PD), which is the most common cause of parkinsonism, is a progressive, neurodegenerative disorder characterized by a constellation of motor and nonmotor symptoms. The prevalence of PD increases with age and it affects approximately 1% to 2% of individuals over the age of 60. Beyond advancing age, some risk factors for PD include male sex, pesticide exposure, solvent exposure, and family history of PD. The motor symptoms of PD result from the selective loss of dopaminergic neurons in the substantia nigra-pars compacta that project to the striatum. The pathological hallmark of PD is the presence of eosinophilic cytoplasmic neuronal inclusions known as Lewy bodies containing α-synuclein.

Clinically, PD is most commonly recognized by its motor phenomena: rigidity, bradykinesia, rest tremor, and postural instability. Functionally, patients may describe difficulty with fine motor tasks (such as doing buttons), difficulty getting dressed, trouble getting up from a chair, a lack of facial expression, changes in speech (softening or hoarseness), decreased arm swing, poor balance, or tremor at rest or when holding a newspaper. Motor symptoms typically present unilaterally and remain asymmetric over time. Parkinsonian gait is characterized by a flexed and stooped posture, with a slow shuffling quality and decreased stride length and heel strike. Patients can also display festination, a phenomenon in which the stooped posture and hypometric stepping results in the center of gravity being located in front of the feet. Some experience freezing of gait, which refers to a brief and sudden inability to initiate or continue walking. Nonmotor manifestations include autonomic dysfunction (orthostatic hypotension, constipation, urinary symptoms, and impaired temperature regulation), psychiatric features (depression, anxiety, apathy, and psychosis), cognitive changes (mild cognitive impairment and dementia), sleep disorders (insomnia, excessive daytime sleepiness, restless legs syndrome, rapid eye movement [REM] sleep behavior disorder), and a myriad

运动系统疾病

沈东超 译　杨洵哲 牛婧雯 审校　姚明 朱以诚 通审

引言

运动系统大致分为锥体系和锥体外系。锥体系的功能是执行运动活动，而锥体外系则为锥体系提供反馈，选择需要的运动模式，而抑制不需要的模式。锥体系是一个包含二级神经元的系统，它起源于额叶的初级运动皮质，并通过白质投射，融合形成内囊；然后穿过脑干（在中脑形成大脑脚，在脑桥形成桥基部，在延髓形成锥体，其中大部分神经元交叉形成皮质脊髓束），终止于脊髓前角的下运动神经元突触。锥体外系主要由基底神经节和小脑组成，在各种传入反馈回路的影响下，为锥体系提供协调和整合信息。基底神经节（图11.1）和小脑（图11.2）的组成部分和通路影响并调节运动皮质的随意运动活动。

运动系统疾病会累及锥体系和锥体外系的组成部分。运动功能障碍的诊治，依赖于通过仔细的病史问诊和重点辅助检查，准确定位受影响的神经解剖区域。锥体系疾病（包括中枢和周围）将在本书的其他章节中描述（第4章、第14章、第18章和第20章）。在这里，我们将重点讨论导致各种运动障碍的锥体外系疾病。

运动障碍简介

运动障碍是一组与基底神经节功能障碍相关的异质性疾病。运动障碍是一组广泛的疾病，以不自主或异常运动为显著特征。与大多数癫痫发作不同，不自主运动发生在患者清醒时，但在睡眠期间消失（极少数例外）。

运动障碍可分为两类：多动性和少动性。多动性现象包括震颤、舞蹈症、肌张力障碍、抽动、肌阵挛和其他不自主运动（表11.1）。少动性障碍包括以自发运动减少（运动不能）、运动缓慢（运动迟缓）和运动幅度小（运动减退）为特征的帕金森综合征，这三个现象通常统称为运动迟缓。这种分类策略对处理患者的异常运动非常重要，然而许多运动障碍可同时表现出多动性和少动性现象。特发性帕金森病是典型的少动性运动障碍，但超过60%的患者伴有多动性震颤。类似地，经典的多动性疾病——亨廷顿病也会表现出运动迟缓。

帕金森综合征

帕金森综合征的特征是运动迟缓、肌肉僵硬、震颤和姿势不稳。它可以由多种退行性疾病、药物、毒素和系统性疾病引起。表11.2总结了帕金森综合征的鉴别诊断。

特发性帕金森病

特发性帕金森病（PD）是帕金森综合征最常见的原因，是一种进行性的神经退行性疾病，以一系列运动和非运动症状为特征。PD的患病率随着年龄的增长而增加，影响1%～2%的60岁以上人群。除了年龄增长外，PD的一些风险因素包括男性、接触农药、溶剂暴露和家族病史。PD的运动症状是由于投射到纹状体的黑质致密部多巴胺能神经元的选择性丧失引起的。PD的病理标志是含有α突触核蛋白的嗜酸性细胞质神经元包涵体（路易体）的存在。

在临床上，PD最常见的表现是其运动症状：僵硬、运动迟缓、静止性震颤和姿势不稳。在功能上，患者可能会描述精细运动任务困难（如扣纽扣）、穿衣困难、起身困难、面部表情缺乏、言语变化（声调变轻或沙哑）、摆臂减少、平衡差、静止时或持报纸时震颤。运动症状通常单侧出现，并且随着时间的推移保持不对称。帕金森步态的特征是屈曲和弯腰姿势、步态缓慢、步幅变小和脚跟触地减少。患者还可能表现出慌张步态，即屈身姿势和步幅缩小导致重心位于脚前方。有些患者会出现步态冻结，即一种突然不能开始或继续行走的现象。非运动症状包括自主神经功能障碍（体位性低血压、便秘、泌尿系统症状和体温调节受损）、精神症状（抑郁、焦虑、淡漠和精神错乱）、认知变化（轻度认知障碍和痴呆）、睡眠障碍［失眠、白天过度嗜睡、不宁腿综合征、快速眼动（REM）期

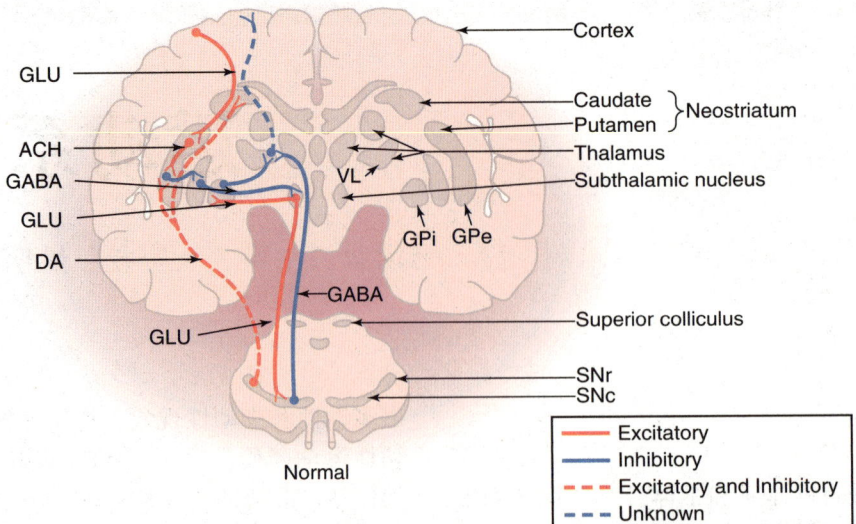

Fig. 11.1 Anatomy of the basal ganglia and their connections. The feedback loop proceeds from cerebral prefrontal areas to the basal ganglia and eventually back from the basal ganglia to the thalamus to the motor cortex. This ultimately regulates the descending corticospinal motor system. *ACH*, Acetylcholine; *DA*, dopamine; *GABA*, γ-aminobutyric acid; *GLU*, glutamate; *GP*, globus pallidum (e, external; i, internal); *SN*, substantia nigra (c, compacta; r, reticulate); *VL*, ventrolateral. (From Jankovic J: The extrapyramidal disorders: Introduction. In Goldman L, Bennett JC, editors: Cecil Textbook of Medicine, ed 21, Philadelphia, 2000, Saunders, p 2078.)

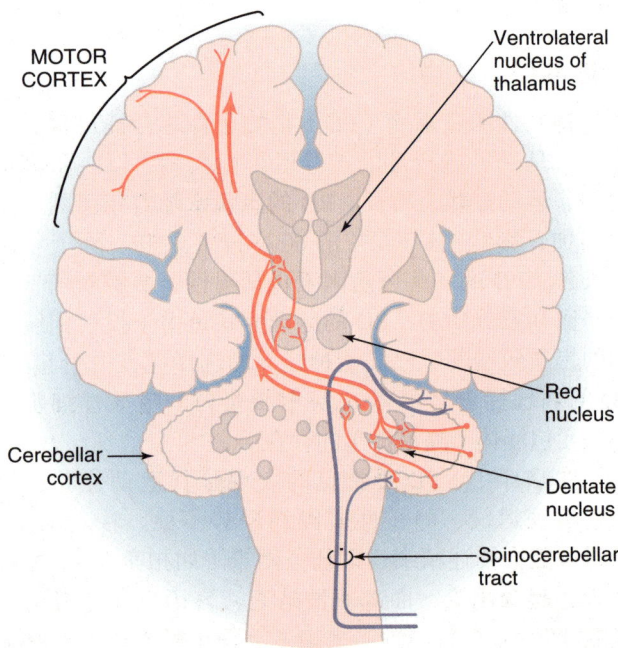

Fig. 11.2 Corticocerebellar loop. The major cerebellar input is from the spinocerebellar tract. Outflow is to the motor cortex via the mesencephalon and thalamus.

of other symptoms (pain, sexual dysfunction, vision changes, fatigue, micrographia, and decreased sense of smell).

PD is a clinical diagnosis based on the presence of gradual progression of characteristic motor symptoms and signs as well as a robust and sustained response to levodopa therapy. While the diagnosis of PD is made on the basis of the presence of a characteristic motor syndrome, it is now recognized that there are earlier stages of PD: preclinical PD (neurodegeneration in the absence of symptoms or signs) and prodromal PD (symptoms and signs, often nonmotor, insufficient to meet diagnostic criteria). Certain "red flags" on history or examination might suggest an atypical or secondary cause of parkinsonism (Table 11.3). Dopamine transporter (DaT) SPECT imaging can assist in distinguishing neurodegenerative forms of parkinsonism from drug-induced parkinsonism and essential tremor with parkinsonian features. The dopamine transporter is responsible for re-uptake of dopamine into presynaptic terminals and is, therefore, an indirect measure of nigro-striatal neuronal density. In PD, nigro-striatal neurons are lost asymmetrically; on dopamine transporter imaging, this is characterized by asymmetric reduction in dopamine transporter signal in the striatum. With drug-induced parkinsonism and essential tremor, dopamine transporter imaging is normal. Dopamine transporter imaging does not distinguish PD from other degenerative forms of parkinsonism.

PD is a slowly progressive disorder associated with accumulating disability. No medications have been proven to slow progression; however, exercise may slow the progression of disease. Treatments of the motor symptoms can reduce disability and improve function. The mainstay of treatment is levodopa, the precursor to dopamine, given with a dopa-decarboxylase inhibitor (e.g., carbidopa) to maximize CNS penetration of levodopa and minimize systemic side effects. Other symptomatic treatments stimulate dopamine receptors in the brain (dopamine agonists) or inhibit the breakdown of levodopa and dopamine (monoamine oxidase type B inhibitors and catechol-O-methyltransferase inhibitors). This approach to symptom management is effective early in the course of the disease; however, as the disease continues to progress, it may be complicated by the development of motor complications, including motor fluctuations and dyskinesias (which manifest as chorea and/or dystonia). Surgical approaches to treatment of motor complications include deep brain stimulation (DBS) and continuous intestinal infusion of levodopa-carbidopa. Unfortunately, some motor features, such as postural instability, are

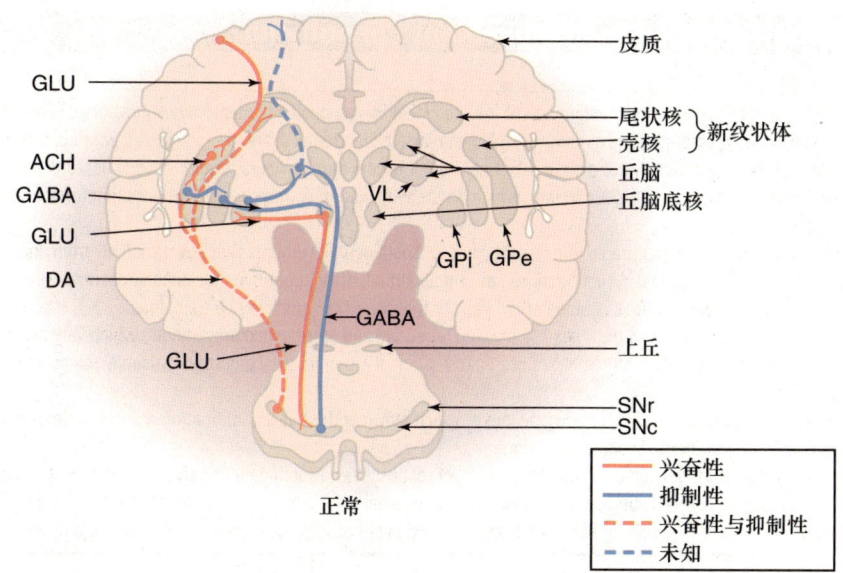

图 11.1 基底神经节及其连接的解剖结构。反馈环路从大脑前额叶区开始，经过基底神经节，最终从基底神经节返回到丘脑，再到运动皮质。最终调节下行皮质脊髓运动系统。ACH，乙酰胆碱；DA，多巴胺；GABA，γ-氨基丁酸；GLU，谷氨酸；GP，苍白球（e，外侧；i，内侧）；SN，黑质（c，致密部；r，网状部）；VL，腹外侧核。（引自 Jankovic J：The extrapyramidal disorders：Introduction. In Goldman L，Bennett JC，editors：Cecil Textbook of Medicine，ed 21，Philadelphia，2000，Saunders，p 2078.）

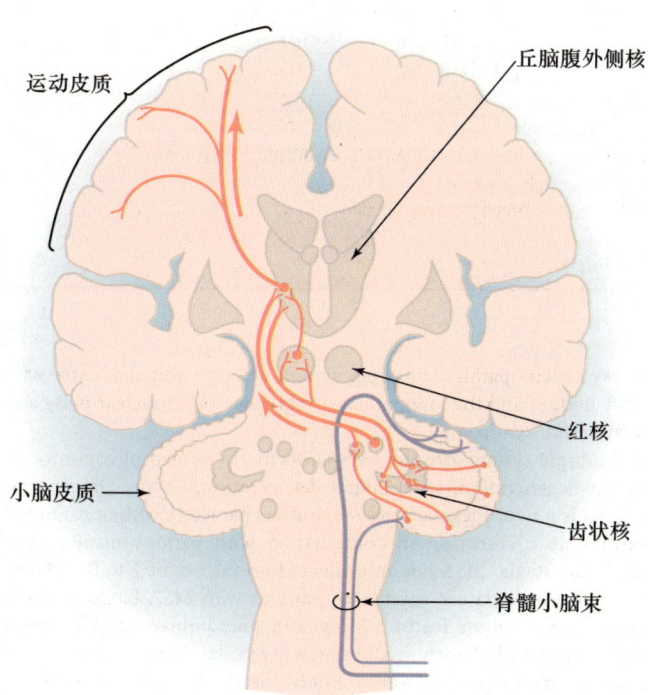

图 11.2 皮质小脑环路。小脑的主要输入来自脊髓小脑束，输出通路经中脑和丘脑传导到运动皮质

睡眠行为障碍]和其他各种症状（疼痛、性功能障碍、视力变化、疲劳、写字过小症和嗅觉减退）。

PD 的临床诊断主要基于特征性运动症状和体征的逐渐进展，以及对左旋多巴治疗显著而持久的反应。尽管 PD 的诊断是基于特征性运动综合征的存在，但现在对 PD 的更早期阶段也有了一定的认识，包括临床前

PD（没有症状或体征的神经退行性变）和前驱 PD（存在症状和体征，通常为非运动性，但不足以满足诊断标准）。病史或辅助检查中的某些"红旗征"可能提示帕金森综合征的非典型或继发性原因（表 11.3）。多巴胺转运体（DaT）SPECT 成像可以帮助区分神经退行性帕金森综合征与药物引起的帕金森综合征以及具有帕金森特征的特发性震颤。多巴胺转运体负责多巴胺在突触前末梢的再摄取，因此可间接反映黑质-纹状体神经元密度。在 PD 中，黑质-纹状体神经元不对称丧失；在多巴胺转运体成像中，这表现为纹状体多巴胺转运体信号的不对称减少。在药物引起的帕金森综合征和特发性震颤中，多巴胺转运体成像是正常的。多巴胺转运体成像不能区分 PD 与其他退行性帕金森综合征。

PD 是一种缓慢进展的疾病，伴随残疾逐渐累积。没有药物被证明可以减缓疾病进程，但体育锻炼可能会减缓疾病的进展。运动症状的治疗可以减少残疾并改善功能。治疗的主要方法是左旋多巴，它是多巴胺的前体，与多巴脱羧酶抑制剂（如卡比多巴）一起给药，以最大限度地增加左旋多巴在中枢神经系统中的渗透并减少全身副作用。其他对症治疗方法包括刺激大脑中的多巴胺受体（多巴胺激动剂）或抑制左旋多巴和多巴胺的分解（单胺氧化酶 B 抑制剂和儿茶酚-O-甲基转移酶抑制剂）。这种对症治疗在疾病早期有效，但随着疾病的进展，可能会因运动并发症的出现而变得复杂，包括症状波动和异动症[表现为舞蹈症和（或）肌张力障碍]。治疗运动并发症的外科治疗方法包括脑深部电刺激（DBS）和连续肠内输注左旋多巴-卡比多巴。不幸的是，某些运

TABLE 11.1 Definition of Common Movement Phenomena

Movement	Definition
Parkinsonism	Generic term referring to some combination of features including a paucity of spontaneous movement (akinesia), slow movements (bradykinesia), and low amplitude movements (hypokinesia) as well as tremor (at rest), rigidity, and postural instability.
Tremor	Rhythmic oscillatory movement of a body part. Rest tremor occurs at rest. Action tremor encompasses postural tremor (present during maintenance of a posture), kinetic tremor (which occurs with voluntary movement), and intention tremor (when the tremor worsens upon approaching a target).
Chorea	Irregular, purposeless, abrupt, rapid, brief, arrhythmic, unsustained movements that flow randomly from one part of the body to another.
Dystonia	Sustained or intermittent muscle contractions causing abnormal, often repetitive movements, postures, or both. Dystonic movements are typically patterned, twisting, sustained at the peak of the movement, and may be tremulous.
Tics	Abrupt, usually brief, suppressible, "jerky" and often repetitive and stereotyped movements, which vary in intensity and are repeated at irregular intervals. Key features of tics are the presence of a premonitory urge that is usually temporarily relieved following the movement.
Ataxia	Impairment in coordination of voluntary movement, which may manifest as incoordination of limb movements, gait impairment, eye movement abnormalities, or speech impairment.
Akathisia	Sensorimotor disorder defined by a subjective sense of restlessness affecting all or part of the body with a marked difficulty staying still.
Myoclonus	Simple, rapid, involuntary movement causing movement of a part of the body across a joint. While it can be similar in appearance to a tic, myoclonus is typically a simpler movement fragment and is not associated with a premonitory urge or post-movement sense of relief.

TABLE 11.2 Differential Diagnosis of Parkinsonism

Degenerative/inherited causes	Idiopathic Parkinson's Disease
	Multiple system atrophy
	Progressive supranuclear palsy
	Dementia with Lewy body
	Corticobasal degeneration
	Frontotemporal dementia with Parkinsonism
	Huntington's disease
	Wilson disease
	Dopa-responsive dystonia
	Pantothenate kinase–associated neurodegeneration
Secondary causes	Dopamine receptor blocking medications (e.g., antipsychotics, metoclopramide, prochlorperazine)
	Presynaptic dopamine depleting medications (tetrabenazine)
	Other medications (e.g., valproic acid, calcium-channel blockers, lithium)
	Cerebrovascular disease
	Toxins (MPTP, manganese, carbon monoxide)

MPTP, 1-Methyl-4-phenyl-1,2,3,6-tetrahydropyridine.

unresponsive to medical or surgical therapy. Rehabilitative therapies play an important role throughout the disease course.

A number of monogenic causes of Parkinsonism have been identified. Mutations in α-synuclein *(SNCA)* and leucine-rich repeat kinase 2 *(LRRK2)* are associated with autosomal dominant parkinsonism. Autosomal dominant causes account for less than 2% of all adult-onset Parkinson's disease cases with higher frequencies in certain populations due to founder effects. Autosomal recessive monogenic causes include mutations in genes encoding parkin *(PRKN)*, PTEN-induced kinase 1 *(PINK1)*, and DJ-1 *(PARK7)* and are relatively common in familial cases with onset before the age of 45. Mutations in glucocerebrosidase (GBA) are the most commonly identified mutations in PD. An improved understanding of these genetic causes suggests an important role of impairment in lysosomal pathways and protein degradation in PD pathogenesis.

Atypical Parkinsonism

The atypical parkinsonian or "Parkinson plus" syndromes refer to a heterogeneous group of sporadic neurodegenerative disorders characterized by parkinsonism, reduced or absent response to dopaminergic therapy, and characteristic nonmotor features. The most common are the synucleinopathies: multiple system atrophy and dementia with Lewy bodies; and the tauopathies: progressive supranuclear palsy and corticobasal syndrome.

Multiple system atrophy (MSA), formerly termed olivopontocerebellar degeneration, striatonigral degeneration, or Shy-Drager syndrome, is a neurodegenerative syndrome characterized by prominent autonomic dysfunction in combination with parkinsonism and/or cerebellar ataxia. MSA has an estimated prevalence of 2 to 5/100,000. Current nomenclature subdivides patients with MSA based on their predominant motor feature: MSA with predominant parkinsonism (MSA-P) and MSA with predominant cerebellar ataxia (MSA-C), but a mixed phenotype is common. Bradykinesia and rigidity are prominent features of the parkinsonism in MSA-P, though these tend to be symmetric, compared to the asymmetry of early idiopathic PD. Both forms of MSA have prominent autonomic dysfunction manifesting as orthostatic hypotension, urinary retention, delayed gastrointestinal motility, or erectile dysfunction in men. Patients may have a transient response to dopaminergic therapy for motor symptoms, though it is often incomplete; limited interventions are available for management of the associated ataxia. Symptomatic therapy can be utilized to manage orthostatic hypotension, constipation, and urinary symptoms

表 11.1 常见运动现象的定义

运动	定义
帕金森综合征	泛指自发运动减少（运动不能）、运动缓慢（运动迟缓）、运动幅度小（运动减退），以及静止性震颤、肌肉僵硬和姿势不稳等特征的某种组合
震颤	身体某部分的节律性摆动。静止性震颤在静止时发生。动作性震颤包括姿势性震颤（维持姿势时出现）、运动性震颤（运动时出现）和意向性震颤（向目标运动时加重）
舞蹈症	不规则、无目的、突发、快速、短暂、无节律、不持续的动作，从身体的某一部分流动至另一部分
肌张力障碍	持续或间歇性的肌肉收缩导致异常的、通常是重复的动作、姿势或两者兼有。肌张力障碍运动通常是有模式的、扭曲的，并在动作高峰时保持，可能会有震颤
抽动症	突然、快速、可抑制的、"急促的"且通常是重复和刻板的动作，强度变化不定，并以不规则的间隔重复。抽动症的关键特征是存在一种预感性冲动，通常在动作后暂时缓解
共济失调	自主运动协调障碍，可能表现为肢体运动、步态、言语和眼球运动的协调障碍
静坐不能	一种感觉运动障碍，定义为主观上的静止不能感，累及全身或部分身体，难以保持静止
肌阵挛	简单、快速、不自主的运动，导致身体某部分跨越关节的运动。虽然其外观可能类似于抽动症，但肌阵挛通常比抽动症更简单，不伴有预感性冲动或动作后的缓解感

表 11.2 帕金森综合征的鉴别诊断

退行性/遗传性原因	特发性帕金森病 多系统萎缩 进行性核上性麻痹 路易体痴呆 皮质基底节变性 伴有帕金森综合征的额颞叶痴呆 亨廷顿病 肝豆状核变性 多巴反应性肌张力障碍 泛酸激酶相关的神经退行性疾病
继发性原因	多巴胺受体阻滞剂（如抗精神病药、甲氧氯普胺、丙氯拉嗪） 突触前多巴胺耗竭剂（丁苯那嗪） 其他药物（如丙戊酸钠、钙通道阻滞剂、锂） 脑血管疾病 毒素（MPTP、锰、一氧化碳）

MPTP，1-甲基-4-苯基-1,2,3,6-四氢吡啶。

动症状，如姿势不稳，对药物或手术治疗均无反应。康复治疗在整个疾病过程中起到至关重要的作用。

目前已经确定了多种单基因帕金森综合征的病因。α 突触核蛋白（*SNCA*）和富亮氨酸重复激酶 2（*LRRK2*）的基因突变与常染色体显性遗传帕金森综合征有关。常染色体显性遗传所致病例在所有成年发病的帕金森综合征中不到 2%，但由于奠基者效应，在某些人群中的频率更高。常染色体隐性遗传的单基因病因包括编码 parkin（*PRKN*）、PTEN 诱导激酶 1（*PINK1*）和 DJ-1（*PARK7*）的基因突变，在 45 岁之前发病的家族病例中相对常见。葡萄糖脑苷脂酶（GBA）突变是 PD 中最常见的突变。对这些遗传机制更深入的理解，提示溶酶体途径和蛋白质降解受损在 PD 发病机制中起到重要作用。

非典型帕金森综合征

非典型帕金森综合征或帕金森叠加综合征是指一组异质性、散发性神经退行性疾病，以帕金森综合征、对多巴胺能治疗反应不佳或缺乏以及特征性非运动症状为特征。最常见的包括以多系统萎缩和路易体痴呆为代表的突触核蛋白病，以及以进行性核上性麻痹和皮质基底节综合征为代表的 tau 蛋白病。

多系统萎缩（MSA），以前被称为橄榄脑桥小脑变性、纹状体黑质变性或 Shy-Drager 综合征，是一种以突出的自主神经功能障碍叠加帕金森综合征和（或）小脑性共济失调为特征的神经退行性综合征。MSA 的估计患病率为（2～5）/10 万。当前的命名法根据其主要运动症状将 MSA 患者分为以帕金森综合征为主要表现的 MSA（MSA-P）和以小脑性共济失调为主要表现的 MSA（MSA-C），但混合表型也很常见。MSA-P 中的帕金森综合征主要表现为运动迟缓和僵硬，但这些症状往往是对称的，与早期特发性 PD 的非对称性形成对比。这两种形式的 MSA 都表现出显著的自主神经功能障碍，如体位性低血压、尿潴留、胃肠蠕动减慢或男性勃起功能障碍。患者的运动症状可能对多巴胺能治疗有暂时的反应，但通常是不完全的；针对共济失调的可用的干预措施十分有限。可对体位性低血压、便秘和尿路症状进行对症治疗（见第 7 章）。死亡通常

TABLE 11.3 "Red Flags" in the Diagnosis of Parkinson's Disease

Clinical or Historical "Red Flag"	Suggested Diagnosis
Early postural instability and falls	PSP, MSA, CBD, DLB, vascular
Early dysphagia	PSP, CBD
Early or spontaneous hallucinations	DLB
Early dementia or dementia predating PD	DLB
Early or severe dysautonomia	MSA
Pyramidal tract and/or cerebellar signs	MSA
Antipsychotic exposure	Tardive or drug-induced
Acute onset and/or non-progressive	Vascular

CBD, Corticobasal degeneration; *DLB*, dementia with Lewy body; *MSA*, multiple system atrophy; *PSP*, progressive supranuclear palsy.

(see Chapter 7). Death typically occurs around 6 to 8 years after the onset of motor symptoms, most often due to respiratory dysfunction or complications of swallowing difficulties.

Dementia with Lewy bodies (DLB) is characterized by the presence of parkinsonism, early dementia (preceding or within 1 year of the onset of motor symptoms), spontaneous visual hallucinations, and fluctuating levels of alertness. Unlike Alzheimer disease, DLB tends to affect visuospatial and executive domains of cognitive function with relative sparing of memory early in the course. The motor symptoms of DLB may be indistinguishable from PD, and patients can have a reasonable response to dopaminergic therapy; however, cautious use is appropriate, given the risk for worsening psychotic symptoms. Patients are also characteristically sensitive to antipsychotics, though atypical antipsychotics with low potency D2 receptor blockade (quetiapine, clozapine, pimavanserin) can generally be used to manage psychotic symptoms. Rivastigmine and other cholinesterase inhibitors are frequently used to treat the cognitive symptoms of PD; these may also offer some benefit for the treatment of hallucinations.

Progressive supranuclear palsy (PSP) is characterized by eye movement abnormalities, early postural instability and falls, axial parkinsonism, dysphagia, dysphonia, and dementia. The supranuclear palsy refers to the characteristic eye movement abnormalities in PSP with a vertical greater than horizontal gaze palsy and preserved oculocephalic reflex; early ocular features can include delayed saccadic initiation (rapid eye movement to focus of interest), slowed vertical eye movements, and the loss of the fast phase of optokinetic nystagmus. There is prominent axial parkinsonism in PSP with truncal rigidity and hyperextension and relatively symmetric appendicular bradykinesia and rigidity; these are typically unresponsive to dopaminergic therapy. Patients may also have prominent dystonia, including frontalis dystonia with associated lid lag giving patients a characteristic surprised appearance. PSP can be rapidly progressive with death often within 5 years of motor symptom onset related to dysphagia, falls, or complications of dementia.

Finally, corticobasal syndrome (CBS) is a rare and heterogeneous disorder characterized by the presence of strikingly asymmetrical parkinsonism, dystonia, and/or myoclonus with associated cortical signs including upper motor neuron features, apraxia, neglect, cortical sensory changes (e.g., agraphesthesia), alien limb phenomena, and dementia. Patients may additionally have oculomotor features that overlap with progressive supranuclear palsy or cognitive features that overlap with frontotemporal dementia. The disease is rapidly progressive, and treatment is symptomatic; motor features do not typically respond to dopaminergic therapy.

Secondary Parkinsonism

There are many causes of secondary parkinsonism, including medications, toxins, and cerebrovascular disease (see Table 11.2). Medications associated with parkinsonism include any medication that reduces dopaminergic tone in the brain, either through direct blockade of postsynaptic dopamine receptors (e.g., antipsychotics and certain antiemetics) or through depletion of presynaptic dopamine stores (e.g., vesicular monoamine transporter-2 inhibitors). Metoclopramide, a medication commonly used to treat gastroparesis, is a frequent cause because its dopamine blocking effects may be overlooked. Although classically characterized by symmetrical parkinsonism and absence of rest tremor, drug-induced parkinsonism can be clinically indistinguishable from PD. Hyposmia, which is common in PD, may be a helpful clue in distinguishing between drug-induced parkinsonism and PD but it should be recalled that hyposmia is also common among the elderly population. Treatment consists of withholding the offending agent, recognizing that it may take months for the symptoms to resolve. Even then, patients exposed to dopamine blocking agents may develop a tardive parkinsonism (i.e., a drug-induced parkinsonism that persists even after the offending agent is removed). DAT SPECT imaging can be useful in distinguishing drug-induced or tardive parkinsonism from a neurodegenerative parkinsonism.

Cerebrovascular disease is a common cause of secondary parkinsonism. Tremor is uncommon in vascular parkinsonism; lower extremity bradykinesia and gait difficulties dominate the clinical picture. Patients may have a history of clinical strokes with acute deteriorations followed by plateaus; however, many patients have vascular risk factors and a history of gradual decline. Neuroimaging is helpful in these cases.

Tremor

Tremor is characterized by a rhythmic oscillatory movement of a body part. Tremor is classified based on location and state (rest or action). Rest tremor is present when the affected body part is fully supported and not actively contracting; however, it is absent during sleep. Types of action tremor include postural tremor, kinetic tremor, and intention tremor. Postural tremor is present during maintenance of a posture against gravity, such as when extending the arms horizontally. Kinetic tremor is present with voluntary movement of the body part. An intention tremor refers to worsening of tremor on approach of a target (e.g., finger to nose) and is characteristic of cerebellar disease. Tremor has multiple etiologies, including medications, alcohol and drug intoxication and withdrawal, systemic disease (e.g., hyperthyroidism), structural brain lesions, or as a component of a neurodegenerative disease.

Essential Tremor

Essential tremor is among the most common movement disorders and the most common cause of tremor. Essential tremor has a worldwide prevalence of 2% to 4% with increasing incidence with aging. While essential tremor is often familial with an apparent autosomal dominant pattern of inheritance, no causative genetic mutation has

表 11.3　帕金森病诊断中的"红旗征"	
临床或病史"红旗征"	建议的诊断
早期姿势不稳和跌倒	PSP、MSA、CBD、DLB、血管性
早期吞咽困难	PSP、CBD
早期或自发性幻觉	DLB
早期痴呆或早于帕金森病的痴呆	DLB
早期或严重的自主神经功能障碍	MSA
锥体束和（或）小脑体征	MSA
抗精神病药物暴露	迟发性或药物引起
急性发作和（或）非进展性	血管性

CBD，皮质基底节变性；DLB，路易体痴呆；MSA，多系统萎缩；PSP，进行性核上性麻痹。

发生在运动症状出现后的 6～8 年，最常见的原因是呼吸功能衰竭或吞咽困难的并发症。

帕金森综合征、早发痴呆（在运动症状出现前或出现 1 年内）、自发性幻视和波动性认知障碍是路易体痴呆（DLB）的特征。与阿尔茨海默病不同，DLB 的认知障碍在早期以视觉空间和执行等认知域更容易受累，而记忆相对保留。DLB 的运动症状可能与 PD 无法区分，患者可能对多巴胺能治疗有一定的反应；然而，鉴于该类药物有加重精神症状的风险，需谨慎使用。患者对抗精神病药物特别敏感，但低效能的阻断 D_2 受体的非典型抗精神病药物（如喹硫平、氯氮平、哌马色林）通常可用于控制精神症状。卡巴拉汀和其他胆碱酯酶抑制剂常被用来治疗 PD 的认知症状，这些药物也可能对幻觉有效。

进行性核上性麻痹（PSP）以眼球运动异常、早期姿势不稳及跌倒、中轴性帕金森综合征、吞咽困难、发音障碍和痴呆为主要特征。核上性麻痹是指 PSP 中的特征性眼球运动异常，表现为垂直方向较水平方向更为严重的凝视麻痹，而头眼反射保留；早期眼部特征可包括扫视启动（快速眼动至兴趣点）延迟、垂直扫视变慢和视动性眼震的快速相消失。PSP 患者会有明显的中轴性帕金森综合征，表现为躯干僵硬和过伸，以及相对对称的肢体运动迟缓和僵硬，这些通常对多巴胺能治疗无反应。患者还可能出现明显的肌张力障碍，包括前额肌张力障碍伴有眼睑退缩，使患者呈现出一种特有的惊讶表情。PSP 可进展迅速，常在运动症状出现后 5 年内因吞咽困难、跌倒或痴呆并发症而死亡。

最后，皮质基底节综合征（CBS）是一种罕见且具有异质性的疾病，其特征是显著的非对称性帕金森综合征、肌张力障碍和（或）肌阵挛，伴有皮质体征，包括上运动神经元体征、失用症、忽视、皮质感觉改变（如触觉失认）、异己肢体现象和痴呆。患者可能还会出现与进行性核上性麻痹重叠的眼动障碍或与额颞叶痴呆重叠的认知障碍。该病进展迅速，仅有对症治疗，运动症状通常对多巴胺能治疗无反应。

继发性帕金森综合征

继发性帕金森综合征有许多原因，包括药物、毒素和脑血管疾病（见表 11.2）。任何可减少大脑中多巴胺能的药物均能导致帕金森综合征，作用机制包括直接阻断突触后多巴胺受体（如抗精神病药和某些止吐药）或耗竭突触前多巴胺储存（如囊泡单胺转运体-2 抑制剂）。甲氧氯普胺是一种常用于治疗胃轻瘫的药物，临床应用中常因忽视了其多巴胺阻断效应而导致帕金森综合征。尽管具有对称性帕金森综合征和缺乏静止性震颤等特征，药物引起的帕金森综合征在临床上仍可能无法与 PD 区分。嗅觉减退在 PD 中很常见，这可能是区分药物引起的帕金森综合征和 PD 的有用线索，但应记住嗅觉减退在普通老年人群中也很常见。治疗包括停止引起症状的药物，但症状可能需要几个月才能消失。即便这样，接触过多巴胺阻断药物的患者也可能会产生迟发性帕金森综合征（即药物引起的帕金森综合征在停药后仍持续存在）。DAT SPECT 成像有助于区分药物引起的或迟发性帕金森综合征与神经退行性帕金森综合征。

脑血管疾病是继发性帕金森综合征的常见原因。震颤在血管性帕金森综合征中不常见，而下肢运动迟缓和步态异常是其主要临床特征。患者可能有临床卒中史，急性恶化后会有一段稳定期；然而，许多患者仅有血管危险因素，症状逐渐缓慢进展。神经影像学将有助于鉴别这些病例。

震颤

震颤以部分身体的节律性振荡运动为特征，根据发生位置和状态（静止或运动）进行分类。静止性震颤发生于受累的身体部位具有完全支撑且没有主动收缩时，但在睡眠时消失。动作性震颤包括姿势性震颤、运动性震颤及意向性震颤。姿势性震颤在维持对抗重力的姿势时出现，例如水平伸展手臂时。运动性震颤在身体部位的主动运动时出现。意向性震颤是指接近目标（如指鼻试验）时震颤加重，是小脑疾病的特征。震颤有多种病因，包括药物、酒精及药物中毒和戒断、系统性疾病（如甲状腺功能亢进）、脑结构性病变，或作为神经退行性疾病的一部分。

特发性震颤

特发性震颤是最常见的运动障碍之一，也是最常见的震颤原因。特发性震颤在全球的患病率为 2%～4%，并随着年龄的增长而增加。尽管特发性震颤通常是家族性的，且呈常染色体显性遗传模式，但尚未发现明

TABLE 11.4	Treatment Options for Essential Tremor
First line	Propranolol
	Primidone
Second line	Topiramate
	Zonisamide
	Benzodiazepines
	Other β-blockers
	Gabapentin/Pregabalin
Medication failure	Botulinum toxin injections
	Deep brain stimulation

TABLE 11.5 Medications Associated With Tremor	
Asthma Medications	**Neuroactive Medications**
β-Agonists (albuterol)	Lithium carbonate
Theophylline	Stimulants (prescribed and illicit)
Antiseizure Medications	Selective serotonin reuptake inhibitors
Valproic acid	Tricyclic antidepressants
Phenytoin	**Other**
Carbamazepine	Levothyroxine
Immunomodulators	Caffeine
Corticosteroids	
Cyclosporine	
Tacrolimus	

been identified, and there are other non-monogenic causes of essential tremor. Cerebellar dysfunction has been implicated in the pathogenesis of essential tremor. Clinically, it is a heterogeneous disorder characterized by relatively symmetric 4- to 12-Hz postural and kinetic tremor of the upper extremities. It may cause functional impairment (e.g., difficulty with handwriting, drinking, or using utensils) and may even be disabling. Involvement of the head and voice are common. Tremor tends to improve with alcohol ingestion. Cognitive dysfunction, psychiatric manifestations (e.g., depression, anxiety), and balance impairment can also be seen. Mild parkinsonian features (e.g., tremor at rest, rigidity with activation) may develop and can make distinguishing incipient PD challenging. Propranolol and primidone are first-line treatments for essential tremor and are of similar benefit (Table 11.4).

Other Tremors
Beyond essential tremor and parkinsonian tremor, there are a number of other less common etiologies of tremor and tremor syndromes. All individuals may have some fine physiologic shaking of the hands or fingers with posture or action. At times when this tremor becomes visibly or functionally notable, it is termed enhanced physiologic tremor. Enhanced physiologic tremor is most commonly due to an underlying physical or psychological stressor. Common causes include anxiety, hyperthyroidism, excessive caffeine intake, stimulant or corticosteroid use, beta agonist use (e.g., albuterol), and valproic acid use among other medications (Table 11.5). Appropriate screening for medications and contributing medical or psychiatric causes should be undertaken in anyone presenting with suspected enhanced physiologic tremor. Enhanced physiologic tremor may be clinically indistinguishable from mild or early essential tremor. If no causative etiologies can be identified or mitigated, the approach to treatment is similar with β-blockers such as propranolol being used most commonly.

Tremor is also commonly seen in association with other movement phenomena including dystonia and cerebellar features. Dystonic tremor is irregular and is associated with abnormal posturing. Cerebellar tremor is an intention tremor that is characteristically low frequency, high amplitude, and worsens as one approaches a target. The distribution of tremor is dependent upon the cause with common locations of both dystonic and cerebellar tremors including the head/neck, trunk, and limbs. The presence of dystonia or cerebellar features is necessary to diagnose a dystonic or cerebellar tremor, and treatment typically focuses on management of the alternative movement. These movements and their associated differential diagnoses are discussed elsewhere in this chapter.

Chorea
Chorea is characterized by purposeless, abrupt, rapid, brief, arrhythmic, unsustained movements that flow randomly from one part of the body to another. The term "choreoathetosis" describes the combination of chorea and athetosis, a slow form of chorea manifested by writhing movements predominantly involving distal extremities. *Ballism* is a severe form of chorea with large amplitude, flinging movements usually affecting the proximal musculature. Chorea is often associated with a variety of secondary clinical features detailed in Table 11.6.

The differential diagnosis for chorea is broad, reflecting a wide variety of processes affecting the basal ganglia network and specifically the striatum. Generally, chorea either represents the primary manifestation of an inherited disorder or is acquired secondary to basal ganglia insults due to various comorbid medical conditions, medications or toxins, or structural abnormalities. Table 11.7 summarizes the differential diagnosis of chorea categorized by genetic and acquired causes.

Huntington's Disease
Huntington's disease (HD) is an autosomal dominant, progressively disabling, and fatal neurodegenerative disease; it is the most common cause of inherited adult-onset chorea. The causative mutation is an expansion of an unstable cytosine-adenine-guanine (CAG) trinucleotide repeat of the IT-15 gene (also known as the HTT or HD gene) on the short arm of chromosome 4, which results in production of abnormal *huntingtin* protein. The neuropathology of HD is characterized by selective neuronal vulnerability, particularly involving the caudate and putamen of the striatum. Microscopically, the pathologic hallmark of the disease is the preferential loss of medium-sized spiny neurons projecting from the striatum to the external pallidum.

The motor symptoms of HD may start at any age, with the peak incidence between 35 and 40 years of age with death occurring 10 to 20 years after development of manifest symptoms. Age of onset and rate of progression of the disease are inversely associated with CAG repeat length with the longest repeats associated with juvenile-onset disease and a more rapid disease progression.

HD is characterized clinically by the triad of a movement disorder, progressive cognitive decline (dementia), and psychiatric features. Chorea is the prototypical motor manifestation of HD occurring in 90% of patients. Other motor manifestations include dystonia, bradykinesia, and rigidity. Cognitive impairment is invariable in HD and typically progresses from selective deficits in psychomotor, executive, and visuospatial abilities to more global impairment with higher cortical functions usually spared. Psychiatric manifestations include depression, irritability, apathy, anxiety, and obsessive-compulsive symptoms.

The juvenile variant of HD, in which motor symptoms start before age 20, typically has an akinetic-rigid phenotype and only rarely chorea; patients may also have seizures. Paternal inheritance of the HD gene is the rule for onset before the age of 10 and paternal inheritance predominates (about 3:1 paternal:maternal) for onset before the age of 20. This can be explained by a phenomenon called anticipation; the

表 11.4 特发性震颤的治疗选择	
一线治疗	普萘洛尔 扑米酮
二线治疗	托吡酯 唑尼沙胺 苯二氮䓬类药物 其他 β 受体阻滞剂 加巴喷丁/普瑞巴林
药物治疗失败	肉毒毒素注射 脑深部电刺激

表 11.5 与震颤相关的药物	
哮喘药物 β 受体激动剂（沙丁胺醇） 茶碱	**神经活性药物** 碳酸锂 兴奋剂（处方的和非法的） 选择性 5-羟色胺再摄取抑制剂
抗癫痫药物 丙戊酸 苯妥英 卡马西平	三环类抗抑郁药 **其他** 左甲状腺素 咖啡因
免疫调节剂 皮质类固醇 环孢素 他克莫司	

确的致病性基因突变，此外还有其他非单基因遗传导致的特发性震颤。小脑功能障碍参与特发性震颤的发病。该病是一种临床异质性疾病，以上肢相对对称的 4～12 Hz 的姿势性和运动性震颤为特征。它可导致功能障碍（例如，书写困难、喝水或使用餐具困难），甚至致残。头部和发声受累也很常见。震颤往往在饮酒后有所改善。患者还可能出现认知功能障碍、精神症状（例如抑郁、焦虑）和平衡障碍，甚至轻度的帕金森特征（例如，静止性震颤、活动时僵硬），为其与早期帕金森病的鉴别带来了挑战性。普萘洛尔和扑米酮是特发性震颤的一线治疗方法，效果相似（表 11.4）。

其他震颤

除了特发性震颤和帕金森震颤外，还有许多其他较少见的震颤和震颤综合征。正常人群也会有一些轻微的生理性手部或手指震颤，当这种震颤变得显著或影响功能时，称为增强的生理性震颤。增强的生理性震颤通常由潜在的身体或心理压力导致，常见原因包括焦虑、甲状腺功能亢进症、摄入过量咖啡因、使用兴奋剂或皮质类固醇、使用 β 受体激动剂（如沙丁胺醇）和丙戊酸等（表 11.5）。对出现疑似增强的生理性震颤患者，均应进行适当的药物筛查和相关医疗或精神病原因的筛查。增强的生理性震颤在临床上可能无法与轻度或早期的特发性震颤相区分。如果无法确定或缓解病因，治疗与特发性震颤是类似的，可以使用 β 受体阻滞剂如普萘洛尔。

震颤还常与其他运动现象相关联，包括肌张力障碍和小脑症状。肌张力障碍性震颤的振荡是不规则的，并伴有姿势异常。小脑性震颤以低频高振幅的意向性震颤为特征，在接近目标时会加重。震颤的分布取决于病因，常见的部位包括头/颈、躯干和四肢。诊断肌张力障碍性或小脑性震颤需要同时存在肌张力障碍或小脑症状，治疗通常侧重于改善其他运动症状。此类运动症状及其相关的鉴别诊断将在本章的其他地方进行讨论。

舞蹈症

舞蹈症的特征是无目的、突然、快速、短暂、不规则、不持久的运动，从身体的一个部位随机累及另一个部位。术语"舞蹈徐动症"描述了舞蹈症和徐动症的组合，后者是一种慢性舞蹈症，表现为主要涉及远端肢体的扭动运动。投掷样运动是一种严重的舞蹈症，具有大幅度的甩动运动，通常影响近端肌肉。舞蹈症常与各种继发性临床特征相关，详见表 11.6。

舞蹈症的鉴别诊断十分广泛，反映了影响基底神经节网络（特别是纹状体）的多种病因过程。舞蹈症通常可分为遗传性或继发性，后者可由各种共病、药物、毒素或结构异常损伤基底神经节导致。表 11.7 总结了舞蹈症的鉴别诊断，按遗传性和获得性原因分类。

亨廷顿病

亨廷顿病（HD）是一种常染色体显性遗传的、逐渐致残和致死性的神经退行性疾病，是成人发病的遗传性舞蹈症的最常见原因。发病原因是 4 号染色体短臂上 IT-15 基因（也称为 HTT 或 HD 基因）的不稳定胞嘧啶-腺嘌呤-鸟嘌呤（CAG）三核苷酸重复扩增，导致异常的亨廷顿蛋白产生所致。HD 的神经病理特征是选择性的神经元易感性，纹状体的尾状核和壳核极易受累。从纹状体投射到外侧苍白球的中型棘状神经元优先丧失是特征性的病理改变。

HD 的运动症状可以在任何年龄开始，发病高峰在 35～40 岁，发病后 10～20 年死亡。发病年龄和疾病进展速度与 CAG 重复长度成反比，重复越多则发病越年轻且疾病进展更快。

HD 的临床特征表现为运动障碍、进行性认知下降（痴呆）及精神症状的三联征。舞蹈症是 HD 的典型运动表现，发生于 90% 的患者。其他运动表现包括肌张力障碍、运动迟缓及僵硬。HD 患者均会出现认知障碍，通常从精神运动、执行和视觉空间能力的选择性受损开始，发展到更广泛的损害，而高层皮质功能保持相对完好。精神症状包括抑郁、易怒、冷漠、焦虑和强迫症状。

青少年变异型的 HD，患者的运动症状始于 20 岁之前，通常表现为无动力-僵硬型，而很少出现舞蹈症，此外还可能有癫痫发作。10 岁前发病的 HD 呈父系遗传，20 岁前发病者父系遗传占主导地位（父:母遗传比例约为 3:1）。这一现象被称为遗传早现；因为

TABLE 11.6 Secondary Features Associated With Chorea

Athetosis	Slow, writhing movements of distal limbs
Ballism	Rapid, flinging movements of proximal limbs
Parakinesis	Incorporation of an involuntary movement into a voluntary movement (e.g., crossing and uncrossing of legs, adjusting glasses)
Motor impersistence	Inability to maintain tongue protrusion, "milk maid's grip"
Partially suppressible	Brief ability to voluntary reduce the severity of movements
Deep tendon reflex changes	"Hung up" or "pendular" reflexes
Gait disorders	Irregular or dancelike gait

TABLE 11.7 Differential Diagnosis of Chorea

Genetic disorders	Autosomal dominant	Huntington's disease
		Spinocerebellar ataxia (SCA 17 >1-3)
		DRPLA
		Neuroferritinopathy
		Benign hereditary chorea
	Autosomal recessive	Neuroacanthocytosis
		Wilson's disease
		Ataxia (Friedreich, ataxia-telangiectasia, ataxia with oculomotor apraxia)
		Disorders associated with brain iron accumulation (PKAN)
	X-linked	McLeod syndrome
		Lesch-Nyhan syndrome
Acquired/sporadic	Medications	Direct side effects (e.g., levodopa)
		Tardive dyskinesia
	Immune mediated	Sydenham chorea
		Systemic lupus erythematosus
		Anti-phospholipid antibody syndrome
		Vasculitis
		Paraneoplastic (*CRMP5* gene, anti-Hu)
	Infectious	HIV/AIDS
		Variant CJD
		Neurosyphilis
	Endocrine	Hyperthyroidism
		Chorea gravidarum
	Metabolic	Hyperglycemia
		Electrolyte disturbances
		Acquired hepatocerebral degeneration
	Vascular	Basal ganglia infarcts/hemorrhage
	Miscellaneous	Polycythemia vera
		Post-cardiac bypass pump
		Multiple sclerosis
		Sporadic neurodegenerative disorders

CJD, Creutzfeldt-Jakob disease; *DRPLA*, dentatorubropallidoluysian atrophy; *PKAN*, pantothenate-kinase-associated neurodegeneration; *SCA*, spinocerebellar ataxia.

CAG trinucleotide repeat is unstable and with paternal transmission the number of repeats tends to expand.

Treatment of HD is currently symptomatic. Vesicular monoamine transporter-2 inhibitors and antipsychotic drugs can be used for the management of chorea. No disease modifying treatments have been identified; *huntingtin* lowering approaches are currently under study.

Other Choreas

Beyond HD, the differential diagnosis of chorea remains quite broad with other inherited etiologies and a number of acquired causes (see Table 11.7). Approximately 10% of individuals with an autosomal dominant HD-like disorder will not carry the causative mutation for HD. Among these "phenocopies," only a small minority will have an identifiable genetic mutation. The most common genetic causes in the Caucasian population include spinocerebellar ataxia (SCA) 17, Friedreich's ataxia, HD-like 2, and familial prion disease (HD-like 1). Alternative diagnoses include dentatorubropallidoluysian atrophy (DRPLA), SCA 1-3, Wilson's disease (described elsewhere in this chapter), neuroacanthocytosis syndromes, and neuroferritinopathy. Young-onset, non-progressive chorea, particularly in the setting of a family history and the absence of cognitive or behavioral changes, should raise concern for benign hereditary chorea, caused by a mutation in the *NKX2* gene; beyond chorea, the condition is associated with an increased risk of pulmonary and thyroid cancers.

Medication side effects are likely the most common acquired and overall cause of chorea. Levodopa-induced dyskinesias can be seen in patients with degenerative parkinsonian syndromes, and tardive

表 11.6	与舞蹈症相关的次要特征
手足徐动症	远端肢体缓慢、扭动的运动
投掷样运动	近端肢体快速、挥动的运动
运动倒错	将不自主运动融入自主运动中（如交叉和打开双腿、调整眼镜）
运动保持困难	无法保持舌头伸出，"挤奶手征"
部分可抑制	短时间内能自主减轻运动的严重程度
深反射变化	"悬挂"或"钟摆"样反射
步态障碍	不规则或舞蹈样步态

表 11.7	舞蹈症的鉴别诊断		
遗传性疾病	常染色体显性遗传		亨廷顿病
			脊髓小脑性共济失调（SCA 17 > 1 ~ 3）
			DRPLA
			神经铁蛋白病
			良性遗传性舞蹈症
	常染色体隐性遗传		神经棘红细胞增多症
			肝豆状核变性
			共济失调（Friedreich 共济失调、共济失调-毛细血管扩张症、眼动失用性共济失调）
			与脑铁沉积相关的疾病（PKAN）
	X 连锁		McLeod 综合征
			Lesch-Nyhan 综合征
获得性/散发性	药物		直接副作用（如左旋多巴）
			迟发性运动障碍
	免疫介导		Sydenham 舞蹈症（小舞蹈症）
			系统性红斑狼疮
			抗磷脂抗体综合征
			血管炎
			副肿瘤性舞蹈症（CRMP-5 基因、抗 Hu）
	感染		HIV/AIDS
			变异型 CJD
			神经梅毒
	内分泌		甲状腺功能亢进症
			妊娠期舞蹈症
	代谢性		高血糖症
			电解质紊乱
			获得性肝脑变性
	血管性		基底神经节梗死/出血
	其他		真性红细胞增多症
			心脏旁路术后
			多发性硬化
			散发性神经退行性疾病

CJD，克-雅病；DRPLA，齿状核-红核-苍白球-路易体萎缩症；PKAN，泛酸激酶相关的神经退行性病变；SCA，脊髓小脑性共济失调。

CAG 三核苷酸重复是不稳定的，通过父系传递时重复次数往往会增加。

目前 HD 仅可对症治疗。囊泡单胺转运体-2 抑制剂和抗精神病药物可用于控制舞蹈症症状。尚无可以改变疾病进程的疗法，降低亨廷顿蛋白的治疗方法正在研究中。

其他舞蹈症

除了 HD 外，舞蹈症的鉴别诊断仍然非常广泛，包括其他遗传性病因和许多获得性病因（见表 11.7）。约 10% 具有 HD 样常染色体显性遗传病的个体并不携带 HD 的致病突变。在这些"拟表型"中，只有一小部分可检测出基因突变。在高加索人群中最常见的遗传因素包括脊髓小脑性共济失调（SCA）17 型、Friedreich 共济失调、HD 样 2 型和家族性朊病毒病（HD 样 1 型）。其他鉴别诊断包括齿状核-红核-苍白球-路易体萎缩症（DRPLA）、SCA 1 ~ 3 型、肝豆状核变性（将在本章其他地方描述）、神经棘红细胞增多症以及神经铁蛋白病。年轻起病的、非进行性舞蹈症，特别是在有家族史但无认知或行为障碍的情况下，还应考虑到由 NKX2 基因突变引起的良性遗传性舞蹈症的可能；除舞蹈外，该病还与肺癌和甲状腺癌风险增加相关。

药物副作用可能是舞蹈症最常见的获得性和系统性原因。在退行性帕金森综合征患者中可以出现左旋多巴引起的运动障碍，在长期使用抗多巴胺能药物的

dyskinesia can be encountered in patients on chronic antidopaminergic therapy. These entities are described elsewhere in the chapter.

Sydenham chorea is the most common acquired cause of chorea in children and follows a throat infection with group A streptococcus. Chorea typically develops within a few weeks of the pharyngeal infection, though can be delayed by more than 6 months. Though the chorea may be generalized, the face and tongue are most commonly involved. Psychiatric symptoms are also common and can include irritability, emotional lability, or obsessive-compulsive symptoms. Various biomarkers including elevated antistreptolysin O (ASO) and anti-deoxyribonuclease B titers are associated with Sydenham chorea but are not required to make a diagnosis. The behavioral and motor symptoms associated with Sydenham disease are typically mild and self-limited. Symptomatic treatment of chorea can be considered; corticosteroids may also be considered in moderate to severe cases and likely shorten the duration of symptoms. Chorea is a major criterion for acute rheumatic fever, and all patients with suspected Sydenham chorea should be evaluated for carditis. Definitive antibiotic therapy to treat the GAS pharyngeal infection is recommended even if there are no ongoing signs or symptoms of pharyngitis. Chronic prophylactic antibiotic therapy is recommended for all patients with Sydenham chorea until age 21; treatment for 10 years or until the age of 40 is generally recommended in those with residual cardiac disease following rheumatic fever.

Other acquired forms of chorea include chorea gravidarum in pregnancy, paraneoplastic chorea, and autoimmune etiologies. Paraneoplastic chorea is most commonly associated with CRMP-5 antibodies in the setting of small-cell lung cancer. Autoimmune causes of chorea include the antiphospholipid antibody syndrome and systemic lupus erythematous. In these cases, identification of the underlying etiology and initiation of appropriate therapy represent the definitive management.

Wilson's Disease

Wilson's disease (WD) is a rare, autosomal recessive disorder of impaired copper metabolism resulting in copper accumulation, neurologic dysfunction, and hepatic dysfunction. Typically, neurologic symptoms in WD begin in the second or third decade although late onset can occur. Patients develop a variety of abnormal movements including chorea, dystonia, parkinsonism, and tremor. The most common form of tremor in WD is an irregular, and somewhat jerky, dystonic tremor. A classical "wing-beating tremor" or "flapping tremor" in combination with dysarthria strongly suggests the diagnosis of WD. Dysarthria is frequently combined with slow tongue movements and orofacial dyskinesia including "risus sardonicus," which is characterized by involuntary grimacing with the mouth open and the upper lip contracted. Beyond abnormal movements, patients may also have seizures, cognitive impairment, and psychiatric features including abnormal behavior (typically increased irritability or disinhibition), personality changes, anxiety, and depression.

WD can present with acute liver failure or chronic liver disease that may clinically be indistinguishable from other hepatic conditions. The absence of clinical or biochemical evidence of liver disease does not exclude WD. A history of jaundice, a positive family history of neuropsychiatric disease, and increased sensitivity to neuroleptics can be diagnostic clues for WD in such patients. Untreated it is invariably fatal; early treatment is associated with better clinical outcomes; therefore, a high level of suspicion should be maintained. Diagnosis is confirmed by the presence of Kayser-Fleischer corneal rings in the setting of increased urinary copper excretion or elevated copper on liver biopsy. Bilateral symmetric high signal intensity in the putamen, caudate, thalamus, and midbrain on T2-weighted MR images can be seen and the classic imaging sign is the "face of the giant panda" (Fig. 11.3). Serum ceruloplasmin is usually low in symptomatic patients, but this is not definitive, and confirmatory testing with ophthalmologic screen, 24-hour urinary copper, liver biopsy, or genetic testing for homozygous mutations in the *ATP7B* gene is necessary. Treatment consists of drugs that facilitate copper excretion, such as zinc, and the copper chelators D-penicillamine, trientine, and tetrathiomolybdate.

Drug-Induced Movement Disorders

The term *tardive dyskinesia (TD)* was initially coined to describe patients with rhythmic, repetitive (stereotypic), persistent movements after long exposure to antipsychotic drugs. Over time, other abnormal, persistent, involuntary movements have been reported after exposure to these drugs and other dopamine receptor blocking agents (DRBAs). Because of differences in treatment and approach, it is helpful to use the term TD to refer to the classic description of rhythmic, repetitive, stereotypic movements of the face, mouth, and tongue manifesting as lip smacking, chewing motions, and tongue protrusion. The term *tardive syndrome* more broadly refers to other phenomena, including rocking movements, tremor, myoclonus, and other forms of dystonia. Akathisia refers to the inability to remain still with an urge to move, giving the appearance of restlessness. It is a sensory phenomenon and a common and disabling form of tardive syndrome. Common movements seen in patients include repetitive self-touching, marching in place, rocking from one leg to the other, pumping the legs up and down, and crossing and uncrossing the legs.

TD and tardive syndromes are characterized by the late appearance of abnormal movements after prolonged exposure to a DRBA. Whenever the diagnosis is suspected, a careful and comprehensive review of treatment history should be done. Risk factors for the development of tardive syndromes include advancing age, female gender, and the use of high-potency antipsychotics. While removal of the offending agent is critical to prevent worsening, symptoms might persist in up to two thirds of patients and treatment can be challenging. Dopamine depleting agents can be considered for treatment and two vesicular monoamine transporter-2 inhibitors have recently been approved for the treatment of TD.

Dystonia

Dystonia is a heterogenous group of disorders that are defined by sustained or intermittent muscle contractions causing abnormal, often repetitive movements, postures, or both. Dystonic movements are typically patterned, twisting, and may be tremulous.

Dystonia may involve nearly any region of the body, emerge at any age, appear static or progressive, and can co-occur with other neurologic or medical problems. The classification of dystonia is challenging. Newer classification systems address the different clinical manifestations with four dimensions: body region affected, age at onset, temporal aspects, and any associated symptoms. Classification according to the presence or absence of associated features addresses whether dystonia occurs by itself (isolated dystonia, previously known as primary dystonia) or is part of a more complex syndrome that combines other features (combined dystonia, previously known as secondary dystonia or dystonia-plus). This new classification system provides a more clinically useful approach for diagnosis than previously used strategies.

Adult-onset focal dystonias are by far the most common. Cervical dystonia is the most common type of focal dystonia, followed by focal dystonias involving the face and jaw muscles (blepharospasm, oromandibular dystonia or the combination); laryngeal and limb dystonias are rare. Adult-onset limb dystonias are usually task-specific with dystonic contraction only occurring during specific voluntary actions (e.g., writer's cramp, musician's dystonia). However, this task

患者中可以出现迟发性运动障碍。这些情况将在本章其他地方进行描述。

Sydenham 舞蹈症是儿童最常见的获得性舞蹈症，通常在 A 组链球菌咽部感染后的数周内发生，但也可能延迟超过 6 个月。尽管舞蹈症可能是全身性的，但以面部和舌部受累最为常见。精神症状也很常见，包括易怒、情绪不稳定或强迫症状。多种生物标志物，包括抗链球菌溶血素 O（ASO）和抗脱氧核糖核酸酶 B 的滴度升高均与 Sydenham 舞蹈症相关，但不是诊断所必需的。与 Sydenham 病相关的行为和运动障碍通常是轻度的且具有自限性。可以考虑对症治疗；在中重度病例中也可以考虑使用皮质类固醇，这可能缩短症状的持续时间。舞蹈症是诊断急性风湿热的主要标准，所有疑似 Sydenham 舞蹈症的患者都应进行心肌炎评估。即使没有咽炎的持续症状，也建议针对 A 组链球菌咽部感染给予明确的抗生素治疗。对于所有 Sydenham 舞蹈症患者，均建议在 21 岁之前进行长期预防性抗生素治疗；对于在风湿热后有心脏后遗症的患者，通常建议治疗 10 年或直到 40 岁。

其他获得性舞蹈症包括妊娠期舞蹈症、副肿瘤性和自身免疫性舞蹈症。副肿瘤性舞蹈症最常见于伴有 CRMP-5 抗体的小细胞肺癌患者。自身免疫性舞蹈症包括抗磷脂抗体综合征和系统性红斑狼疮。这些情况的疾病管理应首先确定潜在病因，并启动适当的治疗。

肝豆状核变性

肝豆状核变性（WD）是一种罕见的常染色体隐性遗传的铜代谢障碍，因铜积累导致神经功能障碍和肝功能障碍。WD 的神经症状通常在 10 岁或 20 岁后发病，尽管也可能发病更晚。患者可出现各种异常运动，包括舞蹈症、肌张力障碍、帕金森综合征以及震颤。WD 中最常见的震颤形式是不规则的、略显颤抖的肌张力障碍性震颤。经典的"振翅样震颤"或"扑翼样震颤"结合构音障碍强烈提示 WD 的诊断。构音障碍经常伴有缓慢的舌部运动和口面部运动障碍（包括"讽刺笑容"），其特征是伴有张口和上唇收缩的不自主咧嘴。除了异常运动外，患者还可能有癫痫发作、认知障碍及精神症状，包括行为异常（通常是易怒或脱抑制）、人格改变、焦虑及抑郁。

WD 可表现为急性肝衰竭或慢性肝病，在临床上可能与其他肝病无法区分。没有肝病的临床或生化证据并不能排除 WD。黄疸病史、神经精神疾病的阳性家族史和对神经安定药的敏感性增加，可以作为此类患者诊断 WD 的线索。如果不给予治疗，WD 必然是致命的；早期治疗可获得更好的临床预后；因此，必须对相关患者保持高度的怀疑。可通过尿铜排泄增加、肝活检铜升高及存在 Kayser-Fleischer 角膜环（K-F 环）来确诊。常可在患者的 T2 加权 MR 图像上见到尾状核、壳核、丘脑和中脑双侧对称的高信号，经典的影像学标志是"巨熊猫脸征"（图 11.3）。有症状的患者其血清铜蓝蛋白通常较低，但这不是决定性证据，需要经过眼科筛查、24 h 尿铜、肝活检或 ATP7B 基因的纯合突变基因检测以确认。主要通过促进铜排泄的药物进行治疗，如锌和铜螯合剂 D-青霉胺、曲恩汀和四硫钼酸钾。

药物诱发的运动障碍

迟发性运动障碍（TD）一词最初是用来描述患者长期使用抗精神病药后出现的节律性、重复性（刻板）、持续性运动。随着时间的推移，在使用这些药物和其他多巴胺受体阻断剂（DRBA）后，也有其他异常的、持续的不自主运动被陆续报道。由于这些异常运动的治疗方法有所不同，现将 TD 一词用于描述面部、口腔和舌部的节律性、重复性、刻板运动，表现为舔嘴唇、咀嚼动作和伸舌。迟发性综合征被更广泛地用于指代其他运动现象，包括摇摆运动、震颤、肌阵挛和其他形式的肌张力障碍。静坐不能是指无法保持静止，有想要移动的冲动，表现为坐立不安。这是一种感觉现象，是迟发性综合征的常见和致残形式。患者常见的动作包括反复的自我触摸、原地踏步、双腿交替抖动、双腿上下活动以及双腿交叉开合运动。

TD 和迟发性综合征的特征是在长期暴露于 DRBA 后出现的迟发异常运动。在疑诊该病时，应仔细和全面梳理患者的治疗史。迟发性综合征的发病危险因素包括年龄增加、女性和使用高效能抗精神病药物。虽然去除致病药物对防止疾病恶化至关重要，但高达 2/3 的患者其症状会持续存在，为治疗带来挑战性。可以考虑使用多巴胺耗竭剂进行治疗，而且 2 种囊泡单胺转运体-2 抑制剂最近被批准用于 TD 的治疗。

肌张力障碍

肌张力障碍是一组异质性疾病，定义为持续性或间歇性肌肉收缩，导致异常的、通常是重复性的运动、姿势或两者兼有。肌张力障碍运动通常是有模式的、扭曲的，并且可能伴有震颤。

肌张力障碍可以累及身体的几乎任何区域，出现在任何年龄，表现为静止性或进行性，并且可以与其他神经科或内科问题共存。肌张力障碍的分类非常具有挑战性。新的分类系统从四个维度对不同临床表现进行阐释：受累的身体区域、发病年龄、时间维度方面和是否伴有任何相关症状。根据是否存在相关特征进行分类是指，肌张力障碍是单独发生（孤立性肌张力障碍，旧称原发性肌张力障碍）还是作为伴有其他特征的更复杂综合征的一部分（组合性肌张力障碍，旧称继发性肌张力障碍或肌张力障碍叠加）。与既往分类系统相比，这种新的分类系统更有助于临床诊断。

成人发病的局灶性肌张力障碍最为常见。颈部肌张力障碍是最常见的局灶性肌张力障碍类型，其次是面部和下颌肌肉的局灶性肌张力障碍（眼睑痉挛、口下颌肌张力障碍或两者兼有）；喉和肢体肌张力障碍较为罕见。成人发病的肢体肌张力障碍通常是任务特异性的，仅在特定自主动作时发生肌张力障碍性收缩

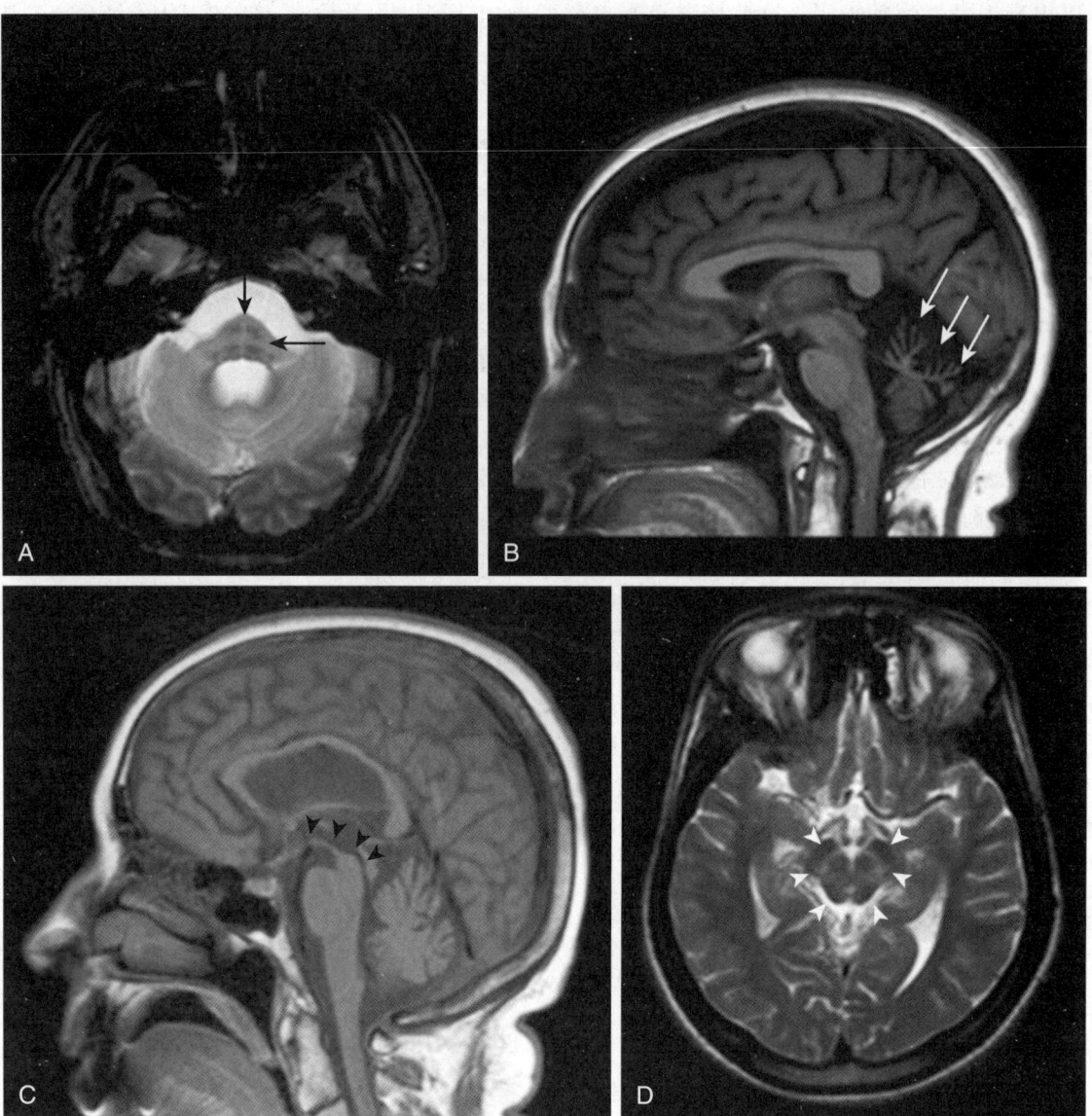

Fig. 11.3 Representative MRI findings of different movement disorders. (A) "Hot cross bun" in multiple system atrophy (MSA) *(black arrows)*. (B) Marked cerebellar and vermis atrophy in spinal cerebellar atrophy (SCA) 6 *(white arrows)*. (C) "Hummingbird" sign in progressive supranuclear palsy (PSP) due to prominent midbrain atrophy *(black arrowheads)*. (D) "Face of giant panda" sign in Wilson's disease *(white arrowheads)*.

specificity may be lost over time and even occur at rest. Focal adult-onset limb dystonia that is not task specific can be the earliest manifestation of parkinsonism and Parkinson's disease.

Recent advances in our understanding of the genetics of dystonia syndromes allow for unique classification and prognosis. Mutations in the *TOR1A* gene *(DYT1)* encoding torsinA are the most common cause of early onset generalized dystonia. Patients present with childhood-onset limb dystonia that often progresses to generalized dystonia within a few years. DYT1 is an autosomal dominant disorder with reduced penetrance (30%).

Dopa-responsive dystonia is a rare but important cause of childhood onset dystonia. It is inherited in autosomal dominant fashion with reduced penetrance (30%) with females more commonly affected than males. It is characterized by lower extremity dystonia, parkinsonism, and diurnal variability with the symptoms worsening as the day progresses and improving with sleep. As the name suggests, it is exquisitely sensitive to levodopa therapy. The condition is often misdiagnosed and untreated; therefore, patients with childhood-onset dystonia should have a trial of levodopa. Other autosomal dominant disorders characterized by dystonia include myoclonus dystonia syndrome and rapid-onset dystonia parkinsonism. In addition, multiple other genetic causes of dystonia have been identified.

Treatment of dystonia consists of a combination of oral medications including anti-epileptics, anticholinergics, benzodiazepines, GABAergic drugs, and botulinum toxin injections for focal or segmental dystonia. Deep brain stimulation is commonly used for refractory cases.

Tics and Tourette Syndrome

Tics are rapid, repetitive, nonrhythmic, and typically briefly suppressible movements or vocalizations associated with a premonitory urge to perform the action and a post-event sense of relief. Tics are quite

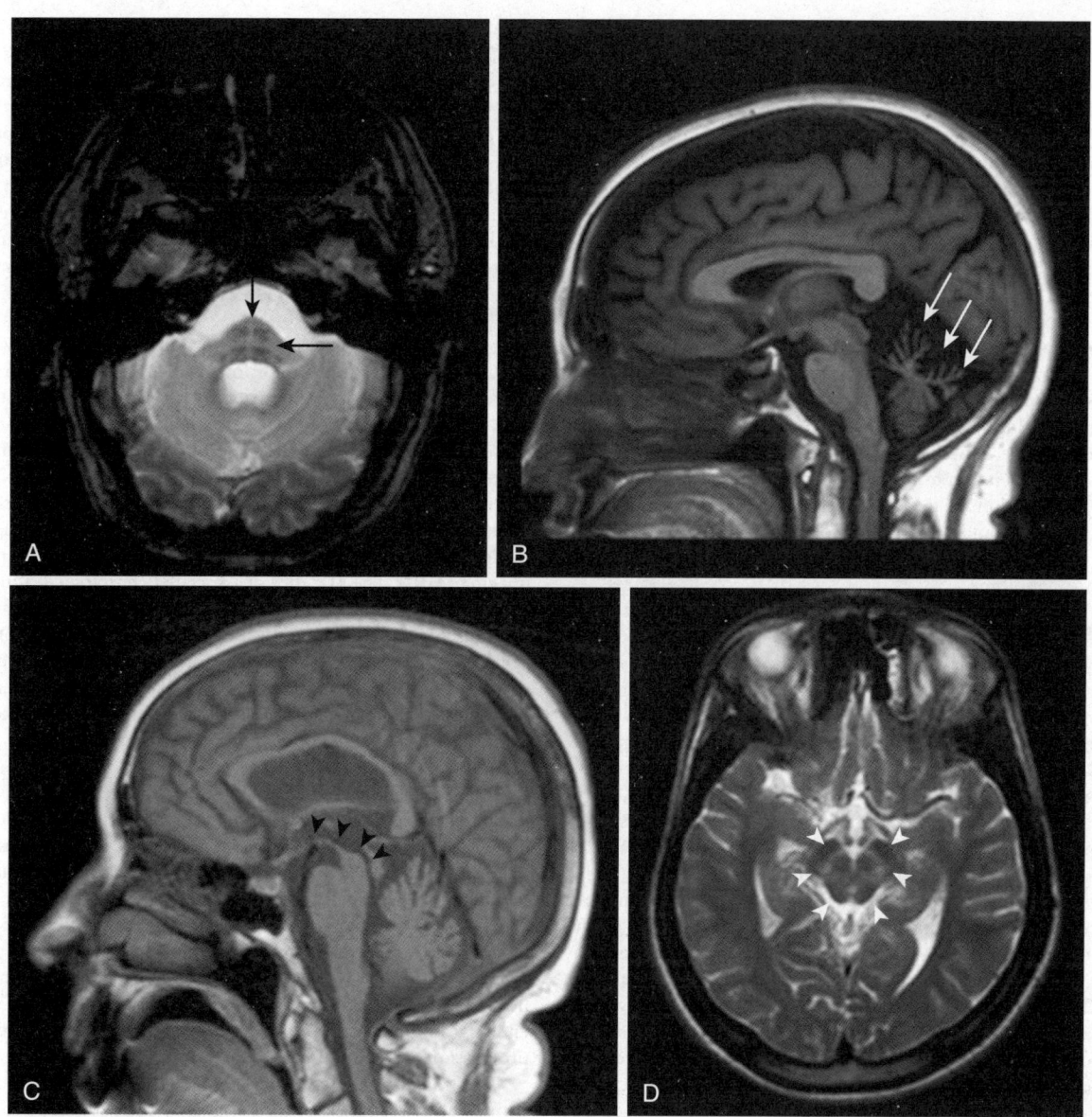

图 11.3 不同运动障碍的代表性 MRI 表现。(A) 多系统萎缩 (MSA) 的"面包十字征"(黑色箭头)。(B) 脊髓小脑萎缩共济失调 (SCA) 6 型中明显的小脑及蚓部萎缩(白色箭头)。(C) 进行性核上性麻痹 (PSP) 中由于显著的中脑萎缩而出现的"蜂鸟征"(黑色箭头)。(D) 肝豆状核变性的"巨熊猫脸征"(白色箭头)

（如书写痉挛、音乐家肌张力障碍）。然而随着时间的推移，这种任务特异性可能会消失，患者甚至会在静止时出现症状。非任务特异性的成人发病的肢体肌张力障碍可能是帕金森综合征和帕金森病的最早表现。

基于我们对肌张力障碍综合征遗传学理解的进展，衍生出了独特的分类和预后体系。编码 torsinA 的 *TOR1A* 基因突变（*DYT1*）是早发全身性肌张力障碍的最常见原因。患者在儿童期出现肢体肌张力障碍，通常在几年内发展为全身性肌张力障碍。DYT1 是一种具有不完全外显（30%）的常染色体显性遗传病。

多巴反应性肌张力障碍是儿童期肌张力障碍的一种罕见但重要的原因。它呈常染色体显性遗传，具有不完全外显现象（30%），女性患者比男性更常见。其特征是下肢肌张力障碍、帕金森综合征和昼夜变异，症状在一天中逐渐加重，睡眠时改善。顾名思义，它对左旋多巴治疗极其敏感。该病常被误诊而延误治疗，因此儿童期发病的肌张力障碍患者均应进行左旋多巴治疗试验。其他以肌张力障碍为特征的常染色体显性遗传病包括肌阵挛-肌张力障碍综合征和快速发作的肌张力障碍帕金森综合征。此外还明确了多种其他遗传性肌张力障碍的病因。

肌张力障碍的治疗包括口服药物（如抗癫痫药、抗胆碱能药、苯二氮䓬类药物、GABA 能药物）和针对局灶性或节段性肌张力障碍的肉毒毒素注射的联合治疗。脑深部电刺激常用于治疗难治性病例。

抽动症和抽动秽语综合征

抽动症是快速、重复、非节律性且通常短暂可抑制的运动或发声，伴有预感冲动去执行该动作和事件完成后的缓解感。抽动症非常常见，影响高达 20% 的

common, affecting up to 20% of school-age children, though the vast majority will have transient tics, lasting less than 12 months. Tics are broadly subdivided into motor tics, which involve movement of one or more parts of the body or musculature, and vocal tics, which involve creation of a sound. These can be further subdivided into simple tics (e.g., excessive blinking, head turning, grunting, and throat clearing) and complex tics (e.g., jumping, moving, and complex vocalizations or patterns of movement).

Tourette syndrome (TS) is the most common chronic tic disorder and involves a combination of motor and vocal tics, present daily, and for at least 1 year. Patients may have comorbid psychiatric diagnoses including attention-deficit/hyperactivity disorder, obsessive-compulsive disorder, or anxiety, which are often more disabling than the tics themselves. Tics commonly improve in late adolescence and in the majority of individuals there is partial or complete resolution of symptoms by adulthood. Treatment of tics can be considered when they are bothersome, functionally impairing, or causing harm to the individual. A combination of behavioral approaches (comprehensive behavioral intervention for tics), oral medications (α-adrenergic agonists, antipsychotics, and vesicular monoamine transporter-2 inhibitors), and botulinum toxin injections can be effective at minimizing the impact of symptoms.

Paroxysmal Dyskinesias

The paroxysmal dyskinesias are a group of rare hyperkinetic movement disorders characterized by recurrent, stereotyped episodes of abnormal involuntary movements (most commonly dystonia, chorea, or a combination of both). The three classically recognized types, paroxysmal kinesigenic dyskinesia (PKD), paroxysmal non-kinesigenic dyskinesia (PNKD), and paroxysmal exercised-induced dyskinesia (PED), were defined on the basis of triggers. Several causal genetic mutations have recently been identified. However, cases may also be secondary to structural abnormalities, and seizures should always be considered in the differential. PKD episodes are triggered by sudden movement, are often preceded by a premonitory sensation, last seconds, and occur with high frequency. The most common genetic cause is a mutation in the *PRRT2* gene. PKD is typically responsive to low-dose carbamazepine. PNKD episodes are triggered by caffeine, alcohol, and stress, may be preceded by a premonitory sensation, last minutes to hours, and occur less frequently than PKD episodes. The most common genetic cause is a mutation in the MR-1 gene. Treatment of PNKD includes avoidance of identified triggers and treatment with benzodiazepines. With both PKD and PNKD, onset typically occurs in childhood and boys are more likely to be affected. PED episodes are triggered by sustained exercise, last minutes to hours, and typically involve the lower extremities. The most common genetic cause is a mutation in the *SLC2A1* gene and when such a mutation is identified, symptoms may be responsive to the ketogenic diet.

Restless Leg Syndrome

Restless leg syndrome (RLS) is a common sensorimotor disorder that predominantly, but not exclusively, affects the legs. RLS is characterized by an urge to move the legs, predominantly when at rest, accompanied by leg discomfort that improves with ambulation. There are diurnal fluctuations with symptoms typically present initially only at night. The prevalence of RLS is variable and highest among European populations (5% to 12%). It is strongly heritable, with one half of patients having at least one affected first-degree relative. The three conditions most strongly associated with RLS are pregnancy, iron deficiency, and end-stage renal disease. Most patients with RLS also have periodic limb movements of sleep, which are periodically recurring limb movements that occur during sleep.

Although the mechanism of the disease is incompletely understood, a hypodopaminergic pathology is suspected in RLS based on the clinical observation that dopaminergic medications improve symptoms. Treatment includes the use of nonpharmacologic strategies like exercise and removal of offending drugs (e.g., antidepressants). Iron replacement should be undertaken when indicated. If medical management is needed, dopamine agonists or alpha-2-delta calcium-channel ligands (gabapentin, pregabalin, and gabapentin enacarbil) can be considered as first-line treatment. The use of opioids and/or benzodiazepines can be entertained in certain refractory cases.

Cerebellar Ataxias

The ataxias are a heterogeneous group of conditions reflecting impaired cerebellar function or impairment in cerebellar afferent and efferent pathways. Clinically, patients may present with incoordination, disorganized gait, poor balance, falls, dysarthria, impaired hand coordination, tremor, swallowing difficulties, and eye movement abnormalities. Comprehensive assessment is critical in elucidating potential etiologies and must include an understanding of the rate of onset/progression, ascertainment of family history, thorough examination for specific diagnostic signs, and brain magnetic resonance imaging (MRI). The presence of associated neurologic features can be useful for differentiating ataxic etiologies and guiding additional investigations. Structural lesions affecting the cerebellum or its connections can present with ataxia including abnormalities of brain development, stroke, tumor, infection, trauma, and inflammatory and demyelinating diseases. Table 11.8 summarizes the differential diagnosis of the ataxic disorders divided by genetic and acquired causes.

Inherited/Genetic Ataxias

Progressive ataxia in coordination and gait disturbance are the cardinal features of the inherited ataxias. Autosomal dominant SCAs may present with a pure cerebellar syndrome or be associated with parkinsonism, spasticity, cognitive, or behavioral features. They are usually adult-onset disorders with variable genetic mutations, including trinucleotide repeats, mutations in noncoding regions, and point mutations. Genetic testing is available for many of the common spinocerebellar ataxias and new mutations are being identified in a rapid and ongoing basis. Currently there are no treatments to address disease progression and symptomatic treatment is limited.

The fragile X mental retardation *(FMR1)* gene contains a CCG trinucleotide repeat expansion of greater than 200 in the fully penetrant mutation associated with mental retardation in boys. Recently a premutation associated with repeats of 55-200 in the *FMR1* gene has been found to be the cause of the adult-onset neurodegenerative disorder, fragile X–associated tremor/ataxia syndrome (FXTAS). Clinically, affected males have a progressive cerebellar tremor and ataxia. Fragile X–associated tremor/ataxia syndrome has been under-recognized and may be the most common genetic cause of late-onset ataxia. Treatment is largely symptomatic and the disease results in progressive disability.

Autosomal recessive ataxias are rare conditions with onset in childhood. Friedreich ataxia (FA) is the most common and best characterized of these disorders. It results from an unstable GAA expansion on chromosome 9. Clinically it is characterized by childhood-onset gait ataxia and clumsiness. The ataxia reflects a combination of spinocerebellar degeneration and peripheral sensory loss. Overt weakness secondary to pyramidal tract dysfunction is a late complication. Nonneurologic manifestations include cardiomyopathy, diabetes mellitus, and skeletal deformities, which add to the morbidity and mortality of the disease. Since identification of the mutation, late-onset forms of the disease with less systemic involvement and milder symptoms have

学龄儿童，尽管绝大多数抽动均为暂时性的，持续时间少于 12 个月。抽动症大致可分为运动抽动（涉及身体某部分或肌肉的运动）和发声抽动（涉及发声），还可以进一步分为简单抽动（如过度眨眼、转头、咕噜声和清嗓子）和复杂抽动（如跳跃、移动和复杂的发声或运动模式）。

抽动秽语综合征（TS）是最常见的慢性抽动障碍，以运动抽动和发声抽动的组合为主要临床表现，症状每日出现且持续存在至少 1 年。患者可能有共患的精神疾病，包括注意力缺陷/多动障碍、强迫症或焦虑症，这些通常比抽动本身更具致残性。抽动通常在青少年晚期改善，大多数人的症状在成年后可部分或完全缓解。当抽动症为患者带来困扰、有功能受损或对个体造成伤害时，可以考虑启动治疗。行为疗法（综合行为干预抽动）、口服药物（α 肾上腺素能激动剂、抗精神病药和囊泡单胺转运体 -2 抑制剂）和肉毒毒素注射可以有效地减轻症状。

发作性运动障碍

发作性运动障碍是一组罕见的多动性运动障碍，其特征是反复发作的、刻板的异常不自主运动（最常见的是肌张力障碍、舞蹈症或两者兼有）。根据诱因将其分为三种经典类型：发作性运动性运动障碍（PKD）、发作性非运动性运动障碍（PNKD）和发作性运动诱发的运动障碍（PED）。最近已确定了几种致病基因突变，但该病也可能继发于结构异常，应该与癫痫进行鉴别。PKD 发作由突然运动触发，发作前常有先兆感觉，发作持续数秒，频率较高，最常见的遗传因素是 *PRRT2* 基因突变。PKD 通常对低剂量卡马西平有反应。PNKD 发作多由咖啡因、酒精和压力触发，发作前可能有先兆感觉，发作持续数分钟到数小时，发作频率低于 PKD，最常见的致病基因是 *MR-1* 基因突变。PNKD 的治疗包括避免已确定的诱因和使用苯二氮䓬类药物。PKD 和 PNKD 通常在儿童期发病，男孩更易受到影响。PED 发作由持续运动触发，持续数分钟到数小时，通常累及下肢，最常见的致病基因是 *SLC2A1* 基因突变，当确定存在这种突变时，生酮饮食可能会改善症状。

不宁腿综合征

不宁腿综合征（RLS）是一种常见的感觉运动障碍，主要累及但不局限于腿部。RLS 的特征是静止时有移动双腿的冲动，腿部不适可在行走时缓解。症状有昼夜波动，通常最初仅在夜间出现。RLS 的患病率差异较大，在欧洲人群中最高（5%～12%）。RLS 具有很强的遗传性，约有一半的患者至少有一位一级亲属也会罹患该病。RLS 最强相关的三种危险因素是妊娠、铁缺乏和终末期肾病。大多数 RLS 患者在睡眠期间也会发生周期性肢体运动。

尽管对该病的发病机制尚未完全明确，但基于临床观察到多巴胺能药物可改善症状，推测 RLS 的病理机制中可能涉及低多巴胺能。治疗方法包括使用非药物策略，如运动和去除致病药物（如抗抑郁药），在必要时应进行铁补充。如果需要药物治疗，可以考虑使用多巴胺激动剂或 α-2-δ 钙通道配体（加巴喷丁、普瑞巴林和加巴喷丁酯）作为一线治疗。在某些难治性病例中，可以考虑使用阿片类药物和（或）苯二氮䓬类药物。

小脑性共济失调

共济失调是一组异质性疾病，反映了小脑功能受损或小脑传入和传出通路受损。患者的临床表现可能包括协调不良、步态紊乱、平衡差、跌倒、构音障碍、手部协调受损、震颤、吞咽困难以及眼球运动异常。全面评估对于揭示潜在病因至关重要，包括了解发病/进展速度、确定有无家族史、详细查体以发现诊断特异性体征以及脑磁共振成像（MRI）。相关神经特征的存在可以帮助区分共济失调的病因，并指导进一步检查。影响小脑或其连接的结构性病变均可表现为共济失调，包括脑发育异常、卒中、肿瘤、感染、创伤、炎症及脱髓鞘疾病。表 11.8 按遗传和获得性病因总结了共济失调的鉴别诊断。

遗传性 / 基因性共济失调

遗传性共济失调的主要特征包括进行性共济失调和步态障碍。常染色体显性遗传的脊髓小脑性共济失调（SCA）可表现为纯小脑综合征或伴有帕金森综合征、痉挛、认知或行为障碍。该类疾病通常成年期发病，包括多种基因突变类型，如三核苷酸重复、非编码区突变和点突变。许多常见类型的 SCA 均可通过基因检测确诊，并且不断有新突变被发现。目前尚无治疗方法可阻止疾病进展，对症治疗手段也十分有限。

脆性 X 神经发育迟滞基因（*FMR1*）突变包含超过 200 次的 CCG 三核苷酸重复扩增且呈完全外显，与男孩智力低下相关。最近发现，55～200 次重复的 *FMR1* 基因前突变是成年发病的神经退行性疾病、脆性 X 相关震颤/共济失调综合征（FXTAS）的病因。受累男性的临床表现包括进行性小脑震颤和共济失调。FXTAS 可能是晚发性共济失调的最常见遗传原因，但其尚未得到充分认识。该疾病会导致进行性残疾，以对症治疗为主。

儿童期发病的共济失调罕见常染色体隐性遗传，Friedreich 共济失调（FA）是其中最常见且研究最为充分的疾病，它是由 9 号染色体上不稳定的 GAA 扩增引起。儿童期发病患者的临床表现包括步态共济失调和笨拙。共济失调由脊髓小脑变性和周围神经感觉丧失所致，锥体束功能障碍导致的严重无力是其晚期并发症。非神经系统症状包括心肌病、糖尿病和骨骼畸形，进一步增加了疾病的发病率和死亡率。自从该突变被发现以来，也有部分神经系统症状较轻、系统受累较

TABLE 11.8		Differential Diagnosis of Cerebellar Ataxia
Genetic disorders	Autosomal dominant	Spinocerebellar ataxias
		Episodic ataxia
		DRPLA
	Autosomal recessive	Friedreich ataxia
		Ataxia-telangiectasia
		Ataxia with oculomotor apraxia
		Ataxia with vitamin E deficiency
	X-linked	Fragile X–associated tremor/ataxia syndrome
	Mitochondrial	Polymerase gamma (POLG)
Acquired/ sporadic	Medications/toxins	Alcohol
		Phenytoin
		Fluorouracil
		Heavy metals
		Carbon monoxide
	Developmental	Chiari malformations
		Dandy-Walker malformations
		Pontocerebellar hypoplasia
	Immune mediated	Paraneoplastic (anti-Hu/Yo/Ri)
		Pediatric postviral
		Behçet's disease
	Infectious	HIV/AIDS
		PML
		CJD
		Lyme disease
	Metabolic	Thiamine deficiency (Wernicke encephalopathy)
		Vitamin E/B_{12} deficiency
		Thyroid disease
	Vascular	Cerebellar stroke/hemorrhage
	Neoplastic	Primary and metastatic tumors
		Paraneoplastic (anti-Hu/Yo/Ri)
	Miscellaneous	MSA-cerebellar
		Multiple sclerosis

CJD, Creutzfeldt-Jakob disease; *DRPLA*, dentatorubropallidoluysian atrophy; *MSA*, multiple system atrophy; *PML*, progressive multifocal leukoencephalopathy.

been identified. Therefore, Friedreich ataxia should be considered in the differential of adult-onset sporadic ataxias.

Ataxia with vitamin E deficiency is a childhood-onset ataxia with a Friedreich ataxia phenotype. Treatment with high-dose vitamin E may slow the progression of neurologic symptoms. Ataxia with vitamin E deficiency should be considered in any child with signs and symptoms of Friedreich ataxia that do not carry the Friedreich ataxia mutation. Abetalipoproteinemia and Refsum disease may resemble Friedreich ataxia and because of the availability of directed testing, they should be considered in the differential. Mitochondrial disorders, ataxia telangiectasia, and ataxia with oculomotor apraxia are other common causes of early-onset ataxia with cerebellar atrophy.

Sporadic/Acquired Ataxias

Insidious onset of cerebellar ataxia without a family history can be a diagnostic challenge. Alcohol abuse, toxins, chronic infections, multiple system atrophy, and mitochondrial disorders are diagnostic considerations. Sporadic autoimmune ataxias amenable to treatment include glutamic acid decarboxylase (GAD) ataxia and steroid-responsive encephalopathy associated with autoimmune thyroiditis.

Acute or subacute onset ataxia is most often associated with cerebrovascular disease, demyelinating illness, or direct or indirect effects of cancer. Paraneoplastic cerebellar degeneration is one of the more common paraneoplastic syndromes usually associated with gynecologic, breast, lung cancer, or lymphoma. A variety of antineuronal antibodies have been implicated; however, anti-Hu/Yo/Ri are most frequently seen. The cerebellar syndrome often predates the identification of the cancer. Treatment of the underlying cancer and plasma exchange are sometimes beneficial.

Vitamin B_{12} and vitamin E deficiency secondary to malabsorption can present with ataxic gait as a result of posterior column sensory deficits. In the appropriate clinical situation, Wernicke encephalopathy due to thiamine deficiency needs to be considered as an acute cause of gait ataxia.

Superficial siderosis is characterized by deposition of free iron and hemosiderin along the pial and subpial structures of the brain and spinal cord, resulting in damage to the cerebellar cortex, cochlear nerves, cerebral cortex, and spinal cord. Patients present with the triad of sensorineural hearing loss, cerebellar ataxia, and spasticity.

Functional Movement Disorders

Functional movement disorders (FMD), which fall into the broader category of functional neurologic disorders, are a heterogeneous group of abnormal involuntary movements that do not adhere to the physiologic characteristics of the other movement phenomena described in this chapter. FMD have traditionally been considered *conversion disorders*, where the body converts an underlying psychological stressor into a physical symptom. However, while there is clearly a link between psychological stressors and prior trauma with the development FMD, this traditional understanding is likely an oversimplification of the pathophysiology, which is not well understood. The prevalence of FMD is not well established, though it has been reported to be as high as 10% of patients seen in movement disorders specialty clinics.

Patients with FMD can present with movements that mimic any of the phenomena described in this chapter (e.g., tremor, dystonia, myoclonus). However, the examination will also typically demonstrate features inconsistent with other causes and suggestive of FMD, including variability (e.g., in the distribution, type of movement, amplitude), entrainment (where the frequency of the abnormal movement entrains to match that of an alternative volitional movement), and distractibility. Abrupt onset of symptoms, the presence of a triggering event, and rapid onset may also be suggestive of a diagnosis of FMD. A clinical diagnosis of FMD can be made based on the presence of these typical features. Electrodiagnostic testing can be helpful in identifying functional tremor and functional myoclonus.

Management of FMD can be challenging but generally starts with patient and family education and requires a multidisciplinary approach. Cognitive-behavioral therapy with counseling is the best evidence-based approach for the management of FMD. Rehabilitative therapies have a role for most patients. Pharmacotherapy has a limited role in the management of FMD though can be useful in the treatment of any comorbid psychiatric conditions.

Acknowledgment

We gratefully acknowledge the contributions of the previous-edition chapter author, Kevin Biglan, to this chapter.

SUGGESTED READINGS

Abdo WF, van de Warrenburg BP, Burn DJ, et al: The clinical approach to movement disorders, Nat Rev Neurol 6:29–37, 2010.

Albanese A, Bhatia K, Bressman SB, et al: Phenomenology and classification of dystonia: a consensus update, Mov Disord 28:863–873, 2013.

表 11.8	小脑性共济失调的鉴别诊断	
遗传性疾病	常染色体显性遗传	脊髓小脑共济失调 发作性共济失调 DRPLA
	常染色体隐性遗传	Friedreich 共济失调 共济失调-毛细血管扩张症 眼动失用性共济失调 维生素 E 缺乏性共济失调
	X 连锁	脆性 X 相关震颤/共济失调综合征
	线粒体	聚合酶 γ（POLG）
获得性/散发性	药物/毒素	酒精 苯妥英 氟尿嘧啶 重金属 一氧化碳
	发育性	Chiari 畸形 Dandy-Walker 畸形 脑桥小脑发育不全
	免疫介导	副肿瘤性（抗 Hu/Yo/Ri） 儿童病毒感染后 白塞病
	感染性	HIV/AIDS PML CJD 莱姆病
	代谢性	维生素 B$_1$ 缺乏（Wernicke 脑病） 维生素 E/B$_{12}$ 缺乏 甲状腺疾病
	血管性	小脑卒中/出血
	肿瘤性	原发性和转移性肿瘤 副肿瘤性（抗 Hu/Yo/Ri）
	其他	MSA-小脑型 多发性硬化

CJD，克-雅病；DRPLA，齿状核-红核-苍白球-路易体萎缩；MSA，多系统萎缩；PML，进行性多灶性白质脑病。

少的晚发型被报道。因此，Friedreich 共济失调应被纳入成人发病的散发性共济失调的鉴别诊断中。

维生素 E 缺乏性共济失调是一种具有 Friedreich 共济失调表型的儿童期发病的共济失调。高剂量维生素 E 治疗可减缓神经系统症状的进展。对于任何表现出 Friedreich 共济失调症状和体征，但没有 Friedreich 共济失调相关基因突变的儿童，均应考虑到维生素 E 缺乏性共济失调的可能。无 β 脂蛋白血症和 Refsum 病可类似于 Friedreich 共济失调，且由于具有直接的指向性检测，也应被纳入鉴别诊断。早发性共济失调伴小脑萎缩的其他常见病因还包括线粒体疾病、毛细血管扩张性共济失调和眼动失用性共济失调。

散发性/获得性共济失调

隐匿起病的、无家族史的小脑性共济失调的诊断极具挑战。酒精滥用、毒素、慢性感染、多系统萎缩和线粒体疾病等因素均需考虑。可治疗的散发性自身免疫性共济失调包括谷氨酸脱羧酶（GAD）共济失调和对类固醇敏感的自身免疫性甲状腺炎相关脑病。

急性或亚急性发病的共济失调最常见于脑血管疾病、脱髓鞘疾病或肿瘤的直接或间接影响。副肿瘤性小脑变性是最常见的副肿瘤综合征之一，常与妇科肿瘤、乳腺癌、肺癌或淋巴瘤相关，涉及各种抗神经元抗体，最常见的是抗 Hu/Yo/Ri 抗体。小脑综合征通常早于肿瘤被发现。治疗潜在的肿瘤和血浆置换有时是有用的。

继发于吸收不良的维生素 B$_{12}$ 和维生素 E 缺乏可因后索感觉缺失而导致共济失调步态。在适当的临床情况下，急性共济失调步态的鉴别需要考虑维生素 B$_1$ 缺乏引起的 Wernicke 脑病。

表面铁沉积症的特征是自由铁和含铁血红蛋白沿脑和脊髓的脊膜及脊膜下结构沉积，导致小脑皮质、耳蜗神经、大脑皮质和脊髓受损。患者表现为感音神经性听力丧失、小脑性共济失调以及肢体痉挛三联征。

功能性运动障碍

功能性运动障碍（FMD）属于更广泛的功能性神经障碍范畴，是一组异质性的异常不自主运动，不符合本章所描述的其他运动现象的生理特征。传统上，FMD 被认为是转换障碍，即身体将潜在的心理压力转换为躯体症状。然而，虽然心理压力和此前的创伤史与 FMD 的发展之间存在显然关联，但这种传统理解可能是对病理生理学的过度简化，机制尚不完全清楚。FMD 的患病率尚未明确，但据报道在运动障碍专科诊所就诊的患者中，FMD 的比例高达 10%。

FMD 患者可以表现出本章中所描述的任何运动现象（如震颤、肌张力障碍、肌阵挛）。然而，在查体时通常也会显示出与其他原因不一致且提示 FMD 的特征，包括变异性（如在分布、运动类型、幅度方面）、夹带效应（异常运动的频率与其他自主运动同步）和注意力分散时症状减轻。症状的突然发作、存在触发事件和快速发病也可能提示 FMD 的诊断。可以根据这些典型特征的存在进行临床诊断。电生理诊断测试有助于识别功能性震颤和功能性肌阵挛。

FMD 的管理具有挑战性，通常需要从患者和家庭教育开始，需要多学科协作。认知行为疗法结合心理咨询是管理 FMD 的最佳循证方法。康复治疗对大多数患者是有作用的。药物治疗在 FMD 管理中的作用有限，但在治疗任何共病精神状况时可能是有用的。

致谢

我们衷心感谢上一版章节作者 Kevin Biglan 对本章的贡献。

推荐阅读

Abdo WF, van de Warrenburg BP, Burn DJ, et al: The clinical approach to movement disorders, Nat Rev Neurol 6:29–37, 2010.

Albanese A, Bhatia K, Bressman SB, et al: Phenomenology and classification of dystonia: a consensus update, Mov Disord 28:863–873, 2013.

Bandmann O, Weiss KH, Kaler SG: Wilson's disease and other neurological copper disorders, Lancet Neurol 14(1):103–113, 2015.

Caron NS, Dorsey ER, Hayden MR: Therapeutic approaches to huntington disease: from the bench to the clinic, Nat Rev Drug Discov 17(10):729–750, 2018.

Ferreira JJ, Mestre TA, Lyons KE, et al: MDS evidence-based review of treatments for essential tremor, Mov Disord 34(7):950–958, 2019.

Hallett M: Functional (psychogenic) movement disorders—clinical presentations, Parkinsonism Relat Disord 22(Suppl 1):S149–152, 2016.

McColgan P, Tabrizi SJ: Huntington's disease: a clinical review, Eur J Neurol 25(1):24–34, 2018.

McFarland NR: Diagnostic approach to atypical parkinsonian syndromes, Continuum (Minneap Minn) 22(4 Movement Disorders):1117–1142, 2016.

Postuma RB, Berg D, Stern M, et al: MDS clinical diagnostic criteria for Parkinson's disease, Mov Disord 30(12):1591–1601, 2015.

Pringsheim T, Okun MS, Müller-Vahl K, et al: Practice guideline recommendations summary: treatment of tics in in people with Tourette syndrome and chronic tic disorders, Neurology 92(19):896–906, 2019.

Ramirez-Zamora A, Zeigler W, Desai N, et al: Treatable causes of cerebellar ataxia, Mov Disord 30(5):614–623, 2015.

Schuepbach WM, Rau J, Knudsen K, et al: Neurostimulation for Parkinson's disease with early motor complications, N Engl J Med 368(7):610–622, 2013.

Seppi K, Weintraub D, Coelho M, et al: The movement disorder society evidence-based medicine review update: treatments for the non-motor symptoms of Parkinson's disease, Mov Disord 26(Suppl 3):S42–S80, 2011.

Verschuur CVM, Suwijn SR, Boel JA, et al: Randomized delayed-start trial of levodopa in Parkinson's disease, N Engl J Med 380(4):315–324, 2019.

Winkelmann J, Allen RP, Högl B, et al: Treatment of restless legs syndrome: evidence-based review and implications for clinical practice (revised 2017), Mov Disord 33(7):1077–1091, 2018.

Bandmann O, Weiss KH, Kaler SG: Wilson's disease and other neurological copper disorders, Lancet Neurol 14(1):103–113, 2015.

Caron NS, Dorsey ER, Hayden MR: Therapeutic approaches to huntington disease: from the bench to the clinic, Nat Rev Drug Discov 17(10):729–750, 2018.

Ferreira JJ, Mestre TA, Lyons KE, et al: MDS evidence-based review of treatments for essential tremor, Mov Disord 34(7):950–958, 2019.

Hallett M: Functional (psychogenic) movement disorders—clinical presentations, Parkinsonism Relat Disord 22(Suppl 1):S149–152, 2016.

McColgan P, Tabrizi SJ: Huntington's disease: a clinical review, Eur J Neurol 25(1):24–34, 2018.

McFarland NR: Diagnostic approach to atypical parkinsonian syndromes, Continuum (Minneap Minn) 22(4 Movement Disorders):1117–1142, 2016.

Postuma RB, Berg D, Stern M, et al: MDS clinical diagnostic criteria for Parkinson's disease, Mov Disord 30(12):1591–1601, 2015.

Pringsheim T, Okun MS, Müller-Vahl K, et al: Practice guideline recommendations summary: treatment of tics in in people with Tourette syndrome and chronic tic disorders, Neurology 92(19):896–906, 2019.

Ramirez-Zamora A, Zeigler W, Desai N, et al: Treatable causes of cerebellar ataxia, Mov Disord 30(5):614–623, 2015.

Schuepbach WM, Rau J, Knudsen K, et al: Neurostimulation for Parkinson's disease with early motor complications, N Engl J Med 368(7):610–622, 2013.

Seppi K, Weintraub D, Coelho M, et al: The movement disorder society evidence-based medicine review update: treatments for the non-motor symptoms of Parkinson's disease, Mov Disord 26(Suppl 3):S42–S80, 2011.

Verschuur CVM, Suwijn SR, Boel JA, et al: Randomized delayed-start trial of levodopa in Parkinson's disease, N Engl J Med 380(4):315–324, 2019.

Winkelmann J, Allen RP, Högl B, et al: Treatment of restless legs syndrome: evidence-based review and implications for clinical practice (revised 2017), Mov Disord 33(7):1077–1091, 2018.

12

Congenital, Developmental, and Neurocutaneous Disorders

Kristin A. Seaborg, Jennifer M. Kwon

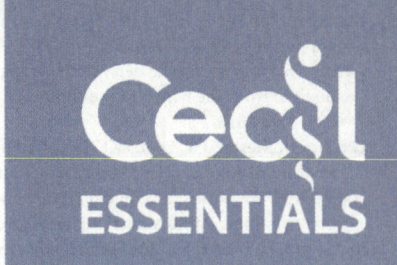

INTRODUCTION

This chapter describes some important congenital nervous system malformations, neurodevelopmental disorders, and neurocutaneous syndromes. Advances in imaging and molecular genetic testing have improved our understanding of these disorders. Neuroimaging facilitates early diagnosis and management of malformations of the brain and spinal cord. Advances in genetic sequencing and microarray analysis are improving our understanding of single-gene disorders, such as fragile X syndrome and neurofibromatosis, as well as genetically complex disorders, such as autism and attention-deficit/hyperactivity disorder (ADHD).

CONGENITAL MALFORMATIONS

Malformations of the central nervous system develop during fetal life. Table 12.1 summarizes the timeline of early neural and cortical development and the defects that may occur during these stages. Malformations developing early in embryogenesis can be more severe than those arising after the basic structures of the nervous system are in place.

Disorders of Dorsal Induction

Definition/Embryology

Dorsal induction is when neural tube closure occurs at 18 to 26 days post-conception. The central portion closes first, then the rostral and caudal portions. Failure to completely close the neural tube can occur anywhere along the neuro axis, leading to neural tube defects (NTDs) in 6.5/10,000 live births, the prevalence varying by geography, and genetic and environmental factors. Use of folic acid at the time of conception and during pregnancy can significantly reduce NTD rates.

If the rostral end of the neural tube fails to close, anencephaly can result, characterized by incomplete development of the brain and skull, and affected infants may not survive. If the caudal end of the neural tube fails to close, the result is spina bifida, described next.

Spina Bifida

Definition/epidemiology. Failure of complete closure of the caudal end of the neural tube during the 24th to 26th days post-conception results in spina bifida, the most common type of NTD, occurring in 3.5 of 10,000 live births. Abnormal caudal closure with overlying bony and skin defects can cause "open" NTDs, such as myelomeningocele (MMC). MMC is the most severe form of spina bifida and is characterized by the protrusion of the spinal cord and meninges through a defect in the vertebral column. "Closed" defects of the caudal spinal cord, or spina bifida occulta, are associated with malformation of one or more vertebrae and typically have limited neurologic symptoms.

Pathology. The deficits associated with meningomyelocele are not only secondary to the abnormal caudal closure of the neural tube but also from the ongoing exposure and chemical damage of the neural tube contents to amniotic fluid, trauma, and leakage of CSF. CSF leak through the open meningomyelocele impairs rostral vesicle expansion, leading to underdevelopment of the posterior fossa with cerebellar tonsil herniation into the upper spinal canal, called the Arnold-Chiari or Chiari 2 malformation.

Clinical presentation. Many of the stigmata of MMC can be detected on first trimester fetal ultrasound. MMC causes severe distal spinal cord dysfunction, including paralysis and sensory loss in the lower extremities as well as bowel and bladder dysfunction. Progressive loss of neurologic function and development of congenital clubfoot is commonly observed during pregnancy. Nearly all children with MMC have a Chiari 2 malformation and obstructive hydrocephalus.

Children with spina bifida occulta, or a "closed" caudal neural tube defect, may have symptoms including lower extremity spasticity and bladder abnormalities and the overlying skin may show nevi, lipomas, abnormal dimples, or whorls of hair. The most common location for spina bifida is within the lumbosacral region.

Diagnosis. Prenatal diagnosis of MMC cannot be reliably determined by ultrasound until the second trimester of pregnancy. Maternal serum testing for α-fetoprotein (AFP), which is secreted from an open spinal dysraphism (incomplete fusion), can be done in conjunction with second trimester ultrasound. Further evaluation of specific characteristics of the fetal anomaly can be done with fetal MRI.

Treatment/prognosis. Previously, infants born with MMC had surgical closure of the defect within the first 2 days of life to minimize neurologic complications. In 2011, the Management of Meningomyelocele Study (MOMS) demonstrated that prenatal surgery for MMC repair decreased the rate of enlarged cerebral ventricles and ventriculoperitoneal shunting by 1 year of age by 42% and improved the rate of independent ambulation by 21%. This study represented a turning point in management of MMC and subsequently led to affected fetuses with normal karyotype, isolated spinal bifida with upper border between T1 and S1, and evidence of hindbrain herniation to be referred for prenatal closure of MMC during the second trimester of pregnancy.

Chiari Malformation Type I

Definition/epidemiology. Though not technically a disorder of ventral induction or a neural tube defect, Chiari I malformation (CM1) is the consequence of similar pathologic processes occurring during formation of the posterior fossa. CM1 is characterized by cerebellar tonsils that are downwardly displaced more than 5 mm past the foramen magnum. CM1 is much more common (1/1000 births) than Chiari 2 and associated with fewer neurologic sequelae.

先天性、发育性和神经皮肤疾病

付瀚辉 译 杨泃哲 谭颖 审校 姚明 朱以诚 通审

引言

本章主要介绍了一些重要的神经系统先天性畸形、神经发育异常和神经皮肤综合征。影像学和分子遗传学诊断技术的发展提高了我们对相关疾病的认识。神经影像学推动了脑和脊髓畸形的早期诊断和治疗。基因测序和微阵列分析的进步加深了我们对单基因疾病（如脆性X染色体综合征和神经纤维瘤病）以及复杂基因疾病[如孤独症和注意缺陷多动障碍（ADHD）]的理解。

先天性畸形

中枢神经系统畸形在胎儿期形成。表12.1总结了早期神经和皮质发育的时间轴以及各时期可能出现的缺陷。胚胎发育早期发生的畸形通常比神经系统基本结构发育完成后出现的畸形更为严重。

背侧诱导障碍
定义和胚胎学

背侧诱导是指受精后18~26天内神经管闭合的过程。神经管中间部分先闭合，然后向头部和尾部延伸。神经管闭合不全可能发生在神经轴的任何位置，约每1万活产儿中有6.5例可出现神经管缺陷（NTD），其患病率因地理、遗传和环境因素而异。受孕期和妊娠期服用叶酸可显著降低NTD发生率。

神经管头部闭合缺陷可导致无脑症，特征是大脑和颅骨发育不完全，可能导致新生儿无法存活。神经管尾部闭合缺陷导致脊柱裂，下文将详细描述。

脊柱裂

定义和流行病学　受精后24~26天神经管尾部如未完全闭合将会导致脊柱裂，这是最常见的神经管缺陷类型，每1万新生儿中约有3.5例。尾部闭合异常伴随骨骼和皮肤缺陷可导致"开放型"NTD，如脊髓脊膜膨出（MMC）。MMC是最严重的脊柱裂形式，脊髓和脑脊膜通过椎骨缺陷暴露在外。"闭合型"尾部神经管缺陷，又称隐性脊柱裂，通常伴有一个或多个椎骨畸形，神经系统症状轻微。

病理学　与脊髓脊膜膨出相关的神经损伤不仅由于神经管尾部闭合不全，还可能源于神经管组织持续暴露于羊水的化学损伤、创伤以及脑脊液漏。脑脊液通过开放的脊髓脊膜膨出漏出会影响头部脑泡延展，导致颅后窝发育不良伴小脑扁桃体疝入上椎管，称为Arnold-Chiari或Chiari 2型畸形。

临床表现　孕早期超声可以发现MMC的许多特征。MMC会导致严重的脊髓远端功能障碍，包括下肢瘫痪和感觉丧失，以及肛门括约肌和膀胱控制障碍。胎儿在妊娠期常发生神经系统功能缺陷和先天性马蹄内翻足。几乎所有MMC患儿合并Chiari 2型畸形和梗阻性脑积水。

隐性脊柱裂或"闭合型"尾部神经管缺陷的患儿可能出现下肢痉挛和膀胱功能异常，相应区域皮肤可出现色素痣、脂肪瘤、异常凹陷或发旋。脊柱裂最常见的部位为腰骶部。

诊断　MMC的产前诊断直到孕中期才能通过超声基本明确。孕中期超声可以联合母体血清甲胎蛋白（AFP）进行，后者由开放性脊柱裂（神经管不完全融合）所分泌。胎儿MRI可用于进一步评估胎儿相关异常特征。

治疗和预后　既往建议出生后发现MMC的患儿在出生后2日内进行外科手术干预以尽量减少神经系统并发症。2011年脊髓脊膜膨出管理研究（MOMS）表明，产前修复手术可以使MMC患儿1岁时脑室扩大和脑室腹腔分流的发生率降低42%，独立行走率提高21%。这项研究标志着MMC治疗的转折点，此后在正常核型胎儿中，对于上缘在T1~S1的孤立型脊柱裂和后脑疝的胎儿，推荐在孕中期手术修复关闭MMC。

Chiari 1 型畸形

定义和流行病学　Chiari 1型畸形（CM1）虽然不属于典型的腹侧诱导障碍（译者注：CM1实际应属于背侧诱导障碍，原文有误）或神经管缺陷，但也在颅后窝发育过程中受到了类似的病理机制影响。CM1的特征是小脑扁桃体向下移位超过枕骨大孔5 mm。CM1（每1000例新生儿中发生1例）较之于Chiari 2型畸形发生率更高，神经系统后遗症更少。

TABLE 12.1 Stages of Prenatal Neural Development (Simplified)

	Stage	Structures Forming	Post-Conceptual Age	Anomalies Seen[a]
Neural tube, brain vesicle development	Dorsal induction	Neural tube closure	18-26 days (3-5 weeks)	Anencephaly, spina bifida, myelomeningocele, Chiari 2 malformation
	Ventral induction	Brain vesicle and face development	5-10 weeks	Holoprosencephaly agenesis of the corpus callosum, septo-optic dysplasia
Cortical development	Proliferation	Development of neuroblasts and glioblasts	2-4 months (neuroblasts)	Microcephaly, megalencephaly
	Migration	Formation of six cortical layers	Peak occurrence at 2-4 months, though occurs from 8 weeks to 8 months	Lissencephaly, periventricular heterotopias
	Post-migrational organization	Cortex formed		Polymicrogyria, schizencephaly

[a]Some anomalies (such as microcephaly, polymicrogyria) can arise from different stages. So even though it may seem intuitive to think of microcephaly as a disorder of neuronal proliferation, there are some forms of microcephaly that develop well after migration.

Pathology. CM1 results from underdeveloped bones of the skull base and reduced volume of the posterior fossa. This leads to displacement of cerebellar tonsils into the spinal canal. Obstruction of CSF outflow through the tight foramen magnum may lead to development of fluid-filled cavities in the spinal cord called syringomyelia (see later). Symptoms can occur with compression of brain stem structures.

Clinical presentation. The clinical presentation of CM1 is variable. Eighty percent of patients report occipital headaches or posterior neck pain. Younger patients can have symptoms from compression of the brain stem, including disordered sleep, vertigo, dysphagia, tinnitus, and ocular symptoms. Some CM1s are found incidentally during MRI evaluation for other reasons. Incidentally found CM1s are less likely to develop syringomyelia, intractable symptoms, or progressive neurologic findings (10%).

Diagnosis/differential. MRI is the most effective method for diagnosis. CSF flow studies may be helpful to establish clinical significance of the CM1. Since any cause of increased intracranial pressure can lead to tonsillar herniation, it is important to exclude idiopathic intracranial hypertension and CNS mass lesions.

Treatment. Asymptomatic patients without syringomyelia may be managed by observation. If patients have severe headaches, neurologic deficits, or syringomyelia, posterior fossa decompression with or without duraplasty is indicated to reestablish CSF flow across the craniovertebral junction.

Prognosis. CM1 is generally not disabling and outcome after surgical decompression leads to resolution of clinical symptoms in over 80% of patients. For symptomatic patients, posterior fossa bone-only decompression without dural opening is associated with a lower rate of complications.

Syringomyelia

Definition/epidemiology. Syringomyelia or syrinx is a cystic cavitation in the parenchyma of the spinal cord or is a dilation in the central spinal canal (hydromyelia). The estimated prevalence of 8/100,00 is likely an underestimate. Syrinx is a common and important neurologic sequela of CM1 in up to 30 to 70% of pediatric patients.

Pathology. Syringomyelia may occur as either a congenital or acquired condition. Congenital syrinx is associated with a neural tube defect and forms during embryogenesis. Acquired syringomyelia is caused by disruption of the normal CSF circulation and is seen with CM1, tethered cord syndrome, spinal cord tumors, or trauma.

Clinical. The classic presentation is a dissociated sensory loss (loss of pain and temperature sensation with preservation of light touch and proprioception) in the neck, arms, or legs. A cervical lesion produces a capelike dissociated sensory loss of the arms and shoulders, atrophy of the hands and arms, with increased tone in the legs. Scoliosis is a common finding in patients with a terminal syrinx.

Diagnosis/differential. Diagnosis is confirmed by MRI, which will also differentiate syrinx from neoplasms, infections, and other spinal cord lesions. MRI of the lumbo-sacral spine should be included to rule out tethered cord.

Treatment. Surgical correction of the cause—CM1, CM2, neoplasm, tethered cord—is the most effective way to treat syringomyelia. A small syrinx may be an asymptomatic incidental finding on MRI and can be observed without intervention.

Prognosis. Syringomyelia is most often a chronic, slowly progressive condition with periods of symptom exacerbation and remission. Patients typically experience symptomatic improvement after corrective surgery. Conservative treatment without surgical correction may be considered in young children and asymptomatic patients.

Disorders of Ventral Induction
Definition/Epidemiology

Ventral induction is the second phase of central nervous system development; the brain vesicles and the face begin to form between the fifth week after conception and mid-gestation. Insults during this phase affect brain and facial development.

Common malformations that arise during this period include holoprosencephaly (HPE), agenesis of the corpus callosum (ACC), agenesis of septum pellucidum, and septo-optic dysplasia (SOD). ACC is most commonly seen. The prevalence in the general population is 0.7% and higher in those with developmental disabilities. The estimated incidence of HPE and SOD are both 1 in 10,000.

Pathology/Embryology

Ventral induction ensues with the cleavage and formation of three primary brain vesicles: prosencephalon, mesencephalon, and rhombencephalon. By embryonic day 49 or gestational week 8, the prosencephalon cleaves into the telencephalon and diencephalon and then the telencephalon subsequently divides into two hemispheres.

Abnormal prosencephalon cleavage leads to HPE, a spectrum of abnormalities ranging from alobar HPE (cortex with a single ventricle)

表 12.1	胚胎神经发育分期（简化版）			
	时期	形成结构	胚胎龄	异常表现 a
神经管，脑泡发育	背侧诱导	神经管闭合	18～26天（3～5周）	无脑畸形、脊柱裂、脊髓脊膜膨出、Chiari 2 型畸形
	腹侧诱导	脑泡和面部发育	5～10周	前脑无裂畸形、胼胝体发育不全、透明隔-视神经发育不良
皮质发育	增殖	成神经细胞和成胶质细胞发育	2～4个月（成神经细胞）	小头畸形、巨头畸形
	迁移	皮质 6 层结构形成	主要发生在 2～4个月，8 周到 8 个月均可能	无脑回畸形，脑室周围灰质异位
	迁移后组织	皮质形成		多小脑回畸形、脑裂畸形

a 一些异常（如小头畸形、多小脑回畸形）可以在不同阶段出现。因此即使直观认为小头畸形是神经元增殖异常所致，也有一些小头畸形发生于迁移完成后。

病理学 CM1 是由于颅底骨发育不全和颅后窝体积减小所致，这导致了小脑扁桃体移位到椎管内。脑脊液从狭窄的枕骨大孔流出时受阻，将会导致脊髓形成充满液体的空腔，称为脊髓空洞症（见后文）。在脑干结构受压时出现相应症状。

临床表现 CM1 的临床表现多样。80% 的患者有枕部头痛或后颈部疼痛。年轻患者可能会出现脑干受压症状，包括睡眠障碍、眩晕、吞咽困难、耳鸣以及眼部症状。CM1 可在 MRI 检查时被偶然发现，这些意外发现的 CM1 一般不会导致脊髓空洞症、顽固的症状或进展性神经系统异常（10%）。

诊断与鉴别诊断 MRI 是最有效的诊断方法。脑脊液动力学研究可能有助于明确 CM1 的临床意义。鉴于任何引起颅内压增高的疾病都可能导致小脑扁桃体疝，应除外特发性颅内高压和中枢神经系统占位性病变。

治疗 无症状的脊髓空洞症患者可随诊观察。如果患者合并严重头痛、神经功能缺损症状或脊髓空洞症，可考虑颅后窝减压手术伴或不伴硬脑膜成形术，以重建颅颈交界处的脑脊液流动。

预后 CM1 一般不会导致残疾，手术减压可改善 80% 以上患者的临床症状。对于有症状的患者，单纯颅后窝骨减压术（不破坏硬脑膜）的并发症发生率较低。

脊髓空洞症

定义和流行病学 脊髓空洞症是指脊髓中的囊性空腔或中央管的扩张（脊髓积水）。估计患病率为 8/10 000，但这一数字可能被低估。在儿童患者中，脊髓空洞症是 CM1 常见且重要的神经系统后遗症，占 30%～70%。

病理学 脊髓空洞症可以是先天性或者获得性。先天性脊髓空洞症在胚胎发育过程中形成，与神经管缺陷有关。获得性脊髓空洞症是由于正常脑脊液循环被中断引起，可见于 CM1、脊髓拴系综合征、脊髓肿瘤或外伤。

临床表现 典型临床表现是颈部和上下肢的分离性感觉障碍（痛觉和温度觉丧失，轻触觉和本体感觉保留）。颈部病变会产生肩膀和手臂的呈斗篷样分离性感觉障碍、手和上肢萎缩及下肢肌张力增高。脊髓空洞症终末期患者常出现脊柱侧凸。

诊断与鉴别诊断 MRI 可用于脊髓空洞症的确诊，同时可鉴别肿瘤、感染和其他脊髓病变。应进行腰骶部 MRI 扫描以除外脊髓拴系。

治疗 手术矫正病因（如 CM1、CM2、肿瘤、脊髓拴系）是治疗脊髓空洞症的最有效方法。小的脊髓空洞症可能是无症状的，通过 MRI 偶然发现，可随诊观察而无须干预。

预后 脊髓空洞症是一种慢性、缓慢进展的疾病，有症状加重和缓解期。患者的症状通常在矫正手术后改善。对于幼儿和无症状患者，可以考虑保守治疗而不进行手术矫正。

腹侧诱导障碍

定义和流行病学

腹侧诱导是中枢神经系统发育的第二阶段，脑泡和面部在受精后第 5 周到孕中期开始形成。这一阶段的损害主要影响脑和面部的发育。

此阶段常见的畸形包括前脑无裂畸形（HPE）、胼胝体发育不全（ACC）、透明隔发育不全和透明隔-视神经发育不良（SOD）。其中 ACC 最常见，在人群中的患病率为 0.7%，在发育障碍患者中更高。HPE 和 SOD 的发病率均约为 1/10 000。

病理学与胚胎学

腹侧诱导伴随三种原始脑泡的分裂和形成：前脑泡、中脑泡和菱脑泡。在胚胎发育第 49 天或妊娠第 8 周，前脑分裂为端脑和间脑，端脑以后演变为大脑两半球。

前脑分裂异常导致 HPE，这是一类异常范围从无脑叶 HPE（单脑室的皮质）到半叶型和叶型 HPE

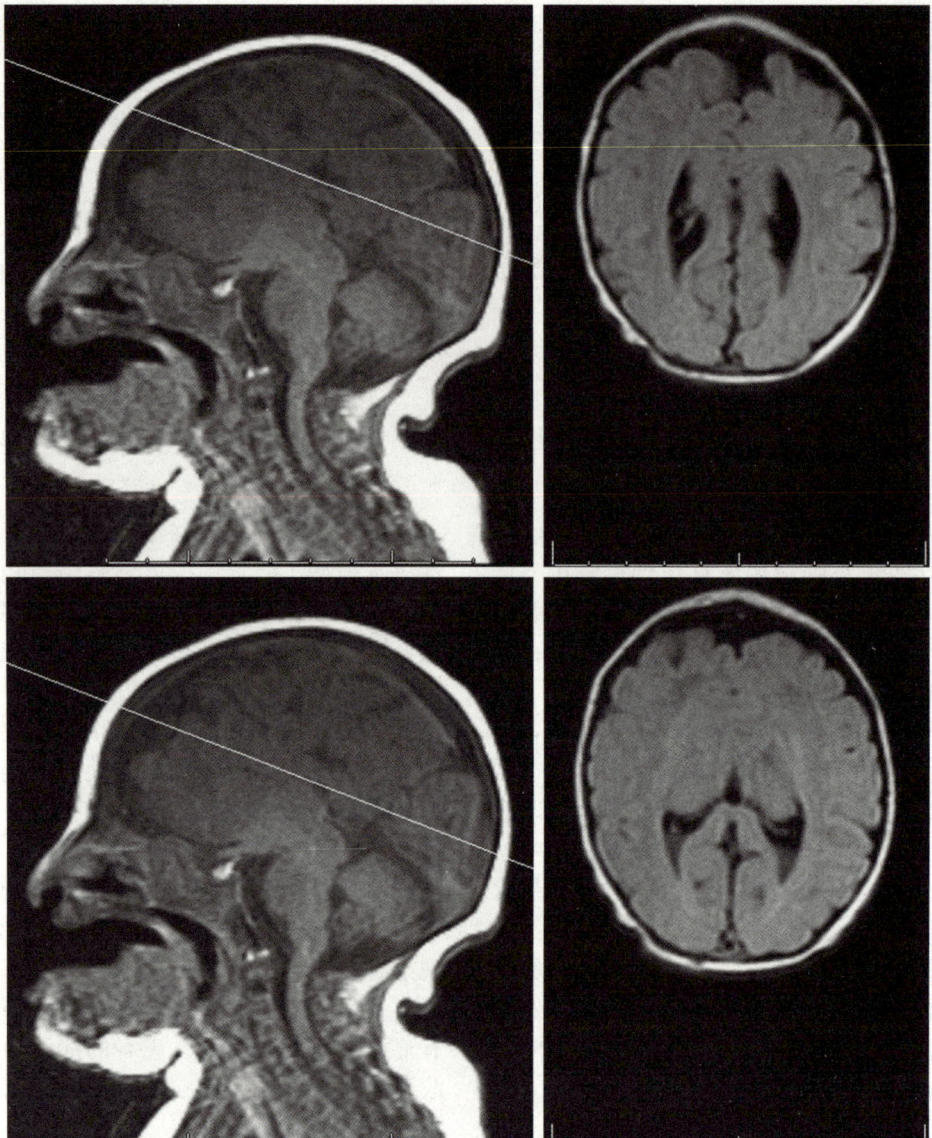

Fig. 12.1 Semilobar HPE. MRI (sagittal T1 image taken at midline paired with an axial FLAIR image whose location is indicated by the scout line) of 13 day old with hypotelorism and microcephaly. There is presence of partial fusion of the frontal lobes with lack of interhemispheric fissure/falx and septum pellucidum. The body and genu of corpus callosum is likewise poorly formed. There is appropriate separation of the thalami.

to semilobar and lobar HPE (cerebral hemispheres are mostly separated except for the frontal lobes) (Fig. 12.1). In all cases, there is some fusion between the two cerebral hemispheres, often accompanied by facial anomalies. ACC and SOD represent more discrete abnormalities localized to specific midline structures and occur later in prosencephalic development.

Clinical Presentation

Children with HPE, ACC, and SOC have varying degrees of developmental disability and other congenital anomalies. Because prosencephalon cleavage occurs at the same time as facial formation, facial anomalies ranging in severity can occur, including hypotelorism, solitary median incisor, cleft palate, proboscis, or cyclopia.

The clinical spectrum of SOD includes optic nerve hypoplasia, pituitary hypofunction, and midline brain abnormalities. Individuals with SOD often present for evaluation of visual abnormalities, poor growth, hypoglycemia, or precocious puberty. Seizures and developmental delay are the most common neurologic manifestations of SOD.

ACC may occur either in isolation or in association with other congenital syndromes. When present in isolation, individuals with ACC may be neurologically intact. If associated with other brain malformations, there may be developmental delay and intellectual disability.

Diagnosis/Differential

Neuroimaging is the primary method for diagnosing HPE, ACC, and SOD. The diagnosis of HPE can be made by prenatal ultrasound between 10 and 14 weeks' gestation. Ophthalmology exam can detect hypoplastic optic nerves in SOD. Because HPE, ACC, and SOD are associated with a number of genetic syndromes, genetic testing is indicated to guide management.

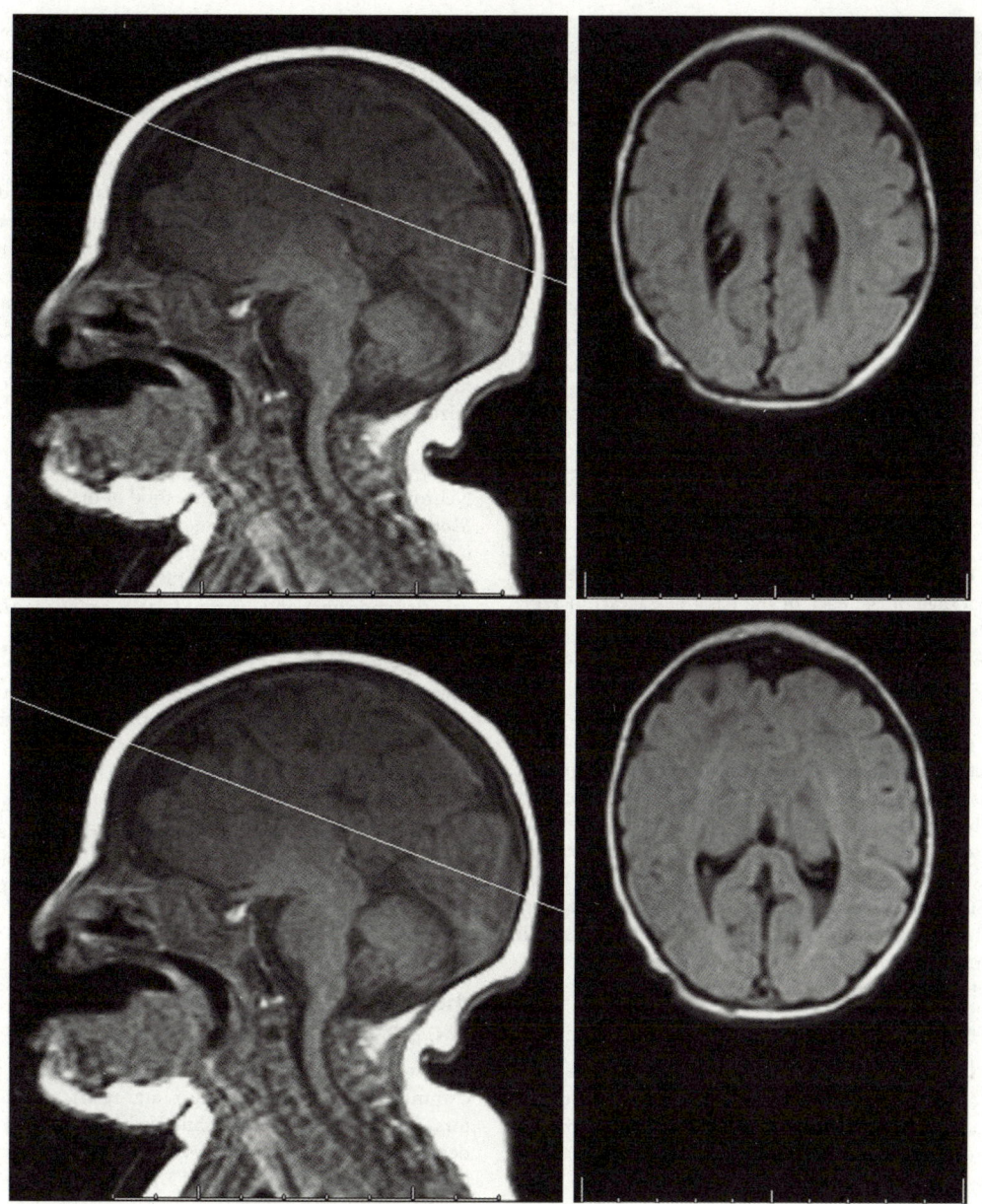

图 12.1　半叶型 HPE。13 天大患儿合并小头畸形和眼距过短的 MRI 表现（正中线矢状位采集的 T1 图像和定位线所示位置的轴位 FLAIR 图像）。额叶部分融合，大脑纵裂（大脑镰）和透明隔未见。胼胝体膝部和体部形成不良，丘脑分离距离适当

（除额叶外，大脑半球大部分分离）的畸形谱系（图 12.1）。所有病例的两侧大脑半球之间都有部分融合，伴有面部畸形。ACC 和 SOD 表现出局限于特定中线结构的更分散的异常，发生于前脑发育的后期。

临床表现

HPE、ACC 和 SOD 患儿均有不同程度的发育障碍和其他先天畸形。由于前脑分裂和面部发育形成处于同一时期，因此可能合并不同严重程度的面部畸形，包括眼距过近、单一中切牙、腭裂、长鼻或独眼畸形。

SOD 的临床表现包括视神经发育不全、垂体功能减退和脑中线结构异常。SOD 患者常因视力异常、生长不良、低血糖或性早熟而首诊。癫痫和发育迟缓是 SOD 最常见的神经系统表现。

ACC 可孤立存在或与其他先天性综合征共存。单独发生时，ACC 患者的神经功能可能正常。如果与其他脑畸形共存，可能会出现发育迟缓和智力障碍。

诊断与鉴别诊断

神经影像学是诊断 HPE、ACC 和 SOD 的主要方法。HPE 可以通过孕 10～14 周的产前超声诊断。眼科检查可用于检测 SOD 的视神经发育不全。由于 HPE、ACC 和 SOD 与多种遗传综合征相关，因此建议行基因筛查以指导后续管理。

TABLE 12.2 Complications and Management of Severe Neurologic Impairment

Complication	Management
Epilepsy	Antiepileptic medications, vagal nerve stimulation, ketogenic diet
Dysphagia	Thickened feeds or enteral feeds via G tube
Respiratory insufficiency	Positive pressure ventilation while asleep, tracheostomy and mechanical ventilation if necessary
Spasticity	Physical therapy, intramuscular or intrathecal baclofen, oral benzodiazepines
Musculoskeletal	Serial monitoring for neuromuscular scoliosis, hip dislocations, and joint contractures. Often requires orthopedic surgeries.
Cognitive impairment	Individualized education plans, therapies

Treatment

Surgical treatment can improve craniofacial anomalies (e.g., cleft lip, choanal atresia [blockage of the back of the nasal passages]) in HPE and hormone replacement can treat pituitary insufficiency in SOD. Table 12.2 shows additional complications and management of the associated complications of severe neurologic impairment.

Prognosis

Prognosis for affected individuals depends on the degree of medical impairment and associated comorbidities. Most fetuses with alobar HPE die perinatally, but those with semilobar and lobar HPE have improved survival with aggressive management of associated problems such as dysphagia and epilepsy.

Children with SOD have variable outcomes depending on the presence of comorbid brain abnormalities. Prognosis for individuals with ACC depends upon whether ACC is an isolated defect (excellent prognosis) or associated with a neurologic or genetic syndrome.

Malformations of Cortical Development
Definition/Epidemiology

Malformations of cortical development (MCD) are a group of disorders that are characterized by disrupted migration and organization of neuronal progenitor cells, resulting in the abnormal appearance of cortical sulci and gyri.

The primary categories of MCD include lissencephaly (refers to smooth appearance of the brain surface), polymicrogyria, schizencephaly, focal cortical dysplasia (FCD), and periventricular nodular heterotopia. The recognized incidence of MCD is increasing with the use of MRI in children with epilepsy and congenital neurologic deficits. It is estimated that 25% to 40% of medication-resistant childhood epilepsy is secondary to MCD. The more severe forms of lissencephaly occur in approximately 1.2/100,000 births. All other forms of MCD are more common than lissencephaly.

Pathology

Neuronal migration is a complex, highly regulated process integral to formation of normal cortical architecture that occurs throughout gestation but peaks from 2 to 4 months. More than 100 genes play various roles in neuronal migration.

Schizencephaly is characterized by the presence of a cleft in the brain that extends from the surface of the pia mater to the cerebral ventricles that may occur as a consequence of a defect in neuronal migration, a genetic mutation, or a structural CNS insult in utero.

Focal cortical dysplasia (FCD) is typically the least severe type of MCD and often is clinically silent until patients present with focal seizures. FCD most often occurs as a postmigrational defect leading to cortical disorganization and focal lesions.

Clinical Presentation

MCD can have highly variable clinical presentations depending on postconceptual timing of cortical disruption and degree of cortical involvement. Lissencephaly has a severe presentation with marked motor disability and seizures, including infantile spasms. Polymicrogyria and schizencephaly, depending on the extent and location, can have less severe presentations. Most children with severe MCD present early in infancy with microcephaly, seizures, feeding difficulties, and developmental delays. The most common presentation of FCD is onset of focal seizures in early childhood.

Diagnosis/Differential

Neuroimaging is the primary method of diagnosing all types of MCD. Moderate- to high-resolution MRI scans are used for diagnosis in infants and young children. Prenatal ultrasound or fetal MRI may identify early features of some MCD. Most MCD are associated with genetic syndromes and warrant further genetic testing.

Treatment

Seizures are treated with antiepileptic medications and, when indicated, epilepsy surgery. Severe neurologic impairment leads to other complications (see Table 12.2).

Prognosis

Children with severe lissencephaly syndromes have a severe course and high mortality rates. Long-term prognosis for all other types of MCD depends on the degree of neurologic impairment and underlying etiology.

DEVELOPMENTAL DISORDERS

Autism Spectrum Disorder
Definition/Epidemiology

Autism spectrum disorder (ASD) is characterized by impaired social communication and interactions and restricted and repetitive behaviors. Approximately 1 in 69 children are affected by ASD with an incidence four times higher in boys than girls. The early symptoms of ASD can be identified between 1 and 3 years of age.

Pathology

A combination of genetic and epigenetic factors are thought to increase the risk of developing ASD. Many genetic syndromes, such as fragile X syndrome and Rett syndrome (see later), have autistic features as part of their clinical presentation. In addition, environmental factors such as advanced maternal or paternal age, maternal diabetes mellitus, or low birthweight increase the risk of ASD.

Clinical Presentation

The early symptoms of ASD are apparent during early childhood and a reliable diagnosis can be obtained by age 2 years. Patients usually present with delayed language development or language regression and limited social interaction. Children with ASD have impaired joint attention and often display repetitive, stereotypic behaviors.

Diagnosis/Differential

Several rating scale instruments and standardized interview tools have been developed to help diagnose ASD. The most commonly used tools

表 12.2 严重神经系统并发症和处理	
并发症	处理
癫痫	抗癫痫药物、迷走神经刺激、生酮饮食
吞咽困难	增稠食物、鼻饲
呼吸功能障碍	睡眠中正压通气，如有必要行气管切开和机械通气
肢体痉挛	物理治疗、肌内或鞘内注射巴氯芬、口服苯二氮䓬类药物
肌肉骨骼异常	对神经肌肉型脊柱侧凸、髋关节脱位和关节挛缩进行定期监测，常需矫形手术
认知障碍	制订个体化训练和治疗方案

治疗

手术治疗可以改善 HPE 的颅面畸形（例如唇裂、鼻后孔闭锁），激素替代疗法可以治疗 SOD 的垂体功能不全。表 12.2 列举了其他严重神经系统并发症和处理原则。

预后

患者的预后取决于受损严重程度和合并症。大多数无脑叶 HPE 的胎儿在产前死亡。半叶型和叶型 HPE 的胎儿在积极处理相关问题（如吞咽困难和癫痫）后生存率有所提高。

SOD 患儿的预后取决于是否合并脑部异常。ACC 患儿的预后取决于 ACC 是否单独的缺陷（预后最好）或者合并有其他神经系统或遗传综合征。

皮质发育畸形

定义和流行病学

皮质发育畸形（MCD）是一组由神经祖细胞迁移和组织功能障碍导致的皮质沟与回外观异常的疾病。

MCD 的主要分类包括无脑回畸形（指脑表面光滑）、多小脑回畸形、脑裂畸形、局灶性皮质发育不良（FCD）和脑室周围结节异位。随着 MRI 在癫痫和先天性神经缺陷儿童中的应用，MCD 的发现率逐年增加。据估计，25%~40% 的难治性儿童癫痫是由 MCD 引起。更为严重的无脑回畸形在新生儿中的发生率约为 1.2/100 000。所有其他形式的 MCD 均较无脑回畸形更常见。

病理学

神经元迁移是一个复杂的、高度调控的过程，与正常皮质结构的形成过程相整合，贯穿整个妊娠期，但主要集中于妊娠 2~4 个月期间。超过 100 个基因在神经元迁移中发挥不同的作用。

脑裂畸形的特征是脑中存在贯通软脑膜到侧脑室的裂隙样结构，可由神经元迁移缺陷、基因突变或宫内中枢神经系统结构损伤所致。

局灶性皮质发育不良（FCD）是 MCD 中最轻的类型，通常无症状，直到患者出现局灶性癫痫发作。FCD 主要源于迁移后缺陷，导致皮质组织紊乱和局灶病变。

临床表现

MCD 患儿临床表现多样，具体取决于皮质畸形产生的时期和皮质受累的严重程度。无脑回畸形患儿通常有严重运动障碍和癫痫，包括婴儿痉挛。多小脑回畸形和脑裂畸形的临床表现取决于病变程度和位置，症状通常较轻。大多数严重 MCD 患儿会在婴儿早期出现小头畸形、癫痫发作、喂养困难和精神发育迟滞。FCD 最常见的表现是在儿童早期局灶性癫痫发作。

诊断与鉴别诊断

神经影像是所有类型 MCD 的主要诊断工具，MRI 扫描可用于婴幼儿的诊断。产前超声或胎儿 MRI 可用于发现某些类型 MCD 的早期表现。大多数 MCD 和遗传综合征有关，需进一步基因检测。

治疗

抗癫痫药物是治疗癫痫发作的主要方法，对于药物难治性癫痫患者，可以考虑外科手术治疗。严重的神经系统损害会导致其他并发症（见表 12.2）。

预后

患有严重无脑回畸形综合征的儿童病情严重、死亡率高。所有其他类型 MCD 的长期预后取决于神经系统损伤的程度和潜在病因。

发育障碍

孤独症谱系障碍

定义和流行病学

孤独症谱系障碍（ASD）是一类以社交沟通能力损害以及局限和刻板重复行为为特征的疾病。大约每 69 名儿童中有 1 名患有 ASD，男孩的发病率是女孩的 4 倍。ASD 的早期症状可以在 1~3 岁显现。

病理学

遗传和表观遗传因素共同作用增加了 ASD 的发病风险。许多遗传综合征，如脆性 X 染色体综合征和 Rett 综合征（见后文），在其临床表现中包含孤独症特征。此外，环境因素如母亲或父亲高龄、母亲患糖尿病或低出生体重也增加了 ASD 的风险。

临床表现

ASD 的早期症状见于儿童早期，至 2 岁时可获得可靠诊断。患者通常表现为语言发育迟缓、语言倒退和有限的社交互动。ASD 患儿具有联合注意缺陷的症状，通常表现出重复的、刻板的行为。

诊断与鉴别诊断

多种评分量表工具和标准化的访谈工具已被开发用于协助诊断 ASD。最常用的工具包括"孤独症诊断观察

are the Autism Diagnostic Observation Schedule (ADOS) and the Autism Diagnostic Interview-Revised (ADI-R). Both use standardized questions and observation scores based on the DSM-5 criteria for ASD.

Treatment
Prompt diagnosis and early initiation of intensive behavioral interventions such as applied behavioral analysis (ABA) and early childhood therapies are among treatments for ASD. In addition, some individuals with ASD require treatment for comorbid ADHD, anxiety, or epilepsy.

Prognosis
In 2014, a review of all studies examining the effectiveness of ABA intervention demonstrated that ABA delivered over an extended time leads to improvement in cognitive ability, language, and adaptive skills. Approximately 10% of children with ASD may develop skills for independent living and work. Early diagnosis and prompt referral to intensive ABA therapy are associated with improved prognostic outcomes.

Attention-Deficit/Hyperactivity Disorder
Definition/Epidemiology
ADHD is a common neurodevelopmental disorder occurring in 5% of children and 2.5% of adults. It is three times more common in males than females and often associated with additional neurodevelopmental and psychiatric disorders. ADHD is marked by inattention, impulsivity, and hyperactivity causing impaired functioning.

Pathology
There are no consistent pathologic brain findings or neurotransmitter abnormalities found in individuals with ADHD. However, ADHD is a highly heritable disorder. Several genetic disorders are associated with ADHD, including fragile X syndrome and 22q11 microdeletion (DiGeorge syndrome).

Environmental factors are known to play a role. Low birthweight, prematurity, and in utero exposure to maternal cigarette smoking, alcohol, and illicit substances are associated with a higher ADHD risk.

Clinical Presentation
Patients with ADHD typically present before age 12 years with complaints of 6 months or more of developmentally inappropriate behaviors, hyperactivity, inappropriate inattention, and impulsivity resulting in significant impairment in at least two different settings (e.g., home, school, work, or with peers).

On neuropsychiatric testing, patients with ADHD often have deficits in response inhibition, vigilance, working memory, and planning. These patients often struggle in school and have a history of behavioral outbursts due to poor impulse control.

Diagnosis/Differential
The diagnosis of ADHD can be made with the help of standardized rating scales that assess for symptoms of inattention, hyperactivity, and impulsivity in several different settings. The Vanderbilt Assessment Scale and Connors' Parent and Teacher Rating Scales are examples of standardized tools that help distinguish ADHD from inattention due to learning disability, hearing impairment, or mood disorders.

Treatment
Stimulant medications such as methylphenidate and amphetamines are the primary class of medication used in ADHD. They can improve cognition, executive and nonexecutive function, and memory. Other nonstimulant medications such as atomoxetine, guanfacine, and clonidine can be used when stimulant side effects are bothersome or when comorbid treatment of anxiety or sleep disorders is desired.

Prognosis
ADHD generally responds to treatment but there are often residual school difficulties. Core symptoms of childhood ADHD generally persist into adulthood, leading to higher risk of adverse occupational, economic, and social outcomes. Improvement in symptoms depends on age at diagnosis, associated intellectual disability, and effectiveness of clinical follow-up.

Rett Syndrome
Definition/Epidemiology
Rett syndrome is an X-linked dominant disorder caused by a mutation of the methyl-cytosine binding protein (MECP2), a transcriptional repressor. It is the second most common cause of severe intellectual disability in girls after Down syndrome, affecting 1 in 9000 to 10,000 girls. In boys, MECP2 mutations are lethal or result in severe encephalopathy.

Pathology
The loss of MECP2 function prevents regulation of gene expression during critical developmental periods in infancy.

A few patients who meet clinical criteria for Rett syndrome do not have MECP2 mutations. Other genes, such as *CDKL5*, *FOXG1*, and *MEF2C*, have been associated with Rett syndrome, and, like MECP2, encode proteins that are essential for early brain development.

Clinical Presentation
Patients with classic Rett syndrome develop normally during their first 6 to 18 months and then have stagnation in development, followed by loss of communication skills and deceleration in head growth. Other findings are "wringing" hand movements at midline, hyperventilation, air swallowing, abdominal distension, and chronic constipation. Between 60% and 80% develop seizures.

Diagnosis/Differential
Diagnosis can be confirmed by MECP2 mutational testing. As noted previously, other genes can cause Rett or Rett-like syndrome. Angelman syndrome, mitochondrial disorders, and neuronal ceroid lipofuscinosis may also present similarly.

Treatment
Girls with Rett syndrome usually require a multidisciplinary approach to address the complications associated with their severe neurologic impairment (see Table 12.2). Comorbidities often seen in Rett syndrome include seizures, spasticity with joint contractures, and prolonged QTc interval.

Prognosis
Most girls survive into adulthood but will not acquire speech or functional skills and will remain dependent for their care.

Fragile X Syndrome
Definition/Epidemiology
Fragile X syndrome (FXS) is an X-linked disorder caused by expanded CGG triplet repeats in the first exon of the fragile X mental retardation gene *(FMR1)*. An X-linked recessive disorder, girls can be symptomatic though they may have milder intellectual disability compared to boys. FXS is the most common single-gene cause of inherited cognitive disability and affects 1.4/10,000 females and 1.9/10,000 males. The prevalence of the female carrier status is estimated to be as high as 1 in 250 to 300.

量表（ADOS）"和"孤独症诊断访谈-修订版（ADI-R）"。两者均使用基于DSM-5标准的标准化问题和观察评分。

治疗

及时诊断和早期强化行为干预［如应用行为分析（ABA）］和儿童早期治疗是ASD的治疗方法之一。此外，一些ASD患者需要治疗共病的注意缺陷多动障碍（ADHD）、焦虑或癫痫。

预后

2014年一项有关ABA干预有效性的综述表明，长期进行ABA干预可以改善认知、语言和适应性技能。约10%的ASD儿童可发展出独立生活和工作的能力。早期诊断和及时转至强化ABA治疗与预后改善相关。

注意缺陷多动障碍（ADHD）

定义和流行病学

ADHD是一种常见的神经发育障碍，见于5%的儿童和2.5%的成人中。男性的发病率是女性的3倍，通常与其他神经发育和精神障碍相关。ADHD的特征是注意力不集中、冲动和多动而导致功能受损。

病理学

在ADHD患者中未发现明确的脑病理改变或神经递质异常。然而，ADHD是一种高度遗传的疾病。多种遗传疾病与ADHD相关，包括脆性X染色体综合征和22q11微缺失（DiGeorge综合征）。

环境因素也起着重要作用。低出生体重、早产以及子宫内暴露于母亲吸烟、饮酒和非法药物中，都会增加ADHD的风险。

临床表现

ADHD患者通常在12岁之前出现行为不适应、过度活跃、注意力不集中和冲动行为，持续6个月或更长时间，至少在两个不同的环境中（例如家庭、学校、工作或与同伴相处）造成显著的功能障碍。

在神经精神测试中，ADHD患者通常表现出反应抑制、警觉性、工作记忆和计划能力的缺陷。这些患者通常在学校表现不佳，并有因冲动控制能力差而导致的暴发行为史。

诊断与鉴别诊断

ADHD的诊断通过利用标准化评分量表评估不同环境中的注意力不集中、多动和冲动症状来进行。常用的工具包括"范德比尔特评估量表"和"康纳斯父母和教师评分量表"，这些工具有助于区分ADHD与学习障碍、听力障碍或情绪障碍引起的注意力不集中。

治疗

兴奋剂药物如哌甲酯和苯丙胺是治疗ADHD的主要药物，有助于改善认知功能、执行和非执行功能以及记忆力。当兴奋剂类药物的副作用无法耐受或需要同时治疗焦虑或睡眠障碍时，可以使用其他非兴奋剂药物如托莫西汀、胍法辛和可乐定。

预后

ADHD通常对治疗有反应，但往往遗留学习障碍。儿童ADHD的核心症状通常持续到成年，很可能对患儿的职业发展、经济和社会状态造成负面影响。症状的改善取决于诊断的年龄、相关智力障碍以及有效的临床随诊。

Rett综合征

定义和流行病学

Rett综合征是一种X连锁显性疾病，由编码甲基-胞嘧啶结合蛋白（MECP2）的基因突变引起，MECP2是一种转录抑制因子。Rett综合征是女孩中第二常见的严重智力障碍性疾病（第一为唐氏综合征），每9000～10 000例女孩中1例患病。在男孩中，MECP2基因突变是致死性的或导致严重的脑病。

病理学

MECP2功能的丧失阻碍了在婴儿关键发育阶段基因表达的调控。

一些符合Rett综合征临床标准的患者没有MECP2基因突变。其他基因如CDKL5、FOXG1和MEF2C，与Rett综合征相关，并且像MECP2基因一样编码参与早期大脑发育的重要蛋白。

临床表现

患有经典Rett综合征的患者在最初6～18个月发育正常，然后出现发育停滞，继而出现沟通能力倒退和头围增长缓慢。其他表现包括中线"绞手"动作、过度换气、吞咽空气、腹胀和慢性便秘。60%～80%的患者会发生癫痫。

诊断与鉴别诊断

可以通过MECP2基因突变检测确认诊断。如前所述，其他基因也可以引起Rett或类似Rett的综合征。Angelman综合征、线粒体疾病和神经元蜡样脂褐质沉积症也可有类似表现。

治疗

患有Rett综合征的女孩通常需要多学科共同管理来解决其严重神经障碍的并发症（见表12.2）。Rett综合征中常见的共病包括癫痫、关节挛缩和QT间期延长。

预后

大多数女孩可以存活到成年，但无法获得语言和功能性技能，终身需他人照料。

脆性X染色体综合征

定义和流行病学

脆性X染色体综合征（FXS）是由脆性X精神发育迟滞基因（FMR1）第一外显子中的CGG三核苷酸重复序列扩增引起的一类X连锁疾病。作为一种X连锁隐性遗传病，女孩可能有症状，但智力损害轻于男性。FXS是最常见的单基因遗传性认知障碍性疾病，女性患病率为1.4/10 000，男性患病率为1.9/10 000。女性携带者高达1/300～1/250。

Pathology

A normal *FMR1* gene contains between 6 and 44 CGG trinucleotide repeats and produces fragile X mental retardation protein (FMRP), which is important in brain development. Affected individuals have greater than 200 repeats, which causes silencing of *FMR1* gene transcription with loss of FMRP.

Clinical Presentation

Boys with FXS typically have moderate to severe cognitive disability and typical facies with relative macrocephaly, long and narrow face, high-arched palate, and prominent ears. Other physical features include pubertal macro-orchidism, joint hypermobility, hypotonia, and pes planus.

Some with FXS have comorbid epilepsy, with onset between 2 and 10 years of age. Other common findings are sleep disturbances, anxiety, and ADHD. Approximately 30% of males and 25% of females with fragile X have a comorbid diagnosis of autism.

Individuals with the "premutation" range of 55 to 200 CGG repeats often develop ataxia, tremor, and cognitive dysfunction in adulthood at a median age of onset of 60 years (fragile X associated tremor/ataxia syndrome or FXTAS).

Diagnosis/Differential

Diagnosis is confirmed by identifying increased CGG repeats in the *FMR1* gene. Other conditions can be mistaken for FXS, including Sotos syndrome, Prader-Willi syndrome, and Klinefelter syndrome. Adult-onset disorders presenting like FXTAS include parkinsonism, other ataxia syndromes, and tremor.

Treatment

Treatment focuses on management of comorbid conditions such as epilepsy, autism, ADHD, and disordered sleep. Use of stimulants or selective serotonin reuptake inhibitors (SSRIs) may effectively decrease inattention, hyperactivity, and psychiatric symptoms. Behavioral and educational services validated for autism are helpful in FXS. Earlier diagnosis and earlier developmental interventions may improve outcomes.

Prognosis

Patients with FXS respond to training and education over time, but their intellectual disability may make it difficult for them to live independently. FXTAS is associated with gradual and progressive neurologic deterioration over many years.

NEUROCUTANEOUS DISORDERS

Neurocutaneous disorders are congenital, often hereditary disorders characterized by pathognomonic cutaneous and central nervous system lesions that uniquely distinguish each disease. Many neurocutaneous disorders are associated with abnormal, noncancerous growth of tissues, often in a disorganized manner. Here we discuss neurofibromatosis 1 and 2 and tuberous sclerosis complex.

Neurofibromatosis 1
Definition/Epidemiology

Neurofibromatosis type 1 (NF1) is an autosomal dominant disorder caused by mutations in the *NF1* gene on chromosome 17. NF1 is characterized by altered skin pigmentation, tumors, and abnormalities of bones, connective tissue, and brain (Fig. 12.2). It is the most common neurocutaneous disorder, occurring in 1/2500 to 1/3000 individuals worldwide.

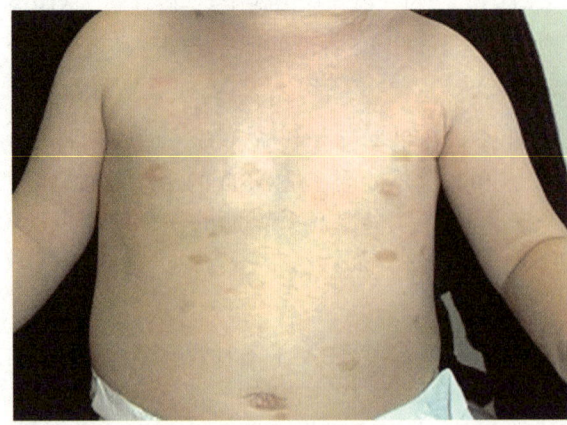

Fig. 12.2 Multiple café-au-lait spots in a child with neurofibromatosis type 1. (From Shah KN: The diagnostic and clinical significant of café-au-lait macules, Pediatr Clin N Am 57:1131-1153, 2010, Fig. 3.)

Pathology

The *NF1* gene codes for neurofibromin, which regulates tissue growth and tumor formation, explaining the occurrence of cutaneous neurofibromas, plexiform neurofibromas, and gliomas in NF1. Malignant tumors can occur secondary to malignant transformation of previously benign tumors. Approximately 50% of NF1 cases are due to spontaneous mutations.

Clinical Presentation

Patients can present with NF1 variably. All NF1 patients can be diagnosed before 20 years of age based on clinical criteria shown in Table 12.3. Patients can have learning disabilities, macrocephaly, and epilepsy. Important complications of NF1 include scoliosis, gastrointestinal neurofibromas, pheochromocytomas, and renal artery stenosis.

Diagnosis/Differential

The diagnostic criteria outlined previously are highly sensitive and specific. *NF1* DNA testing for mutations in NF1 can confirm the diagnosis. Schwannomatosis and neurofibromatosis type 2 may be mistaken for NF1.

Treatment

Regular multidisciplinary surveillance is recommended with frequent skin exams and assessment of neurocognitive development. Ophthalmology exams are strongly recommended until age 8 years because the risk of optic pathway gliomas is highest during this time. Many optic pathway tumors can be followed conservatively without surgery unless there are visual changes, when treatment with chemotherapeutic agents is recommended.

Large cutaneous neurofibromas and smaller fibromas can be removed but often recur. Subcutaneous plexiform neurofibromas grow along nerves and extend into surrounding tissue, causing pain or deformities. They have a high lifetime risk of malignant transformation and should be excised if possible. Drugs that target the biological pathways involved in tumor growth are being actively investigated.

Neurofibromatosis 2
Definition/Epidemiology

Neurofibromatosis type 2 (NF2) is a rare autosomal dominant adult-onset disease affecting 1/33,00 individuals and characterized by bilateral vestibular schwannomas and nonmalignant brain tumors.

病理学

正常人群 *FMR1* 基因 CGG 三核苷酸重复序列的拷贝数为 6～44 个，可产生对大脑发育有重要作用的脆性 X 精神发育迟滞蛋白（FMRP）。患病个体的 CGG 重复序列拷贝数可超过 200 个，导致 *FMR1* 基因转录沉默，无法合成 FMRP。

临床表现

患有 FXS 的男孩通常有中到重度的认知障碍和典型的面容特征，如大头畸形、长而窄的面部、高腭弓和招风耳。其他躯体特征包括青春期的巨睾丸症、关节过度活动、肌张力减退和扁平足。

一些 FXS 患者可合并癫痫，2～10 岁发病。其他常见表现包括睡眠障碍、焦虑和 ADHD。约 30% 的男性和 25% 的女性 FXS 患者合并孤独症。

FMR1 基因的 CGG 重复数在 55～200 个之间被称为"前突变"，"前突变"携带者通常在中位年龄 60 岁时出现共济失调、震颤和认知功能障碍［脆性 X 染色体相关震颤/共济失调综合征（FXTAS）］。

诊断与鉴别诊断

通过检测 *FMR1* 基因 CGG 重复拷贝数而确诊。其他易被误诊为 FXS 的情况包括 Sotos 综合征、Prader-Willi 综合征和 Klinefelter 综合征。成年起病的 FXTAS 需鉴别帕金森综合征、其他共济失调综合征和震颤。

治疗

治疗主要针对并发症的管理，如癫痫、孤独症、ADHD 和睡眠障碍。使用兴奋剂或选择性 5-羟色胺再摄取抑制剂（SSRI）可以有效减少注意力不集中、多动和精神症状。面向孤独症的行为训练和教育服务对 FXS 患者有益。早期诊断和干预可能改善预后。

预后

FXS 患者可以通过不断训练和教育获得症状改善，但由于智力障碍可能无法独立生活。FXTAS 可逐渐出现进行性的神经功能退化。

神经皮肤综合征

神经皮肤综合征是一组先天性、通常是遗传性的疾病，每类疾病均有特征性的病理性皮肤和中枢神经系统病变。许多神经皮肤综合征与异常无序的、非肿瘤性组织增生有关。本章讨论神经纤维瘤病 1 型和 2 型以及结节性硬化症。

神经纤维瘤病 1 型

定义和流行病学

神经纤维瘤病 1 型（NF1）是一类由 17 号染色体上 *NF1* 基因突变引起的常染色体显性遗传病。NF1 具有特征性的皮肤色素沉着、肿瘤、骨骼畸形、结缔组织和脑部异常（图 12.2）。它是最常见的神经皮肤综合

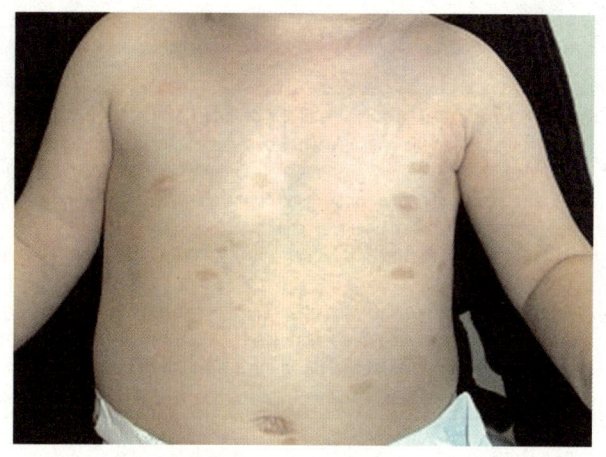

图 12.2 NF1 患儿皮肤多发生奶-咖啡斑。（引自 Shah KN: The diagnostic and clinical significant of café-aulait macules, Pediatr Clin N Am 57: 1131-1153, 2010, Fig. 3.）

征，全球范围内发病率为 1/3000～1/2500。

病理学

NF1 基因编码神经纤维瘤蛋白，其功能是调节组织生长和肿瘤形成，这解释了 NF1 中皮肤神经纤维瘤、丛状神经纤维瘤和神经胶质瘤的发生。一些良性肿瘤可能在后期演化为恶性肿瘤。约 50% 的 NF1 病例是由自发突变引起。

临床表现

NF1 患者的临床表现多样。所有 NF1 患者都可以根据表 12.3 中的临床诊断标准在 20 岁之前诊断。患者可能出现学习障碍、大头畸形及癫痫。NF1 的主要并发症包括脊柱侧凸、胃肠神经纤维瘤、嗜铬细胞瘤及肾动脉狭窄。

诊断与鉴别诊断

前述的诊断标准具有较高的特异性和敏感性。*NF1* 基因检测突变可用于确诊。神经鞘瘤病和神经纤维瘤病 2 型可被误诊为 NF1。

治疗

建议定期进行多学科监测，包括经常进行皮肤检查和神经认知发育评估。强烈推荐在 8 岁之前进行眼科检查，因为在此期间患视路胶质瘤的风险最高。多数情况下视路肿瘤可以保守观察，如出现视力症状，建议使用化疗药物进行治疗。

大的皮肤神经纤维瘤和较小的纤维瘤可以手术切除，但易复发。皮下丛状神经纤维瘤沿神经生长，并可延伸到周围组织，导致疼痛或畸形。这种类型肿瘤终生有较高的恶变风险，因此有条件的话应予切除。针对肿瘤生长通路的靶向药物正在积极研发过程中。

神经纤维瘤病 2 型

定义和流行病学

神经纤维瘤病 2 型（NF2）是一种成人起病的、罕见的常染色体显性遗传病，患病率为 1/3300。其特征为双侧前庭神经鞘瘤和非恶性颅内肿瘤。

TABLE 12.3 NIH Diagnostic Criteria for NF1 and NF2

NF1	NF2

Clinical diagnosis based on presence of two of the following:
1. Six or more café-au-lait macules over 5 mm in diameter in prepubertal individuals and over 15 mm in greatest diameter in postpubertal individuals
2. Two or more neurofibromas of any type or one plexiform neurofibroma
3. Freckling in the axillary or inguinal regions
4. Two or more Lisch nodules (iris hamartomas)
5. Optic glioma
6. A distinctive osseous lesion such as sphenoid dysplasia or thinning of long bone cortex, with or without pseudarthrosis
7. First-degree relative (parent, sibling, or offspring) with NF1 by the above criteria
	The criteria are met by an individual who satisfies condition 1 or 2:
	1. Bilateral masses of the eighth cranial nerve seen with appropriate imaging techniques (e.g., CT or MRI)
	2. A first-degree with NF2 and either:
	  a. Unilateral mass of the eighth cranial nerve, or
	  b. Two of the following:
	    • Neurofibroma
	    • Meningioma
	    • Glioma
	    • Schwannoma
	    • Juvenile posterior subcapsular lenticular opacity

Pathology

The *NF2* gene on chromosome 22q12 is a tumor suppressor gene so mutations lead to loss of the protein merlin and a predisposition for tumor formation. Approximately 50% with NF2 have sporadic mutations.

Clinical Presentation

NF2 is characterized by multiple nonmalignant nervous system tumors including meningiomas, ependymomas, and gliomas. Bilateral vestibular schwannomas are the characteristic tumors of NF2, affecting 95% of patients. NF2 is typically diagnosed around 20 to 30 years with the onset of hearing loss and identification of unilateral or bilateral vestibular schwannomas.

Individuals with NF2 can have café au lait lesions, but rarely in the size or numbers noted in NF1. Many with NF2 have ophthalmologic findings including cataracts, retinal changes, and amblyopia.

Diagnosis/Differential

Like NF1, patients with NF2 are initially diagnosed based on highly specific clinical criteria (see Table 12.3). Molecular testing can confirm the diagnosis.

NF2 is frequently misdiagnosed as NF1, especially if there are café-au-lait spots. Patients with NF2 may also be misdiagnosed as having an isolated meningioma or unilateral vestibular schwannoma if other findings are not sought.

Treatment

Removal of the schwannomas and other tumors is usually indicated later in life when the tumors are larger and causing significant symptoms. There may be postsurgical complications and tumors may recur.

While traditional treatment has focused on surgical interventions, as described in NF1, attention has turned to development of drugs targeting tumor growth pathways.

Tuberous Sclerosis Complex
Definition/Epidemiology

Tuberous sclerosis complex (TSC) is an autosomal dominant disorder of early cellular differentiation, proliferation, and migration. TSC results in hamartomatous lesions involving multiple organs at different stages. The incidence of TSC is 1/6000. Mutations in two genes, *TSC1* and *TSC2*, are known to cause TSC in the majority of cases, and about 70% of cases are sporadic.

Pathology

TSC1 and *TSC2* are on different chromosomes but both encode proteins (hamartin and tuberin, respectively) that act as tumor suppressors, inhibiting the mammalian target of rapamycin (mTOR) pathway, which is essential in cell growth and proliferation. Mutations of these genes lead to unregulated growth and proliferation.

Clinical Presentation

The skin findings of TSC are common. Ninety percent have hypomelanotic macules, or "ash leaf spots." Facial angiofibromas are benign 1- to 5-mm dome-shaped skin-colored papules that first appear between 2 and 5 years of age. Shagreen patches are large plaques in the lumbosacral region with an "orange-peel" texture to the skin and are specific to TSC.

CNS involvement affects almost all individuals with TSC. Common conditions are epilepsy, autism, developmental delay, and intellectual disability. Brain imaging may reveal subcortical tubers, subependymal nodules, and subependymal giant cell astrocytomas (SEGAs) in some. Forty percent to 50% of infants develop a severe form of seizures called infantile spasms.

Diagnosis/Differential

The diagnosis of TSC is confirmed by identifying a pathogenic mutation of TSC1 or TSC2. Because 10% to 25% of affected patients have no mutation, identified clinical criteria have been established as well.

The spectrum of tumors seen in TSC may also be seen in isolation. Biopsy may be needed to distinguish facial angiofibromatomas from acne and other skin lesions.

Treatment

Treatment is primarily directed toward the sequelae of TSC-associated conditions. Several studies have shown that infants with TSC and infantile spasms have a superior response to treatment with vigabatrin.

SEGAs are typically slow growing, benign lesions that may be monitored with serial neuroimaging if asymptomatic. However, SEGAs located near the foramen of Monro can lead to obstructive hydrocephalus. Surgical intervention with gross total resection may be curative, but treatment with mTOR inhibitors such as everolimus is often helpful.

Prognosis

TSC associated with *TSC1* mutations is more often familial and has a milder clinical phenotype. Patients with *TSC2* mutations are more

表 12.3　NIH 神经纤维瘤病 1 型和 2 型的诊断标准	
神经纤维瘤病 1 型（NF1）	神经纤维瘤病 2 型（NF2）
诊断需要至少满足以下任意 2 项： 1. 6 个或以上的牛奶咖啡斑： 　● 青春期前直径＞5 mm 　● 青春期后直径＞15 mm 2. 2 个或以上的神经纤维瘤，或 1 个丛状神经纤维瘤 3. 腋窝或腹股沟区域的雀斑 4. 2 个或以上的 Lisch 小结（虹膜错构瘤） 5. 视路胶质瘤 6. 特征性骨病变，如蝶骨发育不良或长骨皮质变薄，伴或不伴假关节 7. 一级亲属（父母、兄弟姐妹或子女）符合上述 NF1 诊断标准	符合条件 1 或 2： 1. 影像学（如 CT 或 MRI）发现双侧第Ⅷ对脑神经肿物 2. 一级亲属患有 NF2，并且满足以下两个条件之一： 　a. 单侧第Ⅷ脑神经肿物，或者 　b. 符合以下任意 2 项： 　　● 神经纤维瘤 　　● 脑膜瘤 　　● 胶质瘤 　　● 神经鞘瘤 　　● 青少年后囊下晶状体浑浊

病理学

22q12 染色体上的 NF2 基因是一个抑癌基因，因此突变会导致 Merlin 蛋白的缺失和肿瘤形成倾向。大约 50% 的 NF2 病例是散发突变。

临床表现

NF2 的特征是多发的非恶性神经系统肿瘤，包括脑膜瘤、室管膜瘤及胶质瘤。双侧前庭神经鞘瘤是 NF2 的特征性肿瘤，见于 95% 的患者中。NF2 通常在 20～30 岁诊断，表现为听力丧失和单侧或双侧前庭神经鞘瘤。

NF2 患者可能有牛奶咖啡斑，但其大小或数量通常不及 NF1。许多 NF2 患者有眼科症状，包括白内障、视网膜改变和弱视。

诊断与鉴别诊断

与 NF1 类似，NF2 患者主要依据其具有较高特异性的诊断标准（见表 12.3）进行诊断。分子检测可以协助确诊。

NF2 常被误诊为 NF1，尤其是有牛奶咖啡斑时。如果忽略了其他表现，NF2 患者也可能被误诊为孤立的脑膜瘤或单侧前庭神经鞘瘤。

治疗

通常建议在肿瘤较大并引起显著症状时进行神经鞘瘤和其他肿瘤的切除。术后可能会有并发症和肿瘤复发。

尽管传统治疗主要集中在手术干预上，如 NF1 中所述，靶向肿瘤生长通路的药物也在研发中。

结节性硬化症

定义和流行病学

结节性硬化症（TSC）是一类常染色体显性遗传病，与早期细胞分化、增殖和迁移异常有关。TSC 导致不同阶段多器官的错构瘤病变。TSC 的发病率为 1/6000。已知 TSC1 和 TSC2 基因突变是大多数病例的致病基因，大约 70% 的病例是散发性突变。

病理学

TSC1 和 TSC2 位于不同的染色体上，但它们都编码肿瘤抑制蛋白（分别为 Hamartin 和 Tuberin），这些蛋白抑制哺乳动物雷帕霉素靶蛋白（mTOR）通路，该通路对细胞生长和增殖非常重要。TSC1 和 TSC2 基因突变可导致不受控的生长和增殖。

临床表现

皮肤症状是 TSC 的常见表现。90% 的患者有色素减退斑或"灰叶斑"。面部血管纤维瘤是良性 1～5 mm 圆顶状的皮肤色丘疹，通常在 2～5 岁首次出现。鲨鱼皮斑是位于腰骶部的大斑块，皮肤呈"橘皮"质地，是 TSC 的特征性表现。

几乎所有 TSC 患者都有中枢神经系统受累。常见的合并症包括癫痫、孤独症、发育迟缓和智力障碍。脑影像学可能发现皮质下结节、室管膜下结节和室管膜下巨细胞星形细胞瘤（SEGA）。40%～50% 的婴儿会发展为一种严重的癫痫形式，称为婴儿痉挛。

诊断与鉴别诊断

发现 TSC1 或 TSC2 致病基因突变可确诊 TSC。因为 10%～25% 的患者未发现基因突变，因此也建立了临床诊断标准。

TSC 中的肿瘤也可能单独出现。需要进行活检以鉴别面部血管纤维瘤与痤疮和其他皮肤病变。

治疗

治疗主要针对 TSC 相关并发症。研究表明，患有 TSC 和婴儿痉挛的婴儿对氨己烯酸治疗有较好的反应。

SEGA 通常是生长缓慢的良性病变，如果无症状，可通过定期神经影像监测。然而位于室间孔附近的 SEGA 可能导致梗阻性脑积水。通过外科手术全切病变可能治愈，此外使用 mTOR 抑制剂（如依维莫司）治疗也常有效。

预后

TSC1 突变相关的 TSC 常更显示出家族聚集性，并且临床表现较轻。TSC2 突变的患者更可能是自发突变，

likely to have a sporadic mutation with more severe clinical complications. The variability in outcome depends on the extent and type of presenting symptoms. Patients with refractory seizures, developmental delays, and CNS lesions have a poorer prognosis. The development of renal angiolipomas, especially multiple tumors, is also associated with poorer outcome.

Sturge-Weber Syndrome
Definition/Epidemiology
Sturge-Weber syndrome (SWS) is a vascular malformation syndrome characterized by vascular lesions of the skin, brain, and eyes. It occurs in 1/20,000 to 1/50,000 live births with no clear evidence of heritability. SWS is the third most common neurocutaneous syndrome after NF1 and TSC.

Pathology
SWS is caused by somatic mutations in the *GNAQ* gene that plays an important role in vascular development. The gain-of-function mutation in *GNAQ* is found in affected tissues associated with vascular lesions. Leptomeningeal vascular malformations are ipsilateral to the port-wine birthmark and are associated with cortical injury secondary to venous stasis and insufficient tissue perfusion.

Clinical Presentation
SWS is characterized by leptomeningeal angiomatosis of the posterior hemisphere, facial cutaneous vascular malformations known as port-wine birthmarks, choroid angioma of the eye, seizures, and glaucoma.

Diagnosis/Differential
The diagnosis is usually made by observing a port-wine birthmark in the distribution of the ophthalmic branch of the trigeminal nerve, with neuroimaging confirmation of the intracranial abnormality. While 10% to 35% of children with a facial port-wine birthmark on the forehead or upper eyelid will have SWS, as many as 80% of children with a port-wine birthmark do not have intracranial lesions. SWS should be distinguished from other disorders involving abnormal intracranial vessels and seizures, including moyamoya disease, other vascular malformations, and tuberous sclerosis.

Treatment
Aggressive treatment of seizures with antiepileptic medications and consideration for surgical excision of epileptogenic areas may be indicated. Facial birthmarks may be treated with laser ablation for cosmetic purposes. Careful screening and treatment for glaucoma is necessary.
   The use of daily aspirin to prevent strokes is controversial.

Prognosis
Prognosis for patients with SWS depends on the degree of underlying intellectual and developmental disability, control of seizures, and extent of visual impairment usually due to glaucoma.

SUGGESTED READINGS

Adzik NS, Thom EA, Spong CV, et al: A randomized trial of prenatal versus postnatal repair of myelomeningocele, N Eng J Med 364:993–1004, 2011.

Alexander H, Tsering D, Myseros JS, et al: Management of Chiari I malformations: a paradigm in evolution, Childs Nerv Syst 35(10):1809–1826, 2019.

Ardern-Homes S, Fischer G, North K: Neurofibromatosis type 2: presentation, major complications, and management, with a focus on the pediatric age group, J Child Neurol 32(1):9–22, 2017.

Calloni SF, Caschera L, Triulzi FM: Disorders of ventral induction/spectrum of holoprosencephaly, Neuroimag Clin N Am 29:411–421, 2019.

Ciaccio C, Fontana L, Milani D, Tabano S, Miozzo M, Esposito S: Fragile X syndrome a review of clinical and molecular diagnoses, Ital J Pediatr 43, 2017.

Fakhoury M: Autistic spectrum disorders: a review of clinical features, theories, and diagnosis, Int J Devl Neuroscience 43:70–77, 2015.

Gold W, Krishnarajy R, Ellaway C, Christodoulou J: Rett syndrome: a genetic update and clinical review focusing on comorbidities, ACS Chem Neurosci 9:167–176, 2018.

Guerrini R, Dobyns W: Malformations of cortical development: clinical features and genetic causes, Lancet Neurol 13:710–726, 2014.

Hirbe A, Gutmann D: Neurofibromatosis type 1: a multidisciplinary approach to care, Lancet Neurol 13:834–843, 2014.

Kabagambe S, Jensen G, Chen Y, et al: Fetal surgery for myelomeningocele: a systematic review and meta-analysis of outcomes in fetoscopic versus open repair, Fetal Diagn Ther 43:161–174, 2018.

Perlman S: Von Hippel-Lindau disease and Sturge-Weber syndrome, Handbook of Child Neurology 148, 2018, Neurogenetics, Part II.

Raspa M, Wheeler A, Riley C: Public Health Literature Review of Fragile X syndrome, Pediatrics 139:S153, 2017.

Rosenberg R, Kiely Law J, Yenokyan G, McGready J, Kaufmann W, Law PA: Characteristics and concordance of autism spectrum disorders among 277 twin pairs, Arch Pediatr Adolesc Med 163(10):907–914, 2009.

Rosser R: Neurocutaneous disorders, Continuum 24(1, Child Neurology): 96–129, 2018.

Thapar A, Cooper M: Attention deficit hyperactivity disorder, Lancet 387:1240–1250, 2015.

Vandertop WP: Syringomyelia, Neuropediatrics 45:3–9, 2014.

Weitlauf AS, McPheeters ML, Peters B, et al: Therapies for children with autism spectrum disorder: behavioral interventions update. AHRQ Comparative Effectiveness Reviews. Report no. 14-EHC036-EF, Agency for Healthcare Research and Quality, 2014.

伴随更严重的临床并发症。预后的差异取决于临床症状的范围和类型。难治性癫痫、发育迟缓和中枢神经系统病变的患者预后较差。出现肾血管脂肪瘤，尤其是多发性肿瘤，预后也较差。

Sturge-Weber 综合征

定义和流行病学

Sturge-Weber 综合征（SWS）是一种血管畸形综合征，其特征是皮肤、脑和眼睛的血管病变，发生于 1/50 000～1/20 000 的新生儿，无明确的遗传性证据。SWS 是继 NF1 和 TSC 之后第三常见的神经皮肤综合征。

病理学

SWS 是由 *GNAQ* 基因的体细胞突变引起，*GNAQ* 基因在血管发育中起重要作用。在伴有血管病变的受累组织中发现了 *GNAQ* 基因的功能获得性突变。软脑膜血管畸形的同侧出现葡萄酒色胎记，此处常由于静脉淤滞和脑组织灌注不足而继发皮质损害。

临床表现

SWS 的临床表现包括大脑半球后侧的软脑膜血管瘤、面部皮肤血管畸形（包括葡萄酒色胎记）、眼部脉络膜血管瘤、癫痫和青光眼。

诊断与鉴别诊断

诊断通常是发现三叉神经眼支分布区的葡萄酒色胎记，并通过神经影像明确颅内异常表现。额头或上眼睑有葡萄酒色胎记的儿童患 SWS 的比例是 10%～35%，而 80% 有葡萄酒色胎记的儿童没有颅内病变。SWS 应与其他涉及颅内血管异常和癫痫发作的疾病鉴别，包括烟雾病、其他血管畸形和结节性硬化症。

治疗

应积极用抗癫痫药物控制癫痫发作，对于药物控制不佳的情况，考虑手术切除致痫灶。面部胎记可以通过激光进行美容治疗。需要仔细筛查和治疗青光眼。

是否每天使用阿司匹林进行卒中预防存在争议。

预后

SWS 患者的预后取决于智力和发育障碍的程度、癫痫发作的控制以及视觉损害的程度（通常由于青光眼引起）。

推荐阅读

Adzik NS, Thom EA, Spong CV, et al: A randomized trial of prenatal versus postnatal repair of myelomeningocele, N Eng J Med 364:993–1004, 2011.

Alexander H, Tsering D, Myseros JS, et al: Management of Chiari I malformations: a paradigm in evolution, Childs Nerv Syst 35(10):1809–1826, 2019.

Ardern-Homes S, Fischer G, North K: Neurofibromatosis type 2: presentation, major complications, and management, with a focus on the pediatric age group, J Child Neurol 32(1):9–22, 2017.

Calloni SF, Caschera L, Triulzi FM: Disorders of ventral induction/spectrum of holoprosencephaly, Neuroimag Clin N Am 29:411–421, 2019.

Ciaccio C, Fontana L, Milani D, Tabano S, Miozzo M, Esposito S: Fragile X syndrome a review of clinical and molecular diagnoses, Ital J Pediatr 43, 2017.

Fakhoury M: Autistic spectrum disorders: a review of clinical features, theories, and diagnosis, Int J Devl Neuroscience 43:70–77, 2015.

Gold W, Krishnaraj R, Ellaway C, Christodoulou J: Rett syndrome: a genetic update and clinical review focusing on comorbidities, ACS Chem Neurosci 9:167–176, 2018.

Guerrini R, Dobyns W: Malformations of cortical development: clinical features and genetic causes, Lancet Neurol 13:710–726, 2014.

Hirbe A, Gutmann D: Neurofibromatosis type 1: a multidisciplinary approach to care, Lancet Neurol 13:834–843, 2014.

Kabagambe S, Jensen G, Chen Y, et al: Fetal surgery for myelomeningocele: a systematic review and meta-analysis of outcomes in fetoscopic versus open repair, Fetal Diagn Ther 43:161–174, 2018.

Perlman S: Von Hippel-Lindau disease and Sturge-Weber syndrome, Handbook of Child Neurology 148, 2018, Neurogenetics, Part II.

Raspa M, Wheeler A, Riley C: Public Health Literature Review of Fragile X syndrome, Pediatrics 139:S153, 2017.

Rosenberg R, Kiely Law J, Yenokyan G, McGready J, Kaufmann W, Law PA: Characteristics and concordance of autism spectrum disorders among 277 twin pairs, Arch Pediatr Adolesc Med 163(10):907–914, 2009.

Rosser R: Neurocutaneous disorders, Continuum 24(1, Child Neurology): 96–129, 2018.

Thapar A, Cooper M: Attention deficit hyperactivity disorder, Lancet 387:1240–1250, 2015.

Vandertop WP: Syringomyelia, Neuropediatrics 45:3–9, 2014.

Weitlauf AS, McPheeters ML, Peters B, et al: Therapies for children with autism spectrum disorder: behavioral interventions update. AHRQ Comparative Effectiveness Reviews. Report no. 14-EHC036-EF, Agency for Healthcare Research and Quality, 2014.

13

Cerebrovascular Disease

Mitchell S. V. Elkind

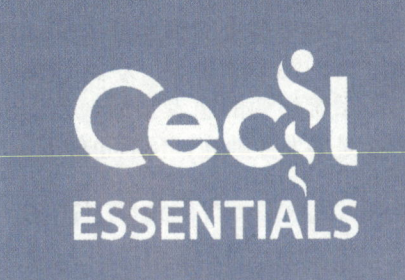

INTRODUCTION

Stroke is a major public health problem throughout the world due to its high prevalence and mortality and its association with significant disability among survivors. Stroke is the fifth leading cause of death in the United States and a leading cause of death in other countries, particularly in Asia. It is the leading cause of serious disability and results in enormous costs measured in both health care dollars and lost productivity. Major strides have been made in understanding the epidemiology, etiology, and pathogenesis of cerebrovascular disease, which have led to dramatic change in the approach to diagnosis and treatment of stroke in the past decade.

DEFINITIONS AND EPIDEMIOLOGY

The term *cerebrovascular disease* encompasses a host of disorders that share pathology localized to the vessels of the brain and spinal cord, including ischemic stroke, transient ischemic attack (TIA), intracerebral hemorrhage (ICH), subarachnoid hemorrhage (SAH), cerebral venous and sinus thrombosis, and disorders of the vessels themselves unassociated with cerebral injury (Table 13.1). Strokes, the major type of cerebrovascular disease, may be classified as either ischemic (i.e., due to lack of blood flow) or hemorrhagic. With widespread use of sensitive brain imaging, such as diffusion-weighted MRI (DWI), cerebral injury from ischemia can be seen among patients whose symptoms last only a few minutes. The definition of a transient ischemic attack has thus evolved from one in which symptoms lasted less than 24 hours, to one in which the duration of symptoms is not as relevant, and the focus is instead on whether there is evident brain injury on imaging (or pathology in those instances in which a patient dies). A definition from an expert panel in 2013 defined an *ischemic stroke* as "an episode of neurological dysfunction caused by focal cerebral, spinal, or retinal infarction." A *stroke due to ICH* was defined as "rapidly developing clinical signs of neurologic dysfunction due to a focal collection of blood within the brain parenchyma or ventricular system which is not due to trauma."

Because advanced imaging techniques permit the detection of abnormalities consistent with infarction or microhemorrhage that are unassociated with any clinical symptoms, the current definitions distinguish between "stroke," which involves clinical symptoms, and "cerebral infarction" and "microhemorrhages" (or "microbleeds"), which need not be associated with symptoms of cerebral injury. So-called "silent strokes," however, are not so silent; they can be associated with cognitive decline, dementia, gait disorders, functional disability, and an increased risk of clinical strokes. Because subclinical infarcts are approximately five times more common than clinically evident strokes, including them (and microbleeds) within the rubric of *cerebrovascular disease* substantially increases the recognized burden of cerebrovascular pathology.

Ischemic strokes may be further classified into etiologic subgroups, based on the mechanism of the ischemia and the type and localization of the vascular lesion. Cardioembolism as the source occurs in 15% to 30% of cases, large vessel atherosclerotic infarction varies from 14% to 40%, and small-vessel lacunar infarcts account for 15% to 30%. Stroke from other determined causes, such as arteritis or dissection, account for less than 5% of cases. In 30% to 40% of ischemic infarcts the cause cannot be determined. Intracranial hemorrhage may also be subdivided into subtypes, based on the site and vascular origin of the blood: subarachnoid, when the bleeding originates in the subarachnoid spaces surrounding the brain; and intracerebral, when the hemorrhage is into the brain parenchyma. Other forms of intracranial bleeding, such as subdural hemorrhage and epidural hemorrhage, are generally associated with trauma and not usually considered manifestations of stroke.

In the United States, there are 6.4 million stroke survivors (prevalence of 3%), and there are approximately 600,000 new (incident) and 200,000 recurrent strokes per year. Of these strokes, about 87% are ischemic infarctions, 10% primary hemorrhages, and 3% SAHs. Among adults age 65 to 74, stroke incidence is 670 to 970/100,000 per year. Stroke incidence rates are approximately twice as high for African Americans as for white individuals. In northern Manhattan, Caribbean Hispanic individuals had an incidence rate intermediate between that of white individuals and African Americans. Temporal trends in stroke incidence suggest that stroke incidence and mortality rates have declined since 1950; however, disparities in stroke incidence and mortality have persisted. Stroke rates in the young have also increased. From 1995 to 2012, stroke hospitalization rates for men age 18 to 44 years have doubled. Overall, due to the graying of the global population and the increased prevalence of stroke risk factors in younger people, the mean global lifetime risk of stroke has increased almost 9% over the past 25 years (through 2016) to 25%, meaning that 1 in 4 people will experience a stroke at some point during their lifetime.

Stroke incidence increases with age, but strokes do occur in young adults and children and may be missed if the diagnosis is not considered. Although stroke incidence rates are higher for men than women at most ages, among young adults the rates are similar or higher among women, probably related to pregnancy, hormonal contraception, and other hormone-related differences. At older ages, incidence rates among women are again greater, and because women tend to live longer than men, overall about 55,000 more women than men have a stroke each year.

MODIFIABLE RISK FACTORS

Well-established modifiable stroke risk factors include hypertension, cardiac disease (particularly atrial fibrillation), diabetes,

脑血管疾病

周梦圆 译　陈玮琪　杨沫 审校　王伊龙 通审

引言

卒中是全球主要的公共卫生问题，因其高发病率、高死亡率以及高致残率而备受关注。在美国，卒中是第五大死亡原因，在其他国家，尤其是亚洲，卒中也是主要的死亡原因之一。卒中是导致严重残疾的主要原因，并带来了巨大的经济成本，这些成本既包括医疗费用的支出，也包括生产力的损失。过去十年里，人们对脑血管疾病的流行病学、病因学和发病机制的研究取得了重大进展，这些进展极大地改变了卒中的诊断和治疗方式。

定义与流行病学

脑血管疾病这一术语涵盖了一系列与脑和脊髓血管病变相关的疾病，包括缺血性卒中、短暂性脑缺血发作（TIA）、脑出血（ICH）、蛛网膜下腔出血（SAH）、脑静脉和静脉窦血栓形成，以及与脑损伤无关的血管本身疾病（表13.1）。卒中作为脑血管疾病的主要类型，可分为缺血性和出血性两种。随着脑部成像技术的广泛应用，如弥散加权磁共振成像（DWI），即使在患者症状仅持续几分钟的情况下，也能观察到缺血引起的脑部损伤。因此，短暂性脑缺血发作的定义已经从症状持续时间少于24 h演变为不再过分关注症状持续时间，而是重点关注影像学检查中是否存在明显的脑损伤（或在患者死亡的情况下是否存在病理学改变）。2013年专家小组给出的定义将缺血性卒中描述为"由局部脑、脊髓或视网膜梗死引起的神经功能障碍发作"。而由ICH引起的卒中则被定义为"由于脑实质或脑室系统内非创伤性局部血液积聚而导致的迅速进展的神经功能障碍"。

随着医学成像技术的飞速发展，高级成像技术能够检测到与梗死灶或微出血相关的异常，而这些异常可能并不伴随任何临床症状。因此，当前的医学定义对"卒中"（涉及临床症状）与"脑梗死"和"微出血"进行了明确的区分，后者并不一定存在脑损伤的相应临床表现。然而，所谓的"无症状卒中"并非真正无声无息；它们可能与认知功能减退、痴呆、步态障碍、功能障碍以及临床卒中风险增加有关。这些无症状梗死灶（以及微出血）在临床上的意义不容忽视，因为它们的发生率大约是症状性卒中的5倍。将这些亚临床情况纳入脑血管疾病的范畴，极大地增加了已知的脑血管病理负担。

缺血性卒中可根据缺血的机制、血管病变的类型和位置进一步进行病因学分类。15%～30%缺血性卒中病因为心源性栓塞，大动脉粥样硬化性梗死占14%～40%，小血管腔隙性梗死占15%～30%。其他已知原因的卒中，如动脉炎或动脉夹层，占比不到5%。30%～40%的缺血性卒中病因无法确定。脑出血可根据出血部位和责任血管分为以下亚型：当出血发生于蛛网膜下腔时，称为蛛网膜下腔出血；当出血进入大脑实质时，称为脑内出血。其他形式的颅内出血，如硬膜下出血和硬膜外出血，通常与创伤相关，因此不被归类为卒中。

在美国，有640万卒中幸存者（患病率为3%），每年约有60万新发病例（首次卒中）和20万复发卒中。在这些卒中事件中，约87%为缺血性卒中，10%为原发性脑出血，3%为蛛网膜下腔出血。在65～74岁的成年人中，卒中发病率为每年（670～970）/10万。非裔美国人的卒中发病率大约是白人的2倍。在曼哈顿北部，加勒比西班牙裔个体的卒中发病率介于白人和非裔美国人之间。卒中发病率的时间趋势表明，自1950年以来，卒中发病率和死亡率有所下降；然而，不同种族间卒中发病率和死亡率的差异一直存在。青年卒中发病率也有所增加。1995—2012年，18～44岁男性的卒中住院率增加了1倍。总体而言，由于全球人口老龄化和年轻人卒中危险因素的增加，过去25年（截至2016年）全球卒中的平均终生风险增加了近9%，达到25%，这意味着每4个人中就有1人在其一生中的某个时刻会经历卒中。

卒中发病率随年龄增长而增加，但卒中也会发生在年轻人和儿童中，如果不考虑诊断，可能会被漏诊。尽管在大多数年龄段，男性的卒中发病率高于女性，但在年轻人中，女性的发病率与男性相似，甚至更高，这可能与怀孕、激素避孕和其他激素相关差异有关。在老年人群中，女性发病率再次升高，而且由于女性往往比男性寿命更长，因此每年女性卒中患者比男性大约多55 000人。

可控的危险因素

公认的、可控制的卒中危险因素包括高血压、心脏疾

TABLE 13.1 Common Forms of Cerebrovascular Disease

Ischemic cerebrovascular disease
　Symptomatic
- Ischemic stroke
  - Cerebral infarction
  - Spinal cord infarction
  - Retinal infarction
- Transient ischemic attack
- Transient monocular blindness *(amaurosis fugax)*

　Asymptomatic
- Cerebral infarction/spinal cord infarction/retinal infarction

Hemorrhagic cerebrovascular disease
- Intracerebral hemorrhage
- Subarachnoid hemorrhage
- Intraventricular hemorrhage
- Subdural hemorrhage
- Epidural hemorrhage
- Cerebral microbleeds

Other forms of cerebrovascular disease
- Cerebral vein thrombosis
- Dural sinus thrombosis

Disorders of cerebral autoregulation
- Posterior reversible encephalopathy syndrome
- Hypertensive encephalopathy
- Reversible cerebral vasoconstriction syndrome

Vascular abnormalities
- Aneurysms
- Arteriovenous malformations
- Cavernous malformations
- Fibromuscular dysplasia

TABLE 13.2 Stroke Risk Factors

Nonmodifiable risk factors	Age
	Sex
	Race/ethnicity
	Family history
	Genetic disorders
Well-established modifiable risk factors	Hypertension/blood pressure
	Diabetes mellitus/hyperglycemia
	Cardiac disorders
	Atrial fibrillation
	Valvular heart disease
	Recent myocardial infarction
	Cardiomyopathy/heart failure
	Bacterial endocarditis
	Hyperlipidemia
	Cigarette smoking
	Carotid stenosis
	Transient ischemic attack (TIA)
	Physical inactivity
	Hypercoagulable states (e.g., antiphospholipid antibody syndrome, cancer-associated hypercoagulopathy)
	Alcohol abuse
	Substance abuse (e.g., cocaine, intravenous drug abuse)
Other potential risk factors	Migraine
	Sleep apnea
	Cardiac disorders
	Paroxysmal supraventricular tachycardia
	Patent foramen ovale/atrial septal aneurysm
	Aortic atheroma
	Atrial cardiopathy
	Infections (e.g., varicella zoster virus, influenza)
	Inflammation
	Others

hyperlipidemia, cigarette use, physical inactivity, alcohol abuse, asymptomatic carotid stenosis, and a history of TIAs (Table 13.2).

Hypertension is the most powerful modifiable stroke risk factor and is associated with both ischemic and hemorrhagic strokes. Risk of stroke decreases with lower systolic and diastolic blood pressures, and this graded decrement in risk persists down to levels as low as 115/75 mm Hg. There is no clearly defined threshold level below which stroke risk levels off.

Cardiac disease is associated with an increased risk of ischemic stroke. Atrial fibrillation (AF) is the cardiac disease most often associated with stroke risk and accounts for up to 24% of cerebral infarction in the elderly. Other cardiac diseases, including valvular heart disease, myocardial infarction (MI), coronary artery disease (CAD), and congestive heart failure (CHF) are also associated with stroke risk. Recent evidence also suggests that other atrial arrhythmias, such as paroxysmal supraventricular tachycardia, may also increase risk of stroke, even in the absence of atrial fibrillation. Other possible sources of cardiac emboli include patent foramen ovale, aortic arch atherosclerotic disease, atrial septal aneurysms, and valvular strands.

Hyperlipidemia is a stroke risk factor, though its relationship to stroke is more complicated than for heart disease, primarily because of the many types of stroke. Lipid abnormalities, such as elevations in low-density lipoprotein (LDL) and decreased levels of high-density lipoprotein, are strongly associated with ischemic stroke of atherosclerotic origin. Somewhat paradoxically, however, low levels of LDL are associated with an increased risk of hemorrhagic stroke.

The role of alcohol as a stroke risk factor also depends on stroke subtype, as well as the quantity consumed. Alcohol consumption has been shown to be a risk factor for both ICH and SAH in a linear fashion, whereas a J-shaped relationship exists between alcohol and ischemic stroke, such that modest consumption (up to two drinks daily in men, and one daily in women) may be protective against stroke and heavy consumption (five or more drinks per day) increases risk.

Asymptomatic carotid artery disease, particularly with 70% or greater stenosis, is associated with increased stroke risk (approximately 2% per year). The risk of stroke also depends, however, on the rate of progression of the stenosis, collateral circulation, and the stability of the atherosclerotic plaque.

TIAs are a strong predictor of subsequent stroke. The first several days after a TIA have the greatest stroke risk, with clinical series demonstrating a 5% risk at 2 days and 10% risk at 90 days. Patients with transient monocular blindness *(amaurosis fugax)* have a better outcome than those with hemispheric ischemic attacks. The stroke risk after TIA depends on the underlying cause of the ischemia, including the presence and severity of underlying atherosclerotic disease or AF. Age, hypertension, the presence of diabetes, clinical syndromes including aphasia and hemiparesis, and duration of at least 10 minutes

表 13.1　脑血管疾病的常见形式
缺血性脑血管病 　症状性 　　● 缺血性卒中 　　　● 脑梗死 　　　● 脊髓梗死 　　　● 视网膜梗死 　　● 短暂性脑缺血发作 　　● 短暂性单眼失明（一过性黑矇） 　无症状性 　　● 脑梗死、脊髓梗死、视网膜梗死 出血性脑血管疾病 　● 脑出血 　● 蛛网膜下腔出血 　● 脑室出血 　● 硬膜下出血 　● 硬膜外出血 　● 脑微出血 其他形式的脑血管疾病 　● 脑静脉血栓形成 　● 硬脑膜窦血栓形成 大脑自动调节功能障碍 　● 可逆性后部脑病综合征 　● 高血压性脑病 　● 可逆性脑血管收缩综合征 血管异常 　● 动脉瘤 　● 动静脉畸形 　● 海绵状血管畸形 　● 纤维肌性发育不良

表 13.2　卒中危险因素	
无法调整的危险因素	年龄 性别 种族/民族 家族史 遗传性疾病
明确的可调整的危险因素	高血压/血压 糖尿病/高血糖 心脏疾病 　心房颤动 　心脏瓣膜病 　近期心肌梗死 　心肌病/心力衰竭 　细菌性心内膜炎 高脂血症 吸烟 颈动脉狭窄 短暂性脑缺血发作（TIA） 缺乏运动 高凝状态（如抗磷脂抗体综合征、肿瘤相关高凝状态） 饮酒 药物滥用（如可卡因、静脉注射药物滥用）
其他潜在的危险因素	偏头痛 睡眠呼吸暂停 心脏异常 　阵发性室上性心动过速 　卵圆孔未闭/房间隔动脉瘤 　主动脉粥样硬化 　心房疾病 感染（如水痘带状疱疹病毒、流行性感冒） 炎症 其他

病（尤其是心房颤动）、糖尿病、高脂血症、吸烟、缺乏运动、酗酒、无症状颈动脉狭窄以及 TIA 病史（表 13.2）。

高血压是最有力的可控的卒中危险因素，与缺血性和出血性卒中均相关。随着收缩压和舒张压下降，卒中风险也随之降低，且这种风险的下降会一直持续到血压低至 115/75 mmHg 的水平。但目前尚无明确界定的阈值水平可以使卒中风险趋于平稳。

心脏疾病与缺血性卒中风险增加相关。心房颤动（AF）是与卒中风险相关性最大的心脏疾病，占老年人群脑梗死病因多达 24%。其他心脏疾病，包括心脏瓣膜病、心肌梗死（MI）、冠状动脉疾病（CAD）和充血性心力衰竭（CHF）也与卒中风险增加有关。最近的证据表明，其他房性心律失常，如阵发性室上性心动过速，即使在没有心房颤动的情况下也可能增加卒中风险。其他可能的心脏栓子来源包括卵圆孔未闭、主动脉弓动脉粥样硬化、房间隔动脉瘤和瓣膜条索。

高脂血症是卒中的风险因素之一，尽管它与卒中的关系比心脏疾病更为复杂，这主要是因为卒中有多种类型。血脂异常，如低密度脂蛋白（LDL）升高和高密度脂蛋白水平降低，与动脉粥样硬化性缺血性卒中均有很强的相关性。然而，有些矛盾的是，低密度脂蛋白水平低也与出血性卒中风险增加相关。

酒精作为卒中危险因素的影响，也取决于卒中亚型和摄入量。酒精摄入已被证实与 ICH 和 SAH 呈线性关系，而酒精与缺血性卒中之间则存在"J"形关系，即适量饮酒（男性每天最多 2 杯，女性每天 1 杯）可能对卒中有保护作用，而大量饮酒（每天 5 杯或更多）则会增加卒中风险。

无症状颈动脉疾病，尤其是狭窄程度达到 70% 或以上的情况，与卒中风险增加有关（每年约 2%）。然而，卒中风险还取决于狭窄的进展速度、侧支循环以及动脉粥样硬化斑块的稳定性。

TIA 是即将发生卒中的强有力的预测因素。TIA 发生后的最初几天，卒中发生风险最高；临床病例系列显示，2 天内风险为 5%，90 天内风险为 10%。患有短暂性单眼失明（一过性黑矇）的患者比患有半球缺血性发作的患者预后更好。TIA 后的卒中风险取决于导致缺血的原因，包括潜在动脉粥样硬化疾病或 AF 的存在和严重程度。年龄、高血压、糖尿病、包括失语和偏瘫在内的临床症状以及持续时间 ≥ 10 min，预示着 TIA

predict TIA patients at higher risk of stroke. Patients with TIA with evidence of infarction on MRI are also at higher risk. Other potential stroke risk factors include migraine, oral contraceptive use, drug abuse, sleep apnea, infection, and inflammation.

PATHOLOGY

Understanding the pathology of cerebrovascular disease requires an appreciation of the vascular anatomy of the brain, the vascular pathologies that can affect brain vessels, and the response of brain tissue to ischemia and hemorrhage.

Clinical Implications of Vascular Anatomy

The brain is perfused by four major vessels, the paired carotid and vertebral arteries. These originate extracranially as branches off the aorta and great vessels and course through the neck and base of the skull to reach the intracranial cavity (Fig. 13.1). The carotid and its branches constitute the anterior circulation and the vertebral arteries and its branches the posterior circulation. Anterior and posterior circulations communicate with one another through the posterior communicating arteries. The left and right sides of the anterior circulation communicate with each other through the anterior communicating artery. The major vessels at the base of the brain and these communicating vessels constitute the circle of Willis, the anastomotic network that allows for collateral blood flow when individual vessels are stenotic or occluded. Because variants in the circle of Willis are common, collateral flow may not be sufficient in many cases of blockage, and the risk of ischemic stroke therefore depends on a patient's individual anatomy.

The right common carotid artery usually begins as a branch from the innominate artery, whereas the left common carotid artery originates directly from the aortic arch. The common carotid arteries bifurcate into the internal and external carotid arteries, usually at the level of the fourth cervical vertebra. The internal carotid arteries have no branches in the neck and face and enter the cranium through the carotid canal. There are four main segments of each internal carotid artery: cervical, petrous, cavernous, and supraclinoid. The siphon is the term used to describe the hairpin turn made by the cavernous and supraclinoid segments, and it is at this level that the ophthalmic artery originates, providing the first major branch of the internal carotid artery and supplying blood flow to the optic nerve and retina. Thus, internal carotid artery disease commonly causes ocular ischemia, leading to a transient ischemic attack (*amaurosis fugax*) or infarction of the optic nerve or retina, a warning sign of impending cerebral stroke. The internal carotid arteries then give off the superior hypophyseal, posterior communicating, and anterior choroidal arteries, before terminating intracranially by dividing into the middle and anterior cerebral arteries. In addition to the eye, the paired carotid systems supply approximately 80% of the hemispheric blood flow, including the frontal, parietal, and anterior temporal lobes. In up to 15% of individuals, the posterior cerebral artery (PCA) also arises directly from the internal carotid artery (the so-called fetal origin PCA), so that the entire hemisphere including the occipital lobe is supplied by the internal carotid artery. The anterior choroidal artery supplies a number of structures in addition to the choroid plexus, including the inferior portion of the posterior limb of the internal capsule, the hippocampus, and portions of the globus pallidus, posterior putamen, lateral geniculate, amygdala, and ventrolateral thalamus.

The middle cerebral artery (MCA) is the largest branch of the internal carotid artery. Its first portion, or stem, is often referred to as the M1 segment, and this usually bifurcates into superior and inferior divisions or, less often, trifurcates into three major divisions (upper, middle, and lower). The MCA stem gives rise to the medial and lateral

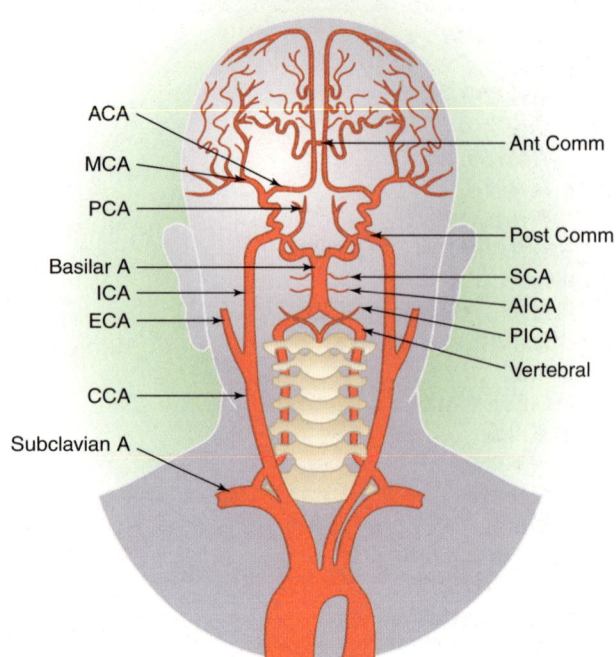

Fig. 13.1 Coronal view of the extracranial and intracranial arterial supply to the brain. Vessels forming the circle of Willis are highlighted. *A*, Artery; *ACA*, anterior cerebral artery; *AICA*, anterior inferior cerebellar artery; *Ant Comm*, anterior communicating artery; *CCA*, common carotid artery; *ECA*, external carotid artery; *ICA*, internal carotid artery; *MCA*, middle cerebral artery; *PCA*, posterior cerebral artery; *PICA*, posterior inferior cerebellar artery; *Post Comm*, posterior communicating artery; *SCA*, superior cerebellar artery. (Modified from Lord R: Surgery of occlusive cerebrovascular disease, St. Louis, 1986, Mosby.)

lenticulostriates, which supply the extreme capsule, claustrum, putamen, most of the globus pallidus, part of the head and the entire body of the caudate, as well as the superior portions of the anterior and posterior limbs of the internal capsule. The divisions of the MCA supply almost the entire lateral cortical surface of the brain, including the insula, operculum, and frontal, parietal, temporal, and occipital cortices.

The anterior cerebral artery (ACA) also has a proximal, or A1, segment, which ends at the junction with the anterior communicating artery. The ipsilateral ACA then continues as the distal, or A2, segment. An important branch is the recurrent artery of Heubner, which supplies the head of the caudate nucleus, and several cortical branches supply the medial and orbital surfaces of the frontal lobe.

The vertebral arteries generally originate from the subclavian arteries, course through the transverse foramina of the cervical vertebrae, pierce the dura, and enter the cranial cavity through the foramen magnum. The two vertebral arteries join to form the basilar artery at the level of the pontomedullary junction. Anterior and posterior spinal arteries and the posterior inferior cerebellar artery (PICA), which supplies the inferior surface of the cerebellum, arise from the distal segments of the vertebrals. The lateral medulla is supplied by the multiple, perforating branches of PICA or the direct penetrating branches of the vertebral artery. Occlusion of the distal vertebral artery may, therefore, cause infarction of the lateral medulla (Wallenberg syndrome), characterized by vertigo, imbalance, Horner syndrome, dysphagia, and sensory loss.

After originating as the union of the right and left vertebral arteries, the basilar artery travels up the ventral pons. Paramedian and

患者后续发生卒中的风险较高。MRI 上显示有梗死证据的 TIA 患者风险也较高。其他潜在的卒中危险因素包括偏头痛、口服避孕药使用、药物滥用、睡眠呼吸暂停、感染和炎症。

病理学

了解脑血管疾病的病理需要了解大脑血管解剖学、可能影响脑血管的血管病理学，以及脑组织对缺血和出血的反应。

血管解剖学的临床意义

大脑由四条主要血管——双侧的颈动脉和椎动脉供血。这些血管起源于主动脉和大血管，穿过颈部和颅底到达颅内（图 13.1）。颈动脉及其分支构成前循环，椎动脉及其分支构成后循环。前循环和后循环通过后交通动脉相互连接。前循环左右两侧通过前交通动脉相互连接。大脑底部的主要血管和这些交通血管构成了 Willis 环，这是一个吻合网络，当某一供血动脉狭窄或闭塞时，侧支循环可通过 Willis 环使血液重新分配和代偿，以维持脑的血液供应。由于 Willis 环的变异很常见，在许多血管闭塞的情况下，侧支血流可能不足，因此缺血性卒中的风险取决于患者的个体血管解剖结构。

右颈总动脉通常起源于无名动脉，而左颈总动脉则直接起源于主动脉弓。颈总动脉通常在第四颈椎水平分叉为颈内动脉和颈外动脉。颈内动脉在颈部和面部没有分支，通过颈动脉管进入颅腔。每条颈内动脉都有 4 个主要部分：颈部、岩部、海绵窦部和前床突上部。"虹吸管"一词用于描述海绵窦部和前床突上部的发夹式转弯，眼动脉起源于这一水平，成为颈内动脉的第一大分支，为视神经和视网膜提供血流。因此，颈内动脉疾病通常会导致眼部缺血，导致短暂性脑缺血发作（一过性黑矇）或者视神经或视网膜梗死，这是即将发生脑卒中的预警信号。颈内动脉在颅内终末端之前相继发出垂体上动脉、后交通动脉和脉络膜前动脉，最后分为大脑中动脉和大脑前动脉。除了双眼，成对的颈动脉系统供应约 80% 的大脑半球血流，包括额叶、顶叶和前颞叶。约 15% 的个体，大脑后动脉（PCA）直接从颈内动脉发出（即胚胎型 PCA），因此对于这部分患者，包括枕叶在内的整个大脑半球都由颈内动脉供应。脉络膜前动脉除了供应脉络丛外，还供应许多其他结构，包括内囊后肢的下部、海马、苍白球、壳核后部、外侧膝状体、杏仁核和丘脑腹外侧。

大脑中动脉（MCA）是颈内动脉的最大分支。其第一部分或主干通常被称为 M1 段，该段通常分为上、下两个分支，或者少数情况下分为三个主要分支（上、中、下支）。MCA 主干发出内侧和外侧纹状体动脉，

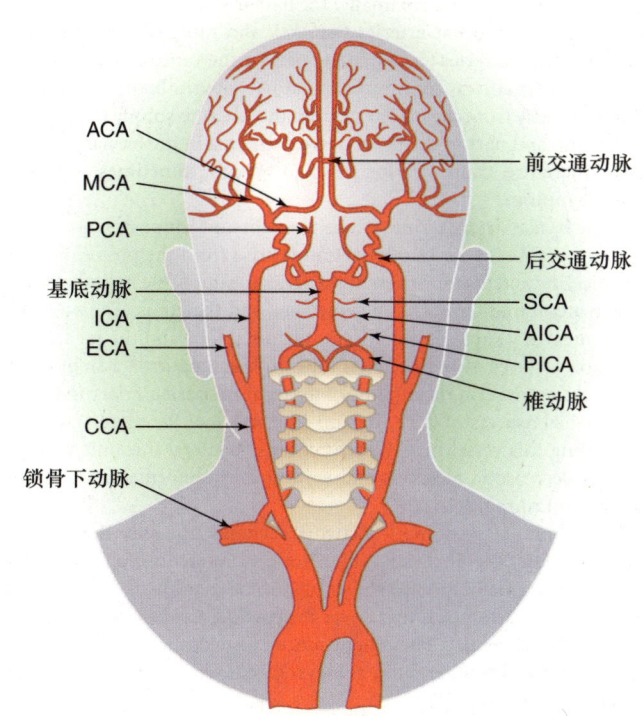

图 13.1 大脑颅外和颅内动脉供应的冠状视图，突出了 Willis 环（大脑动脉环）的血管。ACA，大脑前动脉；AICA，小脑前下动脉；CCA，颈总动脉；ECA，颈外动脉；ICA，颈内动脉；MCA，大脑中动脉；PCA，大脑后动脉；PICA，小脑后下动脉；SCA，小脑上动脉。（改编自 Lord R: Surgery of occlusive cerebrovascular disease, St. Louis, 1986, Mosby.）

供应最外囊、屏状核、壳核、大部分苍白球、尾状核的头部和体部以及内囊前、后肢的上部。MCA 的分支几乎供应整个大脑外侧皮质表面，包括岛叶、岛盖、额叶、顶叶、颞叶和枕叶皮质。

大脑前动脉（ACA）也有一个近端或 A1 段，该段终止于与前交通动脉的交界处。然后，同侧 ACA 继续作为远端或 A2 段。一个重要的分支是 Heubner 回返动脉，它供应尾状核的头部，数个皮质分支供应额叶的内侧面和眶面。

椎动脉通常起源于锁骨下动脉，穿过颈椎的横突孔、硬脑膜，并通过枕骨大孔进入颅腔。两条椎动脉在脑桥延髓交界处水平汇合形成基底动脉。脊髓前动脉、脊髓后动脉以及小脑后下动脉（PICA）均起源于椎动脉的远端，供应小脑的下表面。延髓外侧由 PICA 的多个穿支或椎动脉的直接穿支供应。因此，远端椎动脉的闭塞可能导致延髓背外侧梗死（Wallenberg 综合征），其特征是眩晕、共济失调、Horner 综合征、吞咽困难和感觉丧失。

基底动脉在双侧椎动脉的交汇点起源，向上穿过脑桥的腹侧。脑桥旁正中动脉、短旋动脉和长旋动脉

circumferential penetrating arteries exit the basilar to dive into the pontine parenchyma. Proximally, the basilar gives off the paired anterior inferior cerebellar arteries (AICAs), and more distally the superior cerebellar arteries (SCAs); these perfuse the ventrolateral aspect of the cerebellar cortex. An internal auditory (labyrinthine) artery arises either directly from the basilar or from the AICA to supply the cochlea, labyrinth, and part of the facial nerve. Ischemia in the basilar territory may, therefore, cause hearing loss and vertigo, sometimes as an isolated symptom.

The basilar artery terminates in the right and left posterior cerebral arteries (PCAs). A series of penetrators arise from the posterior communicating and posterior cerebral arteries to supply the hypothalamus, dorsolateral midbrain, lateral geniculate, and thalamus. The posterior cerebral artery supplies the inferior temporal lobe and the medial and inferior surfaces of the occipital lobe. In some patients a single large penetrating vessel at the midline of the terminal basilar artery may supply medial aspects of both thalami (the artery of Percheron); emboli occluding this vessel may, therefore, cause bilateral thalamic infarcts, with a decrease in alertness and vertical gaze abnormalities, without significant motor deficit.

The brain's anastomotic network includes not only the connections through the circle of Willis, but also intercommunicating systems extracranially and more distal connections intracranially through meningeal anastomoses that cover the cortical and cerebellar surfaces (pial-pial collaterals). These networks all protect the brain from ischemia by providing alternative routes to circumvent obstructions in the main arteries.

Venous anatomy is more variable than arterial. Superficial veins drain into the transverse, superior sagittal, and cavernous sinuses. The deep venous drainage is via the great vein of Galen, which drains into the straight sinus, and in turn drains into the torcula along with the sagittal sinus. Blood drains from the torcula to the transverse sinus, then to the sigmoid sinus, and thereafter the jugular vein. Anterior venous drainage is via the cavernous sinus, which communicates with the contralateral cavernous sinus, the transverse sinus via the superior petrosal sinus, and the inferior petrosal sinus, which drains directly into the jugular bulb.

Vascular Pathogenesis

There are multiple mechanisms leading to brain ischemia. Hemodynamic infarction occurs as a result of reduced perfusion, usually in the setting of arterial stenosis due to atherosclerosis. In some cases, stenosis may be due to arterial dissection, vasculitis, fibromuscular dysplasia, or other arteriopathies. Embolism occurs when a thrombus originating from a more proximal source (e.g., arterial or cardiac) travels through the arteries and occludes a cerebral artery. Paradoxical embolism occurs when a thrombus crosses from the venous circulation to the left side of the heart through a patent foramen ovale or, less commonly, an intrapulmonary arteriovenous shunt. Other particles that may embolize include neoplasms, fat, air, or other foreign substances. Air emboli can follow injuries or procedures involving the lungs, the dural sinuses, or jugular veins. Fat embolism usually results from a bone fracture. Septic emboli arise from bacterial endocarditis.

Intracranial hemorrhage results from the rupture of a vessel anywhere within the cranial cavity. Intracranial hemorrhages may be classified by location (e.g., extradural, subdural, subarachnoid, intracerebral, intraventricular), by the type of ruptured vessel (e.g., arterial, capillary, venous), or by cause (e.g., primary, secondary). Trauma is often involved in the generation of extradural hematoma from laceration of the middle meningeal artery or vein, and subdural hematomas from traumatic rupture of veins that traverse the subdural space.

Intracerebral, or intraparenchymal, hemorrhage is characterized by bleeding into the substance of the brain, usually originating from a small penetrating artery. Hypertension has been implicated as the cause of weakening in the walls of arterioles and the formation of microaneurysms (i.e., Charcot-Bouchard aneurysms). The most common sites for hypertensive arterial hemorrhage are the putamen, pons, cerebellum, and thalamus. Blood under arterial pressures destroys or displaces brain tissue. Amyloid angiopathy, due to the vascular deposition of β-amyloid protein similar to that seen in Alzheimer disease has been implicated as an important cause of lobar hemorrhage in elderly patients. Other causes of intracerebral hemorrhage include arteriovenous malformations, infectious aneurysms, cavernous angiomas, moyamoya disease, bleeding disorders, anticoagulation, illicit drug abuse, trauma, and tumors.

Subarachnoid hemorrhage occurs when blood is localized to the surrounding membranes and cerebrospinal fluid. It is most frequently caused by leakage of blood from a cerebral aneurysm. The combination of congenital and acquired factors leads to a degeneration of the arterial wall and the release of blood, under arterial pressures, into the subarachnoid space and cerebrospinal fluid. Aneurysms may be distributed at different sites throughout the base of the brain, particularly at the origin or bifurcations of arteries of the circle of Willis. Other secondary causes that may lead to SAH include trauma, arteriovenous malformations, bleeding disorders or anticoagulation, amyloid angiopathy, or cerebral sinus thrombosis.

The most common intrinsic disorder of the cerebral blood vessels is atherosclerosis, which shares similarities in pathology with atherosclerosis throughout the body. Arteriosclerotic plaques may develop at any point along the carotid artery and the vertebrobasilar system, but the most common sites are the bifurcation of the common carotid artery, the origins of the MCAs and ACAs, and the origins of the vertebral from the subclavian arteries (Fig. 13.2). In the past it was thought that intracranial atherosclerotic disease required significant stenosis (>50%) to cause symptoms. However, recent pathologic and radiologic studies provide evidence that substenotic lesions can also cause strokes due to plaque rupture and acute thrombosis, as is the case elsewhere in the body.

Small-vessel disease refers to the occlusion of a penetrant branch of a larger artery, usually due to microatheroma or to lipohyalinosis, a degenerative disorder of the vessel characterized by deposition of fatty and proteinaceous material. Hematologic disorders and coagulopathies, including leukemia, Waldenström's macroglobulinemia, polycythemia, primary and secondary antiphospholipid antibody syndrome, and genetic defects of the coagulation cascade, may also lead to occlusive thrombi and emboli.

The cerebral circulation differs from the systemic circulation in some important ways. The brain is protected by the anastomoses described previously. In addition, *cerebral autoregulation* maintains a constant cerebral perfusion pressure over a range of systemic blood pressures (Fig. 13.3). Cerebral arterioles have a well-developed muscular coat that allows constriction in response to increased blood pressure and dilation with hypotension. The arterioles are also exquisitely sensitive to changes in peripheral arterial concentrations of carbon dioxide ($Paco_2$) and oxygen (Pao_2). When the partial pressure of CO_2 decreases, such as during hyperventilation, the arterioles constrict and blood flow is reduced. In healthy individuals, cerebral autoregulation maintains a constant cerebral blood flow over mean arterial pressures of 60 to 140 mm Hg. In patients with chronic hypertension, the autoregulatory curve is shifted to the right, so that even minor reductions in blood pressure may not be tolerated. At blood pressures above these limits, moreover, as in severe hypertension, autoregulatory capacity may be overwhelmed, leading to breakthrough edema and hemorrhage.

离开基底动脉，进入脑桥实质供血。近端，基底动脉发出成对的小脑前下动脉（AICA），远端则发出小脑上动脉（SCA）；这些动脉为小脑皮质的腹外侧部分提供血流。内听（迷路）动脉直接起源于基底动脉或AICA，供应耳蜗、迷路和面神经的一部分。因此，基底动脉区的缺血可能导致听力下降和眩晕，有时会作为孤立的症状出现。

基底动脉终止于双侧大脑后动脉（PCA）。一系列穿支血管起源于后交通动脉和PCA，为下丘脑、中脑背外侧、外侧膝状体和丘脑供血。PCA为颞叶下部以及枕叶内侧和下表面供血。在一些患者中，基底动脉末端中线位置的单根穿通动脉（Percheron动脉）可能会为双侧丘脑内侧部分供血；该动脉栓塞可导致双侧丘脑梗死，导致警觉性降低和垂直注视麻痹，但没有明显的运动障碍。

大脑的血管吻合网络不仅包括通过Willis环的连接，还包括颅外的相互沟通系统和颅内更远端覆盖大脑皮质和小脑表面的脑膜支吻合（软脑膜-软脑膜侧支）。这些血管网络通过提供替代血管通路来绕过主要的阻塞动脉，从而保护大脑免受缺血的影响。

静脉解剖比动脉变异性更大。大脑浅静脉汇入横窦、上矢状窦和海绵窦。大脑深静脉通过Galen静脉，引流入直窦，再与矢状窦一起汇入窦汇。窦汇血液随后流入横窦、乙状窦和颈静脉。大脑前部静脉引流是通过海绵窦（与对侧海绵窦相通），再通过岩上窦、岩下窦与横窦相通，直接流入颈静脉球。

血管发病机制

导致脑缺血的机制有很多种。血流动力学梗死是由于灌注降低导致的，通常由动脉粥样硬化引起的动脉狭窄导致。在某些情况下，狭窄可能是由于动脉夹层、血管炎、纤维肌性发育不良或其他动脉病变引起的。栓塞发生于更近端来源（例如，动脉或心脏）的血栓通过动脉并阻塞脑动脉时。血栓通过未闭合的卵圆孔或较少见的肺内动静脉分流从静脉循环进入左心，造成大循环动脉栓塞，称为反常栓塞。其他可能发生栓塞的栓子包括肿瘤、脂肪、空气或其他异物。空气栓塞可能发生在涉及肺、硬脑膜窦或颈静脉的损伤或手术之后。脂肪栓塞通常是由骨折引起的。感染中毒性栓子来源于细菌性心内膜炎。

颅内出血是由颅内任何部位的血管破裂引起的。颅内出血可根据位置（例如，硬膜外、硬膜下、蛛网膜下腔、脑实质内、脑室内）、破裂血管的类型（例如，动脉、毛细血管、静脉）或原因（例如，原发性、继发性）进行分类。创伤通常涉及由脑膜中动脉或静脉撕裂引起的硬膜外血肿，以及穿过硬膜下腔的静脉创伤性破裂引起的硬膜下血肿。

脑出血，或称为脑实质出血，其特征为出血进入脑实质，通常起源于小的穿支动脉。高血压被认为是导致小动脉壁损伤和微动脉瘤形成（即Charcot-Bouchard动脉瘤）的原因。高血压性动脉出血最常见的部位是壳核、脑桥、小脑和丘脑。血液在动脉的压力下流出，进而损伤脑组织或者使脑组织移位。淀粉样脑血管病，由β淀粉样蛋白沉积于血管壁所致，已被证实是老年患者脑叶出血的重要原因。脑出血的其他原因包括动静脉畸形、感染性动脉瘤、海绵状血管瘤、烟雾病、出血性疾病、抗凝治疗、非法药物滥用、创伤和肿瘤。

蛛网膜下腔出血（SAH）是指血液局限于软脑膜和蛛网膜之间以及脑脊液中。最常见的原因是动脉瘤破裂。先天性和后天性因素共同作用导致动脉壁退化，在动脉压力作用下，血液释放到蛛网膜下腔和脑脊液中。动脉瘤可能分布在大脑底部的不同部位，特别是Willis环动脉的起源或分叉处。导致SAH的其他原因包括外伤、动静脉畸形、出血性疾病或抗凝治疗、淀粉样血管病或脑静脉窦血栓形成。

脑血管最常见的疾病是动脉粥样硬化，其病理学特征与全身动脉粥样硬化相似。动脉粥样硬化斑块可发生在颈动脉和椎基底动脉系统的任何部位，但最常见的部位是颈总动脉分叉处、MCA和ACA起源处，以及椎动脉自锁骨下动脉的起始处（图13.2）。既往认为颅内动脉粥样硬化性疾病需要明显的狭窄（＞50%）才能引起症状。然而，最近的病理学和放射学研究证据表明，由于斑块破裂和急性血栓形成，轻微狭窄病变也可能导致卒中，这与身体其他部位的情况相同。

脑小血管病是指较大动脉的穿支动脉闭塞，通常是由于微动脉粥样硬化或脂肪玻璃样变引起的，这是一种以脂肪和蛋白质类物质沉积为特征的血管退行性疾病。血液疾病和凝血障碍，包括白血病、原发性巨球蛋白血症、红细胞增多症、原发性和继发性抗磷脂抗体综合征以及凝血级联反应的遗传缺陷，也可能导致闭塞性血栓和栓塞。

脑部血液循环在某些重要方面与全身循环不同。首先，大脑受到之前描述的血管吻合系统的保护。其次，在全身血压波动时大脑血管自动调节维持恒定的脑灌注压（图13.3）。脑小动脉具有发育良好的肌层，可以在血压升高时收缩，在血压降低时扩张。脑小动脉对外周动脉二氧化碳（$PaCO_2$）和氧气（PaO_2）浓度的变化极为敏感。当二氧化碳分压降低时（例如过度通气），小动脉收缩，血流量减少。在健康个体中，大脑的自动调节功能可以在60～140 mmHg的平均动脉压范围内维持恒定的脑血流量。然而，在慢性高血压患者中，自动调节曲线会向右移动，因此即使是血压的微小降低大脑可能也无法耐受。此外，当血压超过

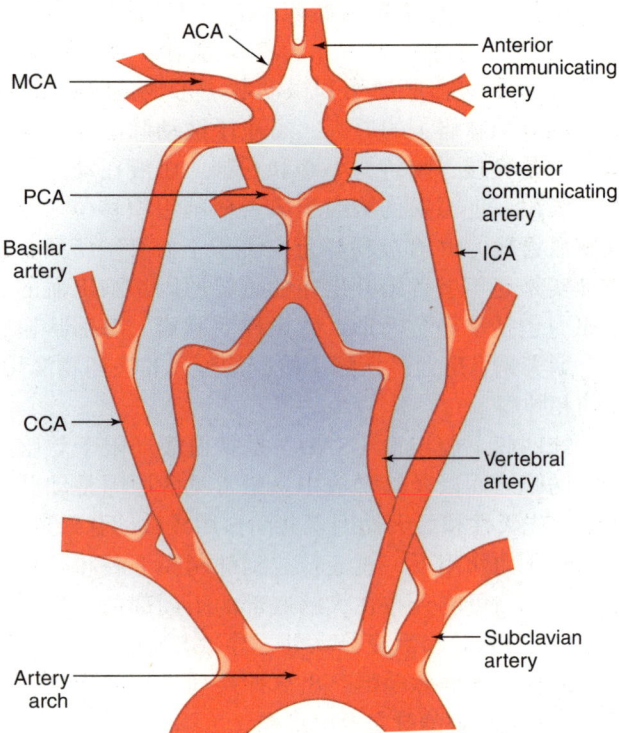

Fig. 13.2 Sites of predilection for atheromatous plaque. *ACA,* Anterior cerebral artery; *CCA,* common carotid artery; *ICA,* internal carotid artery; *MCA,* middle cerebral artery; *PCA,* posterior cerebral artery. (From Caplan LR: Stroke: a clinical approach, ed 2, Boston, 1993, Butterworth-Heinemann.)

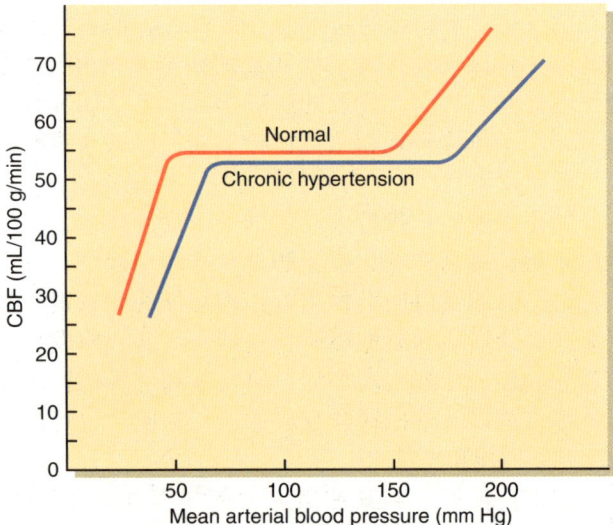

Fig. 13.3 Autoregulatory cerebral blood flow (CBF) response to changes in mean arterial pressure in normotensive and chronically hypertensive persons. Note the shift of the curve toward higher mean pressures with chronic hypertension. (From Pulsinelli WA: Cerebrovascular diseases-principles. In Goldman L, Bennett JC, editors: Cecil textbook of medicine, ed 21, Philadelphia, 2000, Saunders, p 2097.)

In the setting of infarction or hemorrhage, cerebral autoregulation is also impaired, resulting in cerebral dependence on systemic blood pressure to maintain adequate perfusion. Thus, decreasing the blood pressure in the setting of acute ischemia may be hazardous.

Specific disorders may originate from autoregulatory dysfunction: posterior reversible encephalopathy syndrome (PRES) and the reversible cerebral vasoconstriction syndrome (RCVS). In posterior reversible encephalopathy syndrome, there is loss of autoregulatory control with leakage of fluid across the blood-brain barrier, primarily in the posterior regions of the brain. Patients present with elevated blood pressures, headaches, seizures, and loss of visual function. Reversible cerebral vasoconstriction syndrome, a recently recognized syndrome, remains incompletely characterized, and shares features with posterior reversible encephalopathy syndrome. The two disorders overlap in 10% or more of cases. Patients with RCVS are typically young women who present with acute, severe headache, have minimal or no neurologic deficits, and may have evidence of non-aneurysmal, superficial SAH as well as vasospasm of the cerebral arteries. Sympathetic innervation of the vessels is also less in the posterior circulation than anteriorly, leading to a reduced ability of the posterior circulation to adapt to changes in blood pressure, and may contribute to the propensity for edema to form in the occipital lobes during hypertensive crises.

In addition, focal cerebral activity, such as occurs when activating brain regions responsible for moving a limb, is accompanied by increased metabolic activity in the appropriate region, and is accommodated by slight increases in local blood flow and oxygen delivery. Exploitation of this increased local energy demand and delivery is what allows imaging of functional brain activity using MRI, which can detect subtle changes in regional cerebral blood flow. These changes in blood flow are mediated by the neurovascular unit, a complex structure characterized by the local interaction of neural, glial, and vascular elements in the brain. Intracerebral capillaries also lack adventitia, with astrocytes serving as the vascular component of the neurovascular unit. Tight junctions at the capillary level play an important role in the blood-brain barrier, which limits permeability between the vascular compartment and the brain tissue.

Injury to Brain Tissue

The adult brain weighs about 1500 g, or 2% of total body weight, but accounts for 20% of the total body oxygen consumption. Because the brain cannot store much energy, dysfunction results after only a few minutes of deprivation when either oxygen or glucose content is reduced below critical levels. In the resting state, normal total cerebral blood flow is 50 mL/min per 100 g of brain tissue.

Neuronal dysfunction occurs at cerebral blood flow levels below 50 mg/dL, and irreversible neuronal injury begins at levels below 30 mg/dL. Both the degree and duration of reductions in cerebral blood flow are related to the likelihood of permanent neuronal injury. When blood supply is completely interrupted for 30 seconds, brain metabolism is altered; after 1 minute, neuronal function may cease. After 5 minutes, anoxia initiates a chain of events that may result in cerebral infarction; however, if oxygenated blood flow is restored quickly enough, the damage may be reversible, as with a TIA.

Research into the cellular basis of cerebral ischemia has led to the concept of the "ischemic cascade." As perfusion of the brain decreases, a chain of events at the neuronal level begins with failure of the membrane sodium/potassium (Na/K) pump, the depolarization of the neuronal membrane, the release of excitatory neurotransmitters such as glutamate and glycine that hyperstimulate their receptors, and the opening of calcium channels. Calcium enters the neuron through various voltage-sensitive and receptor-mediated channels (e.g., the *N*-methyl-D-aspartate receptor). The influx of calcium is at the root of further neuronal injury, leading to damage to organelles and further destabilization of neuronal metabolism and function. These events may lead to neuronal death, which may be delayed, even after

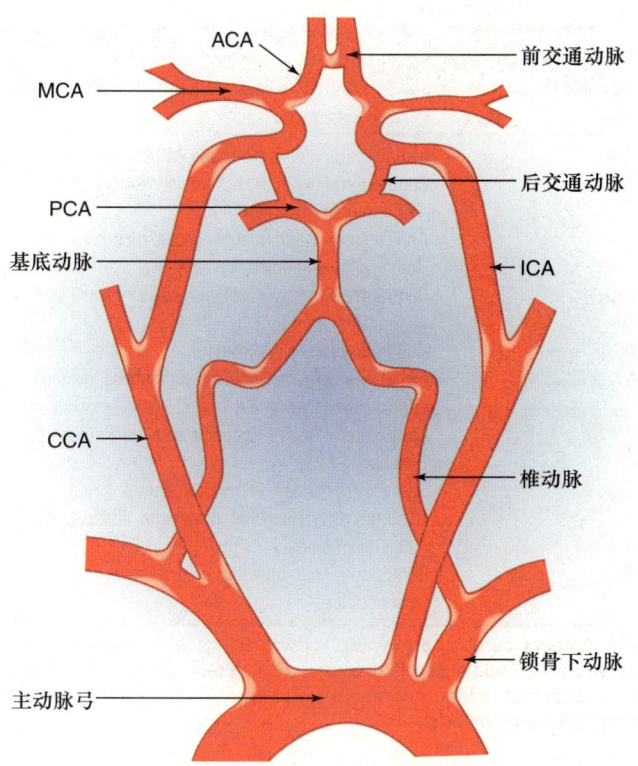

图13.2 动脉粥样硬化斑块的常见部位。ACA，大脑前动脉；CCA，颈总动脉；ICA，颈内动脉；MCA，大脑中动脉；PCA，大脑后动脉。（引自 Caplan LR: Stroke: a clinical approach, ed 2, Boston, 1993, ButterworthHeinemann.）

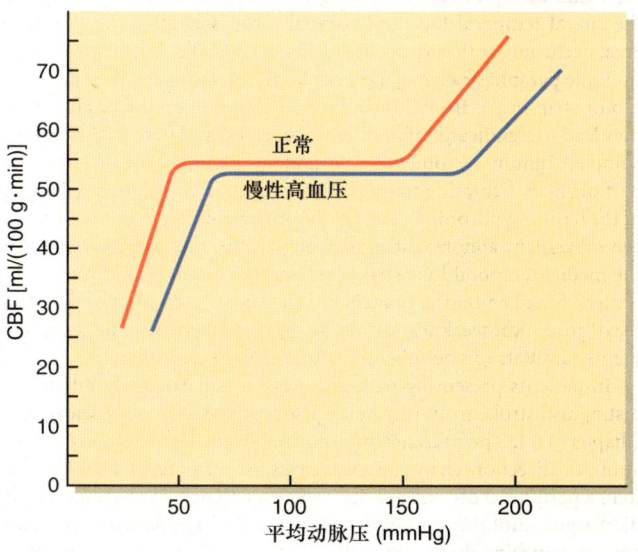

图13.3 正常血压和慢性高血压个体的平均动脉压变化时，脑血流量（CBF）的自动调节反应。请注意，在慢性高血压患者中，曲线向更高的平均压力偏移。（引自 Pulsinelli WA: Cerebrovascular diseases-principles. In Goldman L, Bennett JC, editors: Cecil textbook of medicine, ed 21, Philadelphia, 2000, Saunders, p 2097.）

极限血压水平时，例如严重高血压，大脑自动调节功能可能会被击垮，导致突破性脑出血和水肿。

在梗死或出血的情况下，大脑自动调节功能也会受损，导致大脑依赖系统血压来维持足够的灌注。因此，在急性缺血的情况下进行降血压治疗可能是危险的。

大脑自动调节功能障碍可能导致特定的疾病：可逆性后部脑病综合征（PRES）和可逆性脑血管收缩综合征（RCVS）。在PRES中，大脑失去了自动调节功能，导致脑脊液经血脑屏障发生渗漏，主要集中在大脑的后部区域。患者会出现血压升高、头痛、癫痫发作和视力丧失。RCVS是一种最近才被认识的综合征，其特点尚未完全明确，并且与PRES有共同之处。这两种疾病在10%或更多的病例中存在重叠。RCVS患者通常是年轻女性，表现为急性、严重的头痛，几乎没有或完全没有神经功能损伤，并且合并非动脉瘤性凸面SAH以及脑动脉痉挛。与大脑前循环相比，大脑后循环的血管受交感神经支配较少，导致后循环适应血压变化的能力下降，这可能是高血压危象期间枕叶容易形成水肿的原因。

此外，当激活负责肢体运动的大脑区域时，会产生局部脑活动，并伴有相应脑区代谢活动增加，且局部血流和氧气输送轻微增加。这种局部能量需求和供应的增加，使得通过MRI进行功能性脑活动成像成为可能，其可检测到局部脑血流的细微变化。这些血流变化由神经血管单元介导，神经血管单元是一个复杂的结构，以神经元、胶质细胞和血管的局部相互作用为特征。由于脑内毛细血管缺乏外膜层，因此星形胶质细胞作为神经血管单元中的血管成分发挥作用。毛细血管水平的紧密连接在血脑屏障中起着重要作用，限制了血管腔与脑组织之间的通透性。

脑组织损伤

成人大脑的重量约为1500 g，占总体重的2%，但占全身总耗氧量的20%。由于大脑无法储存太多能量，当氧气或葡萄糖含量降至临界水平以下时，仅几分钟就会导致脑功能障碍。在静息状态下，正常脑血流量为每100 g脑组织50 ml/min。

当脑血流量低于50 mg/dl（译者注：原文有误，应为50 ml/min）时，就会发生神经功能障碍，当低于30 mg/dl（译者注：应为30 ml/min）时，开始出现不可逆的神经元损伤。脑血流减少的程度和持续时间都与永久性神经元损伤有关。当血液供应完全中断30 s时，大脑代谢发生改变；1 min后，神经元功能可能停止。5 min后，缺氧会引发一系列可能导致脑梗死的事件；然而，如果含氧血液流动能够迅速恢复，损伤或许是可逆的，如TIA。

脑缺血的细胞基础研究提出了"缺血级联反应"的概念。随着大脑灌注的减少，神经元发生一系列改变，包括神经元膜上的钠/钾（Na/K）泵失活、神经元膜去极化、兴奋性神经递质释放（如谷氨酸和甘氨酸，这些神经递质会过度刺激其受体），以及钙离子通道开放。钙通过各种电压敏感性通道和受体介导通道（如N-甲基-D-天冬氨酸受体）进入神经元。钙离子内流是神经元进一步损伤的根本原因，导致细胞器损伤以及神经元代谢和功能的进一步不稳定。这些事件可能导致神经元死亡，即使在血流恢复后也可能造成迟发

restoration of blood flow, and are a target of experimental neuroprotective strategies.

Recent research has distinguished between the "core" infarct and an "ischemic penumbra," or shadow. The core represents a central region of necrosis, or tissue that dies very quickly after blood flow ceases. The penumbra represents the surrounding region of brain tissue, in which neurons are dysfunctional but potentially salvageable. Recanalization of occluded vessels with blood flow into infarcted tissue, particularly when delayed, results in "reperfusion injury." Increased use of MRI has shown that petechial hemorrhagic infarction is very common, occurring in the majority of strokes, even when not suspected clinically.

CLINICAL PRESENTATION

The signs and symptoms of strokes are varied and depend on the type of stroke, the region of the nervous system affected by the lack of flow or hemorrhage, and the patient's handedness (Table 13.3). In general, embolic ischemic strokes are characterized by the sudden onset of a neurologic deficit, usually painless. Thrombotic strokes may have a stuttering or progressive course due to fluctuating hypoperfusion and gradual occlusion. Arterial dissections, as well as hemorrhages, are more often associated with headaches than ischemic stroke of other causes. Hemorrhagic strokes and large hemispheric infarcts can lead to decrease in consciousness due to increased intracranial pressure.

Most emboli occur in the territory of the MCAs. Lesions of the dominant (almost always left) hemisphere are characterized by variable combinations of right hemiparesis, right hemisensory loss, right visual loss, impaired gaze to the right side of space, and language disturbance. When the superior division of the MCA is affected, the language impairment is predominantly motor: the patient either cannot speak or produces sparse, agrammatic speech, despite an ability to fully comprehend spoken and written material. When the inferior division is affected, the patient may produce fluent, prosodic (normal stress and intonation), but nonsensical speech and be unable to follow instructions. Larger infarcts of the dominant hemisphere produce a total loss of language function, leaving the patient mute and uncomprehending.

Lesions of the nondominant (right) hemisphere produce deficits of the left side of the body. Language is preserved but the patient may demonstrate impaired attention, particularly to the left side of space; fail to appreciate the presence of people or objects to their left; and may even fail to recognize the left side of their own body (asomatognosia). This neglect phenomenon may extend even to a lack of awareness of any deficit of function on their part (anosognosia). These patients may thus be found at home, lying on the floor paralyzed yet unaware that anything is the matter; their unawareness can delay their presentation to the hospital for treatment and similarly limit their participation in rehabilitation. Lesions in the right hemisphere may also cause dysprosody, the nondominant equivalent of aphasia, which is characterized by a lack of the emotional and gestural components of speech, despite preservation of its semantic content; many of these patients have a flat affect or appear to be depressed.

Infarcts in the territory of the anterior cerebral arteries often cause weakness limited to the legs, due to location of the representation of the legs in the medial part of the hemispheres. They may have incontinence, lack initiative (abulia), and have gaze palsies. In some cases their deficits may be more extensive and mimic those of MCA infarctions. Posterior cerebral artery infarcts lead to visual loss, often without any motor deficit. With involvement of the medial temporal lobes supplied by the PCAs, there may also be behavioral disturbances, including delirium and amnesia.

Brain stem infarcts cause specific syndromes due to the affected neural pathways and nuclei. Midbrain infarcts often produce vertical gaze deficits and impaired consciousness if the reticular activating system is involved.

TABLE 13.3 Clinical Manifestations of Ischemic Stroke

Occluded Vessel	Clinical Signs
ICA	Ipsilateral blindness (variable), MCA syndrome
MCA	Contralateral hemiparesis, hemisensory loss (face or arm more than leg)
	Aphasia (dominant) or anosognosia (nondominant)
	Homonymous hemianopsia (variable)
ACA	Contralateral hemiparesis, hemisensory loss (leg more than arm)
	Abulia (especially if bilateral)
VA or PICA	Ipsilateral facial sensory loss, hemiataxia, nystagmus, Horner syndrome
	Contralateral loss of temperature or pain sensation
	Dysphagia
SCA	Gait ataxia, nausea, vertigo, dysarthria
BA	Quadriparesis, dysarthria, dysphagia, diplopia, somnolence, amnesia
PCA	Contralateral homonymous hemianopsia, amnesia, sensory loss

ACA, Anterior cerebral artery; *BA*, basilar artery; *ICA*, internal carotid artery; *MCA*, middle cerebral artery; *PCA*, posterior cerebral artery; *PICA*, posterior inferior cerebellar artery; *SCA*, superior cerebellar artery; *VA*, vertebral artery.

Many cerebral infarctions do not cause weakness and may therefore be missed by the less astute clinician who assumes that a stroke always leads to paralysis. These syndromes include fluent (or Wernicke) aphasia, cortical visual loss, and Wallenberg syndrome (lateral medullary syndrome caused by occlusion of the vertebral or posterior inferior cerebellar artery). Because the inferior division of the MCA supplies the lateral temporal lobe and parietal lobes, including the Wernicke area, occlusion of that vessel may cause a prosodic, fluent speech with multiple paraphasic errors and poor comprehension, while sparing the motor strip in the frontal lobe. Emboli traveling up the basilar artery may lead to significant infarction in the territory of both PCAs, causing complete blindness, sometimes without awareness of the deficit on the part of the patient, due to infarction of both occipital lobes (the "top of the basilar syndrome"). Behavioral abnormalities, memory loss, and eye movement abnormalities may also occur, due to involvement of the medial temporal lobe structures and the midbrain eye movement centers. Small emboli to branches of the superior division of the MCA may cause focal weakness of the hand, particularly fine finger movements, simulating a peripheral compression neuropathy.

In patients presenting with dizziness, it is particularly difficult to distinguish stroke from vestibular neuronitis or Meniere's disease (see Chapter 10). The presence of a normal head-thrust test, skew deviation, or direction-changing nystagmus are all signs of stroke, rather than a peripheral cause. Patients in the emergency ward should not be discharged until they can walk without imbalance; patients with nausea and vomiting due to cerebellar infarction may develop fatal brain stem compression due to swelling (so-called "fatal gastroenteritis").

The signs and symptoms of *subarachnoid hemorrhage* differ from other stroke types due to the absence of focal deficits. Instead, patients present with abrupt onset of severe headache (i.e., "the worst headache of my life"), vomiting, altered consciousness, and sometimes coma, typically without localizing signs.

Thrombosis of cerebral veins or the larger draining dural sinuses present with a combination of headache due to elevated intracranial pressure, seizures, and focal deficits due to hemorrhage. Rarely the

性损伤，因此钙离子通道是神经保护研究的重要靶点。

近期研究将"核心"梗死与"缺血半暗带"或阴影进行区分。核心梗死区代表坏死的中心区域，即血流停止后迅速死亡的脑组织。缺血半暗带则代表周围的脑组织区域，其中的神经元功能失调但可能具有挽救价值。闭塞血管的再通，尤其是迟发再通时，血液流入梗死组织，会导致"再灌注损伤"。MRI 的更多应用显示点状出血性梗死非常常见，即使没有临床症状，但是在大多数卒中事件中均存在。

临床表现

卒中的症状多种多样，取决于卒中类型、缺血或出血导致的神经系统受累区域以及患者的惯用手（表 13.3）。一般而言，栓塞性缺血性卒中的特点是神经功能突然丧失，不伴疼痛。血栓性卒中可能会由于脑血流灌注不足和逐渐闭塞而出现口吃或病程逐渐加重。动脉夹层和脑出血往往比其他原因引起的缺血性卒中更容易引起头痛。由于颅内压升高，出血性卒中和大脑半球大面积梗死可能导致意识下降。

大多数栓塞发生在 MCA 区域。优势半球（几乎总是左侧）的病变表现为右侧偏瘫、右侧感觉丧失、右侧视力丧失、向右凝视障碍和语言障碍的不同组合。当 MCA 的上支受累时，语言障碍主要是运动性失语：患者或不能说话，或只能发出稀疏、语法错误的言语，尽管他们能够完全理解口头和书面材料。当下支受累时，患者可能会说出流利、抑扬顿挫（正常的重音和语调）但毫无意义的言语，且无法按照指令行事。优势半球较大的梗死会导致语言功能完全丧失，使患者变得沉默且无法理解。

非优势半球（右侧）病变会导致身体左侧出现缺陷。语言功能得以保留，但患者可能表现出注意力受损，尤其是对左侧空间的注意力；无法意识到左侧的人或物体；甚至可能无法识别自己身体的左侧（躯体失认）。这种忽视现象甚至可能扩展到患者对自己的功能丧失缺乏认知（病感失认）。因此，这些患者可能会在家中被发现瘫痪倒地却不自知，而这可能会延误治疗，同时也会限制他们开展康复治疗。右侧大脑半球的病变也可能导致言语声律障碍，相当于失语症的非显性症状，其特点是尽管保留了语义内容，但言语中缺乏情感和手势，多数患者表现为情感淡漠或看上去情绪低落。

大脑前动脉区域的梗死通常会导致腿部力量减弱，因为控制腿部运动的皮质在大脑半球的内侧。患者可能会出现大小便失禁、缺乏主动性（意志缺失）和凝视麻痹。在某些情况下，他们的症状可能会更加广泛，类似 MCA 梗死的表现。大脑后动脉（PCA）梗死会导致视力丧失，但通常不会出现运动障碍。如果 PCA 供应的内侧颞叶受累，还可能出现行为障碍，包括谵妄和遗忘症。

表 13.3 缺血性卒中的临床表现	
闭塞血管	临床征象
ICA	同侧失明（可变），MCA 综合征
MCA	对侧偏瘫，偏身感觉丧失（面部或手臂多于腿部） 失语症（优势半球）或病感失认症（非优势半球） 同向偏盲（可变）
ACA	对侧偏瘫，偏身感觉丧失（腿部多于手臂） 意志缺失（尤其如果是双侧）
VA 或 PICA	同侧面部感觉丧失、偏身共济失调、眼球震颤、霍纳综合征 对侧温度觉或痛觉丧失 吞咽困难
SCA	步态共济失调、恶心、眩晕、构音障碍
BA	四肢麻痹、构音障碍、吞咽困难、复视、嗜睡、遗忘症
PCA	对侧同向偏盲、遗忘症、感觉丧失

ACA，大脑前动脉；BA，基底动脉；ICA，颈内动脉；MCA，大脑中动脉；PCA，大脑后动脉；PICA，小脑后下动脉；SCA，小脑上动脉；VA，椎动脉。

脑干梗死由于受损的神经通路和神经核团不同，会导致特定的综合征。中脑梗死如果累及网状激活系统，往往会导致垂直凝视麻痹和意识障碍。

许多脑梗死不会引起肢体无力，因此，如果临床医生不够警觉，或者认为卒中总是会导致瘫痪，那么这些脑梗死可能会被漏诊。这些综合征包括流利性（或 Wernicke）失语症、皮质盲和 Wallenberg 综合征（由椎动脉或小脑后下动脉闭塞引起的延髓背外侧综合征）。由于 MCA 的下支为颞叶外侧和顶叶（包括 Wernicke 区）供血，该血管的闭塞可能导致出现抑扬顿挫、流畅的言语，但错语和赘语多，理解能力下降，而大脑额叶的运动带功能则未受影响。沿基底动脉向上游走的栓子可能导致双侧 PCA 区域的严重梗死，导致完全失明，有时由于双侧枕叶梗死（基底动脉尖综合征），患者甚至无法意识到自己的功能障碍。由于内侧颞叶和中脑眼球运动中心的受累，患者还可能出现行为异常、记忆力丧失和眼球运动障碍。MCA 上支的小栓子可能导致手部无力，尤其是精细的手指运动，类似外周压迫性神经病。

在出现眩晕症状的患者中，区分卒中与前庭神经元炎或梅尼埃病（见第 10 章）是一大难题。正常的甩头试验、反向偏斜或变向性眼震均是卒中的表现，而非外周原因所致。急诊室的患者在能够稳定行走之前不应出院。由于小脑梗死而出现恶心和呕吐的患者可能会因小脑肿胀而导致致命的脑干受压（所谓的"致命性胃肠炎"）。

蛛网膜下腔出血（SAH）的症状和体征与其他类型的卒中不同，因为没有局灶性功能缺损。相反，患者会突然出现严重头痛（即"我生命中最严重的头痛"）、呕吐、意识改变，有时还会出现昏迷，但通常没有定位体征。

脑静脉或较大的引流硬脑膜窦的血栓形成，会表现为颅内压升高引起的头痛、癫痫发作和出血引起的局灶性神经功能缺损的组合形式。罕见的霹雳样头痛

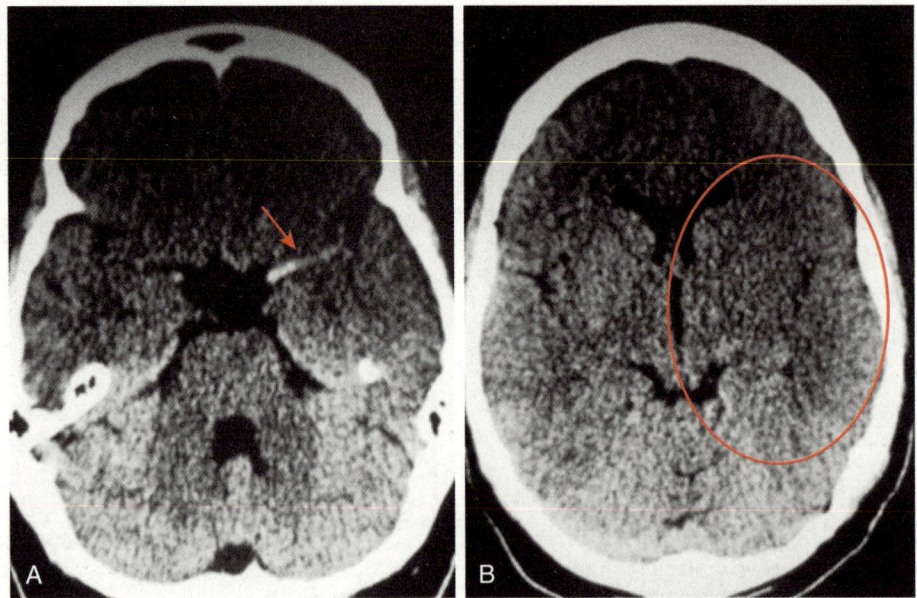

Fig. 13.4 Early signs of infarction on computed tomography of the brain. (A) Hyperdense middle cerebral artery sign *(red arrow)*, and (B) hypoattenuation of the left caudate and lentiform nuclei, loss of the insular ribbon, and sulcal effacement *(outlined in red)*.

syndrome of *thunderclap headache*, or sudden severe headache without any focal signs similar to that occurring in SAH, may be due to venous thrombosis. Occlusion of the cerebral venous sinuses may occur in association with hyperviscosity or a hypercoagulable state, including pregnancy or hormonal contraceptive use. Imaging findings include bilateral hemorrhagic infarctions in a parasagittal distribution and extensive white matter edema. Contrast-enhanced CT may demonstrate the *empty delta* sign, indicating a filling defect in the sagittal sinus. Magnetic resonance venography (MRV) and T1-weighted MRI images confirm the presence of thrombus; cerebral angiography is seldom needed to confirm the diagnosis.

DIAGNOSIS AND DIFFERENTIAL DIAGNOSIS

The potential benefit of thrombolytic therapy within 4.5 hours of onset of acute ischemic stroke requires urgent differentiation of ischemic stroke from hemorrhage and other causes of sudden neurologic symptoms. Headache, vomiting, seizures, and coma are more common in hemorrhagic stroke, though these are never reliable enough to preclude imaging. The distinction is straightforward in most cases once a head CT is performed. The hyperdense signal of blood in the parenchyma on CT almost invariably distinguishes hemorrhage from ischemia. In exceptional cases the typical hyperdensity of ICH is absent owing to severe anemia or to its subacute state, during which blood may be indistinguishable from brain tissue. Certain imaging findings on initial CT further support a presumed diagnosis of infarction, such as a hyperdense vessel sign indicative of thrombus in the vessel, or loss of the gray-white junction and sulci in the cortex, and loss of the demarcation of the insular cortex and deep gray nuclei, both of which are early indicators of ischemia and edema (Fig. 13.4). CT angiography often identifies the site of vascular occlusion.

Imaging in the setting of suspected acute ischemia does not definitively diagnose ischemia but rather excludes hemorrhage; if clinical symptoms are consistent with cerebral ischemia, then thrombolytic treatment is indicated within the appropriate time window. Primary stroke centers must perform and interpret CT scans within 30 minutes of the arrival of a patient with suspected stroke. MRI can also effectively exclude acute hemorrhage, and diffusion-weighted imaging sequences are more sensitive to the earliest changes of ischemia (Fig. 13.5), but the speed and availability of CT make it the initial imaging modality of choice at most centers. MRI scanning may then be used to provide additional information. Specific MRI sequences have greater sensitivity to blood than CT and may identify hemorrhagic infarction missed by CT.

Clinical features at stroke onset may suggest a subtype of cerebral infarction but require confirmatory laboratory data. Cerebral embolism is suggested by sudden onset and a syndrome of circumscribed focal signs attributable to cerebral surface infarction, such as pure aphasia or pure hemianopia. Unless the source of embolization is obvious on hospital admission, blood cultures, electrocardiographic monitoring, and echocardiography are indicated.

A diagnosis of atherosclerotic infarction is suggested if there were previous TIAs, particularly when the symptoms are stereotypical. Doppler ultrasonography, CT angiography or magnetic resonance angiography can usually identify the stenosis. In equivocal cases, conventional angiography may be needed. Small penetrating vessel infarcts, or *lacunar infarcts*, usually spare cortical functions, such as language and cognition, but cause loss of elementary neurologic function, such as strength, sensation, and coordination. Up to 25% of patients with lacunar infarcts have large-vessel disease or a cardioembolic source, so it is important to carry out a complete etiologic evaluation in all stroke patients.

Up to 50% of patients with transient deficits lasting less than 24 hours have evidence of infarction on imaging, and the risk of stroke and other vascular events is as high after TIA as after completed stroke. In the acute setting, when decisions about thrombolysis must be made, it is virtually impossible to know which patients with ischemia will have symptoms resolve without infarction (thus, having a TIA) and which will have a completed infarction. Patients with either stroke or TIA need immediate attention to secondary prevention strategies. In terms of choosing treatments, the important issue is to identify the cause of the cerebral ischemia, rather than its duration. Entities other than cerebral ischemia can masquerade as strokes and TIAs. Among patients diagnosed with stroke in emergency departments, 20% or

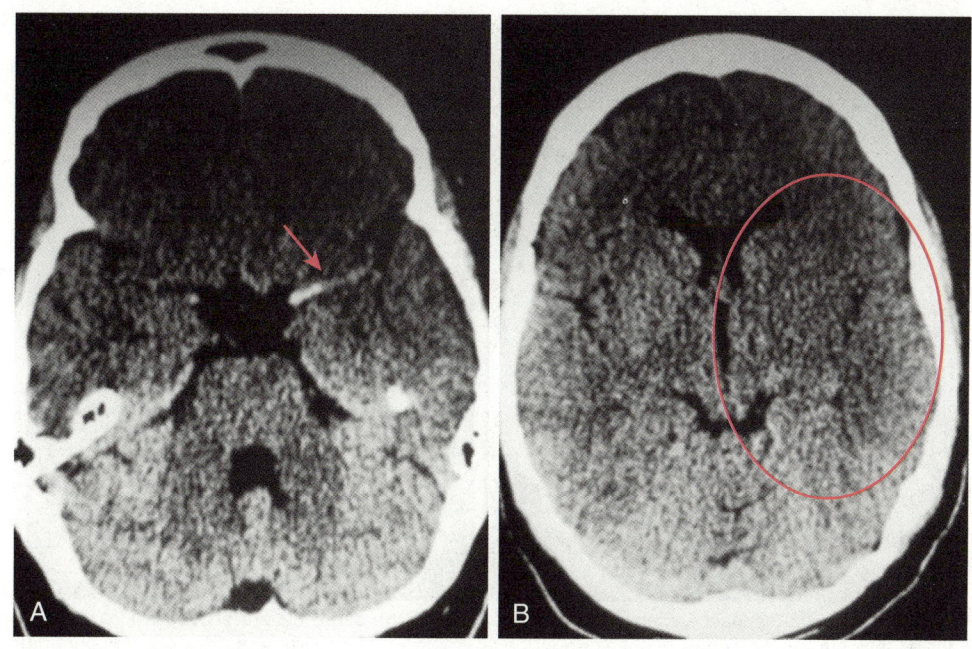

图 13.4 脑计算机断层成像中梗死的早期征象。（A）大脑中动脉高密度征（红色箭头）；（B）左侧尾状核和豆状核的低密度影，岛带消失，脑沟变浅（红色勾勒区）

综合征，或突然出现的严重头痛而无任何局灶性体征，类似于 SAH 时的症状，可能是由静脉血栓形成引起的。脑静脉窦的闭塞可能与血液高黏滞状态或高凝状态有关，包括妊娠或使用激素类避孕药。影像学检查结果包括双侧出血性梗死，呈矢状旁分布，并有广泛的脑白质水肿。增强 CT 可显示空三角征，表明矢状窦内存在充盈缺损。磁共振静脉成像（MRV）和 T1 加权图像可证实血栓的存在，通常很少需要脑血管造影来确诊。

诊断与鉴别诊断

急性缺血性卒中发作后 4.5 h 内进行溶栓治疗具有潜在获益，因此需要迅速区分缺血性卒中、出血性卒中以及导致突发神经症状的其他原因。头痛、呕吐、癫痫发作和昏迷在出血性卒中更为常见，但仅靠这些症状不足以诊断，必须进一步进行影像学检查。大多数情况下，头部 CT 检查观察到脑实质内血液的高密度信号可以直接区分出血和缺血。在特殊情况下，由于严重贫血或脑出血亚急性期，ICH 的典型高密度可能不存在，从而导致无法区分血液与脑组织。初始 CT 上的某些影像学征象可进一步支持脑梗死诊断，如血管高密度征表明血管内有血栓，或大脑皮质的灰白质交界或脑沟消失、岛叶皮质和深部灰质核团之间的界限消失，这两者都是缺血和水肿的早期标志（图 13.4）。CT 血管成像（CTA）通常能确定血管闭塞的部位。

在疑似急性缺血的情况下进行影像学检查并不能明确诊断缺血，而是排除出血；如果临床症状与脑缺血一致，那么应在时间窗内进行溶栓治疗。一级卒中中心必须在疑似卒中患者到达后 30 min 内进行 CT 扫描并解读影像。

MRI 也能有效排除急性出血，而弥散加权成像序列对缺血的早期变化更为敏感（图 13.5），但 CT 更加快捷且普及，因此 CT 是大多数中心首选的首次成像方式。随后可以使用 MRI 检查获取额外信息。特定的 MRI 序列对血液的敏感性高于 CT，并可能识别出 CT 遗漏的出血性梗死。

卒中发作时的临床特征可能提示脑梗死的亚型，但需要实验室数据来证实。脑栓塞常表现为突然发作和由脑表面梗死引起的局灶性症状综合征，如单纯失语或偏盲。除非入院时对栓塞来源十分确定，否则应进行血培养、心电图监测和超声心动图检查。

如果之前有过 TIA，特别是症状刻板发作时，则提示为动脉粥样硬化性梗死。经颅多普勒超声、CTA 或磁共振血管成像（MRA）通常可以识别血管狭窄。在不确定时，则需要进行血管造影术。小穿支血管梗死或腔隙性梗死通常不会损伤皮质功能，如语言和认知，但会导致基本神经功能丧失，如力量、感觉和协调功能。高达 25% 的腔隙性梗死患者合并大血管疾病或心源性栓塞，因此对所有卒中患者进行全面的病因学评估非常重要。

高达 50% 症状持续时间小于 24 h 的 TIA 患者可以在影像学上发现梗死病灶，并且在 TIA 后发生卒中和其他血管事件的风险均与缺血性卒中发生后一样。在急性情况下，当必须做出溶栓决定时，几乎不可能知道哪些缺血患者的症状会消失，且没有梗死灶（即发生 TIA），哪些会出现完全性梗死。卒中或 TIA 患者都需要立即采取二级预防措施。在选择治疗方法时，重要的是要确定脑缺血的原因，而不是其持续时间。除了脑缺血之外，还有其他疾病可能模拟卒中和 TIA。在急诊科被诊断为卒中的患者中，至少 20% 的患者是假

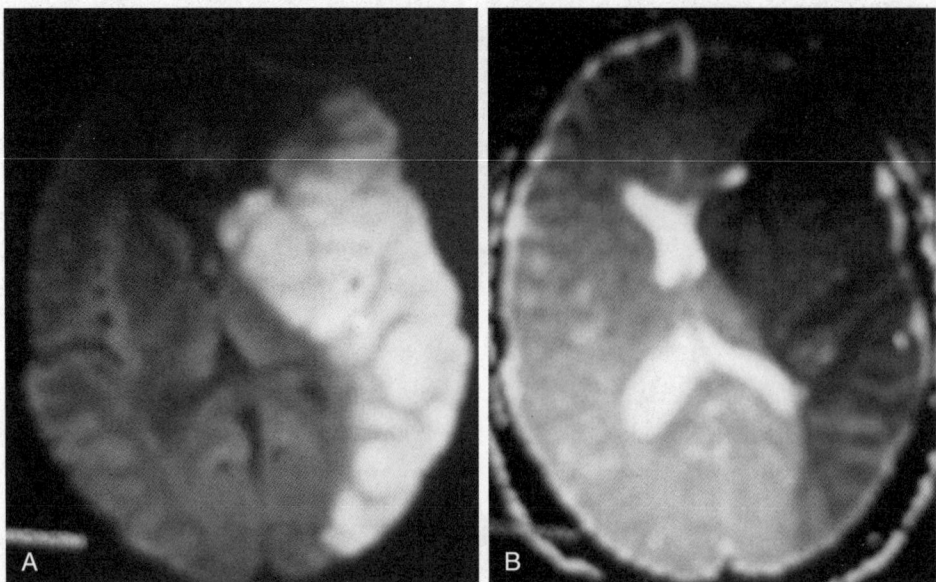

Fig. 13.5 Magnetic resonance imaging scan of the brain of the same patient shown in Fig. 13.4. (A) Diffusion-weighted image shows bright signal in the left middle cerebral artery territory. (B) Apparent diffusion coefficient shows dark signal in the same area, confirming acute infarction.

more have a stroke *mimic*, including seizure, migraine, systemic infection, brain tumor, and toxic-metabolic encephalopathy. Other sources of misdiagnosis are listed in Table 13.4.

In patients with a prior history of cerebral infarct or hemorrhage, new *metabolic derangements*, including infections, may precipitate a recrudescence of the original stroke syndrome. Hypoglycemia, hyponatremia, urinary tract infection, pneumonia, and initiation of a psychotropic medication can each precipitate this phenomenon. The patient returns to normal over hours to days when the new insult is treated or reversed. Such metabolic and infectious causes of neurologic deterioration should be excluded in patients with a history of earlier brain injury before diagnosing a new stroke. Focal signs may also occur with metabolic disturbances in patients without prior history of stroke.

External signs of injury are usually present in brain *trauma*, but they need not be present after acceleration-deceleration injury, such as from a motor vehicle accident. The most frequent sites of brain contusions are the frontal and temporal poles, which are not typical locations for strokes.

Seizures may occasionally complicate acute stroke, but they may also mimic stroke. Unlike stroke, seizures are often characterized by obtundation, an amnestic state, clonic activity, incontinence, or tongue biting. The postictal deficit, often called a *Todd paralysis*, resembles stroke because weakness or language and other cortical deficits may occur. The deficits after seizure usually resolve within hours after the seizure but occasionally persist for up to a week, making the distinction from stroke difficult. Seizures may also develop months or years after an infarct or hemorrhage, and the postictal state in these patients may recapitulate the initial stroke syndrome.

Migraine with persistent aura often mimics stroke or TIA. Aura alone, without headache (i.e., acephalgic migraine), is sometimes experienced by those who previously suffered from migraine with aura. Migraine aura typically produces a visual disturbance that marches across the vision of both eyes as an advancing, enlarging blind spot that takes 20 to 30 minutes to resolve. Subsequent unilateral, pounding headache suggests the diagnosis but may not occur. Less often, migrainous auras take the form of sensory symptoms. The speed of the march is generally slower than the rapid spread of symptoms in stroke.

As many as 10% of *brain tumors* present with acute transient symptoms reflecting intratumoral hemorrhage or focal seizures. Seizures often precede focal signs. Imaging usually demonstrates an enhancing mass even when symptoms are mild.

TABLE 13.4 Stroke Mimics and Differential Diagnosis

Common Mimics
Metabolic encephalopathy (e.g., hypoglycemia, hyponatremia)
Systemic infection
Seizure
Migraine
Brain tumors

Other Mimics
Transient focal neurologic symptoms associated with amyloid angiopathy
Positional vertigo
Cardiac events
Syncope
Trauma (especially acceleration-deceleration without evidence of external injury)
Subdural hematoma
Herpes simplex virus encephalitis
Transient global amnesia
Dementia
Demyelinating disease
Cervical spine disease/radiculopathy/fracture
Myasthenia gravis
Parkinsonism
Hypertensive encephalopathy
Conversion disorder
Intoxication/substance abuse

TREATMENT

Stroke prevention and treatment are directed toward: (1) preventing the first stroke (primary prevention); (2) limiting damage from the stroke; (3) optimizing functional recovery following stroke; and (4)

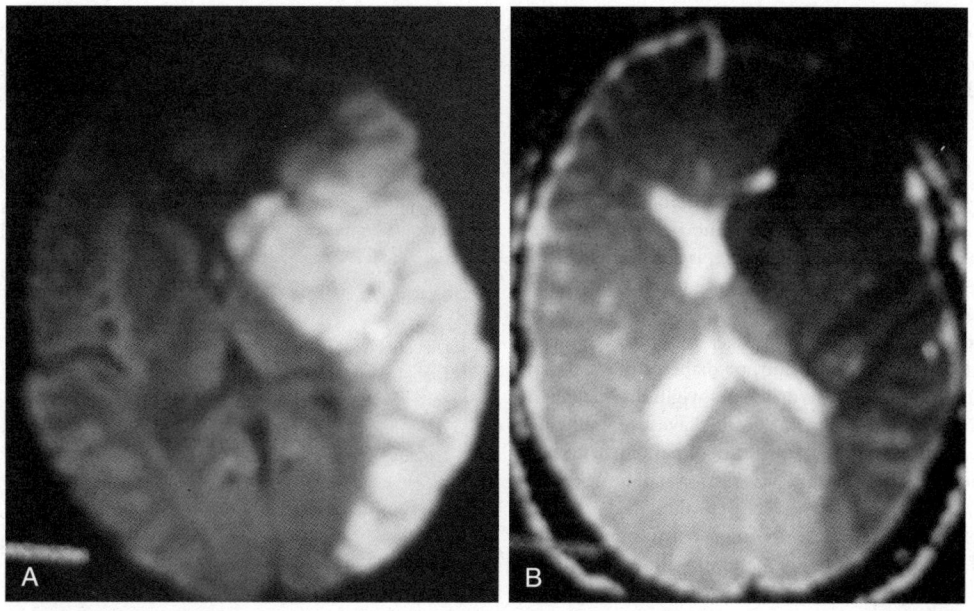

图 13.5 图 13.4 患者的大脑磁共振成像。(**A**) 弥散加权成像显示左侧大脑中动脉供血区高信号。(**B**) 同一区域表观弥散系数显示低信号，证实为急性脑梗死

性卒中，包括癫痫发作、偏头痛、全身感染、脑肿瘤和中毒-代谢性脑病。误诊的其他原因见表 13.4。

对于既往有脑梗死或脑出血病史的患者，新发代谢障碍，包括感染，可能会导致原卒中综合征的复发。低血糖、低钠血症、尿路感染、肺炎以及使用精神类药物都可能诱发这种现象。当新发损伤得到治疗或逆转时，患者会在数小时至数天内恢复正常。在诊断新发卒中之前，应排除有既往脑损伤病史的患者出现神经功能恶化的代谢性和感染性原因。即使在没有卒中病史的患者中，代谢障碍也可能出现局灶性体征。

脑外伤通常伴有外伤体征，但在加速-减速性损伤（如机动车事故）后，这些体征可能不会出现。脑挫伤最常见的部位是额极和颞极，这两个部位不是卒中的典型部位。

癫痫发作有时会并发急性卒中，但也可能模仿卒中症状。与卒中不同，癫痫发作通常以反应迟钝、失忆、阵挛、二便失禁或咬舌为特征。癫痫发作后的后遗症，称为 Todd 瘫痪，与卒中相似，可能出现虚弱、语言障碍和其他皮质缺损症状。通常在癫痫发作后几小时内消失，但偶尔也会持续长达一周，这使得与卒中难以区分。此外，缺血性卒中或出血性卒中后数月或数年也可能出现癫痫发作，且这些患者的癫痫发作后状态可能会重复初次卒中的症状。

伴有持续性先兆的偏头痛常类似卒中或 TIA。曾有先兆偏头痛的患者有时会仅有先兆而没有头痛（非头痛性偏头痛）。偏头痛先兆通常会产生视觉障碍，表现为双眼视野中逐渐扩大、移动的盲点，持续 20～30 min 方可缓解。随后出现单侧搏动性头痛有助于确诊，但也可能不出现。较不常见的是，偏头痛先兆会表现为感觉症状。先兆的进展速度通常比卒中症状进展的速度要慢。

多达 10% 的脑肿瘤会出现急性短暂性神经功能缺损症状，这些症状反映了肿瘤内出血或局灶性癫痫发

表 13.4　卒中模拟病和鉴别诊断
常见卒中模拟病
代谢性脑病（如低血糖症、低钠血症）
系统性感染
癫痫发作
偏头痛
脑肿瘤
其他卒中模拟病
淀粉样血管病相关的短暂性局灶性神经症状
体位性眩晕
心脏事件
晕厥
创伤（特别是没有外部损伤证据的加速-减速性损伤）
硬脑膜下血肿
单纯疱疹病毒性脑炎
短暂性全面性遗忘
痴呆
脱髓鞘疾病
颈椎疾病/神经根病/骨折
重症肌无力
帕金森综合征
高血压脑病
转换障碍
中毒或物质滥用

作。癫痫发作常先于局灶征象。即使症状轻微，影像学也常显示肿瘤强化。

治疗

卒中的预防和治疗旨在：①预防首次卒中（一级预防）；②减轻卒中造成的损害；③优化卒中后的功能康复；④避免复发（二级预防）。治疗和预防的具体措

avoiding recurrence (secondary prevention). Specific measures for treatment and prevention depend on the patient's risk factors and stroke mechanism. The diagnostic evaluation of the stroke patient dictates optimal therapy.

Primary Prevention of Stroke

Randomized trials have demonstrated that specific interventions prevent first stroke among patients with specific risk factors (Table 13.5). Treatment of hypertension, for example, is associated with up to a 45% reduction in the risk of stroke. Among patients with atrial fibrillation, the use of warfarin is associated with a 60% to 70% relative reduction in risk of stroke, though younger patients without any accompanying heart disease, hypertension, or diabetes may be managed with antiplatelet agents alone. Hydroxymethylglutaryl-coenzyme A (HMG-CoA) reductase inhibitors, or statins, have been shown in some primary prevention studies, and in studies of patients with heart disease, to reduce the risk of a first stroke as well as that of heart disease. The effects on stroke risk are more modest than the effects on heart disease, possibly reflecting the greater heterogeneity among causes of stroke compared to heart disease. For patients with asymptomatic carotid stenosis of at least 60%, carotid endarterectomy reduces the risk of stroke, though the effect is much more modest than in symptomatic patients, and the number of patients needed to treat to prevent one stroke is greater. Because many of the large randomized trials of endarterectomy for asymptomatic patients were conducted in the era before the current recommended use of statins and antiplatelet agents, it is no longer clear that surgery is superior to medical therapy. New trials are therefore addressing medical versus surgical and endovascular treatment in patients with asymptomatic stenosis.

Antiplatelet therapy is not of established benefit for prevention of a first stroke. In a large primary prevention study, for example, aspirin use was associated with an increased risk of both ischemic and hemorrhagic stroke, despite reducing the risk of ischemic heart disease. However, other studies have shown that aspirin reduces the risk of ischemic stroke among women over the age of 45.

The Mediterranean diet also protects against cardiovascular disease, including stroke. It is characterized by high intake of fruits, vegetables, and legumes; olive oil as the principal source of fat; moderate consumption of fish and poultry, with minimal intake of red meat and dairy; and an option of mild to moderate consumption of red wine, mostly with meals. Compared to a low-fat diet, this combination of nutrients decreased 5-year stroke risk by approximately 30% in a randomized trial.

Observational studies provide evidence that certain behaviors prevent stroke. Smoking cessation leads to a reduction by 5 years in stroke risk to levels similar to nonsmokers. Consumption of alcohol in moderation, up to two drinks daily for men and one daily for women, is associated with a lower level of stroke risk than in those who do not drink. Physical activity, weight loss when appropriate, and management of diabetes are also recommended.

Acute Treatment of Ischemic Stroke

For patients with ischemic stroke evaluated within 3 hours of symptom onset with no evidence of hemorrhage on a brain CT or MRI, recombinant tissue plasminogen activator (rt-PA), a thrombolytic agent, improves functional outcomes at 3 months compared to placebo. Among the 624 ischemic stroke patients treated within 3 hours in the original landmark study, the proportion of patients achieving normal or near-normal neurologic and functional status by 3 months was significantly higher among those receiving rt-PA, though there was no definite benefit at 24 hours. The proportion of patients who achieved independence in their performance of activities of daily living was increased from 38% to 50%, an absolute benefit of 12%. The absence of an immediate (24-hour) benefit, coupled with the finding of a benefit at 3 months, is consistent with the hypothesis that thrombolytic treatment works to reduce the size of the infarct penumbra by reperfusing tissue before permanent infarction of the entire territory occurs, despite some irreversible injury to a core component.

Patients treated with rt-PA had a 10-fold increase in incidence of hemorrhagic conversion of the infarction (from 0.6% in placebo-treated patients to 6.0% in rt-PA–treated patients). Overall, however, the rates of neurologic deterioration and mortality within the first day after stroke were similar between the groups. Rt-PA was approved for patient use by the US Food and Drug Administration (FDA) in 1996, and it is now considered standard of care for ischemic stroke patients presenting within 3 hours. Specific guidelines for eligibility and exclusion must be met when using rt-PA to reduce the risk of complications (Table 13.6).

Because of the potential to reduce cerebral perfusion below the limits permitted by autoregulation in the setting of acute brain injury, current guidelines recommend that blood pressure not be reduced acutely after ischemic stroke, and systolic blood pressure levels as high as 220 mm Hg are allowed. Before and following thrombolytic treatment, however, systolic blood pressure should be kept below 180 mm Hg to reduce the risk of hemorrhagic conversion. In addition, antiplatelet and anticoagulant medications must be withheld for 24 hours after rt-PA.

Subsequent meta-analyses and individual trials have demonstrated that the benefit of thrombolytic therapy decreases as the time interval between symptom onset (the presumed beginning of ischemia) and treatment increases, but that the therapeutic time window persists as long as 4.5 hours after stroke in selected patients (i.e., those under age 80 years without a combined history of prior ischemic stroke and diabetes mellitus).

In considering the duration of stroke symptoms, neurologists use the time that the patient was last known to be well as the time of onset of the stroke, rather than the time that the patient was discovered to have stroke symptoms. Because stroke is usually painless, patients may not be aware of the onset of symptoms. In patients with aphasia, anosognosia, or diminished consciousness, the patient may not be able to provide details regarding the time of onset of their symptoms, and a witness is required. In patients who wake with stroke,

TABLE 13.5 Evidence-Based Primary Prevention of Ischemic Stroke

Risk Factor	Treatment
Hypertension	Anti-hypertensives
Myocardial infarction	HMG-CoA reductase inhibitors
Hyperlipidemia	HMG-CoA reductase inhibitors
Atrial fibrillation	Anticoagulation (warfarin, other agents)
	Left atrial exclusion (selected patients)
Diabetes mellitus/vascular disease	ACE inhibitor
Diabetes mellitus type II, obesity	Metformin
	Bariatric surgery
Asymptomatic carotid stenosis (60-99%)	Carotid endarterectomy
Diet	Mediterranean diet
High vascular risk populations	Antiplatelet therapy
	HMG-CoA reductase inhibitors

HMG-CoA, Hydroxymethylglutaryl-coenzyme A.

施取决于患者的危险因素和卒中机制。卒中患者的诊断评估决定了最佳治疗方案。

卒中的一级预防

随机试验表明，针对具有特定危险因素的患者采取特定干预措施可以预防首次卒中（表13.5）。例如，治疗高血压可使卒中风险降低45%。在心房颤动患者中，使用华法林可使卒中风险相对降低60%～70%，但无心脏疾病、高血压或糖尿病的年轻患者可仅使用抗血小板药物治疗。在某些一级预防的研究和心脏疾病研究中，羟甲基戊二酰辅酶A（HMG-CoA）还原酶抑制剂或他汀类药物已被证明可降低首次卒中和心脏疾病的风险。这些药物对卒中风险的作用比对心脏疾病的作用要小得多，这可能反映了与心脏疾病相比，导致卒中的原因存在更大的异质性。对于无症状性颈动脉狭窄率超过60%的患者，颈动脉内膜切除术降低了卒中的风险，尽管效果比有症状的患者要小得多，而且为了预防一次卒中需要治疗的患者数量更多。由于许多针对无症状患者的动脉内膜切除术的大型随机试验是在目前推荐使用他汀类药物和抗血小板药物之前进行的，因此目前尚不清楚手术是否优于药物治疗。因此，新的试验正在研究无症状狭窄患者中药物与手术和血管内治疗的优劣。

抗血小板治疗在预防首次卒中方面的作用尚未明确。例如，在一项大型一级预防研究中，尽管阿司匹林的使用降低了缺血性心脏病的风险，但却增加了缺血性和出血性卒中的风险。然而，其他研究表明，阿司匹林可降低45岁以上女性缺血性卒中的风险。

地中海饮食也有助于预防心血管疾病，包括卒中。这种饮食的特点是高摄入水果、蔬菜和豆类；橄榄油作为主要脂肪来源；适量摄入鱼类和禽类，少量摄入红肉和乳制品；以及可选择轻度至中度饮用红葡萄酒，大多在用餐时饮用。与低脂饮食相比，这种营养素组合在随机试验中使5年卒中风险降低了约30%。

观察性研究证据表明，某些行为可以预防卒中。戒烟可使卒中风险在5年内降低到与非吸烟者相似的水平。适度饮酒，即男性每天最多2杯，女性每天1杯，与不喝酒的人相比，卒中风险较低。此外，建议进行体育活动、适当减肥和糖尿病管理。

缺血性卒中急性期治疗

对于在症状出现后3 h内且头部CT或MRI证实无出血的缺血性卒中患者，与安慰剂相比，溶栓药物——重组组织型纤溶酶原激活剂（rt-PA）可改善3个月的功能预后。在最早具有里程碑意义的研究中，纳入624名在3 h内接受治疗的缺血性卒中患者，接受rt-PA治疗的患者在3个月内达到正常或接近正常的神经和功能状态的比例显著高于对照组，尽管在24 h内没有明确的获益。患者独立进行日常生活活动的比例

表13.5　缺血性卒中基于循证的一级预防

危险因素	治疗
高血压	降压
心肌梗死	HMG-CoA还原酶抑制剂
高脂血症	HMG-CoA还原酶抑制剂
心房颤动	抗凝（华法林、其他药物）左心房封堵（选择患者）
糖尿病/血管疾病	ACE抑制剂
2型糖尿病，肥胖	二甲双胍　减肥手术
无症状性颈动脉狭窄（60%～99%）	颈动脉内膜切除术
饮食	地中海饮食
血管高危人群	抗血小板治疗　HMG-CoA还原酶抑制剂

HMG-CoA，羟甲基戊二酰辅酶A。

从38%增加到50%，绝对获益为12%。没有立即（24 h）的获益，但在3个月时获益，这与溶栓治疗在整个区域发生永久梗死之前通过再灌注组织来减少梗死周围区域大小的假说一致，尽管核心部分存在一些不可逆的损伤。

接受rt-PA治疗的患者中，梗死出血性转化的发生率增加了10倍（从接受安慰剂治疗患者的0.6%增加到接受rt-PA治疗患者的6.0%）。然而，总体而言，卒中后第一天内两组间的神经恶化和死亡率相似。rt-PA于1996年获得美国食品和药物管理局（FDA）批准用于患者治疗，现已成为3 h内发病的缺血性卒中患者的标准治疗方案。在使用rt-PA时，必须满足特定的条件和排除标准，以降低并发症的风险（表13.6）。

由于急性脑损伤时可能将脑灌注降低到自动调节所允许的范围以下，当前指南建议不要在缺血性卒中后快速降低血压，并允许收缩压高达220 mmHg。然而，在溶栓治疗前后，应将收缩压维持在180 mmHg以下，以降低出血性转化的风险。此外，在使用rt-PA后的24 h内，必须停用抗血小板药物和抗凝药物。

后续的meta分析和个体试验表明，溶栓治疗的益处会随着症状发作（假定为缺血开始）与治疗之间的时间间隔增加而减少，但在特定的患者中（即80岁以下且既往没有缺血性卒中和糖尿病病史的患者），治疗时间窗可延长至卒中后4.5 h。

在考虑卒中症状持续时间时，神经科医生会使用患者最后一次被确认正常的时间作为卒中发作的时间，而不是患者被发现出现卒中症状的时间。由于卒中通常是无痛的，患者可能未意识到症状的开始。在患有失语症、病感失认症或意识减退的患者中，患者可能无法提供关于症状发作时间的详细信息，因此需要见证人。此外，对于醒后卒中的患者，如果症状开

TABLE 13.6 Eligibility and Exclusion Criteria for Treatment of Acute Ischemic Stroke With Intravenous Rt-PA
Eligibility
Age ≥18 years
Diagnosis of ischemic stroke causing measurable neurologic deficit
Well-documented onset of symptoms <4.5 hours before beginning treatment
Major Exclusion Criteria
Stroke or head trauma within the preceding 3 months
Major surgery within the preceding 2 weeks
History of intracerebral hemorrhage
Systolic blood pressure >185 mm Hg
Diastolic blood pressure >110 mm Hg
Rapidly improving or minor neurologic symptoms and signs
Symptoms suggestive of subarachnoid hemorrhage
Gastrointestinal or urinary tract bleeding within 3 weeks
Arterial puncture at a noncompressible site within 1 week
Platelet count <100,000/mm^3
INR >1.7
Relative Exclusion Criteria (Must Weigh Risks and Benefits)
Seizure at stroke onset
Myocardial infarction within 6 weeks
Infective endocarditis
Hemorrhagic eye disorder
Blood glucose <30 mg/dL (2.7 mmol/L)
Blood glucose >400 mg/dL (21.6 mmol/L)
Patients requiring very aggressive therapy for blood pressure reduction

moreover, it is difficult if not impossible to determine the time at which the symptoms started, and so the time that the patient went to bed is usually considered the starting point of the time window to decide eligibility for thrombolytic therapy. Recent clinical trials, however, provide evidence that when advanced imaging techniques are used, patients can be selected for treatment with intravenous rt-PA up to 9 hours after last known well. In one study, when the MR DWI showed changes consistent with ischemia but the fluid attenuated inversion recovery (FLAIR) sequences did not, the duration of ischemia was presumed to be less than 4.5 hours, and patients were considered eligible for randomization to rt-PA or placebo; among those treated with IV rt-PA, outcomes were significantly better. Another trial used the mismatch between areas of permanent injury and those of diminished perfusion, representing "at risk" tissue, from CT or MRI, to establish an ischemic penumbra that could be salvaged up to 9 hours after onset.

Interventional techniques to revascularize occluded vessels have also been demonstrated to benefit selected patients with ischemic stroke. For patients with MCA occlusions presenting up to 6 hours after symptom onset, there is evidence that intra-arterial thrombolytic agents delivered via catheter into the face of the occluding thrombus can improve functional outcomes, despite an increase in risk of hemorrhage similar to that seen with intravenous rt-PA. More recently, the FDA has approved the use of mechanical devices called stent-retrievers specifically engineered to facilitate clot extraction in the setting of ischemic stroke in the middle cerebral artery in selected patients. These devices, used during an angiographic procedure, provide a wire mesh that can surround the thrombus in the vessel and then be used to pull the clot out. They may be used up to 24 hours after stroke onset and can achieve a recanalization rate of up to 80%. Patients are selected for the procedure by using infarction-perfusion mismatch imaging to identify those with areas of uninfarcted, salvageable brain tissue. Meta-analyses of several randomized trials in these patients have shown marked benefits, with about two to three patients needed to treat to achieve clinically significant functional improvement.

Treatment with heparin and various heparinoids for acute stroke are not of benefit and are not recommended in acute stroke. In some patients with massive hemispheric strokes, surgical decompression (hemicraniectomy) can be life-saving with acceptable functional outcomes, particularly for younger patients.

Since stroke is characterized by a cascade of events that can cause further neuronal injury for hours or days after stroke, experimental animal stroke studies have tested strategies that might limit this injury (i.e., neuroprotection), including drugs targeting N-methyl-D-aspartate (NMDA) receptors, glycine receptors, calcium channels, adhesion molecules, free radicals, albumin, inflammation, and membrane constituents. However, none of these have been of benefit in human clinical trials.

Treatment of Intracerebral Hemorrhage

Treatment of ICH is primarily supportive. Many patients require management in the intensive care setting to manage elevated blood pressure and secondary complications, such as respiratory failure, aspiration, and hemodynamic instability in severely neurologically compromised patients. In many cases, patients also require management of intracranial pressure using osmotic agents, such as mannitol or hypertonic saline, or therapeutic hyperventilation. In some patients, surgical evacuation of hematomas may be life-saving, although trials have thus far failed to show that most ICH patients benefit from surgical decompression. Among more than 1000 participants randomized in a large international study, there was no evidence of benefit of surgical over medical therapy, apart from a potential benefit in the subgroup of patients with small superficial hemorrhages. Most hemorrhages that occur deep within the hemispheres probably cause the majority of their damage immediately after the ictal hemorrhage, so that evacuation does not save tissue and may introduce further damage.

One of the major recent insights into the pathogenesis of cerebral injury associated with ICH has been the recognition that a large proportion of hemorrhages continue to expand during the early hours after onset. As a result, there has been increased interest in the use of prothrombotic agents to reduce this expansion and to limit secondary cerebral injury. Though preliminary studies on the potential benefits of infusing factor VII as a prothrombogenic agent showed promise, subsequent and more definitive studies did not confirm a benefit in the majority of patients, although it remains possible that subgroups of patients, including those with warfarin-associated hemorrhage, may benefit.

For cerebellar hemorrhages, surgical decompression may be life-saving, and it is essential to recognize the signs and symptoms of incipient brain stem compression and herniation (i.e., headache, vertigo, nausea, vomiting, and truncal ataxia without focal weakness, declining sensorium, and gaze-palsy). Neuroimaging studies that support the need for surgical decompression include hematoma greater than 3 cm, fourth ventricular shift, cisternal obliteration, and ventricular enlargement. Lumbar puncture is contraindicated with ICH, particularly with cerebellar hemorrhages, because life-threatening tonsillar herniation and midbrain compression may occur. Great caution must be taken in these patients subjected to ventriculostomy for the purposes of reducing intracranial pressure because upward cerebellar herniation may occur.

The management of aneurysmal SAH is complicated, and recurrent bleeding risks and mortality are high. Antifibrinolytic agents, such as ε-aminocaproic acid, used to preserve the thrombus around

表 13.6 使用静脉注射 rt-PA 治疗急性缺血性卒中的资格与排除标准

资格条件
年龄 ≥ 18 岁
经确诊为缺血性卒中导致的神经功能障碍
症状出现至开始静脉溶栓治疗的时间在 4.5 h 以内

主要排除标准
近 3 个月内发生颅内出血或脑外伤
近 2 周内有重大手术史
脑出血病史
收缩压 > 185 mmHg
舒张压 > 110 mmHg
迅速改善或轻微的神经症状和体征
蛛网膜下腔出血的症状
近 3 周内胃肠道或尿路出血
近 1 周内在难以压迫部位进行动脉穿刺
血小板计数 < 100 000/mm³
INR > 1.7

相对排除标准（需综合考虑治疗的风险与获益）
卒中发病时出现癫痫发作
近 6 周内心肌梗死
感染性心内膜炎
出血性眼部疾病
血糖 < 30 mg/dl（2.7 mmol/L）
血糖 > 400 mg/dl（21.6 mmol/L）
患者需要非常积极的降压治疗

始的时间难以确定或无法确定，则通常将患者上床睡觉的时间视为决定溶栓治疗资格的时间窗的起点。然而，最近的临床试验证据表明，当使用高级成像技术时，患者可以在最后一次被确认正常后的 9 h 内接受静脉 rt-PA 治疗。在一项研究中，当 MR DWI 显示与缺血一致的变化，但液体衰减反转恢复（FLAIR）序列没有显示时，因而假定缺血持续时间小于 4.5 h，患者被认为有资格随机接受 rt-PA 或安慰剂治疗；在接受静脉 rt-PA 治疗的患者中，治疗效果明显更佳。另一项试验通过永久性损伤区域与灌注减少区域之间的不匹配，这些不匹配区域代表"有风险"的组织，通过 CT 或 MRI 来确定可挽救的缺血半暗带，该区域在症状发作后 9 h 内可进行治疗。

血管再通术已被证实对部分缺血性卒中患者有益。对于症状发作后长达 6 h、出现 MCA 闭塞的患者，有证据表明，尽管出血风险增加与静脉 rt-PA 相似，但通过导管将溶栓剂输送至闭塞性血栓的表面可改善功能预后。最近，FDA 批准了支架取栓机械装置的使用，该装置专门用于部分 MCA 缺血性卒中患者的血栓清除。这些装置在血管造影过程中使用，提供一个金属丝网，可以围绕血管中的血栓，然后拉出血栓。它们可在卒中发作后 24 h 内使用，并可实现高达 80% 的再通率。通过梗死-灌注不匹配成像来识别未梗死、可挽救的脑组织区域，以选择适合该手术的患者。针对这些患者的几项随机试验的 meta 分析证实需治疗 2～3 名患者即可实现临床上显著的功能改善。

对于急性卒中，使用肝素和各种肝素衍生物进行治疗并无获益，因此不推荐用于急性卒中。在一些患有大面积梗死的患者中，手术减压（去骨瓣减压术）可以挽救生命，并带来可接受的功能结果，特别是对于年轻患者。

由于卒中存在系列级联反应，可能在卒中发生后的数小时或数天内进一步导致神经元损伤，卒中动物模型研究了可能限制这种损伤（即神经保护）的策略，包括针对 N-甲基-D-天冬氨酸（NMDA）受体、甘氨酸受体、钙通道、黏附分子、自由基、白蛋白、炎症和膜成分的药物。然而，临床研究中以上药物均以失败告终。

脑出血的治疗

ICH 主要依靠对症支持治疗。大部分患者需要在重症监护室中进行治疗，以控制高血压和并发症，如呼吸衰竭、吸入性肺炎和严重神经功能障碍患者的血流动力学不稳定。在许多情况下，患者还需要使用渗透剂（如甘露醇或高渗盐水）或治疗性过度通气来管理颅内压。尽管在某些患者中，进行血肿清除可能是挽救生命的，但到目前为止，尚无证据证实 ICH 患者可从外科减压手术中获益。在一项 1000 多名患者的大型国际随机化研究中，除了小部分浅表少量出血的患者可能获益外，没有证据表明手术治疗优于药物治疗。大多数发生在大脑半球深部的出血可能在出血后立即造成大部分损伤，因此清除血肿并不能挽救脑组织，反而可能引发进一步的损伤。

近年来对 ICH 相关脑损伤发病机制的探索发现，很大一部分出血在发病后几小时内仍在继续扩大。因此，人们对使用促凝血剂来减少这种扩大并限制继发性脑损伤的关注度日益增加。尽管初步研究表明，因子 Ⅶ 作为促凝血剂注入可能具有潜在益处，但后续更明确的研究并未证实大多数患者从中获益，但是华法林相关出血的亚组患者可能获益。

对于小脑出血，外科减压可能是挽救生命的，而且识别脑干压迫和脑疝的早期症状和体征（即头痛、眩晕、恶心、呕吐和躯干共济失调，不伴有局部无力、感觉减退和凝视麻痹）至关重要。支持外科减压需求的神经影像学研究包括血肿大于 3 cm、第四脑室移位、脑池消失和脑室扩大。ICH，特别是小脑出血时，禁止进行腰椎穿刺，因为可能发生危及生命的小脑扁桃体疝和中脑压迫。对于这些患者，在进行脑室造瘘以降低颅内压时必须格外小心，警惕可能发生小脑上疝。

动脉瘤性 SAH 的管理很复杂，再出血风险和死亡率都很高。使用抗纤溶药物（如 ε-氨基己酸）来稳定动脉瘤周围的血栓，从而防止再出血的临床研究以

an aneurysm and thereby prevent rebleeding, have been unsuccessful. Therefore, definitive therapy is elimination of the ruptured aneurysm. This may be accomplished surgically or with interventional embolization techniques, such as with coils deposited in the aneurysm. Even after securing the aneurysmal site of bleeding, however, several other complications may ensue, of which vasospasm leading to cerebral infarction is one of the most common. Vasospasm appears to represent a reaction of the blood vessels to the blood in the surrounding subarachnoid space. Transcranial Doppler screening may be used daily to detect early changes of vasospasm; continuous EEG monitoring and multimodality monitoring of vital signs are other emerging ways to detect cerebral dysfunction while still reversible. The calcium-channel antagonist nimodipine, which crosses the blood-brain barrier, has become standard of care in SAH patients for up to 3 weeks after hemorrhage. It improves outcomes, although it is not clear that this is through a reduction in vasospasm, as originally hypothesized. Hydration, hyperosmolar therapy, hypertensive therapy, and angioplasty of vascular spasm may also be used to reduce risk of infarction. Other complications of SAH include cerebral edema, seizures, ventricular dilatation, the syndrome of inappropriate ADH secretion (SIADH), and cardiac failure. Hydrocephalus may require ventricular shunting.

Rehabilitation and Recovery

A team approach to stroke rehabilitation, starting with a stroke recovery unit with experienced physiatrists and physical therapists, has proven beneficial for the optimum recovery of patients. A specialized stroke unit is particularly helpful in avoiding complications such as infections, contractures, and decubiti, and in maximizing independence for patients. Speech and occupational therapists help patients improve their swallowing, communication, and daily living skills.

Constraint-induced therapy is a specific type of physical therapy that involves having a hemiparetic patient wear a large mitt to prevent use of the unaffected limb for several hours daily, forcing the patient to use the affected limb for most tasks. In a randomized trial, constraint-induced therapy with intensive task-directed therapy was associated with functional improvement compared to standard physical therapy. It remains unclear, however, whether the use of constraints or the intensive nature of the therapy itself was responsible for the improvements in function. Intensive task-directed therapy is both difficult for the patient and expensive, however, and may not be practical for large numbers of patients. Recent studies have suggested that home therapy, guided by therapists using videoconferencing with patients (i.e., "telerehabilitation") may be more feasible for patients.

Depression is a frequent accompaniment of stroke, reflecting both the physical disability and altered brain chemistry. Depression may respond to selective serotonin reuptake inhibitors (SSRIs) and tricyclic antidepressants. Escitalopram administered prophylactically to stroke patients was effective in preventing the development of depression, though other studies have not confirmed this. There is also evidence from other trials that SSRI treatment facilitates functional recovery after stroke.

Secondary Stroke Prevention

The optimal secondary prevention strategy for an individual patient depends on the stroke mechanism. For stroke or TIA caused by carotid stenosis of 70% or more of the vessel diameter, carotid endarterectomy (CEA) by a skilled surgeon with an acceptable complication rate (<5%) is preferable to medical therapy in good surgical candidates. For patients at high risk of surgical complications, including those over age 80, those with cardiac or pulmonary disease, or those with radiation-induced arteriopathy, stenting reduces the risks of cardiac complications. Trials that tested whether carotid angioplasty and stenting are more effective or safer than carotid endarterectomy in patients at low surgical risk have not demonstrated any benefit over open surgery. Among patients with symptomatic intracranial stenosis (lesions not amenable to surgery), a recent randomized trial demonstrated that best medical therapy, including aggressive risk factor control, was associated with a lower recurrence risk.

Anticoagulation is indicated in patients with definite cardioembolic sources of stroke, such as mechanical valves or atrial fibrillation. In patients with atrial fibrillation, anticoagulation with warfarin was superior to aspirin, with a relative risk reduction of about 68%. Recommended options for secondary prevention among patients with atrial fibrillation now include warfarin with an INR between 2.0 and 3.0, or use of one of the newer antithrombotic agents, such as dabigatran, rivaroxaban, edoxaban, or apixaban, which are associated with a lower risk of bleeding complications. For patients who cannot tolerate anticoagulants because of a risk of ICH or bleeding elsewhere, newer treatment modalities, including interventions to exclude the left atrial appendage from the circulation using a device delivered endovascularly has been approved after a clinical trial demonstrated that it was as effective at preventing stroke as anticoagulation with warfarin, with a low risk of bleeding or other complications.

Recent evidence suggests that some patients with unexplained stroke may have cardiac emboli from conditions related to atrial dysfunction but without frank atrial fibrillation; this entity has been labelled *atrial cardiopathy* and may be detected using cardiac biomarkers such as an enlarged heart on echocardiography, frequent ectopy on monitoring, P wave abnormalities on the electrocardiogram, or serum biomarkers. An ongoing clinical trial is testing whether patients with unexplained stroke and atrial cardiopathy would benefit from anticoagulation just as patients with atrial fibrillation do.

Other causes of cardiogenic emboli require different treatments. Closure of patent foramen ovale using umbrella-like devices has now been shown in several randomized trials to reduce the risk of recurrent stroke in selected patients (younger patients without other stroke risk factors). Among patients with patent foramen ovale, there is limited evidence that anticoagulation is any more effective than antiplatelet agents such as aspirin, and anticoagulation is not routinely recommended in the absence of a known hypercoagulable disorder or evidence of thrombi elsewhere. Infected prosthetic valves need replacement if emboli persist on antibiotics, there are large valvular vegetations, or if patients develop heart failure. Emboli from myxomatous tumors of the atria frequently require surgical removal of tumor. The need for anticoagulation among patients with other less well-established sources of emboli, such as calcific valvular disease or aortic arch plaque, is unproven, and current guidelines do not support its use in this setting.

All patients with ischemic stroke without a definite indication for anticoagulation, and in whom no contraindication is present, should receive long-term antiplatelet therapy, which reduces the risk of recurrence by 20% to 25%. Agents currently approved for this purpose include aspirin, dipyridamole, and clopidogrel, a thienopyridine derivative ADP receptor inhibitor. Head-to-head trials have failed to demonstrate a benefit of one of these agents over another; the combination of aspirin and dipyridamole was more effective than either agent alone, but long-term treatment with the combination of aspirin and clopidogrel was no more effective than aspirin alone and increased the risk of significant bleeding. More recent trials suggest that there may be benefit to the combination of aspirin and clopidogrel when used for up to approximately 30 days after stroke or TIA. The benefits to dual antiplatelet agents after about 30 days, however, are outweighed by the increased risk of significant bleeding. Aspirin doses as low as 30 mg

失败告终。因此，有效的治疗方案是消除破裂的动脉瘤。这可以通过手术或介入栓塞术（如在动脉瘤内放置线圈）来实现。然而，即使在确保动脉瘤出血部位安全后，也可能出现其他几种并发症，其中血管痉挛导致的脑梗死是最常见的并发症之一。血管痉挛似乎是血管对周围蛛网膜下腔血液的反应。经颅多普勒超声筛查可每日进行，以检测血管痉挛的早期变化；连续脑电图监测和多模态生命体征监测是检测可逆性脑功能障碍的新兴方法。钙通道拮抗剂尼莫地平能够穿透血脑屏障，是SAH患者出血后长达3周内的标准治疗方案。目前尚不清楚其是否通过减少血管痉挛来改善预后。补水、高渗疗法、高血压疗法和痉挛血管的血管成形术或可用于降低梗死的风险。SAH的其他并发症包括脑水肿、癫痫发作、脑室扩张、抗利尿激素分泌不当综合征（SIADH）和心力衰竭。脑积水可能需要进行脑室分流术。

康复治疗

以卒中康复单元为起点，配备经验丰富的理疗师和物理治疗师的团队卒中康复方式，已被证明有利于患者康复。卒中单元对于避免感染、挛缩和压疮等并发症特别有效，并能最大限度地改善患者预后。语言治疗师和职业治疗师则帮助患者改善吞咽、沟通和日常生活技能。

强制疗法是一种特殊的物理治疗方法，涉及让偏瘫患者每天佩戴大手套数小时，以防止使用未受影响的肢体，从而迫使患者在大多数任务中使用受影响的肢体。在随机试验中，与标准物理治疗相比，结合密集任务导向疗法的强制疗法在功能改善方面更具优势。然而，目前尚不清楚是约束的使用还是治疗的密集性本身导致了功能的改善。密集任务导向疗法对患者来说既困难又昂贵，因此可能不适用于大多数患者。最近的研究表明，由治疗师通过视频会议指导患者（即"远程康复"）的家庭治疗对患者而言可能更为可行。

抑郁是卒中的常见伴随症状，既反映了身体残疾，也反映了大脑化学物质的改变。抑郁可能对选择性5-羟色胺再摄取抑制剂（SSRI）和三环类抗抑郁药有反应。预防性给予卒中患者艾司西酞普兰可有效预防抑郁症的发展，但是其他研究并未证实这一点。此外，也有试验证据表明，SSRI治疗可促进卒中后的功能恢复。

卒中的二级预防

卒中最佳二级预防策略取决于卒中的发生机制。对于颈动脉狭窄≥70%引起的卒中或TIA，在手术风险较低的患者中，由技术熟练的外科医生实施的并发症发生率（<5%）可接受的颈动脉内膜切除术（CEA）要优于药物治疗。对于手术并发症风险较高的患者，包括80岁以上患者、患有心脏或肺部疾病的患者或患有放射性动脉狭窄的患者，支架置入术可降低心脏并发症的风险。研究测试了颈动脉血管成形术和支架置入术在手术风险较低的患者中是否比颈动脉内膜切除术更有效或更安全，但并未显示出比开放手术更有优势。最近的一项随机试验表明，在症状性颅内狭窄（病变不适合手术）的患者中，包括积极控制危险因素在内的最佳药物治疗与较低的复发率相关。

对于存在明确心源性栓塞来源的卒中患者，如机械瓣膜或心房颤动，应使用抗凝治疗。在心房颤动患者中，华法林抗凝治疗优于阿司匹林，相对风险降低约68%。目前，心房颤动患者二级预防的推荐方案包括华法林抗凝治疗，使国际标准化比值（INR）保持在2.0～3.0，或使用新型抗凝药物，如达比加群、利伐沙班、艾多沙班或阿哌沙班，这些药物与较低的出血并发症风险相关。对于因ICH或其他部位出血风险而不能耐受抗凝治疗的患者，已批准采用新的治疗方法，包括使用血管内输送装置将左心耳从循环中排除的干预措施。临床试验表明，该方法预防卒中的效果与华法林抗凝治疗相当，且出血或其他并发症的风险较低。

最近的研究表明，部分不明原因卒中患者可能因心房功能障碍相关疾病而出现心脏栓塞，但并未出现明确的心房颤动；这一情况被称为心房心肌病，可通过心脏生物标志物进行检测，如超声心动图显示心脏增大、频繁异位搏动监测、心电图P波异常或血清生物标志物。目前正在进行的一项临床试验正在测试不明原因卒中和心房心肌病患者是否能像心房颤动患者一样从抗凝治疗中获益。

心源性栓塞的其他原因需要不同的治疗方法。几项随机试验已证明，使用伞状装置封堵卵圆孔未闭可降低特定患者（无其他卒中危险因素的年轻患者）卒中复发的风险。在卵圆孔未闭患者中，抗凝治疗似乎比抗血小板药物（如阿司匹林）更加有效的证据有限，并且在没有已知高凝状态或其他部位血栓证据的情况下，通常不推荐进行抗凝治疗。如果在使用抗生素后感染性人工瓣膜仍持续存在栓塞、瓣膜赘生物较大或发生心力衰竭，则需要更换人工瓣膜。心房黏液瘤引起的栓塞通常需要手术切除肿瘤。对于其他栓塞来源不明确的患者，如钙化性瓣膜病或主动脉弓斑块，是否需要抗凝治疗尚未得到证实，且当前指南不支持在此情况下使用抗凝治疗。

所有无明确抗凝指征且不存在禁忌证的缺血性卒中患者均应接受长期抗血小板治疗，以降低20%～25%的复发风险。目前批准的药物包括阿司匹林、双嘧达莫和氯吡格雷（一种噻吩吡啶衍生物ADP受体抑制剂）。头对头试验未能证明这些药物中哪一种比其他药物更有效；阿司匹林和双嘧达莫的组合比单独使用任何一种药物都更有效，但阿司匹林和氯吡格雷的长期联合治疗并不比单独使用阿司匹林更有效，而且增加了严重出血的风险。最近的试验表明，在卒中或TIA后约30天内使用阿司匹林和氯吡格雷的组合可能有益。然而，在大约30天后，双联抗血小板药物的益处被严重出血风险增加所抵消。阿司匹林每日剂量低至30 mg daily appear effective and have fewer side effects, such as gastrointestinal bleeding, than higher doses, although there is some evidence that the efficacious dose of aspirin may depend on body weight. The FDA recommends doses between 50 and 325 mg daily for stroke prevention.

Clinical trials provide evidence for increased use of anti-hypertensive agents in patients with stroke and TIA. There are theoretical concerns about lowering blood pressure in patients with existing cerebrovascular disease due to the possibility that in patients with arterial disease of cerebral vessels and reduced autoregulation, a reduction in blood pressure could worsen perfusion and precipitate clinical events or affect cognition. Randomized trials provide evidence, however, that blood pressure reduction among patients with cerebrovascular disease reduces risks of recurrent stroke by 28% independently of a history of hypertension. Guidelines currently focus on the use of blood pressure agents to achieve recommended target blood pressure levels, rather than on specific agents, which should be individualized depending on a patient's comorbidities.

Trials using hydroxymethylglutaryl-coenzyme A (HMG-CoA) reductase inhibitors, or statins, among cardiac and other vascular disease high-risk patients have demonstrated benefits in stroke risk reduction. The Stroke Prevention by Aggressive Reduction in Cholesterol Levels (SPARCL) trial provided more direct evidence of the benefit of statin therapy in secondary prevention of stroke among patients presenting with stroke or TIA. SPARCL randomized patients with recent stroke or TIA to atorvastatin 80 mg daily or placebo. Over 5 years, atorvastatin reduced the risk of the primary outcome, recurrent stroke, from 13.1% to 11.2%, an absolute risk reduction of about 2%. More recently, the Treat Stroke to Target trial demonstrated that among patients with ischemic stroke and atherosclerotic disease, those treated to an LDL level of less than 70 mg/dL had a lower risk of recurrent cardiovascular events.

Among those with diabetes, diet and exercise, oral hypoglycemic drugs, and insulin are recommended to obtain glycemic control. Although glycemic control reduces risks of microvascular complications, the benefit in reducing macrovascular complications is less certain. In one trial, tight glycemic control of a prospective cohort of newly diagnosed diabetics was not found to significantly reduce stroke risk. The peroxisome proliferator-activated receptor-γ (PPAR-γ) agonist pioglitazone, a potent insulin-sensitizing agent, was shown in another trial to reduce risk of recurrent stroke among patients with stroke or TIA and insulin resistance, although an increase in weight gain and fractures has limited its use. Recent evidence also suggests that bariatric surgery, a way to reduce obesity and treat the metabolic syndrome, reduces risks of cardiovascular events, including stroke.

Behavioral risk factors are difficult to control but are also important. Smoking is addictive, and cessation may necessitate psychologic counseling and medical aids, such as nicotine patches or varenicline. Physical activity should be encouraged, because a sedentary lifestyle is associated with elevations in blood pressure and stroke risk. Alcohol consumption in excess of two drinks daily should be discouraged, though there is evidence that moderate alcohol consumption may have protective effects against stroke risk. It should be noted, however, that there is only limited evidence that control of these risk factors reduces recurrent stroke risk.

PROGNOSIS

The immediate period after an ischemic stroke carries the greatest risk of death, with fatality rates ranging from 8% to 20% in the first 30 days. Age and stroke severity are the most important predictors of prognosis. Case fatality rates are worse for hemorrhagic strokes, ranging from 30% to 80% for intracerebral hemorrhage and 20% to 50% for subarachnoid hemorrhage.

Stroke survivors continue to have a 3- to 5-fold increased risk of death, compared with the age-matched general population. Annual aggregate estimates of death have been 5% for minor stroke and 8% for major stroke. Survival is influenced by age, hypertension, cardiac disease, and diabetes. Patients with lacunar infarcts appear to have a better long-term survival than do those with the other infarct subtypes.

Recurrent stroke is frequent. The immediate period after a stroke carries the greatest risk for early recurrence; rates range from 3% to 10% during the first 30 days. Thirty-day recurrence risks vary by infarct subtypes; the greatest rates are in patients with atherosclerotic infarction and the lowest rates in patients with lacunes. After the early phase, the risk of stroke recurrence continues to threaten the quality of life of a stroke survivor. Long-term stroke recurrence rates range in different studies from 4% to 14% per year, with aggregate annual estimates of 6% for minor stroke and 9% for major stroke. These rates have been decreasing with the advent of the improved protection strategies outlined previously. Recurrent stroke contributes to the burden of dementia and functional decline after stroke. Importantly, cardiac events are also increased in stroke survivors, and pose a major threat of death.

For a deeper discussion on this topic, please see Chapter 58, "Supraventricular Cardiac Arrhythmias," in *Goldman-Cecil Medicine*, 26th Edition.

SUGGESTED READINGS

Albers GW, Marks MP, Kemp S, et al: Thrombectomy for stroke at 6 to 16 hours with selection by perfusion imaging, N Engl J Med 378:708–718, 2018.

Amarenco P, Bogousslavsky J, Callahan 3rd A, et al: The Stroke Prevention by Aggressive Reduction in Cholesterol Levels (SPARCL) investigators. High-dose atorvastatin after stroke or transient ischemic attack, N Engl J Med 355:549–559, 2006.

Amarenco P, Kim JS, Labreuche J, et al: A comparison of two LDL Cholesterol targets after ischemic stroke, N Engl J Med 382:9–19, 2020.

GBD Lifetime Risk of Stroke Collaborators, Feigin VL, Nguyen G, et al: Global, regional, and country-specific lifetime risks of stroke, 1990 and 2016, N Engl J Med 379:2429–2437, 2018.

George MG, Tong X, Bowman BA: Prevalence of cardiovascular risk factors and strokes in younger adults, J Am Med Assoc Neurol 74:695–703, 2017.

Goyal M, Menon BK, van Zwam WH, et al: Endovascular thrombectomy after large-vessel ischaemic stroke: a meta-analysis of individual patient data from five randomised trials, Lancet 387:1723–1731, 2016.

Hemphill 3rd JC, Greenberg SM, Anderson CS, et al: Guidelines for the management of spontaneous intracerebral hemorrhage: a guideline for healthcare professionals from the American Heart Association/American Stroke Association, Stroke 46:2032–2060, 2015.

Holmes Jr DR, Kar S, Price MJ, et al: Prospective randomized evaluation of the watchman Left atrial appendage closure device in patients with atrial fibrillation versus long-term warfarin therapy: the PREVAIL trial, J Am Coll Cardiol 64(1):1–12, 2014.

Howard G, Lackland DT, Kleindorfer DO, et al: Racial differences in the impact of elevated systolic blood pressure on stroke risk, J Am Med Assoc Intern Med 173:46–51, 2013.

Kamel H, Elkind MSV, Bhave PD, et al: Paroxysmal supraventricular tachycardia and the risk of ischemic stroke, Stroke 44:1550–1554, 2013.

Kamel H, Okin P, Elkind MSV, Iadecola C: Atrial fibrillation and mechanisms of stroke: time for a new model, Stroke 47(3):895–900, 2016.

Johnston SC, Easton JD, Farrant M, et al: Clopidogrel and aspirin in acute ischemic stroke and high-risk TIA, N Engl J Med 379:215–225, 2018.

Kernan WN, Ovbiagele B, Black HR, et al: Guidelines for the prevention of stroke in patients with stroke and transient ischemic attack: a guideline for healthcare professionals from the American Heart Association/American Stroke Association, Stroke 45:2160–2236, 2014.

Lackland DT, Elkind MSV, D'Agostino R, et al: Inclusion of stroke in cardiovascular risk prediction instruments: a statement for healthcare professionals from the American Heart Association/American Stroke Association, Stroke 43:1998–2027, 2012.

似乎有效，且副作用（如胃肠道出血）少于较高剂量，尽管有证据表明阿司匹林的有效剂量可能取决于体重。美国 FDA 建议的卒中预防剂量为每日 50～325 mg。

临床试验为卒中和 TIA 患者使用降压药物提供了证据。在脑血管疾病患者中降低血压存在理论上的担忧，因为对于脑血管动脉疾病和自动调节功能降低的患者，降低血压可能会降低脑灌注，并诱发临床事件或影响认知功能。然而，随机试验证据表明，脑血管疾病患者降低血压可降低 28% 的卒中复发风险，这一效果与高血压病史无关。目前，指南的重点是使用降压药物以达到推荐的目标血压水平，而不是特定药物，具体药物应根据患者的合并症进行个性化选择。

在心脏病和其他血管疾病高危患者中使用 HMG-CoA 还原酶抑制剂或他汀类药物的试验已证明其在降低卒中风险方面的获益。"积极降低胆固醇水平预防卒中（SPARCL）"试验为他汀类药物在卒中或 TIA 患者卒中二级预防中的获益提供了更直接的证据。SPARCL 试验将近期发生卒中或 TIA 的患者随机分配至阿托伐他汀每日 80 mg 组或安慰剂组。在 5 年多的时间里，阿托伐他汀将主要结局（卒中复发）的风险从 13.1% 降至 11.2%，绝对风险降低约 2%。最近，"卒中治疗达标"试验表明，在缺血性卒中和动脉粥样硬化性疾病患者中，将 LDL 水平控制在 70 mg/dl 以下时复发心血管事件的风险较低。

对于糖尿病患者，建议通过饮食和运动、口服降糖药物和胰岛素来控制血糖。虽然血糖控制可降低微血管并发症的风险，但在减少大血管并发症方面尚不确定。在一项试验中，对新诊断的糖尿病患者进行严格的血糖控制并未显著降低卒中风险。另一项试验表明，过氧化物酶体增殖物激活受体-γ（PPAR-γ）激动剂吡格列酮是一种强效的胰岛素增敏剂，可降低卒中或 TIA 合并胰岛素抵抗患者的卒中复发风险，但体重增加和骨折的风险限制了其使用。最近的证据还表明，减肥手术（一种减少肥胖和治疗代谢综合征的方法）可降低包括卒中在内的心血管事件风险。

行为风险因素难以控制，但也十分重要。吸烟会上瘾，戒烟可能需要心理咨询和医疗辅助，如尼古丁贴片或伐尼克兰。应鼓励进行体育活动，因为久坐不动的生活方式与血压升高和卒中风险增加有关。虽然适度饮酒可能有预防卒中风险的保护作用，但应劝阻每日饮酒超过 2 杯的行为。然而，值得注意的是，只有有限的证据表明控制这些风险因素能降低卒中复发风险。

预后

缺血性卒中早期死亡风险最高，在发病后 30 天内死亡率为 8%～20%。年龄和卒中严重程度是影响预后的最重要因素。出血性卒中的病死率更高，脑内出血的病死率为 30%～80%，蛛网膜下腔出血的病死率为 20%～50%。

与年龄匹配的普通人群相比，卒中幸存者后续面临 3～5 倍的死亡风险。轻型卒中的年总死亡率估计为 5%，重度卒中为 8%。生存情况受年龄、高血压、心脏病和糖尿病的影响。腔隙性梗死患者的长期生存率似乎优于其他梗死亚型患者。

卒中复发很常见。卒中早期复发的风险最大；在最初的 30 天内，复发率为 3%～10%。30 天内的复发风险因梗死亚型而异；动脉粥样硬化性梗死患者的复发率最高，腔隙性梗死患者的复发率最低。在早期阶段过后，卒中复发的风险继续威胁着卒中幸存者的生活质量。不同研究中的长期卒中复发率为每年 4%～14%，轻型卒中的年总复发率估计为 6%，重度卒中为 9%。随着前面提到的治疗方案改进，这些比率一直在下降。卒中复发加重了卒中后的痴呆和功能衰退。更重要的是，卒中幸存者中心脏事件的发生率也有所增加，并对死亡构成重大威胁。

有关此专题的深入讨论，请参阅 *Goldman-Cecil Medicine* 第 26 版第 58 章"室上性心律失常"。

推荐阅读

Albers GW, Marks MP, Kemp S, et al: Thrombectomy for stroke at 6 to 16 hours with selection by perfusion imaging, N Engl J Med 378:708–718, 2018.

Amarenco P, Bogousslavsky J, Callahan 3rd A, et al: The Stroke Prevention by Aggressive Reduction in Cholesterol Levels (SPARCL) investigators. High-dose atorvastatin after stroke or transient ischemic attack, N Engl J Med 355:549–559, 2006.

Amarenco P, Kim JS, Labreuche J, et al: A comparison of two LDL Cholesterol targets after ischemic stroke, N Engl J Med 382:9–19, 2020.

GBD Lifetime Risk of Stroke Collaborators, Feigin VL, Nguyen G, et al: Global, regional, and country-specific lifetime risks of stroke, 1990 and 2016, N Engl J Med 379:2429–2437, 2018.

George MG, Tong X, Bowman BA: Prevalence of cardiovascular risk factors and strokes in younger adults, J Am Med Assoc Neurol 74:695–703, 2017.

Goyal M, Menon BK, van Zwam WH, et al: Endovascular thrombectomy after large-vessel ischaemic stroke: a meta-analysis of individual patient data from five randomised trials, Lancet 387:1723–1731, 2016.

Hemphill 3rd JC, Greenberg SM, Anderson CS, et al: Guidelines for the management of spontaneous intracerebral hemorrhage: a guideline for healthcare professionals from the American Heart Association/American Stroke Association, Stroke 46:2032–2060, 2015.

Holmes Jr DR, Kar S, Price MJ, et al: Prospective randomized evaluation of the watchman Left atrial appendage closure device in patients with atrial fibrillation versus long-term warfarin therapy: the PREVAIL trial, J Am Coll Cardiol 64(1):1–12, 2014.

Howard G, Lackland DT, Kleindorfer DO, et al: Racial differences in the impact of elevated systolic blood pressure on stroke risk, J Am Med Assoc Intern Med 173:46–51, 2013.

Kamel H, Elkind MSV, Bhave PD, et al: Paroxysmal supraventricular tachycardia and the risk of ischemic stroke, Stroke 44:1550–1554, 2013.

Kamel H, Okin P, Elkind MSV, Iadecola C: Atrial fibrillation and mechanisms of stroke: time for a new model, Stroke 47(3):895–900, 2016.

Johnston SC, Easton JD, Farrant M, et al: Clopidogrel and aspirin in acute ischemic stroke and high-risk TIA, N Engl J Med 379:215–225, 2018.

Kernan WN, Ovbiagele B, Black HR, et al: Guidelines for the prevention of stroke in patients with stroke and transient ischemic attack: a guideline for healthcare professionals from the American Heart Association/American Stroke Association, Stroke 45:2160–2236, 2014.

Lackland DT, Elkind MSV, D'Agostino R, et al: Inclusion of stroke in cardiovascular risk prediction instruments: a statement for healthcare professionals from the American Heart Association/American Stroke Association, Stroke 43:1998–2027, 2012.

López-López JA, Sterne JAC, Thom HHZ, et al: Oral anticoagulants for prevention of stroke in atrial fibrillation: systematic review, network meta-analysis, and cost effectiveness analysis, BMJ 359:j5058, 2017.

Ma H, Campbell BCV, Parsons MW, et al: Thrombolysis guided by perfusion imaging up to 9 hours after onset of stroke, N Engl J Med 380:1795–1803, 2019.

Mayer SA, Brun NC, Begtrup K, et al: Efficacy and safety of recombinant activated factor VII for acute intracerebral hemorrhage, N Engl J Med 358:2127–2137, 2008.

Mendelow AD, Gregson BA, Fernandes HM, et al: Early surgery versus initial conservative treatment in patients with spontaneous supratentorial intracerebral haematomas in the International Surgical Trial in Intracerebral Haemorrhage (STICH): a randomised trial, Lancet 365:387–397, 2005.

Nogueira RG, Jadhav AP, Haussen DC, et al: Thrombectomy 6 to 24 hours after stroke with a mismatch between deficit and infarct, N Engl J Med 378:11–21, 2018.

Powers WJ, Rabinstein AA, Ackerson T, et al: 2018 Guidelines for the early management of patients with acute ischemic stroke: a guideline for healthcare professionals from the American Heart Association/American Stroke Association, Stroke 50:e344–e418, 2019.

Robinson RG, Jorge RE, Moser DJ, et al: Escitalopram and problem-solving therapy for prevention of poststroke depression: a randomized controlled trial, J Am Med Assoc 299:2391–2400, 2008.

Ropper AH: Tipping point for patent foramen ovale closure, N Engl J Med 377:1093–1095, 2017.

Rothwell PM, Eliasziw M, Gutnikov SA, et al: Analysis of pooled data from the randomised controlled trials of endarterectomy for symptomatic carotid stenosis, Lancet 361:107–116, 2003.

Saver JL, Fonarow GC, Smith EE, et al: Time to treatment with intravenous tissue plasminogen activator and outcome from acute ischemic stroke, J Am Med Assoc 309:2480–2488, 2013.

Singhal AB, Biller J, Elkind MS, et al: Recognition and management of stroke in young adults and adolescents, Neurology 81:1089–1097, 2013.

SPS3 Study Group, Benavente OR, Coffey CS, et al: Blood-pressure targets in patients with recent lacunar stroke: the SPS3 randomised trial, Lancet 382(9891):507–515, 2013.

Thomalla G, Simonsen CZ, Boutitie F, et al: MRI-guided thrombolysis for stroke with unknown time of onset, N Engl J Med 379:611–622, 2018.

Winstein CJ, Stein J, Arena R, et al: Guidelines for adult stroke rehabilitation and recovery: a guideline for healthcare professionals from the American Heart Association/American Stroke Association, Stroke 47:e98–e169, 2016.

Yan G, Wang J, Zhang J, et al: Long-term outcomes of macrovascular diseases and metabolic indicators of bariatric surgery for severe obesity type 2 diabetes patients with a meta-analysis, PloS One 14(12):e0224828, 2019.

López-López JA, Sterne JAC, Thom HHZ, et al: Oral anticoagulants for prevention of stroke in atrial fibrillation: systematic review, network meta-analysis, and cost effectiveness analysis, BMJ 359:j5058, 2017.

Ma H, Campbell BCV, Parsons MW, et al: Thrombolysis guided by perfusion imaging up to 9 hours after onset of stroke, N Engl J Med 380:1795–1803, 2019.

Mayer SA, Brun NC, Begtrup K, et al: Efficacy and safety of recombinant activated factor VII for acute intracerebral hemorrhage, N Engl J Med 358:2127–2137, 2008.

Mendelow AD, Gregson BA, Fernandes HM, et al: Early surgery versus initial conservative treatment in patients with spontaneous supratentorial intracerebral haematomas in the International Surgical Trial in Intracerebral Haemorrhage (STICH): a randomised trial, Lancet 365:387–397, 2005.

Nogueira RG, Jadhav AP, Haussen DC, et al: Thrombectomy 6 to 24 hours after stroke with a mismatch between deficit and infarct, N Engl J Med 378:11–21, 2018.

Powers WJ, Rabinstein AA, Ackerson T, et al: 2018 Guidelines for the early management of patients with acute ischemic stroke: a guideline for healthcare professionals from the American Heart Association/American Stroke Association, Stroke 50:e344–e418, 2019.

Robinson RG, Jorge RE, Moser DJ, et al: Escitalopram and problem-solving therapy for prevention of poststroke depression: a randomized controlled trial, J Am Med Assoc 299:2391–2400, 2008.

Ropper AH: Tipping point for patent foramen ovale closure, N Engl J Med 377:1093–1095, 2017.

Rothwell PM, Eliasziw M, Gutnikov SA, et al: Analysis of pooled data from the randomised controlled trials of endarterectomy for symptomatic carotid stenosis, Lancet 361:107–116, 2003.

Saver JL, Fonarow GC, Smith EE, et al: Time to treatment with intravenous tissue plasminogen activator and outcome from acute ischemic stroke, J Am Med Assoc 309:2480–2488, 2013.

Singhal AB, Biller J, Elkind MS, et al: Recognition and management of stroke in young adults and adolescents, Neurology 81:1089–1097, 2013.

SPS3 Study Group, Benavente OR, Coffey CS, et al: Blood-pressure targets in patients with recent lacunar stroke: the SPS3 randomised trial, Lancet 382(9891):507–515, 2013.

Thomalla G, Simonsen CZ, Boutitie F, et al: MRI-guided thrombolysis for stroke with unknown time of onset, N Engl J Med 379:611–622, 2018.

Winstein CJ, Stein J, Arena R, et al: Guidelines for adult stroke rehabilitation and recovery: a guideline for healthcare professionals from the American Heart Association/American Stroke Association, Stroke 47:e98–e169, 2016.

Yan G, Wang J, Zhang J, et al: Long-term outcomes of macrovascular diseases and metabolic indicators of bariatric surgery for severe obesity type 2 diabetes patients with a meta-analysis, PloS One 14(12):e0224828, 2019.

14 Traumatic Brain Injury and Spinal Cord Injury

Geoffrey S.F. Ling, Jeffrey J. Bazarian

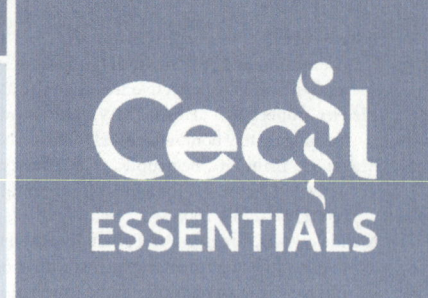

INTRODUCTION

Traumatic brain injury (TBI) and traumatic spinal cord injury (TSCI) are leading causes of traumatic death and disability. It is estimated that almost 60 million people worldwide sustain a TBI each year. According to the World Health Organization, TBI is projected to become the third largest cause of disease burden worldwide by the year 2020. In the United States, TBI results in over 2.5 million emergency department (ED) visits; the vast majority (over 80%) are mild TBI or concussion. However, approximately 52,000 patients in the United States die from severe TBI as a direct consequence, making it the leading cause of traumatic death and disability. Furthermore, yearly, about 11,000 patients are severely disabled by TSCI. The vast majority are due to falls, motor vehicle accidents, sports-related occurrences, and assaults. Among the almost 5.5 million TBI and TSCI survivors, most require prolonged rehabilitation.

TYPES OF INJURY

Certain lesions require neurosurgical intervention while others do not. TBI conditions for which emergency neurosurgery is needed are penetrating wounds, intracerebral hemorrhage with mass effect including subdural and epidural blood, and bony injury such as displaced fracture and vertebral subluxation. However, focal, hypoxic-anoxic, diffuse axonal and diffuse microvascular injuries typically do not require surgery.

MANAGEMENT

Traumatic Brain Injury

Patients with mild TBI typically recover quickly and fully. To optimize outcome, it is critical to first remove the TBI victim from play or work to prevent further injury. Diagnosis of mild TBI or concussion begins simply with identifying affected patients. This is often difficult because these patients suffer transient alteration of consciousness with only a minority completely losing consciousness. Most have memory impairment. As a result, patients are typically unaware that they are injured. Thus, it is important that colleagues, coaches, athletic trainers, parents, and other observers have a heightened suspicion when a potential head injury event occurs. If so, then a sideline point-of-injury screening tool should be administered, such as the standardized assessment of concussion (SAC) or sports concussion assessment tool version 5 (SCAT 5). SAC is a neuropsychological battery that tests orientation, immediate memory, concentration, and memory recall. An abnormal score is less than 25. If the SAC score is abnormal, the patient is at high risk for having suffered a concussion and thus should be brought to medical attention for further evaluation, diagnosis, and treatment. The SCAT-5 includes the SAC and also other neurologic tests such as balance.

In the early stage of management, it is important that patients at risk of having incurred a mild TBI or concussion have a provider skilled in managing TBI perform a detailed history, physical examination, and neurologic examination, especially assessment of cognitive function. The history should determine the duration of altered sensorium, amnesia or loss of consciousness a patient may have suffered.

The decision to obtain neuroimaging is based on the index of suspicion of intracranial hemorrhage or skull fracture. Both CT and MRI are inadequate in ruling out mild TBI, which is a clinical diagnosis. If a patient lost consciousness or has persistent altered mentation, abnormal Glasgow Coma Score (GCS), focal neurologic deficit or is clinically deteriorating, then neuroimaging should be obtained.

In general, patients with mild TBI do not require hospitalization; almost all do well after adequate convalescence. It is essential that patients have adequate time for recovery; they should not return to play or work until fully recovered. A second head injury before full recovery may be catastrophic due to the "second impact syndrome" (SIS), which leads to worse clinical outcome, including death.

The patient must be allowed to rest with minimal cognitive burden. There are no specific medications to foster recovery. Treatment is focused on ameliorating symptoms according to published evidence-based guidelines, such as VA/DoD Clinical Practice Guidelines for the Management of Concussion/mild TBI. In general, headache, the most common complaint, can be treated with acetaminophen or a nonsteroidal anti-inflammatory agent. Triptans can be considered if there are features of migraine. Dizziness can be treated with physical therapy. Meclizine should be reserved only for symptoms that are severe enough to impair activities of daily function. Insomnia can be treated with proper sleep hygiene. A sedative can be used acutely and should be limited to non-benzodiazepine agents such as zolpidem. Visual and auditory symptoms should be evaluated by appropriate medical specialists.

The patient is able to return to play or work after at least 24 hours of recovery and when cleared to do so by an advanced practice health care provider experienced in the management of concussion. In many states, statutes specify these requirements. In general, patients are able to return to play when their symptoms no longer require treatment. At this point, many practitioners will subject the patient to provocative testing such as having the patient perform exertion (e.g., run) followed by cognitive testing. If this does not cause symptoms to recur and the patient performs well cognitively, then he/she is allowed to return to full activity.

For moderate to severe TBI the initial care goals are the "ABCs" of airway, breathing, and circulation. Next is "D" for disability

颅脑损伤和脊髓损伤

李雨贤 译 杨沫 陈玮琪 审校 王伊龙 通审

引言

颅脑损伤（TBI）和外伤性脊髓损伤（TSCI）是外伤性死亡和残疾的主要原因。据估计，全世界每年有近6000万人发生颅脑损伤。据世界卫生组织预测，到2020年，颅脑损伤将成为全球疾病负担的第三大病因。在美国，颅脑损伤导致250多万人到急诊科（ED）就诊，其中绝大多数（超过80%）为轻度颅脑损伤或脑震荡。然而，美国约有52 000名患者直接死于严重颅脑损伤，使得颅脑损伤成为外伤性死亡和残疾的主要原因。此外，每年约有1.1万名患者因外伤性脊髓损伤而严重致残，其中绝大多数是由于跌倒、机动车事故、运动相关事故和袭击造成。近550万名颅脑损伤和外伤性脊髓损伤幸存者中的大多数需要长期康复治疗。

损伤类型

某些损伤病灶需要神经外科干预，而另一些则不需要。需要进行急诊神经外科手术的颅脑损伤情况包括：贯通伤、具有占位效应的颅内出血（包括硬膜下和硬膜外出血）和骨性损伤（如骨折移位和椎体半脱位）。但是，局灶性、缺氧性、弥漫性轴索和弥漫性微血管损伤通常不需要手术治疗。

管理

颅脑损伤

轻度颅脑损伤患者通常可快速完全康复。为获得更佳的治疗结局，关键是首先让颅脑损伤患者脱离导致损伤的训练或工作环境，以防止进一步损伤。轻度颅脑损伤或脑震荡的诊断仅通过识别受影响的患者开始。这通常比较困难，因为这些患者会出现短暂的意识改变，只有少数患者会完全丧失意识。大多数患者有记忆障碍。因此，患者通常不知道自己受伤。因此，当发生疑似头部损伤事件时，同事、教练、运动训练师、家长和其他观察者必须提高警惕。如果发生，则应使用（运动场地）边线损伤点筛查工具，如脑震荡标准化评估（SAC）或运动脑震荡评估工具第5版（SCAT-5）。SAC是一种神经心理测试，可测试定向力、瞬时记忆力、注意力和回忆能力。其评分低于25分为异常。如果SAC得分异常，则患者发生脑震荡的风险很高，因此应就医接受进一步评估、诊断和治疗。SCAT-5包括SAC和其他神经测试，如平衡测试等。

在管理的早期阶段，有轻度颅脑损伤或脑震荡风险的患者必须由擅长管理颅脑损伤的医护人员进行详细的病史采集、体格检查和神经系统检查，尤其是认知功能评估。病史采集应确认患者可能发生的感觉改变、失忆或意识丧失的持续时间。

是否进行神经影像学检查取决于对颅内出血或颅骨骨折的怀疑程度。轻度颅脑损伤依靠临床诊断，CT和MRI均不足以排除轻度颅脑损伤。如果患者意识丧失或出现持续性意识改变、格拉斯哥昏迷评分（GCS）异常、局灶性神经功能缺损或临床病情恶化，则应进行神经影像学检查。

一般来说，轻度颅脑损伤患者不需要住院治疗；经过充分的恢复后，几乎所有患者预后良好。患者必须有足够的康复时间；在完全康复之前，不应重返赛场或工作岗位。由于"二次撞击综合征（SIS）"，在完全康复前头部再次受伤可能会造成灾难性的后果，导致更差的临床结局，甚至死亡。

必须让患者在尽可能低的认知负担下休息。目前还没有促进康复的特效药物。治疗的重点主要集中于根据已发布的循证指南——如"美国退伍军人事务部和国防部（VA/DoD）有关脑震荡、轻度颅脑损伤管理的临床实践指南"来改善症状。一般来说，头痛是最常见的症状，可使用对乙酰氨基酚或非甾体抗炎药对其进行治疗。如有偏头痛的特征，可以考虑应用曲普坦类药物。头晕可通过物理疗法治疗。美克洛嗪只能用于症状严重到影响日常活动的情况。失眠可以通过良好的睡眠卫生习惯进行治疗。急性期可使用镇静剂，但应仅限于非苯二氮䓬类药物，如唑吡坦。视觉和听觉症状应由适当的医学专家进行评估。

患者在康复至少24 h后，经有脑震荡治疗经验的高级执业医师同意，方可重返赛场或工作岗位。许多州的法规都明确规定了这些要求。一般来说，当患者的症状不再需要治疗时就可以重返赛场。此时，许多医生会对患者进行激发性测试，如让患者进行体力活动（如跑步）后进行认知测试。如果上述测试不会导致症状复发，而且患者的认知能力表现良好，则其可以恢复全面活动。

对于中度至重度颅脑损伤，初始的护理目标是"ABC"，即气道、呼吸和循环，其次是"D"即残疾

TABLE 14.1 Glasgow Coma Score

Best Eye Response	Best Verbal Response	Best Motor Response
1 = No eye opening	1 = No verbal response	1 = No motor response
2 = Eye opening to pain	2 = Incomprehensible sounds	2 = Extension to pain
		3 = Flexion to pain
3 = Eye opening to verbal command	3 = Inappropriate words	4 = Withdrawal from pain
	4 = Confused	5 = Localizing pain
4 = Eyes open spontaneously	5 = Orientated	6 = Obeys commands

GCS = Eye Response + Verbal Response + Motor Response.

(neurologic). Every patient should undergo a detailed neurologic examination to ascertain the level of neurologic disability. An initial GCS should be assigned to each patient. The GCS (Table 14.1) categorizes patients with TBI and provides a quantifiable measure of impairment.

Patients with severe TBI are those who present with GCS scores of eight or less. To optimize outcome, medical management should adhere to currently accepted clinical guidelines such as the Brain Trauma Foundation "Clinical Guidelines for Severe TBI." An important early intervention is airway protection, usually by endotracheal intubation. If elevated intracranial pressure (ICP) is suspected, elevate the patient's head to 30° and keep it midline, ideally with a rigid neck collar (at least until the cervical spine can be evaluated for stability). Mannitol should be given intravenously at a dose of 0.5 to 1.0 g/kg. Hyperventilation may also be used with a goal of P_{CO_2} 34 to 36 mm Hg. ICP should be kept less than 20 mm Hg with the cerebral perfusion pressure (CPP) greater than 60 mm Hg. A head CT without contrast should be done as soon as possible to identify lesions that will require surgery and to determine the extent of injury.

If ICP remains poorly controlled, one can consider administering an intravenous bolus of 23% hypertonic saline (50 cc) followed by continuous infusion of 2% or 3% hypertonic saline (75 to 125 cc/hr) through a central venous catheter. If these interventions are unsuccessful, pharmacologic coma or surgical decompression should be considered. Pharmacologic coma can be induced with pentobarbital. This is given as a loading dose of 5 mg/kg intravenously, followed by an infusion of 1 to 3 mg/kg/hr. Alternatively, propofol can be used, which is administered as a loading dose of 2 mg/kg intravenously, followed by an infusion up to 200 μg/min. Continuous EEG monitoring is helpful as the limit of drug induced coma is achieving ICP control or cerebral electrical burst-suppression. Persistently elevated ICP after all these efforts is ominous. Consideration should be given to frontal or temporal lobe decompression and hemicraniectomy.

To meet CPP goals, patients must first be adequately hydrated. The goal of TBI fluid management is to increase the osmolar gradient between systemic vasculature and brain, not dehydration. For this purpose, hyperosmolar intravenous solutions are used, such as normal saline. Other options are hypertonic saline (e.g., 3% sodium solutions). If meeting CPP goals is difficult with intravenous fluids alone, vasoactive pharmacologic agents such as norepinephrine and phenylephrine can be administered. These two agents are preferred because they are considered to have the least effect on cerebral vasomotor tone. Since barbiturates and propofol are myocardial depressants, aggressive cardiovascular management will probably be necessary when pharmacologic coma is induced.

Agitation can be treated with dexmedetomidine, lorazepam or haloperidol. If inadequate, then infusions of midazolam or propofol may be used. Pain should be controlled. Acetaminophen and nonsteroidal anti-inflammatory agents are adequate for mild discomfort. However, for moderate to severe pain, narcotic analgesics such as fentanyl or morphine should be used. A benefit of opioids is that they can be reversed by naloxone to allow reassessment of neurologic status.

Hypoxia, seizures, and fever must be avoided. Maintaining P_{O_2} at approximately 100 mm Hg is sufficient. An antiepileptic drug (AED), such as phenytoin or levetiracetam, is administered for the first 7 days after injury as it will reduce early onset seizures. After 7 days it should be stopped. It can be restarted if seizures recur. Fever should be reduced with antipyretics such as acetaminophen, using a cooling blanket if needed. Other important management considerations include prevention of gastric stress ulcer, deep vein thrombosis (DVT), and decubitus ulcers. Feeding should be instituted as soon as practical to maintain nutrition.

After the initial few hours, efforts should be made to reduce hyperventilation, which is indicated only for initial emergency management. After 12 hours, metabolic compensation negates the ameliorative effects of respiratory alkalosis caused by the hypocapnic state induced by hyperventilation.

Repeated neurologic examination and continuous ICP and CPP measurement are indicated. Generally, the peak period of cerebral edema is from 48 to 96 hours after TBI. Thereafter, the edema resolves spontaneously and clinical improvement should follow.

A complication of TBI is post-concussive syndrome (PCS). Diagnosis can be made using the Post-Concussion Symptom Scale (PCSS) and Graded Symptom Checklist (GSC). The most common symptoms of PCS are headache, difficulty concentrating, appetite changes, sleep abnormalities, and irritability. PCS has a variable presentation and duration depending on the patient and the severity of TBI. In general, PCS lasts for a few weeks post-injury. However, uncommonly, it can persist beyond a year or more. Treatment is symptomatic. For headache, nonsteroidal anti-inflammatory agents, migraine drugs, and biofeedback can be effective. For cognitive dysfunction, neuropsychological testing may be helpful in determining appropriate intervention, which may include cognitive-behavioral therapy.

Traumatic Spinal Cord Injury

The emergency management of traumatic injury to the spinal cord has greatly improved with adherence to the American Association of Neurological Surgeons "Guidelines for the Management of Cervical Spine and Spinal Cord Injuries." Therapy begins with the "ABCs" of airway, breathing, and circulation. A secure airway is absolutely vital. In patients suffering from high cervical lesions, spontaneous ventilation will be lost. Lesions below C5 may also impair ventilatory capability. If the airway or ventilatory efforts are compromised, emergency intubation is required. In a patient in whom cervical spine trauma has not been assessed, the preferred method is nasotracheal intubation using fiberoptic guidance. Other approaches are nasotracheal (blind) or orotracheal intubation, so long as cervical spine alignment is maintained by traction.

Maintaining intravascular volume is essential in TSCI. Hypotension may be due to either neurogenic shock or hypovolemia. For neurogenic shock, vasopressive pharmacologic agents such as phenylephrine may be needed. If tachycardia is present, then hypovolemia is the more likely etiology and fluid resuscitation with normal saline is the appropriate initial management.

After addressing the "ABCs," a neurologic history and examination should be obtained. An accompanying TBI must be considered. Up to 50% of TSCI patients have an associated TBI. Neuroimaging is

表 14.1　格拉斯哥昏迷评分（GCS）		
最佳睁眼反应	最佳语言反应	最佳运动反应
1 = 无睁眼	1 = 无语言反应	1 = 无运动反应
2 = 疼痛刺激睁眼	2 = 发出无意义的声音	2 = 疼痛时伸直
3 = 语言指令睁眼	3 = 只能说出不适当的词语	3 = 疼痛时屈曲
4 = 自发睁眼	4 = 言语错乱	4 = 疼痛时回缩躲避
	5 = 定向正常回答	5 = 可定位疼痛位置
		6 = 可依指令动作

GCS = 睁眼反应 + 语言反应 + 运动反应。

（神经系统）。每位患者都应接受详细的神经系统检查，以确定神经功能损伤的程度。应为每位患者进行初始 GCS（表 14.1）。GCS 可对颅脑损伤患者进行分类，并提供了一种可量化的损伤程度测量方法。

重度颅脑损伤患者是指 GCS 为 8 分或 8 分以下的患者。为获得更佳治疗结局，医疗管理应遵循目前公认的临床指南，如美国脑创伤基金会的"重度颅脑损伤临床指南"。气道保护是非常重要的早期干预措施，通常需要进行气管插管。如果怀疑颅内压（ICP）升高，应将患者头部抬高至 30° 并保持在中线位，且最好使用硬质颈托防护（至少在颈椎稳定性得到评估之前）。可静脉注射甘露醇，剂量为 0.5 ~ 1.0 g/kg。也可使用过度通气，目标是 PCO_2 达到 34 ~ 36 mmHg。颅内压应保持在 20 mmHg 以下，脑灌注压（CPP）应大于 60 mmHg。应尽快进行头部 CT 平扫检查，以确定需要进行手术的病灶，并确定损伤程度。

如果颅内压控制不佳，可以考虑静脉团注 23% 高渗盐水（50 ml），然后通过中心静脉导管持续输注 2% 或 3% 高渗盐水（75 ~ 125 ml/h）。如果上述治疗措施无效，则应考虑药物镇静或手术减压。药物镇静可用戊巴比妥诱导。首先给予 5 mg/kg 负荷剂量静脉注射，然后以 1 ~ 3 mg/(kg·h) 的速度静脉输注。或可使用丙泊酚替代，负荷剂量 2 mg/kg 静脉注射，然后以最高 200 μg/min 的速度静脉输注。持续脑电监测非常重要，因为药物镇静的目标是达到颅内压控制或脑电暴发抑制。在以上所有措施后，颅内压仍持续升高是预后不良的征兆。应考虑额叶或颞叶减压和去骨瓣减压术。

要达到 CPP 目标，必须首先给予患者充分水化。颅脑损伤液体管理的目标是增加外周血管和大脑之间的渗透压梯度，而非脱水。为此，可使用等渗（译者注：原文为高渗，但生理盐水应为等渗溶液）静脉注射液，如生理盐水。其他选择还有高渗盐水（如 3% 氯化钠溶液）。如果仅靠静脉输液难以达到 CPP 目标，可以使用去甲肾上腺素和去氧肾上腺素等血管活性药物。这两种药物被认为对脑血管张力的影响最小，因此为首选药物。由于巴比妥类药物和丙泊酚都是心肌抑制剂，因此在诱导药源性昏迷时可能需要进行积极的心血管系统监测。

躁动可使用右美托咪定、劳拉西泮或氟哌啶醇治疗。如效果不佳，则可应用咪达唑仑或丙泊酚。应控制疼痛。对乙酰氨基酚和非甾体抗炎药足以缓解轻微不适。但对于中度到重度疼痛，则应使用麻醉镇痛剂，如芬太尼或吗啡。阿片类物质的一个优势是可以通过纳洛酮逆转，以便重新评估神经系统状态。

必须避免低氧、癫痫发作和发热。将 PO_2 维持在 100 mmHg 左右为宜。受伤后的前 7 天可服用抗癫痫药物（AED），如苯妥英或左乙拉西坦，以减少早期癫痫发作。7 天后应停止用药。如果癫痫发作再次出现，可以重新开始用药。应使用退热药如对乙酰氨基酚退热，必要时使用冰毯降温。其他重要的管理注意事项包括预防应激性胃溃疡、深静脉血栓形成（DVT）和褥疮。在可行的情况下应尽早开始进食以维持营养水平。

过度通气仅适用于最初的紧急处理，在最初的几小时之后，应采取措施减少过度通气。12 h 后，代谢代偿抵消了过度通气性低碳酸血症所致呼吸性碱中毒的改善作用。

应反复进行神经系统检查，并持续测量 ICP 和 CPP。一般来说，颅脑损伤后 48 ~ 96 h 是脑水肿的高峰期。此后，水肿会自行消退，临床症状也会随之改善。

脑震荡后综合征（PCS）是颅脑损伤的一种并发症。可使用脑震荡后症状量表（PCSS）和分级症状检查表（GSC）进行诊断。PCS 最常见的症状是头痛、难以集中注意力、食欲改变、睡眠异常和易激惹。PCS 的表现和持续时间因患者的不同和颅脑损伤的严重程度而异。一般来说，PCS 会在受伤后持续几周，但偶尔可持续一年或更长时间。治疗方法是对症治疗。对于头痛，非甾体抗炎药、偏头痛药物和生物反馈疗法可能有效。对于认知功能障碍，神经心理测试可能有助于确定适当的干预措施，其中可能包括认知行为疗法。

外伤性脊髓损伤

随着美国神经外科医师协会"颈椎和脊髓损伤管理指南"的实施，脊髓外伤的急诊管理得到了极大的进步。治疗从气道、呼吸和循环的"ABC"开始。气道管理至关重要。高颈段损伤的患者将失去自主通气功能。C5 以下的病变也会影响通气功能。如果气道或通气功能受到影响，则需要紧急插管。对于颈椎外伤尚未得到评估的患者，首选方法是在纤维支气管镜引导下行经鼻气管插管。其他方法包括经鼻气管插管（盲插）或经口气管插管，同时需通过牵引保持颈椎力学对线即可。

维持血管内容量对外伤性脊髓损伤至关重要。低血压可能由神经源性休克或血容量不足引起。对于神经源性休克，可能需要使用血管加压药物，如去氧肾上腺素。如果出现心动过速，则更可能为血容量不足所致，初始管理宜使用生理盐水进行扩容液体复苏。

完成"ABC"的处理后，应了解神经系统病史并进行检查。必须考虑是否伴随颅脑损伤。多达 50% 的

often indicated, but not all patients need radiographic study. A normal neurologic assessment obviates the need for imaging studies. However, a complaint of burning hands or of pain over the spine, numbness, tingling or weakness indicates spinal cord injury. A detailed neurologic examination is needed to identify the level of the injury and the completeness of any deficits and to document the degree of neurologic dysfunction at the earliest time possible. The level of the injury is the lowest spinal cord segment with intact motor and sensory function. The prognosis for neurologic improvement is better if the lesion is incomplete rather than complete. Following the acute injury, serial examinations must be made frequently.

If spinal cord injury is suspected, the patient should be immediately and appropriately immobilized with a rigid collar or backboard or both. Radiologic evaluation should begin with plain radiographs of the bony spine. Abnormalities on radiographs should lead to further neuroimaging. Bony vertebrae should be examined with CT and the spinal cord with MRI. Intervertebral and paravertebral soft tissue are best studied with MRI. A chest radiograph should also be obtained in order to visualize the lower cervical and thoracic vertebrae. Presence of a pleural effusion in the setting of a possible thoracic spine injury suggests a hemothorax.

If the C-spine radiographs are normal but the patient complains of neck pain, then ligamentous injury may be present. Ligamentous injury is evaluated by flexion-extension C-spine radiographs. However, in the acute period, pain may prevent an adequate study. These patients should be kept in a rigid cervical collar for a few days until the pain and neck muscle spasm resolves. At that time, imaging may be performed. If abnormal, the patient will need surgical evaluation.

Spinal Cord Syndromes

There are three main spinal cord syndromes: anterior cord, Brown-Sequard, and central cord. Anterior cord syndrome is associated with deficits referable to bilateral anterior and lateral spinal cord columns. There is loss of touch sensation, pain, temperature, and motor function below the level of the lesion. The posterior column functions of proprioception and vibratory sensation remain intact. In Brown-Sequard syndrome, the deficits are due to injury to a lateral half of the cord. There is functional loss of ipsilateral motor, touch, proprioception and vibration, and contralateral pain and temperature. Central cord results in a "man in a barrel" syndrome: motor paralysis of both upper extremities with sparing of the lower extremities. Weakness is greater proximally than distally. Pain and temperature sensations are generally reduced but proprioception and vibration are spared.

Spinal Shock

Spinal shock may occur after acute injury causing a temporary loss of spinal reflexes below the level of injury. Neurologic examination will reveal loss of muscle stretch reflexes, bulbocavernosus reflex (testing anal sphincter tone in response to stimulating the glans penis or clitoris), and the anal wink. In high cervical injuries, the lower reflexes (bulbocavernosus and anal wink) may be preserved. There may also be the "Schiff-Sherrington" phenomenon, in which reflexes are affected above the level of injury. Additionally, there may be loss of autonomic reflexes leading to neurogenic shock, ileus, and urinary retention.

Acute and Subacute Management

In the intensive care unit, the patient will need continued treatment. TSCI patients require close cardiovascular and respiratory monitoring. Other issues are genitourinary, bowel, infectious disease, nutrition, skin, and prophylaxis against ulcers and deep vein thrombosis formation.

Patients suffering from spinal cord injury are at risk for neurogenic shock and dysautonomia with resulting peripheral vasodilation and hypotension. Lesions at T3 or above compromise sympathetic tone with hypotension accompanied by bradycardia: the classic neurogenic shock triad of bradycardia, hypotension, and peripheral vasodilation.

Dysautonomia is treated by ensuring adequate circulating volume. The goal is to fluid resuscitate to a euvolemic state. Blood can be used if the patient is anemic (i.e., hematocrit less than 30). If blood is not required, then either colloid (e.g., albumin solutions) or crystalloid (e.g., normal saline) may be used. Central venous pressure (CVP) should be maintained at 4 to 6 mm Hg. Hypervolemia should be avoided, as this will exacerbate peripheral edema. Once an adequate circulating volume has been achieved, vasopressive agents can be used (e.g., phenylephrine, norepinephrine or dopamine). The mean arterial pressure (MAP) should be 85 mm Hg or greater. Symptomatic bradycardia can be treated with atropine.

Patients with TSCI are at risk for ventilatory compromise. Patients whose injuries are at C5 or higher typically require mechanical ventilation with an appropriate tidal volume (6 to 10 mL/kg), FIO_2 and mandatory machine driven rate. The FIO_2 inspired oxygen concentration should give a PO_2 between 80 and 100 mm Hg. The rate should be set to give a PCO_2 of 40 mm Hg. Positive end-expiratory pressure (PEEP) should also be used to minimize atelectasis. If the patient does not show signs of ventilatory recovery within 2 weeks of intubation, a tracheostomy should be considered. Lesions below C5 may also be associated with inadequate spontaneous ventilation. Mid-cervical lesions may be associated with intact but compromised diaphragm function. If suspected, a "sniff" test under fluoroscopy can be performed to determine if both hemidiaphragms are functioning properly. If not, intubation/tracheostomy with volume-controlled ventilation may be needed. If intact, then pressure support (PS) ventilation sufficient to maintain an appropriate tidal volume with oxygenation and PEEP should be set as described previously.

Patients with cervical lesions at C6 and below, including the thoracic cord, do not require mechanical ventilation. However, their ventilatory effort may be inadequate because the thoracic cord innervates intercostal muscles, which are accessory muscles of respiration. Such patients have decreased cough and inability to increase ventilation when needed, leading to atelectasis and inability to clear secretions, which can cause pneumonia. Such patients need assistance with clearing their airway: chest percussion, suctioning, and encouragement in coughing.

Thromboembolic disease is a leading cause of morbidity and mortality in patients with TSCI: up to 80% will develop DVT without prophylaxis. All patients with TSCI should receive anticoagulation and have mechanical compression devices applied to their legs. As soon as possible, sequential compression devices (SCD) or compression stockings should be placed on patients. As soon as hemostasis is assured, low-molecular-weight heparin (LMWH) should be initiated. Unfractionated heparin may also be used in conjunction with SCD but LMWH is preferred. An inferior vena cava filter may be placed in those patients in whom anticoagulation therapy is contraindicated but should not be the primary means of preventing DVT.

Mid-low thoracic spinal cord injury can lead to ileus. A nasogastric tube should be placed to decompress the stomach. Parental nutrition should be started as soon as possible. Enteral feeding should be delayed until gastrointestinal motility returns, usually 2 to 3 weeks. Pharmacologic agents that promote motility are metoclopramide, erythromycin, and cisapride. Gastric ulcer should be prevented with medication: H2 receptor antagonists, proton pump inhibitors, antacids or sucralfate. Pancreatitis and trauma-related bowel perforation occur: loss of abdominal muscle tone and visceral sensation may mask usual clinical findings of pain, guarding, or rigidity.

Bladder tone may be lost due to spinal shock. A Foley catheter should be placed and maintained for a minimum of 5 to 7 days to

外伤性脊髓损伤患者伴有颅脑损伤。神经影像学检查通常有指示意义，但并非所有患者均需要进行。神经系统评估正常的患者无须进行影像学检查。但是，如果主诉手部烧灼感，或脊柱疼痛、麻木、刺痛或无力，则表明存在脊髓损伤。需要进行详尽的神经系统检查，以确定损伤平面和所有的缺损症状，并尽早记录神经系统功能障碍的程度。损伤平面是指运动和感觉功能完好的最低脊髓节段。损伤不完全时神经功能改善的预后会较完全损伤更好。急性损伤后续必须频繁进行连续检查。

如果怀疑脊髓损伤，应立即用硬颈托或背板或两者同时使用，对患者进行适当的制动。放射学评估应从骨性脊柱X线平片开始。X线检查发现异常应行进一步的神经影像学检查。骨性椎体使用CT检查，脊髓使用MRI检查。椎间和椎旁软组织最好使用MRI检查。还应拍摄胸部X线片以观察低颈段椎体和胸椎。在胸椎可能受伤的情况下出现胸腔积液提示存在血胸。

如果颈椎X线平片正常，但患者主诉颈部疼痛，则可能存在韧带损伤。韧带损伤可通过颈椎过伸过屈位X线片进行评估。但在急性期疼痛可能会妨碍充分检查。这些患者应佩戴硬颈托数日，直到疼痛和颈部肌肉痉挛缓解。那时可进行影像检查。如果存在异常，患者需要进行手术评估。

脊髓综合征

脊髓综合征主要有三种：脊髓前索综合征、布朗-塞卡综合征（脊髓半切综合征）和脊髓中央管综合征。脊髓前索综合征与双侧脊髓前角和侧角的损伤有关。病变水平以下的触觉、痛觉、温度觉和运动功能丧失。脊髓后索的本体感觉和振动觉功能保持完好。在脊髓半切综合征中，功能障碍是由于脊髓半侧受伤所致。同侧的运动、触觉、本体感觉和振动觉丧失，对侧的痛觉和温度觉丧失。脊髓中央管损伤会导致"桶人"综合征：双上肢瘫痪，下肢活动不受影响。近端较远端肢体无力更显著。痛觉和温度觉通常会减弱，但本体感觉和振动觉保留。

脊髓休克

急性损伤后可能会发生脊髓休克，导致损伤部位以下的脊髓反射暂时消失。神经系统检查会发现肌牵张反射、球海绵体肌反射（测试肛门括约肌张力对刺激龟头或阴蒂的反应）和肛门反射丧失。在高颈段损伤中，低位反射（球海绵体肌反射和肛门反射）可能会保留。也可能出现"希-谢二氏"现象（"Schiff-Sherrington" phenomenon），即受伤部位以上的反射受到影响。此外，自主神经反射的丧失可能会导致神经源性休克、肠梗阻和尿潴留。

急性和亚急性期管理

在重症监护病房，患者需要接受持续性治疗。外伤性脊髓损伤患者需要密切监测心血管和呼吸系统。其他需关注的问题包括泌尿生殖系统、肠道、感染性疾病、营养、皮肤，以及预防褥疮和深静脉血栓形成。

脊髓损伤患者有可能出现神经源性休克和自主神经功能紊乱，从而导致外周血管扩张和低血压。T3或以上的病变会损害交感神经张力，导致低血压伴心动过缓，即典型的神经源性休克三联征：心动过缓、低血压和外周血管扩张。

治疗自主神经功能紊乱的方法是保证足够的循环血容量。目标是通过液体复苏达到正常血容量状态。如果患者贫血（即血细胞比容低于30），可以使用血液制品。如果不需要血液制品，则可使用胶体液（如白蛋白溶液）或晶体液（如生理盐水）。中心静脉压（CVP）应保持在4～6 mmHg。应避免高血容量，因为这会加重外周水肿。一旦达到足够的循环容量，就可以使用血管加压药物（如去氧肾上腺素、去甲肾上腺素或多巴胺）。平均动脉压（MAP）应大于或等于85 mmHg。症状性的心动过缓可用阿托品治疗。

外伤性脊髓损伤患者有通气功能障碍的风险。损伤平面在C5或以上的患者通常需要适当潮气量（6～10 ml/kg）、FiO_2和强制机械通气频率的机械通气。FiO_2吸入氧浓度应使PO_2在80～100 mmHg之间。通气频率应设定为使PCO_2达到40 mmHg。还需应用呼气末正压（PEEP）参数以尽量减少肺不张。如果患者在插管后2周内没有通气恢复的迹象，则应考虑进行气管切开术。C5以下的病变也可能与自主通气不足有关。颈髓中段病变可能与膈肌结构完整但功能障碍有关。如果怀疑膈肌功能障碍，可在荧光透视检查下进行吸鼻试验（"sniff" test），以确定左右单侧膈肌功能是否正常。如果不正常，则可能需要插管或气管切开术和容量控制通气。如果功能正常，则应使用压力支持（PS）通气，以保证适当的潮气量和氧合，PEEP按照前述设置。

颈髓病变部位在C6及以下和胸髓的患者不需要机械通气。然而，由于胸髓支配肋间肌，而肋间肌是呼吸的辅助肌肉，因此它们的通气动力可能不足。这类患者咳嗽减少，无法在需要时增加通气，导致肺不张和无法清除分泌物，从而引发肺炎。这类患者需要加强气道护理：胸部叩击、吸痰和鼓励咳嗽。

血栓栓塞性疾病是外伤性脊髓损伤患者发病和死亡的主要原因：高达80%的患者在未采取预防措施的情况下会发生深静脉血栓。所有外伤性脊髓损伤患者都应接受抗凝治疗，并在腿部使用机械加压装置。应尽快为患者穿上序贯加压装置（SCD）或弹力袜。一旦确保止血，应立即开始使用低分子量肝素（LMWH）。在使用SCD的同时也可使用普通肝素，但首选LMWH。对于有抗凝治疗禁忌证的患者，可放置下腔静脉滤器，但不应将其作为预防深静脉血栓的主要手段。

中低位胸髓损伤可导致肠梗阻。应置入鼻胃管行胃肠减压。应尽快开始肠外营养。肠内营养应推迟到胃肠动力恢复为止，通常为2～3周。促进胃肠蠕动的药物有甲氧氯普胺、红霉素和西沙必利。应使用药物预防胃溃疡：H_2受体拮抗剂、质子泵抑制剂、抗酸剂或硫糖铝。胰腺炎和外伤相关肠穿孔可能发生：腹肌张力和内脏感觉的丧失可能会掩盖常规的疼痛、肌紧张或肌强直等临床表现。

膀胱张力可能会因脊髓休克而丧失。应放置福莱导尿管（Foley catheter）并保持至少5～7天，以排空

TABLE 14.2 American Spinal Injury Association Impairment Scale

Grade	Injury Type	Definition
A	Complete	No motor or sensory function below the lesion
B	Incomplete	Sensory but no motor function
C	Incomplete	Some motor strength (<3)
D	Incomplete	Motor strength >3
E	None	Sensory & motor normal

drain the bladder and to evaluate circulatory volume and renal status. Once spinal shock resolves, autonomic dysreflexia may occur from bladder distention: skin flushing and hypertension. Clinical examination by palpation and percussion will reveal a distended bladder, which can be treated with intermittent catheterization or bladder training. Phenoxybenzamine may be helpful in this condition. Urinary tract infection is a significant risk of Foley catheters and should be monitored for, particularly if spinal cord injury affects normal sensation.

Nutrition should be given. Until enteral feeding can begin, parenteral nutrition should be used. A caloric level of 80% of the Harris-Benedict prediction should be used for quadriplegic patients. The full Harris-Benedict predicted amount should be used for patients with thoracic spine injuries and below. Skin care is essential to prevent decubitus ulcers. Mechanical kinetic beds, regular log rolling (every 2 hours), and padded orthotics are all useful in minimize this complication.

Orthotics, physical therapy, and occupational therapy (for cervical cord injury) are useful. Therapy should begin as soon as the spine is stabilized, with the goal of minimizing contractures and beginning the rehabilitation. Once therapy begins, energy expenditure will increase requiring additional nutrition. If intermittent compression devices need to be removed during therapy, heparin dose may need to be increased.

PROGNOSIS

Traumatic Brain Injury

The most useful prognostic indicator following TBI is the neurologic exam at presentation. Clearly, the better the neurologic exam, the higher the likelihood of improved recovery. The initial GCS score is a very reliable prognostic indicator. The lower the initial GCS score, the less likely it is that a patient will have meaningful neurologic or functional recovery. However, some patients with very low presenting GCS scores can have a meaningful recovery.

Traumatic Spinal Cord Injury

For TSCI, the completeness of the injury is the most useful prognosticator. The American Spine Injury Association Impairment Scale grades spinal cord injury on the basis of completeness (Table 14.2). A grade "A" or complete motor and sensory deficit below the lesion is the most ominous prognosis. If such a lesion persists greater than 24 hours, there is little reasonable likelihood of meaningful recovery. On the other hand, partial injuries, even severe, have substantial probability of recovery.

FUTURE

TBI and TSCI are serious neurologic conditions with significant implications on society. Prevention remains the most effective way of reducing the incidences of these diseases. Introduction of practice guidelines have contributed to improved outcome from TBI and TSCI. Sadly, morbidity remains a serious problem. Medical management is largely confined to supportive efforts primarily directed towards minimizing secondary injury, optimizing perfusion and oxygenation, and preventing nonneurologic morbidity. Surgical intervention helps restore structural stability, minimize further injury, and reduce the lesion. However, neither reverses neuronal death nor fully prevents secondary injury processes. There are significant medical research efforts to improve our understanding of the pathogenesis of these diseases and find ways to mitigate them. As new pharmacologic, medical, and surgical approaches are introduced, there will be increasing opportunities to restore these patients.

SUGGESTED READINGS

Carney N, Totten AM, O'Reilly C, et al: Guidelines for the management of severe traumatic brain injury, fourth edition, Neurosurgery 80:6–15, 2017.

Department of Veteran Affairs. Management of concussion-mild traumatic brain injury (mTBI). 2016. VA/DoD clin practice guidelines[Internet]. 2016 Sep 22 [cited 2016 Sep 24]. Available from http://www.healthquality.va.gov/guidelines/Rehab/mtbi/.

Marshall S, Bayley M, McCullagh S, et al: Updated clinical practice guidelines for concussion/mild traumatic brain injury and persistent symptoms, Brain Inj 29:688–700, 2015.

McCrory P, Meeuwisse W, Dvorak J, et al: Consensus statement on concussion in sport—the 5th international conference on concussion in sport held in Berlin, October 2016, Br J Sports Med, bjsports-2017, 2017.

Waters BC, Hadley MN, Hurlbert RJ, et al: Guidelines for the management of acute cervical spine and spinal cord injuries: 2013 update, Neurosurgery 60(Suppl 1):82–91, 2013.

表 14.2	美国脊柱损伤协会损伤量表	
分级	损伤类型	定义
A	完全	病变部位以下无运动和感觉功能
B	不完全	有感觉但无运动功能
C	不完全	有一定运动力量（<3）
D	不完全	运动力量>3
E	无	感觉和运动功能正常

膀胱，并评估循环容量和肾脏情况。脊髓休克缓解后，膀胱失张力可能会导致自主神经反射异常，表现为皮肤潮红和高血压。通过触诊和叩诊进行临床检查会发现膀胱胀满，可通过间歇性导尿或膀胱训练来治疗。酚苄明对这种情况可能有帮助。尿路感染是使用福莱导尿管的一大风险，应加以注意，尤其是在脊髓损伤影响正常感觉的情况下。

应进行营养供给。在开始肠内营养之前，应进行肠外营养。四肢瘫痪患者的热量水平应为哈里斯-本尼迪克特公式预测值的 80%。胸椎及以下损伤患者应给予哈里斯-本尼迪克特公式预测值的热量。皮肤护理对于预防褥疮至关重要。机械动力床、定时轴线翻身（每 2 h 一次）和加保护垫的矫形器都有助于最大限度地减少这种并发症。

矫形器、物理疗法和作业疗法（针对颈髓损伤）均有效。治疗应在脊柱稳定后立即开始，目的是尽量减少挛缩并开始康复。开始治疗后能量消耗将会增加，需要额外的营养。如在治疗过程中需要移除间歇性加压装置，则可能需要增加肝素剂量。

预后

颅脑损伤

颅脑损伤最有用的预后指标是发病时的神经系统检查。显然，神经系统检查结果越好，康复的可能性就越大。初始 GCS 评分是一个非常可靠的预后指标。初始 GCS 评分越低，患者获得有意义的神经或功能恢复的可能性就越小。然而，一些 GCS 评分很低的患者也可能获得有意义的康复。

外伤性脊髓损伤

对于外伤性脊髓损伤而言，损伤是否完全是最有用的预后预测指标。"美国脊柱损伤协会损伤量表"根据脊髓损伤的完全性进行分级（表 14.2）。A 级或病变部位以下的运动和感觉完全缺失是最差的预后征象。如果这种功能缺失持续超过 24 h，则几乎不可能获得有意义的恢复。另一方面，如果是部分性损伤，即使是严重损伤，也有很大的恢复可能性。

未来展望

颅脑损伤和外伤性脊髓损伤是严重的神经系统疾病，对社会具有重大影响。预防仍然是降低这些疾病发病率的最有效方法。实践指南的引入有助于改善颅脑损伤和外伤性脊髓损伤的治疗效果。遗憾的是，其发病率仍然是一个严重问题。治疗措施在很大程度上局限于支持性治疗，主要目的是尽量减少继发性损伤、增加灌注和氧合以及预防非神经系统并发症的发生。手术干预有助于恢复结构稳定性、减少进一步损伤和缩小病变范围。然而，手术干预既不能逆转神经元死亡，也不能完全避免二次损伤。许多重要的医学研究工作正在进行，将提高我们对这些疾病发病机制的认识，并寻找治疗这些疾病的方法。随着新的药物、治疗方法和手术方法的引入，这些患者将获得越来越多的康复希望。

推荐阅读

Carney N, Totten AM, O'Reilly C, et al: Guidelines for the management of severe traumatic brain injury, fourth edition, Neurosurgery 80:6–15, 2017.

Department of Veteran Affairs. Management of concussion-mild traumatic brain injury (mTBI). 2016. VA/DoD clin practice guidelines[Internet]. 2016 Sep 22 [cited 2016 Sep 24]. Available from http://www.healthquality.va.gov/guidelines/Rehab/mtbi/.

Marshall S, Bayley M, McCullagh S, et al: Updated clinical practice guidelines for concussion/mild traumatic brain injury and persistent symptoms, Brain Inj 29:688–700, 2015.

McCrory P, Meeuwisse W, Dvorak J, et al: Consensus statement on concussion in sport—the 5th international conference on concussion in sport held in Berlin, October 2016, Br J Sports Med, bjsports-2017, 2017.

Waters BC, Hadley MN, Hurlbert RJ, et al: Guidelines for the management of acute cervical spine and spinal cord injuries: 2013 update, Neurosurgery 60(Suppl 1):82–91, 2013.

15

Epilepsy

Andrew S. Blum

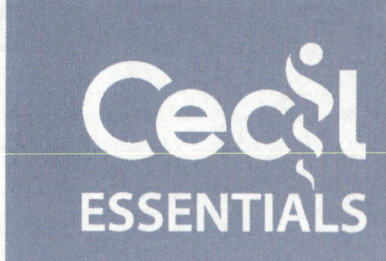

DEFINITIONS AND EPIDEMIOLOGY

Epileptic seizures are defined as transient signs and/or symptoms, often including changes in behavior, due to abnormal neuronal activity (often excessively synchronous) in the brain. A wide range of symptoms accompanies seizures depending upon the CNS networks involved, including involuntary movements, abnormal sensations and behaviors, and impaired consciousness.

Seizures often occur amidst many acute medical or neurologic illnesses that compromise brain function (Table 15.1). Common secondary causes of seizures include metabolic derangements (e.g., hypoglycemia or hyponatremia), intoxications (e.g., alcohol, cocaine), withdrawal states (e.g., alcohol, benzodiazepine), acute traumatic brain injury, and hypoxic-ischemic conditions (e.g., cardiac arrest, embolic stroke). Such *provoked* seizures are usually self-limited and generally do not recur after the underlying disorder abates. Thus, provoked seizures do not constitute epilepsy.

Epilepsy, by contrast, is a chronic CNS disease characterized by a predisposition to *spontaneous* epileptic seizures. The diagnosis of epilepsy is applied when there are at least two unprovoked seizures occurring longer than 24 hours apart or one unprovoked seizure and a presumed high probability of further seizures based upon additional data, such as an epileptiform electroencephalography (EEG) or brain imaging revealing a likely structural substrate for recurrent seizures. Individuals with epilepsy have increased seizure susceptibility (lowered seizure threshold). Epilepsy represents a highly heterogeneous set of distinct epilepsy syndromes, with differing etiologies. Genetic factors and prior CNS injury (of diverse mechanisms) account for many of the causes of epilepsy. There have been successive efforts to classify both seizures and epilepsies over the past 5 decades. Classification of epilepsy syndromes depends upon many factors, including seizure type, etiology, genetics, EEG findings, neuroimaging, and response to therapy. The diagnosis of epilepsy encompasses its neurobiological, cognitive, psychological, and social consequences.

Epilepsy presents a host of challenges for patients and their families. Most seizures in people with epilepsy occur unpredictably. This aspect worsens quality of life for patients with epilepsy. When functionally impairing seizures occur during waking hours (diurnal seizures), then activity restrictions may ensue, including restriction from driving, operating heavy machinery, climbing heights, and unobserved swimming or bathing. These activity restrictions erode independence. The psychological impact of intermittent involuntary loss of bodily control and its aftermath, and the dependence imposed by activity restrictions contribute to the increased incidence of comorbid depression and anxiety in people with epilepsy (up to 50%).

In many people with epilepsy, seizures predominate in sleep due to increased synchronization of neuronal activity. Seizures that occur exclusively in sleep constitute nocturnal epilepsy. In women with epilepsy (WWE), seizures sometimes occur more often during the week around menses or at ovulation (catamenial epilepsy). Sleep deprivation, alcohol consumption, intercurrent infections, certain medications, and marked emotional stress can further lower the seizure threshold and increase the risk of seizures in people with epilepsy (see Table 15.1).

As indicated earlier, provoked seizures are highly prevalent, accompanying many acute medical or neurologic conditions. Ten percent of the population in developed countries will have a seizure at some time during their lifetime. In contrast, approximately 1% of the population has current epilepsy (prevalence) and 3% to 4% have epilepsy at some time during their life (lifetime prevalence). In the United States, there are approximately 125,000 new cases of epilepsy diagnosed each year (incidence). Epilepsy occurs across the age spectrum. However, its incidence and prevalence are biphasic, more common in childhood (primarily because of perinatal injury, infections, and genetic factors) and with advancing age (because of stroke, tumors, and dementia) (Fig. 15.1). In developing countries, the frequency of epilepsy is higher, largely due to the increased burden of CNS infections such as neurocysticercosis.

PATHOLOGY

Prior to the 1990s, the underlying cause of a patient's epilepsy was frequently unsolved. The advent of MRI and, more recently, genetic and immunologic investigations has substantially improved our ability to identify the causes of many epilepsies. About 70% of adults and 40% of children with new-onset epilepsy have focal onset seizures, usually implying a focal cerebral injury or lesion. In parallel with the diversity of seizure types and epilepsies, there is a similarly wide variety of epilepsy-associated pathologies. The most common lesions are hippocampal sclerosis, neuronal and glial tumors, vascular malformations, neuronal migration disorders (e.g., cortical dysplasia), hamartomas, encephalitis, paraneoplastic and related autoimmune mechanisms, cerebral trauma, embolic stroke, and hemorrhage.

Hippocampal sclerosis (sometimes referred to as mesial temporal sclerosis) remains one of the more common and distinctive pathologies and can occur in isolation or secondary to another coincident epileptogenic lesion (dual pathology). It consists of loss of pyramidal cells and gliosis in several hippocampal subfields. Hippocampal sclerosis is associated with temporal lobe epilepsy and often with short-term memory dysfunction. The group of neuronal migration disorders has also been brought to light with wider use of brain imaging, especially MRI. Focal cortical dysplasia (FCD) represents one of the more common examples of such pathologies. These involve zones of dystrophic gray matter located out of place such as in the subcortical white matter, often with distorted neuronal architecture. Microscopy sometimes reveals atypical cells that exhibit both glial and neuronal markers (e.g.,

癫痫

刘韵 译　赵一龙　王婷婷 审校　王伊龙 通审

定义和流行病学

癫痫发作是指由大脑神经元异常放电（通常为高度同步化）引起的短暂性症状和（或）体征，常包括行为改变。根据所累及的中枢神经系统网络不同，癫痫发作会伴随多种症状，包括不自主运动、感觉和行为异常及意识障碍。

癫痫发作通常在伴有脑功能损伤的多种急性内科或神经系统疾病中发生（表15.1）。常见的继发性原因有代谢紊乱（如低血糖或低钠血症）、中毒（如酒精、可卡因）、戒断状态（如酒精、苯二氮䓬类药物）、急性颅脑损伤和缺血缺氧状态（如心脏停搏、栓塞性卒中）。此类诱发的癫痫发作通常呈自限性，在潜在原发疾病缓解后一般不会复发。因此，诱发性癫痫发作不属于癫痫范畴。

相反，癫痫是主要以自发性癫痫发作为特征的慢性中枢神经系统疾病。癫痫的诊断需要有至少两次非诱发性癫痫发作，且两次发作间隔时间超过24 h，或一次非诱发性癫痫发作且基于其他检查结果高度推测可能再次出现癫痫发作，如癫痫样脑电图（EEG）或脑部成像提示可能存在导致癫痫反复发作的结构基础。癫痫患者具有较高的发作易感性（发作阈值降低）。癫痫是一组高度异质性的癫痫综合征，病因各不相同。遗传因素和既往中枢神经系统损伤病史（多种损伤机制）是导致癫痫的主要病因。过去五十年，人们一直致力于对癫痫发作和癫痫综合征进行分类。癫痫综合征的分类取决于多种因素，包括发作类型、病因、遗传学、EEG检查、神经影像学和治疗效果。而癫痫的诊断涵盖了患者的神经生物学、认知、心理和社会等多种因素。

癫痫给患者及其家人带来了一系列挑战。绝大多数癫痫患者的发作不可预知，造成其生活质量明显下降。当功能损伤性癫痫在患者清醒时发作（日间癫痫发作），需要限制患者的活动，包括驾驶、操作重型机械、登高及无人照看下游泳或洗澡等。这些活动的限制削弱了患者的独立性。间歇性不自主的身体失控及其后果所造成的心理影响，以及限制活动所带来的依赖性心理，导致癫痫患者抑郁和焦虑的共病发病率增加（高达50%）。

许多癫痫患者主要是在睡眠中癫痫发作，这是由于神经元放电的同步性增加。这种仅在睡眠中发作的癫痫被称为夜间癫痫发作。女性癫痫患者（WWE）的癫痫发作常在月经前后或排卵期（月经性癫痫）更加频繁。睡眠剥夺、饮酒、并发感染、特定药物以及明显的情绪压力会进一步降低癫痫发作阈值，增加癫痫患者的发作风险（见表15.1）。

如前文所述，诱发性癫痫发作非常普遍，伴有多种急性内科或神经系统疾病。在发达国家，10%的人群在其一生中的某个时刻可能会经历癫痫发作。相比之下，约1%的人群目前患有癫痫（患病率），3%～4%的人群在其一生中罹患过癫痫（终生患病率）。在美国，每年约有125 000例新发的癫痫病例（发病率）。癫痫发生于各个年龄段。但其发病率和患病率呈双峰性，在儿童（主要由于围生期损伤、感染和遗传因素）和老年人（由于脑卒中、肿瘤和痴呆）中更为常见（图15.1）。在发展中国家，由于中枢神经系统感染性疾病（如脑囊虫病）的负担较重，癫痫的发生率会更高。

病理学

20世纪90年代之前，大多数癫痫患者的潜在病因尚未明确。MRI的问世以及新近的遗传学和免疫学研究大大提高了我们识别多种癫痫病因的能力。约70%成人和40%儿童的新发癫痫患者呈现局灶性发作，通常提示有局灶性脑外伤或病变。与癫痫发作类型及癫痫综合征的多样化一致，癫痫相关病理变化也是多种多样。最常见的病理变化包括海马硬化、神经元和神经胶质细胞瘤、血管畸形、神经元迁移障碍（如皮质发育不良）、错构瘤、脑炎、副肿瘤及相关自身免疫机制、脑外伤、栓塞性脑卒中和出血等。

海马硬化（有时称为内侧颞叶硬化）仍是较常见且具有特征性的病理变化之一，可以单独发生或继发于其他同时存在的致痫性病变（双重病理改变）。其病理表现包括多个海马亚区锥体细胞的缺失和神经胶质增生。海马硬化与颞叶癫痫相关，常伴有短期记忆功能障碍。随着脑成像技术（尤其是MRI）的广泛使用，海马硬化区可清晰地观察到神经元迁移障碍。局灶性皮质发育不良（FCD）是出现这种病理变化的常见疾病之一。病变累及发育不良的皮质下灰质异位区（如皮质下白质），伴有神经元结构扭曲。显微镜下偶见同时出现神经胶质

TABLE 15.1 Causes of Symptomatic Seizures[a]
Acute Electrolyte Disorders
Acute hyponatremia (<120 mEq/L)
Acute hypernatremia (>155 mEq/L)
Hyperosmolality (>310 mOsm/L)
Hypocalcemia (<7 mg/dL)
Hypomagnesemia (<0.8 mEq/L)
Hypoglycemia (<30 mg/dL)
Hyperglycemia (>450 mg/dL)
Drugs
Quinolone antibiotics, isoniazid, carbapenems, penicillins (in renal insufficiency)
Theophylline, aminophylline, ephedrine, phenylpropanolamine, terbutaline
Tramadol, lidocaine, meperidine (in renal insufficiency), fentanyl
Tricyclic antidepressants (especially clomipramine), bupropion, clozapine, neuroleptics
Cyclosporine, chlorambucil
Cocaine (crack), phencyclidine, amphetamines; alcohol withdrawal, benzodiazepine and barbiturate withdrawal
Central Nervous System Disease
Hypertensive encephalopathy, eclampsia
Hepatic and uremic encephalopathy
Sickle cell disease, thrombotic thrombocytopenic purpura
Systemic lupus erythematosus
Meningitis, encephalitis, brain abscess
Acute head trauma, stroke, brain tumor

[a]The metabolic derangements and drugs listed in here also lower the seizure threshold in people with epilepsy.

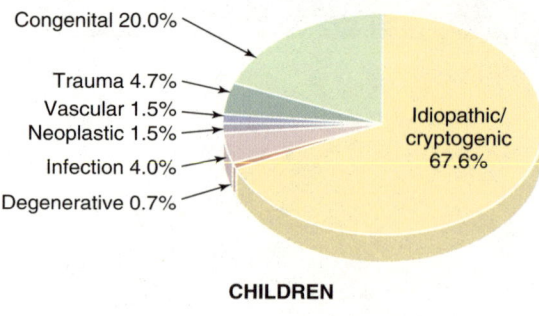
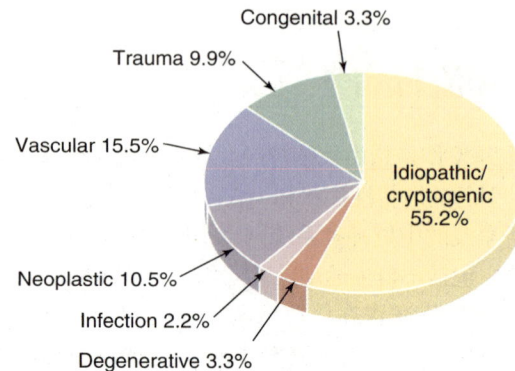

Fig. 15.1 Etiology of epilepsy, according to age, in all newly diagnosed cases in Rochester, Minnesota, 1935-1984. (Modified from Hauser WA, Annegers JF, Kurland LT: Incidence of epilepsy and unprovoked seizures in Rochester, Minnesota: 1935-1984, Epilepsia 34:453-468, 1993.)

balloon cells of type IIb FCDs). Not all patients with cerebral lesions develop epilepsy nor do all lesions in a single patient equally contribute to the epileptic phenotype; how or why a particular lesion becomes epileptogenic remains poorly understood.

Hereditary influences have long been associated with epilepsy. During the past several decades, many gene mutations have been linked with specific epilepsy syndromes, including those with either focal or generalized seizure types. Many such gene mutations affect ion channel proteins, which, not surprisingly, lead to neuronal dysfunction and epilepsy. These have been collectively termed channelopathies. Two important examples of channelopathies are genetic (generalized) epilepsy with febrile seizures plus (GEFS+) and Dravet syndrome. These genetically related syndromes have markedly different phenotypes. GEFS+ is typically associated with a partial loss of function mutation in the voltage-gated sodium channel gene, *SCN1A*, whereas a complete loss of function mutation in the same gene results in Dravet syndrome. Less commonly, mutations in other ion channel genes can also lead to the same phenotypes. GEFS+ can begin at any age, although it is usually evident in childhood, with various seizure types in different affected family members; some have febrile seizures after age 6 years (febrile seizures plus), whereas others may have myoclonic, absence, or partial seizures. In contrast, Dravet syndrome typically presents at 6 to 8 months of age with prolonged hemi-clonic seizures associated with an intercurrent fever. Children with Dravet syndrome often develop cognitive deficits, spasticity or ataxia, and occasionally nocturnal clonic seizures plus other seizure types.

The newly recognized group of paraneoplastic and autoimmune epilepsies constitute a very different etiologic process and pathology. These conditions arise either in the context of a systemic malignancy that triggers an aberrant immune attack on specific CNS targets or arise spontaneously (autoimmune). In many cases, MRIs may show multifocal signal changes in various cortical and limbic CNS regions. These syndromes can increasingly be diagnosed by serum or CSF assays for specific antibodies reactive to specific CNS antigens. Some antigens are intracellular (e.g., Hu), while others are membrane bound (e.g., the NMDA receptor).

CLASSIFICATION AND CLINICAL MANIFESTATIONS

Seizures

Various classification strategies have been used over decades to help sort out the diversity of seizure types and epilepsies. In 2017, the International League Against Epilepsy (ILAE) published their most recently revised seizure and epilepsy classification, which makes salient changes to its predecessors, including changes to core terminology. The new system offers important advantages, but since several terms from earlier systems persist in common clinical use, this section will occasionally reference both sets of terms, new and old, where felt helpful.

Seizure classification will be addressed first. Seizures are classified by their clinical symptoms and signs. The manifestations of a seizure depend upon whether its onset includes broad bilateral cortical regions or only a part of the cerebral cortex and reflect the functions of the involved cortical areas and the subsequent pattern of spread within the brain. Seizures are now initially subdivided into three broad types: those with onset limited to a specific region of cerebral cortex (*focal seizures*), those with onset involving the cerebral cortex diffusely and bilaterally (*generalized seizures*), and a new third group in the 2017 classification for *seizures of unknown onset*. (Note that in the 1981 classification, focal seizures were also called partial seizures. The term

表 15.1 症状性癫痫发作的病因 [a]
急性电解质紊乱
急性低钠血症（< 120 mmol/L）
急性高钠血症（> 155 mmol/L）
高渗血症（> 310 mOsm/L）
低钙血症（< 7 mg/dl）
低镁血症（< 0.4 mmol/L）
低血糖症（< 30 mg/dl）
高血糖症（> 450 mg/dl）
药物
喹诺酮类抗生素、异烟肼、碳青霉烯类、青霉素类（肾功能不全时）
茶碱、氨茶碱、麻黄碱、苯丙醇胺、特布他林
曲马多、利多卡因、哌替啶（肾功能不全时）、芬太尼
三环抗抑郁药（尤指氯米帕明）、安非他酮、氯氮平、神经阻滞剂
环孢素、苯丁酸氮芥
可卡因（crack）、苯环利定、苯丙胺类；酒精戒断，苯二氮䓬类和巴比妥类药物戒断
中枢神经系统疾病
高血压性脑病、子痫
肝性脑病和尿毒症脑病
镰状细胞病、血栓性血小板减少性紫癜
系统性红斑狼疮
脑膜炎、脑炎、脑脓肿
急性脑创伤、卒中、脑肿瘤

[a] 表中所列出的代谢紊乱和药物也可降低癫痫患者的癫痫发作阈值。

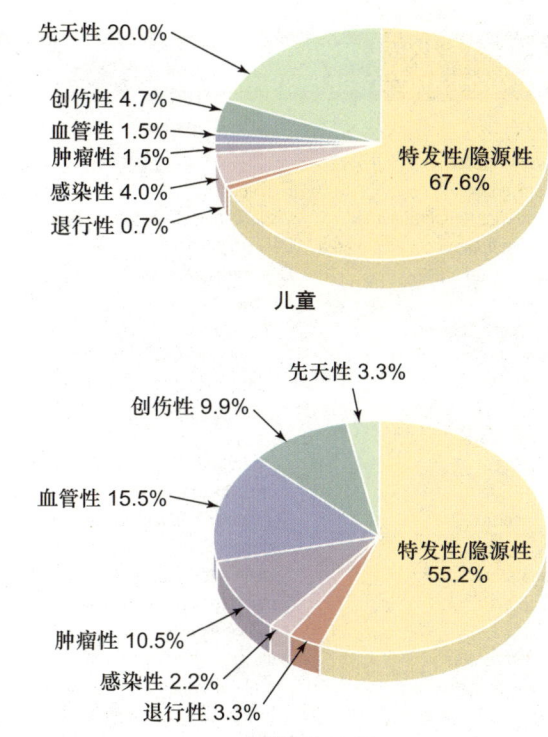

图 15.1 1935—1984 年明尼苏达州罗彻斯特市所有新诊断的病例中，根据年龄划分的癫痫病因。（改编自 Hauser WA，Annegers JF，Kurland LT：Incidence of epilepsy and unprovoked seizures in Rochester，Minnesota：1935-1984，Epilepsia 34：453-468，1993.）

和神经元标志的非典型细胞（例如 FCD Ⅱb 型气球样细胞）。并非所有脑损伤患者都会发展为癫痫，也不是患者的所有病灶都能同等地诱发癫痫表型；特定部位的病变如何或者为何变成致痫性病灶，仍然尚未明确。

一直以来人们认为癫痫与遗传因素有关。过去的几十年中，已发现许多基因突变与特定的癫痫综合征相关，包括局灶性或全面性癫痫发作类型。许多基因突变影响离子通道蛋白，不出所料地会导致神经元功能障碍和癫痫，此类疾病统称为通道病。通道病的两个重要癫痫表型是伴热性惊厥的遗传性（全面性）癫痫（GEFS+）和 Dravet 综合征。这些遗传相关的综合征具有明显不同的表型。GEFS+ 通常与电压门控钠离子通道基因 *SCN1A* 的部分功能缺失突变有关，而该基因的完全功能缺失突变则引起 Dravet 综合征。其他离子通道基因突变也可导致相同的癫痫表型，但并不常见。GEFS+ 可以在任何年龄段发病，但在儿童中多见，不同的家族成员发作类型各不相同，有些在 6 岁以后出现热性惊厥（热性惊厥附加症），而其他人可能有肌阵挛、失神或部分性癫痫发作。相比之下，Dravet 综合征通常在 6～8 个月大的患儿中出现，伴有持续性单侧阵挛发作和间歇性发热。Dravet 综合征患儿通常会出现认知缺陷、痉挛或共济失调、偶发性夜间阵挛性发作和其他类型的癫痫发作。

新近发现的一组副肿瘤性和自身免疫性癫痫具有截然不同的病因学和病理学特征。这些疾病是在系统性恶性肿瘤对特定的中枢神经系统靶标触发异常的免疫攻击时发生，或者自发产生（自身免疫性）。许多病例中，MRI 可见中枢神经系统皮质和边缘区域多发局灶性信号改变。血清或脑脊液中针对中枢神经系统特定抗原的特异性抗体检测逐渐用于诊断此类综合征。一些抗原位于细胞内（如 Hu），而其他抗原则与细胞膜结合（如 NMDA 受体）。

分类与临床表现

癫痫发作

几十年来，多种分类策略被用来协助区分癫痫发作类型和癫痫的多样性。2017 年，国际抗癫痫联盟（ILAE）发布了最新修订的癫痫发作和癫痫分类，较之前的版本有显著变化，包括核心术语的变更。新分类体系具有明显的优势，但由于早期分类体系中的一些术语仍在临床中普遍使用，因此本章认为有帮助时，会同时引用新旧两套术语。

首先讨论癫痫发作的分类。癫痫发作根据其临床症状和体征进行分类。癫痫发作的临床症状取决于其发作是广泛双侧皮质区还是局限于大脑皮质的某一脑区，并反映所累及皮质脑区的功能及随后在脑内的传播模式。癫痫发作分为三种类型：发作仅局限于大脑皮质的特定区域（局灶性癫痫发作），发作广泛累及双侧大脑皮质（全面性癫痫发作），以及 2017 新分类中的第三类，即未知起源的癫痫发作。（注意在 1981 年分类中，局灶性发作也被称为部分性发作。"部分性发

TABLE 15.2 Localization of Seizures by Symptoms and Ictal Manifestations

Locus	Manifestation
Temporal Lobe	
Uncus/amygdala	Foul odor
Middle/inferior temporal gyrus	Visual changes: micropsia, macropsia
Parahippocampal-hippocampal area	Déjà vu; jamais vu
Amygdala-septal area	Fear, pleasure, anger, dreamy sensation
Auditory association cortex	Voices, music
Insular, anterior temporal cortex	Lip smacking, drooling, abdominal symptoms, cardiac arrhythmia
Frontal Lobe	
Motor cortex	Contralateral clonic movements of face, fingers, hand, foot
Premotor cortex	Contralateral arm extension, hypermotor behaviors
Language areas	Speech arrest, aphasia
Lateral cortex	Contralateral eye deviation
Bifrontal	Absence-like seizure
Parietal lobe cortex	Sensory symptoms
Occipital lobe cortex	Visual hallucinations (often in color), teichopsias, metamorphopsias

"partial seizure" has been set aside in the updated version, though this descriptor is still frequently encountered in practice.) Among focal seizure types, the next criterion relates to the retention or impairment of awareness. (In the 1981 version, "simple partial seizure" was used to indicate a *focal seizure with retained awareness*, the currently used term. Similarly, a "complex partial seizure" in 1981 parlance now corresponds to a *focal seizure with impaired awareness*.)

The next criterion relates to specific focal seizure related symptoms, motor or nonmotor, that predominate early on (Table 15.2), reflecting the distinct functions of the various CNS regions that are engaged. Focal seizures are dynamic, with evolving patterns of spread within the brain. Thus, focal seizures with preserved awareness (previously "simple partial seizures" or "auras") often progress into more widespread focal seizures with impaired awareness (previously "complex partial seizures") and can spread further still to become *focal to bilateral tonic-clonic seizures* in the 2017 nomenclature (previously "secondarily generalized tonic-clonic seizures").

Generalized seizures at onset are subdivided into those with motor or nonmotor symptoms. Seizures of unknown onset are also subdivided in similar fashion. If the information is insufficient or if the seizure can't be classified, then it can be designated as "unclassified."

In an individual, seizures are typically stereotyped, although some patients have more than one seizure type and a specific seizure type often has varying intensities. The behaviors that occur during the seizure are termed the *seizure semiology*. The seizure itself is referred to as the *ictus* and the period of the actual seizure is termed the *ictal phase*. The period after the seizure has ended until the patient is fully recovered is the *postictal phase* (usually minutes to hours, but occasionally days to rarely 1 to 2 weeks) and the time between seizures (which can be seconds to years) is the *interictal phase*. Most routine outpatient EEGs are performed during the interictal phase. Long-term video-EEG monitoring, however, may also record examples of the ictal and early postictal phases. Specific seizure types are further illustrated later, followed by a description of several attendant epilepsy syndromes.

Focal Seizures

In some focal seizures, the abnormal neuronal firing may be so confined to a small non-eloquent patch of cortex that there is no clinical manifestation of the seizure, which can only be detected with EEG. This is termed a *subclinical* or *electrographic seizure*.

Focal Seizures With Preserved Awareness (Previously Simple Partial Seizures)

This seizure type occurs when the electrical discharge involves a small but clinically functional area. This manifests as a symptom without impairment of consciousness. The symptom may be a sensation, an autonomic symptom (e.g., nausea or other epigastric sensation), abnormal thought (e.g., fear, déjà vu), or involuntary movement. This type of seizure is also commonly called an *aura* and can serve as a warning symptom to the patient that a more intense seizure may follow. Auras occur in about 60% of patients with focal epilepsy. During a focal seizure with preserved awareness, the patient can interact normally with the environment except for any limitations imposed by the seizure itself on specific functions. Thus, some subdivide this category into subgroups with impairment (e.g., a jerking limb) or without impairment (e.g., only an internal sensation). Those focal seizures with preserved awareness but with impairment may be more apt to impede safe driving.

Focal Seizures With Impaired Awareness (Previously Complex Partial Seizures)

The degree of impaired awareness within this category varies considerably. The patient's eyes are almost always open during the ictus. The eyes may close after the seizure ends and the patient typically experiences some degree of postictal confusion, fatigue, and sometimes headache (often ipsilateral to the seizure focus). Focal seizures with impaired awareness typically last 1 to 2 minutes with a postictal state lasting a few minutes up to several hours. The specific signs and symptoms that occur during such a focal seizure characteristically reflect the location of seizure onset (see Table 15.2). The location of the focus is important because it can predict the nature of the pathology and directs diagnostic testing. As well, surgical treatment options are largely governed by the location of the seizure focus.

Focal to Bilateral Tonic-Clonic Seizures (Previously Secondarily Generalized Tonic-Clonic Seizures)

A focal-onset seizure that spreads throughout the brain leading to a convulsion is termed a *focal to bilateral tonic-clonic seizure*. Typically, the tonic phase consists of extensor posturing lasting 20 to 60 seconds followed by progressively longer periods of CNS inhibition manifesting as the clonic phase that lasts up to another minute before resolving. In some patients, a few clonic jerks precede the tonic-clonic sequence; in others, only a tonic or clonic phase occurs.

As a focal seizure transitions into a bilateral tonic-clonic seizure, the arm contralateral to the seizure focus may extend first, while the ipsilateral arm flexes at the elbow. This is termed the *figure-4 sign* and can aid in lateralization of the seizure focus. A loud *tonic-cry* may occur at the onset of a convulsion as air is forcibly expelled through tightly contracted vocal cords. The eyes are open and commonly described to roll upward. During a convulsion, breathing stops and cyanosis may develop. Foaming at the mouth may occur. Oral trauma, especially tongue laceration, is typical; this most commonly affects the lateral aspect of the mid-tongue. Urinary incontinence is common. Fecal incontinence is less so. First aid involves turning the patient onto their side as the seizure ends to allow saliva to drool from the mouth, decreasing the likelihood of aspiration. The tonic-clonic phase rarely lasts longer than 2 minutes, though witnesses commonly describe such

表 15.2 通过症状和临床表现进行癫痫病灶定位

部位	临床表现
颞叶	
钩回/杏仁核	恶臭感
颞中回/颞下回	视觉改变：视物显小症、视物显大症
海马旁回-海马区	似曾相识感、旧事如新感
杏仁核-隔区	恐惧、快乐、愤怒、梦幻感
听觉皮质	声音、音乐
岛叶、前颞叶皮质	咂嘴、流涎、腹部症状、心律失常
额叶	
运动皮质	对侧面部、手指、手和脚的阵挛性运动
运动前区皮质	对侧手臂伸展，运动过度
语言区	言语中止，失语症
外侧皮质	对侧眼球偏斜
双额叶	失神样发作
顶叶皮质	感觉症状
枕叶皮质	幻视（常为彩色）、闪光暗点、视物变形

作"这一术语在新版本中已被弃用，但在临床中经常遇到）。局灶性癫痫发作根据意识的保留或受损进一步分类。（1981 年分类中"简单部分性发作"是指新分类的"意识清楚的局灶性癫痫发作"。同样，1981 年分类中"复杂部分性发作"对应于当前使用的"意识受损的局灶性癫痫发作"。）

下一个分类标准与早期占主导地位的特定局灶性癫痫发作的相关症状（运动性还是非运动性）有关（表 15.2），反映了不同中枢神经系统区域功能受累。局灶性癫痫发作是动态变化的，在大脑内的扩散模式会不断改变。因此意识保留的局灶性癫痫发作（既往称"单纯部分性发作"或"先兆"）通常进展为意识受损的更广泛的局灶性癫痫发作（既往称"复杂部分性发作"），并且进一步扩散，演变为 2017 年新分类中"局灶扩展至双侧强直-阵挛发作"（既往称"继发性全面性强直-阵挛发作"）。

全面性癫痫发作一开始就被细分为伴有运动症状或非运动症状的发作。未知起源的癫痫发作也以类似的方式进行分类。如果信息不足或无法对癫痫发作进行分类，则可以将其归为"未分类"。

癫痫患者发病通常具有刻板性，但也可以同时具有多种发作类型，并且某一特定的发作类型往往具有不同的强度。在癫痫发作期间发生的行为称为癫痫发作症状。癫痫发作本身称为痫性发作，而实际发作的时期称为发作期。发作结束后直到患者完全恢复至正常的时段称为发作后期（通常为数分钟至数小时，偶尔为数天，极少为 1～2 周），两次癫痫发作之间的时段（可以是从数秒到数年）称为发作间期。多数常规门诊 EEG 检测是在发作间期进行的。长程视频 EEG 监测也可以记录发作期和发作后早期。下文将进一步描述特定的癫痫发作类型，并介绍几种伴随的癫痫综合征。

局灶性癫痫发作

在某些局灶性癫痫发作中，异常神经元放电可能局限在小范围非功能皮质区，以至于没有癫痫发作的临床表现，仅可通过 EEG 检测到。这种情况被称为亚临床癫痫发作或电图性癫痫发作。

意识清楚的局灶性癫痫发作（简单部分性发作）

此类癫痫发作涉及一个较小但具有临床功能的脑区放电。出现不伴有意识障碍的临床表现，包括感觉、自主神经症状（如恶心或其他上腹部异常感）、异常思维（如恐惧、似曾相识感）或不自主运动。此类型的癫痫发作也常称为"先兆"，作为预警症状提示患者可能随后会发生更强烈的发作。先兆在约 60% 的局灶性癫痫患者中发生。在意识清楚的局灶性癫痫发作期间，患者能与周围环境正常交流，但发作本身可能会限制患者的特定功能。因此，有人将这一类别细分为有损害（如肢体抽搐）和无损害（如仅有内部感觉）两个亚组。意识清楚但有损害的局灶性癫痫发作可能更易妨碍安全驾驶。

意识受损的局灶性癫痫发作（复杂部分性发作）

这类患者的意识障碍程度差异较大。发作期间患者的眼睛始终保持睁开。发作结束后，患者可能会闭眼，也通常会经历一定程度的发作后意识模糊、疲劳，有时会出现头痛（通常与致痫灶同侧）。意识受损的局灶性癫痫发作通常持续 1～2 min，发作后状态则持续几分钟到数小时不等。发作期间出现的特定症状和体征，特征性地提示癫痫发作的起源部位（见表 15.2）。致痫灶的定位至关重要，因为它能预测病灶的病理性质，并指导诊断性检测。此外，手术治疗方案很大程度上取决于致痫灶的部位。

局灶扩展至双侧强直-阵挛发作（继发性全面性强直-阵挛发作）

局灶性发作扩散至整个大脑，导致惊厥的癫痫发作称为局灶扩展至双侧强直-阵挛发作。通常先是持续 20～60 s 的肢体过伸的强直期，随后是逐渐延长的中枢神经系统抑制期即阵挛期，持续长达 1 min 后缓解。有些患者在强直-阵挛发作之前会出现几次阵挛性抽搐，而有些患者只出现强直期或阵挛期。

当局灶性癫痫发作过渡到双侧强直-阵挛发作时，患者致痫灶对侧的上肢先出现伸展，而致痫灶同侧的上肢肘关节呈屈曲状，这种体征被称为"4 字征"，有助于判断致痫灶的偏侧性。在惊厥发作时，由于空气通过紧绷的声带被强行排出，可能会发出响亮的强直性哭喊声。发作时患者双眼睁开，经常表现为眼球上翻。在惊厥发作过程中可能会出现呼吸停止、发绀，也可能出现口吐白沫。口腔外伤（尤其是舌裂伤）最常见，多见于舌中部侧面。尿失禁也较常见，大便失禁较少见。急救包括在发作结束后将患者侧卧，以便唾液从口腔流出，减少误吸的可能。强直-阵挛期持续时间较少超过 2 min，尽

convulsions as lasting 5 to 10 minutes or even longer. The CNS mechanisms that terminate such seizures are a matter of great research interest. Failure of seizure termination leads to convulsive status epilepticus. The postictal phase is marked by a transient deep stupor, followed in 15 to 30 minutes by a lethargic, confused state. Occasionally, this period of immediate post convulsive stupor is accompanied by profound suppression of EEG activity (postictal generalized EEG suppression, PGES). As recovery progresses, many patients complain of headache, muscle soreness, mental dulling, lack of energy, or mood changes lasting hours to days. Rarely, patients may report feeling not fully back to normal for 1 to 2 weeks. Convulsions result in many striking, transient physiologic changes, including hypoxemia, lactic acidosis, elevated catecholamine levels, and increased serum concentrations of creatine phosphokinase, prolactin, corticotropin, and cortisol. Complications include oral trauma, vertebral compression fractures, shoulder dislocation, aspiration pneumonia, and, very rarely, sudden death, which may relate to acute pulmonary edema, cardiac arrhythmia, or respiratory failure. Recent research has explored whether transient PGES may predict a greater risk of sudden unexplained death in epilepsy (SUDEP). The contributors and mechanisms of SUDEP are still incompletely understood.

Focal seizures of all intensities may be followed by transient neurologic dysfunction reflecting postictal depression of the epileptogenic cortical area. Thus, focal weakness may follow a focal motor seizure or numbness may follow a sensory seizure. These reversible neurologic deficits are collectively referred to as *Todd paralysis* and last minutes to hours, rarely more than 48 hours. Examination of a patient immediately after a seizure may show transient focal abnormalities that help implicate the site or side of seizure origin.

Generalized Seizures

Generalized seizures begin diffusely and involve both cerebral hemispheres simultaneously from the outset. Generalized seizures should be distinguished from focal to bilateral tonic-clonic seizures because, while in many instances they have similar clinical features, they may respond better to different treatments. These are subdivided into motor and nonmotor categories.

Nonmotor generalized seizures include *typical absence seizures* (historically termed "petit mal"). These occur mainly in children and are characterized by sudden, momentary lapses in awareness with staring. Sometimes eye fluttering occurs with a slight loss of neck tone. Many absence seizures last less than 15 seconds. If the absence lasts longer than 20 seconds, automatisms are usually present, making differentiation from focal seizures with impaired awareness and motor automatisms difficult. The EEG has a characteristic pattern of generalized 3-per-second spikes and slow waves (Fig. 15.2) during a typical absence seizure. Behavior and awareness typically return to normal immediately after the seizure ends. There is no postictal period and usually no recollection that a seizure occurred.

Atypical absence seizures somewhat clinically resemble typical absence seizures (discussed previously). These also involve staring or mental slowing but instead are associated with a slower generalized spike and slow wave discharge (2.5 Hz or less) on EEG. Also, atypical absence seizures may last longer than typical absence seizures, up to many minutes. Fluctuating levels of awareness, gradual onset and offset, and occasional hypotonia are notable features of atypical absence seizures that differentiate them from typical (3 Hz) absence seizures.

Among the motor group of generalized onset seizures, several patterns will be highlighted, including myoclonic, tonic-clonic, tonic, and atonic seizures. *Myoclonic seizures* manifest as rapid, recurrent, brief muscle jerks that can occur unilaterally or bilaterally, synchronously or asynchronously, without loss of consciousness. Myoclonic seizures may affect the limbs, face, eyes or eyelids and may be of variable amplitude. Myoclonic seizures have a corresponding discharge on EEG. Other types of noncortical myoclonus that lack an EEG correlate, such as benign nocturnal (hypnic) jerks, or subcortical and spinal myoclonus, are not considered epileptic seizures. Repeated myoclonic seizures may crescendo and evolve into a generalized tonic-clonic seizure (called myoclonic-tonic-clonic seizures). Although myoclonic seizures can occur at any time, clusters of such shortly after awakening are typical.

Generalized onset tonic-clonic seizures may begin with a few myoclonic jerks or abruptly with a tonic phase lasting 20 to 60 seconds, followed then by a clonic phase of similar duration, then by a postictal state. Although there are usually no focal features, head turning occasionally occurs; this movement does not suggest a specific localization. If the onset of this seizure type is missed, it is often impossible to clinically distinguish a generalized onset tonic-clonic seizure from a focal to bilateral tonic-clonic seizure.

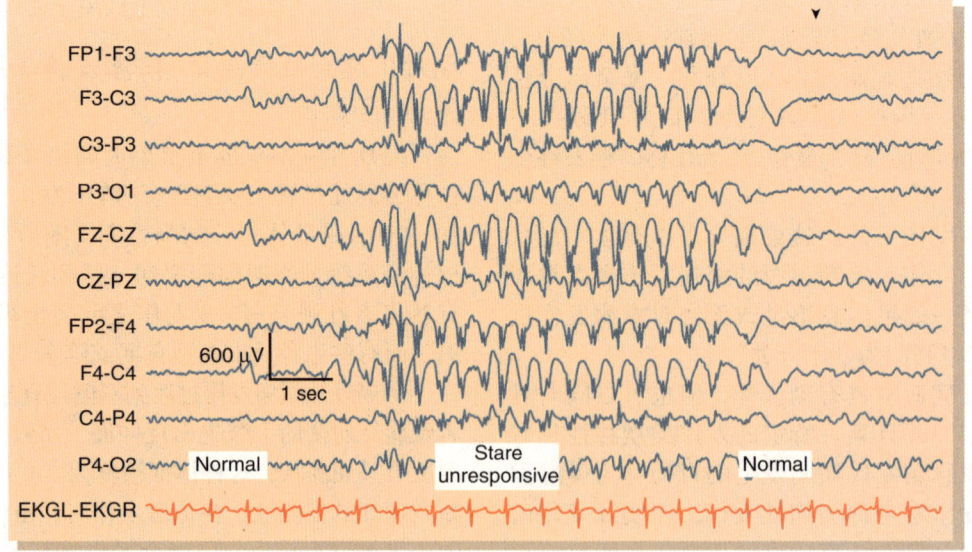

Fig. 15.2 Absence (petit mal) epilepsy. The electroencephalogram shows the typical pattern of generalized 3-Hz spike-wave complexes associated with a clinical absence seizure.

管目击者通常描述此类抽搐持续 5 ～ 10 min 甚至更长。探索终止此类癫痫发作的中枢神经系统机制是当今研究的热门领域。癫痫发作无法终止会导致惊厥性癫痫持续状态。发作后期出现短暂深度昏迷状态，15 ～ 30 min 后出现嗜睡、意识模糊状态。发作后即刻昏迷阶段偶尔出现 EEG 活动的显著抑制，称为发作后全面性脑电抑制（PGES）。随着症状逐渐恢复，很多患者会自诉头痛、肌肉酸痛、精神迟钝、无力或情绪变化，持续数小时，极少数情况下会持续 1 ～ 2 周仍未完全恢复正常。惊厥会导致许多明显的短暂性生理改变，包括低氧血症、乳酸性酸中毒、儿茶酚胺水平升高，以及肌酸磷酸激酶、催乳素、促肾上腺皮质激素和皮质醇的血清水平升高。并发症有口腔创伤、椎体压缩性骨折、肩关节脱位、吸入性肺炎及非常罕见的猝死，其可能与急性肺水肿、心律失常或呼吸衰竭有关。新近研究探讨了短暂性 PGES 是否可以预测不明原因癫痫猝死（SUDEP）的风险更高。然而 SUDEP 的病因和机制尚未完全明确。

不同强度的局灶性癫痫发作之后都可能出现短暂的神经功能障碍，可能与致痫皮质区的发作后抑制有关。因此，局灶性运动性癫痫发作后可能会出现局部无力，感觉性癫痫发作后可能会出现麻木。这些可逆性神经功能缺损统称为 Todd 瘫痪，症状持续数分钟至数小时，很少超过 48 h。发作后立即对患者进行检查，可能会发现短暂的局部神经功能异常，有助于确定致痫灶的部位和侧别。

全面性癫痫发作

全面性癫痫发作起源于双侧大脑半球且呈弥漫性。全面性癫痫发作应与局灶扩展至双侧强直-阵挛发作相鉴别，尽管在多数情况下它们具有相似的临床特征，但它们可能对不同的治疗产生较好疗效。全面性癫痫发作可进一步细分为运动性和非运动性两类。

非运动性全面性癫痫发作包括典型失神发作（曾被称为"癫痫小发作"），儿童多见，其特点为突然、短暂的意识丧失伴有凝视。有时会出现眼睛飘动和颈部张力轻微减低。多数失神发作持续时间不到 15 s。如果失神发作持续时间超过 20 s，则通常会出现自动症，这使得其与伴有意识受损和运动性自动症的局灶性癫痫发作在临床上难以区分。典型失神发作的 EEG 显示特征性的广泛性 3 次/秒的棘波和慢波（图 15.2）。发作结束后患者的行为和意识通常立即恢复正常，无发作后期，事后对发作不能记忆。

非典型失神发作在临床上类似于典型失神发作（前文已述）。此类发作也表现为凝视或精神运动迟缓，但 EEG 显示为较慢的广泛性棘慢波放电（2.5 Hz 或更低）。此外，非典型失神发作的持续时间可能比典型失神发作更长，可持续数分钟。意识水平波动、起病和恢复缓慢，以及偶有肌张力减低是非典型失神发作的显著特征，使其与典型（3 Hz）失神发作相区别。

在运动性全面性癫痫发作中，将重点介绍几种类型，包括肌阵挛发作、强直-阵挛发作、强直发作和失张力发作。肌阵挛发作表现为单侧或双侧、同步或非同步的快速、短暂、重复的肌肉抽动，且不伴有意识丧失。肌阵挛发作可不同程度地波及肢体、面部、眼睛和眼睑。EEG 可观察到与发作一致的异常放电。其他类型的非皮质肌阵挛，如良性夜间（入睡前）肌阵挛、皮质下和脊髓型肌阵挛，均无 EEG 相关异常放电现象，不视为癫痫发作。反复肌阵挛发作可逐渐增强并演变为全面性强直-阵挛发作（称为肌阵挛-强直-阵挛发作）。尽管肌阵挛发作可在任何时间发生，但多在睡醒后不久出现丛集性发作。

全面性强直-阵挛发作先有数次肌阵挛性抽动，或突然发作进入持续 20 ～ 60 s 的强直期，随后进入持续相似时间的阵挛期，最后进入发作后期。患者通常没有局灶性体征，有时会发生头部转动，但该动作并不表明特定的病灶位置。如果遗漏发作起始症状，通常无法在临床上区分全面性强直-阵挛发作和局灶扩展至双侧强直-阵挛发作。

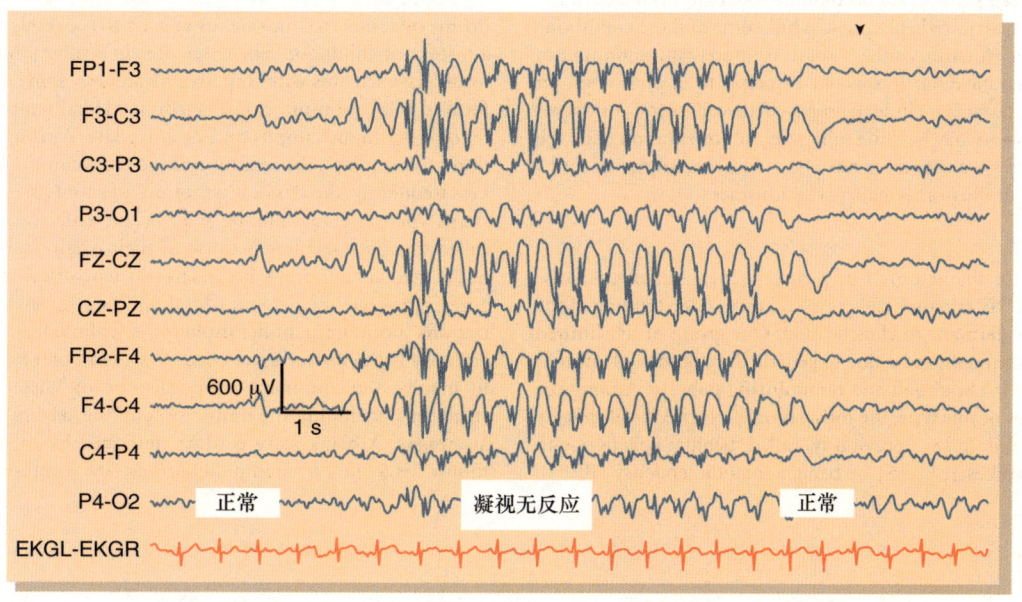

图 15.2 失神癫痫（癫痫小发作）。EEG 显示与临床失神发作相关的典型广泛性 3 Hz 棘慢复合波

Tonic Seizures, Atonic Seizures, and Epileptic Spasms

Generalized onset *tonic seizures* are characterized by a sudden marked increase in tone, usually involving bilateral limbs and torso. They are more apt to occur during sleep and are typically brief, under 20 seconds. If standing, these seizures may lead to falls with associated injuries, including head injuries. Generalized onset *atonic seizures* are denoted by a sudden loss of tone affecting the head, limbs or torso. If standing, the patient may fall due to loss of tone, with associated risk of injuries. Head protective gear may be helpful. Such seizures are brief, usually less than 15 seconds. They are often referred to as drop attacks or drop seizures. *Epileptic spasms* are very brief attacks that may cluster and are classically denoted by sudden flexion of the trunk and simultaneous flexion or extension of the limbs. Epileptic spasms manifest as flexor or extensor tonus, myoclonus, or a mixed pattern. The spasms last 1 to 20 seconds each and often occur in clusters for up to 20 minutes. Epileptic spasms often occur in infancy with several forms of early life epilepsies (see later).

EPILEPSIES

Epilepsy classification is governed by the seizure type(s) expressed by that form of epilepsy. This is primarily driven on clinical grounds but is supported by EEG findings, imaging or other metrics. The epilepsies are now divided into four major categories: focal epilepsy, generalized epilepsy (also known as idiopathic or genetic generalized epilepsy), combined generalized and focal epilepsy, and unknown epilepsy. Within each category are epilepsy syndromes. Reflex epilepsy syndromes may reside in either the generalized or the focal epilepsies. Epilepsy syndromes involve a cluster of features such as seizure types, EEG findings, imaging findings, age of onset, prognosis, comorbidities, family history, and genetics. Epilepsy etiology is a major feature in epilepsy classification. There are six main etiologies: structural, genetic, infectious, metabolic, immune, and unknown. Examples of structural epilepsies include post-stroke epilepsy, post-traumatic, tumor-related, postinfectious, and cortical maldevelopment. Genetic causes of epilepsy are being rapidly discovered. While some do run in pedigrees, many are found de novo in the affected patient. Absence of a clear family history does not exclude a genetic etiology. One family of genetic causes relates to channelopathies, or mutations in ion channels or receptors that regulate neuronal excitability. Another subset refers to gene mutations that disrupt neural development. Another subset relates to genes that disrupt metabolism (e.g., glucose transporter, or mitochondrial genes). The immune etiologies are some of the most recently recognized. Assays for various autoantibodies targeting distinct CNS antigens, both intracellular and cell surface, are becoming more commonplace in the work-up of certain acquired epilepsies. While some of these conditions are paraneoplastic in nature, others are more purely autoimmune in origin. These often have seizures as one principle facet of a symptom complex, which may also include neuropsychiatric, dystonic, or cognitive symptoms. These may be quite fulminant in presentation (e.g., the anti-NMDA receptor antibody syndrome). Some examples of common, distinctive, or illustrative epilepsy syndromes follow.

Focal Epilepsy

Focal epilepsies are characterized by recurrent focal seizures. As discussed previously, six etiologic categories aid our understanding of the epilepsies and are germane to classification. One group of self-limited focal epilepsies is thought to be due to genetic developmental anomalies that manifest in childhood and remit during puberty. Among the several syndromes of this type, the most common is *childhood epilepsy with centrotemporal spikes* (previously called benign epilepsy with centrotemporal spikes [BECTS] or benign rolandic epilepsy [BRE]). Seizures usually begin between the ages of 3 and 12 years in an otherwise normal child. The seizures are focal and consist of brief hemifacial motor or sensory events with preserved awareness. Typically, there is twitching of one side of the face, speech arrest, drooling, and paresthesias of the face, gums, tongue, or inner cheeks. The affected child often points to their face and goes to a parent and holds on until it is over; the child then quickly resumes normal activity. Seizures may progress to include hemiclonic movements or hemitonic posturing. Focal to bilateral tonic-clonic seizures occasionally occur, usually during sleep. The parents may report only the convulsions, as the focal onset can be missed unless the child is carefully questioned. The EEG reveals distinctive, stereotyped epileptiform discharges over the central and midtemporal regions that are dramatically activated by sleep with a normal underlying background. Prognosis for this syndrome is good, as it is for most of the other self-limited focal epilepsy syndromes; the seizures disappear and the EEG normalizes by mid to late adolescence. Outcome is unaffected by treatment, but antiepileptic drugs (AEDs) can prevent recurrent attacks.

Another example within this group is the Panayiotopoulos syndrome (also known as early onset occipital epilepsy). This self-limited syndrome is associated with focal autonomic seizures, classically involving pallor, hypersalivation, and vomiting, occasionally with eye deviation and tonic-clonic activity. Most seizures arise from sleep, often within the first hour of sleep. Seizures are lengthy, 20 to 60 minutes. The EEG in the Panayiotopoulos syndrome shows high amplitude and sleep activated, unilateral or bilateral occipital spikes. Seizures may continue for 2 to 3 years after presentation but then abate. Prognosis is good.

Many focal epilepsies can be understood by their specific locale of focal seizure onset. Temporal lobe epilepsy is an example, as is frontal lobe epilepsy. Within each of these designations, one may be able to define the epilepsy further, as in mesial temporal lobe epilepsy, or supplementary motor frontal lobe epilepsy. Distinct etiologies may account for individual forms but the seizure semiology may be similar if the seizure onset zone is shared. For instance, a structural mesial temporal lobe epilepsy secondary to a ganglioglioma may involve identical seizures as would hippocampal sclerosis associated with long-standing mesial temporal lobe epilepsy. These acquired focal epilepsies are often classified based upon the cerebral lobe involved during the initial phase of the seizure. Temporal lobe epilepsy is the most frequent, followed by frontal, then by rarer cases of parietal and occipital lobe epilepsies. Most cases of focal epilepsy entail a single seizure focus. However, the focus can sometimes involve a large, multilobar circuit. Some patients have multiple foci, each associated with a different seizure semiology.

Temporal lobe epilepsy (TLE) is the most common epilepsy syndrome of adults, accounting for at least 40% of epilepsy cases. There is a history of childhood febrile seizures in a subset. Most patients have focal onset seizures with impaired awareness, some of which evolve to focal to bilateral tonic-clonic seizures. Medial temporal lobe seizures involve the hippocampus and/or amygdala. A rising epigastric sensation or vague cephalic sensation is the most commonly reported aura. Less frequently, the classical symptoms of a foul smell, déjà vu, or other stereotyped altered thinking may occur. Olfactory auras have been called uncinate seizures because of their origin in or near the uncus of the medial temporal lobe. In lateral (neocortical) temporal lobe seizures, language impairment (dominant hemisphere), recurring vocalizations (nondominant hemisphere), eye blinking, or formed visual or auditory hallucinations can occur. As a temporal lobe seizure spreads to involve the dominant temporal lobe or bilateral temporal lobe structures, including the limbic system, the seizure evolves to impair awareness. A blank stare is often described by witnesses. Automatic motor behaviors, termed *automatisms*, are common in seizures that

强直发作、失张力发作和癫痫性痉挛

全面性强直发作以肌张力突然显著增高为特征，通常累及双侧肢体和躯干，常发生在睡眠期间，通常较为短暂，一般持续时间少于20 s。如果患者站立时发作，可能会跌倒并导致头部外伤。全面性失张力发作表现为患者头部、肢体或躯干肌张力突然丧失。站立时发作患者会因肌张力丧失而跌倒，并有受伤的风险。佩戴头部防护装置可能会有所帮助。这类癫痫发作较为短暂，通常持续时间不足15 s，也称为跌倒发作或猝倒发作。癫痫性痉挛发作时间非常短暂，可能呈簇状发作，其典型特征是躯干突然屈曲，同时伴有四肢的屈曲或伸直。癫痫性痉挛可有屈肌或伸肌强直、肌阵挛或混合型。每次痉挛持续1～20 s，也可长达20 min呈簇状发作。癫痫性痉挛通常发生在婴儿期，伴随多种形式的早期癫痫（见下文）。

癫痫

癫痫的分类取决于此类癫痫所表现出的发作类型，主要基于临床依据，同时也需要EEG结果、影像学或其他指标的支持。目前，癫痫被分为四大类：局灶性癫痫、全面性癫痫（也称为特发性或遗传性全面性癫痫）、全面性合并局灶性癫痫，以及不明分类的癫痫。每一大类中都包含多种癫痫综合征。反射性癫痫综合征既可存在于全面性癫痫，也可存在于局灶性癫痫中。癫痫综合征包括一系列特征，如癫痫发作类型、EEG和影像学结果、发病年龄、预后、并发症、家族史和遗传史。癫痫病因是癫痫分类的主要特征，有六大癫痫病因：结构性、遗传性、感染性、代谢性、免疫性和未知病因。结构性癫痫包括脑卒中后癫痫、脑外伤后癫痫、肿瘤相关性癫痫、感染后癫痫和皮质发育不良性癫痫等。遗传性病因现在仍在探索中，某些癫痫确实有家系遗传，仍有很多遗传性癫痫首次在患者中发现。缺乏明确的家族史并不能排除遗传性病因。其中一类遗传性病因涉及离子通道病，即调节神经元兴奋性的离子通道或受体发生突变。另一类是破坏神经发育的基因发生突变。还有一类与扰乱代谢的基因有关（如葡萄糖转运体或线粒体基因）。免疫性病因是近年才得到认可。针对中枢神经系统不同抗原（包括细胞内抗原和细胞表面抗原）的各种自身抗体的检测在获得性癫痫检查中越来越普遍。虽然其中某些抗体本质上是副肿瘤性，但更多的抗体源于自身免疫性疾病。癫痫综合征通常以癫痫发作为典型表现，伴有神经精神症状、肌张力障碍或认知障碍等，这些症状在发作时可能相当剧烈（如抗NMDA受体抗体综合征）。以下是较为常见或具有代表性的癫痫综合征的示例。

局灶性癫痫

局灶性癫痫以反复出现的局灶性癫痫发作为特征。如上文所述，六大病因分类有助于我们理解癫痫并进行分类。其中，自限性局灶性癫痫是由遗传发育异常所致，儿童期发病，青春期缓解。在这类癫痫综合征中，最常见的是伴中央颞部棘波的儿童癫痫［既往称伴中央颞部棘波的良性癫痫（BECTS）或良性运动性癫痫（BRE）］，通常发生在3～12岁的儿童中，患儿其他方面表现正常。癫痫发作呈局灶性，表现为短暂的一侧面部运动或感觉症状，但意识保持清醒。典型症状为一侧面部抽搐、语言停顿、流涎，以及面部、牙龈、舌或内颊的感觉异常。发病时患儿通常会指着自己的脸，走向父母，直到发作结束，患儿会迅速恢复正常活动。发作可能进展成一侧阵挛性运动或一侧强直性姿势。偶尔会出现局灶扩展至双侧强直-阵挛发作，通常发生在睡眠期间。家长可能只描述惊厥，除非仔细询问患儿，否则会忽略局灶性发作的起病症状。EEG可显示正常的背景活动下，睡眠诱发中央和中颞区明显的、刻板的癫痫样放电。与其他大多数自限性局灶性癫痫综合征一样，该病预后良好，到青春期中后期发作消失，EEG恢复正常。预后不受治疗影响，但抗癫痫药物（AED）可以预防其反复发作。

另一种是Panayiotopoulos综合征（也称早发性枕叶癫痫）。这种自限性综合征与局灶性自主神经癫痫发作有关，典型症状有面色苍白、流涎和呕吐，偶有眼球偏斜和强直-阵挛性活动。绝大多数此类癫痫发作可由睡眠诱导，通常在入睡后的第1个小时内发生。发作时间长，持续20～60 min。EEG显示高振幅、睡眠诱发的单侧或双侧枕部棘波。发作可能在发病后持续2～3年，但随后会缓解。预后良好。

局灶性癫痫可根据其发作起始的特定部位进行分类，例如颞叶癫痫和额叶癫痫。在这种分类中，人们可以进一步细分癫痫，如内侧颞叶癫痫或辅助运动区额叶癫痫等。不同病因可能导致不同的癫痫发作形式，但如果癫痫发作起始区相同，临床表现可能相似。例如，继发于神经节胶质瘤的结构性内侧颞叶癫痫可能与海马硬化导致的长期内侧颞叶癫痫症状相同。这些获得性局灶性癫痫通常根据癫痫发作初期所累及的脑叶进行分类。颞叶癫痫最为常见，其次是额叶癫痫，顶叶和枕叶癫痫较为少见。绝大多数局灶性癫痫源于单个致痫灶。但致痫灶本身可波及多脑叶反馈通路。某些患者可有多个致痫灶，每个致痫灶都与不同的癫痫发作症状相关。

颞叶癫痫（TLE）是成人最常见的癫痫综合征，占癫痫病例的40%以上。部分患者有儿童期热性惊厥史。大多数患者表现为意识受损的局灶性发作，其中一些可进展为局灶扩展至双侧强直-阵挛发作。内侧颞叶癫痫可累及海马和（或）杏仁核区，最常见的先兆症状是上腹部胃气上升感或脑内模糊感。较少见的经典症状有恶臭感、似曾相识感或刻板思维改变。嗅觉先兆可被称为钩回发作，因为它们源于内侧颞叶钩回或其附近。外侧颞叶（新皮质）发作可出现言语障碍（优势半球）、反复发声（非优势半球）、眨眼或成形的视幻觉或听幻觉。当颞叶发作扩散累及优势半球或双侧颞叶结构，包括边缘系统时，癫痫发作可伴有意识受损，目击者经常描述患者有茫然的凝视。

involve the limbic system (usually in the temporal lobe). Automatisms include oroalimentary signs (e.g., lip-smacking, repetitive swallowing) and repetitive hand movements (manual automatisms).

Frontal lobe epilepsy (FLE) can be more difficult to diagnose because the scalp EEG may be normal or not reveal a classic epileptic discharge, even with ictal recordings. There are at least four different premotor frontal lobe seizure semiologic patterns, with differing localization. *Supplementary motor* seizures (superior frontal gyri, posterior aspect) consist of contralateral versive posturing of the head and arms in a so-called "fencer posture"; the contralateral arm is extended, the head is turned strongly to that side, and the ipsilateral arm is flexed and held either up above the head or across the chest. *Lateral frontal* seizures manifest as contralateral head and eye deviation. *Hypermotor* seizures (frontal, poorly localized) consist of wild asynchronous movements and are often confused with psychogenic nonepileptic attacks. Almost all hypermotor seizures last less than 40 seconds and typically occur one to five times per night during sleep and less often during waking. *Frontal absence* seizures are rare and due to diffuse, bisynchronous frontal epileptic activity. These consist of staring and mimic typical or atypical absence seizures. Seizures arising in the posterior frontal lobe motor cortex (precentral gyrus) are classically clonic with a Jacksonian march.

Reflex epilepsies are distinguished by seizures that are precipitated by a specific stimulus such as touch, a musical tune, a specific movement, reading, flashing lights, or certain complex visual images. Apart from the photosensitive response in juvenile myoclonic epilepsy (see later), which is relatively common, reflex seizures are rare and are classified as a type of parietal or occipital lobe epilepsy because these regions mediate sensory functions.

Focal post-traumatic epilepsy is a common etiologic type of structural epilepsy. The likelihood of developing post-traumatic epilepsy relates directly to the severity of the head injury. The relative risk for developing epilepsy after a penetrating wound to the brain (e.g., bullet or shrapnel) is up to 600 times that of the general population. Severe closed head injuries result in epilepsy in 20% of patients. Severe closed head injuries are defined by the presence of intracranial hemorrhage of various types, unconsciousness or amnesia lasting more than 24 hours, or persistent abnormalities on neurologic examination, such as hemiparesis or aphasia. Although most patients with epilepsy following severe traumatic brain injury develop seizures within 1 to 2 years of their head injury, new-onset epilepsy may appear after 20 years or longer from the insult. Mild closed head injuries (uncomplicated brief loss of consciousness, no skull fracture, absence of focal neurologic signs, and no contusion or hematoma) may minimally increase the risk of seizures. Post-traumatic epilepsy is always focal or multifocal.

Idiopathic or Genetic Generalized Epilepsy

Both terms, "idiopathic" and "genetic," for this subset of the generalized epilepsies have advocates and critics among experts. *Idiopathic* in this context is meant to imply "self or genetic" in origin. Genetic often suggests that these forms of epilepsy are inherited and track within a family tree. However, often there is no helpful family history and so some of these instances probably arise de novo in affected individuals. The idiopathic (or genetic) generalized epilepsies (IGEs) are likely polygenic, resulting from a combination of mutations and polymorphisms in genes involved in thalamocortical circuitry. Different members within a family carrying these traits often exhibit dissimilar phenotypes. However, only rare IGE genes have been identified. A person with IGE has a 10% chance of passing the condition to a child. Most people with IGE have normal intelligence. Four entities comprise this group and are described later.

Childhood absence epilepsy (CAE; pyknolepsy, petit mal epilepsy) begins between 4 and 10 years of age with a peak at 7 years. Children with CAE have frequent absences (often dozens per day) and are sometimes initially thought to have attentional problems or to be daydreamers. The absences occur throughout the day. Some children with CAE have occasional generalized tonic-clonic seizures (GTCs). CAE is usually self-limited and seizures and EEG abnormalities resolve by young adulthood in most. The absence seizures of CAE are typically provoked by hyperventilation, a useful procedure in the office setting and during an EEG. The ictal EEG findings of CAE include abrupt and bilaterally synchronous 3-Hz spike and wave discharges, lasting 4 to 20 seconds with loss of responsiveness. Interictal EEGs show brief generalized spike and wave discharges in isolation or in brief bursts lasting a few seconds. Occipital intermittent rhythmic delta activity (OIRDA) is a less frequent finding.

Juvenile myoclonic epilepsy (JME) begins between ages 5 to 34 years old, with peak onset in the mid-teens, and is highly prevalent. JME exhibits a distinctive age-related expression of diverse seizure types, some of which have a clear nonrandom relationship to the sleep-wake cycle. As the name suggests, myoclonic seizures are a core feature; essentially all with JME have myoclonic seizures, though they may be occasionally subtle. Clusters of myoclonic seizures occur most commonly in the morning, usually soon after awakening. The clustered myoclonic seizures typically persist for up to 30 minutes. Myoclonic jerks predominantly affect the arms and last less than 1 second each. Consciousness is preserved with these events. Affected patients may often fail to mention their morning jerks unless specifically asked. Generalized tonic-clonic seizures often occur as well, often arising a bit later in adolescence or into the early 20s. This seizure type often brings the patient to neurologic attention. In JME, GTC seizures are more common after sleep deprivation or alcohol consumption the prior night. People with JME are usually photosensitive. That is, the seizures and EEG discharges are activated by flickering lights between 5 to 20 Hz (*photoparoxysmal* or *photoconvulsive* responses). This is a type of reflex seizure. Between 20% and 40% of patients with JME also have absence seizures. Absences in JME arise several years prior to the appearance of myoclonic seizures. The EEG in JME is like that of CAE, but the generalized discharges are slightly faster (classically 4 to 6 Hz) and often have polyspike components over a normal waking background rhythm. Unlike CAE, seizures in JME persist into adulthood and can be lifelong.

Less common IGE phenotypes include *juvenile absence epilepsy (JAE)* and epilepsy with *generalized tonic-clonic seizures alone (EGTCS)*. In JAE the predominant seizure type is absence with peak onset in the early teenage years and, unlike CAE, persists into adulthood. Absences are numerous. GTC seizures occur frequently as well, but myoclonic seizures are less common in JAE. In EGTCS, the predominant seizure type is a GTC seizure. These GTCs often occur within 1 to 2 hours of awakening but can occur anytime. EGTCS arises between 5 and 40 years of age, most often in the teens, and is not a self-limited epilepsy.

Combined Generalized and Focal Epilepsy

This category includes those epilepsies in which patients may have both focal and generalized seizures. Similarly, EEGs of these patients may exhibit both focal and generalized epileptiform patterns. This new epilepsy category includes a subgroup presently called developmental and epileptic encephalopathies, that were previously termed the symptomatic generalized epilepsies (ILAE, 1989 classification). Individuals with these epilepsies have multifocal or diffuse brain dysfunction since early in life. There is an associated encephalopathy with variable developmental delay. Important examples of the developmental and epileptic encephalopathies are Lennox-Gastaut syndrome (LGS), infantile spasms, and Dravet syndrome.

自动运动行为，又称自动症，常见于累及边缘系统（通常在颞叶）的癫痫发作。自动症包括口咽部自动症（如咂嘴、反复吞咽）或重复的手部动作（手自动症）。

额叶癫痫（FLE）诊断较为困难，因为即使有发作记录，头皮 EEG 可能显示正常或记录不到典型的癫痫样放电。根据受累部位，至少有 4 种不同的运动前区额叶癫痫的发作类型。辅助运动区癫痫发作（额上回，后部）包括头部和上肢组成的对侧偏转姿势，又称"击剑姿势"，表现为致痫灶对侧上肢外展，头部快速转向该侧，致痫灶同侧上肢屈曲并抬起至头部上方或横跨于胸前。额叶外侧癫痫发作表现为头部和眼球向致痫灶对侧偏斜。过度运动性癫痫发作（额叶，具体定位不明）表现为疯狂的非同步运动，常与心因性非癫痫发作混淆。几乎所有的过度运动性癫痫发作持续时间不超过 40 s，通常在夜间睡眠时发生 1～5 次，清醒时较少发生。额叶失神发作较为罕见，由双侧额叶广泛同步放电引起，表现为凝视和类似典型或非典型的失神发作。起源于额叶后部运动皮质（中央前回）的癫痫发作为典型的阵挛性发作，呈贾克森扩布（Jacksonian march）。

反射性癫痫的特点是由特定刺激（如触摸、乐曲、特定的运动、阅读、闪光灯或某些复杂的视觉图像）诱发的癫痫发作。除青少年肌阵挛性癫痫（见下文）中相对常见的光敏反应外，反射性发作较为罕见，属于顶叶或枕叶癫痫，因为这两个脑区具有感觉功能。

局灶性外伤后癫痫是结构性癫痫的常见病因类型。外伤后癫痫的发生概率与头部损伤的严重程度直接相关。脑贯通伤（如子弹或弹片）后发生癫痫的相对风险是普通人群的 600 倍。严重闭合性颅脑损伤导致 20% 的患者发生癫痫。严重闭合性颅脑损伤定义为存在各种类型的颅内出血、昏迷或遗忘持续超过 24 h，或神经系统检查持续异常（如偏瘫或失语）。大多数严重的创伤性颅脑损伤患者在受伤后 1～2 年内发生癫痫发作，但新的癫痫发作也可能在 20 年或更长时间后出现。轻度闭合性颅脑损伤（无并发症的短暂性意识丧失，无颅骨骨折，无局灶性神经系统体征，无挫伤或血肿）可能仅轻微增加癫痫发作的风险。外伤后癫痫通常为局灶性或多灶性。

特发性或遗传性全面性癫痫

"特发性"和"遗传性"两个术语用于描述全面性癫痫的子集，在专家中有支持者和批评者。特发性是指起源于"自身或遗传"。遗传性通常指该类型的癫痫具有遗传性，并可在家谱中追踪。然而某些情况下家族史并无帮助，因为一些遗传性癫痫可能在患者中新发出现。特发性全面性癫痫（IGE）或遗传性全面性癫痫可能是多基因遗传，是丘脑-皮质神经环路基因突变和多态性的综合结果。家族中携带该类型基因的不同成员往往表现出不同的表型。然而，仅有少数 IGE 基因被发现。IGE 患者遗传给后代的概率约为 10%。绝大多数 IGE 患者智力正常。以下为该组类型中的四个亚型。

儿童失神癫痫（CAE；密集性癫痫，癫痫小发作）在 4～10 岁发病，发病高峰在 7 岁。CAE 患儿表现为频繁失神发作（通常每天数十次），发病初期有时有注意力问题或似白日做梦。失神发作在一天中任何时间段均可能发生。有些 CAE 患儿偶尔有全面性强直-阵挛发作（GTC）。CAE 具有自限性，大多数癫痫发作和 EGG 异常可在成年早期缓解消失。CAE 的失神发作通常由过度通气诱发，其在诊室环境和 EEG 检查中较为有用。CAE 发作时 EEG 表现为突发的双侧同步 3 Hz 棘慢波放电，持续 4～20 s，伴有反应能力丧失。发作间期 EEG 显示孤立或短暂暴发的持续数秒的广泛性棘慢波放电。枕区间歇性节律性 δ 活动（OIRDA）比较少见。

青少年肌阵挛性癫痫（JME）在 5～34 岁发病，发病高峰在青少年中期，具有较高患病率。JME 表现为与年龄相关的不同的癫痫发作类型，其中某些发作类型与睡眠-觉醒周期有显著的非随机关系。顾名思义，肌阵挛发作是 JME 的核心特征，几乎所有 JME 患者都会出现肌阵挛发作，尽管有时可能不易察觉。群集性肌阵挛发作最常见于早晨，通常在醒后不久发生。群集性肌阵挛发作通常持续时间长达 30 min。肌阵挛性抽搐主要累及上肢，且每次发作持续时间不足 1 s。发作过程中意识保持清醒。除非刻意询问，患者往往不会主动提及这种晨起抽搐。全面性强直-阵挛发作也时常发生，通常见于青春期或 20 岁出头的人群。这种发作类型通常引起神经科医生的关注。若 JME 患者在前一晚睡眠剥夺或饮酒，则次日特别容易发生 GTC。JME 患者通常具有光敏性，给予 5～20 Hz 的闪光刺激会诱发癫痫发作和 EEG 异常放电（光阵发或光惊厥反应），这是一种反射性发作。20%～40% 的 JME 患者也有失神发作。JME 失神发作比肌阵挛发作早发生数年。JME 的 EEG 与 CAE 相似，但在正常清醒期背景节律中，其广泛性放电略快（通常为 4～6 Hz），并且常有多棘波成分。与 CAE 不同，JME 发作可持续到成年期，并且可能是终身发作。

较少见的 IGE 类型包括青少年失神癫痫（JAE）和单纯全面性强直-阵挛癫痫（EGTCS）。JAE 主要表现为失神发作，发病高峰在青少年早期，并且与 CAE 不同，发作会持续到成年期。该类型失神发作较为频繁，GTC 也经常发生，但 JAE 中肌阵挛发作较为少见。在 EGTCS 中，GTC 为主要的发作类型，一般好发于醒后 1～2 h 内，也可随时发生。EGTCS 的发病年龄在 5～40 岁，最常见于青少年，是一种非自限性的癫痫类型。

全面性合并局灶性癫痫

此类是指同时出现局灶性和全面性发作的癫痫患者。这些患者 EEG 可能同时表现为局灶性和全面性癫痫样放电模式。这类癫痫中有一亚组称为发育性癫痫性脑病，既往称为症状性全面性癫痫（ILAE，1989 年分类）。患者自幼就出现多灶性或弥漫性脑功能障碍，伴有不同程度的发育迟缓。其中重要的范例有 Lennox-Gastaut 综合征（LGS）、婴儿痉挛症和 Dravet 综合征。

LGS is a more common form of combined generalized and focal epilepsy. LGS presents from 2 to 10 years of age. It is characterized by the presence of multiple seizure types, usually a combination of tonic or atonic seizures, myoclonic seizures, and atypical absences, and with a characteristic EEG pattern of 2.5 Hz or slower generalized spike and slow wave discharges, in the setting of intellectual disability. Sixty percent have preexisting encephalopathy and developmental delay and up to 25% had infantile spasms earlier in their course. Tonic-clonic and focal seizures also occur. Sleep EEG recordings reveal bursts of diffuse 10- to 20-Hz rhythms with or without coincident tonic seizures. LGS is a chronic condition requiring supervision; many patients ultimately live in group homes. If drop seizures are present, and the patient is ambulatory, a protective helmet should be considered.

Infantile spasms are often a precursor to LGS. Infantile spasms usually begin during the first year of life, rarely beyond 18 months. *West syndrome* is the combination of epileptic spasms in infancy, hypsarrhythmia (a chaotic, disorganized epileptiform EEG pattern), and arrest of psychomotor development. The term infantile spasms is often used synonymously with West syndrome. Numerous etiologies can give rise to infantile spasms. Diagnostic evaluation may uncover an etiology in up to two thirds of cases. Common etiologies include CNS malformations such as cortical dysplasia, neurocutaneous disorders such as tuberous sclerosis complex, various metabolic disorders of infancy (e.g., phenylketonuria), congenital infections, genetic causes (e.g., chromosomal disorders, specific genetic abnormalities), plus other peri- and postnatal CNS insults. Infantile spasms have a poor prognosis with over 90% developing intellectual disability and most progressing to LGS; a small percent of usually cryptogenic cases have a more favorable outcome.

Dravet syndrome (previously severe myoclonic epilepsy of infancy) is both a genetic epilepsy and a developmental and epileptic encephalopathy. Children with Dravet syndrome have refractory epilepsy including multiple seizure types. Seizures commonly present within the first year of life, rarely during the second year. Affected children have normal development up to their presentation with seizures but then experience neurodevelopmental delay. Their initial seizure is typically a prolonged febrile tonic-clonic seizure, either unilateral or bilateral. More often, this is in the context of a febrile illness or recent vaccination, or less frequently with bathing. No precipitants are found in one third. Within weeks to months of this first seizure, more seizures follow, febrile or afebrile, often including bouts of status epilepticus. These may include hemiclonic seizures amongst others; these can even alternate sides. Seizures can be readily triggered by a variety of stimuli. Treatment-resistant seizures are accompanied by psychomotor impairment beginning months after the sentinel seizure. Cognitive, behavioral, language, gait, and other motor impairments accrue. EEGs show both focal and generalized epileptiform patterns and may vary with age. Mutations in the voltage-gated sodium channel, alpha-1 gene (SCN1A) are responsible for this syndrome in 70% to 80% of cases. Recognition of Dravet syndrome is important because voltage-gated sodium channel blocking AEDs (e.g., lamotrigine, phenytoin) can cause clinical deterioration, whereas others are particularly beneficial (e.g., topiramate, levetiracetam, valproate, benzodiazepines).

Other Seizure Conditions

Febrile seizures affect 3% to 5% of children younger than the age of 6 years. About 30% of children have more than one episode; recurrence is more likely if the first seizure occurs before 1 year of age or there is a family history of febrile seizures. Several distinct gene mutations predispose to febrile seizures. Although most affected children have no long-term consequences and appear to outgrow this age-restricted trait, febrile seizures increase the risk of later epilepsy. This risk is low for most children (2% to 3%) but increases to 10% to 15% in those with prolonged or focal febrile seizures *(complicated febrile seizures)*, a family history of nonfebrile seizures, or neurologic abnormalities that predate their first febrile seizure.

DIAGNOSIS

Accurate diagnosis is the cornerstone of epilepsy care. The diagnostic evaluation has three objectives: (1) to determine whether the patient's spell(s) are epileptic seizures, (2) to identify a specific underlying cause, and (3) to establish if the seizures are provoked and isolated, or if epilepsy is present and, if so, to determine the type of epilepsy, ideally the specific epilepsy syndrome.

History and Examination

The patient's and witnesses' descriptions of the events are central to diagnosis. The patient's recall of their seizure may be spotty due to associated amnesia surrounding the episode, and so the witnesses' descriptions are often more helpful. Attention should be paid to details of the patient's behavior before, during, and after the seizure. The setting of the seizure can suggest acute causes such as drug withdrawal, CNS infection, trauma, stroke, or other contributing or provoking factors. Recent-onset seizures in an adult may suggest a new intracranial process. A prior history of seizures suggests epilepsy. Any focal feature before, during, or after the seizure may suggest a possible structural brain lesion requiring appropriate investigation. The pattern of the seizures and the patient's age are often important clues to the seizure and epilepsy type.

The physical examination is normal in most patients with epilepsy. Examination should seek overt or subtle focal neurologic signs: slight unilateral lower facial paresis, clumsy fine finger movements, or mild hyperreflexia. These can be present in patients with epilepsy with a contralateral seizure focus. Careful skin examination is indicated to detect features of neurocutaneous syndromes such as a facial port-wine stain involving the upper eyelid in Sturge-Weber syndrome, hypopigmented macules (ash-leaf spots), shagreen patch (pink, elevated skin nodules with "orange peel" appearance found in the lumbar area), facial angiofibromas in tuberous sclerosis, and café-au-lait spots and axillary freckling in neurofibromatosis. Asymmetry in the size of the hands, feet, or face may signify a long-standing abnormality of the cerebral hemisphere contralateral to the smaller side. Absence seizures can be triggered during an office examination in untreated children with CAE with hyperventilation for 2 to 3 minutes.

Laboratory Tests—EEG

EEG is the most helpful diagnostic test for seizures and epilepsy. EEG findings help confirm the diagnosis, classify the seizures, identify the epilepsy syndrome, and impact therapeutic decisions. Epilepsy remains a largely clinical diagnosis, informed by EEG and other test findings. In combination with suitable clinical findings, *epileptiform* EEG discharges, termed *spikes* or *sharp waves*, strongly support a diagnosis of epilepsy. In patients with recurrent seizures, focal epileptiform discharges are consistent with epilepsies with focal onset seizures, whereas generalized epileptiform activity usually indicates a generalized form of epilepsy (associated with seizures of generalized onset). Most EEGs are obtained between seizures, and such interictal abnormalities alone cannot prove or disprove a diagnosis of epilepsy. Up to 50% of patients with epilepsy show epileptiform abnormalities on their initial EEG. The chance of capturing epileptiform activity is enhanced by sleep deprivation the night before the test, which increases the likelihood of recording drowsiness and light sleep during the EEG. Serial EEGs also increase the yield of a positive test. Some neurologists rely

Lennox-Gastaut 综合征（LGS）是一种较常见的全面性癫痫伴局灶性发作形式。LGS 发病多见于 2～10 岁。其特点为具有多种癫痫发作类型，通常是强直或失张力发作、肌阵挛发作和非典型失神发作的组合；此外，脑电图表现为特征性 2.5 Hz 或更慢的广泛性棘慢波放电，同时伴有智力缺陷。60% 患儿在癫痫发作之前已患有脑病和发育迟缓，高达 25% 的患者在发病早期曾患有婴儿痉挛。患者也会发生强直-阵挛发作和局灶性发作。睡眠期 EEG 显示阵发性弥漫性 10～20 Hz 节律，伴或不伴强直性发作。LGS 是一种需要监护的慢性疾病，许多患者最终住在集体住所。如果患者能够行走活动，若存在跌倒发作时，则考虑佩戴头盔进行防护。

婴儿痉挛症通常是 LGS 的先兆。婴儿痉挛症在患者出生后一年内起病，极少超过 18 个月。West 综合征是婴儿期癫痫性痉挛、EEG 高度节律失调（杂乱无序的癫痫样放电）和精神运动发育停滞三联征，常作为婴儿痉挛症的同义词。婴儿痉挛症的病因很多，诊断评估可能会为 2/3 的病例找到病因。常见的病因包括中枢神经系统畸形（如皮质发育不良）、神经皮肤病（如结节性硬化症）、各种婴儿期代谢障碍（如苯丙酮尿症）、先天性感染、遗传因素（如染色体病、特定遗传异常）以及其他围生期和产后中枢神经系统损伤。婴儿痉挛症的预后较差，超过 90% 的病例会发展为智力障碍，绝大多数会进展为 LGS，极少数的隐源性病例可有良好的预后。

Dravet 综合征（既往称婴儿重症肌阵挛性癫痫）既是一种遗传性癫痫，也是一种发育性癫痫性脑病。Dravet 综合征患儿表现为多种发作类型的难治性癫痫。癫痫发作通常在出生后第一年内发生，极少在第二年发生。患儿在发生癫痫发作前发育正常，但随后会出现神经发育迟缓。初次发作通常是一次长时程的热性惊厥（强直-阵挛发作），可为单侧或双侧。Dravet 综合征通常在发热性疾病或近期接种疫苗后发生，较少在洗澡时发生。1/3 的患者未发现诱因。首次癫痫发作后的数周到数月内会出现更多的发作，包括癫痫持续状态，伴有热性或无热性发作。这些发作可能包括偏侧阵挛发作，甚至可以交替侧别发生。各种刺激因素都能诱发癫痫发作。难治性癫痫伴随精神运动障碍，通常在首次发作后数月开始出现。认知、行为、语言、步态和其他运动障碍也会逐渐累及。EEG 显示局灶性和全面性癫痫样波型，可随年龄变化。70%～80% 的 Dravet 综合征病例是由电压门控钠通道 α-1 基因（*SCN1A*）突变引起。鉴别 Dravet 综合征很重要，因为电压门控钠通道阻滞剂类抗癫痫药物（如拉莫三嗪、苯妥英钠）可能会导致患者病情恶化，而其他药物（如托吡酯、左乙拉西坦、丙戊酸、苯二氮䓬类药物）可以发挥其正常疗效。

不明分类的癫痫

热性惊厥主要见于 6 岁以下儿童，患病率为 3%～5%。约 30% 的儿童可有不止一次发作，如果首次发作是发生在 1 岁之前或有热性惊厥的家族史，则复发的可能性更大。某些基因突变可增加罹患热性惊厥的风险。尽管大多数患儿没有远期不良影响，并且随着年龄的增长不再具有这种年龄限制性特征，但热性惊厥可增加日后发生癫痫的风险。对于大多数儿童来说，这种风险相对较低（2%～3%），但对于发作持续时间较长或局灶性热性惊厥（复杂热性惊厥）、有非热性癫痫发作家族史或在首次热性惊厥发作之前已有神经系统异常的患儿来说，这种风险会增加到 10%～15%。

诊断

准确的诊断是癫痫治疗的基石。诊断评估有三个目的：①确定患者是否是癫痫发作；②探究具体的潜在原因；③确定癫痫发作是诱发性、单次发作，或是否存在癫痫，如果存在，确定癫痫类型，最好是确定具体的癫痫综合征。

病史与体格检查

患者和目击者关于事件的描述对诊断至关重要。患者对发作的回忆可能会因癫痫发作期的失忆而变得模糊不清，因此目击者的描述往往更有帮助。应当注意患者在癫痫发作前、发作期间和发作后的具体行为细节。癫痫发作的背景可能提示急性原因，如药物戒断、中枢神经系统感染、创伤、卒中、其他促成或诱发因素。成人近期出现的癫痫发作提示颅内有新发病变。如果患者既往有癫痫发作史则提示癫痫。癫痫发作前、发作期间或发作后出现的任何局灶性体征可能提示脑结构性病变，需要进行相应的检查。癫痫发作的形式和患者的年龄常常是诊断癫痫发作和癫痫类型的重要依据。

大多数癫痫患者的体格检查正常。体检时应注意明显的或轻微的局灶性神经系统体征，如轻度单侧下面部瘫痪、手指精细运动笨拙或轻度反射亢进等。这些体征可能出现在对侧致痫灶的癫痫患者中。仔细的皮肤检查有助于发现神经皮肤综合征的特征，如 Sturge-Weber 综合征可见累及上眼睑的面部葡萄酒色斑，结节性硬化症可见色素减退斑（灰叶斑）、鲨鱼皮斑（腰部突起的粉红色皮肤结节，外观类似"橘皮"）和面部血管纤维瘤，神经纤维瘤病可见牛奶咖啡斑和腋下雀斑。手、足或面部的大小不对称提示发育较小侧的对侧大脑半球已存在长期病变。未治疗的儿童失神癫痫（CAE）可在诊室检查期间通过 2～3 min 的过度换气诱发失神发作。

实验室检查——EEG

EEG 是对癫痫发作和癫痫最有帮助的诊断性检查。EEG 结果有助于确定诊断、区分发作类型、识别癫痫综合征及做出治疗决策。癫痫是一种基于 EEG 和其他检查结果的临床诊断。结合相应的临床表现，EEG 存在棘波或尖波癫痫样放电则强烈支持癫痫诊断。反复癫痫发作的患者中，EEG 出现局灶性癫痫样放电提示局灶性癫痫，而出现广泛性癫痫样放电通常提示全面性癫痫（与全面性癫痫发作相关）。大多数 EEG 检查在癫痫发作间期进行，仅凭这种发作间期的异常无法明确或排除癫痫诊断。多达 50% 的癫痫患者在最初 EEG 上可显示癫痫

on prolonged EEG monitoring studies to record much more data including more sleep samples. Supplemental T1 and T2 electrodes can occasionally benefit the yield of the EEG. A small proportion of patients with epilepsy have normal interictal EEGs despite all efforts to record an abnormality.

The interpretation of the interictal EEG is confounded by two factors. Epileptiform discharges occur in about 2% of normal people; many of these may be asymptomatic markers of a genetic trait, especially in children. Also, the interpretation of the EEG is subjective. Normal benign variant waveforms and artifacts can be occasionally misinterpreted as epileptiform activity and erroneously considered to indicate seizure susceptibility.

Epilepsy can be definitively established by recording a characteristic ictal discharge during a representative clinical attack. This is uncommon during routine EEGs but can often be accomplished with *video-EEG long-term monitoring (LTM)*. This can be performed in the outpatient setting (ambulatory video-EEG LTM) or in the inpatient setting at many epilepsy centers throughout the world. The inpatient setting permits AED tapering as needed in a safe setting to increase the odds of eliciting one or more seizures for characterization, whereas this is not the case for ambulatory LTM. Inpatient video-EEG monitoring is indicated in people who have ongoing seizures despite treatment with appropriate AEDs. About one third of patients admitted for LTM are found not to have epilepsy. The majority of these patients have psychogenic nonepileptic attacks. A much smaller subset of patients with nonepileptic seizures have other physiologic mimics of epileptic seizures (e.g., certain movement disorders). In the approximately 30% of people with treatment-resistant epilepsy (those with seizures despite trials of multiple AEDs, alone or in combination), inpatient video-EEG monitoring to more precisely define the seizure focus is a critical step toward determining candidacy for various epilepsy surgery options. Phase I LTM involves scalp EEG recordings. A subset of patients require phase II LTM studies in which electrodes are neurosurgically implanted in or on the brain to more precisely localize the seizure onset zone and map critical functional cortical regions nearby. Recently, stereotactically placed depth leads have been gaining popularity for such investigations in many tertiary epilepsy centers in the United States.

Laboratory Tests—Neuroimaging

Brain MRI complements EEG findings by identifying structural pathology that is causally related to the development of epilepsy. MRI is the best test to detect epileptogenic cerebral lesions including hippocampal sclerosis, neuronal migration disorders, tumors, focal atrophy, arteriovenous malformations, and cavernous malformations. It is important to obtain a complete imaging study that includes T1-weighted, T2-weighted, and inversion-recovery sequences in coronal and axial planes. Contrast can also be helpful for some epilepsy pathologies. Imaging in the coronal plane perpendicular to the long axis of the hippocampus has improved detection of hippocampal atrophy and increased T2 signal, findings that correlate with the pathologic finding of hippocampal sclerosis and an epileptogenic temporal lobe. Additional sequences that should be routine include T2-weighted gradient echo (GRE), to detect hemosiderin indicating prior hemorrhage associated with vascular malformations or trauma, and diffusion-weighted images (DWI) for cytotoxic edema, sometimes present with acute cerebral injury from prolonged seizures or status epilepticus. In 2019, many tertiary centers in the United States offered 3T MRI. This provides improved resolution over lower strength MRIs and can aid in detecting smaller lesions such as very small cortical dysplasias.

An MRI should be obtained in all patients with suspected epilepsy with the exception that many pediatric epileptologists view MRI as optional for patients with definite childhood epilepsy with centrotemporal spikes or definite generalized genetic epilepsies (e.g., CAE and JME). CT scan with contrast is an alternative study for those who cannot have MRI but has lower resolution than MRI for detecting small lesions. Any patient with seizures and abnormal neurologic findings or focal slow-wave abnormalities on EEG should have neuroimaging. Repeat neuroimaging should be considered if there is an unexplained change in seizure pattern, to evaluate for a new lesion, or in those with possible low-grade neoplastic lesions.

Positron emission tomography (PET) and single-photon emission computed tomography (SPECT) use physiologically active, radio-labeled tracers to image the brain's metabolic activity and are useful adjunctive imaging methods for certain patients seeking a surgical treatment option for their epilepsy. SPECT is most useful when an ictal and interictal study are combined to identify an extratemporal seizure focus. Abnormalities on PET or SPECT can be present when brain MRI is normal and thus add value in that scenario. PET has been most useful in treatment-resistant, MRI-negative, temporal lobe epilepsy.

Other Tests

Routine blood tests rarely offer diagnostic assistance in otherwise healthy patients with epilepsy. Serum electrolytes, liver function tests, and complete blood count are useful with acute new-onset seizures and as baseline studies before AED therapy is started. A mildly increased serum WBC count without a marked "left shift" is a common, but nonspecific, transient finding after convulsive seizures or status epilepticus. Serum CPK can also transiently increase postictally but is also nonspecific and no longer commonly obtained outside of the setting of suspected myonecrosis or rhabdomyolysis. Adolescents and adults with unexplained seizures should be screened for substance abuse (especially cocaine) with blood or urine studies. Genetic testing should be considered in specific cases with suspected phenotypes, especially if a positive genetic test would alter therapy, such as in SCN1A-associated epilepsies (e.g., Dravet syndrome). Lumbar puncture is indicated if there is a suspicion of meningitis, encephalitis, autoimmune or paraneoplastic process, or a CNS glucose transporter abnormality. Repeated generalized seizures and status epilepticus can increase cerebrospinal fluid protein measures slightly and produce a mild pleocytosis for 24 to 48 hours; cerebrospinal fluid pleocytosis should be attributed to seizures only in retrospect after excluding an intracranial inflammatory process. An electrocardiogram (ECG) should be obtained in any young person with a first generalized seizure if there is a family history of arrhythmia, sudden unexplained death, or episodic unconsciousness. An ECG should also be obtained in any patient with a personal history of cardiac arrhythmia or valvular disease.

DIFFERENTIAL DIAGNOSIS

Not every paroxysmal event is a seizure, and misidentification of other conditions leads to ineffective, unnecessary, and potentially harmful treatments plus delay to reach the correct diagnosis. Misdiagnosis accounts for a subset of patients who have not responded to AED treatment. The conditions confused with epilepsy depend on the age of the patient and the nature and circumstances of the attacks (Table 15.3). Nonepileptic paroxysmal disorders that are confused with epileptic seizures have sudden, discrete abnormal behaviors, variable responsiveness, changes in muscle tone, and various postures or movements.

Psychogenic nonepileptic seizures (PNES) frequently are misdiagnosed as intractable epilepsy in adults. PNES are felt to be due to unconscious emotional conflicts impacting the patient's physical state, mimicking a seizure (i.e., a somatoform manifestation of psychologic distress). Roughly 10% of patients with PNES also have epilepsy.

样放电异常。检查前一晚的睡眠剥夺可增加 EEG 捕获癫痫样活动的概率，同时也增加了记录困倦和轻度睡眠的可能性。连续 EEG 检查也会增加发现阳性结果的概率。神经科医生可通过长时程 EEG 监测记录更多数据，包括更多睡眠时的数据。增加 T1 和 T2 电极有时能提高 EEG 的检出率。虽然竭尽全力去记录异常脑电表现，但仍有一小部分癫痫患者发作间期的 EEG 显示正常。

发作间期 EEG 的判读受两个因素的影响。一方面，约 2% 的正常人 EEG 可出现癫痫样放电，这些人可能是具有遗传特征的无症状携带者，尤其是儿童。另外，EEG 的判读具有主观性。正常良性变异波和伪迹有时会被误判为癫痫样异常放电，并被错误地视为癫痫发作易感性的证据。

如果在典型临床发作过程中 EEG 记录到特征性发作放电，即可明确癫痫诊断。其在常规 EEG 检查中并不多见，但可通过视频 EGG 长程监测（LTM）实现。LTM 可在门诊中进行（动态视频-EGG LTM），也可在世界各地癫痫中心的住院病房中开展。住院病房可允许在安全的环境中根据需要逐渐减少 AED 以增加诱发一次或多次癫痫发作的概率，而门诊 LTM 则不具备这种条件。住院视频 EEG 监测适用于正在接受适当 AED 治疗但仍出现持续性癫痫发作的患者。大约 1/3 的 LTM 患者未发现癫痫。这些患者中大多数有心因性非癫痫性发作。极少部分非癫痫性发作的患者有其他类似于癫痫发作的生理性特征（如某些运动障碍）。对于约 30% 的难治性癫痫患者（单独或联合使用多种 AED 后仍出现癫痫发作的患者）来说，住院视频 EEG 监测能更精确地定位致痫灶，这是确定癫痫手术的关键步骤。Ⅰ 期 LTM 为头皮 EEG 记录。一部分患者需要 Ⅱ 期 LTM 研究，通过神经外科手术将电极植入大脑内部或表面，以更精确地定位发作起始区，并绘制附近的关键皮质功能区。近年来在美国的许多三级癫痫中心中，立体定向植入深部电极被越来越多地应用于此类研究。

实验室检查——神经影像学

脑 MRI 通过发现与癫痫发生有因果关系的脑结构病理学改变，对 EEG 检查结果进行补充。作为发现致痫灶的最佳检查方法，MRI 能发现引起癫痫的脑损伤，如海马硬化、神经元移行障碍、肿瘤、局灶性萎缩、动静脉畸形和海绵状血管畸形等。获得完整的 MRI 资料很重要，包括冠状位和轴位的 T1 加权像、T2 加权像及反转恢复序列。造影剂的使用有助于发现某些癫痫病理改变。垂直于海马长轴的冠状位成像能更好地发现海马萎缩和 T2 信号增强，这些影像学结果与海马硬化及颞叶致痫灶的病理学发现相关。常规的增补序列包括 T2 加权梯度回波（GRE），用于检测与血管畸形或创伤相关的陈旧性出血中含铁血黄素，以及弥散加权成像（DWI），用于检测长时间癫痫发作或癫痫持续状态引起急性脑损伤时的细胞毒性水肿。2019 年美国某些三级医院提供 3T MRI，这种成像技术比低场强 MRI 具有更高的分辨率，有助于发现更小的病灶，如微小皮质发育不良。

所有疑似癫痫的患者都应进行 MRI 检查，但一些儿科癫痫专家认为，对于明确伴有中央颞区棘波的儿童癫痫或遗传性全面性癫痫（如 CAE 和 JME），MRI 不是必需的检查。对于无法进行 MRI 检查的患者，可以选择 CT 增强扫描，但其分辨率低于 MRI，难以发现较小的病灶。任何有癫痫发作和神经系统检查异常或 EEG 显示局灶性慢波异常的患者都应进行神经影像学检查。如果癫痫发作波型出现不明原因的变化，应考虑重复进行神经影像学检查，以评估新病变或可能存在的低级别肿瘤病变。

正电子发射断层成像（PET）和单光子发射计算机断层成像术（SPECT）是使用具有生理学活性的放射性标记的示踪剂对脑代谢活动进行成像的技术，对某些寻求癫痫手术治疗的患者来说是一种有用的辅助成像方法。通过发作期和发作间期的对比研究来明确颞外癫痫发作的致痫灶时，SPECT 检查最为有用。当脑部 MRI 检查结果正常时，PET 或 SPECT 检查可能存在异常，这种情况下增加了其检测价值。PET 最适用于难治性、MRI 阴性的颞叶癫痫。

其他检查

在其他方面均健康的癫痫患者，血常规检查很少能够提供诊断帮助。血清电解质、肝功能检测和全血细胞计数对急性新发癫痫发作和开始 AED 治疗前的基线检查非常有用。惊厥发作或癫痫持续状态后，血清白细胞计数轻度增加但没有明显"核左移"是常见且非特异性的短暂表现。血清肌酸磷酸激酶（CPK）也可在发作后短暂升高，但同样是非特异性的表现，除非怀疑肌坏死或横纹肌溶解症，血清 CPK 现在已不再是常规检查。青少年和成人发生原因不明的癫痫发作时，应做血液或尿液检查来筛查物质滥用（特别是可卡因）。在具有疑似表型的特殊病例中应考虑基因检测，特别是基因检测结果阳性会改变治疗方案的病例，如 SCN1A 相关癫痫（Dravet 综合征）。如怀疑脑膜炎、脑炎、自身免疫性或副肿瘤反应或中枢神经系统（CNS）葡萄糖转运蛋白异常，应进行腰椎穿刺检查。反复全面性癫痫发作和癫痫持续状态可导致轻度脑脊液蛋白质含量增加和细胞数增多，可持续 24～48 h，只有在排除颅内炎性病变后，脑脊液细胞数增多才可归因于癫痫发作。存在心律失常、不明原因猝死或发作性意识丧失家族史的年轻人，在首次全面性癫痫发作时应进行心电图（ECG）检查。任何有心律失常或心脏瓣膜病史的患者，也应进行 ECG 检查。

鉴别诊断

并非所有发作性事件都是癫痫发作，对其他疾病的误诊会导致无效、不必要甚至可能有害的治疗，还可能延误正确诊断。误诊可能导致部分患者对 AED 治疗无效。许多疾病易与癫痫混淆，具体情况取决于患者年龄及发作的性质和情形（表 15.3）。这些非癫痫发作性疾病一般表现为突发、间断的行为异常，以及变化不一的反应、肌张力改变和各种不同的姿势或动作。

心因性非癫痫发作（PNES）经常被误诊为成年人难治性癫痫。PNES 是由影响患者身体状态的无意识的情绪冲突引起，类似癫痫发作（即心理痛苦的躯体表现）。大

TABLE 15.3 Nonepileptic Episodic Disorders That May Resemble Seizures
Movement disorders: tic disorders, subcortical myoclonus, paroxysmal choreoathetosis, episodic ataxias, hyperekplexia (startle disease)
Migraine: confusional, vertebrobasilar, visual auras
Syncope (particularly convulsive syncope)
Behavioral and psychiatric: psychogenic nonepileptic seizures, hyperventilation syndrome, panic/anxiety disorder, dissociative states
Cataplexy (usually associated with narcolepsy), parasomnias
Transient ischemic attack (especially aphasic or limb-shaking)
Alcoholic blackouts
Hypoglycemia

Definitive diagnosis requires video-EEG documentation, although a history of atypical and nonstereotyped attacks, emotional or psychological precipitants, psychiatric illness, lack of response to AEDs, and repeatedly normal interictal EEGs suggests PNES as an alternate consideration. A substantial fraction of patients with PNES have experienced prior physical or sexual abuse. PNES are more common in females than in males and occur across a broad range of ages.

Panic attacks (anxiety attacks) with hyperventilation can superficially resemble focal seizures with affective, autonomic, or special sensory symptoms. Hyperventilation typically causes perioral and fingertip tingling. Prolonged hyperventilation results in muscle twitching or spasms (tetany); affected patients may faint.

Syncope refers to the symptom complex associated with a transient reduction in global cerebral perfusion associated with cardiovascular dysfunction. Loss of consciousness typically lasts only a few seconds, uncommonly a minute or more, and recovery is usually rapid. If the cerebral ischemia is sufficiently severe, the syncopal episode may include tonic posturing of the trunk or clonic jerks of the arms and legs and even incontinence *(convulsive syncope)*. Convulsive syncope is a form of syncope, not seizure; it is a frequent mimic of epileptic seizures.

Some forms of *migraine* can be mistaken for seizures, especially if the headache is atypical or mild and/or when confusion occurs. The visual aura, present in some migraineurs, is typically black, gray, and white; a colored aura more often indicates an epileptic seizure. Basilar artery migraine, usually in children and young adults, can include lethargy, mood changes, confusion, disorientation, vertigo, bilateral visual disturbances, and loss of consciousness. This uncommon form of migraine may also mimic a seizure.

TIAs can occasionally mimic seizure and vice versa. The postictal phase of a seizure can be quite stroke-like in nature and typically resolves as do TIA-related symptoms. Seizures involving the language cortex often produce speech arrest—aphasia—as is more commonly encountered in association with TIA/stroke.

TREATMENT

If the cause of a provoked seizure is corrected, AEDs are usually not necessary. Adults with a single, unprovoked seizure and normal clinical, EEG, and imaging findings frequently do not have subsequent seizures. AEDs are usually not indicated if only one seizure has occurred in those instances. However, patients with abnormal focal findings on neurologic exam or abnormal radiologic or EEG findings are at higher risk for repeated seizures and may therefore be more often recommended AED treatment. In individual patients, social considerations may dictate treatment after a single seizure. Patients who have had repeated unprovoked seizures (>24 hours apart) are recommended for AED prophylaxis.

Medication Therapy

The goal in epilepsy care is complete seizure freedom. In the United States, as of 2019, there were 22 AEDs in standard use for epilepsy with several other medications sometimes used adjunctively. There is no ideal AED; all have potential toxic side effects and idiosyncratic reactions. For over one half of people with epilepsy, the appropriate AED for their type(s) of seizures can be highly effective and well tolerated. However, for 25% to 30% of people with epilepsy, no AED alone or in combination is completely effective (termed treatment-resistant or medically refractory epilepsy). Once the seizure type and epilepsy syndrome are determined, an initial and, if needed, subsequent AED, should be chosen based on both anticipated efficacy and toxicity profiles. All AEDs can cause sedation, cognitive dysfunction, and/or incoordination in some patients, especially at high blood levels. Various rare, sometimes life-threatening, reactions can occur with all the AEDs. Some common scenarios follow.

Genetic Generalized Epilepsy (CAE, JME, and Others)

- In all genetic generalized epilepsies, valproate or lamotrigine are first-line agents and result in complete seizure control in 85% to 90% of patients.
  - Valproate may promote weight gain in many patients and has been associated with hair loss in approximately 5%. It causes tremor in many in a dose-related manner. It poses an increased risk of teratogenicity relative to other AEDs. It can be associated with hyperammonemia and rare thrombocytopenia and liver function test abnormalities.
  - Lamotrigine has a small but significant risk of a severe rash (e.g., toxic epidermal necrolysis, Stevens Johnson syndrome [SJS]) for about the first several months after initiation. A slow dose escalation substantially lowers this risk. Much less severe allergic reactions (e.g., rash) can occur in 3% to 5%. Lamotrigine's metabolism is substantially inhibited by valproate, so in combination, lower doses of lamotrigine are required. Occasionally lamotrigine worsens myoclonus, but it is effective in most cases of JME.
- Second-line options include clobazam, topiramate, levetiracetam, and zonisamide. Levetiracetam is often used as an early option for JME, given its efficacy in myoclonic seizures.
- In childhood absence epilepsy with exclusively absence seizures, ethosuximide should be the first treatment choice. If any convulsions have occurred, valproate or lamotrigine should be used.
- If there is a history of more than 5 minutes of crescendo absences or myoclonus (often described as a "foggy" state) culminating in a convulsion, then oral benzodiazepines (lorazepam or diazepam) can occasionally help abort the cluster and prevent an impending convulsion.
- Absences and myoclonus can be exacerbated by carbamazepine, oxcarbazepine, and GABAergic compounds including gabapentin, pregabalin, and tiagabine. These AEDs should be avoided in the genetic generalized epilepsies.

Focal Epilepsy

- Almost all of the AEDs (except ethosuximide) can be effective in focal epilepsy. The choice of the first AED should be mainly guided by individualized side effect considerations, teratogenicity where appropriate, and pharmacokinetics.
- Phenytoin remains one of the most commonly used AEDs in focal epilepsy in developed countries. Patients presenting with initial seizures or status epilepticus to the emergency room are commonly "loaded" intravenously with phenytoin and subsequently continued. However, phenytoin has substantial short- and long-term

表 15.3	类似癫痫发作的非癫痫发作性疾病

运动障碍：抽动障碍、皮质下肌阵挛、阵发性舞蹈手足徐动症、发作性共济失调、过度惊吓反应症（惊跳病）
偏头痛：意识模糊，椎基底动脉型，视觉先兆
晕厥（特别是惊厥性晕厥）
行为和精神疾病：心因性非癫痫发作、过度换气综合征、惊恐/焦虑障碍、分裂状态
猝倒症（通常伴有发作性睡病）、异态睡眠
短暂性脑缺血发作（特指失语性或肢体抖动性）
酒精性遗忘
低血糖症

约 10% 的 PNES 患者同时患有癫痫。即使有非典型和非刻板发作史、情绪或精神性诱因、精神疾病、对 AED 无效及多次发作间期 EEG 正常，提示 PNES 可作为考虑因素，但确诊仍需要视频 EEG 记录。大部分 PNES 患者有过躯体或性虐待经历。PNES 多见于女性，任何年龄段都可发病。

惊恐发作（焦虑发作）伴有过度换气，临床表现类似于伴有情感、自主神经或特殊感觉症状的局灶性癫痫发作。患者因过度换气导致口周和指尖麻刺感。长时间过度换气会导致肌肉抽搐或痉挛（手足搐搦），受影响的患者可能会出现昏厥。

晕厥是指与心血管功能障碍相关的短暂性全脑灌注不足所致的一组症状。意识丧失通常仅持续数秒，很少超过 1 min，可快速恢复。如果脑缺血非常严重，则晕厥发生时可伴有躯干强直性姿势或肢体阵挛性抽搐，甚至二便失禁（惊厥性晕厥）。惊厥性晕厥是常见的类似于癫痫发作的一种晕厥形式，而非癫痫发作。

某些偏头痛类型可能被误认为是癫痫发作，尤其是当头痛不典型或比较轻微和（或）出现意识模糊时。一些偏头痛患者的视觉先兆通常是黑色、灰色和白色，而出现颜色先兆更常提示癫痫发作。基底动脉型偏头痛通常在儿童和年轻成人中发生，会出现嗜睡、情绪变化、意识模糊、定向障碍、眩晕、双侧视觉障碍和意识丧失。这种罕见的偏头痛类型也可能与癫痫发作相混淆。

短暂性脑缺血发作（TIA）有时可以模仿癫痫发作，反之亦然。癫痫发作后期的特征类似脑卒中，通常会像 TIA 相关症状一样自行消退。累及语言皮质的癫痫发作通常会导致言语中止-失语，其在 TIA 或脑卒中中更为常见。

治疗

如果诱发性癫痫发作病因得到纠正，则通常不需要使用 AED。成年人出现单次非诱发性癫痫发作且临床、EEG 和影像学检查结果均正常，一般不会再次出现癫痫发作。只发生一次癫痫发作时通常不需要使用 AED。然而，对于神经系统检查、影像学或 EEG 检查结果显示异常局灶性病变，并提示反复癫痫发作风险较高的患者，推荐使用 AED 治疗。个别患者中，社会因素可能决定单次癫痫发作后的治疗。对于反复非诱发性癫痫发作（间隔 > 24 h）的患者，建议使用 AED 预防性治疗。

药物治疗

癫痫治疗的目标是完全控制发作。在美国，截至 2019 年已有 22 种 AED 被用于癫痫治疗，另有其他几种药物可作为辅助用药。目前没有理想的 AED，所有 AED 均具有潜在的毒副作用和特异性反应。对超过一半的癫痫患者来说，适用于其癫痫发作类型的 AED 非常有效且耐受性良好。然而，对于 25%～30% 的癫痫患者来说，单独或联合使用任何一种 AED 都不会完全有效（称为难治性癫痫或药物难治性癫痫）。一旦确定癫痫发作类型和癫痫综合征，应根据预期疗效和毒副作用选择初始 AED，必要时再选择后续 AED。所有 AED 都可能导致患者出现镇静、认知功能障碍和（或）动作失调，尤其当血药浓度较高时。所有 AED 都有可能发生各种罕见、有时危及生命的副作用。一些常见情况如下所述。

遗传性全面性癫痫（CAE、JME 和其他）

- 丙戊酸钠或拉莫三嗪是所有遗传性全面性癫痫的首选药物，85%～90% 的患者发作都能得到完全控制。
  - 丙戊酸钠可能会导致一些患者体重增加，约 5% 患者会出现脱发。它可能导致许多患者出现震颤，与剂量有关。与其他 AED 相比，丙戊酸钠具有较高的致畸风险。其可能与高氨血症、罕见的血小板减少症和肝功能检查异常有关。
  - 拉莫三嗪在用药后几个月内可出现较为少见但严重的皮疹[如中毒性表皮坏死溶解症、史-约综合征（SJS）]。缓慢递增剂量可以显著降低该风险。较轻微的过敏反应（如皮疹）发生率在 3%～5%。拉莫三嗪的代谢可被丙戊酸钠显著抑制，因此两者联合使用时应减少拉莫三嗪剂量。拉莫三嗪偶尔加重肌阵挛发作，但对大多数 JME 患者有效。
- 二线药物包括氯巴占、托吡酯、左乙拉西坦和唑尼沙胺。鉴于左乙拉西坦对肌阵挛性癫痫发作的疗效，常作为 JME 的早期治疗用药。
- 对于仅表现为失神发作的儿童失神癫痫，乙琥胺是其首选治疗药物。如果出现惊厥发作，则应选择丙戊酸钠或拉莫三嗪。
- 如果有超过 5 min 的逐次增强的失神发作或肌阵挛（通常描述为"朦胧"状态）并最终引起惊厥发作的病史，口服苯二氮䓬类药物（劳拉西泮或地西泮）可终止这一系列发作，并预防惊厥发生。
- 卡马西平、奥卡西平及包括加巴喷丁、普瑞巴林和噻加宾在内的 GABA 能化合物会加重失神发作和肌阵挛。遗传性全面性癫痫患者应避免使用这些 AED。

局灶性癫痫

- 几乎所有 AED（除乙琥胺外）均对局灶性癫痫有效。应基于个体毒副反应、致畸性（如适用）和药代动力学特性选择一线 AED。
- 苯妥英钠是发达国家用于治疗局灶性癫痫最常用的 AED 之一。初次发作或癫痫持续状态患者

toxicity and its levels are difficult to regulate due to saturation kinetics and multiple drug interactions. Its toxicities include hirsutism, coarsening of features, and gingival hyperplasia, especially in children and adolescents. Long-term risks include osteomalacia, peripheral neuropathy, and cerebellar degeneration with risk of permanent incoordination. Peak level toxicities include nystagmus, ataxia, lethargy, and, if the level rises above 50, acute cerebellar degeneration and cardiac arrhythmias. Phenytoin poses an allergic risk to a subset, including the rare risk of SJS.

- Carbamazepine, oxcarbazepine, topiramate, levetiracetam, lamotrigine, and zonisamide are currently used as first-line therapy for partial seizures. Carbamazepine and oxcarbazepine can cause hyponatremia and allergic reactions, rarely severe in type (SJS). Topiramate can lead to weight loss but also has undesirable dose-dependent cognitive side effects and predisposes to renal stones (1%). Levetiracetam can cause undesirable mood changes, sometimes only transiently, sedation, and rare allergic risk, but is usually well tolerated. Lamotrigine needs to be titrated slowly due to its allergic risk (discussed previously). Zonisamide, which also can cause weight loss and predisposes to renal stones, has a long half-life (48 to 72 hours) so is a good option for less consistently compliant patients or those less successful with more than once-daily dosing. It can cause allergic reactions (including rarely severe ones).
- Patients of Asian ancestry should be tested for the HLA-B*1502 allele and patients of Northern European ancestry tested for the HLA-A*3101 allele prior to initiating treatment with carbamazepine, oxcarbazepine, and eslicarbazepine. Patients with these alleles are at increased risk of SJS and toxic epidermal necrolysis when exposed to these drugs.
- Adjunctive treatments for focal seizures include clobazam, valproate, pregabalin, lacosamide, gabapentin, perampanel, and primidone. The proportion of gabapentin that is absorbed decreases with increasing dose, limiting its effectiveness. For most, pregabalin may be a better choice.
- Phenobarbital is the most widely used AED in the world due to its low cost. However, it causes sedation, cognitive impairment, and poses a risk of bone loss and therefore should probably be avoided except in difficult to control epilepsy. The exception is in neonatal seizures where it remains one of the most commonly accepted AEDs.

Developmental and Epileptic Encephalopathies

- All AEDs have a role in the treatment of this category of epilepsies, but seizure freedom is rarely achieved. At a minimum, control of the more severe seizures, including drop seizures and convulsions, should be a central goal of therapy. AED polytherapy is usually required.
- Valproate is commonly the initial medication instituted.
- Added efficacy can occur with clobazam, lamotrigine, topiramate, levetiracetam, rufinamide, and zonisamide.
- Felbamate may be effective, but its use should be limited to epileptologists due to its significant risk of fatal aplastic anemia and liver failure.
- The vagus nerve stimulator (see later) has a specific role in reducing the severity of seizures in these conditions.
- Dravet syndrome and possibly the related syndrome of GEFS+ respond best to topiramate, levetiracetam, and benzodiazepines. Some voltage-gated sodium channel blocking AEDs, including lamotrigine and phenytoin, worsen Dravet syndrome.

Dosing of AEDs must be done with great care. Only a few AEDs are safe to load or start at a full therapeutic dose. Most should be started with a gradual dose escalation. Management guidelines are: (1) the type of seizures and epilepsy should be defined and the preferred medication for such should be given in usual starting doses and then increased until seizure control is complete or side effects occur (Table 15.4); (2) If seizures persist despite toxic levels, or if major side effects occur, another AED should be tried; (3) Do not stop one agent until another has been added (overlap during transitions). Otherwise, status epilepticus may occur; (4) If seizures persist after one to two AEDs have been given to toxic levels, consider referral to a specialized epilepsy center for further evaluation and treatment; (5) Toxic levels of some AEDs (e.g., phenytoin and carbamazepine) can cause seizures; (6) Extended release and longer acting AEDs are preferred for most patients; (7) Patients should be counseled to adhere to the medication regimen. Pill boxes should be encouraged. Medication noncompliance is a leading cause of poor seizure control.

Epilepsy Surgery

In most patients, epilepsy is controlled with AEDs. When seizures cannot be controlled by adequate trials of two appropriate single agents and/or by the combination of two agents, the epilepsy is termed

TABLE 15.4 Frequently Prescribed Antiepileptic Drugs

Nonproprietary AED Name	Adult Total Dose Per Day	Dose Frequency (in Hours)	"Therapeutic" Concentrations
Carbamazepine	600-1400 mg	6-8 (12 for sustained release)	4-12 µg/mL
Clobazam	10-40 mg	12	Unknown
Ethosuximide	500-1500 mg	8-12	40-100 µg/mL
Gabapentin	900-3600 mg	6-8	2-20 µg/mL
Lacosamide	200-600 mg	12	Unknown
Lamotrigine[a]	100-800 mg	12	2-18 µg/mL
Levetiracetam	500-3000 mg	12	10-45 µg/mL
Oxcarbazepine	900-2400 mg	8-12	10-35 µg/mL
Phenobarbital	60-240 mg	24	15-40 µg/mL
Phenytoin	200-600 mg	24	10-20 µg/mL
Pregabalin	100-600 mg	12	Unknown
Topiramate	50-400 mg	12	2-20 µg/mL
Valproate	500-5000 mg	8 (12-24 for sustained release)	50-125 µg/mL
Zonisamide	100-600 mg	24	10-40 µg/mL

[a]Slow initial dose titration mandatory for lamotrigine and often indicated for other agents. Daily dose targets are adjusted depending on co-administered AEDs.

可在急诊室静脉注射苯妥英钠，随后继续用药。然而苯妥英钠本身具有较大的短期和长期毒副作用，同时由于其饱和动力学及多种药物的相互作用，其剂量难以调控。苯妥英钠毒性反应包括多毛症、面部特征粗化和牙龈增生，特别在儿童和青少年中多见。长期毒性反应包括骨软化症、周围神经病变和小脑变性伴永久性协调障碍。峰值水平毒性包括眼球震颤、共济失调、嗜睡，如果峰值浓度超过50，可能引发急性小脑变性和心律失常。苯妥英钠对某些人群存在过敏风险，包括发生罕见的SJS风险。

- 卡马西平、奥卡西平、托吡酯、左乙拉西坦、拉莫三嗪和唑尼沙胺是目前治疗部分性发作的一线药物。卡马西平和奥卡西平可能导致低钠血症和过敏反应，很少发生严重过敏反应类型（如SJS）。托吡酯可能导致体重减轻，但也有剂量相关的认知副作用和罹患肾结石的风险（1%）。左乙拉西坦可能引起不良情绪变化，有时仅持续片刻，还可引起镇静和罕见的过敏风险，但通常耐受性较好。拉莫三嗪因其过敏风险需缓慢递增剂量（前文已讨论）。唑尼沙胺也可能引起体重减轻和罹患肾结石风险，由于其半衰期（48～72 h）较长，适合依从性较差或难以坚持每日服药一次以上的患者。唑尼沙胺也可引起过敏反应（包括罕见的严重过敏反应）。
- 在卡马西平、奥卡西平和艾司利卡西平开始治疗前，亚裔患者应检测HLA-B*1502等位基因，北欧裔患者应检测HLA-A*3101等位基因。携带这些等位基因的患者使用这些药物会增加罹患SJS和中毒性表皮坏死溶解症的风险。
- 局灶性癫痫发作的辅助治疗药物包括氯巴占、丙戊酸钠、普瑞巴林、拉考沙胺、加巴喷丁、吡仑帕奈和扑米酮。加巴喷丁的吸收率随着剂量增加而减少，限制了其疗效。对于大多数患者来说，普瑞巴林可能是更好的选择。
- 苯巴比妥因其低廉的成本成为全球使用最广泛的AED。由于其可导致镇静、认知障碍，并存在骨质流失的风险，因此除了难以控制的癫痫外，应避免使用。例外情况是在新生儿惊厥中，苯巴比妥是最常使用的抗癫痫药物之一。

发育性癫痫性脑病

- 所有AED对治疗这类癫痫均有一定的作用，但很少能完全控制。最基本的治疗目标应当是控制更严重的癫痫发作，包括跌倒发作和惊厥。通常需要多种AED联合治疗。
- 丙戊酸钠是常见的初始用药。
- 氯巴占、拉莫三嗪、托吡酯、左乙拉西坦、芦非酰胺和唑尼沙胺可能会增加疗效。
- 非尔氨酯可能有效，但由于其较高的致命性再生障碍性贫血和肝衰竭风险，只能由癫痫科医生决定是否使用。
- 迷走神经刺激器（见下文）在降低癫痫发作的严重程度方面具有特殊的作用。
- Dravet综合征及GEFS+相关综合征对托吡酯、左乙拉西坦和苯二氮䓬类药物反应最好。而包括拉莫三嗪和苯妥英钠在内的一些电压门控钠通道阻滞剂类AED会加重Dravet综合征。

AED用药必须非常谨慎。仅少数AED可安全地以负荷剂量或全剂量开始用药。大多数药物应以逐渐增加剂量开始。药物管理指南包括：①应明确癫痫发作和癫痫的类型，给予常规剂量的首选药物，逐渐增加剂量至癫痫发作完全控制或出现副作用（表15.4）；②如果药物达到中毒剂量时，癫痫发作仍持续存在，或出现严重副作用，应尝试另一种AED；③在增加另一种药物之前不要停止使用上一种药物（药物过渡期间重叠），否则可能出现癫痫持续状态；④如果给予1～2种AED达到中毒剂量，癫痫发作仍然持续存在，应考虑转诊到专门的癫痫中心进行进一步评估和治疗；⑤某些AED（如苯妥英钠和卡马西平）在毒性剂量时可能会导致癫痫发作；⑥绝大多数患者应首选缓释型和长效型AED；⑦建议患者坚持服药，鼓励患者使用药盒。药物依从性差是导致癫痫发作控制较差的主要原因之一。

癫痫手术

绝大多数癫痫患者通过AED控制发作。当癫痫发作无法通过两种合适的单药或联合用药来控制时，称为难

表15.4 常用抗癫痫药

通用名称	成人每日总剂量	给药间隔（h）	"治疗"浓度
卡马西平	600～1400 mg	6～8（缓释制剂为12）	4～12 μg/ml
氯巴占	10～40 mg	12	不确定
乙琥胺	500～1500 mg	8～12	40～100 μg/ml
加巴喷丁	900～3600 mg	6～8	2～20 μg/ml
拉考沙胺	200～600 mg	12	不确定
拉莫三嗪[a]	100～800 mg	12	2～18 μg/ml
左乙拉西坦	500～3000 mg	12	10～45 μg/ml
奥卡西平	900～2400 mg	8～12	10～35 μg/ml
苯巴比妥	60～240 mg	24	15～40 μg/ml
苯妥英钠	200～600 mg	24	10～20 μg/ml
普瑞巴林	100～600 mg	12	不确定
托吡酯	50～400 mg	12	2～20 μg/ml
丙戊酸钠	500～5000 mg	8（缓释制剂为12～24）	50～125 μg/ml
唑尼沙胺	100～600 mg	24	10～40 μg/ml

[a] 必须对拉莫三嗪初始剂量进行缓慢调整，也适用于其他药物。每日剂量范围根据联合应用的AED进行调整。

treatment resistant (or *medically refractory*), a situation encountered in 25% to 30% of patients with epilepsy. Such patients are at risk for many consequences: inability to drive; stigmatization by schools, employers, and society; and threats to personal educational and occupational goals, possible cognitive or memory loss over time, plus seizure-related morbidity and mortality including risk of SUDEP. In appropriately selected cases, epilepsy surgery can abolish seizures with restoration of normal neurologic function. The accurate localization of a safely resectable seizure focus requires intensive investigation at a specialized epilepsy center.

A variety of surgical approaches are presently available. These range from lesionectomies, to lobectomies, to (rarely) hemispherectomies. Palliative approaches such as transection of the corpus callosum can help those with drop attacks. The surgical options are tailored to the needs of each individual patient, depending on the nature of their epileptogenic lesion and proximity to cortical regions that cannot be resected without causing unacceptable neurologic deficits (so-called "eloquent cortex"). Recently, laser-mediated ablative techniques have permitted surgical approaches for certain pathologies, with much less risk to the surrounding normal brain near the surgical target. Laser interstitial thermal therapy (LITT) can permit smaller surgical approaches, shorter inpatient stays, and faster postoperative recoveries. Outcomes seem to approach those of conventional resective approaches, though longer-term outcome data are still needed.

Dietary Therapy

The *ketogenic diet* is a very high fat diet with markedly restricted carbohydrates and adequate protein carefully designed to cause a ketotic state, while still supplying adequate nutrition. It is mainly used in children with developmental and epileptic encephalopathies who have an unsatisfactory response to AED treatment. The ketogenic diet can be effective in these most refractory forms of epilepsy, resulting in seizure freedom in 15% to 20%. However, the diet is hard to maintain and requires a dedicated, cooperative caregiver and a specially trained dietician.

The *modified Atkins diet* (MAD) and *low glycemic-index diet* are scaled-down versions of the ketogenic diet with mainly carbohydrate restriction. These diets are more palatable than the ketogenic diet and can be tolerated by adults. The slight ketosis achieved sometimes results in dramatic seizure reduction in many forms of epilepsy.

Neurostimulators

The *vagal nerve stimulator (VNS)* is a surgically implanted device. The stimulating electrode is placed on the left vagus nerve in the neck. The current version of this device has three treatment modes. Routine round-the-clock stimulation occurs intermittently according to programmed settings. Standard settings deliver stimuli lasting 30 seconds every 5 minutes. However, one can program the VNS to deliver stimuli in a more rapid cycling pattern (greater duty cycle) and/or alter the intensity of the stimulation by modifying other parameters. Swiping a magnet over the device gives an extra "on-demand" stimulation that can sometimes abort a seizure. A third mode called autostimulation delivers stimulation based upon detected tachycardias of sufficient magnitude, since a significant percentage of seizures foster an associated tachycardia. Preapproval studies found that approximately 45% of recipients had a greater than 50% reduction in their seizure frequency (the responder rate) and seizure intensity was also often decreased in many. Postapproval long-term follow-up studies suggest an even more robust response to VNS therapy.

Deep brain stimulation (DBS) of bilateral anterior nuclei of the thalami also has been approved in the United States since 2018 for treatment-resistant epilepsy involving bilateral limbic regions. Like the VNS, this method also relies on preset, round-the-clock, intermittent stimulation to modulate the epileptic circuitry and decrease seizure burden. Studies show that it can lead to a 60% responder rate with several years of follow-up.

Another newer strategy for medically refractory focal epilepsy is *responsive neurostimulation (RNS)*, approved in the United States since 2013. Chronically implanted electrodes at or near the seizure foci are used to rapidly detect seizure onset and treat the seizure and its supporting circuitry within seconds by delivering electrical stimulation directly to the seizure focus. This method can use implanted depth electrodes or strips of electrodes to access either cortical or deeper targets (e.g., hippocampi) and provides a means to treat patients with greater than one seizure focus, thereby offering a non-resective option for patients who would not otherwise be appropriate resective surgical candidates. Detection and stimulation algorithms are tailored to the patient's electrocorticography samples collected over time to improve its performance. Studies have reported a 72% responder rate with 5-year follow-up.

All three neuromodulatory methods appear to variably thwart seizures as they initiate and spread and, perhaps more importantly, gradually reduce the propensity of the epileptic circuitry to generate seizures. These treatments seem to improve clinical outcomes in a slower manner than is commonly seen with AEDs. However, unlike AEDs, the neuromodulatory treatments so far appear to exhibit sustained improved outcomes over years, do not seem to lose efficacy, are nonsedating, and spare neurocognitive function versus most resective surgical methods.

The process by which tertiary epilepsy programs assess the candidacy of medically refractory patients for the above dietary, surgical, or neuromodulatory methods involves careful analysis of several streams of clinical data. Patients' EEG and LTM results are aligned with their brain imaging and neuropsychological test results. Concordant data more strongly implicate the localization of the seizure focus or foci. This is then matched with the most appropriate treatment options in a highly individualized manner.

Status Epilepticus

Status epilepticus can occur with focal or generalized seizure types and is defined as prolonged or rapidly recurring seizures without full intervening recovery. *Acute repetitive seizures* are defined as a cluster of seizures over minutes to hours with intervening recovery.

Convulsive status epilepticus is a medical emergency. Prolonged and continuous generalized convulsive epileptic activity can lead to irreversible brain injury. The most frequent cause is abrupt withdrawal of AEDs (e.g., noncompliance) in a person with epilepsy. Other precipitants include acute withdrawal from alcohol, benzodiazepines or barbiturates, cerebral infections such as encephalitis, trauma, hemorrhage, and brain tumor.

Nonconvulsive status epilepticus includes two main types. *Focal status epilepticus* (also known as complex partial status epilepticus) may resemble a sustained confusional state often associated with motor and autonomic automatisms. Some instances produce bizarre behaviors or stupor. These bouts can even last for hours or days. Occasionally, this is preceded by an overt convulsive seizure that may have incompletely resolved, with or without AED treatment. This can be diagnostically challenging, as the semiology overlaps with a myriad of other forms of encephalopathy or delirium. EEG is crucial for diagnosis and shows nearly continuous epileptiform activity predominating in a brain region or regions, often the temporal lobes.

The other main form of nonconvulsive status epilepticus is *absence status epilepticus* (or petit mal status). This resembles focal status epilepticus and consists of a similar confusional state with some automatisms. EEG reveals continuous runs of generalized 3- to 4-Hz spike and slow wave activity. This usually occurs in children or young adults with known absence epilepsy.

治性癫痫（或药物难治性癫痫），在癫痫患者中占25%~30%。这些患者面临许多不良事件的影响，如不能驾驶，被学校、雇主和社会歧视，个人教育和职业目标受到威胁，随着时间推移可能出现认知或记忆丧失，以及癫痫发作相关的发病率和死亡率，包括不明原因癫痫猝死（SUDEP）的风险。在适合手术治疗的病例中，癫痫手术可以控制癫痫发作，并恢复正常的神经功能。需要在专门的癫痫中心对可安全切除的癫痫病灶进行准确的定位评估。

目前已有多种手术方案可供选择，包括病灶切除术、脑叶切除术和大脑半球切除术（较罕见）。姑息手术如胼胝体切开术可以缓解跌倒发作。手术方案应根据每位患者的需要量身定制，取决于其致痫灶的性质以及是否靠近无法切除的皮质区域（所谓"功能区"，若切除可造成不能接受的神经功能缺损）。近年来，激光介导的消融技术可针对某种病理进行手术治疗，对手术靶点附近正常的脑组织风险较小。激光间质热疗（LITT）可以实现更小的手术切口、更短的住院时间和更快的术后恢复。结果似乎接近传统的切除方法，尽管仍需更多长期疗效数据的支持。

饮食治疗

生酮饮食是一种极高脂肪、低碳水化合物、适当蛋白质的饮食方案，在提供足够营养的同时，可以引起酮症状态。其主要用于对AED治疗反应不佳的发育性癫痫性脑病患儿。生酮饮食对最难治的癫痫类型可能有效，可使15%~20%患者恢复至无癫痫发作状态。然而，这种饮食方案难以维持，需要专门的护理人员和专业的营养师进行配合。

改良阿特金斯饮食（MAD）和低血糖指数饮食主要限制碳水化合物的摄入，是生酮饮食的简化版。这些饮食比生酮饮食更加可口，成年人可以耐受。轻微的酮症状态可以导致各种类型癫痫的发作急剧减少。

神经刺激器

迷走神经刺激器（VNS）是一种手术植入装置。刺激电极置于颈部的左侧迷走神经处。该设备的当前版本有三种治疗模式。常规全天候刺激可根据程序设置间歇进行。标准设置为每5 min提供持续30 s的刺激。然而，可对VNS进行编程使其以更快的循环模式（更高效的工作周期）传递刺激和（或）通过修改其他参数来改变刺激的强度。磁铁划过装置可以提供额外的"按需"刺激，有时可以中止癫痫发作。第三种模式称为自动刺激，可根据检测到的足够强度的心动过速提供刺激，因为有相当大比例的癫痫发作会诱发心动过速。上市前研究发现大约45%的受试者VNS治疗后癫痫发作频率（应答率）降低了50%以上，且许多癫痫发作强度也降低。上市后的长期随访研究表明，VNS治疗的疗效更为显著。

双侧丘脑前核深部脑刺激（DBS）已于2018年在美国获批用于治疗累及双侧边缘区的难治性癫痫。与VNS类似，该方法也依赖预设的全天候间歇刺激来调节癫痫回路，减少癫痫发作。数年的随访研究显示DBS应答率可达60%。

难治性局灶性癫痫的另一种新兴治疗方法是反应性神经刺激术（RNS），自2013年起在美国获得批准。通过在致痫灶或附近长期植入电极可快速检测到癫痫发作，并通过直接向致痫灶施加电刺激，可在数秒内控制癫痫发作及其支持回路。这种方法可以将深度电极或电极条植入皮质或更深的靶点（如海马体），为多个致痫灶的患者提供治疗手段，从而为那些不适合手术切除的患者提供了非切除治疗方案。检测和刺激算法可根据患者的皮质EEG数据定制，以提高其疗效。5年随访研究显示RNS可导致72%的应答率。

这三种神经调控治疗似乎都能够在癫痫发作开始并扩散时对其进行抑制，更重要的是能逐渐减少癫痫回路产生癫痫发作的可能性。这些治疗方法改善临床结局的速度似乎比常见的AED治疗要慢。然而，与AED不同的是，迄今为止神经调控治疗多年来表现出持续改善的结局，不会失去疗效，不会引起镇静作用，并且与大多数手术切除治疗相比，能够保留神经认知功能。

三级癫痫治疗项目评估难治性患者是否适合上述饮食、手术或神经调控方法的过程，涉及对多种临床数据的详尽分析。患者的EEG和LTM结果与其脑部成像和神经心理测试结果相一致。一致的数据更能说明致痫灶或病灶的位置。然后，以高度个体化的方式匹配最适合的治疗方案。

癫痫持续状态

癫痫持续状态发生在局灶性或全面性癫痫发作类型中，其定义为癫痫发作持续时间长或快速复发，中间意识未完全恢复。急性反复癫痫发作定义为数分钟至数小时内的一组癫痫发作，中间意识可恢复正常。

惊厥性癫痫持续状态是一种医学急症。长时间连续的全面性惊厥性癫痫活动可能导致不可逆的脑损伤。最常见的原因是癫痫患者突然停用AED（例如不遵医嘱），其他诱发因素包括急性酒精戒断、停用苯二氮䓬类或巴比妥类药物、脑部感染（如脑炎）、创伤、出血和脑肿瘤等。

非惊厥性癫痫持续状态可分为两大类。局灶性癫痫持续状态（也称为复杂部分性癫痫持续状态）可能类似于持续的意识模糊状态，通常伴有运动和自主神经自动症。有些情况下还会出现古怪行为或昏睡。发作甚至可能持续数小时或数天。偶尔，在此之前会出现明显的惊厥性癫痫发作，可能不完全缓解，无论是否接受AED治疗。这在诊断上具有挑战性，因为其症状与多种其他脑病或谵妄状态重叠。EEG对诊断至关重要，可显示一个或多个脑区（通常是颞叶）主导的几乎连续的癫痫样活动。

另一种非惊厥性癫痫持续状态类型是失神性癫痫持续状态（或小发作持续状态）。与局灶性癫痫持续状态相似，表现为类似的意识模糊状态和自动症。EGG显示连续广泛性3~4 Hz的棘慢波活动。常见于已有失神癫痫的儿童或年轻成人。

With the current widespread use of ICU EEG monitoring in neurocritically ill patients, there is a burgeoning subset whose EEGs show less sustained and less rapid epileptiform discharges than in typical status epilepticus, though often periodic and abundant, with a waxing and waning quality. Such epileptiform discharges may be lateralized or generalized. These patterns fall short of the status epilepticus patterns described previously but may follow recent bouts of status epilepticus, as they resolve. Recently, these patterns have been categorized as falling within the "ictal-interictal continuum." Their clinical significance is less clear and is a current focus of investigation.

Focal motor status epilepticus (or *epilepsy partialis continua, [EPC]*) ranges from highly focal, clonic movements of the face or hand to jerks involving a limb or half the body. The clonus frequency can vary from 0.3 to 3.0 Hz. It is less common. Causes include stroke, trauma, neoplasm, encephalitis, and marked hyperglycemia (e.g., glucose > 450 mg/dL as in nonketotic hyperglycemic states) and in Rasmussen encephalitis, a very rare, usually pediatric epilepsy syndrome. Status epilepticus related to profound hyperglycemia can produce refractory focal status epilepticus that often resolves once hyperglycemia is corrected.

Postanoxic myoclonic status epilepticus is often accompanied by generalized polyspike and slow wave epileptiform discharges on EEG but may be less responsive to common AED treatments for status epilepticus. It typically reflects significant and extensive cortical injury, often associated with a poor prognosis.

Once status epilepticus is diagnosed, treatment is urgent. The longer status epilepticus lasts, the more difficult it is to terminate and the more likely it is to cause brain damage. Aggressive therapy is mandatory for convulsive status epilepticus (Table 15.5). If initial therapy is not rapidly effective, anesthetic agents requiring intubation and ventilation should be used within an hour of onset. Focal status epilepticus can also result in permanent neuronal injury and should also be treated expeditiously, although therapeutic choices are often made to try to stop focal status epilepticus with agents that do not cause respiratory depression to avoid intubation. Absence status is unlikely to result in permanent sequelae and usually responds promptly to benzodiazepine treatment. Investigation into the cause of status epilepticus should be undertaken during its treatment and continued after seizures stop.

GENETIC COUNSELING AND PREGNANCY

Heredity

Patients with epilepsy should be advised about the hereditary risks to their children, although in most people with epilepsy, it does not influence their decision about having children. The most common genetic generalized epilepsies have complex inheritance patterns with about 10% of children of an affected parent developing seizures. There are over 200 mendelian-inherited syndromes with epilepsy, all rare. Screening for genetic causes of epilepsy has become more useful for certain subgroups of patients, particularly those with unknown etiology under the age of 2 years. Gene microarray assays have become more effective tools and have added to older less precise genetic assays such as karyotype or FISH assays. Genetics counselors provide valuable diagnostic and educational assistance in the care of patients who may have a genetic form of epilepsy or who may have specific concerns about the potential risk for their children.

TABLE 15.5 Treatment of Convulsive Status Epilepticus

Time (Min)	Steps

0-5 (Stabilize, ABCs)	Give O$_2$; ensure adequate ventilation
	Monitor: vital signs, ECG, oximetry, seizure duration
	Establish intravenous access;
	Obtain finger stick blood glucose level, If <60 mg/dL, then:
	    Adults: 100 mg thiamine IV, then 50 mL D50W IV
	    Children ≥2 years: 2 mL/kg D25W IV
	    Children <2 years: 4 mL/kg D12.5W IV
	Collect complete blood cell count, electrolytes, Ca, Mg, toxins, and AED levels

5-20 Initial therapy (benzodiazepine)	Choose one of the following 3 options:
	  1. Intravenously administer lorazepam 0.1 mg/kg/dose, max: 4 mg/dose, may repeat dose once, or
	  2. Intravenously administer diazepam 0.15-0.2 mg/kg/dose, max: 10 mg/dose, may repeat dose once, or
	  3. Intramuscularly administer midazolam 10 mg for >40 kg, 5 mg for 13-40 kg, single dose.
	If none of the above are available, then choose one of the following:
	  1. IV phenobarbital 15 mg/kg/dose, single dose. Note that IV phenobarbital following a benzodiazepine ventilatory assistance is usually required.
	  2. Rectal diazepam 0.2-0.5 mg/kg, max: 20 mg/dose, single dose
	  3. Intranasal midazolam, buccal midazolam

20-40 (Second therapy)	If status epilepticus persists, administer one of the following:
	  1. IV fosphenytoin[a] 20 mg PE/kg, max: 1500 mg PE/dose, 1 dose
	  2. IV valproic acid 40 mg/kg, max: 3000 mg/dose, 1 dose
	  3. IV levetiracetam 60 mg/kg, max: 4500 mg/dose, 1 dose
	If none of the above are available, and if not already given, administer IV phenobarbital 15 mg/kg, max dose.
	(Alternative to fosphenytoin above, may use phenytoin at 1 mg/kg/min up to 50 mg/min max rate in adults in a proximal IV. Monitor carefully for hypotension, arrhythmia, local extravasation.)

40-60 (Third therapy)	If the seizures do not stop after the above, choices include repeating second-line therapies not previously given, or intravenous anesthetic doses of thiopental, midazolam, or propofol, with intubation and with continuous EEG monitoring. Vasopressors or supplemental IV fluids are often necessary.

ABCs, Airway, breathing, and circulation; *AED,* antiepileptic drug; *ECG,* electrocardiogram; *EEG,* electroencephalograph.
[a]Always dosed in phenytoin-equivalents (PE).

近年来随着 ICU EEG 监测在神经危重症患者中的广泛应用，出现了一个新的癫痫亚群，其 EEG 表现的癫痫样放电不如典型的癫痫持续状态持续时间长、速度快，但往往具有周期性和丰富性，且时好时坏。这种癫痫样放电可能局限于一侧或广泛存在。这些模式不完全符合之前描述的癫痫持续状态模式，但可能在癫痫持续状态缓解后出现，作为其后续表现。最近，这些模式被归类为"发作期-发作间期连续体（IIC）"，其临床意义尚不明确，是目前研究的重点。

局灶性运动性癫痫持续状态［或称部分性癫痫持续状态（EPC）］波及范围可从面部或手部的高度局灶性、阵挛性运动到累及肢体或半侧身体的抽搐。阵挛频率为 0.3～3.0 Hz 不等。这种症状较为罕见。其原因包括脑卒中、创伤、肿瘤、脑炎、显著高血糖症（例如，在非酮症高血糖状态下血糖＞ 450 mg/dl）以及 Rasmussen 脑炎，后者是一种非常罕见的儿童癫痫综合征。严重高血糖相关的癫痫持续状态可以诱发难治性局灶性癫痫持续状态，一旦高血糖得到纠正，症状通常也会得到缓解。

缺氧后肌阵挛性癫痫持续状态通常伴随 EEG 显示广泛性多棘波和慢波的癫痫样放电，但可能对癫痫持续状态的常规 AED 治疗反应较差，通常反映了严重且广泛的皮质损伤，往往预后不良。

一旦诊断为癫痫持续状态，应立即治疗。癫痫持续状态持续时间越长，终止难度越大，越有可能造成脑损伤。对于惊厥性癫痫持续状态，必须进行积极治疗（表 15.5）。如果初始治疗未能快速起效，应在发作开始后 1 h 内使用需要插管和通气支持的麻醉药物。局灶性癫痫持续状态也能导致永久性神经元损伤，应当同样进行迅速处理，在治疗时尽量选择使用不会引起呼吸抑制的药物，以避免气管插管。失神持续状态一般不会导致永久性后遗症，且通常对苯二氮䓬类药物治疗反应迅速。在治疗癫痫持续状态的同时应探究其病因，并在发作停止后继续明确病因诊断。

遗传咨询和妊娠

遗传

应告知癫痫患者有关其子女遗传该病的风险，尽管对大多数癫痫患者来说，遗传风险不会影响他们生育子女的决定。最常见的遗传性全面性癫痫具有复杂的遗传模式，患者子女中大约有 10% 出现癫痫发作。目前有 200 多种孟德尔遗传综合征都伴有癫痫，但均罕见。对一些患者群体，特别是 2 岁以下病因不明的患儿，筛查癫痫的遗传病因十分有用。基因微阵列分析作为更有效的工具，补充了早期较不精确的遗传检测方法，如核型分析或荧光原位杂交（FISH）分析。遗传咨询师为可能患有遗传性癫痫或担心其子女存在潜在风险的患者提供非常有价值的诊断和教育援助。

表 15.5 惊厥性癫痫持续状态的治疗	
时间（min）	步骤
0～5（稳定，ABC）	给氧，确保充分通气。 监测：生命体征、ECG、血氧饱和度、癫痫发作持续时间。 建立静脉通道。 获取指尖血糖水平，如果＜ 60 mg/dl，则 　成人：静脉注射 100 mg 维生素 B_1，随后静脉注射 50 ml 50% 葡萄糖溶液； 　≥ 2 岁儿童：静脉注射 2 ml/kg 25% 葡萄糖溶液； 　＜ 2 岁儿童：静脉注射 4 ml/kg 12.5% 葡萄糖溶液。 检测全血细胞计数、电解质（钙、镁）、毒素和 AED 浓度。
5～20 初始治疗（苯二氮䓬类药物）	以下三个方案中任选一项： 1. 静脉注射劳拉西泮，剂量为 0.1 mg/kg，每次最大剂量 4 mg，必要时重复一次。 2. 静脉注射地西泮，剂量为 0.15～0.2 mg/kg，每次最大剂量 10 mg，必要时重复一次。 3. 肌内注射咪达唑仑，体重超过 40 kg 患者注射 10 mg，体重 13～40 kg 患者注射 5 mg，单次剂量。 如果上述方案都不可用，可选择以下其中一项： 1. 静脉注射苯巴比妥，剂量为 15 mg/kg，单次剂量。注意在使用苯二氮䓬类药物后静脉注射苯巴比妥时，通常需要呼吸辅助。 2. 地西泮直肠给药，剂量为 0.2～0.5 mg/kg，每次最大剂量 20 mg，单次剂量。 3. 咪达唑仑鼻内给药，咪达唑仑口服。
20～40（第二次治疗）	如果癫痫持续状态持续存在，给予以下其中一种方案： 1. 静脉注射磷苯妥英[a]，剂量为 20 mg PE/kg，每次最大剂量 1500 mg PE，单次剂量。 2. 静脉注射丙戊酸，剂量为 40 mg/kg，每次最大剂量 3000 mg，单次剂量。 3. 静脉注射左乙拉西坦，剂量为 60 mg/kg，每次最大剂量 4500 mg，单次剂量。 如果以上治疗条件均不具备，或尚未给予，则静脉注射苯巴比妥，最大剂量 15 mg/kg。 ［作为上述磷苯妥英的替代方案，成人可端静脉注射苯妥英钠，给药速度按 1 mg/(kg·min)，最大可至 50 mg/min。要密切监测有无低血压、心律失常和药物局部渗漏的情况。］
40～60（第三次治疗）	如果癫痫发作在上述治疗后仍未停止，可以重复选择未使用过的第二次治疗，或者给予静脉麻醉药物如硫喷妥钠、咪达唑仑或丙泊酚，并进行插管和持续 EEG 监测。通常需要给予血管加压药物或静脉补充液体。

ABC，气道、呼吸和循环；AED，抗癫痫药；ECG，心电图；EEG，脑电图。
[a] 始终按苯妥英钠等效剂量（PE）给药。

Teratogenicity

Children of mothers taking AEDs have a birth defect rate of 2% up to 9%, which is up to five times that of the general population. However, seizures, especially convulsive seizures, also pose a substantial risk to both the mother and fetus. Thus, AEDs should not be stopped during pregnancy. There is significant variation in the relative teratogenic risk of the available AEDs and in their specific effects on fetal development. Two AEDs, valproate and carbamazepine, have been incriminated in neural tube closure defects. Since the neural tube closes by 28 days of fetal development, this defect develops before the mother may be aware that she is pregnant. Phenytoin, phenobarbital, primidone, and topiramate have been associated with a spectrum of neurodevelopmental abnormalities. Topiramate has been associated with higher risk of low birthweight and increased oral cleft risk. Large registries suggest that the newer AEDs have less teratogenic risk, but the data are incomplete for some of these newer AEDs. Lamotrigine and levetiracetam are presently associated with the lowest rates of major congenital malformations in these registries (approximately 2%). By contrast, valproate has the worst profile with an approximately 9% incidence. Use of two or more AEDs (polytherapy) increases the teratogenic risk. Pregnancies in women with epilepsy should be planned. During the year prior to conception, an attempt should be made to minimize the teratogenic potential of the AED regimen by considering a change to AEDs with significantly superior teratogenic risk where appropriate, to monotherapy from polytherapy, or tapering off AEDs, if there are reasons to believe that seizures will not recur (see later). The lowest effective dose of the AEDs should be used, but this must be balanced with the risk of breakthrough seizures. Folic acid deficiency is an established risk factor for neural tube defects in the general population. There is little evidence that additional folic acid in a well-nourished woman with epilepsy decreases the AED effects on neural tube closure. However, it is shared practice to advise women with epilepsy of childbearing age to take supplemental folic acid (1 mg per day) as prophylaxis against neural tube defects. Once pregnancy is planned or recognized, the dose of folic acid is commonly increased to 4 mg per day.

Management During and After Pregnancy

Women with epilepsy have generally a 1- to 1.7-fold increased rate of complications of pregnancy, including prematurity, preeclampsia, preterm labor, placental abruption, fetal death, bleeding, and poor fetal growth, except for a 10-fold higher rate of maternal mortality than the general population. They should be managed as high-risk pregnancies. High-quality level 2 ultrasound (and possibly 3D ultrasound), maternal serum α-fetoprotein level (elevated in neural tube closure defects), and amniocentesis for chromosomal analysis are used to identify fetal malformations.

During pregnancy, AED serum levels decrease due to increased hepatic and renal clearance and increased plasma volume. The free fraction of highly protein-bound AEDs (e.g., phenytoin and valproate) typically increases due to decreased albumin concentration and increased competition for binding sites by sex steroids. Thus, it is essential to monitor AED levels (free levels for highly protein-bound AEDs) prior to conception and at regular intervals throughout pregnancy (generally every 4 weeks). Hormonal changes associated with pregnancy lead to progressive induction of hepatic glucuronidation pathways that dramatically reduce lamotrigine levels, sometimes requiring doubling or even tripling the lamotrigine dose over the course of pregnancy to maintain prepregnancy levels. In light of these expected AED level changes, it is very helpful to have prepregnancy baseline AED levels, especially those corresponding to periods of good seizure control, in women aiming for pregnancy.

Emesis, a common problem during early pregnancy, can result in missed and partial doses of AEDs. The pregnant woman should be instructed to retake a full or partial dose of her AEDs if vomiting occurs after medications are taken. After the child is born, the dose of AEDs should be tapered to prepregnancy doses over 3 to 6 weeks, beginning approximately 3 days postpartum, but the duration of taper may vary according to the AED's route of clearance (renal or glucuronidation pathways—3 weeks; cytochrome pathways—6 weeks). The AED levels can be checked 1 to 2 weeks after completing the taper to confirm they are at the patient's baseline. In general, breast-feeding is not contraindicated in women taking AEDs.

During the postpartum period the mother with epilepsy may be at increased risk of seizures, especially if her seizures are activated by sleep deprivation. To lessen this risk, a support person should perform at least one of the newborn's nighttime feedings. Patients whose seizure semiology would put the infant at risk (e.g., dropping or excessively clutching the baby) require childcare modification and/or supervision.

PSYCHOSOCIAL CONCERNS

Ongoing epileptic seizures often have major emotional consequences for the patient and family. Comorbid depression is present in up to 30% to 50% of patients with refractory epilepsy and 20% of patients with controlled epilepsy. Anxiety disorders accompany epilepsy in 15% to 20%. Both are often unrecognized and untreated. In people with epilepsy, quality of life impairment better correlates with depression than with seizure frequency. The unpredictable nature of seizures and the necessary activity restrictions cause dependence, decreased self-worth, embarrassment, stigma, underemployment, and helplessness. Reduced libido and hyposexuality are common in patients with epilepsy and often unrecognized.

Family dynamics may also be disrupted by the presence of epilepsy. Patients and their families often fear seizures (seizure phobia). Family members may think their loved one is dying when they convulse, especially for the first time. Patients with epilepsy are helped most by seizure freedom, but reassurance and optimistic support from family and friends aids immeasurably. Once seizure control is achieved, people with epilepsy should be encouraged to live as normal and full a life as possible, using common sense as a guide. Although activity restrictions may eventually be lifted, patients with past epilepsy (with the exception of CAE and childhood epilepsy with centrotemporal spikes, which completely remit) should be advised to avoid head contact sports and activities or occupations that may prove catastrophic were a seizure to recur (e.g., swimming alone, working at great heights, weapon use).

All states grant automobile driver's licenses to patients with epilepsy provided that no seizures impairing consciousness or bodily control have occurred for specified periods of time (typically 3 months to 1 year). Life and health insurance policies can generally be obtained. The American with Disabilities Act (ADA) provides protection from loss of employment on the basis of disability and this pertains to those with epilepsy. Reasonable accommodations to patients should be made in the workplace setting, although there are several important caveats to these rules. Epilepsy foundations and local social service organizations can assist patients with case coordination, including social and vocational concerns.

PROGNOSIS

Two thirds of those with epilepsy achieve a 5-year remission of seizures within 10 years of diagnosis. About half of these patients can eventually become seizure-free without AEDs. Factors favoring remission include specific genetic generalized forms of epilepsy, a normal neurologic

致畸性

服用 AED 的孕妇所生子女的出生缺陷率为 2%～9%，是普通人群的 5 倍。然而，癫痫发作尤其是惊厥发作，对孕妇和胎儿带来巨大风险。因此妊娠期间不应停用 AED。现有 AED 的相对致畸风险及对胎儿发育的具体影响存在显著差异。丙戊酸钠和卡马西平已被证实与神经管闭合缺陷有关。由于神经管在胎儿发育的第 28 天闭合，这种缺陷在母亲发现自己妊娠之前就已经出现。苯妥英钠、苯巴比妥、扑米酮和托吡酯与一系列神经发育异常有关。托吡酯与较高的低出生体重和唇裂风险有关。大型登记数据表明，新型 AED 的致畸风险较低，但其中一些新药数据尚不完整。目前拉莫三嗪和左乙拉西坦在这些登记数据中表现出最低的先天致畸率（约 2%）。相比之下，丙戊酸钠的致畸风险最高，发生率约为 9%。使用两种或多种抗癫痫药物（多药治疗）会增加致畸风险。癫痫妇女应当计划妊娠。受孕前一年应尝试将 AED 方案中的致畸潜能降至最低，考虑在适当情况下更换致畸风险显著较低的 AED（如适用），从多药治疗改为单药治疗，或在有证据提示癫痫不会复发的情况下逐渐减少 AED 剂量（见下文）。应当使用最低有效剂量的 AED，但必须均衡发生癫痫发作的风险。叶酸缺乏是一种导致普通人群神经管缺陷的明确风险因素。当前尚无充分证据表明营养良好的女性癫痫患者额外补充叶酸能降低 AED 对神经管闭合的影响。目前普遍的做法是建议育龄期女性癫痫患者每日补充 1 mg 叶酸，以预防神经管缺陷。一旦计划或发现妊娠后，叶酸剂量通常增至每日 4 mg。

孕期及产后管理

癫痫患者妊娠并发症的发生率一般比普通人群高 1～1.7 倍，并发症包括早产、先兆子痫、胎盘早剥、胎儿死亡、出血和胎儿生长不良，此外孕产妇死亡率比普通人群高 10 倍。应将其作为高危妊娠进行管理。高质量 2 级超声（和可能的 3D 超声）、母体血清甲胎蛋白水平（神经管闭合缺陷患者中升高）以及用于染色体分析的羊膜穿刺术均可用于检测胎儿畸形。

由于肝、肾清除率以及血浆容量增加，妊娠期间血清 AED 浓度下降。高蛋白结合性 AED（如苯妥英钠和丙戊酸钠）的游离部分通常会增加，这是由于白蛋白浓度下降和性激素对蛋白结合位点竞争增加所致。因此必须在受孕前和怀孕期间定期（通常每 4 周）监测 AED 水平（高蛋白结合性 AED 的游离水平）。妊娠相关激素变化会进行性诱导肝葡萄糖醛酸化途径，从而显著降低拉莫三嗪水平，有时需在怀孕期间将拉莫三嗪的剂量加倍甚至 3 倍以维持妊娠前水平。鉴于这些预期的 AED 水平变化，对于计划妊娠的女性来说，了解妊娠前的 AED 基线水平非常有帮助，特别是癫痫控制良好时血药浓度的基线水平。

呕吐是妊娠早期的一种常见反应，可能导致 AED 漏服或部分服药。如果用药后发生呕吐，应指导孕妇再次服用全量或部分剂量的 AED。孩子出生后，AED 的剂量应在产后约 3 天开始，在 3～6 周内逐步减量至妊娠前水平，但减量持续时间长短可能会根据 AED 的清除途径而有所不同（肾或葡萄糖醛酸化途径为 3 周，细胞色素途径为 6 周）。完成减量后 1～2 周内检测 AED 浓度以确认是否恢复至患者的基线水平。一般来说，服用 AED 的女性可进行母乳喂养。

在产后期间，患有癫痫的母亲可能会增加癫痫发作的风险，尤其是存在睡眠剥夺导致癫痫发作的情况下。为了减少这种风险，陪护人员应至少为新生儿进行一次夜间喂养。患者癫痫发作的症状可能给婴儿带来风险（如坠落或患者过度抱紧婴儿），需要调整和（或）监督患者对儿童的护理方式。

社会心理问题

持续癫痫发作往往对患者和家庭造成严重的情绪影响。30%～50% 的难治性癫痫患者和 20% 已被控制的癫痫患者合并有抑郁症。15%～20% 的癫痫患者伴有焦虑障碍。这两种疾病常被忽视而未给予治疗。相较于癫痫发作频率，癫痫患者生活质量的受损与抑郁症明显相关。癫痫发作的不可预测性和必要的活动限制导致患者出现依赖、自我价值感降低、窘迫、羞耻感、就业率低和无助感。性欲降低和性欲减退在癫痫患者很常见，往往也会被忽视。

家庭关系也可能因癫痫的存在而被破坏。患者及其家人常常害怕癫痫发作（称为癫痫发作恐惧症）。当患者发生抽搐，特别是首次发作时，其家庭成员可能认为患者即将死亡。癫痫患者最需要的是摆脱癫痫发作，但家人和朋友的安慰和乐观支持也对其极为重要。一旦癫痫发作得到控制，应当鼓励患者以常识作为指导，尽可能回归正常和充实的生活。虽然活动限制最终可能被解除，但还是建议既往有癫痫病史的患者（CAE 和儿童癫痫伴中央颞区棘波除外，这两种癫痫可以完全缓解）避免头部接触的运动，以及避免从事可能在癫痫再次发作时造成严重后果的活动或职业（如独自游泳、高空作业、使用武器）。

如果在指定的时间段内（通常为 3 个月到 1 年）没有发生影响意识或身体控制的癫痫发作，所有国家均允许癫痫患者考取机动车驾驶证，患者一般可以获得人寿和健康保险。美国残疾人法案（ADA）为基于残疾的失业提供保护，该法案也适用于癫痫患者。在工作场所应对患者提供合理的便利，尽管这些规定有一些重要的限制条件。癫痫基金会和当地社会服务组织可从社会和职业方面协助患者处理事务。

预后

2/3 的癫痫患者在确诊后 10 年内可以达到 5 年癫痫发作缓解。其中约半数患者最终可在没有服用 AED 的情况下不再复发癫痫。有利于病情缓解的因素包括特定的遗传性全面性癫痫、神经系统检查正常，及儿

examination, and onset in early to middle childhood (excluding neonatal seizures). Approximately 30% of patients continue to have seizures and never achieve a permanent remission despite one or more AEDs. Such treatment-resistant (or medically refractory) patients should be evaluated at an epilepsy center to ensure diagnostic accuracy and to explore the full gamut of available treatments. Seizures are occasionally associated with significant morbidity and mortality. Injuries due to seizures are common. These can include traumatic injuries such as lacerations and fractures, head injuries, aspiration, drowning, and burns, among others. Such injuries can infrequently be life-threatening. Accidental deaths related to seizures (e.g., motor vehicle collisions) further increase the death rate. Aspiration with convulsions is common but can be prevented by turning the head to one side as the convulsion ends. A growing literature suggests that some types of repeated seizures, especially prolonged seizures and status epilepticus, may be associated with certain forms of cognitive decline such as memory impairment, over the lifetime of a patient.

SUDEP occurs in approximately 1 per 1000 patients per year, taking all forms of epilepsy together. In the most refractory epilepsies, the SUDEP rate may approach 10 per 1000 patients per year. SUDEP may result from transient autonomic nervous system dysfunction, which may occur during or immediately after an unwitnessed seizure (often during sleep) with resultant cardiac arrhythmia or respiratory dysfunction (central and/or peripheral forms of apnea). Suffocation can occur after an unwitnessed convulsion if the patient is prone with face down in a pillow or bedding. Whether some patients have a still unknown genetic predisposition toward SUDEP is a current active area of investigation, as are new monitoring technologies to help detect nocturnal seizures or their autonomic sequelae and alert caregivers.

DISCONTINUING ANTIEPILEPTIC DRUGS

Many patients with epilepsy become seizure-free on AED therapy for an extended time. Some patients can successfully discontinue AEDs without relapse. Successful drug withdrawal is most likely with shorter duration of epilepsy before achieving remission, with a longer seizure-free interval before antiseizure drug withdrawal (minimum of 2 years is advised but many advocate for at least 5 years), fewer seizures before achieving remission (≥10 carries higher relapse risk), history of a self-limiting epilepsy syndrome (e.g., absence epilepsy, childhood epilepsy with centrotemporal spikes), and no epileptiform abnormalities on EEG before withdrawal. Other factors of possibly lesser statistical import that may also increase the risk of relapse upon AED taper include an abnormal neurologic exam, brain MRI revealing a pertinent structural correlate, intellectual disability, family history of epilepsy, history of multiple seizure types, or if seizure control was difficult to establish and required polytherapy. Ultimately, this decision is highly individualized as the perceived burden of continuing AED treatment versus the impact of a seizure relapse may vary among individual patients with differing goals and life circumstances.

Acknowledgments

The author would like to acknowledge the work of Michel J. Berg, who contributed this chapter to the previous edition.

SUGGESTED READINGS

Berg AT, Coryell J, Saneto RP, et al: Early-life epilepsies and the emerging role of genetic testing, JAMA Pediatr 171(9):863–871, 2017.

Berg AT, Scheffer IE: New concepts in classification of the epilepsies: entering the 21st century, Epilepsia 52:1058–1062, 2011.

Fazel S, Wolf A, Langstrom N, et al: Premature mortality in epilepsy and the role of psychiatric comorbidity: a total population study, Lancet 382:1646–1654, 2013.

Fisher RS, Cross JH, French JA, et al: Operational classification of seizure types by the International League against epilepsy: position paper of the ILAE commission for classification and terminology, Epilepsia 58(4):522–530, 2017.

French JA, Pedley TA: Clinical practice. Initial management of epilepsy, N Engl J Med 359:166–176, 2008.

Glauser T, Shinnar S, Gloss D, et al: Evidence-based guideline: treatment of convulsive status epilepticus in children and adults: report of the guideline Committee of the American epilepsy society, Epilepsy Curr 16(1):48–61, 2016.

Harden CL, Hopp J, Ting TY, et al: Practice parameter update: management issues for women with epilepsy—focus on pregnancy (an evidence-based review): obstetrical complications and change in seizure frequency, Neurology 73(2):126–132, 2009.

Harden CL, Meador KJ, Pennell PB, et al: Practice parameter update: management issues for women with epilepsy—focus on pregnancy (an evidence-based review): teratogenesis and perinatal outcomes, Neurology 73:133–141, 2009.

Krumholz A, Wiebe S, Gronseth GS, et al: Evidence-based guideline: management of an unprovoked first seizure in adults, Neurology 84(16):1705–1713, 2015.

Kumada T, Miyajima T, Hiejima I, et al: Modified Atkins Diet and Low Glycemic Index Treatment for Medication-Resistant Epilepsy. Current Trends in Ketogenic Diet, J Neurol Neurophysiol S2:007, 2013.

Pack AM: Epilepsy overview and revised classification of seizures and epilepsies, Continuum (Minneap Minn) 25(2):306–321, 2019.

Proposal for revised classification of epilepsies and epileptic syndromes: Commission on classification and terminology of the international League against epilepsy, Epilepsia 30(4):389–399, 1989.

Proposal for revised clinical and electroencephalographic classification of epileptic seizures: From the commission on classification and terminology of the international League against epilepsy, Epilepsia 22(4):489–501, 1981.

Scheffer IE, Berkovic S, Capovilla G, et al: ILAE classification of the epilepsies: position paper of the ILAE Commission for Classification and Terminology, Epilepsia 58(4):512–521, 2017.

童中早期发病（不包括新生儿惊厥）。虽然服用了一种或多种 AED，仍有约 30% 的患者继续发作，未能完全缓解。这些难治性（或药物难治性）患者应该前往癫痫中心进行评估，以确保诊断的准确性，并探索所有可行的治疗方法。癫痫发作偶尔会导致较高的发病率和死亡率。癫痫发作导致的伤害很常见，包括创伤性损伤，如撕裂伤和骨折、头部损伤、误吸、溺水和烧伤等。这些伤害很少会危及生命。与癫痫发作相关的意外死亡（如机动车碰撞）进一步增加死亡率。抽搐时的误吸很常见，但可通过在抽搐结束时将头转向一侧来预防。越来越多的文献表明，某些癫痫类型的反复发作，尤其是长时程发作和癫痫持续状态，可能与患者一生中的某些认知功能下降有关，如记忆力受损。

不明原因癫痫猝死（SUDEP）在所有癫痫患者中的年发生率为 1/1000。绝大多数难治性癫痫的 SUDEP 年发生率为 1/100。SUDEP 可能由于短暂的自主神经系统功能障碍引起，一般发生在未被察觉的癫痫发作期间或之后（通常在睡眠中），导致心律失常或呼吸功能障碍［中枢和（或）外周性呼吸暂停］。如果患者在无人察觉的抽搐后俯卧在枕头或被褥上，可能导致窒息。有些患者是否具有导致 SUDEP 的遗传倾向尚未明确，这是目前正在积极研究的领域。此外，有助于检测夜间癫痫发作或其自主神经后遗症、并能提醒护理人员的新的监测技术也在积极探索中。

抗癫痫药物停用

许多癫痫患者经过长期 AED 治疗后可不再出现癫痫发作。一些患者停用 AED 后也没有再复发。成功停药最有可能出现在以下情况：缓解前癫痫持续时间变短，抗癫痫药物停药前发作间隔延长（建议至少 2 年，但一些专家主张至少 5 年），在达到缓解前癫痫发作减少（≥ 10 次提示复发风险较高），有自限性癫痫综合征病史（如失神癫痫、儿童癫痫伴中央颞区棘波），停药前 EEG 无癫痫样异常。其他可能统计意义较低但仍增加 AED 减量后癫痫复发风险的因素包括：异常的神经系统检查、脑 MRI 显示相关的结构异常、智力障碍、癫痫家族史、多种癫痫发作类型病史，或难以控制的癫痫发作且需要联合治疗。最后，停药决策高度个体化，继续使用 AED 的负担与癫痫复发的影响在不同患者中可能会有所不同，因为他们的目标和生活情况也各不相同。

致谢

作者感谢 Michel J. Berg 在上一版中为本章所做的贡献。

推荐阅读

Berg AT, Coryell J, Saneto RP, et al: Early-life epilepsies and the emerging role of genetic testing, JAMA Pediatr 171(9):863–871, 2017.

Berg AT, Scheffer IE: New concepts in classification of the epilepsies: entering the 21st century, Epilepsia 52:1058–1062, 2011.

Fazel S, Wolf A, Langstrom N, et al: Premature mortality in epilepsy and the role of psychiatric comorbidity: a total population study, Lancet 382:1646–1654, 2013.

Fisher RS, Cross JH, French JA, et al: Operational classification of seizure types by the International League against epilepsy: position paper of the ILAE commission for classification and terminology, Epilepsia 58(4):522–530, 2017.

French JA, Pedley TA: Clinical practice. Initial management of epilepsy, N Engl J Med 359:166–176, 2008.

Glauser T, Shinnar S, Gloss D, et al: Evidence-based guideline: treatment of convulsive status epilepticus in children and adults: report of the guideline Committee of the American epilepsy society, Epilepsy Curr 16(1):48–61, 2016.

Harden CL, Hopp J, Ting TY, et al: Practice parameter update: management issues for women with epilepsy—focus on pregnancy (an evidence-based review): obstetrical complications and change in seizure frequency, Neurology 73(2):126–132, 2009.

Harden CL, Meador KJ, Pennell PB, et al: Practice parameter update: management issues for women with epilepsy—focus on pregnancy (an evidence-based review): teratogenesis and perinatal outcomes, Neurology 73:133–141, 2009.

Krumholz A, Wiebe S, Gronseth GS, et al: Evidence-based guideline: management of an unprovoked first seizure in adults, Neurology 84(16):1705–1713, 2015.

Kumada T, Miyajima T, Hiejima I, et al: Modified Atkins Diet and Low Glycemic Index Treatment for Medication-Resistant Epilepsy. Current Trends in Ketogenic Diet, J Neurol Neurophysiol S2:007, 2013.

Pack AM: Epilepsy overview and revised classification of seizures and epilepsies, Continuum (Minneap Minn) 25(2):306–321, 2019.

Proposal for revised classification of epilepsies and epileptic syndromes: Commission on classification and terminology of the international League against epilepsy, Epilepsia 30(4):389–399, 1989.

Proposal for revised clinical and electroencephalographic classification of epileptic seizures: From the commission on classification and terminology of the international League against epilepsy, Epilepsia 22(4):489–501, 1981.

Scheffer IE, Berkovic S, Capovilla G, et al: ILAE classification of the epilepsies: position paper of the ILAE Commission for Classification and Terminology, Epilepsia 58(4):512–521, 2017.

Central Nervous System Tumors

Bryan J. Bonder, Lisa R. Rogers

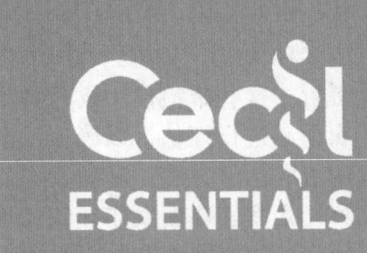

DEFINITION/EPIDEMIOLOGY

Central nervous system (CNS) tumors are of two types, primary or metastatic. Primary tumors arise from a variety of cell types within the parenchyma of the brain, spinal cord or the meninges. Metastatic tumors result from spread of systemic cancer to the brain, spinal cord, or meninges and represent the majority of central nervous system tumors. This chapter reviews both primary and metastatic brain tumors.

The incidence of primary malignant and nonmalignant brain tumors in the United States increases with age and is 5.65/100,000 in persons age 0 to 14, 11.2/100,000 in persons age 15 to 39, and 44.47/100,000 in persons older than 40. High-grade gliomas and meningiomas are the most common types of adult primary brain tumors. Meningiomas are the most common benign intracranial tumor and account for approximately one third of benign brain tumors. The incidence of primary CNS lymphoma (PCNSL) is increasing in all age groups, accounted for only in part by CNS lymphoma associated with HIV and immunocompromised states such as solid organ transplant.

Brain metastases are one of the most common neurologic complications of cancer with an incidence of up to 17%. Because incidence rates are based on tumor registries and many patients with brain metastasis do not undergo surgery, they may be underrepresented in these statistics.

Primary brain tumors are the second most common cancers in children. Medulloblastomas are the most common malignant pediatric brain tumor. In the United States, approximately 300 new cases of pediatric medulloblastomas are diagnosed each year. The cause of most primary CNS tumors is unknown. Aside from exposure to ionizing radiation, no environmental agents are known to be causative. Hereditary syndromes that are associated with an increased risk of CNS tumors include neurofibromatosis 1 and 2, tuberous sclerosis, von Hippel-Lindau disease, Li-Fraumeni syndrome, and Turcot syndrome, but these account for less than 1% of primary CNS tumors. Although the chromosomal abnormalities associated with many of these syndromes are known, the specific mechanisms leading to CNS neoplasia have not been defined.

PATHOLOGY

The most recent World Health Organization classification from 2016 defines brain tumors based on the cell of origin and molecular signature and includes a grading system, which is of use in predicting the biological behavior of the tumor. Most adult primary brain tumors are of neuroepithelial origin and result from neoplastic transformation of astrocytes, oligodendrocytes, or ependymocytes. Astrocytomas are the most common primary parenchymal brain tumor in adults. Meningiomas derive from arachnoidal cap cells in the meningeal covering of the brain. They most frequently occur in older adults. Common locations of meningioma are the cerebral convexity, falx and parasagittal area, olfactory groove, sphenoid wing, and posterior fossa. They are comprised of heterogeneous histopathology patterns, and careful neuropathological assessment is needed for accurate grading.

Primary central nervous system lymphoma is a rare form of non-Hodgkin's lymphoma, typically of B cell origin. It presents within the white matter of the cerebral hemispheres, often in a periventricular location, and is often multiple.

Brain metastasis develops when tumor cells gain access to the systemic circulation and embolize to the brain. Metastases occur most commonly from solid tumors arising in the breast, lung, kidneys, colon, and skin (melanoma). Lung cancer, both non–small and small cell type, is one of the most common tumors to metastasize to the brain and constitutes up to 50% of cases of brain metastasis. In women, breast cancer is the most common source. Malignant melanoma is a less common systemic cancer but carries a high risk of brain metastasis; up to 50% of stage IV melanoma patients develop brain metastasis.

Medulloblastomas are of primitive neuro-ectodermal origin and are highly cellular. Homer Wright rosettes (arrangement of tumor cells around a central area filled with neurofibrillary processes) can be identified in resected specimens in up to 40% of cases. Medulloblastomas are grade IV tumors as they are invasive and rapidly growing, with a tendency to disseminate through the cerebrospinal fluid (CSF).

CLINICAL PRESENTATION

Symptoms and signs caused by brain tumors typically result from compression or invasion of adjacent neural tissue by the tumor or from vasogenic edema resulting from disruption of the blood-brain barrier which can be caused by cerebral vessel compression/invasion from tumor or from "leaky" blood vessels present within the tumor. Neoangiogenesis associated with tumor growth is typically comprised of embryonic vessels that lack a normal blood-brain barrier. Because of the uncompromising rigidity of the cranial vault, both histologically benign and malignant tumors may cause symptoms, even when they are small. Symptoms caused by low-grade primary brain tumors tend to be slowly progressive whereas those in mid- and high-grade histology are acute or subacute (over weeks to months). The exception is the clinical presentation of a low-grade glioma with seizure. Metastatic tumors often present in a subacute fashion but may present acutely when hemorrhage into the tumor occurs. Hemorrhage into metastatic brain tumors is most common with renal cell, lung, papillary thyroid carcinomas, melanoma, and choriocarcinomas.

The clinical symptoms and signs depend on the location of tumor. In most pediatric patients with brain tumors, tumors arise in the posterior fossa and result in diplopia, ataxia, dysphagia, or nausea/vomiting. Most adult brain tumors arise in the cerebral hemispheres and

中枢神经系统肿瘤

李雨贤 译 杨沫 陈玮琪 审校 王伊龙 通审

定义和流行病学

中枢神经系统（CNS）肿瘤分为原发性和转移性两种。原发性肿瘤起源于脑实质、脊髓或脑膜的各种细胞类型。转移性肿瘤是由全身性癌症扩散到脑、脊髓或脑膜所致，在中枢神经系统肿瘤中占大多数。本章对原发性和转移性脑肿瘤做一回顾。

美国原发性恶性和非恶性脑肿瘤的发病率随着年龄的增长而增加，0～14岁的发病率为5.65/10万，15～39岁的发病率为11.2/10万，40岁以上的发病率为44.47/10万。高级别胶质瘤和脑膜瘤是成人原发性脑肿瘤中最常见的类型。脑膜瘤是最常见的颅内良性肿瘤，约占良性脑肿瘤的1/3。原发性中枢神经系统淋巴瘤（PCNSL）的发病率在所有年龄组中均呈上升趋势，与人类免疫缺陷病毒（HIV）和免疫功能低下状态（如实体器官移植）有关的中枢神经系统淋巴瘤只占其中一部分。

脑转移是癌症最常见的神经系统并发症之一，其发病率高达17%。由于发病率以肿瘤登记为统计基础，而许多脑转移患者并未接受手术治疗，因此转移瘤的发病率可能被低估。

原发性脑肿瘤是儿童第二大常见癌症类型。髓母细胞瘤是最常见的小儿恶性脑肿瘤。美国每年约有300例新确诊的儿童髓母细胞瘤。大多数原发性中枢神经系统肿瘤的病因不明。除了暴露于电离辐射外，其余致病的环境因素尚不清楚。与中枢神经系统肿瘤发病风险增加有关的遗传性综合征包括神经纤维瘤病1型和2型、结节性硬化症、希佩尔-林道病、利-弗劳梅尼综合征和特科特综合征，但这些综合征占原发性中枢神经系统肿瘤的比例不到1%。虽然与这些综合征相关的染色体异常多数已经为人所知，但导致中枢神经系统肿瘤的具体机制尚未明确。

病理学

世界卫生组织2016年的最新分类根据起源细胞和分子特征对脑肿瘤进行了定义，并囊括了一个分级系统，该系统有助于预测肿瘤的生物学行为。大多数成人原发性脑肿瘤起源于神经上皮细胞，由星形胶质细胞、少突胶质细胞或室管膜细胞的致瘤性转化所致。星形细胞瘤是成人最常见的原发性脑实质肿瘤。脑膜瘤起源于覆盖在脑表面的脑膜中的蛛网膜帽细胞，其在老年人群中常见。脑膜瘤的常见部位是大脑半球凸面、大脑镰和矢状窦旁、嗅沟、蝶骨翼和颅后窝。脑膜瘤的组织病理学形态不一，需要进行仔细的神经病理学评估才能准确分级。

原发性中枢神经系统淋巴瘤是一种罕见的非霍奇金淋巴瘤，通常为B细胞起源。它出现于大脑半球的白质中，通常位于脑室周围，且往往为多发性。

当肿瘤细胞进入全身循环并栓塞到大脑时，会发生肿瘤脑转移。脑转移最常见于以下部位的实体瘤：乳腺、肺、肾、结肠和皮肤（黑色素瘤）。肺癌，包括非小细胞型和小细胞型两种，是最常见的脑转移肿瘤之一，占脑转移病例的50%。在女性中，乳腺癌是最常见的转移来源。恶性黑色素瘤是一种不常见的全身性癌症，但其脑部转移的风险很高；多达50%的Ⅳ期黑色素瘤患者会发生脑转移。

髓母细胞瘤起源于原始神经外胚层，具有高度细胞性。高达40%的病例可在切除标本中发现霍默-赖特菊形团（肿瘤细胞围绕充满神经纤维的中心区域排列）。髓母细胞瘤属于Ⅳ级肿瘤，因其具有侵袭性且生长迅速，有通过脑脊液（CSF）播散的倾向。

临床表现

脑肿瘤引起的症状和体征通常是由于肿瘤压迫或侵犯邻近的神经组织所致，或者因肿瘤或肿瘤内的"渗漏"血管压迫或侵犯脑血管导致血脑屏障破坏而引起血管源性水肿所致。肿瘤生长相关的新生血管通常由缺乏正常血脑屏障的胚胎血管发育形成。由于颅骨穹窿坚硬不易形变，即使瘤体很小，组织学良性肿瘤和恶性肿瘤均可能引起症状。低级别原发性脑肿瘤引起的症状往往是缓慢进展的，而由病理诊断的中-高级别肿瘤引起的症状则是急性或亚急性的（在数周至数月内）。低级别胶质瘤偶尔伴有癫痫发作。转移瘤通常表现为亚急性，但当肿瘤内出血时也可能表现为急性。转移瘤出血最常见于肾细胞癌、肺癌、甲状腺乳头状癌、黑色素瘤和绒毛膜癌。

临床症状和体征取决于肿瘤的位置。大多数儿童患者脑肿瘤位于颅后窝，会导致复视、共济失调、吞咽困难、恶心或呕吐。大多数成人脑肿瘤位于大脑半

present with symptoms and signs related to the supratentorial structure involved: unilateral limb weakness, aphasia, and speech abnormality or memory loss are common. Tumors in either location may present with generalized symptoms arising from increased intracranial pressure or meningeal irritation. Headache occurs in up to two thirds of patients as a presenting sign. There are no unique characteristics to this headache, but useful clinical clues include a new or different headache pattern, a progressively worsening headache, and one that occurs at night or on awakening. The pain may localize to the side of the tumor in patients with supratentorial tumors, whereas patients with infratentorial tumors frequently describe pain in the retro-orbital, retroauricular, or occipital region. Other generalized symptoms include changes in mood or personality, a decrease in appetite, and nausea. Projectile vomiting, while common in children with posterior fossa tumors, is rare in adults. Meningiomas generally grow slowly; they may also be found incidentally during the evaluation of unrelated neurologic symptoms. Seizures may develop over the course of the illness in up to 15% of patients with any type of primary tumor, often in association with tumor progression.

DIAGNOSIS/DIFFERENTIAL

All patients suspected of having a brain tumor should undergo a contrast-enhanced magnetic resonance imaging (MRI) brain scan. If MRI is not available or is contraindicated because of a non-MRI-compatible pacemaker or other condition, brain computed tomography (CT) with contrast should be obtained. Brain MRI is preferred because it is more useful in imaging the temporal and posterior fossae and it is more sensitive in detecting the extent of parenchymal involvement by tumor of any type. In addition, advanced sequences such as diffusion, perfusion, and spectroscopy can add to the diagnostic accuracy of imaging. Vasogenic edema resulting from leakage of intravascular fluid through a disrupted blood-brain barrier is easily visible on MRI.

High-grade gliomas typically appear as irregularly shaped contrast-enhancing masses surrounded by edema. Central necrosis is characteristic of glioblastoma (Fig. 16.1). Anaplastic gliomas appear similarly, except for less frequent regions of necrosis. Although there are exceptions, most low-grade gliomas do not enhance after intravenous contrast injection (Fig. 16.2). Meningiomas typically demonstrate smooth and homogeneous enhancement originating from the extra-axial space and may also compress adjacent brain. Primary CNS lymphomas typically present as multiple contrast-enhancing lesions within the white matter but in rare instances do not show contrast enhancement. Brain metastases are often located at the gray-white junction of the brain and demonstrate homogeneous enhancement or peripheral enhancement surrounding a necrotic or cystic center. When solitary, a brain metastasis cannot be accurately distinguished from other neoplasm or nonneoplastic entities. Medulloblastomas are usually large by the time they are identified and demonstrate homogeneous enhancement within or superior to the floor of the fourth ventricle (Fig. 16.3). They are often accompanied by hydrocephalus. The desmoplastic variant of medulloblastomas can be located lateral to the fourth ventricle.

The differential diagnosis of contrast-enhancing lesions includes brain abscess, but infection is a consideration only in rare clinical situations. Diffusion-weighted magnetic resonance images can be useful in distinguishing tumor from infection. Low-grade gliomas can be misdiagnosed as cerebral infarction, especially on brain CT. Periventricular enhancement in PCNSL can sometimes be confused with active multiple sclerosis lesions or with brain metastasis. Dural pathologies such as sarcoidosis, meningeal infection, or dural metastasis can mimic a meningioma. Posterior fossa ependymomas in children can mimic medulloblastomas.

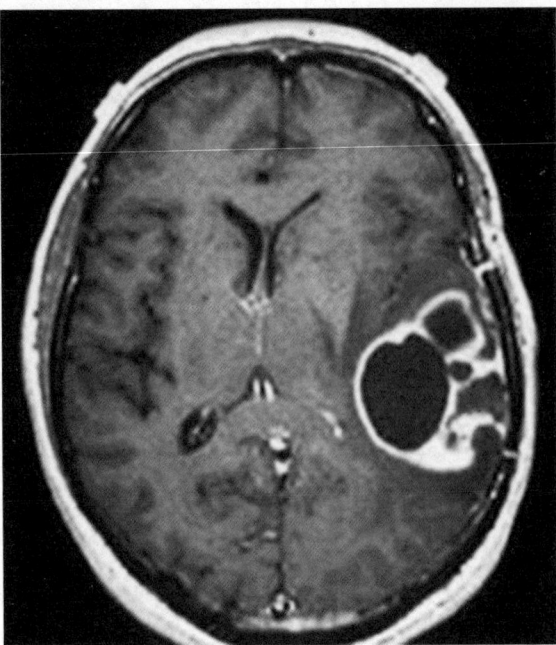

Fig. 16.1 Contrast-enhanced T1-weighted MRI demonstrates irregular contrast enhancement with central necrosis in the left temporal lobe. There is adjacent vasogenic edema and mass effect on midline structures characteristic of a high grade glioma.

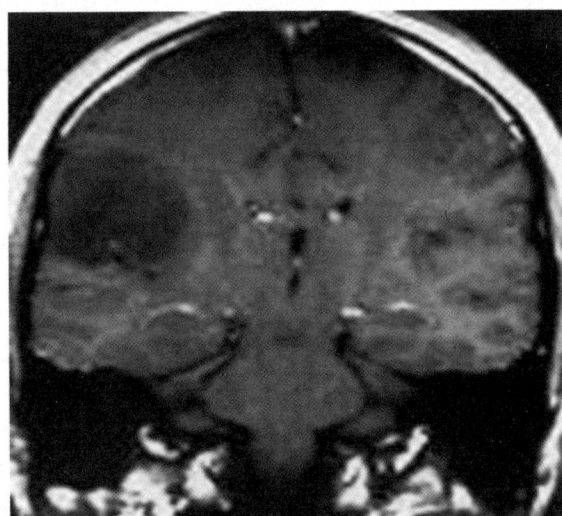

Fig. 16.2 Coronal T-weighted MRI following contrast injection in a low-grade astrocytoma shows low signal intensity and no contrast enhancement, typical of a low-grade glioma.

Leptomeningeal metastasis can be suspected in cancer patients with multiple cranial nerve deficits, asymmetrical limb weakness, unexplained headaches or seizures. Evaluation typically includes imaging of the entire neuraxis with contrast-enhanced MRI. Leptomeningeal tumor will appear as diffuse or nodular enhancement arising from the leptomeninges of the brain or spinal cord. Cranial nerves, when involved, may enhance and appear thickened. The diagnosis can be made by MRI in the appropriate clinical setting, but definitive diagnosis is established by demonstration of tumor cells in cytology examination of CSF. In patients with lymphoma, flow cytometry is preferable to cytology. A large volume (>10 mL) lumbar puncture is frequently

球，并表现出与所累及幕上结构有关的症状和体征，常见有单侧肢体无力、失语、言语异常或记忆力减退。任何一个部位的肿瘤都可能因颅内压增高或脑膜刺激而出现全身症状。高达 2/3 的患者存在头痛表现。这种头痛没有特异性，但有提示作用的临床线索包括新的或不同的头痛模式、逐渐加重的头痛，以及在夜间或醒来时发生的头痛。幕上肿瘤患者的疼痛可能定位于肿瘤侧，而幕下肿瘤的患者则经常描述眶后、耳后或枕部疼痛。其他全身症状包括情绪或性格改变、食欲下降和恶心。喷射性呕吐在颅后窝肿瘤的儿童中很常见，在成人中很少见。脑膜瘤一般生长缓慢，也可能在评估无关的神经系统症状时偶然发现。在任何类型的原发性肿瘤患者中，多达 15% 的患者会在病程中出现癫痫发作，通常与肿瘤进展有关。

诊断和鉴别诊断

所有疑似脑肿瘤的患者都应接受对比增强磁共振成像（MRI）脑部扫描。如果 MRI 不可用，或因 MRI 无法兼容心脏起搏器或其他原因而存在禁忌，则应进行脑部对比增强计算机断层成像（CT）。脑部 MRI 是首选，因为它对颞叶和颅后窝的成像更有帮助，而且对检测各类肿瘤的脑实质受累程度更加敏感。此外，弥散、灌注和波谱等高级序列可提高影像诊断的准确性。血管内液体通过破坏的血脑屏障渗出所致的血管源性水肿在 MRI 上很容易被识别。

高级别胶质瘤通常表现为形态不规则的对比增强占位，且其周围有水肿。中央坏死是胶质母细胞瘤的特征（图 16.1）。间变性胶质瘤表现类似，只是坏死区域较少见。虽然有例外情况，但大多数低级别胶质瘤在静脉注射造影剂后不会出现强化表现（图 16.2）。脑膜瘤通常表现为源于轴外间隙的平滑均匀强化，也可能压迫邻近的脑组织。原发性中枢神经系统淋巴瘤通常表现为白质内多个强化病灶，但在极少数情况下不显示对比增强。脑转移瘤通常位于脑灰白质交界处，表现为均匀强化或者围绕坏死或囊性中心的周围强化。孤立的脑转移瘤无法与其他肿瘤或非肿瘤实体准确区分。髓母细胞瘤被发现时通常体积较大，在第四脑室底部或上方呈均匀强化（图 16.3），其通常伴发脑积水。促纤维增生型髓母细胞瘤可位于第四脑室侧面。

对比增强病变的鉴别诊断包括脑脓肿，但只有在少数的临床情形下才考虑感染。弥散加权磁共振成像有助于区分肿瘤和感染。低级别胶质瘤可能会被误诊为脑梗死，尤其是在脑部 CT 上。PCNSL 的脑室周围强化有时会与活动性多发性硬化病变或脑转移瘤相混淆。硬脑膜病变，如结节病、脑膜感染或硬脑膜转移瘤可拟似脑膜瘤。儿童颅后窝室管膜瘤可类似于髓母细胞瘤。

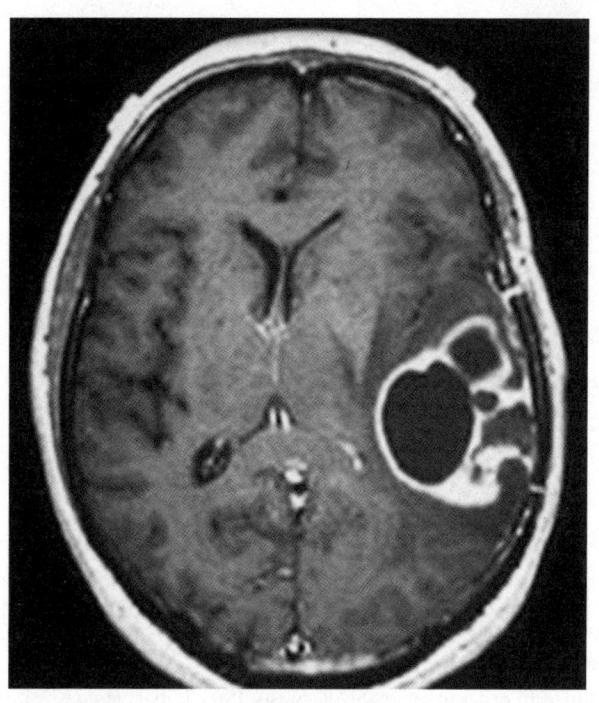

图 16.1 对比增强 T1 加权 MRI 显示左侧颞叶不规则增强伴中央坏死。可见邻近的血管源性水肿和中线结构的占位效应为高级别胶质瘤的特征

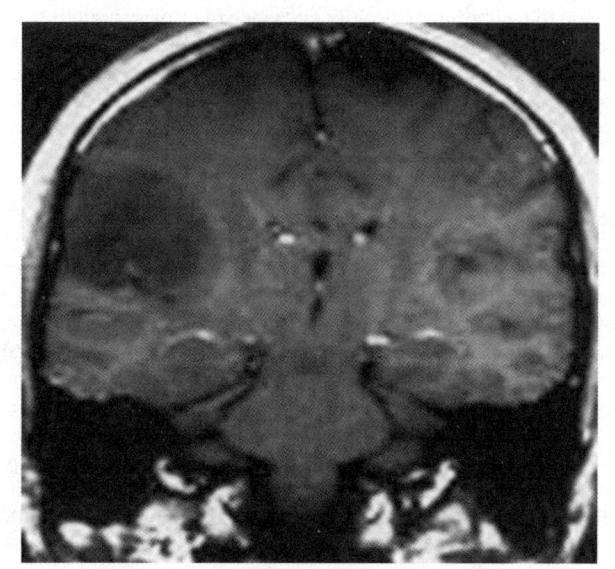

图 16.2 低级别星形细胞瘤注射造影剂后的冠状位 T1 加权 MRI 显示低信号，无对比增强，是低级别胶质瘤的典型表现

癌症患者如出现多发脑神经功能缺损、不对称的肢体无力、不明原因的头痛或癫痫发作，需警惕存在软脑膜转移。评估通常包括使用对比增强 MRI 对整个神经轴进行成像。软脑（脊）膜肿瘤表现为软脑膜或脊膜的弥漫性或结节性强化。脑神经受累时可能会增强和增粗。在特定的临床环境下，可通过 MRI 做出诊断，但明确诊断需要通过脑脊液细胞学检查显示肿瘤细胞。对于淋巴瘤患者，流式细胞术比细胞学检查更为适合。通常需进行腰椎穿刺术以取得较大体积的脑脊液（>10 ml）才能明确诊断。如果最初的细胞学检查为阴性，但高度怀

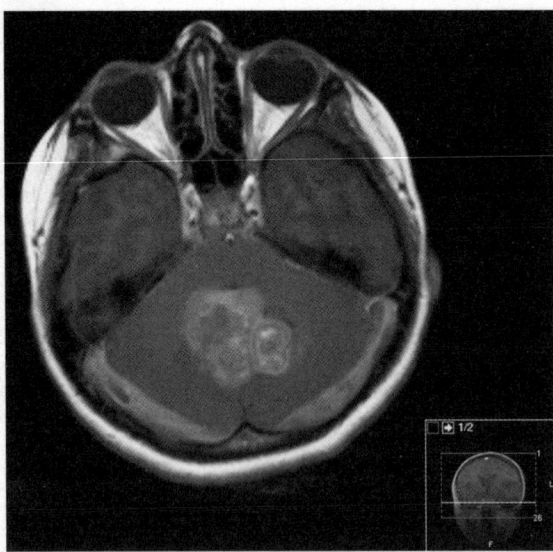

Fig. 16.3 Contrast-enhanced T1-weighted MRI shows a large enhancing tumor in the midline of the cerebellum with compression of the fourth ventricle.

required in order to make the diagnosis. If the initial cytology is negative and suspicion is high, additional lumbar puncture can be considered. Findings of elevated CSF protein and white blood cell count or low glucose should raise suspicion.

In the majority of cases, biopsy or resection is the preferred method to establish the histology and grade of primary brain tumors. Exceptions include patients suspected to have PCNSL; a search for malignant cells in the CSF or by vitreous biopsy can be attempted to avoid surgery. Additionally, surgery is typically avoided in brain stem gliomas because the MRI appearance is characteristic and biopsy is considered dangerous.

TREATMENT

Surgical resection is the initial goal for most patients with benign and malignant primary brain tumors. Surgical resection provides tissue for analysis and often relieves neurologic symptoms; maximal surgical resection, when feasible, improves outcome. One exception is PCNSL, in which clinical deterioration can result from resection. Biopsy alone is adequate unless significant symptoms of mass effect from the tumor are present. In addition, small meningiomas can often be observed.

Standard therapy for newly diagnosed glioblastoma is maximal resection and focal external beam radiation of 60 Gy in combination with temozolomide followed by adjuvant temozolomide for 6 months. In a prospective randomized trial of newly diagnosed glioblastoma patients, the median survival with radiation and temozolomide was 14.6 months versus 12.1 months with radiation alone. In addition, the 2-year survival rate was superior with the combined regimen (26.5%) versus radiation alone (10.4%). O-6-methylguanine DNA methyltransferase (MGMT) is a DNA repair gene that reduces the efficacy of temozolomide and other DNA-damaging treatments for cancer. Methylation of the MGMT promoter in tumor tissue silences this gene and results in improved survival in glioblastoma. There is evidence that tumors harboring isocitrate dehydrogenase (IDH) 1and 2 mutations are correlated with a superior outcome compared with wild-type IDH. The discovery of molecular "drivers" may lead to identification of additional targets for therapy. New approaches using next-generation sequencing and DNA-methylation fingerprinting are being evaluated in trials of glioblastoma.

The introduction of "targeted agents" that are designed to deactivate oncogenic pathways or angiogenesis is a major advance in cancer treatment. Bevacizumab, a monoclonal antibody to vascular endothelial growth factor, is associated with a high response rate and reduction in neurologic symptoms in recurrent glioblastoma, although the effect on overall survival is not significant. Because current treatment results are unsatisfactory, it is suggested that patients with glioblastoma be referred for clinical trial.

Anaplastic gliomas, most commonly anaplastic astrocytoma and anaplastic oligodendroglioma, are treated by maximal surgical resection, followed by focal external beam radiation in association with chemotherapy. However, there is increasing reliance upon the molecular markers of MGMT and IDH1 status to predict survival and to dictate the utility of adding chemotherapy in poor prognosis patients. One type of anaplastic glioma exquisitely sensitive to chemotherapy is the anaplastic oligodendroglioma with co-deletions of 1p and 19q.

The long-term progression-free survival and overall survival of low-grade glioma (grade 2) patients is better than those with glioblastoma or anaplastic glioma, but malignant transformation occurs in up to 50% of such patients and close monitoring with serial MRIs is required. Most patients with low-grade gliomas should be treated initially with maximal safe surgical resection. When grade 2 patients undergo resection, adjuvant therapy with radiation and chemotherapy is reserved for those who are older than 40 years of age or in whom the resection was subtotal. Characterizing low-grade gliomas by molecular markers such as IDH1 and chromosomal analysis for co-deletion of 1p and 19q mutations and (IDH) mutation predicts prognosis. Regardless of the treatment modality selected, serial monitoring for progression with regular MRIs is indicated. If there is disease progression or recurrence, repeat surgery, RT, and chemotherapy are all potential options depending on individual patient characteristics.

The type of therapy selected for a meningioma depends on patient characteristics, tumor features, potential for harm if untreated, and consideration of side effects of the treatment. Maximal surgical resection is important to reduce the risk of relapse. When complete removal is not possible, radiation therapy should be considered postoperatively, especially for grade 2 tumors. Radiation therapy is recommended regardless of the extent of resection for malignant (grade 3) meningiomas. Chemotherapy for this disease has not been proven to be effective.

Symptoms and imaging abnormalities associated with PCNSL often improve with the administration of corticosteroids because of the cytotoxic effects of steroids on lymphoma cells. However, administration of steroids before brain biopsy reduces the yield of tissue biopsy and can confound diagnosis. Therefore, delaying steroids prior to surgery is appropriate in suspected PCNSL because resection is often associated with neurologic deterioration and because there is no clear evidence that resection improves prognosis. A high-dose methotrexate-based regimen incorporating an alkylating agent and rituximab is the preferred induction therapy. Consolidation therapy may include other chemotherapies or low-dose whole brain radiation. High-dose radiation following chemotherapy should be avoided because of the risk of white matter damage. Up to a quarter of patients have ocular or CSF involvement at the presentation of CNS lymphomas, and staging by performing lumbar puncture and consultation with ophthalmology is appropriate prior to beginning therapy.

Contemporary management of brain metastases is individualized and is often best accomplished by a multidisciplinary team including medical oncology, neuro-oncology, radiation oncology, and neurosurgery. Initial systemic evaluation for a suspected new brain metastasis should include contrast-enhanced CT scans of the chest, abdomen, and pelvis and additionally a mammogram if the patient is female. If

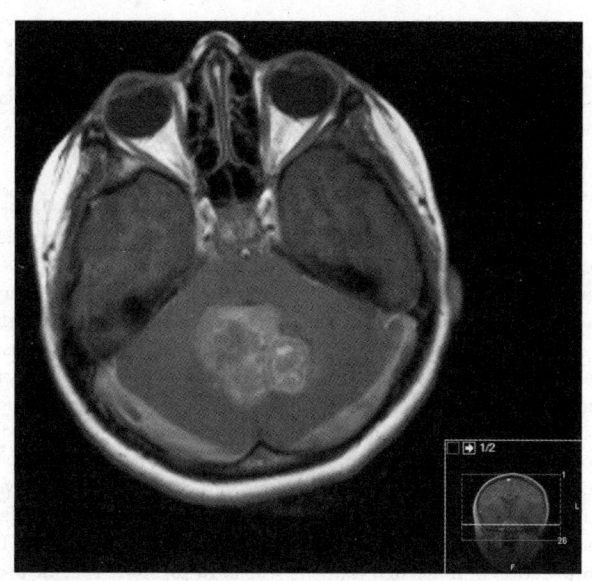

图 16.3 对比增强 T1 加权 MRI 显示小脑中线存在一个巨大的强化肿瘤，并压迫第四脑室

疑，则可考虑复查腰椎穿刺。如果发现脑脊液蛋白质和白细胞计数升高或葡萄糖降低，则需提高怀疑。

在大部分情况下，活检或切除术是确定原发性脑肿瘤组织学和分级的首选方法。例外情况包括怀疑患有 PCNSL 的患者；可尝试在脑脊液中或通过玻璃体活检寻找恶性细胞，以避免手术。此外，脑干胶质瘤通常需避免活检，因为其 MRI 表现具有特征性且活检相对危险。

治疗

手术切除是大多数良性和恶性原发性脑肿瘤患者的初始治疗目标。手术切除可提供用于分析的组织，通常可缓解神经系统症状；在可行的情况下，最大限度地手术切除可改善预后。PCNSL 是一个例外，切除可能导致临床症状恶化。除非肿瘤有明显的占位效应，否则单纯活检即可。此外，小的脑膜瘤通常可继续观察。

新确诊的胶质母细胞瘤的标准治疗方法是最大限度地切除肿瘤，行 60 Gy 的局灶外线束辐射治疗联合替莫唑胺，然后使用替莫唑胺辅助治疗 6 个月。在一项针对新确诊胶质母细胞瘤患者的前瞻性随机对照试验中，放疗联合替莫唑胺的中位生存期为 14.6 个月，而单纯放疗的中位生存期为 12.1 个月。此外，联合疗法的 2 年生存率（26.5%）优于单纯放疗（10.4%）。O-6-甲基鸟嘌呤 DNA 甲基转移酶（MGMT）是一种 DNA 修复基因，可降低替莫唑胺和其他损伤癌细胞 DNA 的癌症治疗的疗效。肿瘤组织中 MGMT 启动子的甲基化可使该基因沉默，从而提高胶质母细胞瘤患者的生存率。有证据表明，携带异柠檬酸脱氢酶（IDH）1 和 2 突变的肿瘤与野生型 IDH 相比，具有更好的预后。分子水平"驱动因素"的发现可能会促进更多治疗靶点的发现。使用二代测序和 DNA 甲基化指纹图谱的新方法正在胶质母细胞瘤的相关临床试验中被评估。

旨在抑制致癌途径或血管生成的"靶向药物"的问世是癌症治疗领域的一项重大进步。贝伐珠单抗是一种针对血管内皮生长因子的单克隆抗体，对复发性胶质母细胞瘤的治疗有较高的反应率，并可减轻神经系统症状，但对总生存期的影响并不显著。由于现有的治疗手段效果并不理想，建议将胶质母细胞瘤患者转介至临床试验。

间变性胶质瘤，最常见的是间变性星形细胞瘤和间变性少突胶质细胞瘤，治疗方法是进行最大限度地手术切除，然后进行局灶外源性放疗联合化疗。而目前我们越来越依赖 MGMT 和 IDH1 的分子标志物来预测患者生存率，并据此评估是否对预后不良的患者使用化疗治疗。1p 和 19q 共缺失的间变性少突胶质细胞瘤是一种对化疗非常敏感的间变性胶质瘤。

低级别胶质瘤（2 级）患者的长期无进展生存期和总生存期优于胶质母细胞瘤或间变性胶质瘤患者，但高达 50% 的此类患者会发生恶变，因此需要通过连续 MRI 进行密切监测。大多数低级别胶质瘤患者初始都应接受最大限度安全的手术切除治疗。2 级患者接受切除术后，放疗和化疗辅助治疗仅限于年龄超过 40 岁或切除术为次全切除的患者。通过 IDH1 等分子标志物以及染色体分析 1p 和 19q 共缺失突变和（IDH）突变来确定低级别胶质瘤的特征，可以预测预后。无论选择哪种治疗方式，都应定期进行 MRI 检查，连续监测病情进展。如果疾病进展或复发，根据患者的个体特征，再次手术、放疗和化疗都是潜在选择。

脑膜瘤治疗方式的选择取决于患者的特点、肿瘤特征、不治疗的潜在危害以及对治疗副作用的考虑。最大限度地手术切除对于降低复发风险至关重要。如果无法完全切除，术后应考虑放疗，尤其是 2 级肿瘤。对于恶性（3 级）脑膜瘤，无论切除程度如何，都建议采用放疗。化疗的疗效尚未得到证实。

由于类固醇对淋巴细胞具有细胞毒性作用，因此与 PCNSL 相关的症状和影像学异常通常会在使用皮质类固醇后得到改善。然而，在脑活检前使用类固醇会影响组织活检的结果，并可能混淆诊断。因此，对于疑似 PCNSL 患者，在手术前延迟使用类固醇药物是合适的，因为切除术通常会导致神经功能恶化，而且没有明确证据表明切除术会改善预后。以大剂量氨甲蝶呤为基础、结合烷化剂和利妥昔单抗的方案是首选的诱导治疗方法。巩固治疗可包括其他化疗方式或小剂量全脑放疗。化疗后应避免大剂量放疗，因为存在白质损伤的风险。多达 1/4 的中枢神经系统淋巴瘤患者在发病时存在眼部或脑脊液受累，因此在开始治疗前应进行腰椎穿刺并请眼科医师会诊，以协助分期。

脑转移瘤的现代化管理需要个体化，通常最好由包括肿瘤内科、神经肿瘤科、肿瘤放射科和神经外科在内的多学科团队共同完成。对疑似新发脑转移瘤的初步系统评估应包括胸部、腹部和盆腔的增强 CT 扫描，如果患者是女性，还应进行乳腺钼靶检查。如果

the lesions are multiple and the underlying diagnosis is not known, tissue from the safest and most readily accessible site should be obtained. Standard therapy for patients with a single brain metastasis is complete resection if the tumor is resectable and the patient has a good performance status and has limited extracranial disease. Some patients with limited systemic cancer show a survival benefit with resection of up to three metastatic tumors. Resection is typically followed by whole brain radiation or stereotactic surgery to the tumor margin. Radiosurgery to all lesions, avoiding resection, is also an option. The addition of whole brain radiation therapy (WBRT) after resection or radiosurgery provides better control of tumor in the brain but does not result in increased survival, and its use should be determined based on the individual clinical circumstances.

Patients presenting with more than three brain metastases should be considered for WBRT. Novel approaches to preserving memory in patients undergoing WBRT include sparing the hippocampus during radiation and/or adding memantine. If the patient does not receive WBRT, close observation with periodic MRI scans is indicated to assess for recurrence at the original site or at other sites in the brain. A variety of systemic treatments show therapeutic efficacy in newly diagnosed and recurrent brain metastasis, depend upon the sensitivity of the brain metastasis to the agent. Examples include small molecule targeted agents for non–small cell lung cancer, immunotherapy for malignant melanoma, and chemotherapy with or without targeted agents for breast cancer.

Leptomeningeal metastasis is treated based on the underlying pathology and the performance status of the patient. Options include radiation to symptomatic sites or bulky disease in the brain or spine on MRI, systemic chemotherapy, or intrathecal chemotherapy.

The extent of resection is prognostic in medulloblastomas. Staging evaluations for the extent of disease include postoperative MRI of the brain and spine and lumbar CSF sampling. Prospective randomized trials and single-arm trials suggest that adjuvant chemotherapy administered during and after craniospinal radiation improves the progression-free survival and overall survival in both average and poor risk groups. The therapy for children younger than 3 years of age excludes craniospinal radiation therapy because of the long-term deleterious effects and includes surgery and chemotherapy alone. Distinct subgroups of medulloblastomas have been identified, and profiling of these subgroups reveals distinct genomic events, some of which represent actionable targets for therapy.

Vasogenic edema associated with parenchymal and meningeal tumor causes neurologic symptoms and signs and can be life-threatening. Treatment with corticosteroids often reduces edema and improves neurologic function. Dexamethasone is the preferred steroid because of its long half-life and low mineralocorticoid activity. Patients with symptoms related to vasogenic edema often improve within 48 hours of dexamethasone administration. Doses used for treatment of tumor-related edema are typically 4 to 24 mg/day of dexamethasone given in divided doses (two to four times daily). Because steroids can be associated with a variety of adverse effects, the lowest dose and duration of administration should be sought. In patients with severe neurologic signs related to brain edema, an intravenous bolus of 10 mg dexamethasone should be considered. If the neurologic signs are life-threatening, including signs of brain herniation, mannitol and dexamethasone should be administered and urgent neurosurgical consultation obtained. Seizures should be aggressively managed with antiepileptic drugs. Liver nonenzyme-inducing antiepileptic drugs (e.g., phenytoin) are favored because of a better safety profile than liver enzyme-inducing drugs and because of the lack of interaction with other medications prescribed to treat the tumor, including steroids and chemotherapy. Prophylactic antiepileptic drugs are generally not recommended for patients with a primary or metastatic brain tumor. One exception is melanoma brain metastases in which patients with multiple supratentorial brain metastases, especially those with hemorrhage, have a high risk of seizures.

PROGNOSIS

The grade of glioma, performance status, and age are important predictors of prognosis. Glioblastoma has the worst prognosis, with a median survival of just over 1 year even with aggressive therapy. Favorable prognosis patients can live more than 2 years. Data from the nationwide Surveillance, Epidemiology, and End Results registry identified an overall median survival of 15 months and 42 months for patients with anaplastic astrocytomas and anaplastic oligodendrogliomas, respectively. This analysis did not include the status of 1p19q chromosomal loss, and the more favorable survival of patients with co-deletions was thus not demonstrated. Low-grade gliomas have a median survival of approximately 5 years, but there is individual variation depending on age, size of tumor, and extent of resection. The incorporation of molecular markers will allow for more specific prognostication in these tumors.

Recurrence rates in meningioma depend upon grade and vary from greater than 25% in grade 1 to greater than 90% in grade 3. Risk factors for recurrence include incomplete resection, higher tumor grade, young age, specific subtypes, brain infiltration, and high proliferative rate.

Median survival in PCNSL has improved with the introduction of high-dose methotrexate regimens in contrast to whole brain radiation that was used decades ago. Depending upon a variety of clinical factors, most importantly age and performance status, it ranges from 1 to 8 years. Elderly patients (>70 years) fare the worst.

Performance status, age, status of the extracranial tumor, and number of brain metastases are some of the factors that predict prognosis in patients with brain metastasis. The prognosis of patients with brain metastases has become increasingly individualized. As newer targeted therapies become available, the particular genetic mutations driving the cancer are also becoming important for determination of prognosis. The median survival ranges from 3 to 6 months in patients with multiple metastases treated with whole brain radiation therapy. Patients with a single metastasis with limited extracranial disease who undergo surgical resection and whole brain radiation therapy have significantly improved survival (40 weeks) as compared with those who undergo whole brain radiation therapy alone (15 weeks). Importantly, the improved survival is accompanied by a longer period of functional independence.

The 5-year progression-free survival in medulloblastomas is 70% to 85%. However, more than one third of patients experience recurrence, and there is no standard therapy at the time of recurrence. Median survival after recurrence is usually less than 1 year.

The advent of molecular markers in the diagnostic evaluation of primary brain tumors, especially gliomas, has significantly altered the approach to predicting prognosis and treatment response. In addition, multi-institution trials have provided robust information regarding the optimal therapy for subgroups of glioma, subdivided by important clinical factors such as patient age, performance status, degree of surgical resection, and incorporation of molecular markers. It is anticipated that prospectively designed trials, stratified on these factors, will yield additional information to aid the clinician in treatment recommendations. Significant advances in the treatment of systemic cancer are providing additional therapies when those cancers spread to the central nervous system.

病灶是多发性的，且基础诊断不明确，则应从最安全、最容易获取的部位取得组织。对于单发脑转移瘤患者，如果肿瘤可切除、患者情况良好且颅外疾病尚可控制，标准治疗方法是完全切除。一些局限性多发转移瘤患者在切除多达 3 个转移瘤后显示出生存获益。切除术后通常会对肿瘤切缘进行全脑放疗或立体定向手术。也可以选择对所有病灶进行放射外科手术取代切除术。切除术或放射外科手术后加用全脑放射治疗（WBRT）可更好地控制脑肿瘤，但并不会提高生存率，应根据个体临床情况决定是否使用。

存在 3 个以上脑转移灶的患者应考虑接受 WBRT。对于接受 WBRT 的患者，保护记忆力的新方法包括在放疗时保护海马区和（或）加用美金刚。如果患者不接受 WBRT，则应定期进行 MRI 扫描以密切观察，评估原发部位或脑部其他部位的复发情况。根据脑转移瘤对药物的敏感性，多种全身治疗方法对新诊断和复发的脑转移瘤均显示出疗效，例如，治疗非小细胞肺癌的小分子靶向药物、治疗恶性黑色素瘤的免疫疗法、治疗乳腺癌的靶向或非靶向化疗药物等。

软脑膜转移瘤的治疗取决于病理基础和患者的功能状态。治疗方法包括对有症状的部位或 MRI 显示的脑部或脊髓巨大肿块病变进行放疗、全身化疗或鞘内化疗。

髓母细胞瘤的切除范围对患者预后具有提示作用。对疾病范围的分期评估包括术后脑部和脊柱的磁共振成像以及腰穿 CSF 取样。前瞻性随机试验和单臂试验表明，在脑脊髓放疗期间和之后进行辅助化疗，可提高一般风险组和低风险组的无进展生存率和总生存率。3 岁以下儿童的治疗仅包括手术和化疗，由于远期的有害效果而排除了脑脊髓放疗。髓母细胞瘤已被鉴定存在不同的亚组，对这些亚组的分析揭示了不同的基因组事件，其中一些为潜在的治疗靶点。

脑实质和脑膜肿瘤引起的血管源性水肿会导致神经系统症状和体征，并可能危及生命。使用皮质类固醇治疗通常可以减轻水肿，改善神经功能。地塞米松是首选的类固醇，因为它的半衰期长且盐皮质激素活性低。有血管源性水肿相关症状的患者通常会在使用地塞米松后 48 h 内好转。治疗肿瘤相关性水肿的剂量通常为地塞米松 4～24 mg/d，分次给药（每天 2～4 次）。由于类固醇药物可能会产生多种不良反应，因此应寻求最低剂量和最短给药持续时间。如果患者出现与脑水肿有关的严重神经系统体征，应考虑静脉团注 10 mg 地塞米松。如果出现危及生命的神经系统体征，如脑疝征象，则应给予甘露醇和地塞米松，并请神经外科紧急会诊。应积极使用抗癫痫药物控制癫痫发作。非肝酶诱导类抗癫痫药物（如苯妥英）的安全性优于肝酶诱导类药物，而且较少与治疗肿瘤的其他药物（包括类固醇和化疗）发生相互作用，因此更受青睐。对于原发性或转移性脑肿瘤患者，一般不建议使用预防性抗癫痫药物。但黑色素瘤脑转移是一个例外，有多个幕上转移灶的患者，尤其是有出血的患者，癫痫发作的风险很高。

预后

胶质瘤的分级、功能状态和年龄是预后的重要预测因素。胶质母细胞瘤的预后最差，即使积极治疗，中位生存期也只有 1 年多。预后良好的患者可存活 2 年以上。国家监测、流行病学和终末结局（SEER）登记数据库显示，间变性星形细胞瘤和间变性少突胶质细胞瘤患者的总中位生存期分别为 15 个月和 42 个月。这项分析未统计 1p 和 19q 染色体缺失的情况，因此并未证明共缺失患者的生存率更高。低级别胶质瘤的中位生存期约为 5 年，但因年龄、肿瘤大小和切除范围不同而存在个体差异。使用分子标志物联合判定预后的准确性相对更高。

脑膜瘤的复发率取决于其级别，从 1 级的多于 25% 到 3 级的多于 90% 不等。复发的风险因素包括切除不彻底、肿瘤级别较高、年龄较小、特定亚型、脑部浸润和高增殖率。

与几十年前使用的全脑放疗相比，随着大剂量氨甲蝶呤治疗方案的引入，PCNSL 的中位生存期有所改善。中位生存期取决于各种临床因素，最重要的是年龄和功能状态，从 1 年到 8 年不等。老年患者（大于 70 岁）的情况最差。

功能状态、年龄、颅外肿瘤状况和脑转移灶的数量是脑转移瘤患者预后的预测因素。脑转移瘤患者的预后评估越来越个体化。随着新的靶向疗法的出现，驱动癌症的特定基因突变也成为判断预后的重要因素。接受全脑放疗的多发转移灶患者的中位生存期为 3～6 个月。与仅接受全脑放疗的患者（15 周）相比，颅外病变有限的单发脑转移瘤患者接受手术切除和全脑放疗的生存期明显提高（40 周）。重要的是，随着生存率的提高，患者功能独立时间进一步延长。

髓母细胞瘤的 5 年无进展生存率为 70%～85%。然而，超过 1/3 的患者会复发，而复发没有标准治疗方法。复发后的中位生存期通常不到 1 年。

分子标志物在原发性脑肿瘤（尤其是胶质瘤）诊断评估中的问世，极大改变了评估预后和治疗反应的方法。此外，多中心试验为胶质瘤不同亚组的最佳治疗提供了可靠信息，胶质瘤根据重要临床因素（如患者年龄、功能状态、手术切除程度以及分子标志物的纳入等）分为不同亚组。可以预见，根据这些因素分层设计的前瞻性试验将获得更多信息，以提供给临床医生更多的治疗决策建议。全身性癌症治疗的重大进步也为扩散至中枢神经系统的转移瘤提供了更多的治疗选择。

SUGGESTED READINGS

American Cancer Society: www.cancer.org. Accessed October 22, 2013.

Backer-Grøndahl T, Moen BH, Torp SH: The histopathological spectrum of human meningiomas, Int J Clin Exp Pathol 5:231–242, 2012.

Barnholtz-Sloan JS, Yu C, Sloan AE, et al: A nomogram for individualized estimation of survival among patients with brain metastasis, Neuro Oncol 14:910–918, 2012.

Buckner, et al: Radiation plus procarbazine, CCNU, and vincristine in low-grade-glioma, NEJM 374:1344–1355, 2016.

CBTRUS: Primary Brain and Central Nervous System Tumors Diagnosed in the United States in 2004–2007, Central Brain Tumor Registry of the United States statistical Report, 2011.

De Braganca KC, Packer RJ: Treatment options for medulloblastoma and CNS primitive neuroectodermal tumor (PNET), Curr Treat Options Neurol 15:593–606, 2013.

Nuño M, Birch K, Mukherjee D, et al: Survival and prognostic factors in anaplastic gliomas, Neurosurgery 73:458–465, 2013.

Olson JJ, Paleologos NA, Gaspar LE, et al: The role of emerging and investigational therapies for metastatic brain tumors: a systematic review and evidence-based clinical practice guideline of selected topics, J Neuro Oncol 96(1):115–142, 2010.

Patil CG, Pricola K, Sarmiento JM, et al: Whole brain radiation therapy (WBRT) alone versus WBRT and radiosurgery for the treatment of brain metastases, Cochrane Database Syst Rev 9:CD006121, 2012.

Rutkowski S, von Hoff K, Emser A, et al: Survival and prognostic factors of early childhood medulloblastoma: an international meta-analysis, J Clin Oncol 28:4961–4968, 2010.

Stupp R, Mason WP, van den Bent MJ, et al: Radiotherapy plus concomitant and adjuvant temozolomide for glioblastoma, N Engl J Med 352(10):987–996, 2005.

Tawbi, et al: Combined nivolumab and ipilimumab in melanoma metastatic to the brain, NEJM 379:722–730, 2018.

van den Bent MJ, Brandes AA, Taphoorn MJ, et al: Adjuvant procarbazine, lomustine, and vincristine chemotherapy in newly diagnosed anaplastic oligodendroglioma: long-term follow-up of EORTC brain tumor group study 26951, J Clin Oncol 31:344–350, 2013.

Wang Z, Bao Z, Yan W, et al: Isocitrate dehydrogenase 1 (IDH1) mutation-specific microRNA signature predicts favorable prognosis in glioblastoma patients with IDH1 wild type, J Exp Clin Cancer Res 32:59, 2013.

推荐阅读

American Cancer Society: www.cancer.org. Accessed October 22, 2013.

Backer-Grøndahl T, Moen BH, Torp SH: The histopathological spectrum of human meningiomas, Int J Clin Exp Pathol 5:231–242, 2012.

Barnholtz-Sloan JS, Yu C, Sloan AE, et al: A nomogram for individualized estimation of survival among patients with brain metastasis, Neuro Oncol 14:910–918, 2012.

Buckner, et al: Radiation plus procarbazine, CCNU, and vincristine in low-grade-glioma, NEJM 374:1344–1355, 2016.

CBTRUS: Primary Brain and Central Nervous System Tumors Diagnosed in the United States in 2004–2007, Central Brain Tumor Registry of the United States statistical Report, 2011.

De Braganca KC, Packer RJ: Treatment options for medulloblastoma and CNS primitive neuroectodermal tumor (PNET), Curr Treat Options Neurol 15:593–606, 2013.

Nuño M, Birch K, Mukherjee D, et al: Survival and prognostic factors in anaplastic gliomas, Neurosurgery 73:458–465, 2013.

Olson JJ, Paleologos NA, Gaspar LE, et al: The role of emerging and investigational therapies for metastatic brain tumors: a systematic review and evidence-based clinical practice guideline of selected topics, J Neuro Oncol 96(1):115–142, 2010.

Patil CG, Pricola K, Sarmiento JM, et al: Whole brain radiation therapy (WBRT) alone versus WBRT and radiosurgery for the treatment of brain metastases, Cochrane Database Syst Rev 9:CD006121, 2012.

Rutkowski S, von Hoff K, Emser A, et al: Survival and prognostic factors of early childhood medulloblastoma: an international meta-analysis, J Clin Oncol 28:4961–4968, 2010.

Stupp R, Mason WP, van den Bent MJ, et al: Radiotherapy plus concomitant and adjuvant temozolomide for glioblastoma, N Engl J Med 352(10):987–996, 2005.

Tawbi, et al: Combined nivolumab and ipilimumab in melanoma metastatic to the brain, NEJM 379:722–730, 2018.

van den Bent MJ, Brandes AA, Taphoorn MJ, et al: Adjuvant procarbazine, lomustine, and vincristine chemotherapy in newly diagnosed anaplastic oligodendroglioma: long-term follow-up of EORTC brain tumor group study 26951, J Clin Oncol 31:344–350, 2013.

Wang Z, Bao Z, Yan W, et al: Isocitrate dehydrogenase 1 (IDH1) mutation-specific microRNA signature predicts favorable prognosis in glioblastoma patients with IDH1 wild type, J Exp Clin Cancer Res 32:59, 2013.

Demyelinating and Inflammatory Disorders

Anne Haney Cross

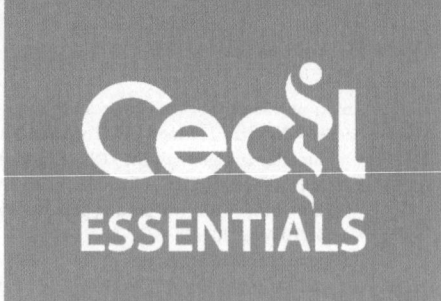

INTRODUCTION

In demyelinating CNS disorders, previously normal myelin is lost due to an acquired, typically inflammatory disease. The prototypic CNS demyelinating disorder is multiple sclerosis (MS). Other disorders of this type include neuromyelitis optica (NMO), acute disseminated encephalomyelitis (ADEM), acute transverse myelitis (TM), and optic neuritis (ON).

MULTIPLE SCLEROSIS

Definition/Epidemiology

Recent data indicate that MS affects between 600,000 and 900,000 people in the United States and over 2.3 million worldwide. Though presumed to be autoimmune, its exact etiology is still not fully understood. MS begins as a relapsing remitting disease in greater than 80% of patients and ultimately becomes progressive in greater than 50% of patients with untreated relapsing-remitting MS (RRMS). Progressive MS patients accumulate neurologic disability unassociated with relapses (although relapses may be superimposed). MS is more common in females, with the current female to male ratio in North America and in Europe estimated at 2:1 to 4:1. An exception is primary progressive MS (see Clinical Presentation), where the female to male ratio is 1:1.

MS is most common in persons of northern European ancestry. Recent genome-wide association studies indicate that many genes affect the risk of MS, although most confer only a small risk of disease (odds ratios less than 1.5). Alleles within the HLA-DR region (DRB1*15:01 > DRB1*13:03 > DRB1*03:01) are the most well established and confer the greatest risk with odds ratios between 1.5 and 4 for most populations of northern European ancestry.

Environmental factors can confer risk for MS, including modifiable factors such as low vitamin D blood level, high body mass index during adolescence/young adulthood, and smoking cigarettes. Seropositivity to the Epstein-Barr virus increases the risk of MS; a symptomatic case of infectious mononucleosis confers greater risk than seropositivity alone. Though relatively high at 1/1000 to 1/500, MS incidence appears to be relatively stable in North America, the United Kingdom, and Europe. Incidence of MS may be increasing in several regions where MS was not previously prevalent, such as Iran, Turkey, Sicily, and South Africa. These reports of increasing incidence may reflect a real increase, improved recognition, or both.

Pathology

Classically, MS causes demyelinating CNS white matter lesions with relative sparing of axons. The most common pathology of active lesions in white matter is perivascular mononuclear cell infiltration (monocyte/macrophages, lymphocytes), with a variable presence of antibody and activated complement. Acutely active white matter lesions display blood-brain barrier breakdown, manifest on MRI by gadolinium enhancement. Despite its categorization as a "white matter disease," gray matter is also damaged in MS. Gray matter MS lesions have been under-recognized because they are difficult to see by MRI and are often not appreciated pathologically without special stains. Such gray matter lesions may occur in the deep gray structures such as the thalamus and in the cerebral cortex. Cortical gray matter lesions can be subpial, extend into cortex from underlying white matter (leukocortical), or wholly within the cortex (intracortical). Cortical lesions are characterized by activated microglia and relatively fewer infiltrating lymphocytes and macrophages than white matter MS lesions. Ectopic lymphoid tissue containing components of secondary lymphoid tissues (B cells, follicular helper T cells, dendritic cells, CXCL13) has been observed in meninges of people with MS, especially those with progressive MS, and is associated with poor prognosis.

Clinical Presentation

MS may manifest with a variety of symptoms and signs. Common presentations include: optic neuritis, diplopia (often caused by internuclear ophthalmoplegia due to a propensity of MS to affect the medial longitudinal fasciculus), other brain stem syndromes, partial transverse myelitis, sensory disturbances, and weakness. Less frequent presentations include seizures, cognitive problems, bladder control problems, and pain. Pain in MS is often of a burning, tingling, or electrical nature. Clinically isolated syndrome (CIS) refers to a single attack that is likely due to CNS demyelination. CIS may be acute or subacute in onset and may involve a single or more than one CNS region. CIS presentations may look identical to MS attacks, but a formal diagnosis of MS cannot be made without dissemination of lesions in space and time. New MS diagnostic criteria allow positive spinal fluid findings (CSF-restricted oligoclonal bands) to substitute for dissemination in time. Ultimately, most CIS patients with typical demyelinating syndromes develop MS. In one study, over 85% of CIS patients with even one silent abnormality on brain or spinal cord magnetic resonance imaging (MRI) eventually developed clinically definite MS.

Three main clinical subtypes of MS are defined based on clinical course: relapsing remitting, secondary progressive, and primary progressive. RRMS is characterized by clinical stability between individual attacks from which the person may or may not fully recover. Secondary progressive MS (SPMS) patients have gradual neurologic deterioration and may also have superimposed attacks ("active" SPMS). Secondary progressive MS develops following an initial relapsing-remitting course in a substantial proportion of individuals with RRMS. This proportion may be declining with the advent of disease-modifying therapies.

脱髓鞘性和炎症性疾病

朱亚辉 译 王婷婷 赵一龙 审校 王伊龙 通审

引言

在中枢神经系统脱髓鞘疾病中，先前正常的髓鞘由于获得性疾病（通常为炎症性疾病）而脱失。典型的中枢神经系统脱髓鞘疾病是多发性硬化（MS）。其他同类型疾病包括视神经脊髓炎（NMO）、急性播散性脑脊髓炎（ADEM）、急性横贯性脊髓炎（TM）和视神经炎（ON）。

多发性硬化（MS）

定义和流行病学

最新数据显示，MS 在美国的患病人数为 60 万至 90 万，全世界的患病人数超过 230 万。虽然推测 MS 是自身免疫性疾病，但其确切病因尚未完全明确。80% 以上的 MS 患者最初表现为复发-缓解病程，而 50% 以上未经治疗的复发-缓解型 MS（RRMS）患者最终发展成为进展型。进展型 MS 患者累积的神经系统残疾与复发无关（尽管复发可能会叠加）。MS 在女性中更为常见，目前在北美和欧洲，女性与男性患者的比例约为 2∶1 至 4∶1。原发进展型 MS 例外（见临床表现），其男/女患者比例为 1∶1。

MS 在北欧裔的人群中最为常见。最近的全基因组关联研究表明，许多基因会影响 MS 的患病风险，尽管大多数基因只带来很小的患病风险[比值比（OR）< 1.5]。HLA-DR 的等位基因（DRB1*15∶01 > DRB1*13∶03 > DRB1*03∶01）最为确定，为大多数北欧裔人群带来最大的患病风险，OR 值为 1.5～4。

环境因素可以增加罹患 MS 的风险，包括可改变的因素，如血液中维生素 D 水平低、青春期/青年期体重指数高，以及吸烟。EB 病毒血清阳性会增加罹患 MS 的风险，有症状的传染性单核细胞增多症比单纯的血清阳性风险更大。虽然 MS 的发病率相对较高，为 1/1000～1/500，但在北美、英国和欧洲似乎相对稳定。在伊朗、土耳其、西西里和南非等以前 MS 并不流行的地区，MS 的发病率可能正在上升。这些报告可能反映了实际发病率的增高，或对疾病识别能力的提高，或者两者兼而有之。

病理学

MS 通常会导致中枢神经系统白质脱髓鞘病变，轴突则相对保留。活动性白质病变最常见的病理变化是血管周围单核细胞浸润（单核细胞/巨噬细胞、淋巴细胞），并伴有不同水平的抗体及活化补体。急性活动性白质病变表现为血脑屏障破坏，在磁共振成像（MRI）上表现为钆增强。尽管 MS 被归类为"白质疾病"，但灰质也会受累。MS 的灰质病变一直未被充分认识，因为 MRI 上很难看到这些病灶，而且如果没有特殊的染色方法，病理上也难以鉴别。这种灰质病变可累及丘脑等深部灰质结构和大脑皮质。皮质灰质病变可能发生在皮质下，从皮质下白质延伸到皮质（白质-皮质病变），或者完全在皮质内（皮质内病变）。皮质病变的特点是小胶质细胞活化，与 MS 白质病变相比，其浸润的淋巴细胞和巨噬细胞相对较少。在 MS 患者，特别是进展型 MS 患者的脑膜中可见含有继发性淋巴组织成分（B 细胞、滤泡辅助性 T 细胞、树突状细胞、CXCL13）的异位淋巴组织，其与预后不良有关。

临床表现

MS 的临床症状和体征多种多样，常见的临床表现包括：视神经炎、复视（通常由于 MS 易累及内侧纵束而导致的核间性眼肌麻痹引起）、其他脑干综合征、部分横贯性脊髓炎、感觉障碍和无力。不常见的临床表现包括癫痫发作、认知障碍、膀胱控制功能障碍和疼痛。MS 的疼痛通常表现为烧灼感、刺痛或电击感。临床孤立综合征（CIS）是指可能由中枢神经系统脱髓鞘引起的单次发作，临床上可表现为急性或亚急性起病，累及单个或多个中枢神经系统区域。CIS 的临床表现可能与 MS 发作相同，但如果病变没有表现出空间和时间多发性，就不能正式诊断为 MS。新的 MS 诊断标准允许用脊髓液阳性结果（脑脊液寡克隆带）来替代时间多发性。最终，大多数具有典型脱髓鞘综合征的 CIS 患者都会发展为 MS。一项研究表明，超过 85% 的 CIS 患者即使在脑或脊髓 MRI 上仅有一个无症状性病灶，最终也会发展为临床确诊的 MS。

根据临床病程，MS 可分为三大临床亚型：复发-缓解型、继发进展型和原发进展型。复发-缓解型 MS（RRMS）的临床特征是发作间期症状稳定，伴完全或不完全缓解。继发进展型 MS（SPMS）患者的神经系统功能逐渐恶化，也可能出现叠加发作（"活动性"SPMS）。相当一部分复发-缓解型 MS 患者在最初的复发-缓解病程后发展为继发进展型 MS。随着疾病修饰治疗的出现，

TABLE 17.1 The 2017 Revised McDonald Criteria

Clinical[a]	Lesions With Objective Clinical Evidence	Additional Data Needed for MS Diagnosis
≥2 attacks	≥2	None
≥2 attacks	1 lesion, plus clear cut historical evidence of a prior attack in a different anatomic location	None
≥2 attacks	1	DIS demonstrated by an additional clinical attack implicating a different anatomic location, or >1 new T2w lesion in at least one other region typical of MS (periventricular, cortical or juxtacortical, brain stem/cerebellar, spinal cord)
1 attack	≥2 lesions	DIT demonstrated by a 2nd clinical attack, or new T2w and/or gad+ lesion on follow-up MRI, or simultaneous presence of gad+ and nonenhancing lesion on MRI at any time, or positive cerebrospinal fluid findings (oligoclonal bands restricted to CSF)
1 attack	1 lesion (CIS)	DIS demonstrated by a 2nd clinical attack implicating a different CNS region, or ≥1 new T2w lesion in MS-typical region of CNS; DIT demonstrated by a 2nd clinical attack plus either new T2w MRI lesion *or* CSF-restricted oligoclonal bands
Gradual neurologic progression suggestive of MS (PPMS)	1 year or more of disease progression plus two of three of following criteria: evidence for DIS in the brain based on ≥1 T2w lesions characteristic of MS, evidence of DIS in the spinal cord based on ≥2 T2w cord lesions, positive CSF (elevated IgG index or oligoclonal bands not present in serum)	

[a]These criteria were developed in Caucasian adults aged 18 to 50 years with CIS presentations typical of CNS inflammatory demyelinating disease. Care should be taken when applying these criteria to persons not fitting this description. Alternative diagnoses that might better explain the disorder must always be considered and reasonably excluded.
DIS, Dissemination in space; *DIT,* dissemination in time.
Modified from Thompson AJ, Banwell BL, Barkhof F, et al: Diagnosis of multiple sclerosis: 2017 revisions of the McDonald Criteria, Lancet Neurol 17:162–173, 2018.

About 10% of MS patients have primary progressive MS (PPMS), which from onset is characterized by gradual downhill progression without any clinical attacks. The International Advisory Committee on Clinical Trials of MS has proposed additional clinical descriptors that include disease activity (based on relapse rate and new imaging findings) and progression over the prior year.

Diagnosis

The diagnosis of MS requires dissemination of CNS disease in time and in space, and no other disease should provide a better explanation. MRI, spinal fluid analyses, evoked potentials (EPs) and ocular coherence tomography (OCT) are tools that may aid in the diagnosis. The latest McDonald criteria (Table 17.1) allow CSF-restricted oligoclonal bands to substitute for dissemination in time in the diagnosis of MS in the setting of a CIS typical of demyelination. The new diagnostic criteria allow more rapid diagnosis of MS and earlier treatment.

MRI

The finding of classic imaging features on brain and spinal cord MRI greatly aids the certainty of diagnosis. MS lesions are characterized by increased intensity on T2-weighted (T2w) and T2-FLAIR (fluid attenuated inversion recovery) images (Fig. 17.1A). Lesions are usually ovoid and often localize to the periventricular or juxtacortical regions, the corpus callosum, the brain stem, and the cervical spinal cord. On sagittal images, lesions in the corpus callosum are usually flame-shaped (Fig 17.1C). On T1w images, MS lesions may be isointense or hypointense. T1w hypointensity in a chronic inactive lesion denotes underlying tissue damage, including axonal loss (Fig. 17.1D). Enhancement of lesions following administration of gadolinium containing contrast agents indicates blood-brain barrier breakdown; such a lesion is considered to be active (Fig. 17.1B). Enhancing lesions are also often T1w hypointense, but this hypointensity resolves more than 50% of the time. A ring pattern (often an incomplete ring) of enhancement is common. Most enhancing MS lesions display no mass effect. Occasional "tumefactive" MS lesions are difficult to distinguish from tumors and may require biopsy.

Spinal Fluid Analysis

Evidence of increased intrathecal immunoglobulin synthesis is present in more than 90% of people with MS. Elevated concentrations of CSF IgG and IgM, CSF-restricted oligoclonal bands of immunoglobulin (Fig. 17.2), and a high intrathecal IgG synthesis rate are seen. The IgG index, which is derived from the ratio of CSF to serum IgG and takes BBB integrity into account, is elevated in MS. A mild lymphocytic pleocytosis is frequently seen in CSF during MS relapses.

Evoked Potentials

EPs detected by surface electrode recording were used in the past to detect subclinical demyelination in the brain stem (auditory EPs), spinal cord (somatosensory EPs), and optic nerves (visual EPs). The advent of high-resolution MRI has led to far less use of EPs to aid MS diagnosis.

Optical Coherence Tomography

OCT is a safe and rapid means to image the retina and detect evidence of prior optic neuritis. OCT uses infrared light to measure thickness of the retinal nerve fiber layer (RNFL), which contains axons that form the optic nerve. A thinned temporal region of the RNFL can be used as evidence of prior subclinical optic neuritis.

Differential Diagnosis

The diagnosis of MS requires the exclusion of diseases that might better explain the clinical scenario. The differential diagnosis of MS is broad (Table 17.2). Some diseases that can mimic MS have relapses and others display progressive courses. "Red flags" that are atypical for MS, such as systemic (arthritis, rash, mouth or genital sores, or pulmonary) symptoms, bilateral hearing loss, peripheral neuropathy, or

表 17.1　2017 年修订的 McDonald 标准

临床表现[a]	有客观临床证据的病灶	多发性硬化诊断所需的附加数据
≥2 次临床发作	≥2 个病灶	无
≥2 次临床发作	1 个病灶，并有既往发作累及不同解剖部位的明确病史证据	无
≥2 次临床发作	1 个病灶	空间多发性（DIS）：累及不同解剖部位的再次临床发作，或者 MS 典型病灶区域（脑室周围、皮质或皮质旁、脑干/小脑、脊髓）中至少 2 个区域有≥1 个新发 T2w 病灶
1 次临床发作	≥2 个病灶	时间多发性（DIT）：再次临床发作，或者随访 MRI 检查有新发 T2w 病灶和（或）钆增强病灶，或者任何时间 MRI 检查同时出现钆增强和非增强病灶，或者脑脊液检查结果阳性（脑脊液寡克隆带）
1 次临床发作	1 个病灶（CIS）	空间多发性（DIS）：累及不同中枢神经系统区域的再次临床发作，或者中枢神经系统 MS 典型病灶区域出现≥1 个新发 T2w 病变；时间多发性（DIT）：再次临床发作，且 T2w MRI 上有新发病灶或脑脊液寡克隆带阳性
原发进展型 MS	疾病进展至少 1 年，并符合以下 3 项标准中的 2 项：脑内≥1 个符合典型 MS 特征的 T2w 病灶证明空间多发性（DIS），脊髓≥2 个 T2w 病灶证明空间多发性（DIS），脑脊液阳性结果（血清中未出现 IgG 指数升高或寡克隆带）	

[a] 此标准适应于 18～50 岁、具有 CIS 典型中枢神经系统炎性脱髓鞘疾病表现的白种人群，应谨慎应用于其他人群。使用该标准时，须始终考虑并合理排除可能更好解释该病的其他诊断。
CIS，临床孤立综合征。
改编自 Thompson AJ, Banwell BL, Barkhof F, et al: Diagnosis of multiple sclerosis: 2017 revisions of the McDonald Criteria, Lancet Neurol 17: 162-173, 2018.

这一比例可能会下降。约 10% 的 MS 患者是原发进展型 MS（PPMS），其特点是自发病以来病情逐渐恶化，且无临床发作。国际 MS 临床试验咨询委员会提出更多的临床描述指标，包括疾病活动性（基于复发率和新的影像学检查结果）和上一年的疾病进展。

诊断

MS 的诊断需要中枢神经系统疾病具有时间和空间多发性，且没有其他疾病能提供更好的解释。MRI、脊髓液分析、诱发电位（EP）和光学相干断层扫描（OCT）可用于协助诊断。最新的 McDonald 诊断标准（表 17.1）允许在出现具有典型脱髓鞘表现的 CIS 时，用脑脊液寡克隆带检查结果替代时间多发性来诊断 MS。新的诊断标准使 MS 的诊断更加迅速，治疗更加及时。

磁共振成像

脑和脊髓 MRI 检查有典型的影像学特征可极大提高诊断的确定性。MS 的病灶特征是 T2 加权（T2w）和 T2- 液体衰减反转恢复（FLAIR）图像高信号（图 17.1A）。病灶通常呈卵圆形，常位于脑室周围或皮质旁区、胼胝体、脑干和颈髓。矢状位时，胼胝体的病灶通常呈火焰状（图 17.1C）。在 T1w 图像上，MS 病灶可能表现为等信号或低信号。慢性非活动性病灶在 T1w 上呈低信号提示潜在的组织损伤，包括轴索缺失（图 17.1D）。钆增强病灶提示血脑屏障破坏，通常认为是活动性病灶（图 17.1B），其在 T1w 上呈低信号，但这种低信号 50% 以上可能会消退。环状（通常是不完全环状）强化较常见。多数增强的 MS 病灶没有占位效应，偶尔出现"肿瘤样"MS 病灶难以与肿瘤区分，可能需要活检以明确诊断。

脑脊液分析

90% 以上的 MS 患者被证实鞘内免疫球蛋白合成增加，包括脑脊液 IgG 和 IgM 水平升高、脑脊液免疫球蛋白寡克隆带阳性（图 17.2）以及鞘内 IgG 合成率增高。MS 患者的 IgG 指数也会升高，该指数由脑脊液与血清 IgG 的比值得出，可能与血脑屏障（BBB）的完整性有关。MS 复发时，经常出现脑脊液中轻度淋巴细胞增多。

诱发电位

既往通过表面电极检测到的诱发电位（EP）可用于检测脑干（听觉 EP）、脊髓（躯体感觉 EP）和视神经（视觉 EP）的亚临床脱髓鞘情况。随着高分辨率 MRI 的出现，EP 在 MS 诊断中的应用已大大减少。

光学相干断层成像

光学相干断层成像（OCT）是一种安全、快速的视网膜成像方法，能检测出既往视神经炎的证据。OCT 利用红外线测量视网膜神经纤维层（RNFL）的厚度，其包含构成视神经的轴突。RNFL 的颞部变薄可作为既往罹患亚临床视神经炎的证据。

鉴别诊断

MS 的诊断需要排除能更好解释其临床症状的其他疾病。MS 的鉴别诊断范围较广（表 17.2）。一些拟似 MS 的疾病会表现为复发和进展性病程。"红旗征"是 MS 的非典型症状，包括全身性症状（关节炎、皮疹、

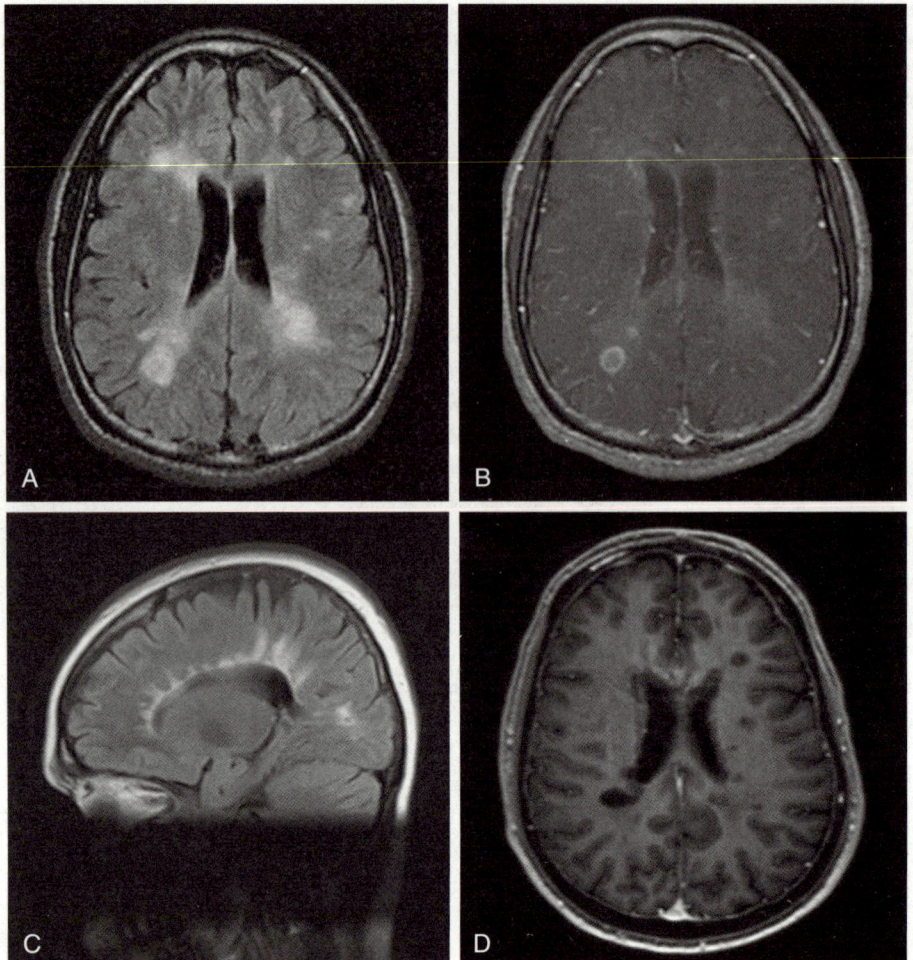

Fig. 17.1 (A) Axial fluid-attenuated inversion recovery (FLAIR) image of the brain from a person with MS revealing classical periventricular and deep white matter high-signal intensity lesions. (B) Axial T1-weighted image following gadolinium contrast administration in the same patient as A. Enhancing lesions after gadolinium contrast administration, indicating loss of integrity of the blood-brain barrier that is seen with active MS lesions. One enhancing lesion in the right parietal region is ring enhancing. (C) Sagittal FLAIR image of the brain of a person with MS demonstrating classical flame-shaped pericallosal lesions radiating outward from the ventricle. (D) Axial T1-weighted image showing areas of T1 low signal intensity ("black holes").

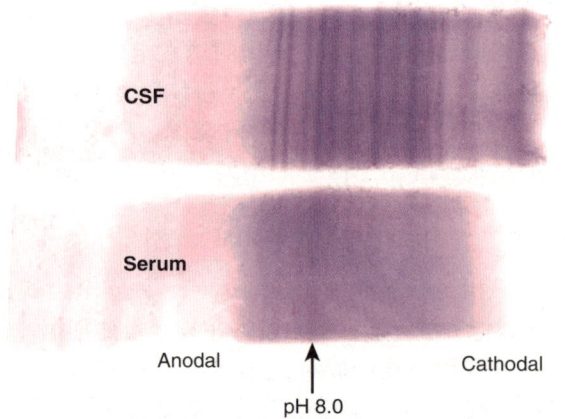

Fig. 17.2 Isoelectric focusing gel of cerebrospinal fluid (CSF) and serum of a patient with multiple sclerosis. The CSF *(upper lane)* shows oligoclonal bands cathodal to the pH 8.0, which are not seen in the serum *(lower lane)*.

atypical age of onset (early childhood or after age 50) should lead the clinician to seek further support for the diagnosis of MS.

Prognosis of Multiple Sclerosis

MS is highly variable. It is occasionally "benign," in which case the disease has little impact on quality of life. It can also be severe with considerable disability or early death. Most people with MS fall in between these extremes. It is currently not possible to predict the future course of MS in an individual patient with full accuracy. Poor prognostic indicators at onset of MS include primary progressive course, male gender, frequent attacks, prominent motor or cerebellar findings, and high initial MRI lesion burden. Expected lifespan of people with MS is reduced overall by 7 to 14 years. Suicide rate is 1.7 to 7.5 times that of the general population. The use of disease modifying therapies likely improves not only relapse rate but also long-term disability and even mortality. In one non-randomized study, early initiation of disease modifying therapies within a year of symptom onset was associated with better long-term outcomes.

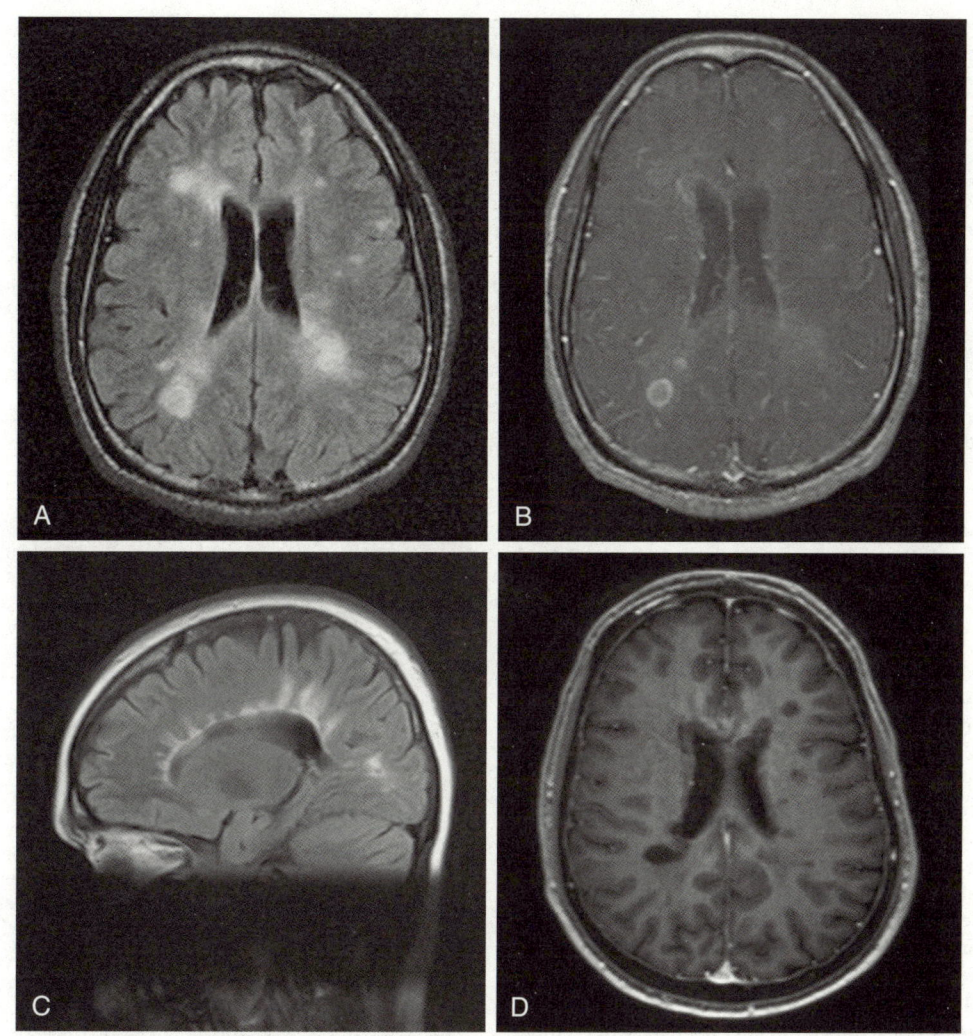

图 17.1 （A）一位 MS 患者的大脑轴位 FLAIR 图像，显示典型的脑室周围和深部白质高信号病灶。（B）同一患者的钆增强后轴位 T1 加权图像。病灶在使用钆造影剂后强化，提示血脑屏障完整性缺失，见于活动性 MS 病灶。右侧顶叶区域病灶呈环形强化。（C）一位 MS 患者的大脑矢状位 FLAIR 图像，显示典型的胼胝体周围火焰状病灶，由脑室向外放射。（D）轴位 T1 加权图像，病灶在 T1 上呈低信号（"黑洞征"）

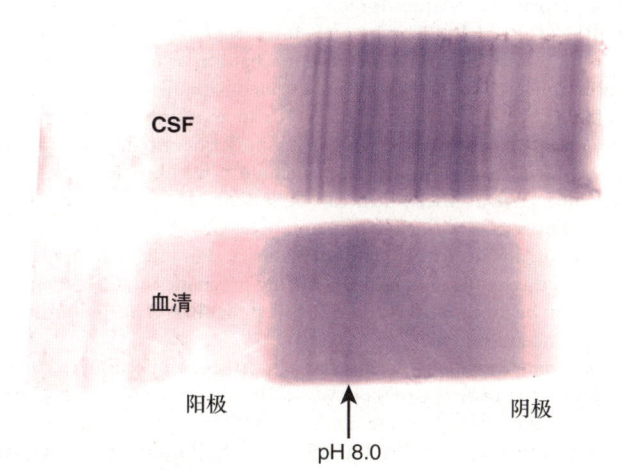

图 17.2　多发性硬化患者脑脊液（CSF）和血清的等电聚焦凝胶。脑脊液（上泳道）显示阴极至 pH 8.0 间的寡克隆带，此寡克隆带在血清（下泳道）中未见

口腔或生殖器溃疡、肺部症状）、双侧听力丧失、周围神经病或非典型发病年龄（儿童早期或 50 岁以后），应引导临床医生进一步寻求支持 MS 诊断的证据。

多发性硬化的预后

MS 具有高度异质性。其可为"良性"，对患者的生活质量影响较小，也可较严重，导致重度残疾或早期死亡。大多数 MS 患者介于两种极端情况之间。目前尚无法准确预测每位 MS 患者的未来病程进展。MS 发病时的不良预后指标包括：原发进展型病程、男性、频繁发作、运动或小脑症状突出、初始 MRI 病灶负荷高。MS 患者的预期寿命会缩短 7～14 年，自杀率是普通人群的 1.7～7.5 倍。应用疾病修饰治疗不仅能降低复发率，还能改善长期残疾情况，甚至降低死亡率。一项非随机研究结果提示，症状出现一年内尽早使用疾病修饰治疗与较好的长期预后有关。

TABLE 17.2 Differential Diagnosis of Demyelinating Diseases

Disease Category[a]	Examples of Disorders[b]
Immune-mediated/autoimmune	Multiple sclerosis, neuromyelitis optica (NMO), anti-MOG disorder, acute demyelinating encephalomyelitis (ADEM), idiopathic optic neuritis, CRION, idiopathic transverse myelitis, Behçet's disease
Infectious	Progressive multifocal leukoencephalopathy (PML), HTLV-I, HIV, CNS abscess, Lyme disease, Whipple disease, neurosyphilis
Metabolic	Vitamin B_{12}, vitamin E or copper deficiency, central pontine and extrapontine myelinolysis
Neurodegenerative	Spinocerebellar ataxias, spine disease (e.g., compressive cervical spondylopathy, central canal stenosis)
Rheumatologic	Sarcoidosis, systemic lupus erythematosus, antiphospholipid antibody syndrome, Sjögren's syndrome
Genetic disorders	Adrenoleukodystrophy/adrenomyeloneuropathy, hereditary spastic paraparesis, CADASIL (a hereditary stroke disorder), Leber optic neuropathy, Perlizeus-Merzbacher, Wilson's disease
Neoplastic/paraneoplastic	CNS lymphoma, meningeal carcinomatosis, paraneoplastic CRMP-5 IgG, anti-amphiphysin-1 Abs
Vascular	CNS vasculitis (e.g., giant cell arteritis, primary CNS vasculitis), spinal dural fistula, Susac syndrome
Iatrogenic	TNF inhibitors, CNS irradiation, immune checkpoint inhibitors

[a]Several of the disorders listed could be placed in more than one category.
[b]This list is not comprehensive.

 For a deeper discussion of these topics, please see Chapter 383, "Multiple Sclerosis and Demyelinating Conditions of the Central Nervous System," in *Goldman-Cecil Medicine*, 26th Edition.

Treatment

MS treatment can be divided into three categories: treatment of symptoms (e.g., spasticity, fatigue, or depression), treatment of acute relapses, and disease modifying therapies. The following discussion will be limited to the latter two categories. However, Table 17.3 lists some frequent MS symptoms and their therapies.

Relapses that alter function or cause severe pain are usually treated with corticosteroids. Severe relapses are often managed with high-dose corticosteroids, such as intravenous methylprednisolone at 500 to 1000 mg daily for 3 to 5 days, followed by a short oral taper. Lower dosed corticosteroid courses may be used for mild relapses. Blood pressure, serum electrolytes and glucose, and patient mood should be monitored during corticosteroid therapy. Based on the multicenter Optic Neuritis Treatment Trial (ONTT), this regimen will lead to more rapid recovery from the attack but is unlikely to alter the degree of eventual recovery.

For severe relapses that do not respond to high-dose IV corticosteroids, a small randomized study showed that plasma exchange can be effective. Rapid functional improvement in over 40% of patients occurred with early initiation of plasma exchange. Subjects in this trial likely included patients with NMO and ADEM, in addition to MS.

MS is one of only a handful of chronic neurologic disorders with effective disease modifying therapies. The beta-interferons (BIFNs) and glatiramer acetate (GA) are US Food and Drug Administration (FDA)-approved for the treatment of patients with relapsing forms of MS to decrease the frequency of clinical exacerbations and delay the accumulation of physical disability. The BIFNs and GA all reduced annualized relapse rate by about 30% in early pivotal studies. Most have been shown in randomized trials to delay progression to definite MS in those with CIS who are at high risk for developing MS.

As of mid-2020, 19 different disease modifying therapies, plus several generics versions of these, with 10 different mechanisms of action are available for MS (Table 17.4). The approved agents have distinct risk profiles. As there are currently no biomarkers that direct the choice of disease modifying therapies for an individual patient, selection of the disease modifying therapy for an individual is based on disease course and severity, comorbidities, and patient preferences.

Five BIFNs are approved for use in relapsing MS and CIS in the United States. They differ in dosage, mode of administration, side

TABLE 17.3 Selected MS Symptoms and Their Management

Symptom/Sign	Treatment(s)
Stiffness/cramps/spasms/spasticity	Baclofen, tizanidine
Fatigue	Amantadine, modafinil, armodafinil
Depression	Selective serotonin reuptake inhibitors, cognitive behavioral therapy
Pain/paresthesias/trigeminal neuralgia	Gabapentin, carbamazepine, oxcarbazepine, pregabalin, amitriptyline
Gait impairment	Fampridine SR
Nystagmus, with visual impairment	Gabapentin
Dizziness/vertigo	Meclizine, dimenhydrinate, benzodiazepines
Urinary urgency/incontinence/neurogenic bladder	Mirabegron, oxybutynin, tolterodine, other anticholinergics, BOTOX injection
Impotence/erectile dysfunction	Sildenafil, tadalafil, testosterone supplementation if low
Tonic spasms	Phenytoin, carbamazepine

effects, and incidence of neutralizing antibody induction. Three are identical to human BIFN-1a. Polyethylene glycol has been covalently attached to one of the three for longer duration of effect. The other two are BIFN-1b, which differs by one amino acid from BIFN-1a. BIFNs are immunomodulators whose exact mechanism of action in MS is not fully established. BIFN therapy is associated with increased circulating soluble VCAM-1, and increased IL-10, an immunoregulatory cytokine. Hepatic transaminases and CBC should be monitored in those taking BIFNs. Common side effects include a "flu-like" feeling for several hours after a dose, which can be lessened by nonsteroidal anti-inflammatory medications or acetaminophen. BIFNs are administered by injection and, as with any injectable drug, skin infection can occur. Although the risk of taking BIFNs during pregnancy and lactation are thought to be minimal, it is recommended that BIFNs be discontinued before conception.

Glatiramer acetate is given as a subcutaneous injection at 20 mg per day or 40 mg three times per week. This drug is a random polymer of four amino acids that are abundant within myelin basic protein, a major protein in CNS myelin. It is considered immunomodulatory not immunosuppressive, although its mechanism of action is not

表 17.2 脱髓鞘疾病的鉴别诊断

疾病类型[a]	疾病举例[b]
免疫介导/自身免疫性	多发性硬化、视神经脊髓炎（NMO）、抗 MOG 抗体病、急性播散性脑脊髓炎（ADEM）、特发性视神经炎、慢性复发性炎症性视神经病变（CRION）、特发性横贯性脊髓炎、白塞病
感染性	进行性多灶性白质脑病（PML）、HTLV-1、HIV、中枢神经系统脓肿、莱姆病、Whipple 病、神经梅毒
代谢性	维生素 B_{12}、维生素 E 或铜缺乏症，脑桥中央和脑桥外髓鞘溶解症
神经退行性	脊髓小脑性共济失调、脊柱疾病（如压迫性颈椎病、中央管狭窄）
风湿性	结节病、系统性红斑狼疮、抗磷脂抗体综合征、干燥综合征
遗传性疾病	肾上腺脑白质营养不良／肾上腺脊髓神经病、遗传性痉挛性截瘫、CADASIL（遗传性卒中疾病）、Leber 视神经病变、佩梅病、Wilson 病
肿瘤/副肿瘤	中枢神经系统淋巴瘤、脑膜癌病、副肿瘤性 CRMP-5 IgG、抗 amphiphysin-1 抗体
血管性	中枢神经系统血管炎（如巨细胞动脉炎、原发性中枢神经系统血管炎）、脊髓硬脊膜瘘、Susac 综合征
医源性	TNF 抑制剂、中枢神经系统辐射、免疫检查点抑制剂

HIV，人类免疫缺陷病毒；HTLV-1，人类嗜 T 淋巴细胞病毒 -1；MOG，髓鞘少突胶质细胞糖蛋白。
[a] 此表列出的一些疾病可以归入多种疾病类型。
[b] 此列表并不全面。

❖ 有关此专题的深入讨论，请参阅 Goldman-Cecil Medicine 第 26 版第 383 章"多发性硬化和中枢神经系统脱髓鞘疾病"。

治疗

MS 的治疗可分为三类：对症治疗（如痉挛、疲劳或抑郁）、急性复发治疗和疾病修饰治疗。下文的讨论将仅限于后两类。表 17.3 列出了常见的 MS 症状及其治疗方法。

通常使用皮质类固醇治疗引起功能改变或剧烈疼痛的复发。严重的复发通常需要使用大剂量皮质类固醇，如静脉注射甲泼尼龙 500～1000 mg/d，持续 3～5 天，续贯短期口服药物治疗并逐渐减停。较轻的复发可使用较小剂量的皮质类固醇。在皮质类固醇治疗期间，应监测血压、血清电解质和血糖，以及患者的情绪。基于多中心视神经炎治疗试验（ONTT）的结果，该治疗方案可以更快地让患者从发作中恢复，但不太可能改变其最终的康复程度。

一项小型随机研究显示，对于大剂量静脉注射皮质固醇无效的严重复发患者，血浆置换可能有效。超过 40% 的患者早期开始血浆置换后功能迅速改善。该试验的受试者除 MS 患者外，可能还包括 NMO 和 ADEM 患者。

MS 是仅有的几种对疾病修饰治疗有效的慢性神经系统疾病之一。β- 干扰素（BIFN）和醋酸格拉默（GA）是美国食品和药物管理局（FDA）批准用于治疗复发型 MS 患者的药物，可降低临床症状恶化的频率，并延缓身体残疾。在早期的关键性研究中，BIFN 和 GA 均可将年复发率降低约 30%。在随机试验中，大多数药物能延缓高危 CIS 患者进展为明确的 MS。

截至 2020 年中期，加上几种仿制药，MS 已有 19 种不同的疾病修饰治疗方法，共有 10 种不同的作用机制（表 17.4）。已批准的药物具有不同的风险特征。由于目前还没有生物标志物来指导患者选择个体化的疾病修饰治疗方法，因此个体化治疗选择需要依据病程和严重程度、合并症以及患者的个人倾向。

在美国，有五种 BIFN 批准用于复发型 MS 和 CIS。其在剂量、给药方式、副作用和诱导中和抗体的发生率

表 17.3 部分多发性硬化的症状及其管理

症状和体征	治疗
僵硬、抽筋、痉挛及痉挛状态	巴氯芬、替扎尼定
疲劳	金刚烷胺、莫达非尼、阿莫非尼
抑郁	选择性 5- 羟色胺再摄取抑制剂、认知行为疗法
疼痛、感觉异常、三叉神经痛	加巴喷丁、卡马西平、奥卡西平、普瑞巴林、阿米替林
步态障碍	氨吡啶 -SR
眼球震颤，伴有视力障碍	加巴喷丁
头晕、眩晕	美克洛嗪、茶苯海明、苯二氮䓬类药物
尿急、尿失禁、神经源性膀胱	米拉贝隆、奥昔布宁、托特罗定、其他抗胆碱能药、保妥适（BOTOX）注射剂
阳痿、勃起功能障碍	西地那非、他达拉非、睾酮低时补充睾酮
强直性痉挛	苯妥英、卡马西平

方面各不相同。其中三种与人类 BIFN-1a 相同。聚乙二醇被共价连接到这三种药物中的一种，以延长药效持续时间。另外两种是 BIFN-1b，与 BIFN-1a 只有一个氨基酸的差别。BIFN 是一种免疫调节剂，其在 MS 中的作用机制尚未完全明确。BIFN 治疗机制与提高血液循环中可溶性 VCAM-1 和免疫调节细胞因子 IL-10 的水平有关。使用 BIFN 治疗时应监测肝转氨酶和全血细胞计数。其常见的副作用包括用药后数小时内有"流感样"感觉，服用非甾体抗炎药或对乙酰氨基酚可减轻这种感觉。BIFN 通过注射给药，与其他注射药物一样，可能会发生皮肤感染。虽然在怀孕和哺乳期间应用 BIFN 的风险极小，但仍建议在怀孕前停用 BIFN。

醋酸格拉默需每天皮下注射 20 mg，或每周注射 3 次，每次 40 mg。该药物是髓鞘碱性蛋白（中枢神经系统髓鞘的主要组成蛋白）中含量丰富的四个氨基酸的随机聚合物。虽然其作用机制尚未完全清楚，但被认为是免疫调节剂而非免疫抑制剂。醋酸格拉默没有已知的药物相互作用，无须进行实验室监测。其副作用

TABLE 17.4 Disease Modifying Medications for MS

Drug (Brand Name), Dosing	Approved	MS Indication	Mechanism of Action
Interferon-β-1b (Betaseron, Extavia), 250 μg SQ qod	1993, 2009	RRMS, CIS	Inhibits "pro-inflammatory" cytokines, such as interferon (IFN)-γ, tumor necrosis factor-α, and lymphotoxin. Increases IL-10. Adhesion molecule and class II MHC induction reduced.
Interferon-β-1a (Avonex) 30 μg IM weekly	1996	RRMS, CIS	
Interferon-β-1a (Rebif) 22 or 44 μg SQ 3×/wk	2002	RRMS	
Interferon-β-1a (Plegridy) 125 μg SQ every 14 days	2014	Relapsing forms of MS	
Glatiramer acetate (Copaxone) 20 mg SQ daily, or 40 mg SQ 3×/wk	1996, 2014	RRMS, CIS	Alters T cell cytokine profile toward that of Th2 immunomodulatory cells
Mitoxantrone (Novantrone) 12 mg/m² IV q 3 months	2000	Worsening RRMS, relapsing SPMS, PRMS	Anthracenedione chemotherapeutic agent
Natalizumab (Tysabri) 300 mg IV q 4 weeks	2004/2006 (removed briefly from market)	Relapsing forms of MS	Monoclonal antibody targeting the alpha-4-integrins, part of the VLA-4 adhesion molecule
Fingolimod (Gilenya) 0.5 mg po daily	2010	Relapsing MS, including children	Modulates sphingosine1-phosphate receptors 1,3,4, and 5; lymphocytes unable to migrate out of lymphoid tissue. May have direct effects in CNS.
Teriflunomide (Aubagio) 7 mg or 14 mg po daily	2012	Relapsing MS	Inhibits dihydroorotate dehydrogenase, thus inhibiting proliferation of activated lymphocytes
Dimethyl fumarate (Tecfidera) 240 mg po BID;	2013	Relapsing forms of MS, including active SPMS and CIS	Activates nuclear factor erythroid 2-related factor 2 (Nrf2) pathway that enhances response to oxidative stress
Diroximel fumarate (Vumerity) 231 mg po BID;	2020		
Monomethyl fumarate (Bafiertam) 95 mg po BID	2020		
Alemtuzumab (Lemtrada) IV infusion	2014	Relapsing forms of MS	Monoclonal antibody that lyses cells expressing CD52
Ocrelizumab (Ocrevus) IV infusion 600 mg every 24 weeks	2017	Relapsing forms of MS, primary progressive MS	Lytic monoclonal antibody targeting B cells expressing CD20
Oral cladribine (Mavenclad) 1.75 mg/kg po yearly ×2	2019	Relapsing forms of MS, including active SPMS	Cytotoxic to T and B lymphocytes through impairment of DNA synthesis
Siponimod (Mayzent) usually 2 mg po daily;	2019	Relapsing forms of MS, including active SPMS and CIS	Modulates sphingosine 1-phosphate receptors 1 and 5, lymphocytes are unable to migrate out of lymphoid tissue. May have direct effects in CNS.
Ozanimod (Zeposia) 0.92 mg po daily	2020		
Ofatumumab (Kesimpta) 20 mg SQ monthly	2020	Relapsing forms of MS, including CIS and active SPMS	Human lytic monoclonal antibody targeting B cells expressing CD20

fully understood. Glatiramer acetate has no known drug interactions. Laboratory monitoring is not needed. Side effects include injection site reactions and a tachycardia reaction that occurs infrequently and seemingly randomly, but always soon after an injection. Lipoatrophy at injection sites may develop with prolonged use. Glatiramer acetate is considered the safest MS disease modifying therapy to use in women who may become pregnant. No increase in risks for malformations or fetal/neonatal toxicity or pregnancy loss has been noted in those who were exposed to branded glatiramer acetate, although exposure has been mostly limited to the first trimester.

Mitoxantrone is an anthracenedione chemotherapeutic agent that is FDA approved for secondary progressive MS, progressive relapsing MS, or worsening relapsing-remitting MS. It is administered by IV infusion every 3 months. Due to dose-limiting cardiotoxicity and drug-induced leukemia (the latter in approximately 1% of MS patients receiving it), mitoxantrone is rarely used any more.

Natalizumab is a humanized monoclonal antibody targeting the α-4-integrins, part of the VLA-4 adhesion-related heterodimer. The dose is 300 mg infused intravenously every 4 weeks. A 2-year phase 3 trial of natalizumab showed 68% reduction in annualized relapse rate, 42% reduction in sustained disability, and over 90% reduction in gadolinium-enhancing lesions compared with placebo. Natalizumab was temporarily removed from the market in 2005 due to its association with progressive multifocal leukoencephalopathy (PML), a severe and sometimes fatal viral disorder caused by the JC virus. Because of its association with PML, this drug is recommended mainly in cases of an inadequate response or intolerance of an alternative MS therapy. Patients should be tested for serum antibodies to the JC virus prior to initiating therapy with natalizumab and, if positive, treatment should proceed with caution. Enrollment in a risk-mitigation program is required, and the drug can only be infused at a certified infusion center. Infusion reactions are not uncommon, and neutralizing antibodies to natalizumab develop in some patients. It is not recommended that natalizumab be used during pregnancy or during breast-feeding.

Fingolimod, an oral disease modifying therapy, is indicated for those with relapsing forms of MS, including CIS, RRMS, and active SPMS MS patients 10 years of age and older. This daily 0.5-mg capsule reduces annualized relapse rate in adults with RRMS by about 50% and disability progression by about 25% versus placebo. Fingolimod modulates sphingosine 1-phosphate receptors 1, 3, 4, and 5 and is believed to work in relapsing MS primarily by the sequestration of lymphocytes in secondary lymphoid tissues. Fingolimod affects several organ systems. Adverse effects include macular edema, pulmonary dysfunction, bradycardia, and increased infection rate (including opportunistic infections such as herpetic and cryptococcal infections and PML). Patients who are varicella zoster virus antibody-negative should be vaccinated prior to initiation. Fingolimod is contraindicated

表 17.4 多发性硬化的疾病修饰药物

药物（商品名），剂量	批准时间（年）	MS 的适应证	作用机制
干扰素-β-1b（Betaseron, Extavia），皮下注射，每次 250 μg，隔日 1 次	1993, 2009	RRMS、CIS	抑制"促炎"细胞因子，如干扰素-γ、肿瘤坏死因子-α 和淋巴毒素。增加 IL-10。减少黏附分子和 II 类 MHC 诱导
干扰素-β-1a（Avonex），肌内注射，每次 30 μg，每周 1 次	1996	RRMS、CIS	
干扰素-β-1a（Rebif），皮下注射，每次 22 μg 或 44 μg，每周 3 次	2002	RRMS	
干扰素-β-1a（Plegridy），皮下注射，每次 125 μg，每 14 天一次	2014	复发型 MS	
醋酸格拉默（Copaxone），皮下注射，每天 20 mg；或每次 40 mg，每周 3 次	1996, 2014	RRMS、CIS	改变 T 细胞的细胞因子谱，使其趋向于 Th2 免疫调节细胞
米托蒽醌（Novantrone），静脉注射，12 mg/m²，每 3 个月一次	2000	恶化的 RRMS、复发的 SPMS、PRMS	蒽醌类化疗药
那他珠单抗（Tysabri），静脉注射，每次 300 mg，每 4 周一次	2004/2006（短暂退出市场）	复发型 MS	针对 α-4 整合素（VLA-4 黏附分子的一部分）的单克隆抗体
芬戈莫德（Gilenya），口服，每次 0.5 mg，每日 1 次	2010	复发型 MS，包括儿童	调节鞘氨醇-1-磷酸受体 1、3、4 和 5，使淋巴细胞无法移出淋巴组织。可能对中枢神经系统有直接影响
特立氟胺（Aubagio），口服，每次 7 mg 或 14 mg，每日 1 次	2012	复发型 MS	抑制二氢乳清酸脱氢酶，从而抑制活化淋巴细胞的增殖
二甲基富马酸（Tecfidera），口服，每次 240 mg，每日 2 次	2013	复发型 MS，包括活动性 SPMS 和 CIS	激活核因子红细胞 2-相关因子 2（Nrf2）通路，增强对氧化应激的反应能力
富马酸地洛西美（Vumerity），口服，每次 231 mg，每日 2 次	2020		
富马酸单甲酯（Bafiertam），口服，每次 95 mg，每日 2 次	2020		
阿仑单抗（Lemtrada），静脉输注	2014	复发型 MS	能裂解表达 CD52 细胞的单克隆抗体
奥瑞珠单抗（Ocrevus），静脉输注，每次 600 mg，每 24 周一次	2017	复发型 MS、原发进展型 MS	针对表达 CD20 的 B 细胞的溶解性单克隆抗体
克拉屈滨（Mavenclad），口服，1.75 mg/kg，每年 1 次 × 2 年	2019	复发型 MS，包括活动性 SPMS	通过破坏 DNA 合成而对 T 和 B 淋巴细胞具有细胞毒性
西尼莫德（Mayzent），口服，通常每次 2 mg，每日 1 次	2019	复发型 MS，包括活动性 SPMS 和 CIS	调节鞘氨醇-1-磷酸受体 1 和 5，使淋巴细胞无法移出淋巴组织。可能对中枢神经系统有直接影响
奥扎莫德（Zeposia），口服，每次 0.92 mg，每日 1 次	2020		
奥法木单抗（Kesimpta），皮下注射，每次 20 mg，每月 1 次	2020	复发型 MS，包括 CIS 和活动性 SPMS	针对表达 CD20 的 B 细胞的人溶解性单克隆抗体

CIS，临床孤立综合征；MS，多发性硬化；RRMS，复发-缓解型 MS；SPMS，继发进展型 MS；PRMS，进展复发型 MS。

包括局部注射反应和心动过速，不常发生，似乎具有随机性，一般在注射后不久出现。长期使用可能会出现注射部位脂肪萎缩。醋酸格拉默是对育龄期女性最安全的 MS 疾病修饰治疗药物。在暴露于醋酸格拉默的女性中，尽管暴露时间大多限于妊娠的前三个月，但未增加畸形、胎儿/新生儿毒性或妊娠失败的风险。

米托蒽醌是一种蒽醌类化疗药，已获得 FDA 批准用于治疗继发进展型 MS、进展复发型 MS 或恶化的复发-缓解型 MS。该药每 3 个月静脉输注一次。由于存在剂量限制性心脏毒性和药物诱导性白血病（约 1% 服用该药的 MS 患者会出现后者），米托蒽醌已很少使用。

那他珠单抗是一种针对 α-4 整合素的人源化单克隆抗体，α-4 整合素是 VLA-4 黏附相关异二聚体的一部分。剂量为 300 mg，每 4 周静脉注射一次。一项为期 2 年的那他珠单抗三期试验显示，与安慰剂相比，那他珠单抗的年复发率降低 68%，持续致残率降低 42%，钆增强病灶减少 90% 以上。进行性多灶性白质脑病（PML）是由 JC 病毒引起的一种严重的、偶可致命的病毒性疾病，2005 年，那他珠单抗因与 PML 的发生有关而暂时退市。由于该药与 PML 有关，因此主要推荐用于对其他 MS 治疗反应不充分或不耐受的患者。患者在开始接受那他珠单抗治疗前应检测血清中的 JC 病毒抗体，如果呈阳性，则应谨慎治疗。使用该药必须加入风险缓解计划，而且只能在经过认证的输液中心输注该药物。输液反应并不少见，部分患者会产生那他珠单抗中和抗体。不建议在妊娠期或哺乳期使用那他珠单抗。

芬戈莫德是一种口服的疾病修饰治疗药物，适用于 10 岁及以上的复发型 MS 患者，包括 CIS、RRMS 和活动性 SPMS。与安慰剂相比，每天服用 0.5 mg 的芬戈莫德胶囊可将 RRMS 成人患者的年复发率降低约 50%，将残疾进展率降低约 25%。芬戈莫德可调节鞘氨醇-1-磷酸受体 1、3、4 和 5，主要通过将淋巴细胞封闭在继发性淋巴组织中来治疗复发型 MS。芬戈莫德会影响多个系统器官。其不良反应包括黄斑水肿、肺功能障碍、心动过缓以及感染率升高（包括机会性感染，如疱疹病毒和隐球菌感染，以及进行性多灶性白质脑病）。水痘带状疱疹病毒抗体阴性的患者在使用该药前需接种疫苗。近期发生过心肌梗死、卒中、未控制的心力衰

in the setting of recent myocardial infarction, stroke, uncontrolled heart failure, unstable angina, stroke, transient ischemic attack, or if baseline QTc interval on ECG is 500 ms or greater. Fingolimod can interact with a number of other drugs; it should not be initiated in those taking class IA and class III antiarrhythmic drugs. Medical monitoring for potential bradycardia for at least 6 hours after the first dose is required. Fingolimod may cause fetal harm. Women of childbearing age should use contraception during fingolimod use and for 2 months after its discontinuation.

Siponimod is a second-generation sphingosine 1-phosphate receptor modulator that was FDA-approved in 2019 for adults with relapsing forms of MS, including active SPMS, RRMS, and CIS. Siponimod is more specific than fingolimod, primarily modulating sphingosine 1-phosphate receptors 1 and 5. The maintenance dose is 2 mg per day by mouth but should be reduced to 1 mg/day for those with CYP2C9*1/*3 or *2/*3 genotype, and it is contraindicated for those who are CYP2C9*3/*3 homozygous. In a study of SPMS patients who were notably older (mean age 48 years) and more disabled (median EDSS 6.0) compared with most other MS clinical trials, siponimod reduced 3-month confirmed disability progression by a statistically significant 21% ($P = 0.013$) versus placebo. First-dose monitoring should be done in people with sinus bradycardia, first- or second-degree atrioventricular block, history of myocardial infarction or heart failure. Women of childbearing age who take siponimod should undergo effective contraception, as siponimod has potential for a serious risk to the fetus. Several other sphingosine 1-phosphate receptor modulators are currently being studied in MS.

Ozanimod is a second-generation sphingosine 1-phosphate receptor 1 and 5 modulator that was FDA-approved in 2020 for adults with relapsing forms of MS. In two trials enrolling over 800 subjects with active relapsing MS each, ozanimod was compared to BIFN 1a 30 g IM weekly, showing 48% and 38% relative reductions (each $P < 0.0001$) in annualized relapse rate versus active comparator. As with fingolimod and siponimod, patients should have baseline bloodwork to include CBC and liver function tests, an electrocardiogram to assess for preexisting conduction abnormalities, and baseline and follow-up ophthalmic assessments to assess for macular edema. If live attenuated vaccine immunizations are needed (such as for varicella zoster), these should be administered at least 1 month prior to starting ozanimod (or fingolimod or siponimod). Several other sphingosine 1-phosphate receptor modulators are currently being studied in MS with at least one of these expected to be approved in 2021.

Teriflunomide is a once-daily oral tablet of 7 mg/day or 14 mg/day. Two phase 3 studies in patients with relapsing forms of MS found that the 14-mg/day dose significantly reduced annualized relapse rate by over 30% and disability progression by around 30%. The 7-mg dose had a lesser beneficial effect. Teriflunomide can cause hepatotoxicity, and liver blood work monitoring should continue monthly for 6 months after initiation. Based on animal data, teriflunomide may cause major birth defects and thus pregnancy must be avoided during treatment. If necessary, teriflunomide can be rapidly eliminated from the body using cholestyramine; otherwise, it persists for long periods. Teriflunomide may reactivate latent tuberculosis, is associated with peripheral neuropathy, and can increase blood pressure. Teriflunomide is closely related to the drug leflunomide, approved for rheumatoid arthritis in 1998.

Dimethyl fumarate is an oral medication taken twice daily and is indicated for all relapsing forms of MS. In phase 3 trials, it reduced MS relapse rates by 44% to 53% and improved MRI outcomes. The white blood cell count may drop and should be monitored. In late 2014, the FDA issued a warning regarding the association of PML with this medication, and since then over 20 people have developed PML in the setting of dimethyl fumarate use. The risk of PML may be greater in those with persistent low lymphocyte counts and those over age 50. Adverse effects include flushing, gastrointestinal side effects, and rash. Dimethyl fumarate should be discontinued prior to conception. Several related fumarates with improved side effect profiles are under investigation for use in MS.

Diroximel fumarate and *monomethyl fumarate* are two second generation oral fumarates each approved in 2020 by the FDA for relapsing forms of MS. These oral fumarates have similar efficacy and safety to dimethyl fumarate, but fewer gastrointestinal side effects.

Alemtuzumab is a lytic monoclonal antibody targeting cells expressing CD52, which includes T and B lymphocytes, monocytes, and other mononuclear white blood cells. In the United States, it is indicated for people with relapsing forms of MS and, because of its health risks, is reserved for those with inadequate response to two or more disease-modifying drugs for MS. In the CARE-MS I and II studies in RRMS patients, alemtuzumab infusions were compared to 44 μg BIFN-1a given subcutaneously three times per week. Patients treated with alemtuzumab had a lower annualized relapse rate (by 49% and 53.8%) and disability progression (by 28% and 42%). Alemtuzumab leads to a profound drop in the white blood cell count, which may last for months or even years. In trials, secondary autoimmune diseases developed in a sizeable proportion of alemtuzumab-treated subjects, with autoimmune thyroid disease being most common. Alemtuzumab may increase risk of malignancies, including thyroid cancer, melanoma, and lymphoproliferative disorders. Infusion reactions are common and can be life-threatening. Alemtuzumab is available only through clinicians and infusion centers that have been certified to use it. Women of childbearing potential should use effective contraceptive measures when receiving a course of alemtuzumab and for 4 months following that course of treatment.

Ocrelizumab is a fully humanized lytic monoclonal antibody targeting CD20, a cell surface antigen found on B lymphocytes. Ocrelizumab was FDA-approved in 2017 for patients with relapsing or primary progressive forms of MS. Ocrelizumab is given as an intravenous infusion of 600 mg every 24 weeks. In the phase 3 studies, those in the ocrelizumab group had almost 50% reduction in annualized relapse rate and a 40% reduction in 12-week confirmed disability progression compared to relapsing MS patients given subcutaneous BIFN-1a at 44 micrograms three times per week. In the phase 3 ORATORIO study in primary progressive MS, those receiving ocrelizumab had 24% reduction in 3 month confirmed progression versus placebo. Side effects include infusion reactions, increased infection rate (including herpetic infections) and a possible increased risk of cancers, including breast cancer. Patients should screen negative for hepatitis B before commencing use of ocrelizumab. Risks associated with ocrelizumab in pregnant women are unclear, but transient B cell depletion and lymphocytopenia have been reported in infants born to mothers exposed to other anti-CD20 antibodies during pregnancy. Being of immunoglobulin G1 subtype, ocrelizumab is expected to cross the placental barrier. Women of childbearing potential should use contraception while receiving ocrelizumab and for 6 months after the last infusion.

Ofatumumab is a human monoclonal antibody that targets and lyses cells expressing CD20. It is administered monthly, subcutaneously. In two clinical trials of over 900 relapsing MS patients each, ofatumumab was compared to teriflunomide 14 mg/day po. Annualized relapse rate reductions of 51% and 59% (both $P < 0.001$) were observed in the ofatumumab groups relative to teriflunomide groups. The combined studies showed ofatumumab to confer a 34.4% relative reduction in three-month confirmed disability progression ($P = .002$) versus teriflunomide. Potential risks and side effects are similar to those for

竭、不稳定型心绞痛、短暂性脑缺血发作或者心电图基线QTc间期≥500 ms的患者禁用芬戈莫德。芬戈莫德可与多种其他药物发生相互作用，服用ⅠA类和Ⅲ类抗心律失常药物的患者不应使用芬戈莫德。需要在首次用药后至少6 h内对潜在的心动过缓进行医学监测。芬戈莫德可能会对胎儿造成伤害。育龄期妇女在服用芬戈莫德期间和停药后2个月内应采取避孕措施。

西尼莫德是第二代鞘氨醇-1-磷酸受体调节剂，2019年FDA批准其用于治疗成人复发型MS，包括活动性SPMS、RRMS和CIS。西尼莫德比芬戈莫德更具特异性，主要调节鞘氨醇-1-磷酸受体1和5。维持剂量为每天口服2 mg，但CYP2C9*1/*3或*2/*3基因型患者应减量至每天1 mg，CYP2C9*3/*3患者禁用。一项针对SPMS患者的研究发现，与安慰剂相比，西尼莫德可将3个月确诊的残疾进展减少21%（$P = 0.013$），结果具有显著的统计学意义。与多数其他MS临床试验相比，该研究中的患者年龄明显偏大（平均年龄48岁）、残疾程度更高（EDSS中位数为6.0）。有窦性心动过缓、一度或二度房室传导阻滞、心肌梗死或心力衰竭病史的患者应进行首次剂量监测。服用西尼莫德的育龄期妇女应采取有效的避孕措施，因为西尼莫德可能对胎儿造成严重危害。目前正在研究其他几种鞘氨醇-1-磷酸受体调节剂在MS中的应用。

奥扎莫德是第二代鞘氨醇-1-磷酸受体1和5调节剂，2020年FDA批准其用于治疗成人复发型MS。在两项各招募800多名活动性复发型MS患者的试验中，比较了奥扎莫德与BIFN-1a 30 g（译者注：原文有误，应为μg）肌内注射、每周1次的疗效，结果显示与活性药物对照组相比，二者的年复发率分别相对降低了48%和38%（P值均＜0.0001）。与芬戈莫德和西尼莫德一样，患者在应用奥扎莫德时应进行基线血液检查，包括全血细胞计数和肝功能检测、心电图检查以评估原有的传导异常，以及基线和随访期眼科检查以评估黄斑水肿。如果需要接种减毒活性疫苗（如水痘带状疱疹病毒疫苗），应在开始使用奥扎莫德（或芬戈莫德或西尼莫德）前至少1个月接种。目前正在研究其他几种鞘氨醇-1-磷酸受体调节剂在MS中的应用，预计至少有一种药物将于2021年获得FDA批准。

特立氟胺是片剂，每日口服1次，剂量为7 mg或14 mg。两项针对复发型MS患者的3期研究发现，每日14 mg的剂量可显著降低30%以上的年复发率和30%左右的残疾进展率。7 mg剂量的疗效较差。特立氟胺可引起肝毒性，用药后6个月内应持续每月监测肝功能。根据动物实验数据，特立氟胺可能会导致严重的先天缺陷，因此在治疗期间必须避孕。必要时，可使用考来烯胺将特立氟胺迅速排出体外，否则，特立氟胺会长期存在于体内。特立氟胺可能会重新激活潜伏的结核病，其与周围神经病有关，并可能会升高血压。特立氟胺与1998年获批用于治疗类风湿关节炎的来氟米特密切相关。

二甲基富马酸是口服药物，每日服用2次，适用于所有复发型MS。在3期试验中，该药将MS的复发率降低了44%～53%，并改善了MRI结局。用药过程中可能引起白细胞计数下降，应进行监测。2014年底，FDA就该药与PML的关联性发出警告，此后已有20多人在使用二甲基富马酸时出现PML。淋巴细胞计数持续偏低者和50岁以上患者发生PML的风险可能更大。其不良反应包括面部潮红、胃肠道副作用和皮疹。受孕前应停用二甲基富马酸。目前正在研究几种副作用有所改善的相关富马酸盐在MS中的应用。

富马酸地洛西美和富马酸单甲酯是2020年FDA批准用于复发型MS的两种第二代口服富马酸盐。其疗效和安全性与二甲基富马酸相似，但胃肠道副作用较少。

阿仑单抗是一种溶解性单克隆抗体，靶向表达CD52的细胞，包括T和B淋巴细胞、单核细胞和其他单核白细胞。在美国，该药适用于复发型MS患者，并且由于其健康风险，仅用于对2种或2种以上MS疾病修饰治疗药物反应不充分的患者。在针对RRMS患者的CARE-MSⅠ和Ⅱ研究中，比较了阿仑单抗输注与BIFN-1a 44 μg每周3次皮下注射的疗效，接受阿仑单抗治疗的患者年复发率（49%和53.8%）和残疾进展率（28%和42%）均更低。阿仑单抗会导致白细胞数量急剧下降，并且可能会持续数月甚至数年。在试验中，相当一部分接受阿仑单抗治疗的受试者出现了继发性自身免疫性疾病，其中以自身免疫性甲状腺疾病最为常见。阿仑单抗可能会增加恶性肿瘤的风险，包括甲状腺癌、黑色素瘤和淋巴增生性疾病。输液反应较常见，并且可能危及生命。阿仑单抗只能通过获得认证的临床医生和输液中心获取。有生育能力的女性在接受阿仑单抗治疗时和治疗后的4个月内应采取有效的避孕措施。

奥瑞珠单抗是一种靶向CD20的全人源化裂解性单克隆抗体，CD20是一种存在于B淋巴细胞上的细胞表面抗原。奥瑞珠单抗于2017年获得FDA批准，用于治疗复发型或原发进展型MS患者。奥瑞珠单抗每24周静脉输注600 mg。在3期临床研究中，比较了奥瑞珠单抗与BIFN-1a 44 μg每周3次皮下注射对复发型MS的疗效，研究提示奥瑞珠单抗组患者的年复发率降低了近50%，12周确诊的残疾进展降低了40%。在针对原发进展型MS的ORATORIO 3期研究中，与安慰剂相比，接受奥瑞珠单抗治疗的患者3个月确诊的疾病进展降低了24%。其副作用包括输液反应、感染率增加（包括疱疹病毒感染）以及罹患癌症（包括乳腺癌）的风险可能增加。患者在开始使用奥瑞珠单抗前应进行乙型肝炎筛查，阴性方可用药。与奥瑞珠单抗相关的孕妇风险尚不明确，但有报道称在妊娠期间接触过其他抗CD20抗体的母亲所生育的婴儿会出现一过性B细胞耗竭和淋巴细胞减少。奥瑞珠单抗属于免疫球蛋白G1亚型，可穿过胎盘屏障。育龄期女性在接受奥瑞珠单抗治疗期间以及最后一次输注后的6个月内应采取避孕措施。

奥法木单抗是一种人源性单克隆抗体，能靶向并裂解表达CD20的细胞。每月皮下注射1次。在两项各有900多名复发型MS患者参加的临床试验中，奥法木单抗与特立氟胺每日14 mg口服进行了比较。与特立氟胺组相比，奥法木单抗组的年复发率分别降低了51%

ocrelizumab and include infections, injection reactions, and reduced response to vaccinations.

Oral cladribine was approved by the FDA in 2019 for the treatment of relapsing forms of MS in adults, including RRMS and active SPMS. This drug is recommended for patients who have had an inadequate response to, or are unable to tolerate, an alternative disease modifying treatment of MS. Oral cladribine is a purine antimetabolite that destroys certain immune cells. It is given at a cumulative dosage of 3.5 mg/kg divided into two treatment courses at 1.75 mg/kg per treatment course given a year apart. Oral cladribine may increase the risk of malignancy, and it is contraindicated in those with concurrent malignancy. Patients should be screened for HIV, tuberculosis, and hepatitis B and C prior to use. Varicella zoster virus antibody-negative persons should be vaccinated before initiation. Oral cladribine is contraindicated in pregnant or breast-feeding women and in both women and men of reproductive potential who do not plan to use effective contraception because of risk of fetal harm.

NEUROMYELITIS OPTICA SPECTRUM DISORDER (DEVIC DISEASE)

Definition/Epidemiology

Neuromyelitis optica spectrum disorders (NMOSD) comprise a spectrum of inflammatory CNS disorders causing both demyelination and necrosis that are clinically characterized by attacks of optic neuritis and longitudinally extensive TM that are not necessarily concurrent. Only rarely is NMOSD monophasic. In most cases serum autoantibodies to the aquaporin 4 (AQP4) water channels are found. AQP4 channels are strongly expressed by astrocytes. AQP4 is also expressed outside of the CNS in the kidney, stomach, and other tissues, but curiously no pathology has been recognized in the non-CNS organs expressing AQP4.

NMOSD is much less common than MS, with estimates by the Guthy-Jackson Charitable Foundation of 15,000 patients in the United States. It is even more female-preponderant than MS, with female to male ratio estimated at 7:1. Children and adults both develop NMO. Unlike MS, NMO is *not* associated with HLA-DRB1*15:01, and it affects those of Asian, African, Hispanic, and Polynesian ancestry disproportionately.

Clinical Presentation

NMO presents clinically as an acute attack of optic neuritis and/or TM; it often takes a relapsing course. Gradually progressive NMO is exceedingly rare (helping to distinguish progressive MS from NMO). Other autoimmune diseases often occur together with NMOSD including Sjögren's syndrome, systemic lupus erythematosus, Hashimoto disease, and myasthenia gravis.

Diagnosis/Differential

In 2004, researchers first reported the presence of a serum IgG autoantibody targeting aquaporin 4 in NMO. NMO-IgG/AQP4-IgG is highly specific (>90%) and moderately sensitive (≈75%) for NMOSD. Fulfilling two out of three of the following criteria is reported to be 99% sensitive and 90% specific in the setting of optic neuritis and TM: (1) longitudinally extensive spinal cord lesion, which is greater than or equal to three segments in length (Fig. 17.3); (2) NMO-IgG (anti-AQP4) positivity; and (3) brain MRI not typical or diagnostic for MS.

For a deeper discussion of these topics, please see Chapter 383, "Multiple Sclerosis and Demyelinating Conditions of the Central Nervous System," in *Goldman-Cecil Medicine*, 26th Edition.

Pathology

Histopathologic changes in NMOSD are mostly in the spinal cord and optic nerves; the brain is less involved. Lesions affect both white and gray matter. In the brain, lesions are most common in the hypothalamus and around the fourth ventricle. NMO lesions center on blood vessels where IgG, IgM, and complement activation products are seen. The vessels are abnormally thickened and hyalinized. Active

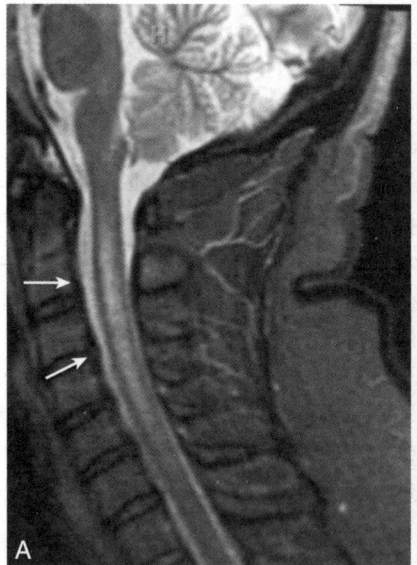 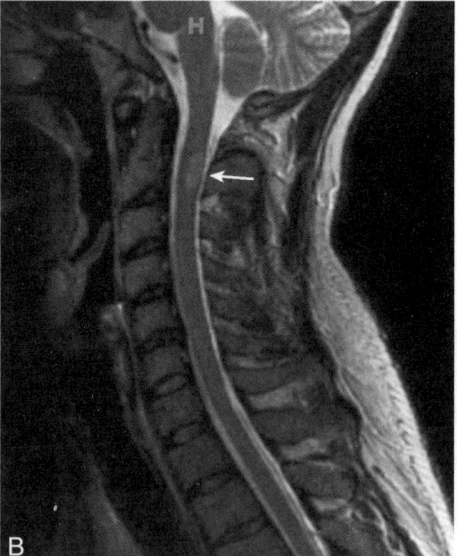

Fig. 17.3 (A) Sagittal T2w image of the upper spinal cord in a 37-year-old female with NMO. She developed quadriparesis over several days and was AQP4-IgG seropositive. Two years later she had right eye optic neuritis, which left her with visual acuity of only 20/200. The spinal cord lesion *(arrows)* had mild mass effect and was contiguous over six vertebral segments. (B) Sagittal T2w image of the upper spinal cord in a 24-year-old male with MS shows a lesion *(arrow)* in the posterior cord at C2. This patient had moderate vibration loss in the legs but was otherwise asymptomatic.

和 59%（P 值均 < 0.001）。综合研究显示，与特立氟胺相比，奥法木单抗可使 3 个月确诊的残疾进展相对减少 34.4%（P = 0.002）。潜在的风险和副作用与奥瑞珠单抗相似，包括感染、注射反应和对疫苗的反应减弱。

口服克拉屈滨于 2019 年被 FDA 批准用于治疗成人复发型 MS，包括 RRMS 和活动性 SPMS。该药推荐用于对其他疾病修饰治疗反应不充分或无法耐受的 MS 患者。口服克拉屈滨是一种嘌呤类抗代谢药，可破坏某些免疫细胞。该药累积剂量为 3.5 mg/kg，治疗分为两个疗程，每个疗程 1.75 mg/kg，相隔一年使用。口服克拉屈滨可能会增加罹患恶性肿瘤的风险，恶性肿瘤患者需禁用。患者在使用前应进行 HIV、肺结核、乙型和丙型肝炎筛查。水痘带状疱疹病毒抗体阴性者应在用药前接种疫苗。由于存在对胎儿造成伤害的风险，孕妇或哺乳期妇女以及不打算采取有效避孕措施的具有生育能力的女性和男性禁用口服克拉屈滨。

视神经脊髓炎谱系疾病（DEVIC 病）

定义和流行病学

视神经脊髓炎谱系疾病（NMOSD）是由可引起脱髓鞘和坏死的中枢神经系统炎症性疾病组成的疾病谱系，临床特征是视神经炎发作和纵向扩展的横贯性脊髓炎，二者未必同时发生。NMOSD 单相病程较为少见。大多数病例中可发现血清中存在针对水通道蛋白 4（AQP4）的自身抗体。星形胶质细胞高表达 AQP4 通道。AQP4 在中枢神经系统以外的肾、胃和其他组织中也有表达，但奇怪的是，尚未在表达 AQP4 的非中枢神经系统器官中发现病理改变。

NMOSD 的发病率远低于 MS，据 Guthy-Jackson 慈善基金会估计，美国有 15 000 名 NMOSD 患者。与 MS 相比，NMOSD 患者中女性居多，女/男比例约为 7：1。儿童和成年人都可能患 NMO。与 MS 不同，NMO 与 HLA-DRB1*15：01 无关，亚裔、非裔、西班牙裔和波利尼西亚裔人群罹患此病的比例更高。

临床表现

NMO 临床表现为视神经炎和（或）横贯性脊髓炎急性发作，通常呈复发性病程。逐渐进展的 NMO 非常罕见（有助于鉴别进展型 MS 与 NMO）。其他自身免疫性疾病经常与 NMOSD 同时发生，包括干燥综合征、系统性红斑狼疮、桥本病和重症肌无力。

诊断和鉴别诊断

2004 年，研究人员首次报道了 NMO 患者血清中存在针对水通道蛋白 4 的 IgG 自身抗体。NMO-IgG/AQP4-IgG 对 NMOSD 具有高度特异性（> 90%）和中度敏感性（≈ 75%）。据报道，在视神经炎和横贯性脊髓炎的背景下满足以下 3 项标准中的 2 项，诊断 NMO 即可具有 99% 的敏感性和 90% 的特异性：①纵向广泛性脊髓病变，长度≥ 3 个椎体节段（图 17.3）；② NMO-IgG（抗AQP4）阳性；③脑 MRI 不符合 MS 诊断标准。

有关此专题的深入讨论，请参阅 *Goldman-Cecil Medicine* 第 26 版第 383 章 "多发性硬化和中枢神经系统脱髓鞘疾病"。

病理学

NMOSD 的组织病理改变主要发生在脊髓和视神经，大脑较少受累。病变同时累及白质和灰质。在大脑中，病变最常见于下丘脑和第四脑室周围。NMO 病灶以血管为中心，可见 IgG、IgM 和补体活化产物。血管异常增粗和透明化。活动性 NMO 病变表现为单核细胞（淋巴细胞、单核细胞）、中性粒细胞和嗜酸性粒细胞浸润。陈旧的病灶表现为脱髓鞘、轴突丢失、少突

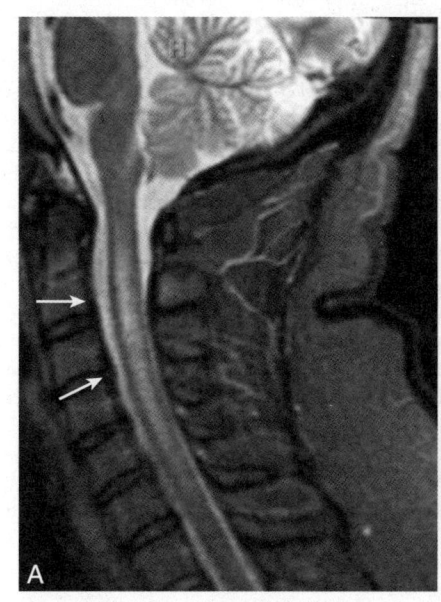
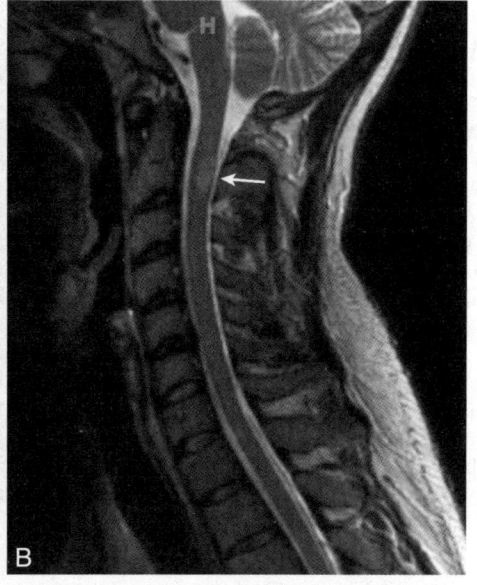

图 17.3 （A）一名 37 岁女性 NMO 患者的脊髓上部 T2w 矢状位图像。该患者在数日内出现四肢瘫痪，血清 AQP4-IgG 阳性。2 年后，其出现右眼视神经炎，视力仅为 20/200。脊髓病灶（箭头）有轻度占位效应，并发生在连续 6 个椎体节段。（B）一名 24 岁男性 MS 患者的脊髓上部 T2w 矢状位图像，C2 后部脊髓有病灶（箭头）。该患者双腿振动觉中度减弱，但无其他症状

NMO lesions show infiltration by mononuclear cells (lymphocytes, monocytes), neutrophils, and eosinophils. Older lesions display demyelination, axon loss, and death of oligodendroglia and neurons. Accumulating data indicate that AQP4-IgG itself is pathogenic, causing complement- and antibody-mediated damage.

Treatment

Acute relapses are treated with high-dose corticosteroids. If these are not quickly effective, plasma exchange is performed. Although NMO is rare, several multicenter randomized, controlled trials of disease modifying therapies have been completed recently with notably positive results.

Eculizumab, a monoclonal antibody that inhibits the complement cascade, was compared to placebo in a randomized, double-blind, multicenter trial in adult NMOSD patients. The trial was stopped early when it showed that relapses occurred in only 3% in the eculizumab group versus 43% in the placebo group (hazard ratio, 0.06; 95% confidence interval, 0.02 to 0.20; $P < 0.001$). Upper respiratory tract infections and headaches were more common in the eculizumab group and a death from pulmonary empyema occurred in this group.

Inebilizumab, a monoclonal antibody to CD19 that depletes B cells, was compared to placebo in adults with NMOSD in a randomized, double-blind, multicenter study. Primary end point was time to onset of an NMOSD attack. This study too was stopped before complete enrollment because of a clear demonstration of efficacy. Twelve percent of 174 participants receiving inebilizumab had an attack versus 39% those receiving placebo (hazard ratio 0.272 [95% confidence interval 0.150 to 0.496]; $P < 0.0001$). Serious adverse effects were no higher in the active treatment group than in the placebo group.

Satralizumab, a monoclonal antibody targeting the IL-6 receptor and thereby inhibiting IL-6 activity, has been reported to show positive results in NMOSD, particularly in those with positive ant-AQP4 antibodies. Notably, beta-interferons are *not* effective for NMOSD and may actually increase the rate of attacks.

Prognosis

NMOSD typically displays worse outcomes than MS. Seropositive NMO patients tend to have more frequent and severe relapses than AQP4-IgG negative patients. The death rate in a retrospective study covering 1950 to 1997 was over 30%. Less than 10% mortality was reported in a more recent retrospective study of Caucasian NMO patients. Death is often due to respiratory failure.

ANTI-MYELIN OLIGODENDROCYTE GLYCOPROTEIN DISORDER

A CNS demyelinating disease identified by its association with serum antibodies to the CNS myelin component, myelin oligodendrocyte glycoprotein (MOG), was recently described. Diagnosis is based on positive serum IgG1antibodies to MOG using cell-based assays, as well as the absence of anti-AQP4 antibodies, and absence of CSF-restricted oligoclonal bands. Anti-MOG disorder shares features with both MS and classical NMO. Anti-MOG disorder occurs in children and adults and affects males and females in similar proportion. In adults, anti-MOG disorder is often characterized by optic neuritis and transverse myelitis (which may occur separately), but the disease is usually less severe than AQP4 antibody positive NMOSD and is often monophasic. An acute disseminated encephalomyelitis-like presentation is common in children. The spectrum of anti-MOG disorder is still being determined, as is the optimum treatment strategy.

ACUTE DISSEMINATED ENCEPHALOMYELITIS

ADEM is an acute, inflammatory, presumed immune-mediated disorder of the CNS that is encountered primarily in children but may occur in adults. An antecedent viral infection or vaccination is common. ADEM presents with multifocal neurologic symptoms and signs. These can include encephalopathy, which may manifest as reduced level of consciousness (even coma) or as behavioral changes (e.g., confusion or irritability). Fever is common. Seizures, optic neuritis, and spinal cord involvement can all occur. Males and females are about equally affected. ADEM is usually monophasic, although relapsing ADEM has been described. On MRI, both white and gray matter CNS regions are affected. Gray matter involvement can include the basal ganglia, a region not typically affected in MS. The periventricular white matter region is often spared, unlike MS. When present, enhancement with gadolinium occurs in all lesions simultaneously. CSF often shows pleocytosis and an elevated protein but no infection. Findings typical of MS, such as oligoclonal bands, are unusual. No randomized prospective treatment trials for acute disseminated encephalomyelitis are reported. Intravenous methylprednisolone followed by a prednisone taper is typically administered with usually good response. Over 80% of cases recover. Because ADEM is only rarely recurrent, long-term immunomodulatory/immunosuppressive therapy is not indicated. A rare hemorrhagic form of ADEM (Weston Hurst syndrome) is more severe and can lead to death or severe disability.

ACUTE TRANSVERSE MYELITIS

TM is an inflammatory spinal cord syndrome presenting with abrupt or subacute onset of motor and/or sensory loss below a specific spinal level. Control of bladder and bowel is often affected, as is autonomic function below the level. Back pain and paresthesias may be prominent. Many cases of acute TM are idiopathic, but treatable causes must be ruled out. An urgent MRI with and without gadolinium should be obtained to look for compressive etiologies needing immediate treatment. After a compressive etiology has been ruled out, a lumbar puncture to assess CSF for cell count, glucose, and protein and cultures and PCRs for infectious causes should be done. The usual tests for MS should be performed, and CSF should be analyzed for evidence of neoplastic cells. Serum AQP4-IgG, anti-MOG using cell-based assays, paraneoplastic panels, and chest CT should be considered. CSF may also be tested for NMO-IgG, angiotensin converting enzyme, and paraneoplastic antibodies when no etiology is forthcoming.

Acute TM can be the presenting episode for MS (in which case the TM is generally incomplete and asymmetrical) or NMO (where the TM affects ≥3 spinal cord segments). Acute TM can also be caused by spinal cord infarction due to occlusion of the anterior spinal artery. Infections by viruses can cause acute or subacute TM. The most common viruses associated with acute TM are varicella zoster, herpes virus type 2, and cytomegalovirus. The retroviruses HTLV-I and HIV can each cause a myelopathy that is usually subacute. West Nile virus can cause a myelopathy that resembles poliomyelitis, with flaccid paralysis due to infection and death of anterior horn cells. Subacute TM may be caused by vitamin B_{12} or copper deficiency or infiltrating or compressive syndromes such as tumors or abscesses. Nitrous oxide anesthesia can precipitate an acute-onset myelopathy in the case of borderline vitamin B_{12} deficiency. Rheumatologic disorders such as Sjögren's disease, systemic lupus erythematosus, and Behçet's disease can all cause TM. Paraneoplastic syndromes associated with anti-CRMP-5 and anti-amphiphysin can cause a tract-specific myelopathy. The history and physical examination should be performed with these disorders in mind.

胶质细胞和神经元死亡。越来越多的数据表明，AQP4-IgG 本身具有致病性，可导致补体和抗体介导的损伤。

治疗

急性复发时可使用大剂量皮质类固醇治疗。如果效果不佳，则进行血浆置换。虽然 NMO 较为罕见，但最近完成的几项疾病修饰治疗的多中心随机对照试验取得了显著的阳性结果。

依库珠单抗是抑制补体级联反应的单克隆抗体。一项随机、双盲、安慰剂对照的多中心试验比较了依库珠单抗与安慰剂对成人 NMOSD 的疗效。研究结果表明，与安慰剂相比，依库珠单抗组仅有 3% 的患者复发，而安慰剂组则有 43% 的患者复发（危险比为 0.06，95% 置信区间为 0.02～0.20，$P < 0.001$），因此试验提前终止。上呼吸道感染和头痛在依库珠单抗组中更为常见，且该组中有一例受试者死于肺积脓。

伊奈利珠单抗是消耗 B 细胞的 CD19 单克隆抗体。一项随机、双盲、安慰剂对照的多中心试验比较了伊奈利珠单抗与安慰剂对成人 NMOSD 的疗效，其主要终点是 NMOSD 的发病时间。由于伊奈利珠单抗疗效明显，该研究也提前终止。在 174 名接受伊奈利珠单抗治疗的患者中，有 12% 的患者发病，而接受安慰剂治疗的患者发病率为 39%（危险比为 0.272，95% 置信区间为 0.150～0.496，$P < 0.0001$）。治疗组的严重不良反应发生率并不高于安慰剂组。

萨特利珠单抗是针对 IL-6 受体从而抑制 IL-6 活性的单克隆抗体。据报道，该药对 NMOSD 有积极疗效，尤其是对抗 AQP4 抗体阳性的患者。值得注意的是，β-干扰素对 NMOSD 无效，实际可能增加其发病率。

预后

NMOSD 的预后通常比 MS 差。血清 AQP4-IgG 阳性的 NMO 患者往往比阴性的患者复发更频繁、更严重。在一项涵盖 1950—1997 年的回顾性研究中，NMOSD 的死亡率超过 30%。最近一项针对白种人 NMO 患者的回顾性研究显示，该病的死亡率不到 10%，其死亡原因通常是呼吸衰竭。

抗髓鞘少突胶质细胞糖蛋白抗体病

最近报道的一种中枢神经系统脱髓鞘疾病，与中枢神经系统髓鞘成分——髓鞘少突胶质细胞糖蛋白（MOG）的血清抗体有关。该病的诊断依据是使用细胞检测法检测血清中的 MOG-IgG1 抗体阳性、抗 AQP4 抗体阴性，且脑脊液寡克隆带阴性。抗 MOG 抗体病与 MS 和典型的 NMO 有相同的特征。抗 MOG 抗体病发生于儿童和成人，男性和女性患者的比例相近。在成人中，抗 MOG 抗体病的特征通常是视神经炎和横贯性脊髓炎（可单独发生），但病情通常不如 AQP4 抗体阳性的 NMOSD 严重，而且通常是单相病程。急性播散性脑脊髓炎样表现常见于儿童。抗 MOG 抗体病的疾病谱以及最佳治疗策略尚未明确。

急性播散性脑脊髓炎

急性播散性脑脊髓炎（ADEM）是急性、炎症性、推测为免疫介导的中枢神经系统（CNS）疾病，主要见于儿童，但也可发生于成人。既往病毒感染或接种疫苗是常见诱发因素。ADEM 表现为多灶性神经系统症状和体征，可以包括脑病，表现为意识减退（甚至昏迷）或行为改变（如精神错乱或易怒），发热较常见，癫痫发作、视神经炎和脊髓受累均可发生。男性和女性患病风险大致相同。ADEM 通常是单相病程，但也有复发性 ADEM 的报道。MRI 上该病 CNS 白质和灰质区域均可受累。灰质受累可包括基底节区，MS 通常不累及该区域。与 MS 不同的是，ADEM 脑室周围白质区域通常不受累。罹患该病时，所有病灶可同时表现为钆增强。脑脊液常显示细胞增多和蛋白质升高，但无感染表现。寡克隆带阳性等 MS 的典型表现并不常见。目前尚无关于 ADEM 随机、前瞻性治疗试验的报道。该病的治疗为静脉注射甲泼尼龙，序贯口服泼尼松并逐渐减停，通常会有良好反应。超过 80% 的 ADEM 病例可痊愈。由于 ADEM 很少复发，因此不需要进行长期免疫调节/免疫抑制治疗。一种罕见的出血性 ADEM（Weston Hurst 综合征）较为严重，可导致死亡或严重残疾。

急性横贯性脊髓炎

横贯性脊髓炎（TM）是炎症性脊髓综合征，表现为突发或亚急性发病的特定脊髓水平以下的运动和（或）感觉缺失。膀胱和肠道的控制功能通常受累，因为该水平以下的自主神经功能受累。背痛和感觉异常可能较明显。许多急性 TM 病例为特发性，但必须排除可治疗的病因。患者应立即进行钆增强和非增强 MRI 检查，以明确是否存在压迫性病因，并采取相应的治疗措施。排除压迫性病因后，患者应进行腰椎穿刺以评估脑脊液中细胞数、葡萄糖和蛋白质水平，并进行脑脊液培养和 PCR 检查以明确感染性病因。此外，患者应进行 MS 的常规检查，寻找脑脊液中肿瘤细胞的证据。也应考虑检测血清 AQP4-IgG、使用细胞检测法检测抗 MOG 抗体、副肿瘤细胞检测和胸部 CT 检查。如果仍找不到病因，也可以检测脑脊液中的 NMO-IgG、血管紧张素转换酶和副肿瘤抗体。

急性 TM 可能是 MS（TM 病灶通常不完全且不对称）或 NMO（TM 病灶累及≥3 个椎体节段）的首发症状。急性 TM 也可由脊髓前动脉闭塞导致的脊髓梗死引起。病毒感染可导致急性或亚急性 TM。与急性 TM 相关的最常见的病毒是水痘带状疱疹病毒、2 型疱疹病毒和巨细胞病毒。逆转录病毒 HTLV-1 和 HIV 可分别引起脊髓病，但通常是亚急性起病。西尼罗河病毒可引起类似脊髓灰质炎的脊髓病，由于感染和前角细胞死亡而导致弛缓性瘫痪。亚急性 TM 可能由维生素 B_{12} 或铜缺乏症或者肿瘤或脓肿等浸润性或压迫性综合征引起。当维生素 B_{12} 缺乏时，氧化亚氮麻醉可诱发急性脊髓病。风湿性疾病，如干燥综合征、系统性红斑狼疮和白塞病都可能导致 TM。与抗 CRMP-5 和抗

Treatment is determined by the most likely etiology. Idiopathic TM is treated much like TM in MS or NMO, with intravenous methylprednisolone at 500 mg to 1000 mg/day, usually followed by a short oral prednisone taper. When response to intravenous methylprednisolone is suboptimal, plasma exchange should be considered.

IDIOPATHIC ACUTE OPTIC NEURITIS

Inflammatory demyelinating optic neuritis can occur as part of MS or NMO, or as an idiopathic entity. Classically, optic neuritis presents over hours with loss of vision together with pain exacerbated by eye movement. Vision loss may range from subclinical to frank blindness. Color vision and contrast sensitivity are disproportionately affected. On examination, a relative afferent pupillary defect is seen in unilateral optic neuritis. Acute demyelinating optic neuritis is often retrobulbar without papillitis. On MRI, the optic nerve can be swollen and enhance after gadolinium contrast. After recovery from the acute episode, the optic disk may appear pale, and the relative afferent pupillary defect may persist. Transient worsening of vision when the body temperature rises due to exercise or fever (Uhthoff phenomenon) may occur following recovery. The differential diagnosis includes other causes of acute monocular or binocular vision loss, such as Leber hereditary optic neuropathy, giant cell arteritis, and acute nonarteritic anterior ischemic optic neuropathy.

The Optic Neuritis Treatment Trial studied patients with acute optic neuritis (either idiopathic or due to MS) who were randomized to one of three treatments, intravenous methylprednisolone versus oral prednisone taper versus oral placebo. Visual acuity initially recovered faster in the intravenous methylprednisolone group, but by 6 months later there was no difference among the three groups. Recovery of vision was good. Patients from this trial were examined 10 years later and acuity in the affected eyes was 20/20 or better in 74% and less than 20/200 in only 3%. However, recurrence of optic neuritis was common and had occurred in either eye in 35% of the patients. Recurrences were more frequent in those who had MS than in those with idiopathic optic neuritis ($P < .001$).

CHRONIC RELAPSING INFLAMMATORY OPTIC NEUROPATHY

First described in 2003, chronic relapsing inflammatory optic neuropathy (CRION) is an inflammatory optic neuropathy characterized by acute relapses, often with more severe visual loss than idiopathic optic neuritis or optic neuritis associated with MS. CRION can commence at any age and has been described worldwide. Prevalence rates and epidemiology are still unclear. As in other types of optic neuritis, eye pain at onset is frequent. Five diagnostic criteria for CRION have been suggested: (1) optic neuritis with at least one relapse, (2) visual loss, (3) AQP4-IgG seronegativity, (4) contrast enhancement on MRI of acutely inflamed optic nerve, and (5) response to immunosuppressive treatment and relapse on withdrawal. Other diseases that might present similarly, such as sarcoidosis and giant cell arteritis, should be ruled out. Acute CRION is treated similarly to other causes of optic neuritis, with high-dose methylprednisolone. Relapses are common upon corticosteroid discontinuation. Successful long-term treatment with "steroid sparing" agents such as methotrexate, azathioprine, or mycophenolate mofetil has been reported. The underlying pathology is not yet known, but the disease appears inflammatory based on clinical presentation, imaging, and specific medication response. Eventual visual outcomes are often poor. One report indicated that visual acuity was less than 20/200 in one third of CRION patients.

SUGGESTED READINGS

Correale J, Gaitán MI, Ysrraelit MC, Fiol MP: Progressive multiple sclerosis: from pathogenic mechanisms to treatment, Brain 140:527–546, 2017.

Kim SH, Huh SY, Lee SJ: A 5-year follow-up of rituximab treatment in patients with neuromyelitis optica spectrum disorder, JAMA Neurol 70:1110–1117, 2013.

Klaver R, De Vries HE, Schenk GJ, et al: Grey matter damage in multiple sclerosis: a pathology perspective, Prion 7:66–75, 2013.

Langer-Gould A, Brara SM, Beaber BE, et al: Incidence of multiple sclerosis in multiple racial and ethnic groups, Neurology 80:1734–1739, 2013.

Lublin FD, Reingold SC, Cohen JA, et al: Defining the clinical course of multiple sclerosis: the 2013 revisions, Neurology 83:277–286, 2014.

Petzold A, Plant GT: Chronic relapsing inflammatory optic neuropathy: a systematic review of 122 cases reported, J Neurol 261:17–26, 2014.

Pittock SJ, Berthele A, Fujihara K, et al: Eculizumab in aquaporin-4-positive neuromyelitis optica spectrum disorder, N Engl J Med 381:614–625, 2019.

Reindl M, Di Pauli F, Rostásy K, Berger T: The spectrum of MOG antibody-associated demyelinating disorders, Nat Rev Neurol 9:455–461, 2013.

Thompson AJ, Banwell BL, Barkhof F, et al: Diagnosis of multiple sclerosis: 2017 revisions of the McDonald criteria, Lancet Neurol 17:162–173, 2018.

West TW, Hess C, Cree BA: Acute transverse myelitis: demyelinating, inflammatory, and infectious myelopathies, Semin Neurol 32:97–113, 2012.

amphiphysin 相关的副肿瘤综合征可导致传导束特异性脊髓病。在进行病史和体格检查时应考虑到这些疾病。

根据最可能的病因确定治疗方法。特发性 TM 的治疗方法与 MS 或 NMO 中的 TM 很相似，都是静脉注射甲泼尼龙，剂量为每天 500～1000 mg/d，通常序贯短期口服泼尼松治疗，而后逐渐减停。当对静脉甲泼尼龙的反应不理想时，应考虑进行血浆置换。

特发性急性视神经炎

炎性脱髓鞘性视神经炎可能是 MS 或 NMO 的部分发作，也可能是一种特发性疾病。通常，视神经炎会在数小时内出现视力减退，并伴有因眼球运动而加剧的疼痛。视力丧失的程度从亚临床到完全失明不等。色觉和对比敏感度受累尤为严重。检查时，单侧视神经炎患者会出现相对性传入性瞳孔障碍。急性脱髓鞘性视神经炎通常为球后性，无视盘炎。磁共振成像时，视神经会肿胀并表现为钆增强。急性发作恢复后，视盘可显苍白，相对性传入性瞳孔障碍可能持续存在。恢复后，当运动或发热导致体温升高时，视力可能会一过性恶化（Uhthoff 现象）。其鉴别诊断包括导致急性单眼或双眼视力丧失的其他原因，如 Leber 遗传性视神经病变、巨细胞动脉炎和急性非动脉炎性前部缺血性视神经病变。

视神经炎治疗试验纳入急性视神经炎（特发性或由 MS 导致）患者，随机被分为三组，即静脉注射甲泼尼龙组、口服泼尼松逐渐减量组与口服安慰剂组。治疗初始阶段，静脉注射甲泼尼龙组的患者视力恢复更快，但治疗 6 个月后，三组之间并没有差异，视力恢复情况均良好。该试验的患者在 10 年后接受了视力检查，74% 的患者患眼视力达到或超过 20/20，只有 3% 的患者视力低于 20/200。然而，视神经炎复发较常见，35% 的患者两眼均有复发。MS 患者的复发率高于特发性视神经炎患者（$P < 0.001$）。

慢性复发性炎症性视神经病变

慢性复发性炎症性视神经病变（CRION）于 2003 年首次被报道，是以急性复发为特征的炎症性视神经病变，视力丧失通常比特发性视神经炎或与 MS 相关的视神经炎更严重。CRION 可在任何年龄段发病，世界各地均有病例报道。患病率和流行病学尚不清楚。与其他类型的视神经炎一样，CRION 发病时常伴有眼痛。CRION 有 5 项诊断标准：①视神经炎至少复发一次；②视力下降；④血清 AQP4-IgG 阴性；④急性炎性视神经的 MRI 检查强化；⑤对免疫抑制治疗有反应，停药后复发。诊断该病时应排除可能出现类似表现的其他疾病，如结节病和巨细胞动脉炎。CRION 急性发作的治疗方法与其他原因引起的视神经炎类似，都是使用大剂量甲泼尼龙。停用皮质类固醇后复发较常见。有报道称，使用"无类固醇"治疗药物（如氨甲蝶呤、硫唑嘌呤或吗替麦考酚酯）进行长期治疗可取得成功。该病潜在的病理机制尚不清楚，但根据临床表现、影像学检查和对特定药物的治疗反应，该病可能是炎症性病变。患者最终的视觉预后通常较差。报告显示，1/3 的 CRION 患者视力低于 20/200。

推荐阅读

Correale J, Gaitán MI, Ysrraelit MC, Fiol MP: Progressive multiple sclerosis: from pathogenic mechanisms to treatment, Brain 140:527–546, 2017.

Kim SH, Huh SY, Lee SJ: A 5-year follow-up of rituximab treatment in patients with neuromyelitis optica spectrum disorder, JAMA Neurol 70:1110–1117, 2013.

Klaver R, De Vries HE, Schenk GJ, et al: Grey matter damage in multiple sclerosis: a pathology perspective, Prion 7:66–75, 2013.

Langer-Gould A, Brara SM, Beaber BE, et al: Incidence of multiple sclerosis in multiple racial and ethnic groups, Neurology 80:1734–1739, 2013.

Lublin FD, Reingold SC, Cohen JA, et al: Defining the clinical course of multiple sclerosis: the 2013 revisions, Neurology 83:277–286, 2014.

Petzold A, Plant GT: Chronic relapsing inflammatory optic neuropathy: a systematic review of 122 cases reported, J Neurol 261:17–26, 2014.

Pittock SJ, Berthele A, Fujihara K, et al: Eculizumab in aquaporin-4-positive neuromyelitis optica spectrum disorder, N Engl J Med 381:614–625, 2019.

Reindl M, Di Pauli F, Rostásy K, Berger T: The spectrum of MOG antibody-associated demyelinating disorders, Nat Rev Neurol 9:455–461, 2013.

Thompson AJ, Banwell BL, Barkhof F, et al: Diagnosis of multiple sclerosis: 2017 revisions of the McDonald criteria, Lancet Neurol 17:162–173, 2018.

West TW, Hess C, Cree BA: Acute transverse myelitis: demyelinating, inflammatory, and infectious myelopathies, Semin Neurol 32:97–113, 2012.

18

Neuromuscular Diseases: Disorders of the Motor Neuron and Plexus and Peripheral Nerve Disease

Carlayne E. Jackson, Ratna Bhavaraju-Sanka

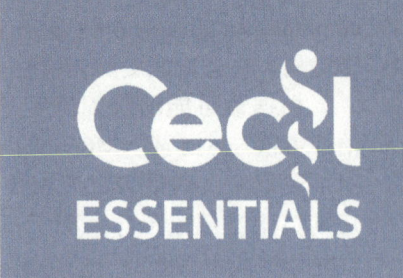

INTRODUCTION

Neuromuscular diseases are classified into four groups, according to which portion of the motor unit is involved (Table 18.1). Motor neuron and peripheral nerve diseases are considered in this chapter; myopathies are considered in Chapter 19, and neuromuscular junction diseases are considered in Chapter 20. The symptoms and signs of the neuromuscular diseases are at times indistinguishable. However, some useful general rules apply to assist with localization based on the distribution of weakness, presence or absence of sensory symptoms, reflex abnormalities, and specific associated clinical features (Table 18.2).

Electromyography and Nerve Conduction Studies

Electromyography (EMG) and nerve conduction studies can also be useful diagnostic tools in localizing the lesion in a patient with a suspected neuromuscular disease. The measurement of electrical activity arising from muscle fibers is performed by inserting a needle electrode percutaneously into a muscle. Normal muscle is electrically silent at rest. Spontaneous activity during complete relaxation occurs in myotonic disorders, in inflammatory myopathies, and in denervated muscles. Spontaneous activity of a single muscle fiber is called a *fibrillation*, and such activity of part of or an entire motor unit is called a *fasciculation*. In myotonia, repeated muscle depolarization and contraction occur despite voluntary relaxation. Abnormalities in motor unit potentials occur during the course of denervation; with the development of reinnervation, the remaining motor units increase in amplitude and become longer in duration and polyphasic. Conversely, in muscle diseases such as the muscular dystrophies and other diseases that destroy scattered fibers within a motor unit, the motor unit action potentials are of lower amplitude and shorter duration and are polyphasic. A reduced recruitment (interference) pattern from maximum voluntary effort occurs in denervation. Conversely, in patients with primary muscle disease, submaximal voluntary effort produces a full recruitment pattern despite marked weakness.

Nerve conduction is studied by stimulating a peripheral nerve (e.g., the ulnar) with surface electrodes placed over the nerve or muscle. The resulting action potential is recorded by electrodes placed over the nerve more proximally in the case of large sensory nerve fibers and over the muscle distally in the case of motor nerve fibers in a mixed motor sensory nerve. For sensory nerves, the sensory nerve action potential (SNAP) is quantitated, and for motor nerves, the compound muscle action potential (CMAP) is quantitated. Abnormalities in sensory and motor nerve studies are suggestive of a peripheral neuropathy while abnormalities in motor nerve studies with normal sensory studies can indicate a myopathy, motor neuronopathy, pure motor neuropathy or radiculopathy.

DISEASES OF THE MOTOR NEURON (ANTERIOR HORN CELL)

Amyotrophic Lateral Sclerosis

Definition and Epidemiology

The most common *acquired* motor neuron disease, amyotrophic lateral sclerosis (ALS), is a progressive, typically fatal disorder. The incidence is approximately 2 to 5 per 100,000 population, and there is a slight male predominance. The peak age of onset is in the sixth decade, although the disease can occur at any time throughout adulthood. The cumulative lifetime risk is about 1 in 400. Epidemiologic studies have incriminated risk factors for ALS including exposure to insecticides, smoking, participation in varsity athletics, and military service in the Gulf War. The cause of ALS is largely unknown, with 95% of cases considered "sporadic," and 5% related to an autosomal dominant disease (familial ALS [FALS]). FALS is an adult-onset disease that is clinically and pathologically indistinguishable from sporadic ALS. FALS is caused by mutations in many genes, including the *C9orf72*, *SOD1*, *TARDBP*, *FUS*, *ANG*, *ALS2*, *SETX*, and *VAPB* genes. Mutations in the *C9orf72* gene are responsible for 30% to 45% of FALS in the United States and Europe. Mutations in *C9orf72* also cause sporadic ALS.

Pathology

ALS results from degeneration of the cortical motor neurons originating in layer five of the motor cortex and descending via the pyramidal tract (resulting in upper motor neuron signs and symptoms) and from degeneration of the anterior horn cells in the spinal cord and their brain stem homologues innervating bulbar muscles (resulting in lower motor neuron signs and symptoms) (Table 18.3).

Clinical Presentation

Clinical symptoms relating to the upper motor neuron degeneration include loss of dexterity, slowed movements, muscle weakness, stiffness, and emotional lability. Signs on neurologic examination that confirm an upper motor neuron lesion include pseudobulbar affect, pathologic hyperreflexia, spasticity, and extensor plantar responses (Babinski sign). Lower motor neuron signs and symptoms caused by anterior horn cell degeneration include weakness, muscle atrophy, fasciculations, and cramps. Fasciculations in the absence of associated muscle atrophy or weakness are usually benign and may be aggravated by sleep deprivation, stress, and excessive caffeine ingestion. Muscle weakness in patients with ALS usually begins distally and asymmetrically and may manifest as a monoparesis, hemiparesis, paraparesis, or quadriparesis. It may also be limited initially to the bulbar region, resulting in difficulty with swallowing, speech, and movements of the

18 神经肌肉疾病：运动神经元和神经丛疾病以及周围神经疾病

陈奕奕 译　高颖 杨营营 审校　王伊龙 通审

引言

根据运动单位的受累部位，神经肌肉疾病分为四类（表18.1）。本章介绍运动神经元和周围神经疾病，第19章介绍肌病，第20章介绍神经肌肉接头疾病。神经肌肉疾病的症状和体征有时难以鉴别，但可以通过一些基本规则进行辅助定位诊断，例如根据无力的分布、是否存在感觉症状、反射的异常和特定的相关临床特征（表18.2）。

肌电图和神经传导检查

对于疑诊神经肌肉疾病的患者，肌电图和神经传导检查是进行病灶定位的重要诊断工具，其原理是通过将针状电极经皮插入肌肉来测量肌纤维产生的电活动。正常的肌肉在安静状态下没有电活动，肌强直性障碍、炎性肌病和失神经支配的肌肉在完全放松时则会出现自发电活动。单个肌纤维自发的电活动称为肌纤维震颤，而部分或整个运动单位的这种电活动则称为肌束震颤。在肌强直时，尽管可以自主放松，肌肉仍然会出现反复的去极化和收缩。在失神经支配的过程中，运动单位电位会出现异常；随着神经再生，剩余运动单位的波幅增加、时限增宽，并具有多相性。相反，在肌病（如肌营养不良和其他破坏运动单位内散在肌纤维的疾病）中，运动单位动作电位的波幅降低、时限缩短，并具有多相性。在失神经支配时，最大力收缩时见募集相（干扰）减少。相反，在原发性肌病患者中，尽管有明显的无力，次大力收缩时可产生完整的募集相。

神经传导是通过放置在神经或肌肉上方的表面电极刺激周围神经（如尺神经）进行检查。对于大的感觉神经纤维，在神经近端放置电极记录动作电位；对于运动感觉混合神经中的运动神经纤维，电极则放置在支配的肌肉远端。神经传导检查可以定量检测感觉神经的感觉神经动作电位（SNAP）和运动神经的复合肌肉动作电位（CMAP）。感觉和运动神经检查均异常提示周围神经病，而感觉神经检查正常、运动神经检查异常可能提示肌病、运动神经元病、纯运动神经病或神经根病变。

运动神经元（前角细胞）病

肌萎缩侧索硬化

定义和流行病学

肌萎缩侧索硬化（ALS）是最常见的获得性运动神经元病，其病程呈进行性发展，具有高度的致死性。发病率为每10万人中2~5人，男性略高于女性。发病高峰年龄在50~60岁，但也见于整个成年期的任何时段。终生累积发病风险约为1/400。流行病学研究显示，ALS的危险因素包括杀虫剂暴露、吸烟、参与大学校队运动以及在海湾战争中服役。ALS病因大多不明，95%的病例认为是"散发性"，5%的病例与常染色体显性遗传病［家族性肌萎缩侧索硬化（FALS）］有关。FALS在成年期发病，在临床和病理上与散发性ALS难以鉴别。FALS由许多基因突变引起，包括 C9orf72、SOD1、TARDBP、FUS、ANG、ALS2、SETX 和 VAPB 基因。在美国和欧洲，30%~45%的FALS是由 C9orf72 基因突变引起。C9orf72 基因突变也会引起散发性ALS。

病理学

ALS是由于起源于运动皮质第五层并通过锥体束下行的皮质运动神经元变性（导致上运动神经元症状和体征），以及脊髓前角细胞和负责延髓支配肌肉的脑干后组运动神经元变性（导致下运动神经元症状和体征）引起（表18.3）。

临床表现

与上运动神经元变性有关的临床症状包括动作灵活性丧失、运动减慢、肌肉无力、僵硬以及情绪不稳。神经系统检查可证实上运动神经元病变的体征包括假性延髓麻痹、病理反射亢进、痉挛状态和伸跖反射（巴宾斯基征）。由前角细胞变性引起的下运动神经元症状和体征包括无力、肌萎缩、肌束震颤和痉挛。不伴有肌肉萎缩或无力的肌束震颤通常是良性的，可能会因睡眠剥夺、应激和过量摄入咖啡因而加重。ALS患者的肌无力通常从远端开始，且不对称，可能表现为单肢轻瘫、轻偏瘫、轻截瘫或四肢轻瘫；最初也可能

face and tongue. For unclear reasons, ocular motility is spared until the very late stages of the illness. Bowel and bladder function and sensation remain spared throughout the course of the disease although patients may develop symptoms of bladder urgency. Up to 60% of patients with ALS may also have a component of frontotemporal dementia characterized by executive dysfunction, poor insight, personality changes (disinhibition, impulsivity, apathy), abnormal eating habits, poor hygiene, and language dysfunction.

Diagnosis/Differential

The diagnosis of ALS remains one of "exclusion," in which other potential causes must be ruled out through a variety of neuroimaging, laboratory, and electrodiagnostic investigations. For example, compression of the cervical spinal cord or cervicomedullary junction from tumors or cervical spondylosis can produce weakness, atrophy, and fasciculations in the upper extremities and spasticity in the lower extremities, closely resembling ALS.

Treatment

Specialized multidisciplinary clinic referral should be considered for patients with ALS to optimize health care delivery and prolong survival. The first US Food and Drug Administration (FDA)–approved therapy for ALS was riluzole 50 mg twice per day, which in clinical trials prolonged survival by 2 to 3 months. The mechanism of this effect is not known with certainty; however, riluzole may reduce excitotoxicity by diminishing presynaptic glutamate release. Edaravone was also recently FDA approved based on studies suggesting a slowing of the rate of functional decline by 33% (measured by the ALS Functional Rating Scale-Revised). Initiation of noninvasive ventilation (NIV) on a spontaneous timed mode has also been shown to prolong survival up to 20 months, to slow the rate of forced vital capacity (FVC) decline (level B) and to improve quality of life. NIV should be initiated when the FVC is less than 50%, the maximal inspiratory pressure is less than −60 cm, or when patients report symptoms that suggest nocturnal hypoventilation (daytime fatigue, frequent arousals, supine dyspnea, morning headaches). A cough-assist device can be used to assist with clearing upper airway secretions and has been shown to minimize the risk of pneumonia in clinical trials. A percutaneous gastrostomy (PEG) tube should be considered for prolonging survival and stabilizing body weight in patients with impaired oral food intake. Symptomatic therapy for spasticity, pseudobulbar affect, muscle cramping, and sialorrhea is also essential in maintaining patient dignity and quality of life (Table 18.4). Augmentative speech devices can assist patients with communication and computer access.

TABLE 18.1 Classification of Neuromuscular Diseases

Site of Involvement	Typical Examples
Anterior Horn Cell	
Without upper motor neuron involvement	Spinal muscular atrophy
	Progressive muscular atrophy
	Bulbospinal muscular atrophy
	Poliomyelitis
	West Nile virus
With upper motor neuron involvement	Amyotrophic lateral sclerosis
	Primary lateral sclerosis
Peripheral Nerve	
Mononeuropathy	Carpal tunnel syndrome
	Ulnar palsy
	Meralgia paresthetica
Multiple mononeuropathies	Mononeuritis multiplex (e.g., polyarteritis nodosa), leprosy, sarcoidosis, amyloidosis
Polyneuropathies	Diabetic neuropathy
	Charcot-Marie-Tooth disease
	Guillain-Barré syndrome
Neuromuscular Junction	
	Myasthenia gravis
	Lambert-Eaton syndrome
Muscle	
	Duchenne muscular dystrophy
	Dermatomyositis

TABLE 18.3 Symptoms and Signs Associated With Amyotrophic Lateral Sclerosis

Symptoms	Signs
Upper Motor Neuron Degeneration	
Loss of dexterity	Pathologic hyperreflexia
Slowed movements	Babinski response
Weakness	Hoffman response
Stiffness	Jaw jerk
Pseudobulbar affect	Spasticity
Lower Motor Neuron Degeneration	
Weakness	Muscle atrophy
Fasciculations	Fibrillation potentials on electromyography
Cramps	Neurogenic atrophy on muscle biopsy

TABLE 18.2 Clinical Features of the Neuromuscular Diseases

Clinical Feature	Anterior Horn Cell	Peripheral Nerve	Neuromuscular Junction	Muscle
Distribution of weakness	Asymmetrical limb or bulbar	Symmetrical, usually distal	Extraocular, bulbar, proximal limb	Symmetrical, proximal limb
Atrophy	Marked and early	Mild, distal	None (or very late)	Slight early; marked later
Sensory involvement	None	Dysesthesias, loss of sensation	None	None
Reflexes	Variable (depending on degree of upper motor neuron involvement)	Decreased out of proportion to weakness	Normal in myasthenia gravis, depressed in Lambert-Eaton syndrome	Decreased in proportion to weakness
Characteristic features	Fasciculations, cramps	Combined sensory and motor abnormalities	Fatigability	Usually painless

局限于延髓区域，导致吞咽、言语困难以及面部和舌运动困难。基于不明的原因，疾病晚期才会出现眼球运动不能。虽然患者可能会出现膀胱急迫症状，但在整个病程中，肠道和膀胱的功能和感觉都不会受到影响。多达 60% 的 ALS 患者可能还伴有额颞叶痴呆的症状，表现为执行功能障碍、自知力差、人格改变（去抑制、冲动、情感淡漠）、饮食习惯异常、卫生条件差和语言功能障碍。

诊断和鉴别诊断

ALS 的诊断仍然是排他性的，必须通过各种神经影像学、实验室检查和电生理检查排除其他潜在病因。例如，肿瘤或颈椎病压迫颈髓或颈-延髓交界处会导致上肢无力、肌萎缩和肌束震颤以及下肢痉挛状态，这与 ALS 非常相似。

治疗

为优化 ALS 患者的医疗服务并延长其生存期，应推荐转诊至专业的多学科诊所。美国食品和药物管理局（FDA）已批准利鲁唑作为首个治疗 ALS 的药物，推荐剂量为每次 50 mg，每日 2 次。临床试验提示其能延长患者生存期 2～3 个月。这种药物的作用机制尚不确切，但利鲁唑可能通过减少突触前谷氨酸释放来减轻兴奋性毒性。近期，基于一项依达拉奉可将患者的功能衰退速度减缓 33%（根据 ALS 功能评定量表-修订版评估）的研究证据，FDA 批准了依达拉奉的应用。研究还表明，以自定发定时模式启动无创通气（NIV）可延长患者生存期长达 20 个月，同时减缓用力肺活量（FVC）的下降（B 级证据），并改善生活质量。当 FVC 低于 50%、最大吸气压力低于 -60 cmH$_2$O，或患者出现夜间通气不足的症状，如日间疲劳、频繁觉醒、仰卧位呼吸困难、晨起头痛时，应启动 NIV。咳嗽辅助装置可用于辅助清除上气道分泌物，并被临床试验证实可使肺炎风险降至最低。对于经口进食受限的患者，经皮内镜下胃造瘘（PEG）管是延长生存期和维持体重的重要措施。对于痉挛状态、假性延髓麻痹、肌肉痉挛和流涎的患者，对症治疗对维持患者的尊严和生存质量也至关重要（表 18.4）。此外，言语辅助设备有助于患者进行交流和计算机操作能力的提升。

表 18.1 神经肌肉疾病的分类

累及部位	典型疾病
前角细胞	
不伴有上运动神经元受累	脊髓性肌萎缩 进行性肌萎缩 延髓脊肌萎缩 脊髓灰质炎 西尼罗病毒感染
伴有上运动神经元受累	肌萎缩侧索硬化 原发性侧索硬化
周围神经	
单神经病	腕管综合征 尺神经麻痹 感觉异常性股痛
多发性单神经病	多发性单神经炎（如结节性多动脉炎）、麻风病、结节病、淀粉样变性
多发性神经病	糖尿病神经病变 夏科-马里-图思病（进行性腓骨肌萎缩症） 吉兰-巴雷综合征
神经肌肉接头	重症肌无力 兰伯特-伊顿综合征
肌肉	进行性假肥大性肌营养不良 皮肌炎

表 18.3 与肌萎缩侧索硬化相关的症状和体征

症状	体征
上运动神经元变性	
动作灵活性丧失	病理反射亢进
运动减慢	巴宾斯基征
无力	霍夫曼征
僵硬	下颌反射
假性延髓麻痹	痉挛状态
下运动神经元变性	
无力	肌萎缩
肌束震颤	肌电图可见纤颤电位
痉挛	肌肉活检可见神经源性萎缩

表 18.2 神经肌肉疾病的临床特征

临床特征	前角细胞	周围神经	神经肌肉接头	肌肉
无力的分布	非对称的肢体或延髓支配肌	对称的，通常是肢体远端	眼外肌、延髓支配肌、近端肢体	对称的，近端肢体
肌肉萎缩	显著，早期	轻度，远端	无（或晚期）	早期轻微，晚期显著
感觉受累	无	感觉迟钝、感觉丧失	无	无
腱反射	可变的（取决于上运动神经元受累程度）	与无力呈不成比例地下降	重症肌无力正常，兰伯特-伊顿综合征下降	与无力呈成比例地下降
典型特征	肌束震颤、痉挛	感觉与运动异常均存在	易疲劳性	通常是无痛性的

TABLE 18.4 Symptom Management for Motor Neuron Diseases
Respiratory Insufficiency
Noninvasive ventilation
Cough-assist devices
Dysarthria
Augmentative speech device
Dysphagia
Percutaneous endoscopic gastrostomy (PEG) placement
Suction machine
Sialorrhea
Amitriptyline 25-75 mg qhs
Glycopyrrolate 1-2 mg q8h
Botulinum toxin
Spasticity
Baclofen 10-20 mg QID
Dantrium 25-100 mg QID
Pseudobulbar Affect
Serotonin reuptake inhibitors
Amitriptyline 25-75 mg QHS
Dextromethorphan/quinidine 20/10 mg BID
Weakness
Ankle-foot orthosis
Wheelchair
Elevated toilet seat

TABLE 18.5 Clinical Spectrum of Motor Neuron Diseases[a]
Upper and Lower Motor Neuron Involvement
Sporadic amyotrophic lateral sclerosis
Familial amyotrophic lateral sclerosis
Upper Motor Neuron Involvement
Primary lateral sclerosis
Hereditary spastic paraparesis
Lower Motor Neuron Involvement
Motor neuronopathy related to malignancy or paraproteinemia
Poliomyelitis
West Nile virus
Postpolio syndrome
Hexosaminidase deficiency
Progressive muscular atrophy
Spinal muscular atrophy
Type I: Infantile onset (Werdnig-Hoffmann disease)
Type II: Late infantile onset
Type III: Juvenile onset (Kugelberg-Welander disease)

[a]Italicized disorders are hereditary.

Prognosis

Mean survival from onset of symptoms is 2 to 5 years, with 10% of patients surviving beyond 10 years. The majority of deaths are related to respiratory muscle failure and aspiration pneumonia.

Other Acquired Motor Neuron Diseases

Other motor neuron diseases involve only particular subsets of motor neurons (Table 18.5). Progressive muscular atrophy (PMA) is a pure lower motor neuron disease that accounts for 8% to 10% of patients with motor neuron disease. Weakness is typically distal and asymmetrical, and bulbar involvement is rare. Patients with PMA generally have a better prognosis than those with ALS, with a survival of 3 to 14 years. Primary lateral sclerosis (PLS) is a pure upper motor neuron syndrome in which patients demonstrate either a slowly progressive spastic paralysis or dysarthria. This is a rare disorder, accounting for 2% of all motor neuron cases. Survival is generally years to decades.

Spinal Muscular Atrophy

Spinal muscular atrophy (SMA) is a hereditary form of motor neuron disease in which only the lower motor neuron is affected. It is an autosomal recessive disorder that may begin in utero, in infancy, in childhood, or in adult life and represents the first class of neurologic disorders in which a developmental defect in neuronal apoptosis most likely produces the disease. The most common forms of SMA are due to a defect in the survival motor neuron 1 *(SMN1)* gene localized to 5q11.2-q13.3. All affected individuals with SMA have mutations in both copies of the *SMN1* gene causing little or no SMN (survival motor neuron) protein production from this gene. The *SMN2* gene can help replace some of the missing SMN protein. Patients who have multiple copies of the *SMN2* gene are usually associated with later onset and less severe disease. Nusinersen was recently approved for intrathecal use and has been shown to significantly slow functional decline and increase life expectancy. It is an antisense oligonucleotide targeted to increase the proportion of SMN2 mRNA transcripts, leading to translation of more full-length SMN protein. In May of 2019 the FDA also approved onasemnogene abeparvovec-xioi (Zolgensma), the first gene therapy to treat children less than 2 years of age with SMA.

Bulbospinal muscular atrophy (BSMA) or Kennedy disease is an X-linked recessive disorder in which the mean age at onset is 30 years; the range is from 15 to 60 years. BSMA is a trinucleotide repeat disorder with a CAG expansion encoding for a polyglutamine tract in the first exon of the androgen receptor gene, on chromosome Xq11-12. The mechanism by which disruption of the androgen receptor gene alters the function of bulbar and spinal motor neurons is not known. An inverse correlation exists between the number of CAG repeats and the age of onset of the disease. Affected individuals exhibit chin fasciculations, midline furrowing and atrophy of the tongue, and proximal weakness. Dysphagia and dysarthria are common, and up to 90% of patients demonstrate gynecomastia and infertility. Two findings distinguishing this disorder from ALS are the absence of upper motor neuron signs and in some patients the presence of a subtle sensory neuropathy.

DISORDERS OF THE BRACHIAL AND LUMBOSACRAL PLEXUS

The roots within the cervical, lumbar, and sacral regions organize into the cervical, lumbar, and sacral plexuses before giving rise to individual peripheral nerves. Diseases of these plexuses (plexopathies) tend to be *focal* in symptoms and signs, whereas many diseases of the peripheral nerves and muscles are *generalized.*

Brachial Plexopathy

The brachial plexus is constituted by mixed nerve roots from C5 to T1 that fuse into upper, middle, and lower trunks above the level of the clavicle and redistribute into lateral, posterior, and medial cords below that landmark. Symptoms include weakness, pain, and sensory loss in the shoulders or arms. Upper trunk lesions may be due to birth injury, trauma, and idiopathic brachial plexitis (see later). Lower trunk lesions may result from birth injury, malignant tumor invasion, thoracic outlet syndrome, or as a complication of sternotomy. If the entire plexus is involved, radiation injury, trauma, and late metastatic disease are the most common causes.

表 18.4　运动神经元病的症状管理
呼吸功能不全
无创通气
咳嗽辅助设备
构音障碍
辅助语音设备
吞咽困难
经皮内镜下胃造瘘（PEG）
吸痰机
流涎
阿米替林，25～75 mg，每日睡前
格隆溴铵，1～2 mg，每8 h一次
肉毒杆菌毒素
痉挛状态
巴氯芬，每次10～20 mg，每日4次
丹曲林钠，每次25～100 mg，每日4次
假性延髓麻痹
5-羟色胺再摄取抑制剂
阿米替林，25～75 mg，每日睡前
右美沙芬/奎尼丁，每次20/10 mg，每日2次
无力
踝-足矫形器
轮椅
加高马桶座椅

表 18.5　运动神经元病的临床谱系[a]
上、下运动神经元受累
散发性肌萎缩侧索硬化
家族性肌萎缩侧索硬化
上运动神经元受累
原发性侧索硬化
遗传性痉挛性截瘫
下运动神经元受累
与恶性肿瘤或副蛋白血症相关的运动神经元病
脊髓灰质炎
西尼罗病毒感染
脊髓灰质炎后综合征
氨基己糖苷酶缺乏症
进行性肌萎缩
脊髓性肌萎缩
Ⅰ型：婴儿期型（韦德尼希-霍夫曼综合征）
Ⅱ型：迟发婴儿型
Ⅲ型：青少年型（库格尔贝格-韦兰德病）

[a] 以斜体显示的疾病为遗传病。

预后

患者平均生存期为出现症状后2～5年，10%的患者可存活10年以上；多死于呼吸肌衰竭或吸入性肺炎。

其他获得性运动神经元病

其他运动神经元病只累及特定的运动神经元亚群（表18.5）。进行性肌萎缩（PMA）是一种单纯下运动神经元病，占运动神经元病患者的8%～10%。患者无力通常在远端且不对称，很少累及延髓支配肌肉。PMA患者的预后通常比ALS患者好，生存期3～14年。原发性侧索硬化（PLS）是一种单纯上运动神经元综合征，患者表现为缓慢进行性痉挛性瘫痪或构音障碍。这是一种罕见的疾病，占所有运动神经元病例的2%，生存期一般为数年至数十年。

脊髓性肌萎缩

脊髓性肌萎缩（SMA）是一种单纯累及下运动神经元的遗传性运动神经元病，遵循常染色体隐性遗传模式。其发病可始于子宫内、婴儿期、儿童期或成年期，属于第一类神经系统疾病，SMA的发病机制常涉及神经元凋亡的发育缺陷。最常见的SMA类型是由位于5q11.2-q13.3的存活运动神经元1（*SMN1*）基因缺陷所致。所有SMA患者均表现为*SMN1*基因双拷贝突变，导致SMN蛋白显著减少或完全缺失。*SMN2*基因能部分补偿SMN蛋白的缺失，有*SMN2*基因拷贝数较多的患者通常发病较晚、病情较轻。诺西那生最近被批准用于鞘内注射，可显著减缓功能衰退并延长预期寿命；这是一种反义寡核苷酸，可增加SMN2 mRNA转录物的比例，促进更多的全长SMN蛋白的产生。

2019年5月，FDA批准了索伐瑞韦（Zolgensma）作为首个可用于2岁以下SMA儿童的基因治疗药物。

延髓脊肌萎缩（BSMA）又称肯尼迪病，是一种X连锁隐性遗传病，发病年龄横跨15～60岁，平均发病年龄30岁。BSMA是一种三核苷酸重复序列疾病，特征为X染色体q11-12区域雄激素受体基因的第一个外显子上有胞嘧啶-腺嘌呤-鸟嘌呤（CAG）重复序列扩增，导致多聚谷氨酰胺束的编码异常。尽管雄激素受体基因受损影响延髓和脊髓运动神经元功能的机制尚不清楚，但CAG重复序列的数量与发病年龄呈负相关。患者表现为颏肌束颤、舌中线形成沟和舌肌萎缩以及近端肢体无力，吞咽困难和构音障碍亦常见，有高达90%的患者会出现男性乳房发育和不孕不育。BSMA与ALS的主要区别在于患者无上运动神经元体征，以及部分患者伴有轻微的感觉神经病变。

臂丛和腰骶丛疾病

颈椎、腰椎和骶椎区域内的神经根组成颈丛、腰丛和骶丛，然后再发出单个的周围神经。这些神经丛疾病（神经丛病）的症状和体征往往是局灶性的，而许多周围神经和肌肉疾病则是全身性的。

臂丛神经病

臂丛神经由C5～T1的混合神经根构成，在锁骨水平以上融合成上、中、下干，在锁骨水平以下重新分布成外侧束、后束和内侧束。臂丛神经病的症状包括肩部或手臂无力、疼痛和感觉丧失。上干病变可能是由于产伤、创伤和特发性臂丛神经炎造成（见后文），下干病变可能是产伤、恶性肿瘤侵犯、胸廓出口综合征或胸骨切开术并发症所致。整个臂丛受累最常见的原因包括放射性损伤、创伤和晚期转移性疾病。

Acute Autoimmune Brachial Neuritis

Acute autoimmune brachial neuritis (or neuralgic amyotrophy or Parsonage-Turner syndrome) is characterized by the abrupt onset of severe pain, usually over the lateral shoulder, but at times extending into the neck or entire arm. The acute pain generally subsides after a few days to a week; by this time, weakness of the proximal arm becomes apparent. The serratus anterior, deltoid, and supraspinatus are the most commonly affected muscles, but other muscles of the shoulder girdle may also be affected. In rare cases, most of the patient's arm and even the ipsilateral diaphragm are involved. Sensory loss is usually slight and generally involves the axillary nerve distribution. Weakness lasts weeks to months and will be accompanied by severe atrophy of the shoulder girdle. No therapy has been shown to alter or shorten the clinical course, although steroids and analgesics may reduce pain. Most patients recover within several months to 3 years. The disorder frequently follows an upper respiratory infection or an immunization, but in many instances no antecedent illness occurs. It is bilateral in one third of cases but is always asymmetrical; it may recur in 5% of patients. Recurrent brachial plexopathies that are painless may be related to an autosomal dominant disorder with mutation in the *SEPTIN9* gene on chromosome 17q25 or hereditary neuropathy with liability to pressure palsies (HNPP), caused by a deletion or point mutation of PMP-22 protein (chromosome 17p).

Lumbosacral Plexopathy

The lumbosacral plexus is formed from the ventral rami of spinal nerves T12 to S4. These divide within the plexus into ventral and dorsal branches that form the femoral, sciatic, and obturator nerves. The plexus is located within the substance of the psoas major muscle. Clinical features include proximal pain and weakness in anterior thigh muscles (femoral) or posterior thigh muscles and the buttocks. Bowel and bladder dysfunction may also occur. Diabetes, malignant invasion, radiation therapy, infection (herpes zoster), psoas abscess, trauma, and retroperitoneal hemorrhage are common causes. An autoimmune form is much less frequent than brachial neuritis.

DISORDERS OF THE PERIPHERAL NERVES

Definition and Epidemiology

Peripheral neuropathy refers to a large group of disorders that can produce focal (mononeuropathy or multiple mononeuropathies) or generalized nerve dysfunction (polyneuropathies) (Table 18.6). Peripheral neuropathies are prevalent neurologic conditions, affecting 2% to 8% of adults, with the incidence increasing with age. They range in severity from mild sensory abnormalities, found in up to 70% of patients with long-standing diabetes, to fulminant, life-threatening paralytic disorders such as Guillain-Barré syndrome (GBS) or acute inflammatory demyelinating polyradiculoneuropathy (AIDP).

Mononeuropathies are disorders in which only a single peripheral nerve is affected. The most common cause is nerve entrapment such as median nerve compression resulting in carpal tunnel syndrome or peroneal nerve injury causing foot drop (Table 18.7). When more than one peripheral nerve is involved, the term *mononeuropathy multiplex* or *multiple mononeuropathies* is often used. Multiple mononeuropathies are most commonly seen in diabetes mellitus and vasculitis but also occur in leprosy, vasculitis, sarcoidosis, hereditary neuropathy with predisposition to pressure palsies, and amyloidosis.

Polyneuropathies are a group of disorders affecting the motor, sensory, and autonomic nerves. These disorders may predominantly affect the nerve axon (axonal neuropathies), myelin sheath (demyelinating neuropathies), or the small- to medium-sized blood vessels supplying the nerves (vasculitic neuropathies). The clinical features of the polyneuropathies reflect the pathology of the underlying process.

TABLE 18.6 Classification and Causes of Peripheral Neuropathy

Type of Neuropathy	Examples
Mononeuropathies	
Compressive	Carpal tunnel syndrome, ulnar palsy
Hereditary	Hereditary neuropathy with predisposition to pressure palsies
Inflammatory	Bell's palsy
Multiple mononeuropathies	Vasculitis (mononeuritis multiplex), diabetes, leprosy, sarcoidosis, amyloidosis
Polyneuropathies	
Hereditary	Charcot-Marie-Tooth disease, familial amyloid polyneuropathy
Endocrine	Diabetes, hypothyroidism
Metabolic	Uremia, liver failure
Infections	Leprosy, diphtheria, human immunodeficiency virus, Lyme disease
Immune mediated	Guillain-Barré syndrome, chronic inflammatory demyelinating polyneuropathy
Toxic	Lead-, arsenic-, alcohol-, drug-induced
Paraneoplastic	Lung cancer

Pathology

In the symmetrical *axonal* polyneuropathies, the underlying pathology is usually a slowly evolving type of axonal degeneration that involves the ends of long nerve fibers first and preferentially. With time, the degenerative process involves more proximal regions of long fibers, and shorter fibers are affected. This pattern of distal axonal degeneration or *dying back* of nerve fibers results from a wide variety of metabolic, toxic, and endocrinologic causes.

In the *demyelinating* polyneuropathies, the underlying pathology involves the myelin sheath. Demyelination of a peripheral nerve at even a single site can block conduction, resulting in a functional deficit identical to that seen after axonal degeneration. In contrast to repair by regeneration, however, repair by remyelination can be rapid. Autoimmune attack on the myelin sheath occurs in the inflammatory demyelinating neuropathies (GBS/AIDP and chronic inflammatory demyelinating polyneuropathy [CIDP]) and some neuropathies associated with paraproteinemias (see later). Inherited disorders of myelin such as Charcot-Marie-Tooth (CMT) disease comprise the other major category of demyelinating neuropathies. Other causes include toxic, mechanical, and physical injuries to nerves. Although these examples have nearly pure demyelination, many neuropathies have both axonal degeneration and demyelination. This mixed pathologic abnormality reflects the mutual interdependency of the axons and the myelin-forming Schwann cells. Vasculitic neuropathies occur as a result of disease of the small or medium-sized blood vessels that leads to ischemia and infarction of isolated peripheral nerves. The term *mononeuritis multiplex* is also used to describe this clinical situation, in which there is multifocal involvement of individual nerves.

Clinical Presentation

The clinical picture of an *axonal* polyneuropathy includes early loss of muscle stretch reflexes at the ankle and weakness that initially involves the intrinsic muscles of the feet, the extensors of the toes, and the dorsiflexors at the ankle. The motor signs are usually mild in

急性自身免疫性臂丛神经炎

急性自身免疫性臂丛神经炎（或称神经痛性肌萎缩或 Parsonage-Turner 综合征）的特点是突然出现剧烈疼痛，通常发生在肩外侧，但有时也会延伸至颈部或整个手臂。急性疼痛一般会在几天到一周后缓解，期间手臂近端会出现明显的无力。前锯肌、三角肌和冈上肌是最常受累的肌肉，但其他肩带肌也可能受累；少数情况下，会累及手臂大部分肌肉甚至同侧膈肌。感觉缺失通常很轻微，通常累及腋神经分布区。肢体无力会持续数周至数月，并伴有严重的肩带肌萎缩。虽然类固醇和镇痛剂可以减轻疼痛，但目前尚没有可以改变或缩短病程的有效治疗。大多数患者可在数月至3年内痊愈。该病常发生在上呼吸道感染或免疫接种后，但在许多情况下并没有前驱疾病。1/3 的病例为双侧受累，但多不对称；5% 的患者可能会复发。无痛性复发性臂丛神经病可能与染色体 17q25 上 SEPTIN9 基因突变导致的常染色体显性遗传病有关，也可能与 PMP-22 蛋白（染色体 17p）缺失或点突变导致的遗传性压力易感性周围神经病（HNPP）有关。

腰骶丛神经病

腰骶丛由脊神经 T12～S4 的腹侧支构成，这些神经在神经丛内分为腹侧支和背侧支，再形成股神经、坐骨神经和闭孔神经。该神经丛位于腰大肌的深部。腰骶丛神经病的临床特征包括大腿前群肌肉（股）或大腿后群肌肉和臀部肌肉的近端疼痛和无力，还可能出现肠道与膀胱功能障碍。糖尿病、恶性肿瘤侵袭、放射治疗、感染（带状疱疹）、腰大肌脓肿、创伤和腹膜后出血是常见的病因。与臂丛神经炎相比，腰骶丛神经病中自身免疫性病因少见。

周围神经疾病

定义和流行病学

周围神经病是一大类可产生局灶性（单神经病或多发性单神经病）或全身性（多发性神经病）神经功能障碍的疾病（表 18.6）。周围神经病是一种常见的神经系统疾病，成年人患病率为 2%～8%，发病率随年龄增长而增加。其严重程度不一，可仅表现为轻微的感觉异常（多达 70% 的长期糖尿病患者会出现这种症状），也可能出现危及生命的严重瘫痪，如吉兰-巴雷综合征（GBS）或急性炎症性脱髓鞘性多发性神经根神经病（AIDP）。

单神经病是指只有单一周围神经受累的疾病。最常见的原因是神经卡压，如正中神经受压导致腕管综合征或腓神经损伤导致足下垂（表 18.7）。当不止一条周围神经受累时，通常称为多发性单神经病或多数性单神经病。多发性单神经病最常见于糖尿病和血管炎，也可见于麻风、结节病、遗传性压力易感性周围神经

表 18.6 周围神经病的分类和病因

神经病类型	示例
单神经病	
卡压性	腕管综合征、尺神经麻痹
遗传性	遗传性压力易感性神经病
炎症性	贝尔麻痹
多发性单神经病	血管炎（多发性单神经炎）、糖尿病、麻风、结节病、淀粉样变性
多发性神经病	
遗传性	夏科-马里-图思病、家族性淀粉样多发性神经病
内分泌	糖尿病、甲状腺功能减退症
代谢性	尿毒症、肝衰竭
感染性	麻风、白喉、人类免疫缺陷病毒、莱姆病
免疫介导性	吉兰-巴雷综合征、慢性炎症性脱髓鞘性多发性神经病
中毒性	铅、砷、酒精、药物诱发
副肿瘤性	肺癌

病和淀粉样变性。

多发性神经病是一组可累及运动神经、感觉神经和自主神经的疾病。这些疾病可能主要累及神经轴索（轴索性神经病）、髓鞘（脱髓鞘性神经病）或滋养神经的中小血管（血管炎性神经病）。多发性神经病的临床特征反映了潜在的病理过程。

病理学

在对称性轴索性多发性神经病中，潜在的病理变化通常是一种缓慢进展的轴索变性，首先且优先累及长神经纤维的末端。随着时间的推移，变性过程会累及长神经纤维更近端的区域，较短的神经纤维也会被累及。这种远端轴索变性或神经纤维逆死性改变可由各种各样的代谢性、中毒性和内分泌性因素导致。

脱髓鞘性多发性神经病的基本病理改变累及髓鞘。即使周围神经只有一个部位发生脱髓鞘，也会阻断信号传导，造成与轴索变性相同的功能障碍。不过，与轴索再生修复相比，髓鞘的修复速度更快。对髓鞘的自身免疫性攻击发生在炎症性脱髓鞘性神经病［GBS/AIDP 和慢性炎症性脱髓鞘性多发性神经病（CIDP）］以及一些与副蛋白血症相关的神经病中（见后文）。脱髓鞘性神经病的另一主要类型是遗传性脱髓鞘疾病［如夏科-马里-图思病（CMT）］。其他脱髓鞘性神经病的病因包括神经中毒、机械损伤和物理损伤。虽然这些疾病几乎都是单纯的脱髓鞘，但许多神经病同时存在轴索变性和脱髓鞘，这种混合性病理改变反映了轴索和形成髓鞘的施万细胞之间的相互依存关系。血管炎性神经病是由于小血管或中血管病变导致孤立的周围神经缺血和梗死而引起的。多发性单神经病一词也用于描述单个神经的多灶性受累这种临床情况。

临床表现

轴索性多发性神经病的临床表现包括踝反射的早期丧失，以及最初累及足内在肌、趾伸肌和踝背屈肌

TABLE 18.7 Common Mononeuropathies

	Precipitating Factors	Motor Signs and Symptoms	Sensory Signs and Symptoms	Treatment
Median Nerve				
Entrapment at the wrist (carpal tunnel syndrome)	Repetitive wrist flexion or sleep	Weakness in thenar muscle	Numbness, tingling, and/or pain in thumb, index finger, middle finger, and medial half of ring finger. Tinel and Phalen signs	Neutral wrist splint, carpal tunnel injections or surgery
Ulnar Nerve				
Entrapment at the elbow	External compression in condylar groove, fracture of humerus	Weakness or atrophy of the interossei and thumb adductor	Sensory loss in the little finger and contiguous half of the ring finger	Elbow pads; ulnar nerve transposition or decompression of cubital tunnel
Radial Nerve				
Entrapment at the spiral groove	Prolonged sleeping on arm after drinking excessive amounts of alcohol: "Saturday night palsy"	Wrist drop with sparing of elbow extension; weakness of finger and thumb extensors	Sensory loss on dorsum of hand	Spontaneous recovery; wrist splint
Femoral Nerve				
	Abdominal hysterectomy, hematoma, prolonged lithotomy position, diabetes	Weakness and atrophy of quadriceps	Sensory loss in anterior thigh and medial calf	Physical therapy
Lateral Femoral Cutaneous Nerve				
Meralgia paresthetica	Obesity, pregnancy, diabetes, constrictive belts	None	Sensory loss, pain, or tingling over anterolateral thigh	Weight loss; spontaneous recovery
Peroneal Nerve				
Entrapment at the fibular head	Habitual leg crossing, knee casts, prolonged squatting, profound weight loss	Weakness of ankle dorsiflexors or evertors and toe extensors	Sensory loss in anterolateral leg and dorsum of foot	Ankle-foot orthosis; remove source of compression
Sciatic Nerve				
	Injection injury, fracture or dislocation of hip	Weakness of hamstrings, ankle plantar flexors or dorsiflexors	Sensory loss in buttock, lateral calf, and foot	Ankle-foot orthosis; physical therapy
Tibial Nerve				
Entrapment in tarsal tunnel	External compression from tight shoes, trauma, tenosynovitis	None	Sensory loss and tingling in sole of foot	Tarsal tunnel injection, eliminate source of compression, medial arch support

contrast to the sensory abnormalities, which may include numbness, tingling, and burning sensations (dysesthesias). The sensory symptoms usually begin symmetrically in the toes and feet and then ascend proximally to the legs in a "stocking" distribution. When the sensory abnormalities reach the level of the knees, the symptoms begin in the hands, in a "glove" distribution. Truncal and abdominal dysesthesias may develop once the sensory abnormalities ascend to the level of the elbows.

The prominent clinical feature of an acquired *demyelinating* polyneuropathy is weakness that affects not only the distal muscles but also the proximal and facial muscles. Unlike in an axonal neuropathy, sensory loss is rarely the presenting symptom. Patients generally have diffuse hyporeflexia or areflexia.

Vasculitic neuropathies typically present with acute or subacute asymmetrical, predominantly distal weakness and sensory loss associated with severe pain.

Diagnosis/Differential

Neuropathic disorders can be broadly divided into those that are acquired and those that are hereditary (Table 18.8). Acquired disorders are the more common and have many causes: metabolic or endocrine disorders (diabetes mellitus, renal failure, porphyria); immune-mediated disorders (GBS, CIDP, multifocal motor neuropathy, anti-myelin-associated glycoprotein neuropathy); infectious causes (human immunodeficiency virus [HIV], Lyme disease, cytomegalovirus [CMV], syphilis, leprosy, diphtheria); medications (HIV drugs, chemotherapies); environmental toxins (heavy metals); or paraneoplastic processes. Diabetes mellitus and alcoholism are the most common causes of polyneuropathy in developed countries. As many as one third of acquired neuropathies are cryptogenic in which the etiology can never be identified. Causes of mononeuritis multiplex include systemic vasculitis (rheumatoid arthritis, systemic lupus erythematosus, Wegener granulomatosis, Churg-Strauss syndrome, polyarteritis nodosa) and primary peripheral system vasculitis (25% of cases).

表 18.7 常见的单神经病

	诱因	运动症状和体征	感觉症状和体征	治疗
正中神经				
腕部卡压（腕管综合征）	反复屈腕或睡眠	鱼际肌无力	拇指、示指、中指和环指桡侧半麻木、刺痛和（或）疼痛。Tinel 征和 Phalen 征	腕部固定夹板，腕管注射或手术
尺神经				
肘部卡压	髁沟外部压迫，肱骨骨折	骨间肌和拇指内收肌无力或萎缩	小指和环指尺侧半感觉丧失	肘垫，尺神经转位术或肘管减压术
桡神经				
桡神经沟卡压	饮酒过量后长时间趴在手臂上睡眠："周六夜麻痹"	腕下垂，肘部伸展功能保留；手指和拇指伸肌无力	手背感觉丧失	自然恢复，腕部夹板
股神经				
	经腹子宫切除术、血肿、长时间截石位、糖尿病	股四头肌无力和萎缩	大腿前部及小腿内侧感觉丧失	物理治疗
股外侧皮神经				
感觉异常性股痛	肥胖、妊娠、糖尿病、束腰带	无	大腿前外侧感觉丧失、疼痛或刺痛感	减重，自然恢复
腓神经				
腓骨头卡压	习惯性跷二郎腿、膝盖打石膏、长时间下蹲、过度减重	踝背屈肌或外翻肌以及趾伸肌无力	小腿前外侧和足背感觉丧失	踝-足矫形器，解除压迫
坐骨神经				
	注射损伤、髋关节骨折或脱位	腘绳肌、踝跖屈肌或背屈肌无力	臀部、小腿外侧和足部感觉丧失	踝-足矫形器，物理治疗
胫神经				
跗管卡压	穿鞋太紧导致外部压迫、创伤、腱鞘炎	无	足底感觉丧失和刺痛感	跗骨注射，消除压迫来源，内侧足弓支撑

群的肌无力。运动体征通常比较轻微，而感觉异常可能包括麻木、刺痛和烧灼感（感觉迟钝）。感觉症状常始于足趾和足部，呈对称性分布，然后沿小腿向近端蔓延，呈"袜套样"分布。当下肢感觉异常扩展至膝水平时，手部亦常受累，表现为"手套状"分布的感觉异常。当上肢感觉异常扩展至肘水平时，可能伴随躯干和腹部的感觉迟钝。

获得性脱髓鞘性多发性神经病的显著临床特征是无力，广泛累及远端、近端乃至面部肌肉。与轴索性神经病不同的是，感觉丧失并非其主要表现，患者常出现弥漫性反射减弱或反射消失。

血管炎性神经病的典型表现是急性或亚急性起病，具有非对称特征，主要表现为远端肢体无力和感觉丧失，并伴有剧烈疼痛。

诊断和鉴别诊断

神经疾病大致可分为获得性和遗传性两大类（表 18.8）。获得性神经疾病更为普遍，病因广泛，包括代谢或内分泌疾病（糖尿病、肾衰竭、卟啉病）、免疫介导性疾病（GBS、CIDP、多灶性运动神经病、抗髓鞘相关糖蛋白神经病）、感染性因素［人类免疫缺陷病毒（HIV）、莱姆病、巨细胞病毒（CMV）、梅毒、麻风、白喉］、药物（HIV 治疗药物、化疗药物）、环境毒素暴露（重金属）或副肿瘤性疾病。在发达国家，糖尿病和酒精中毒是多发性神经病最为常见的病因。多达 1/3 的获得性神经病的病因难以明确，称为隐源性。多发性单神经炎的病因包括系统性血管炎（类风湿关节炎、系统性红斑狼疮、韦格纳肉芽肿、Churg-Strauss 综合征、结节性多动脉炎）和原发性外周系统血管炎（占 25%）。

TABLE 18.8 Hereditary Neuropathic Disorders

	Inheritance Pattern	Genetic Defect	Clinical Features
Hereditary sensorimotor neuropathies	AR, AD, or X-linked		Pes cavus, distal atrophy and weakness, hammer toes
Familial amyloid polyneuropathy	AD	Transthyretin Gelsolin Apolipoprotein AI	Pain, autonomic dysfunction, carpal tunnel syndrome, heart failure.
Fabry disease	X-linked	α-Galactosidase	Cardiac ischemia, renal disease, stroke, cutaneous angiokeratomas, cornea verticillata
Tangier disease	AR	Apolipoprotein A	Low HDL levels, orange tonsils
Refsum disease	AR	Phytanic acid oxidase	Retinitis pigmentosa, cardiomyopathy, deafness, ichthyosis

AD, Autosomal dominant; *AR*, autosomal recessive; *HDL*, high-density lipoprotein.

TABLE 18.9 Differential Diagnosis of Neuropathic Disorders Based on Symptoms

Motor Symptoms Only	Sensory Symptoms Only	Autonomic Symptoms
Porphyria	Cryptogenic sensory polyneuropathy	Amyloid neuropathy
Charcot-Marie-Tooth	Metabolic, drug-related, or toxic neuropathy	Diabetic neuropathy
Chronic inflammatory demyelinating polyneuropathy	Paraneoplastic sensory neuropathy	Fabry disease
Guillain-Barré syndrome		Guillain-Barré syndrome
Lead neuropathy		Hereditary sensory or autonomic neuropathy
Motor neuron disease		Porphyria

Because of the many causes, it is important to approach the patient with neuropathy systematically, beginning with the patient's history and physical examination. It is essential to determine which nerves are involved (motor, sensory, or autonomic) and in what specific combination (Table 18.9). Small-fiber neuropathies often manifest with unpleasant or abnormal sensations such as a burning pain, electric shock–like sensations, cramping, tingling, pins and needles, or prickly feelings such as the limb "feeling asleep." Large-fiber neuropathies can manifest as numbness, tingling, or as gait ataxia. Symptoms suggesting motor nerve involvement include muscle weakness that typically involves the distal foot muscles. Autonomic nerve involvement is suggested by symptoms of orthostatic hypotension, impotence, cardiac arrhythmia, or bladder dysfunction.

The distribution of muscle weakness is important. In axonal neuropathies, the weakness predominantly involves the distal lower extremity muscles, and in demyelinating neuropathies the weakness can involve both proximal and distal muscles as well as facial muscles. Most neuropathies result in *symmetrical* weakness. If asymmetry is present, motor neuron disease, radiculopathy, plexopathy, compressive mononeuropathies, or mononeuritis multiplex should be considered. The intensity and distribution of painful dysesthesias can also be informative. Although many axonal neuropathies are associated with a burning sensation in the feet, pain as the chief complaint suggests specific causes of neuropathy (Table 18.10). A neuropathy that manifests with acute, asymmetrical weakness and severe pain suggests vasculitis.

In patients with severe, asymmetrical proprioceptive deficits, with sparing of motor function, the site of the lesion is usually the sensory neuron/dorsal root ganglion. This specific syndrome has a relatively limited differential diagnosis, including paraneoplastic process with anti-Hu antibodies, Sjögren's syndrome, cisplatinum toxicity, vitamin B_6 toxicity, and HIV infection.

Most neuropathies are relatively insidious in onset, particularly those associated with metabolic or endocrine disorders. Acute neuropathies may be caused by a vasculitic process, toxin exposure, porphyria, or GBS. GBS

TABLE 18.10 Neuropathies Associated With Pain

Alcoholic neuropathy
Amyloidosis
Cryptogenic sensorimotor neuropathy
Diabetic neuropathy
Fabry disease
Guillain-Barré syndrome
Heavy metal toxicity (arsenic, thallium)
Hereditary sensory or autonomic neuropathy
HIV sensorimotor neuropathy
Radiculopathy or plexopathy
Vasculitis

HIV, Human immunodeficiency virus.

is commonly preceded by a viral illness, immunization, or a surgical procedure. The neurologic history must thoroughly explore potential toxic exposures such as prior medications and alcohol use.

Because many neuropathies are hereditary, it is essential to obtain a detailed family history, specifically inquiring about a history of gait instability, use of adaptive equipment, or skeletal deformities of the feet. Hereditary neuropathies may be autosomal recessive, autosomal dominant, or X-linked. In some situations, it may be helpful to actually examine family members because the severity of disease may vary considerably from one generation to the next. The most common hereditary neuropathy is Charcot-Marie-Tooth disease (see later).

A complete neurologic examination should always be performed in a patient complaining of numbness. If the patient shows evidence of upper motor neuron involvement in addition to the sensory loss, vitamin B_{12} or copper deficiency should be considered, even in the absence of apparent anemia. An elevated methylmalonic acid or homocystine level can also help confirm the diagnosis of B_{12} deficiency in patients

表 18.8 遗传性神经病

	遗传模式	遗传缺陷	临床特征
遗传性感觉运动神经病	AR、AD 或 X 连锁		高弓足、远端萎缩无力、锤状趾
家族性淀粉样多发性神经病	AD	甲状腺素转运蛋白 凝溶胶蛋白 载脂蛋白 A1	疼痛、自主神经功能障碍、腕管综合征、心力衰竭
法布里病	X 连锁	α 半乳糖苷酶	心肌缺血、肾病、卒中、皮肤血管角化瘤、角膜涡状营养不良
丹吉尔病	AR	载脂蛋白 A	HDL 水平低、橙黄色扁桃体
雷夫叙姆病	AR	植烷酸氧化酶	视网膜色素变性、心肌病、耳聋、鱼鳞病

AD, 常染色体显性遗传; AR, 常染色体隐性遗传; HDL, 高密度脂蛋白。

表 18.9 基于症状的神经疾病鉴别诊断

仅有运动症状	仅有感觉症状	自主神经症状
卟啉病 夏科-马里-图思病 慢性炎症性脱髓鞘性多发性神经病 吉兰-巴雷综合征 铅中毒性神经病 运动神经元病	隐源性感觉性多发性神经病 代谢性、药物相关或中毒性神经病 副肿瘤性感觉神经病	淀粉样神经病 糖尿病神经病变 法布里病 吉兰-巴雷综合征 遗传性感觉或自主神经病 卟啉病

鉴于神经病的病因复杂,对患者的诊疗应从病史和体格检查入手,系统地评估以明确受累的神经类型(运动神经、感觉神经或自主神经)以及具体的组合模式(表 18.9)。小纤维神经病变常表现为感觉不适或异常,如烧灼痛、电击样感觉、痉挛、麻刺感、针刺感或刺痛感,如肢体"感觉睡着了"。大纤维神经病变则表现为麻木、麻刺感或步态共济失调。运动神经受累的标志性症状是肌肉无力,尤以远端足部肌肉明显。自主神经受累的症状包括体位性低血压、阳痿、心律失常或膀胱功能障碍。

肌无力的分布模式对于疾病的诊断十分重要。轴索性神经病的无力主要累及下肢远端肌肉,而脱髓鞘性神经病的无力可累及近端和远端肌肉以及面部肌肉。对称性无力是多数神经病的特征,非对称性无力则提示特定疾病如运动神经元、神经根病、神经丛病、卡压性单神经病或多发性单神经炎。痛觉迟钝的强度和分布评估也非常关键。虽然许多轴索性神经病都伴有足部烧灼感,但以疼痛为主诉的神经病需要考虑特定的病因(表 18.10)。表现为急性起病、不对称性无力和剧烈疼痛的神经病可能指向血管炎。

对于伴有严重且不对称的本体感觉障碍而运动功能保留的患者,病变部位通常是感觉神经元或背根神经节。这种特殊综合征的鉴别诊断相对有限,包括抗 Hu 抗体阳性的副肿瘤性疾病、干燥综合征、顺铂中毒、维生素 B_6 中毒和 HIV 感染。

大多数神经病起病相对隐匿,尤其是与代谢或内分泌失调相关者。急性起病的神经病可能由血管炎、毒素暴露、卟啉病或 GBS 引起。GBS 发病前常伴有病

表 18.10 与疼痛有关的神经病

酒精性神经病
淀粉样变性
隐源性感觉运动神经病
糖尿病神经病变
法布里病
吉兰-巴雷综合征
重金属中毒(砷、铊)
遗传性感觉或自主神经病
HIV 感觉运动神经病
神经根病或神经丛病
血管炎

HIV, 人类免疫缺陷病毒。

毒性疾病、免疫接种或外科手术史等前驱病史。因此,神经系统的病史采集必须彻底探究潜在的毒素暴露,如既往用药史和饮酒史。

由于许多神经病是遗传性的,因此必须详细了解家族史,尤其关注步态异常、辅助设备使用或足部骨骼畸形史。遗传性神经病可能是常染色体隐性遗传、常染色体显性遗传或 X 连锁遗传。在某些情况下,对家族成员进行检查可能会有所帮助,因为疾病的严重程度可能会因世代不同而有很大差异。最常见的遗传性神经病是夏科-马里-图思病(见后文)。

对于主诉为麻木的患者,应进行全面的神经系统检查。如果患者除了感觉丧失外,还有上运动神经元受累的迹象,即使没有明显贫血,也应考虑维生素 B_{12} 或铜缺乏症。在维生素 B_{12} 水平处于临界状态的患者,甲基丙二酸或同型半胱氨酸水平升高也有助于确诊维生素 B_{12} 缺乏症。出现无力和上运动神经元体征而无相

TABLE 18.11 Peripheral Neuropathy Laboratory Studies	
Standard Tests	Tests Indicated in Selected Cases
B_{12}	Anti-Hu antibody
Complete blood count (CBC)	ESR, ANA, RF, SS-A, SS-B
Glucose tolerance test	Genetic studies for Charcot-Marie-Tooth
RPR	Human immunodeficiency virus (HIV)
Chem 20	Lyme antibody
Serum protein electrophoresis (SPEP) and immunofixation electrophoresis (IFE)	Phytanic acid
	Copper level
Thyroid function tests	24-hr urine for heavy metals
Nerve conduction studies or electromyogram (EMG)	Quantitative sensory testing
	Lumbar puncture
	Nerve biopsy
	Skin biopsy
	Tilt table testing

with borderline levels. The presence of weakness and upper motor neuron signs without associated sensory loss suggests ALS.

If the neuropathy is associated with mental status abnormalities, then pyridoxine intoxication or deficiencies of thiamine, niacin ("dementia, diarrhea, dermatitis"), and vitamin B_{12} should be considered in the differential diagnosis. Lyme disease may result in both peripheral nervous system symptoms (facial nerve palsies, paresthesias, weakness) and central nervous system symptoms (dementia, headache). Acquired immunodeficiency syndrome (AIDS) can also affect both the central and the peripheral nervous systems. GBS and CIDP usually occur at the time of HIV seroconversion, whereas sensory neuropathy, mononeuritis multiplex, and CMV polyradiculopathy generally occur in the context of low CD4 counts in the later stages of the disease. Older antiretroviral drugs (e.g., stavudine) were associated with a significant rate of neuropathy.

Once a preliminary differential diagnosis is developed based on the history and neurologic examination findings, laboratory studies can confirm the diagnosis. Laboratory tests to identify potentially treatable causes of neuropathy are included in Table 18.11. Additional studies can be ordered based on the suspected diagnosis. An impaired glucose tolerance test is found in more than half of patients with cryptogenic sensory peripheral neuropathy and is more sensitive than tests of fasting glucose or hemoglobin A_{1c} (HbA_{1c}). In a patient with acute, asymmetrical weakness and sensory loss, screening for an inflammatory process (ESR, ANA, RA, SS-A, SS-B) is appropriate. In addition, genetic testing is now available for most patients with CMT disease. If a monoclonal protein is identified on serum protein electrophoresis, a skeletal survey, urine immunofixation electrophoresis, and bone marrow biopsy should be ordered to rule out an underlying lymphoproliferative disorder. If the patient has a monoclonal protein associated with autonomic dysfunction, congestive heart failure, or renal insufficiency, a biopsy (rectal, abdominal fat, or sural nerve) should be considered for diagnosis of amyloidosis. Amyloidosis can be acquired or familial with mutations in the transthyretin (TTR) gene. CIDP can be associated with a monoclonal gammopathy, and in this situation patients should be treated with immunosuppressive therapy. Monoclonal gammopathies observed in patients with an axonal peripheral neuropathy are frequently benign (monoclonal gammopathy of unknown significance) and do not necessarily warrant therapy.

A lumbar puncture is indicated only if an acquired demyelinating neuropathy such as GBS or CIDP is being considered. In these cases, one expects to find an "albuminocytologic dissociation" with an elevation in cerebrospinal fluid (CSF) protein and a relatively normal white blood cell (WBC) count. If the CSF WBC count is greater than 50, Lyme disease, HIV-associated disease, or a paraneoplastic process must be considered.

Electrodiagnostic studies consisting of nerve conduction testing and EMG can be a helpful extension of the physical examination. These studies are useful in defining whether the neuropathic process is caused by a primarily axonal or demyelinating process. In general, axonal degeneration decreases the amplitude of the compound muscle action potential out of proportion to the degree of reduction in peripheral nerve conduction velocity, whereas demyelination produces prominent reduction in conduction velocities. Nerve conduction testing can help determine, in the case of a demyelinating neuropathy, whether the process has an acquired or hereditary cause. A uniform slowing of nerve conduction usually suggests a hereditary cause while focal demyelination causing conduction block suggests an acquired demyelinating neuropathy. Electrodiagnostic studies can identify subclinical neuropathy (in patients receiving potentially neurotoxic medications) and can quantitate the extent of axon loss. Finally, these studies can localize the lesion in the case of radiculopathies, dorsal root ganglionopathies, plexopathies, and multiple mononeuropathies.

Sensory nerve biopsies should be obtained for diagnosis of a vasculitic neuropathy because treatment involves potentially toxic medications. Performing a muscle biopsy in addition to the nerve biopsy may improve the diagnostic yield and should be considered because the inflammation is random and focal and easily missed. Nerve biopsies are not indicated in "cryptogenic" neuropathies, diabetic neuropathy, or motor neuron disease. If nerve conduction studies are normal, skin biopsies allow quantification of the number of intraepidermal nerve fibers. A length-dependent decrease in the number of these fibers can help confirm a small-fiber neuropathy.

Treatment

Despite a very thorough history, examination, and laboratory studies, the cause of as many as one third of neuropathies remains unknown. In this situation, the focus of management is pain control. Patients with neuropathy frequently report a burning, searing, and aching sensation in their feet and hands that interferes with sleep. Neuropathic pain is difficult to treat but may respond to various medications having different mechanisms of action (Table 18.12). It is important to "start low and taper slow" and to treat for a minimum of 4 weeks before concluding that an agent is ineffective. In patients with a vasculitic neuropathy, therapy with corticosteroids in addition to a cytotoxic agent can stabilize and, in some cases, improve the neuropathy.

Prognosis

Peripheral neuropathies caused by axonal degeneration are generally progressive unless the underlying cause can be identified and treated. Recovery from axonal degeneration requires nerve regeneration, a process that often requires 2 to 3 years. Prognosis of demyelinating and vasculitic neuropathies is extremely variable, depending on the cause.

COMMON MONONEUROPATHIES

Common mononeuropathies are explored in Table 18.7.

Carpal Tunnel Syndrome

Carpal tunnel syndrome results from compression of the median nerve at the wrist as it passes beneath the flexor retinaculum. Precipitating factors include activities that require repetitive wrist movements:

表 18.11	周围神经病的实验室检查
标准检查	特定疾病中所需检查
维生素 B$_{12}$	抗 Hu 抗体
全血细胞计数（CBC）	ESR、ANA、RF、SS-A 抗体、SS-B
糖耐量试验	抗体
快速血浆反应素（RPR）	夏科-马里-图思基因检查
血生化 20 项	人类免疫缺陷病毒（HIV）
血清蛋白电泳（SPEP）和	莱姆病抗体
免疫固定电泳（IFE）	植烷酸
甲状腺功能检查	铜水平
神经传导检查或肌电图	24 h 尿液重金属检测
（EMG）	感觉定量检查
	腰椎穿刺
	神经活检
	皮肤活检
	倾斜台检查

ESR，红细胞沉降率；ANA，抗核抗体；RF，类风湿因子。

应的感觉丧失，提示 ALS。

如果神经病伴有精神状态异常，鉴别诊断时应考虑吡哆醇中毒或维生素 B$_1$、烟酸（"痴呆、腹泻、皮炎"）和维生素 B$_{12}$ 缺乏症。莱姆病可引起周围神经系统症状（面神经麻痹、感觉异常、无力）和中枢神经系统症状（痴呆、头痛）。获得性免疫缺陷综合征（AIDS）同样累及中枢神经系统和周围神经系统。GBS 和 CIDP 常在 HIV 血清抗体阳转时发病，而感觉性神经病、多发性单神经炎和 CMV 多发性神经根病则多见于疾病后期 CD4 计数水平低下时。一些较老的抗逆转录病毒药物（如司他夫定）与神经病高发有关。

初步鉴别诊断基于病史和神经系统体格检查，确诊则需依赖实验室检查。表 18.11 列出了针对潜在可治疗病因的实验室检查项目，并可根据疑似诊断进一步扩展检查范围。隐源性感觉性周围神经病患者中，半数以上会出现糖耐量减低，其敏感性高于空腹血糖或血红蛋白 A$_{1c}$（HbA$_{1c}$）检测。对于急性起病、非对称性无力和感觉丧失的患者，应筛查炎症反应标志物（红细胞沉降率、抗核抗体、类风湿因子、SS-A 抗体、SS-B 抗体）。此外，多数 CMT 患者可进行基因检测。如果在血清蛋白电泳中发现单克隆蛋白，则应进行骨骼检查、尿液免疫固定电泳和骨髓活检，以排除潜在的淋巴增殖性疾病。如果患者的单克隆蛋白与自主神经功能障碍、充血性心力衰竭或肾功能不全有关，则应考虑进行活检（直肠、腹部脂肪或腓肠神经）以诊断淀粉样变性。淀粉样变性可能是获得性的，也可能是家族性的甲状腺素转运蛋白（TTR）基因突变所致。CIDP 伴有单克隆丙种球蛋白病的患者需要接受免疫抑制治疗；而轴索性周围神经病伴发的单克隆丙种球蛋白病多为良性（意义不明的单克隆丙种球蛋白病），并不一定需要治疗。

只有在考虑获得性脱髓鞘性神经病（如 GBS 或 CIDP）的诊断时，才需要进行腰椎穿刺。脑脊液出现特征性"蛋白-细胞分离"现象，即脑脊液（CSF）中蛋白质升高，而白细胞计数相对正常。如果 CSF 白细胞计数大于 50 个，应排查莱姆病、HIV 相关疾病或副肿瘤性病因。

电诊断性检查是体格检查的有益补充，包括神经传导检查和肌电图。这些检查有助于确定神经的病理性改变主要是由轴索还是脱髓鞘病变引起的。一般来说，轴索变性会降低复合肌肉动作电位的波幅，与周围神经传导速度的降低程度不成比例，而脱髓鞘则会导致传导速度的显著降低。神经传导检查有助于确定脱髓鞘性神经病的病因是获得性还是遗传性：神经传导速度均匀减慢通常提示遗传性病因，而局灶性脱髓鞘引起的传导阻滞则提示是获得性脱髓鞘性神经病。电诊断性检查可识别亚临床神经病（在接受潜在神经毒性药物治疗的患者中），并可量化轴索丢失的程度。这类检查还可以对神经根病、背根神经节病、神经丛病和多发性单神经病患者的病变部位进行定位。

在血管炎性神经病的诊断中，鉴于治疗药物的潜在毒性，应进行感觉神经活检。由于炎症反应是随机的、局灶性的，容易被漏诊，应考虑在进行神经活检的同时进行肌肉活检，以提高诊断阳性率。神经活检并不适用于"隐源性"神经病、糖尿病神经病变或运动神经元病。如果神经传导检查是正常的，可通过皮肤活检量化表皮内神经纤维的数量。神经纤维数量的减少呈现长度依赖性，这有助于确诊小纤维神经病。

治疗

尽管进行过了全面的病史采集、体格检查和实验室检查，仍有 1/3 的神经病患者病因不明。这种情况下，治疗的重点是疼痛症状的缓解。患者常自述手脚有烧灼感、灼热感和疼痛感，影响其睡眠。尽管神经病理性疼痛的治疗颇具挑战性，但患者可能对不同作用机制的药物产生治疗反应（表 18.12）。因此，遵循"从低剂量起始，缓慢减量"的用药原则至关重要，且需在治疗持续至少 4 周后，方可准确评估药物疗效。对于血管炎性神经病患者，联用细胞毒性药物与皮质类固醇药物有助于稳定病情，并在特定情况下促进神经病变的改善。

预后

轴索变性所致周围神经病多呈进行性发展，除非根本病因得以明确并治疗。轴索变性需要通过神经再生来恢复，通常需要 2～3 年的时间。而脱髓鞘性和血管炎性神经病的预后则因病因而异。

常见的单神经病

常见的单神经病见表 18.7。

腕管综合征

腕管综合征是由于正中神经在腕部屈肌支持带下穿过时受压所致。诱发因素包括需要重复运动手腕的

TABLE 18.12 Symptomatic Treatment for Neuropathic Pain
Tricyclic Antidepressants
Amitriptyline 10-150 mg qhs
Nortriptyline 10-150 mg qhs
Imipramine 10-150 mg qhs
Desipramine 10-150 mg qhs
Venlafaxine 75-225 mg qd
Anticonvulsants
Gabapentin 300-1200 mg tid
Carbamazepine 100-200 mg tid
Topiramate 150-200 mg bid
Duloxetine 60-120 mg qd
Pregabalin 150-600 mg qd
Sodium valproate 250-500 mg bid
Alternative Treatments
Tramadol 50-100 mg qid
Lidoderm patches
Capsaicin cream
Transcutaneous nerve stimulation
Acupuncture

mechanical work, gardening, house painting, and typing. Predisposing causes include pregnancy, diabetes, acromegaly, rheumatoid arthritis, chronic renal failure, thyroid disorders, and primary amyloidosis.

Symptoms usually begin in the dominant hand but commonly involve both hands over time. Patients typically report numbness, tingling, and burning sensations in the palm and in the fingers supplied by the median nerve: the thumb, index finger, middle finger, and medial one half of the ring finger. Some patients report that all fingers become numb. Pain and paresthesias are most prominent at night and often interrupt sleep. The pain is prominent at the wrist but may radiate to the forearm and occasionally to the shoulder. Shaking the hand relieves both pain and paresthesias. Percussion of the median nerve at the wrist provokes paresthesias in a median nerve distribution in 60% of patients (Tinel sign), and flexion of the wrist for 30 to 60 seconds provokes pain or paresthesias in 75% of cases (Phalen sign).

The diagnosis is based on clinical symptoms and signs. Electrodiagnostic studies may demonstrate prolongation of the sensory or motor latencies across the wrist in up to 85% of patients. In more severe cases, EMG may demonstrate evidence of denervation in the abductor pollicis brevis.

Treatment initially includes avoidance of repetitive wrist activities and the use of a neutral wrist splint. If these conservative measures fail, injections of lidocaine and methylprednisolone can be given into the carpal tunnel or surgical treatment by section of the transverse carpal ligament can effectively decompress the nerve. Indicators that have been shown to predict failure with conservative management include age older than 50, disease duration longer than 10 months, constant paresthesias, and a positive Phalen sign in less than 10 seconds.

Ulnar Palsy

The ulnar nerve may become entrapped at the elbow because of external compression in the condylar groove. Injury may also occur years after a malunited supracondylar fracture of the humerus with bony overgrowth. Contrary to the findings in carpal tunnel syndrome, muscle weakness and atrophy characteristically predominate over sensory symptoms and signs. Patients notice atrophy of the first dorsal interosseous muscle and difficulty performing fine manipulations of the fingers. Numbness of the little finger, the contiguous one half of the ring finger, and the ulnar border of the hand may be present. Ulnar nerve compression can be confirmed with electrodiagnostic studies demonstrating slowed motor conduction velocity across the elbow. Treatment includes the use of elbow pads to avoid compression or surgical procedures including transposition of the ulnar nerve or decompression of the cubital tunnel.

Peroneal Neuropathy

The peroneal nerve can become compressed as it wraps around the fibular head and passes into the fibular tunnel between the peroneus longus muscle and the fibula. Compression may occur as a result of habitual leg crossing, prolonged bed rest, knee casts, prolonged squatting, anesthesia, or profound weight loss. The nerve can also be compressed as a result of Baker cysts, fibular fractures, blunt trauma, tumors, or hematomas at the knee. Symptoms include "foot drop" with selective weakness of the ankle dorsiflexors and evertors as well as the toe extensors. Reflexes remain normal, and sensory loss generally involves the anterolateral leg and dorsum of the foot. Electrodiagnostic studies demonstrate slowing of the peroneal conduction velocity across the fibular head and may demonstrate denervation if axonal injury is present. Compressive injuries usually resolve spontaneously within weeks to months. Magnetic resonance imaging (MRI) and surgical exploration should be considered if symptoms are progressive.

SPECIFIC ACQUIRED POLYNEUROPATHIES

Guillain-Barré Syndrome: Acute Inflammatory Demyelinating Polyneuropathy

Since the advent of polio vaccination, GBS has become the most frequent cause of acute flaccid paralysis throughout the world. GBS is an immune-mediated disorder that follows an identifiable infectious disorder in approximately 60% of patients. The best-documented antecedents include infection with *Campylobacter jejuni*, infectious mononucleosis, CMV, herpesvirus, and mycoplasma. *C. jejuni* is often associated with more severe axonal cases.

The initial symptoms of GBS often consist of tingling and pins-and-needles sensations in the feet and may be associated with dull low-back pain. By the time of presentation, which occurs hours to 1 to 2 days after the first symptoms, weakness has usually developed. The weakness is usually most prominent in the legs, but the arms or cranial musculature may be involved first. Muscle stretch reflexes are lost early, even in regions where strength is retained. Cutaneous sensory deficits (loss of pain and temperature) are relatively mild; however, large-fiber functions (vibration and proprioception) are more severely impaired. Other clinical features include pain (20%), paresthesias (50%), autonomic symptoms (20%), facial weakness (50%), ophthalmoparesis (9%), bulbar weakness, and respiratory failure (25%). Symptoms associated with GBS typically evolve over a 2- to 4-week period, with approximately 90% of patients showing no evidence of progression beyond 4 weeks. For this reason, patients who are seen within several weeks from onset continue to require hospitalization for close observation. Respiratory muscle strength should be monitored with bedside measurements of the FVC and negative inspiratory function (NIF). Intubation should be initiated when the FVC falls below 15 mL/kg or NIF is less than −20 cm of H_2O.

Treatment may include either intravenous gammaglobulin (0.4 g/kg/day × 5 days) or plasmapheresis—the exchange of the patient's plasma for albumin (200 mL/kg over 7 to 10 days). Clinical studies have confirmed equal efficacy between these two therapies, with no additional benefit conferred with combination therapy. Corticosteroids are

表 18.12　神经病理性疼痛的对症治疗
三环类抗抑郁药
阿米替林，10～150 mg，每日睡前
去甲替林，10～150 mg，每日睡前
丙米嗪，10～150 mg，每日睡前
地昔帕明，10～150 mg，每日睡前
文拉法辛，75～225 mg，每日 1 次
抗惊厥药
加巴喷丁，300～1200 mg，每日 3 次
卡马西平，100～200 mg，每日 3 次
托吡酯，150～200 mg，每日 2 次
度洛西汀，60～120 mg，每日 1 次
普瑞巴林，150～600 mg，每日 1 次
丙戊酸钠，250～500 mg，每日 2 次
替代治疗
曲马多，50～100 mg，每日 4 次
利多卡因贴剂
辣椒碱乳膏
经皮神经电刺激
针灸

活动：机械工作、园艺、房屋粉刷和打字。致病原因包括妊娠、糖尿病、肢端肥大症、类风湿关节炎、慢性肾衰竭、甲状腺疾病和原发性淀粉样变性。

症状通常始于优势手，但随着时间的推移，通常会累及双手。患者常自述手掌和正中神经所支配的手指（拇指、示指、中指和环指桡侧半）有麻木、刺痛和灼烧感，有些患者所有手指均有麻木感。疼痛和感觉异常在夜间最为明显，常导致睡眠中断。疼痛主要发生在手腕处，可放射至前臂，偶尔也会放射至肩部。晃动手部有助于缓解疼痛和感觉异常症状。通过叩击腕部正中神经，可诱发 60% 的患者在正中神经支配区出现感觉异常，此现象被称为 Tinel 征；屈腕 30～60 s 可引起 75% 的患者出现疼痛或感觉异常，这一体征被称为 Phalen 征。

诊断主要依据临床症状和体征。此外，85% 患者的电诊断检查可能提示腕部感觉或运动神经传导潜伏期延长。对于病情更为严重的病例，肌电图可能会提示拇短展肌去神经支配的证据，从而进一步支持诊断。

腕管综合征的初始治疗包括避免腕部重复性活动和采用腕部固定夹板以减轻症状。如果保守治疗未能达到预期效果，可考虑腕管内注射利多卡因和甲泼尼龙，或行腕横韧带切开术，以有效解除神经压迫。预测保守治疗可能失败的指标包括年龄超过 50 岁、病程持续超过 10 个月、持续性感觉异常以及 Phalen 征在 10 s 内即呈阳性。

尺神经麻痹

尺神经在肘部可能会因髁沟的外部压迫而发生卡压现象。此外，由于肱骨髁上骨折后的畸形愈合以及骨质异常增生，尺神经也可能在数年后发生损伤。与腕管综合征不同的是，尺神经麻痹更多地导致肌无力和肌萎缩的特征性症状和体征，而非单纯的感觉障碍。患者常自述第一背侧骨间肌萎缩，并伴有手指精细动作能力下降。此外，可能会出现小指、环指尺侧半以及手部尺侧边缘的麻木感。电诊断检查可显示肘部运动传导速度减慢，从而协助确认尺神经受压的诊断。治疗方法包括使用肘垫以避免受压，或进行手术治疗，包括尺神经转位术或肘管减压术，以缓解神经受压状况。

腓神经病

腓神经在绕过腓骨头、进入腓骨长肌和腓骨之间的腓骨隧道时，易受到压迫。诱发因素包括习惯性跷二郎腿、长期卧床、膝盖石膏固定、长时间下蹲、麻醉或过度减重等。此外，腘窝囊肿、腓骨骨折、钝性创伤、肿瘤或膝关节血肿等病理状况也可能导致腓神经受压。腓神经病的症状特征性表现为"足下垂"，具体为踝背屈肌和外翻肌以及趾伸肌选择性无力；但踝反射仍然正常，感觉丧失一般累及小腿前外侧和足背。电诊断检查可显示腓神经在腓骨头处传导速度减慢，如果存在轴索损伤，则可能呈去神经支配表现。压迫性损伤通常会在数周至数月内自发缓解；如果症状呈进行性加重，则应考虑进行磁共振成像（MRI）和手术探查。

特殊获得性多发性神经病

吉兰-巴雷综合征（GBS）：急性炎症性脱髓鞘性多发性神经病

自脊髓灰质炎疫苗问世以来，GBS 已成为全球范围内引发急性弛缓性瘫痪的首要病因。GBS 作为一种免疫介导的疾病，约 60% 患者发病前有明确的感染史作为前驱事件，最常见的包括空肠弯曲菌感染、传染性单核细胞增多症、CMV、疱疹病毒和支原体感染。其中，空肠弯曲菌感染往往与更严重的轴索性 GBS 亚型有关。

GBS 初期表现为足部刺痛和针刺样感觉，可能伴有腰背部钝痛。随后，在数小时至 1～2 天后，患者会逐渐出现无力症状，其中腿部肌无力通常最为突出，但亦有部分患者首先出现手臂或头面部肌肉的受累。肌肉牵张反射在早期即丧失，即便在肌力保留的区域也不例外。皮肤感觉障碍方面，痛觉和温度觉丧失相对较轻，而大纤维介导的振动觉和本体感觉受损更为严重。此外，GBS 还伴随一系列其他临床特征，包括疼痛（20%）、感觉异常（50%）、自主神经症状（20%）、面瘫（50%）、眼肌麻痹（9%）、延髓麻痹和呼吸衰竭（25%）。这些症状的进展通常会在 2～4 周内达到高峰，约 90% 的患者在 4 周后病情趋于稳定。因此，在发病后数周内就诊的患者仍需住院进行严密观察。为监测呼吸肌功能，应在床旁进行用力肺活量（FVC）和负吸气功能（NIF）检测。当 FVC 降至 15 ml/kg 以下或 NIF 低于 $-20\ cmH_2O$ 时，应及时进行气管插管，给予呼吸支持。

治疗方法包括静脉注射丙种球蛋白（每天 0.4 g/kg，连续 5 天）或进行血浆置换，置换患者血浆中的白蛋白（200 ml/kg，连续 7～10 天）。临床研究证实，这两种疗法的疗效相当，且联合治疗不会带来额外获益。此外，皮质类固醇药物在 GBS 的治疗中被证实无效。治疗指征

not effective in GBS. Indications for therapy include inability to ambulate independently, impaired respiratory function, or rapidly progressive weakness.

Clinical features predicting a poor prognosis or prolonged recovery time include rapidly progressive weakness, need for mechanical ventilation, and low-amplitude CMAPs. The mortality rate remains 5% to 10%, usually due to respiratory complications, cardiac arrhythmia, or pulmonary embolism. With appropriate supportive care and rehabilitation, 80% to 90% of patients recover with little or no disability.

Chronic Inflammatory Demyelinating Polyneuropathy

CIDP has been considered the "chronic form" of GBS, because by definition the symptoms must progress for at least 8 weeks. The clinical features include proximal and distal weakness, areflexia, and distal sensory loss. Autonomic dysfunction, respiratory insufficiency, and cranial nerve involvement can occur but are much less common than in GBS. Treatment for CIDP includes the use of oral immunosuppressive agents such as prednisone, cyclosporine, mycophenolate mofetil, and azathioprine. Intravenous immune globulin and plasmapheresis are also indicated for severe or refractory cases.

Diabetic Neuropathy

Diabetes mellitus is the most frequent cause of peripheral neuropathy worldwide. The diabetic neuropathies take many clinical forms, including symmetrical polyneuropathies and a wide variety of individual plexus or nerve disorders.

Diabetes mellitus often causes a slowly progressive, distal, symmetrical sensorimotor polyneuropathy (DSPN). DSPN is uncommon at the time of diagnosis of diabetes, but its prevalence increases with duration of diabetes with a lifetime prevalence of 55% for type 1 and 45% for type 2. The precise pathogenesis is not defined, but, similar to the ocular and renal complications, diabetic neuropathy can be reduced in incidence and in severity by maintaining blood glucose levels close to normal.

Initial symptoms may consist of numbness, tingling, burning, or prickling sensations affecting the feet and toes. Mild distal weakness and gait instability may subsequently develop. The sensory symptoms can then slowly progress to involve a "stocking-glove pattern." The small-fiber dysfunction often produces spontaneous neuropathic pain in which unpleasant sensations can be evoked by normally innocuous stimuli, such as the bed sheets on the toes at night. Continuous burning or throbbing pain may occur, and prolonged walking is often distressing. In severe cases, patients may develop foot ulcers in insensitive areas that necessitate amputation. Autonomic dysfunction is also frequently associated with DSPN including impotence, nocturnal diarrhea, sweating abnormalities, orthostatic hypotension, and gastroparesis.

Other less common neuropathies associated with diabetes include cranial neuropathies (the sixth, third, and rarely fourth nerves), mononeuropathies, mononeuropathy multiplex, radiculopathies, and plexopathies. Diabetic amyotrophy (also known as *diabetic lumbosacral polyradiculoplexopathy*) is a distinctive disorder characterized by severe thigh pain followed by proximal greater than distal lower extremity weakness that progresses over a period of months. The onset is invariably unilateral, but the condition may progress to involve both lower extremities. Physical therapy and effective pain management are essential; treatment with immune modulators is controversial.

Toxic-Induced Neuropathies

Toxic neuropathies constitute a large number of disorders caused by alcohol, drugs, heavy metals, and environmental substances. The majority of toxic neuropathies manifest as a distal sensorimotor axonal neuropathy that chronically progresses over time unless the offending agent is eliminated. Clinical evaluation should focus on the temporal relationship between exposure and the onset of sensory or motor symptoms as well as symptoms of systemic toxicity.

Critical Illness Polyneuropathy

Critical illness polyneuropathy (CIP) is a common cause of failure to wean from a ventilator in a patient with associated sepsis and multiorgan failure. Clinical features include generalized or distal flaccid paralysis, especially involving the lower extremities, depressed or absent reflexes, and distal sensory loss with relative sparing of cranial nerve function. The diagnosis can be confirmed with nerve conduction studies showing evidence of a severe, generalized axonal neuropathy. CSF protein should be normal and, in addition to conduction studies, distinguishes CIP from GBS.

SPECIFIC HEREDITARY POLYNEUROPATHIES

Charcot-Marie-Tooth Disease

CMT identifies a group of heritable disorders of peripheral nerves that share clinical features but differ in their pathologic mechanisms and the specific genetic abnormalities. CMT is the most common heritable neuromuscular disorder, with an incidence of 17 to 40 cases per 100,000.

CMT disease usually manifests during the first to second decades with symptoms related to insidious foot drop: frequent tripping and inability to jump well or run as fast as other children. Over time, distal upper extremity weakness develops, resulting in difficulty with buttoning, handling keys, and opening jars. Examination reveals distal weakness and wasting of the intrinsic muscles of the feet, the peroneal muscles, the anterior tibial muscles, and the calves ("inverted champagne bottle" legs). A variable degree of impaired large-fiber sensory function is reflected in reduced vibratory sensation at the toes. Muscle stretch reflexes are lost, first at the ankles. Typically, a foot deformity exists, with high arches (pes cavus) and hammer toes, reflecting long-standing muscle imbalance in the feet. Most patients with CMT disease have nearly normal occupational and daily activities, and they have a normal life span. Although no specific treatment has been developed, the foot drop can be treated by appropriate bracing of the ankle with ankle-foot orthoses. Genetic counseling and education of affected patients and their families are important, both for reassurance and to preclude unnecessary diagnostic evaluation of affected members in future generations.

Demyelinating forms of CMT are classified as CMT1 and axonal forms as CMT2. CMT is usually transmitted as an autosomal dominant trait; however, X-linked dominant transmission is responsible for approximately 10% of cases. Rare autosomal recessive forms are designated CMT4, and these patients tend to have an earlier onset and more severe phenotype. CMT1A is the most common form and accounts for 90% of CMT1 and 50% of all CMT cases. CMT1A is associated with the 17p11.2-p12 duplication in the *PMP22* gene expressed by Schwann cells. A deletion or a point mutation of the *PMP22* gene produces a different phenotype, HNPP, which is characterized by recurrent episodes of focal entrapment with attacks of weakness and numbness in the peroneal, ulnar, radial, and median nerves (in descending order of frequency) or in a brachial plexus distribution.

FAMILIAL AMYLOID NEUROPATHIES

Amyloid neuropathy is an autosomal dominant disorder caused by extracellular deposition of the fibrillary protein amyloid in peripheral nerve and sensory and autonomic ganglia, as well as around blood

包括无法独立行走、呼吸功能受损或快速进展性无力。

预后不良或恢复期延长的临床标志为快速进展性无力、机械通气需求和低波幅 CMAP。死亡率在 5%～10%，多死于呼吸系统并发症、心律失常或肺栓塞。经过妥善的支持性护理和康复治疗，80%～90% 的患者可以恢复至无或接近无残疾状态。

慢性炎症性脱髓鞘性多发性神经病（CIDP）

CIDP 被认为是"慢性"型 GBS，依据定义，其症状需持续进展至少 8 周。其临床特征包括近端和远端无力、反射消失和远端感觉丧失。此外，还可出现自主神经功能障碍、呼吸功能不全和脑神经受累，但较 GBS 少见。CIDP 的治疗主要是口服免疫抑制剂，如泼尼松、环孢素、吗替麦考酚酯和硫唑嘌呤。对于重症或难治性病例，可采用静脉注射免疫球蛋白或血浆置换。

糖尿病神经病变

糖尿病是全球范围内导致周围神经病的最主要病因。糖尿病神经病变临床表现多样，包括对称性多发性神经病和各种单一神经丛或神经疾病。

糖尿病常引起缓慢进展的远端对称性感觉运动多发性神经病（DSPN），该病症在糖尿病确诊时并不常见，但其患病率会随着病程延长而增加，在 1 型糖尿病患者中的终生患病率可达 55%，在 2 型糖尿病患者的终生患病率达 45%。尽管 DSPN 的确切发病机制尚不明确，但与糖尿病眼部和肾并发症类似，控制血糖水平接近正常范围可降低糖尿病神经病变的发病率和严重程度。

DSPN 的初期症状可包括足部和脚趾的麻木、刺痛感、灼烧或刺痛感，之后可能会出现轻微的远端无力和步态异常。感觉症状会逐渐进展，形成典型的"袜套-手套样"感觉障碍。小纤维功能障碍可引发自发性神经病理性疼痛，日常轻微刺激（如夜间床单接触脚趾）即可诱发不适，表现为持续的烧灼感或跳痛，影响患者长时程行走功能。严重的患者可能会在感觉迟钝的部位出现足部溃疡，增加截肢风险。此外，DSPN 常伴有自主神经功能障碍，包括阳痿、夜间腹泻、出汗异常、体位性低血压和胃轻瘫。

除 DSPN 外，糖尿病还可引发其他不常见的神经病，包括脑神经病（主要累及第 VI、第 III 脑神经，偶尔累及第 IV 脑神经）、单神经病、多发性单神经病、神经根病和神经丛病。糖尿病肌萎缩（又称糖尿病腰骶多发性神经根神经丛病）是一种特殊类型的神经病变，其临床特征表现为大腿剧烈疼痛后出现下肢无力，近端重于远端，病程可持续数月。通常单侧起病，但病情可能进展到双下肢受累。针对此类患者，物理治疗和有效的疼痛管理至关重要；然而，免疫调节剂的应用尚存在争议。

中毒性神经病变

中毒性神经病变是一类由酒精、药物、重金属和环境物质引起的多种疾病集合。此类病变多表现为远端感觉运动轴索性神经病，如不及时消除致病因素，其病程常呈慢性进行性进展。在临床评估中，需要重点关注暴露与感觉或运动症状及全身中毒症状之间的时间关系。

危重症多发性神经病

危重症多发性神经病（CIP）是感染中毒症伴有多器官功能衰竭患者难以脱离呼吸机的常见原因。临床特征包括全身或远端弛缓性瘫痪，尤以下肢显著，伴随反射减弱或消失，以及远端感觉缺失，而脑神经功能则保持相对完整。神经传导检查发现严重而广泛的轴索性神经病变征象，即可确诊。此外，CSF 蛋白质水平正常可作为辅助依据，可作为神经传导检查以外鉴别 CIP 与 GBS 的重要依据。

特殊的遗传性多发性神经病

夏科-马里-图思病

夏科-马里-图思病（CMT）是一组遗传性周围神经疾病，它们有共同的临床特征，但在病理机制和特定的遗传异常方面呈现异质性。作为最常见的遗传性神经肌肉疾病，其发病率为（17～40）/10 万。

CMT 初发多见于 10～20 岁，初期症状隐匿，以足下垂为特征：患者易绊倒，跳跃和跑步能力减退。随病程进展，患者会出现上肢远端无力，影响扣纽扣、拿钥匙和开罐子等精细动作执行。体格检查可发现远端无力伴足内在肌、腓骨肌、胫骨前肌和小腿肌肉萎缩（"倒立的香槟酒瓶"状腿）。大纤维感觉功能不同程度受损，表现为足趾的振动觉减退。肌肉牵张反射消失，以踝关节为首。高弓足和锤状趾等足部畸形常见，反映出足部肌肉长期失衡。但大多数 CMT 患者能维持正常的职业活动、日常活动和预期寿命。目前，CMT 尚无特异性治疗手段，但足下垂可通过踝-足矫形器提供适当的踝关节支撑来加以管理。为减轻患者及家属的心理负担，以及避免后代不必要的检查，遗传咨询和教育至关重要。

CMT 依据病理机制分为脱髓鞘型（CMT1）与轴索型（CMT2）。CMT 多为常染色体显性遗传，但约有 10% 的病例为 X 连锁显性遗传。罕见的常染色体隐性遗传形式称为 CMT4 型，这类患者往往起病较早，且表型严重。其中，CMT1A 型最为常见，占 CMT1 型的 90% 及所有 CMT 病例的 50%，该亚型与施万细胞表达的 *PMP22* 基因 17p11.2-p12 重复突变有关。*PMP22* 基因的缺失或点突变则会导致不同的疾病表型——HNPP，其特征是腓神经、尺神经、桡神经和正中神经（按发生频率由高到低排列）或臂丛神经分布区反复发作的局灶性卡压，并伴有无力和麻木感。

家族性淀粉样神经病

淀粉样神经病是一种常染色体显性遗传性疾病，由于淀粉样纤维蛋白在周围神经、感觉和自主神经节，以

vessels in nerves and other tissues. The age of onset varies from 18 to 83 years. In all forms of amyloidosis, the initial and major abnormalities affect the small sensory and autonomic fibers. Involvement of small fibers responsible for pain and temperature sensibilities leads to loss of the ability to perceive mechanical and thermal injuries and to an increased risk of tissue damage. As a result, painless injuries present a major hazard of this disorder; in advanced stages, they can lead to chronic infections or osteomyelitis of the feet or hands and the necessity for amputation. Amyloid deposition in the heart can lead to cardiomyopathy. Mutations in transthyretin, apolipoprotein A1, or gelsolin are responsible. Early recognition is essential, as liver transplantation has been shown to halt disease progression. Recently, the FDA approved two new medications, inotersen and patisiran, for treatment of transthyretin-associated familial amyloid polyneuropathy.

SUGGESTED READINGS

Alport AR, Sander HW: Clinical approach to peripheral neuropathy: Anatomic localization and diagnostic testing, Continuum Lifelong Learning Neurol 18(1):13–38, 2012.

Al-Zaidy, SA, Mendell JR: From clinical trials to clinical practice: Practical considerations for gene replacement therapy in SMA type 1. Pediatr Neurol 100:P3–11, 2019.

Bril V, England J, Franklin GM, et al: Evidence-based guideline: treatment of painful diabetic neuropathy, Muscle Nerve 43:910–917, 2011.

Bromberg MB: An approach to the evaluation of peripheral neuropathies, Semin Neurol 25(2):153–159, 2005.

Brown RH, Al-Chalabi: Amyotrophic lateral sclerosis, N Engl J Med 377:162–172, 2017.

Camdessanche JP, Jousserand G, et al: The pattern and diagnostic criteria of sensory neuronopathy: a case-control study, Brain 132(7):1723–1733, 2009.

Chiriboga CA: Nusinersen for the treatment of spinal muscular atrophy, Expert Review of Neurotherapeutics 17(10):955–962, 2017.

Ludolph AC, Brettschneider J, Weishaupt JH: Amyotrophic lateral sclerosis, Curr Opin Neurol 25(5):530–535, 2012.

Mauermann ML, Burns TM: The evaluation of chronic axonal polyneuropathies, Semin Neurol 28(2):133–151, 2008.

Miller RG, Jackson CE, Kasarkis EJ, et al: Practice parameter update: the care of the patient with amyotrophic lateral sclerosis: drug, nutritional, and respiratory therapies (an evidence-based review): report of the Quality Standards Subcommittee of the American Academy of Neurology, Neurology 73(15):1218–1226, 2009.

Miller RG, Jackson CE, Kasarksi EJ, et al: Practice parameter update: the care of the patient with amyotrophic lateral sclerosis: multidisciplinary care, symptom management, and cognitive/behavioral impairment (an evidence-based review): report of the Quality Standards Subcommittee of the American Academy of Neurology, Neurology 73(15):1227–1233, 2009.

Oskarsson B, Gendron TF, Staff NP: Amyotrophic lateral sclerosis: an update for 2018, Mayo Clin Proc 93(11):1617–1628, 2018.

Turner MR, Hardiman O, Benatar M: Controversies and priorities in amyotrophic lateral sclerosis, Lancet Neurol 12(3):310–322, 2013.

及在神经和其他组织的血管周围呈细胞外沉积引起。发病年龄从 18～83 岁不等。在所有淀粉样变性中，最初且主要的异常累及细小的感觉神经纤维和自主神经纤维。负责痛觉和温度觉的小纤维受累后，会引发机械性刺激和热损伤的感知能力丧失，进而增加组织损伤的风险。因此，无痛性损伤是这类疾病的主要危害；疾病晚期可导致足部或手部的慢性感染甚至骨髓炎，最终导致截肢手术。心脏的淀粉样蛋白沉积可诱发心肌病。该病的致病机制包括甲状腺素转运蛋白、载脂蛋白 A1 或凝溶胶蛋白的基因突变。疾病的早期识别至关重要，因为肝移植已被证实可以有效阻止病情进展。近年来，FDA 已批准 inotersen 和 patisiran 两种新型药物，用于治疗甲状腺素转运蛋白相关的家族性淀粉样多发性神经病。

推荐阅读

Alport AR, Sander HW: Clinical approach to peripheral neuropathy: Anatomic localization and diagnostic testing, Continuum Lifelong Learning Neurol 18(1):13–38, 2012.

Al-Zaidy, SA, Mendell JR: From clinical trials to clinical practice: Practical considerations for gene replacement therapy in SMA type 1. Pediatr Neurol 100:P3–11, 2019.

Bril V, England J, Franklin GM, et al: Evidence-based guideline: treatment of painful diabetic neuropathy, Muscle Nerve 43:910–917, 2011.

Bromberg MB: An approach to the evaluation of peripheral neuropathies, Semin Neurol 25(2):153–159, 2005.

Brown RH, Al-Chalabi: Amyotrophic lateral sclerosis, N Engl J Med 377:162–172, 2017.

Camdessanche JP, Jousserand G, et al: The pattern and diagnostic criteria of sensory neuronopathy: a case-control study, Brain 132(7):1723–1733, 2009.

Chiriboga CA: Nusinersen for the treatment of spinal muscular atrophy, Expert Review of Neurotherapeutics 17(10):955–962, 2017.

Ludolph AC, Brettschneider J, Weishaupt JH: Amyotrophic lateral sclerosis, Curr Opin Neurol 25(5):530–535, 2012.

Mauermann ML, Burns TM: The evaluation of chronic axonal polyneuropathies, Semin Neurol 28(2):133–151, 2008.

Miller RG, Jackson CE, Kasarkis EJ, et al: Practice parameter update: the care of the patient with amyotrophic lateral sclerosis: drug, nutritional, and respiratory therapies (an evidence-based review): report of the Quality Standards Subcommittee of the American Academy of Neurology, Neurology 73(15):1218–1226, 2009.

Miller RG, Jackson CE, Kasarksi EJ, et al: Practice parameter update: the care of the patient with amyotrophic lateral sclerosis: multidisciplinary care, symptom management, and cognitive/behavioral impairment (an evidence-based review): report of the Quality Standards Subcommittee of the American Academy of Neurology, Neurology 73(15):1227–1233, 2009.

Oskarsson B, Gendron TF, Staff NP: Amyotrophic lateral sclerosis: an update for 2018, Mayo Clin Proc 93(11):1617–1628, 2018.

Turner MR, Hardiman O, Benatar M: Controversies and priorities in amyotrophic lateral sclerosis, Lancet Neurol 12(3):310–322, 2013.

Muscle Diseases

Johanna Hamel, Jeffrey M. Statland

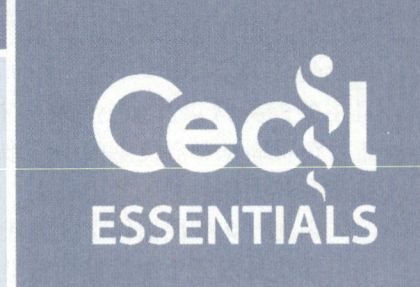

INTRODUCTION

Skeletal muscle fibers are the effector cells of the nervous system, turn thoughts into actions, and are the means by which we interact with our environment. Myopathies are primary diseases of the muscle and can be both inherited and acquired (Table 19.1). Myopathies can result in weakness and muscle wasting, myalgias, cramps, muscle breakdown, or contractures. Inherited disorders affect muscle proteins involved in transmission of signals from the neuromuscular junction, proteins involved in energy production or metabolism, or structural proteins that anchor and transmit force from the contractile apparatus to the extracellular matrix. They do this either by mutations directly to the muscle proteins or by mutations altering cell regulation of transcription or splicing. Acquired myopathies are caused by external factors and can be due to metabolic derangements, toxic exposures or drugs, infections, or autoimmune dysfunction often resulting in inflammation in the muscle. Acquired myopathies can improve with treatments geared towards eliminating or ameliorating the precipitating factors.

With recent advances in our understanding of the genetic and molecular mechanisms in hereditary myopathies, coupled with advances in drug development targeting DNA and RNA, efforts to develop targeted therapies for hereditary muscle diseases accelerated and increased exponentially. The first treatment targeting the underlying genetic mechanism of a muscle disease (Duchenne muscular dystrophy) was approved by the US Food and Drug Administration (FDA) in 2016. Many more disease-specific treatments targeting genetic mechanisms of muscle diseases are currently in clinical trials with a subset expected to become available to patients in the future. This change in paradigm, from supportive to disease-modifying therapies, targeting patients' DNA or RNA that will alter the trajectory of progression, will change the landscape of how we care for patients with muscle diseases. One technology worth mentioning here due to imminent clinical trials and the possibility for transformational change in inherited myopathies is systemic gene replacement therapies. The three concepts that make up systemic gene therapy are: (1) the vector, which is a virus, serotypes of which can specifically target muscle or the heart; (2) the construct, which is the gene that will be packaged into the virus vector; the size can be limited by the capsid size, and so for large genes like dystrophin new engineered genes (i.e., microdystrophin) are used; and (3) the promotor, the on and off switch for the gene, which can also be tissue specific. The first such systemic gene replacement therapy was approved for spinal muscular atrophy, and several companies have phase 3 studies starting for muscular dystrophies. With these fundamental advances on the horizon, early recognition and diagnosis of these rare diseases will be important to achieve the greatest benefit from these treatments. Physicians administering the therapies not only need to be familiar with the disease and its complications but with molecular and genetic mechanisms that are being targeted. These advances provide abundant opportunities and challenges.

ORGANIZATION AND STRUCTURE OF NORMAL MUSCLE

Each muscle is enclosed in a connective tissue sheath made up of collagen and extracellular matrix proteins called the epimysium, which merges at either end to form the tendons, which attach muscle to bone. The epimysium divides internally into the perimysium, which separates the muscle into individual bundles of muscle fibers called fascicles. The endomysium surrounds and provides support for the individual fibers. Each muscle fiber is a single multi-nucleated syncytial cell and can be as long as 10 cm. On cross section, muscle fibers appear polygonal in shape and in adults range from 40 to 80 micrometers in diameter. Medium size arterioles and veins run in the perimysium, with capillaries between the individual muscle fibers. On hematoxylin and eosin stains, cytoplasm appears pink and the nuclei blue (Fig. 19.1A). Each individual muscle fiber has multiple nuclei, which are found beneath the sarcolemma membrane on the periphery of the cell.

The plasma membrane around the muscle fiber is called the sarcolemma, and inside there are a large number of myofibrils made of thick (myosin) and thin (actin) filaments, which make up 70% to 80% of the volume of the cell, and when activated, create force. Electrochemical signals carry the signal from the nerve, through the neuromuscular junction, into the muscle fiber along the sarcolemma and t-tubule system. Muscle ion channels line this network and carry electrochemical signals. Mitochondria and enzymes involved in glycolysis and fatty acid metabolism provide energy for muscle. A network of proteins, the dystrophin-glycoprotein complex (DGC), anchors the myofibrils to the subsarcolemma cytoskeleton and connects to the extracellular matrix (Fig. 19.2). Many inherited myopathies are caused by mutations in these ion channels, metabolic enzymes, or structural anchoring proteins.

SYMPTOMS OF MUSCLE DISEASE

The most common symptom of a patient with muscle disease is a loss of function caused by weakness (for an overview of symptoms see Table 19.2). Other common symptoms, like fatigue, exercise intolerance or myalgias (muscle pain), are less specific than muscle weakness. Muscle cramping is more commonly caused by disorders of the nerves, and not the muscle.

EXAMINATION

The physical examination uses a standard modified Medical Research Council scale of motor strength to determine the pattern and degree of involvement of various muscles (Table 19.3). But just as important as isolated strength testing are functional

19

肌肉疾病

赵梦西 译 杨营营 高颖 审校 王伊龙 通审

引言

骨骼肌纤维是将思想转化为行动的神经系统效应细胞，是我们与环境互动的方式。肌病是主要的肌肉疾病，可以是遗传性或获得性的（表 19.1）。肌病可能导致肌肉无力和萎缩、肌痛、痉挛、肌肉分解或挛缩。遗传性疾病会影响参与神经肌肉接头信号传递的肌肉蛋白、参与能量产生或代谢的蛋白，或将收缩装置的力锚定和传递至细胞外基质的结构蛋白。它们通过肌肉蛋白基因的直接突变或者改变细胞转录或剪接调控的突变来实现这一点。获得性肌病则由外部因素引起，可能是由于代谢紊乱、毒物暴露、药物、感染或自身免疫性功能障碍等，常导致肌肉炎症。获得性肌病可以通过消除或减轻诱发因素的治疗而得到改善。

随着我们对遗传性肌病的遗传和分子机制的理解取得了新进展，加上针对 DNA 和 RNA 的药物研发的进步，针对遗传性肌肉疾病的靶向治疗的研究得到了加速发展并呈指数增长。第一种针对肌肉疾病（进行性假肥大性肌营养不良）潜在遗传机制的治疗方法于 2016 年获得美国食品和药物管理局（FDA）的批准。许多针对肌肉疾病遗传机制的特异性治疗目前正处于临床试验阶段，其中一部分预计将在未来可供患者使用。这一从支持性疗法转向疾病修饰疗法的范式转换，通过针对患者的 DNA 或 RNA 来改变疾病进程，将彻底改变我们对肌肉疾病患者的治疗方式。在这里，有一种技术，因其即将进行的临床试验以及对遗传性肌病带来变革性改变的潜力而值得被提及，即系统基因替代疗法。系统基因疗法包括三个概念：①载体，一种能够特异性靶向肌肉或心脏的病毒血清型；②构建体，即被包装入病毒载体的基因，其大小可能受限于衣壳尺寸，因此对于像抗肌萎缩蛋白这样的大基因，使用了新设计的基因（如微型抗肌萎缩蛋白基因）；③启动子，基因的开关，也可以是组织特异性的。第一种此类系统基因替代疗法已经获批用于治疗脊髓性肌萎缩，且几家公司已经启动了针对肌营养不良症的三期研究。随着这些基础性研究的进展，早期识别与诊断这些罕见疾病将成为从这些治疗中获得最大利益的重要因素。实施这些治疗的医生不仅需要熟悉这些疾病及其并发症，还需要了解所针对的分子和遗传机制。这些进展为我们提供了丰富的机遇和挑战。

正常肌肉的组成和结构

每块肌肉都被一种由胶原蛋白和细胞外基质蛋白构成的结缔组织鞘包裹，称为肌外膜。这种肌外膜在两端融合形成肌腱，将肌肉连接到骨骼上。肌外膜在内部划分为肌束膜，将肌肉分隔成单个的肌束。肌束膜内的肌束由若干单个的肌纤维细胞构成，每个肌纤维都被肌内膜包围并提供支持。每个肌纤维是一个多核的合胞体细胞，其长度可达 10 cm。在横截面上，肌纤维呈多边形，成年人肌纤维的直径范围为 40～80 μm。中等大小的微动脉和静脉在肌束膜中穿行，微血管位于单个肌纤维之间。在苏木精-伊红染色中，细胞质呈粉红色，细胞核呈蓝色（图 19.1A）。每个肌纤维细胞具有多个细胞核，这些细胞核位于肌膜下的细胞外围。

肌纤维周围的质膜称为肌膜，内部有大量由粗（肌球蛋白）和细（肌动蛋白）肌丝组成的肌原纤维，它们占细胞体积的 70%～80%，在激活时会产生力量。电化学信号从神经通过神经肌肉接头，沿着肌膜和 T 小管系统进入肌纤维。肌肉离子通道排列在这一网络中并传递电化学信号。线粒体和参与糖酵解及脂肪酸代谢的酶为肌肉提供能量。一组称为抗肌萎缩蛋白-糖蛋白复合物（DGC）的蛋白质网络将肌原纤维锚定在肌膜下的细胞骨架上，并连接到细胞外基质（图 19.2）。许多遗传性肌病是由这些离子通道、代谢酶或结构锚定蛋白的突变而引起。

肌肉疾病的症状

肌肉疾病患者最常见的症状是由于无力引起的功能丧失（关于症状的概览，参见表 19.2）。其他常见症状如疲劳、运动不耐受或肌痛（肌肉疼痛）等，较肌无力更不具特异性。肌肉痉挛更常见于神经障碍，而非肌肉本身的问题。

检查

体格检查使用标准改良医学研究会运动力量测试量表来确定各种肌肉受累的模式和程度（表 19.3）。但与单独的力量测试同样重要的是功能性运动任务，

TABLE 19.1 Overview of Myopathies

Hereditary Myopathies
Muscular dystrophies
Congenital myopathies
Metabolic/mitochondrial myopathies
Channelopathies

Acquired Myopathies
Inflammatory myopathies
Myopathy with HMGCR antibodies
Endocrine myopathies
Systemic illness/infectious myopathies
Toxic/drug-induced myopathies

motor tasks, particularly in children. Muscles should be inspected for atrophy or hypertrophy and range of motion around the joints for evidence of tendon contractures. Ten broad patterns of muscle weakness occur in myopathies (Table 19.4). Most myopathies have the proximal, limb-girdle pattern. There are other, highly distinctive, patterns. Weakness that is asymmetric and includes the face, proximal arms and shoulders, and distal lower extremities is characteristic of facioscapulohumeral muscular dystrophy. Weakness that starts in the distal finger flexors (patients cannot curl fingers when making a fist) and proximal lower extremities (the quadriceps) is virtually pathognomonic for sporadic inclusion body myositis. A patient in middle age who presents with ptosis and difficulty swallowing is highly characteristic for oculopharyngeal muscular dystrophy.

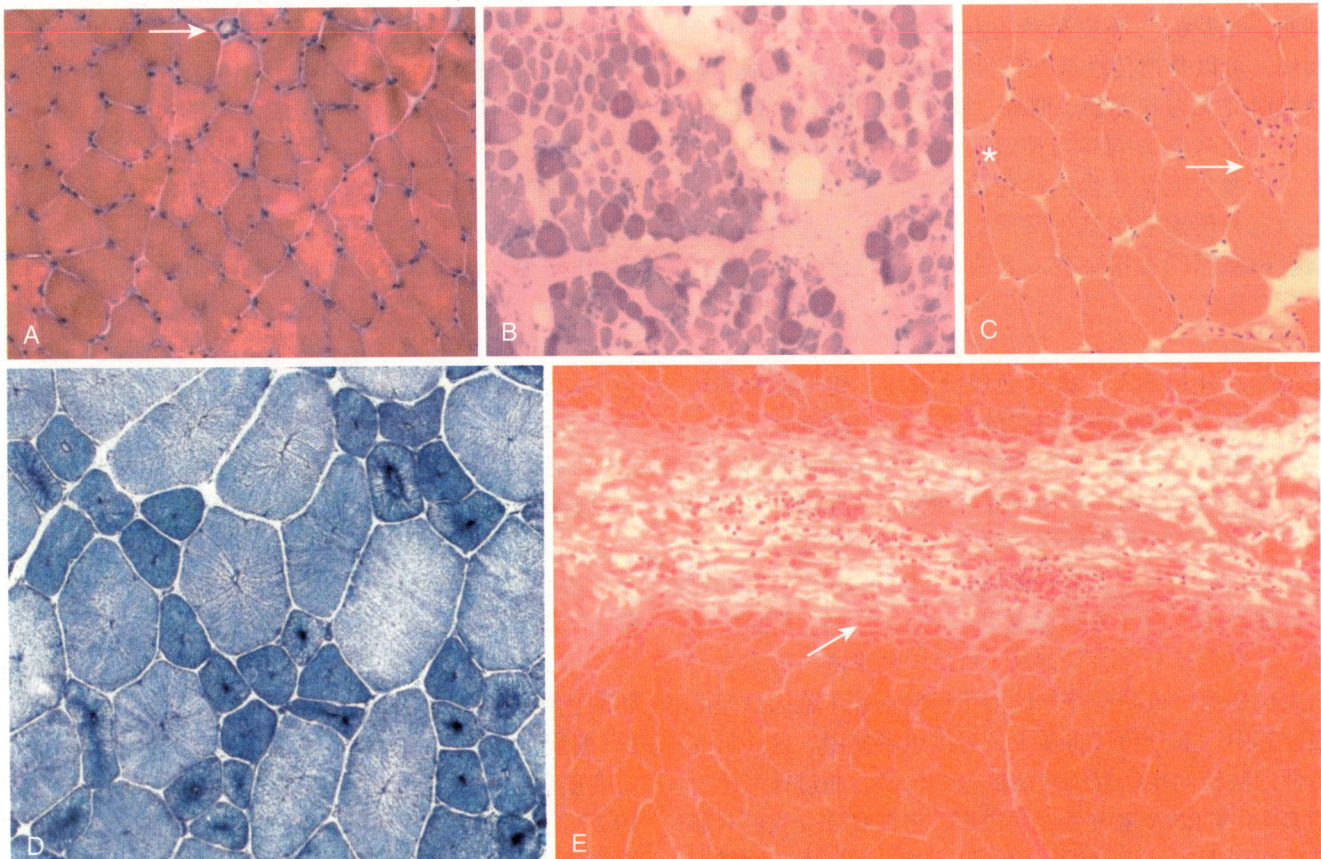

Fig. 19.1 Muscle biopsies hematoxylin and eosin staining. When assessing the health of muscle tissue, the pathologist evaluates the size, shape and internal architecture of muscle fibers, presence of inflammation and mitochondrial dysfunction, and amount of connective tissue. In a chronic myopathic muscle, the muscle fibers are typically more variable in size, rounded, and have central nuclei. Connective tissue can be increased. In an active myopathy, necrotic fibers undergoing phagocytosis and regenerating fibers can be seen. (A) **Normal adult muscle**, medium power. Notice polygonal muscle fibers arranged in fascicles with blue staining nuclei on the periphery. A small arteriole is visible *(white arrow)*. (B) **Chronic myopathy**, Duchenne muscular dystrophy low power. Note the variability in fiber size with rounding of fibers, increase in connective tissue, and fatty deposition. (C) **Acute myopathy**, necrotizing myopathy with HMGCR antibodies. Necrotic fiber *(white arrow)* undergoing phagocytosis and regenerating fiber (*) with plump nuclei. Examples for disease characteristic findings on muscle pathology. (D) **Centronuclear congenital myopathy.** The NADH reaction shows numerous fibers with spoke-like, radial projections with central nuclei. Also notable fiber size variability, identified as moderate type 1 fiber atrophy on other stains. (E) **Dermatomyositis** on low power. Notice the prominent pathognomonic perifascicular atrophy *(white arrow)* of fibers, and perivascular inflammatory infiltrates.

表 19.1　肌病概述
遗传性肌病
肌营养不良症
先天性肌病
代谢性 / 线粒体肌病
离子通道病
获得性肌病
炎症性肌病
HMGCR 抗体肌病
内分泌性肌病
系统性疾病 / 感染性肌病
中毒 / 药物诱导性肌病

特别是在儿童中。应检查肌肉是否有萎缩或肥大，并检查关节周围的活动范围以寻找肌腱挛缩的证据。肌病中存在 10 种常见的肌无力模式（表 19.4）。大多数肌病具有近端、肢带模式。此外，还有一些非常特异的模式。面肩肱型肌营养不良的特征是面部、近端手臂和肩部，以及远端下肢的不对称无力。远端手指屈肌（患者无法在握拳时弯曲手指）和近端下肢（股四头肌）无力是散发性包涵体肌炎的特征性表现。中年患者出现眼睑下垂和吞咽困难是眼咽肌营养不良的高度特异性表现。

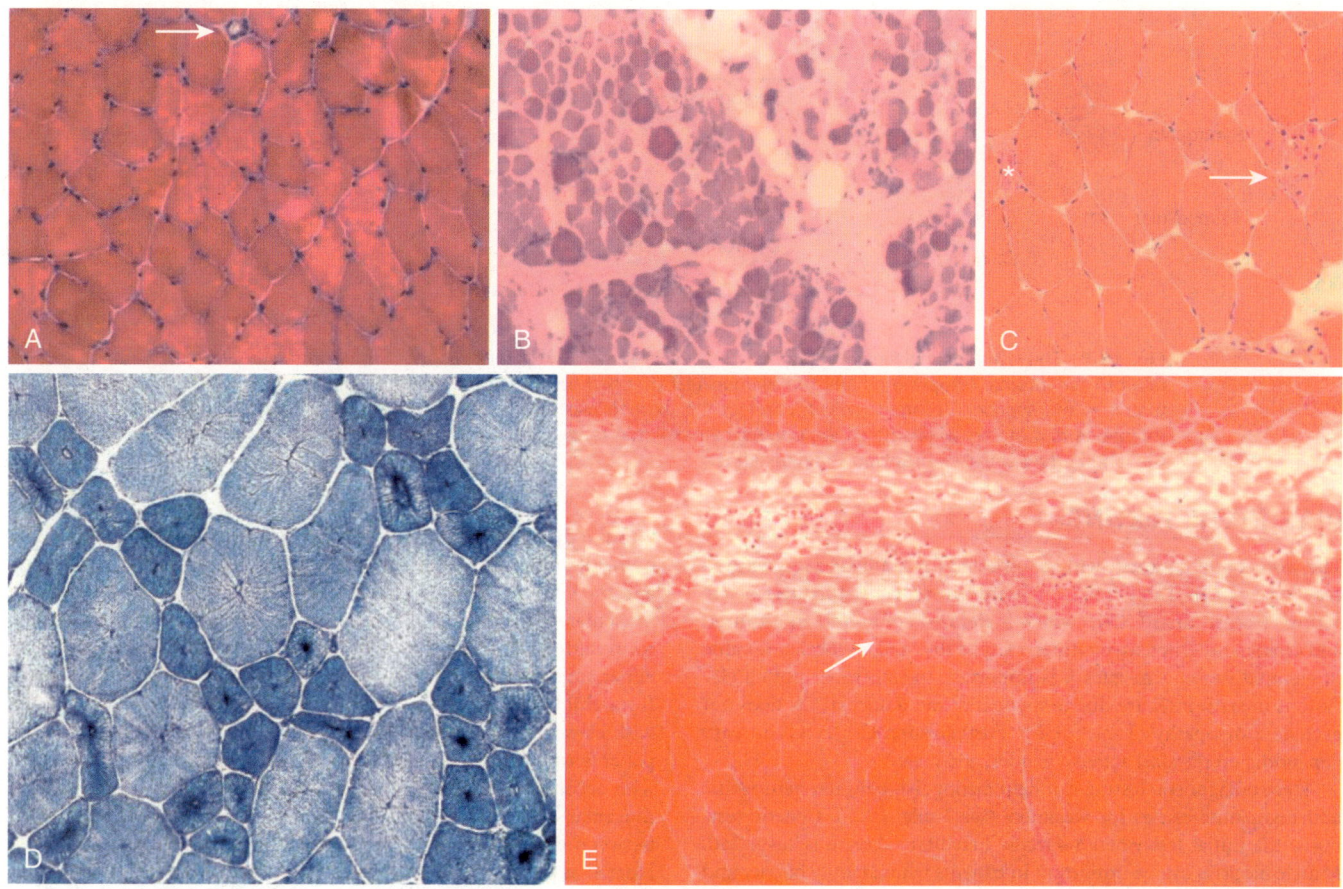

图 19.1　肌肉活检苏木精-伊红染色。病理学家在评估肌肉组织健康状况时，会检查肌纤维的大小、形状及其内部结构，是否存在炎症和线粒体功能障碍，以及结缔组织的数量。在慢性肌病中，肌纤维的大小通常更为多样，形状呈圆形，有中央核。结缔组织可能增多。在活动性肌病中，可以看到正在被吞噬的坏死纤维和再生纤维。（**A**）**正常成年人肌肉**，中倍镜。注意排列成束的多边形肌纤维，外围有蓝染的细胞核。可见一个小动脉（白色箭头）。（**B**）**慢性肌病**，低倍镜下的进行性假肥大性肌营养不良。注意纤维大小的变化和纤维的圆形化，结缔组织增多和脂肪沉积。（**C**）**急性肌病**，伴有 HMGCR 抗体的坏死性肌病。可见正在被吞噬的坏死纤维（白色箭头）和具有丰满细胞核的再生纤维（*）。这些是肌肉病理中疾病特征性表现的示例。（**D**）**中央核先天性肌病**。NADH 反应显示许多纤维具有辐射状投射及中央核，同时纤维的大小差异明显，在其他染色中被鉴定为中度 1 型纤维萎缩。（**E**）低倍镜下的**皮肌炎**。注意纤维显著的特征性束周萎缩（白色箭头），以及血管周围的炎性浸润

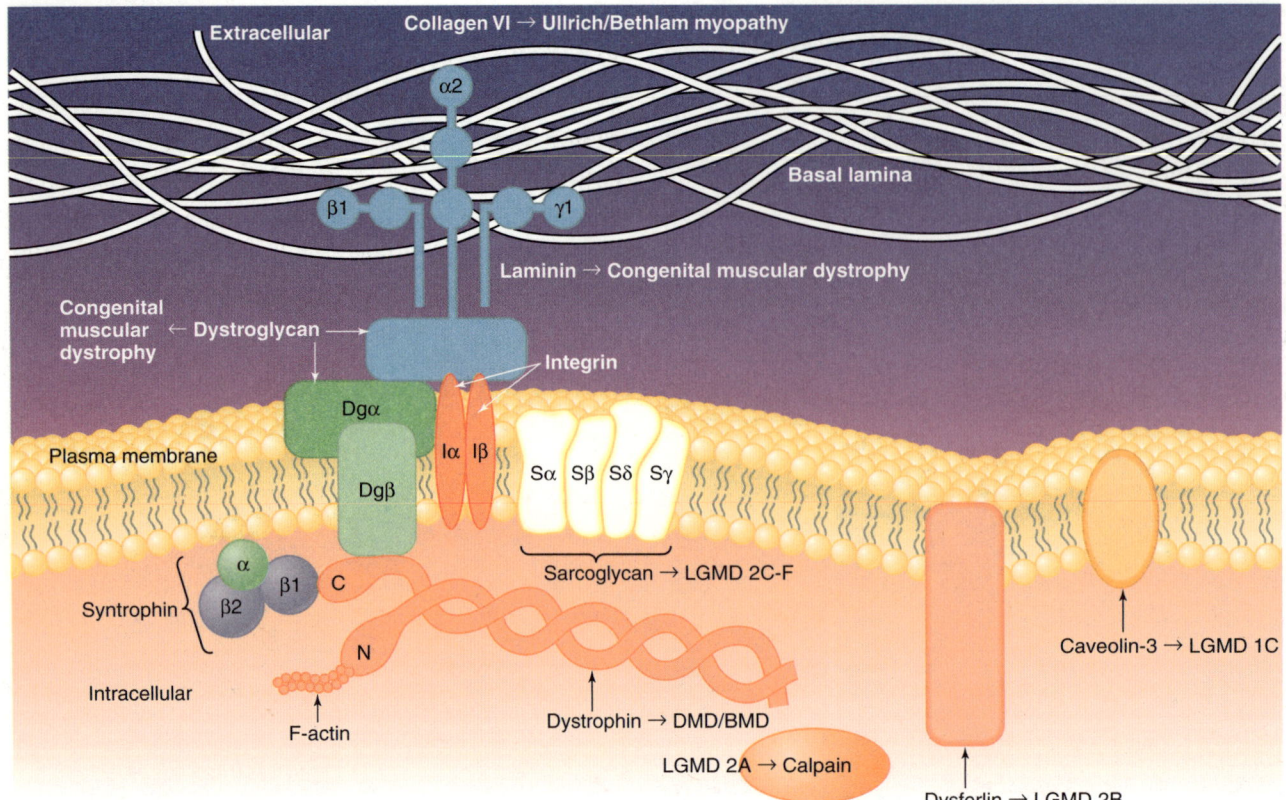

Fig. 19.2 The dystrophin-glycoprotein complex. Muscle structural proteins connect the contractile apparatus to the internal cytoskeleton and the extracellular matrix. Mutations in proteins from the extracellular matrix to the anchoring proteins, which connect the extracellular matrix to the internal cytoskeleton, and mutations to proteins, which attach the internal cytoskeleton to the contractile apparatus, are all involved in the inherited muscular dystrophies and myopathies.

DIAGNOSTIC TESTING

The work-up of a patient with a suspected myopathy is a staged process, outlined in Table 19.2. A useful initial laboratory test is the serum creatine kinase (CK), which is elevated commonly in acquired and often in inherited myopathies. Despite the obvious localizing value of elevated muscle enzymes it is important to remember not all elevations in serum CK are due to myopathy and a normal CK does not exclude a myopathy (Table 19.5). Furthermore, CK levels can vary depending on physical activity, gender, and race.

Electrodiagnostic testing can help distinguish between neurogenic and myopathic causes for weakness (see Table 19.2). Genetic testing is the initial test when a specific hereditary disease is suspected. Muscle biopsies can be important in patients whose family history and physical examination does not suggest a particular myopathic diagnosis and can help resolve variants of uncertain significance on genetic testing. Characteristic morphologic changes (see Fig. 19.1) are hallmarks of the congenital myopathies (e.g., centronuclear myopathy in Fig. 19.1D), inflammatory myopathies (dermatomyositis in Fig. 19.1E), and metabolic myopathies (glycogen storage disorders), but most myopathies result in nonspecific muscle changes, which confirms the localization (muscle), but not the cause.

INHERITED MYOPATHIES

Muscular Dystrophies

The muscular dystrophies are inherited myopathies characterized by progressive weakness. Typically the muscular dystrophies are divided into the dystrophinopathies, the myotonic dystrophies, facioscapulohumeral muscular dystrophy, Emery-Dreifuss muscular dystrophy, and the limb-girdle dystrophies (Tables 19.6, 19.7). The limb-girdle muscular dystrophies (LGMD) are a diverse group of diseases due to mutations in more than 20 genes. The LGMDs are inherited in either autosomal dominant or recessive fashion and present anywhere from childhood after achieving independent walking to later in life, with elevated CK and proximal muscle weakness. Another group of patients who have dystrophic changes in the muscle from birth, often with accompanying changes in the brain on MRI, include congenital muscular dystrophies (see Table 19.7). The traditional distinction between dystrophies and other inherited myopathies is becoming blurred as our genetic understanding advances because mutations for different diseases are often allelic.

Dystrophinopathies
Definition and Epidemiology

Dystrophinopathies are X-linked recessive disorders resulting from mutations of the large dystrophin gene located at Xp21. The incidence of Duchenne muscular dystrophy is 1 in 5300 male births; one third of the cases result from a new mutation. Becker muscular dystrophy is a milder form of dystrophinopathy and is less common than the Duchenne form, with an incidence of 5 per 100,000.

Genetics and Pathology

The majority of patients have deletions or duplications in the dystrophin gene. In the remaining patients, mutations can be small insertions

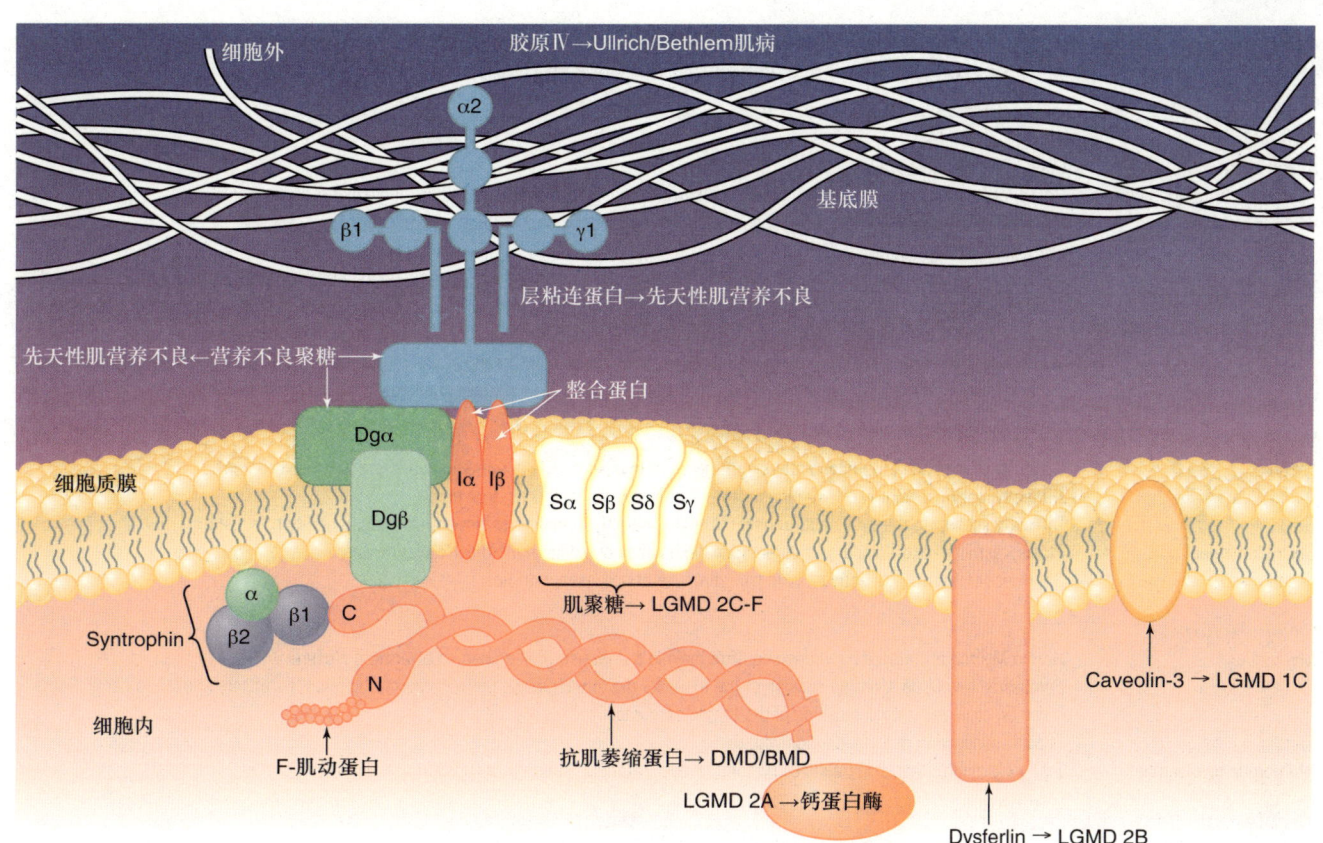

图19.2 抗肌萎缩蛋白-糖蛋白复合物。肌肉结构蛋白将收缩装置连接到内部细胞骨架和细胞外基质。无论是从细胞外基质到连接细胞外基质与内部细胞骨架的锚定蛋白,还是将内部细胞骨架连接至收缩装置的蛋白,这些蛋白的突变都与遗传性肌营养不良和肌病有关

诊断性检查

对疑似肌病患者的检查是一个分阶段的过程,详见表19.2。首选的实验室检查是血清肌酸激酶(CK),它在获得性和遗传性肌病中常常升高。尽管肌酶升高具有重要的诊断意义,但必须记住,并非所有血清CK升高都是由肌病引起的,且正常的CK水平并不排除肌病的可能性(表19.5)。此外,CK水平可能因体力活动、性别和种族而有所不同。

肌电图检查可以帮助区分神经源性和肌源性病因所致的无力(见表19.2)。在怀疑特定遗传性疾病时,基因检测是首选检查。对于家族史和体格检查未提示特定肌病诊断的患者,肌肉活检可能非常重要,并且有助于解释基因检测中意义不明的变异。特征性的形态学变化(见图19.1)是先天性肌病(如图19.1D中的中央核肌病)、炎症性肌病(如图19.1E中的皮肌炎)以及代谢性肌病(糖原贮积症)的标志,但大多数肌病会导致非特异性的肌肉变化,这虽然证实了病变的定位(在肌肉),但并未明确其病因。

遗传性肌病

肌营养不良

肌营养不良是一类遗传性肌病,其特征是进行性无力。通常,肌营养不良分为抗肌萎缩蛋白病、强直性肌营养不良、面肩肱型肌营养不良、埃默里-德赖弗斯肌营养不良和肢带型肌营养不良(表19.6和表19.7)。肢带型肌营养不良(LGMD)是由超过20个基因突变引起的一类多样化疾病。这些疾病可通过常染色体显性或隐性方式遗传,可在自独立行走后到晚年时期的不同年龄段出现症状,伴有CK水平升高和近端肌肉无力。另外一类患者自出生起就有肌营养不良性变化,常伴随MRI显示的脑部变化,包括先天性肌营养不良(见表19.7)。随着我们对遗传学的理解不断深入,传统上对肌营养不良和其他遗传性肌病的区分变得越来越模糊,因为不同疾病的突变往往是等位基因。

抗肌萎缩蛋白病

定义与流行病学

抗肌萎缩蛋白病是一类由位于Xp21上的大型抗肌萎缩蛋白基因突变引起的X连锁隐性遗传疾病。进行性假肥大性肌营养不良的发病率为每5300名男婴中有1例,其中1/3的病例是由于新突变引起的。贝克肌营养不良是抗肌萎缩蛋白病中较轻的一种,其发病率较进行性假肥大性肌营养不良低,每10万人中有5例。

遗传学与病理学

大多数患者的抗肌萎缩蛋白基因存在缺失或重复突变。少数患者可能表现为小插入或缺失、点突变或

TABLE 19.2 Evaluation for a Patient With Suspected Myopathy

Feature	Description
History	
Age of onset	Congenital, childhood, adult
Acute/subacute or chronic	Hereditary myopathies are usually chronic with gradual onset, acquired myopathies can occur more acutely
Progressive or episodic	Dystrophies are usually progressive; congenital static; metabolic/channelopathies episodic
Triggers	Exercise, foods, temperature
Myotonia	Delayed relaxation of muscle: e.g., difficulty letting go when shaking hands, opening doorknobs, myotonia can also affect tongue movements (speech) and chewing. Myotonia improves with repetition (warm-up phenomenon) and gets worse in cold temperature.
Family History	It can be helpful to draw out a pedigree to determine the pattern of inheritance, which can be dominant, recessive, or no family history. Questions about whether family members require assistive devices to walk or wheelchairs, and asking about extra-muscular manifestation of muscular dystrophies can be useful, specifically as diseases may not have been recognized.
Weakness on Exam	
Proximal	Difficulty lifting objects, climbing stairs, getting up from chair, scapular winging, waddling gait, Gower sign
Distal	Difficulty making a tight fist, fastening buttons, opening jars, wrist drop, foot drop
Facial	Difficulty squeezing the eyes shut, transverse smile, inability to pucker or blow out cheeks, inability to whistle
Oculopharyngeal	Ptosis, restricted extra-ocular movements, coughing after drinking, and difficulty swallowing
Respiratory	Shortness of breath with activity, with lying flat, use of accessory muscles
Other Features	
Myotonia	Action Myotonia: Delayed hand opening after making a tight fist, or eye opening after tight closure
	Percussion Myotonia: With percussion of the extensor digitorum muscle in the forearm, the finger extensors relax with delay. Same can be observed with percussion of the thenar eminence
Cardiac	Cardiac conduction defects, cardiomyopathy
Multiorgan involvement	E.g., joint deformities, skin (rash), GI symptoms, eye (cataract), hearing loss, CNS involvement
Laboratory	
Creatine kinase (CK)	Dystrophies/inflammatory myopathy increased >10× normal; congenital 3–5× normal; metabolic >10× normal during attacks
Thyroid/Parathyroid	High TSH, low T4, low PTH, Ca^{2+}
Antibodies	Patients with myositis:
	Myositis specific antibodies: Anti-Jo-1, antisynthetase antibodies, signal recognition particle (SRP) antibodies, Mi-2 antibodies, anti hPMS-1, anti-MDA-5 antibody, anti-p140, anti-p155/140.
	Inclusion Body myositis: Cytoplasmic 5′-nucleotidase 1A (cN1A)
	Patients with proximal muscle weakness of unknown etiology or necrotizing myopathies: Antibodies to 3-hydroxy-3-methylglutaryl coenzyme A reductase (HMGCR)
Genetic Testing	Patients with family history and/or examination suggestive of a hereditary myopathy. A positive test can be confirmatory and avoid additional diagnostic testing.
Electrodiagnostic Studies	Nerve conduction studies are typically normal in muscle diseases. On electromyography, irritated muscle shows fibrillations and positive sharp waves; myopathic motor units are brief, low amplitude, and polyphasic; electrical myotonia is a repetitive muscle fiber potential discharge with waxing and waning frequency and amplitude with characteristic sound similar to an accelerating, decelerating motorcycle engine.
Muscle Biopsy	Chronic: Changes in muscle fiber shape and composition of fiber types, central nuclei, increased amount of connective tissue
	Acute: Necrotic muscle fibers, regenerating fibers
	Other: Presence of inflammatory cells, number or morphology of mitochondria, or abnormal deposits of fat or glycogen

or deletions, point mutations, or splice site variants. Dystrophin is a large subsarcolemmal cytoskeletal protein that, along with the other components of the dystrophin-glycoprotein complex, provides support to the muscle membrane during contraction. Mutations in dystrophin can result in a spectrum of dystrophin dysfunction, from a severely truncated protein that is rapidly degraded, as in Duchenne muscular dystrophy, to a semi-functional protein still expressed such as in the milder form, Becker's muscular dystrophy, or mild dysfunction such as in female carriers. Muscle biopsies are typically not required for diagnosis (example depicted in Fig. 19.1B).

Clinical Presentation

Duchenne muscular dystrophy manifests as early as age 2 to 3 years with delays in motor milestones and difficulty running. Patients can have marked pseudo-hypertrophy of the calf muscles. And when asked to get up from the floor, boys use a Gower maneuver (use hands to push up). The average age of diagnosis is around 4 years of age. The proximal muscles are the most severely affected, and the course is relentlessly progressive. Patients begin to fall frequently by age 5 to 6, have difficulty climbing stairs by age 8 years, and are usually confined to a wheelchair in their early teens. Patients have a reduced life expectancy due to cardiac (dilated cardiomyopathy) and respiratory muscle weakness. The average IQ of boys with Duchenne muscular dystrophy is low, reflecting central nervous system involvement.

Diagnosis and Differential Diagnosis

Diagnosis is based on clinical history, physical examination, serum CK, and is confirmed by genetic testing. Other differential considerations are congenital myopathies, muscular dystrophies, and limb-girdle muscular dystrophies.

表 19.2　对疑似肌病患者的评估	
特征	描述
病史	
发病年龄	先天性、儿童期、成人期
急性、亚急性或慢性	遗传性肌病通常具有慢性且逐渐发病的特点，而获得性肌病则更可能急性发病
进展性或阵发性	肌营养不良通常是进展性的，先天性肌病则是静止性的，代谢性肌病和离子通道病则表现为阵发性发作
诱因	运动、食物、温度
肌强直	肌肉的延迟放松：例如，在握手后难以松手、开门把手困难，肌强直还可以影响舌头运动（言语）和咀嚼。肌强直在重复活动后有所改善（预热现象），在低温下则变得更严重
家族史	绘制家系图以确定遗传模式（显性、隐性或无家族史）可能是有帮助的。询问家族成员是否需要助行器或轮椅，以及询问肌营养不良的肌肉外表现可能很有价值，特别是当这些疾病尚未被识别时
查体中的无力	
近端	举物、爬楼梯、从椅子上站起存在困难，肩胛骨翼状突出，鸭步步态，Gower 征
远端	握拳、系扣子、开启罐子存在困难，腕下垂、足下垂
面部	闭眼困难，横向微笑，无法噘嘴或鼓腮，不能吹口哨
眼咽部	上睑下垂，眼外肌活动受限，饮水后咳嗽，吞咽困难
呼吸系统	活动后、平躺时气短，使用辅助呼吸肌
其他特征	
肌强直	动作性肌强直：握紧拳头后手部打开延迟，或紧闭眼睛后眼睁开延迟 叩击性肌强直：叩击前臂的指伸肌时，手指伸肌放松延迟。同样的现象可在叩击鱼际肌时观察到
心脏	心脏传导缺陷、心肌病
多器官受累	例如，关节畸形、皮肤（皮疹）、胃肠道症状、眼睛（白内障）、听力损失、中枢神经系统受累
实验室检查	
肌酸激酶（CK）	肌营养不良/炎症性肌病增加＞正常的 10 倍，先天性肌病是正常的 3～5 倍，代谢性肌病在发作期间＞正常的 10 倍
甲状腺和甲状旁腺	高 TSH、低 T4、低 PTH、低 Ca^{2+}
抗体	肌炎患者： 肌炎相关特异性抗体：抗 Jo-1 抗体、抗合成酶抗体、信号识别颗粒（SRP）抗体、Mi-2 抗体、抗 hPMS-1 抗体、抗 MDA-5 抗体、抗 p140 抗体、抗 p155/140 抗体 包涵体肌炎：胞质 5′-核苷酸酶 1A（cN1A） 病因不明的近端肌无力或坏死性肌病患者：抗 3-羟基-3-甲基戊二酰辅酶 A 还原酶（HMGCR）抗体
基因检测	有家族史和（或）检查提示遗传性肌病的患者。阳性检测可以确认诊断，并避免额外的诊断测试
电生理诊断研究	肌肉疾病中的神经传导检查通常正常。在肌电图检查中，受累肌肉显示纤颤和正锐波；肌源性运动单位短暂、低幅、多相；电性肌强直是重复的肌纤维电位放电，频率和幅度呈现波动，具有类似发动机加速和减速的特征性声音
肌肉活检	慢性：肌纤维形状和纤维类型的成分发生改变，中央核，结缔组织增加 急性：坏死的肌纤维，再生的纤维 其他：存在炎性细胞，线粒体的数量或形态，或异常的脂肪或糖原沉积

TSH，促甲状腺激素；PTH，甲状旁腺激素。

剪接位点变异。抗肌萎缩蛋白是一种大型膜下细胞骨架蛋白，与抗肌萎缩蛋白-糖蛋白复合物的其他成分一起，在肌肉收缩过程中为肌膜提供支持。抗肌萎缩蛋白的突变可导致一系列的抗肌萎缩蛋白功能障碍谱系疾病，从迅速降解的严重截短蛋白（如进行性假肥大性肌营养不良），到仍有部分功能表达的蛋白（如较轻型的贝克肌营养不良），或者像女性携带者那样的轻度功能障碍。通常诊断不需要进行肌肉活检（示例见图 19.1B）。

临床表现

进行性假肥大性肌营养不良通常在 2～3 岁时出现症状，表现为运动发育迟缓和跑步困难。患者的小腿肌肉显著假性肥大。当要求从地上站起来时，男孩会使用 Gower 动作（用手推起身体）。平均诊断年龄约为 4 岁。近端肌肉受累最为严重，病程呈持续进行性发展。患者在 5～6 岁时开始频繁跌倒，8 岁时爬楼梯困难，通常在青少年早期就需依靠轮椅。由于心脏（扩张型心肌病）和呼吸肌无力，患者的预期寿命减少。患有进行性假肥大性肌营养不良的男孩平均智商较低，这反映了疾病累及中枢神经系统。

诊断和鉴别诊断

诊断基于临床病史、体格检查、血清 CK 水平，并通过基因检测确认。其他需要鉴别的疾病包括先天性肌病、肌营养不良和肢带型肌营养不良。

Treatment

Care for children with Duchenne muscular dystrophy involves a multidisciplinary team along with pulmonologists, orthopedists, and cardiologists, with monitoring of cardiac and respiratory function as well as scoliosis. Prednisone and deflazacort (a synthetic derivative of prednisolone) improve strength and motor function, pulmonary function, and prolong the ability to walk and survival in children with Duchenne muscular dystrophy.

About 15% of patients with Duchenne muscular dystrophy carry a mutation on exon 51. Eteplirsen is a drug that binds to exon 51 and induces "exon skipping," resulting in production of a truncated, but potentially functional dystrophin protein. The drug was approved in the United States by the FDA in 2016 and current trials are carried out to demonstrate a clinical benefit. Subsequently, two therapies were approved for patients with pathogenic variants on exon 53 (about 8% of patients with Duchenne muscular dystrophy). These therapies, golodirsen and vitolarsen, target RNA and result in exon 53 skipping. Ataluren is approved in countries outside of the United States for children with nonsense mutation. The drug allows read-through of premature stop mutations with the goal to produce a more functional dystrophin protein but with mixed results on functional outcome measures. Continued efforts and studies focus on strategies to make the cell produce some form of dystrophin, by targeting RNA or utilizing gene therapy targeting DNA. While these therapies will likely change the trajectory of DMD and care practices, new challenges will arise, such as costs, access (due to the genetic variability of DMD, therapies will target a subset of patients), duration of effect, and long-term safety concerns.

There are no guidelines for the treatment of Becker muscular dystrophy and clinical presentation is highly variable, but monitoring for cardiac and respiratory involvement is warranted. Some female carriers of dystrophin mutations may become symptomatic later in life and may have severe cardiomyopathy.

Prognosis

Patients with Duchenne muscular dystrophy die of respiratory complications in their 20s unless they are provided with respiratory support. Emerging targeted therapies will likely change this trajectory. Congestive heart failure and arrhythmias can occur late in the disease.

TABLE 19.3 Modified Medical Research Council Motor Strength Testing Scale

Grade	Degree of Strength
5	Normal strength through entire range of motion and against resistance
5−	Equivocal, barely detectable weakness
4+	Able to move against gravity and resistance, but examiner can break
4	Able to move against gravity and some resistance
4−	Able to resist gravity but only minimal resistance
3+	Able to overcome gravity and transient resistance, but then quickly gives out
3	Able to overcome gravity but no resistance
3−	Able to resist gravity but not through full range of motion
2	Able to move through range of motion with gravity eliminated
1	Trace muscle contraction
0	No contraction

TABLE 19.4 Characteristic Patterns of Muscle Weakness and Associated Myopathies

Pattern	Weakness	Diseases
Proximal limb-girdle	Symmetrical, pelvic and shoulder girdle muscles. Distal muscles to lesser extent. ±Neck flexor/extensor	Nonspecific: Duchenne muscular dystrophy; limb-girdle muscular dystrophy; inflammatory myopathies; Myopathy with HMGCR antibodies; myotonic dystrophy type 2
Distal	Symmetrical, distal upper or lower extremity. Proximal muscles to lesser degree	Nonspecific: Miyoshi myopathy (calves); Welander myopathy (wrist and finger extensors); Nonaka and Markesbery/Udd myopathy (tibialis anterior); rule out neuropathy
Proximal arm/distal leg	Scapuloperoneal distribution: periscapular muscles (proximal arm) and anterior compartment distal leg (tibialis anterior). Scapular winging. Can be asymmetrical.	When face involved highly suggestive of facioscapulohumeral muscular dystrophy; with elbow contractures Emory-Dreifuss dystrophy; scapuloperoneal dystrophies; certain limb-girdle dystrophies; congenital myopathies
Distal arm/proximal leg	Distal forearm muscles (distal finger flexors) and proximal leg (quadriceps). Other muscles variable. Often asymmetrical.	Highly suggestive of sporadic inclusion body myositis; also consider myotonic dystrophy type 1 with distal leg, neck flexion, respiratory and facial weakness
Ptosis ± ophthalmoparesis	Restriction of eye movements often without diplopia. Often with pharyngeal weakness and variable extremity weakness.	Ocular and pharyngeal weakness highly suggestive of oculopharyngeal muscular dystrophy; mitochondrial myopathies
Neck extensor weakness	Neck extensors, "dropped head syndrome." Variable neck flexor. ±Extremity weakness.	Inflammatory myopathies, in isolation consider isolated neck extensor myopathy; rule out amyotrophic lateral sclerosis and myasthenia gravis
Bulbar weakness	Tongue and pharyngeal weakness	Certain myopathies (e.g., oculopharyngeal muscular dystrophy); significant overlap with neuromuscular junction and motor neuron disease
Episodic pain, weakness, and myoglobinuria	May be triggered by exercise or metabolic stress	Metabolic myopathies; may also occur in deconditioning
Episodic weakness delayed or unrelated to exercise	May be triggered by food, stress, rest after exercise	Characteristic of periodic paralyses
Stiffness and decreased ability to relax	May be episodic, triggered by cold	Characteristic of myotonic disorders

Modified from Jackson CE, Barohn RJ: A pattern recognition approach to myopathy, Continuum (Minneap Minn) 19(6 Muscle Diseases):1674-1697, 2013.

治疗

对于进行性假肥大性肌营养不良儿童的治疗需要多学科团队参与，包括胸肺科医生、骨科医生和心脏病专科医生，需要监测心肺功能和脊柱侧弯。泼尼松和地夫可特（一种泼尼松龙的合成衍生物）可以改善肌力和运动功能、肺功能，并延长进行性假肥大性肌营养不良儿童的行走能力和生存期。

约 15% 的进行性假肥大性肌营养不良患者携有外显子 51 的突变。依特立生（Eteplirsen）是一种可以与外显子 51 结合并诱导"外显子跳跃"的药物，从而产生截短但潜在功能的抗肌萎缩蛋白。该药物于 2016 年在美国获 FDA 批准，目前正在进行临床试验以验证其临床益处。随后，又有两种针对外显子 53 致病性变异（约占进行性假肥大性肌营养不良患者的 8%）的治疗药物获批，分别是戈洛迪森（golodirsen）和维特拉森（vitolarsen），旨在诱导外显子 53 跳跃。阿塔鲁伦（Ataluren）则在美国以外的国家获批用于无义突变的儿童。该药物允许读取"提前终止"突变，以产生功能更强的抗肌萎缩蛋白，但其对功能结局测量指标的效果参差不齐。持续的努力和研究集中在通过靶向 RNA 或利用基因疗法靶向 DNA，来使细胞产生某种形式的抗肌萎缩蛋白。尽管这些疗法可能会改变进行性假肥大性肌营养不良（DMD）的进程和护理实践，但也会带来新的挑战，如成本、获取（由于 DMD 的遗传变异性，这些疗法仅针对一部分患者）、效果持久性和长期安全性问题。

目前对于贝克肌营养不良的治疗没有指南，临床表现高度多样，但需要监测心肺功能。一些肌营养不良蛋白突变的女性携带者可能会在更大年龄时出现症状，并可能发展为严重的心肌病。

预后

进行性假肥大性肌营养不良患者通常在 20 多岁时死于呼吸并发症，除非患者得到呼吸支持。新兴的靶向治疗可能会改变这一进程。晚期可出现充血性心力衰竭和心律失常。

表 19.3　改良医学研究会运动力量测试量表

等级	肌力程度
5	在整个活动范围内对抗阻力均能正常发力
5−	微弱的、勉强可察觉的无力
4+	能够克服重力和阻力，但检查者可以打破
4	能够克服重力和部分阻力
4−	能够克服重力，但只能克服最小阻力
3+	能够克服重力和短暂阻力，但随后就会失去力量
3	能够克服重力，但无法克服任何阻力
3−	能够克服重力，但不能坚持整个活动范围
2	在消除重力的情况下能够完成活动范围
1	有微弱的肌肉收缩
0	无肌肉收缩

表 19.4　肌肉无力及相关肌病的特征模式

模式	无力	疾病
近端肢带型	对称性、骨盆和肩胛带肌受累。远端肌肉受累程度较轻。± 颈部屈肌 / 伸肌	非特异性：进行性假肥大性肌营养不良，肢带型肌营养不良，炎症性肌病，HMGCR 抗体肌病，强直性肌营养不良 2 型
远端型	对称性、远端上肢或下肢受累。近端肌肉受累程度较轻	非特异性：Miyoshi 肌病（小腿），Welander 肌病（腕部和手指伸肌），Nonaka 和 Markesbery/Udd 肌病（胫骨前肌）；需要排除神经病
近端上肢 / 远端下肢	肩胛腓肠肌分布：肩胛周围肌肉（近端上肢）和远端腿前部肌肉（胫骨前肌）。肩胛骨翼状突出。可能不对称	面部受累时高度提示面肩肱型肌营养不良，伴有肘部挛缩提示埃默里-德赖弗斯肌营养不良，肩胛腓肠肌营养不良，某些肢带型肌营养不良，先天性肌病
远端上肢 / 近端下肢	远端前臂肌肉（远端手指屈肌）和近端腿部肌肉（股四头肌）。其他肌肉受累程度不一。常见不对称	高度提示散发性包涵体肌炎，也要考虑 1 型强直性肌营养不良伴远端腿部、颈部屈肌、呼吸肌和面肌无力
上睑下垂 ± 眼肌麻痹	眼球运动受限，通常无复视。常伴咽部无力和不同程度的肢体无力	眼部和咽部无力高度提示眼咽肌营养不良，线粒体肌病
颈部伸肌无力	颈部伸肌无力，"下垂头综合征"。颈部屈肌受累程度不一。± 肢体无力	炎症性肌病，单独考虑孤立性颈伸肌肌病；需排除肌萎缩侧索硬化和重症肌无力
延髓支配肌无力	舌肌和咽肌无力	某些肌病（如眼咽肌营养不良），与神经肌肉接头疾病和运动神经元疾病有显著重叠
阵发性疼痛、无力和肌红蛋白尿	可能由运动或代谢应激引发	代谢性肌病，也可见于失用性肌病（deconditioning）
与运动无关或延迟的阵发性无力	可能由食物、压力、运动后休息引发	周期性瘫痪的特征
僵硬和放松能力降低	可能是阵发性，由寒冷引发	肌强直性疾病的特征

改编自 Jackson CE，Barohn RJ：A pattern recognition approach to myopathy，Continuum（Minneap Minn）19（6 Muscle Diseases）：1674-1697，2013.

TABLE 19.5 Causes for Elevated Serum CK

Myopathies
Muscular dystrophies/Duchenne carrier state
Congenital myopathies
Metabolic myopathies
Inflammatory myopathies

Channelopathies
Motor Neuron Disease (ALS, SMA)
Neuropathies (GBS, CIDP)
Viral Illness

Medications
Statins
Fibric acid derivatives
Chloroquine
Colchicine

Endocrine Abnormalities (Thyroid/Parathyroid)
Surgery
Trauma
Strenuous Exercise
Increased Muscle Mass
Idiopathic—Ethnic Variability

Myotonic Dystrophy
Definition and Epidemiology

Myotonic dystrophies are the most common muscular dystrophies in adults of European ancestry with autosomal dominant inheritance. There are two types of myotonic dystrophy, type 1 (DM1) and type 2 (DM2). The frequency of DM1 in Europe is estimated at 1 in 8000. While DM1 and DM2 are equally frequent in Europe, DM2 seems less common in the United States.

Genetics and Pathology

DM1 is caused by a CTG repeat expansion on the *DMPK* gene whereas DM2 is caused by a CCTG repeat expansion on the *CNBP* gene. Both diseases share the same mechanism of RNA toxicity. Expanded CUG/CCUG repeats accumulate in nuclear foci and sequester important proteins that typically regulate RNA splicing. Loss of function of these proteins results in missplicing of various RNAs of multiple genes, resulting in wide transcriptome changes and multisystemic disease. In DM1, some but not all of the variability in age of symptom onset is explained by repeat length, with earlier onset typically associated with greater disease severity and longer repeat length. The CTG repeat is unstable and increases in somatic tissue throughout a persons' life (somatic instability) and tends to increase from generation to generation (anticipation). Genetic testing confirms the diagnosis and muscle biopsies are not required but characteristic findings

TABLE 19.6 Prevalent Muscular Dystrophies

Disease	Inheritance	Mutations	Age of Onset	Phenotypes	Treatment
Dystrophinopathies	X-linked recessive	Xp21; ≈75% deletion or duplication	Duchenne diagnosis by age 4; Becker variable	Limb-girdle pattern. Duchenne: severe progressive and life limiting. Becker: progressive but not as severe, more variable. Calf pseudo-hypertrophy; isolated cardiomyopathy.	For Duchenne: Prednisone (or deflazacort), Eteplirsen, golodirsen, and vitolarsen; surveillance for respiratory, cardiac, and orthopedic problems
Myotonic dystrophy type 1	Autosomal dominant	19q13; CTG expansion >50 repeats	Any age with marked variability; congenital at birth	Marked clinical variability but typically muscle weakness and wasting affecting face, neck flexion, respiratory and distal muscles (finger flexion, ankle dorsiflexion); myotonia; temporal wasting, frontal balding; multisystemic disease manifestations (e.g., with cognitive deficits, hypersomnolence, cataracts); cardiac conduction deficits	Mexiletine for symptomatic myotonia; yearly surveillance for ocular and respiratory involvement and cardiac conduction deficits
Myotonic dystrophy type 2	Autosomal dominant	3q13; CCTG expansion >75 repeats	30s and older	Limb-girdle pattern; myalgia; myotonia; multisystem involvement (e.g., cataracts, cardiac conduction deficits); diabetes	Mexiletine for symptomatic myotonia; surveillance for ocular, cardiac, and respiratory involvement
Facioscapulohumeral muscular dystrophy	Autosomal dominant	95%: 4q35 (FSHD1), 5% digenic mutation affecting methylation (FSHD2)	Any age	Scapuloperoneal pattern with facial involvement; can have marked asymmetry; significant axial involvement	Screening for extramuscular manifestation
Emery-Dreifuss muscular dystrophy	X-linked recessive; autosomal dominant or recessive	≈70% Xq28 Emerin or FHL1 mutation; 1q21 lamin A/C, both dominant and recessive mutations reported	Joint contractures childhood; progressive weakness 20s–30s	Scapuloperoneal pattern; early joint contractures, particularly at elbows, marked cardiac involvement	Yearly surveillance for cardiac and respiratory involvement; orthopedic evaluation for symptomatic contractures
Oculopharyngeal muscular dystrophy	Autosomal dominant and recessive	14q11 PABPN1 GCG repeats >11 repeats	40s (range 20s–60s)	Ptosis dysphagia; limb-girdle pattern weakness	Swallow study; blepharoplasty for ptosis, cricopharyngeal myotomy for severe swallowing difficulty

强直性肌营养不良

定义和流行病学

强直性肌营养不良（DM）是欧裔成人中最常见的肌营养不良，呈常染色体显性遗传。强直性肌营养不良有两种类型：1 型（DM1）和 2 型（DM2）。在欧洲，DM1 的发病率估计为 1/8000。虽然 DM1 和 DM2 在欧洲同样常见，但 DM2 在美国似乎不太常见。

遗传学和病理学

DM1 是由 *DMPK* 基因上的 CTG 重复扩增引起，而 DM2 则由 *CNBP* 基因上的 CCTG 重复扩增引起。两种疾病共享相同的 RNA 毒性机制。扩增的 CUG/CCUG 重复序列累积在细胞核内，并隔离通常调控 RNA 剪接的重要蛋白质。这些蛋白质功能的丧失导致多种基因的 RNA 错误剪接，引起广泛的转录组序列变化和多系统疾病。在 DM1 中，部分（但并非所有）症状出现年龄的变异性可由重复长度解释，较长的重复长度通常与更早的发病和更严重的疾病程度相关。CTG 重复序列在体细胞中不稳定，并随着人的一生在体细胞中增加（体细胞不稳定性），且在代际间倾向于增加（早现现象）。基因检测可确诊，无须进行肌肉活检，但特征

表 19.5 血清肌酸激酶（CK）升高的原因

肌病
　肌营养不良/进行性假肥大性肌营养不良携带状态
　先天性肌病
　代谢性肌病
　炎症性肌病

离子通道病
运动神经元病（ALS、SMA）
神经病（GBS、CIDP）
病毒性疾病

药物
　他汀类
　纤维酸衍生物
　氯喹
　秋水仙碱

内分泌异常（甲状腺/甲状旁腺）
手术
创伤
剧烈运动
肌肉量增加
特发性——种族差异

ALS，肌萎缩侧索硬化；CIDP，慢性炎症性脱髓鞘性多发性神经病；GBS，吉兰-巴雷综合征；SMA，脊髓性肌萎缩。

表 19.6 常见的肌营养不良

疾病	遗传	突变	发病年龄	表型	治疗
肌营养不良	X 连锁隐性遗传	Xp21；≈ 75% 缺失或重复	进行性假肥大性：发病约为 4 岁；贝克型：发病年龄多变	肢带型模式。进行性假肥大性：严重进行性且生命受限。贝克型：进行性，但不那么严重，变异性更大。小腿假性肥大，孤立性心肌病	关于进行性假肥大性：泼尼松（或地夫可特）、依特立生、戈洛迪森和维特拉森；需监测呼吸、心脏和骨科问题
强直性肌营养不良 1 型	常染色体显性遗传	19q13；CTG 扩增 > 50 次重复	任何年龄，变异较大；先天性于出生时即发病	临床变异性明显，但通常表现为面部、颈部屈肌、呼吸肌和远端肌肉（手指屈肌、踝关节背屈）的肌无力和肌肉萎缩；肌强直；颞部肌肉萎缩，额部脱发；多系统疾病表现（如认知缺陷、嗜睡、白内障）；心脏传导缺陷	美西律可缓解症状性肌强直；需每年监测眼部和呼吸系统受累，以及心脏传导缺陷
强直性肌营养不良 2 型	常染色体显性遗传	3q13；CCTG 扩增 > 75 次重复	30 岁及以上	肢带型模式；肌痛，肌强直，多系统受累（如白内障、心脏传导缺陷、糖尿病）	美西律可缓解症状性肌强直；需监测眼部、心脏和呼吸系统受累
面肩肱型肌营养不良	常染色体显性遗传	95%：4q35（FSHD1）；5% 双基因突变影响甲基化（FSHD2）	任何年龄	肩胛腓肠肌模式伴有面部受累，可出现明显不对称，轴性肌肉明显受累	筛查肌肉外表现
埃默里-德赖弗斯肌营养不良	X 连锁隐性遗传；常染色体显性或隐性遗传	≈ 70% Xq28 Emerin 或 FHL1 突变；1q21 lamin A/C，均有显性和隐性突变	关节挛缩在儿童期出现，20～30 岁出现进展性肌无力	肩胛腓肠肌模式；早期关节挛缩，特别是肘关节，心脏受累明显	需每年监测心脏和呼吸系统受累，骨科评估症状性关节挛缩
眼咽肌营养不良	常染色体显性和隐性遗传	14q11 PABPN1 GCG 扩增 > 11 次重复	40 岁（范围 20～60 岁）	上睑下垂，吞咽困难；肢带型肌无力	吞咽功能检查；对上睑下垂行眼睑成形术，针对严重吞咽困难进行环咽肌切开术

TABLE 19.7 Congenital Muscular Dystrophies

Name/AKA	Gene	Inheritance	Phenotype	CNS Involvement
Merosin-deficient	6q22; laminin alpha-2	Autosomal recessive	Hypotonia; contractures; scoliosis or rigid spine; respiratory involvement; external ophthalmoplegia	MRI diffuse white matter changes; 20%–30% seizures
Bethlem myopathy/ Ullrich muscular dystrophy	21q22; 2q37; COL6 (collagen 6 spectrum disorders)	Autosomal dominant or recessive	Hypotonia; contractures; distal joint laxity; keloid; respiratory involvement	
Dystroglycanopathy	9q34 (POMT1); 14q24 (POMT2); 9q31 (fukutin); 19q13 (FKRP); 22q12 (LARGE); 1q32 (POMGnT1); 7p21 (ISPD)	Autosomal recessive	Spectrum of disorders but characteristic intellectual, eye, and brain involvement; motor early death, to acquiring ambulation	Walker-Warburg syndrome: severe eye involvement, cobblestone lissencephaly, hypoplastic cerebellum and brain stem. Muscle eye brain syndrome: common eye involvement, pachygyria/polymicrogyria, hypoplastic cerebellum and brain stem. Fukuyama: mild eye involvement, cortex mild changes, hypoplastic cerebellum but normal brain stem
SEPN1-related myopathy	1q36 (SEPN1)	Autosomal recessive	Cervicoaxial weakness, rigid spine syndrome, early nocturnal hypoventilation, medial thigh wasting	
LMNA related	1q22 (lamin A/C)	Autosomal dominant and recessive	Cervicoaxial weakness, dropped head, rigid spine syndrome, respiratory and cardiac involvement	

include pyknotic clumps (result of severe fiber atrophy), ring fibers, and type 1 fiber predominance.

Clinical Presentation

DM1 is one of the most variable monogenetic diseases and can present at any age. The wide spectrum of disease ranges from infants with hypotonia, respiratory weakness, and clubfeet at birth (congenital myotonic dystrophy) to late onset of disease at old age with minimal symptoms or signs. Typical features include facial weakness with temporalis muscle wasting, frontal balding, ptosis, and neck flexor weakness. Speech can be dysarthric with bulbar weakness resulting in dysphagia. Inspiratory (difficulty lying flat) and expiratory (weak cough) muscle weakness may be present. Extremity weakness usually begins distally and progresses slowly to affect the proximal limb-girdle muscles. In conjunction with myotonia (see Table 19.2), this phenotype is nearly pathognomonic of DM1. DM2 is considered milder because age of onset occurs typically in the late 30s and there is no congenital or childhood form of the disease. The pattern of weakness predominantly affecting proximal muscles and less facial involvement is different than in DM1. Pain is commonly described by patients with DM2. Both disorders affect multiple organ systems, such as early cataracts (<55 years), cardiac conduction abnormalities, and smooth muscle involvement with symptoms mimicking irritable bowel syndrome. *DMPK* is expressed in the brain and patients with DM1 can experience cognitive deficits including visuospatial and executive dysfunction, apathy, as well as hypersomnolence, which can be one of the most bothersome symptom in some individuals. Central nervous system involvement is thought to be less severe in DM2.

Diagnosis and Differential Diagnosis

The diagnosis is based on clinical examination, demonstration of myotonia clinically and electromyographically, and is confirmed by genetic testing. The classic phenotype and multisystemic presentation typically distinguishes myotonic dystrophy from other adult onset muscular dystrophies and non-dystrophic myotonic disorders.

Treatment

Annual surveillance for cardiac (ECG) and respiratory involvement (pulmonary function testing) is recommended. A sleep study can identify the presence of sleep apnea. Noninvasive ventilation is recommended for respiratory weakness and sleep apnea. With advanced heart block, a pacemaker may need to be placed. Mexiletine, a type IB anti-arrhythmic medication, effectively treats myotonia but is contraindicated in patients with severe arrhythmia. There is currently no treatment to halt disease progression but many therapies targeting the toxic RNA or releasing the sequestered proteins are under investigation.

Prognosis

Patients with DM1 have a reduced life expectancy due to respiratory and cardiac involvement, which on average appears to be less severe in DM2.

Facioscapulohumeral Muscular Dystrophy

Definition and Epidemiology

Facioscapulohumeral muscular dystrophy (FSHD) is the second most common adult muscular dystrophy with an estimated prevalence of 1:15,000.

Genetics and Pathology

FSHD is caused by *DUX4* expression, a gene that is typically silenced but is toxic to muscle when expressed. *DUX4* is expressed when the segment on chromosome 4q35 carrying the gene is hypomethylated. In most patients hypomethylation occurs due to a deletion/contraction of the segment on 4q35 (FSHD1), but in about 5% of patients it is caused by a mutation in a different gene regulating methylation (FSHD2). Both forms are clinically indistinguishable. FSHD1 has an autosomal dominant inheritance whereas FSHD2 as a digenic disease requires mutations on two genes, and sporadic occurrences occur in both. Muscle biopsy is typically not required for the diagnosis but shows nonspecific myopathic changes and inflammatory infiltrates in up to 30% of biopsies.

表 19.7 先天性肌营养不良

名称/别称	基因	遗传	表型	中枢神经系统受累
Merosin 蛋白缺陷型	6q22；层粘连蛋白 α-2	常染色体隐性遗传	低肌张力，关节挛缩，脊柱侧弯或僵直脊柱，呼吸系统受累，眼外肌麻痹	MRI 广泛白质改变，20%～30% 有癫痫发作
贝特莱姆肌病/乌尔里希肌营养不良	21q22；2q37；COL6（胶原 6 谱系疾病）	常染色体显性或隐性遗传	低肌张力，关节挛缩，远端关节松弛，瘢痕疙瘩，呼吸系统受累	
肌营养不良蛋白聚糖病	9q34（POMT1）；14q24（POMT2）；9q31（fukutin）；19q13（FKRP）；22q12（LARGE）；1q32（POMGnT1）；7p21（ISPD）	常染色体隐性遗传	谱系疾病，但有特征性的智力、眼部和大脑受累；从早期运动障碍到获得行走能力	沃克-沃伯格综合征：严重眼部受累，鹅卵石样无脑回畸形，小脑和脑干发育不良 肌眼脑综合征：常见眼部受累，巨脑回/多微脑回，小脑和脑干发育不良 福冈型：眼部受累轻微，皮质改变轻微，小脑发育不良但脑干正常
SEPN1 相关肌病	1q36（SEPN1）	常染色体隐性遗传	颈轴肌无力，僵直脊柱综合征，早期夜间低通气，大腿内侧肌肉萎缩	
LMNA 相关	1q22（lamin A/C）	常染色体显性和隐性遗传	颈轴肌无力，下垂头，僵直脊柱综合征，呼吸和心脏受累	

性发现包括固缩性核团块（严重肌纤维萎缩的结果）、环状纤维和 1 型纤维占优势。

临床表现

DM1 是最多变的单基因疾病之一，可在任何年龄发病。疾病谱广泛，从出生时即有肌张力低下、呼吸无力和畸形足的婴儿（先天性强直性肌营养不良），到老年时期仅有轻微症状或体征的晚发型。典型特征包括面部无力伴颞肌萎缩、额部脱发、上睑下垂和颈屈肌无力。可有构音障碍以及由于延髓性肌无力导致吞咽困难。可能存在吸气（平卧困难）和呼气（咳嗽无力）肌无力。肢体无力通常从远端开始，缓慢进展至累及近端肢带肌肉。结合肌强直（见表 19.2），这种表型几乎是 DM1 的病理性特征。DM2 被认为较轻，通常发病于 30 多岁，且无先天性或儿童型；其主要累及近端肌肉的肌无力模式和面部受累较轻的表现与 DM1 不同。DM2 患者常描述存在疼痛。这两种疾病均影响多个器官系统，如早发性白内障（＜55 岁）、心脏传导异常、类似肠易激综合征的平滑肌受累症状。*DMPK* 在大脑中表达，DM1 的患者可出现认知缺陷，包括视空间和执行功能障碍、淡漠以及过度嗜睡，后者可能是某些个体最令人烦恼的症状。DM2 的中枢神经系统受累被认为较轻。

诊断和鉴别诊断

诊断基于临床检查、临床和肌电图证实的肌强直，并通过基因检测进行确认。经典表型和多系统表现通常将强直性肌营养不良与其他成人发病的肌营养不良和非营养不良性肌强直疾病区分开来。

治疗

建议每年进行心脏（心电图）和呼吸系统（肺功能测试）的监测。睡眠研究可以识别睡眠呼吸暂停的存在。对于呼吸肌无力和睡眠呼吸暂停，推荐使用无创通气。在严重心脏传导阻滞的情况下，可能需要安置起搏器。美西律（一种ⅠB 型抗心律失常药物）对治疗肌强直有效，但在严重心律失常患者中禁用。目前尚无阻止疾病进展的治疗方法，但许多针对毒性 RNA 或释放被隔离蛋白的疗法正在研究中。

预后

由于呼吸系统和心脏受累，DM1 患者的寿命预期减少，而 DM2 的症状似乎不那么严重。

面肩肱型肌营养不良

定义和流行病学

面肩肱型肌营养不良（FSHD）是第二常见的成人肌营养不良，估计患病率为 1∶15 000。

遗传学与病理学

FSHD 是由 *DUX4* 基因的表达引起，这个基因通常是沉默的，但一旦表达则对肌肉有毒性作用。当 4 号染色体 q35 区域上携带该基因的片段发生低甲基化时，*DUX4* 才会表达。在大多数患者中，低甲基化是由于 4q35 片段的缺失/收缩（FSHD1）导致的，但大约 5% 的患者是由于另一个调控甲基化的基因突变（FSHD2）所致。两种形式在临床上无法区分。FSHD1 具有常染色体显性遗传特征，而 FSHD2 作为一种双基因疾病需要 2 个基因的突变，在这两种形式中都可能出现散发病例。肌肉活检通常不需要用于诊断，但在多达 30% 的活检中会显示非特异性肌病变化和炎性浸润。

Clinical Presentation

Although FSHD can affect people at all ages, most patients present in their late teens or early twenties with weakness in a characteristic pattern, often with dramatic side-to-side asymmetry: typically first in the face, shoulders, and arms, and later involving the trunk and distal lower extremities. Patients are unable to squeeze their eyes shut, have a transverse smile, scapular winging, loss of proximal muscle mass with often preserved forearm muscles, and a positive Beevor sign (movement of the umbilicus up or down when asked to tense the abdominal muscles). Extramuscular manifestations of FSHD are rare: retinal vascular changes, which can occasionally lead to symptomatic retinal vasculopathy termed Coat syndrome, high-frequency hearing loss, and atrial arrhythmias.

Diagnosis and Differential Diagnosis

Diagnosis is based on clinical examination and family history and is confirmed by genetic testing. The differential diagnosis includes other myopathies such as inclusion body myositis, limb-girdle muscular dystrophies and acid maltase deficiency.

Treatment

There are currently no pharmacologic disease-modifying therapies available. However, several therapy approaches are being studied with the unifying goal to suppress DUX4. One drug is currently being tested in a multisite clinical trial. In the interim, treatment is supportive with ankle bracing and assistive devices. In selected patients surgical fixation of the scapular can improve function. Monitoring for retinal disease, hearing loss, and respiratory function is indicated.

Prognosis

FSHD is not life limiting, but approximately 20% over the age of 50 will require a wheelchair.

CONGENITAL MYOPATHIES

Congenital myopathies are defined by their appearance on biopsy (see Fig. 19.1D) and have a large number of genetic mutations associated with them. They are usually present at birth with hypotonia and subsequent delayed motor development. If the child survives the perinatal period, most congenital myopathies are relatively nonprogressive and may not be diagnosed until the second or third decade. Clinical findings common in the congenital myopathies are reduced muscle bulk, slender body build, a long and narrow face, skeletal abnormalities (high-arched palate, pectus excavatum, kyphoscoliosis, dislocated hips, and pes cavus), and absent or reduced muscle stretch reflexes.

METABOLIC MYOPATHIES

Metabolic myopathies are muscle diseases due to mutations in enzymes responsible for energy production including glycogen, lipid, and mitochondrial metabolism. Classically, these disorders present in older children or adults with episodes of exercise intolerance, muscle cramping, myalgia, and recurrent rhabdomyolysis associated with myoglobinuria. Newborns and infants can present with severe multisystem disorders that are often fatal.

Glucose and Glycogen Metabolism Disorders
Definition and Epidemiology

Glucose, and its storage from glycogen, is essential for the short-term, predominantly anaerobic energy requirements of muscle. Disorders of glucose and glycogen metabolism (called glycogenosis) have two distinct syndromes: (1) static symptoms of fixed weakness without exercise intolerance or myoglobinuria and (2) dynamic symptoms of exercise intolerance, pain, cramps, and myoglobinuria. Acid maltase deficiency (Pompe disease) is an example of the first and is treatable with enzyme replacement therapy, which is life extending for the childhood variant. McArdle disease is an example of the second. The incidence varies between region and ethnic group. For example, acid maltase deficiency has an incidence as high as 1:14,000 in African Americans. The prevalence of McArdle disease is approximately 1:100,000.

Genetics and Pathology

All are due to mutations in enzymes responsible for glucose or glycogen metabolism. Muscle biopsies usually show subsarcolemmal accumulation of glycogen.

Clinical Presentation

Acid maltase disease typically has a severe infantile form with respiratory and cardiac involvement and a slowly progressive adult myopathy, which can present with respiratory muscle weakness as the initial symptom. McArdle disease presents with severe episodes of muscle cramping and contractures associated with exercise and a fixed myopathy later in life. Many patients note a "second wind" phenomenon, which means that after a brief period of rest patients can resume physical activity with improved tolerance.

Diagnosis and Differential Diagnosis

Diagnosis is made by characteristic appearance on muscle biopsy with subsequent study of the enzyme activity or by searching for specific genetic mutations. The differential diagnosis includes other glycogen storage disorders, disorders of lipid metabolism, or mitochondrial disorders.

Treatment

The only glycogen storage disorder with a therapy approved by the FDA is enzyme replacement for infantile or adult-onset acid maltase deficiency. Therapies targeting the genetic mechanism of acid maltase deficiency are expected to enter clinical trials in the near future.

Prognosis

The spectrum is wide from severe fatal infantile diseases to milder symptoms in adults.

DISORDERS OF FATTY ACID METABOLISM

Disorders of lipid metabolism differ from glucose and glycogen disorders in that the metabolic derangement is in the enzymatic breakdown of fatty acids. Many present in childhood with episodes of encephalopathy precipitated by fasting with hypoketotic hypoglycemia. Serum fatty acid profiles often show reduced carnitine and increased longer chain fractions, depending on whether the mutation is in very long chain, long chain, or medium chain fatty acid metabolism. Adults typically show exercise intolerance and myoglobinuria and may develop a mild limb-girdle pattern myopathy. The most prevalent disorder of fatty acid metabolism is carnitine palmitoyltransferase II (CPT II) deficiency. This disease ranges from a lethal neonatal form to an adult form with muscle pain and recurrent myoglobinuria, often precipitated by exercise, febrile illness, or fasting. The diagnosis is usually made by detection of reduced CPT II activity in skeletal muscle with confirmatory genetic testing.

MITOCHONDRIAL MYOPATHIES

Definition and Epidemiology

Mitochondrial myopathies can present at any age, with varying degrees of severity or weakness, affect multiple organ systems, and have any

临床表现

尽管 FSHD 可以发生在各个年龄段，但大多数患者在青春期后期或二十多岁时出现症状，表现为特征性的肌无力模式，常伴有明显的左右不对称性：通常首先累及面部、肩部和上肢，随后累及躯干和远端下肢。患者无法紧闭双眼，表现为横向微笑、肩胛骨翼状突出、近端肌肉量减少但前臂肌肉常保留完整，以及 Beevor 征阳性（要求收缩腹肌时，脐部会上下移动）。FSHD 的肌肉外表现罕见，包括视网膜血管变化（有时可能导致称为 Coat 综合征的症状性视网膜血管病变）、高频听力损失和房性心律失常。

诊断和鉴别诊断

诊断依据临床检查和家族史，并通过基因检测确诊。鉴别诊断包括其他肌病，如包涵体肌炎、肢带型肌营养不良和酸性麦芽糖酶缺乏症。

治疗

目前尚无可用的疾病修饰治疗药物。然而，多种抑制 *DUX4* 表达的治疗方法正在研究中，其中一种药物正处于多中心临床试验阶段。在此期间，治疗主要为支持性疗法，如使用踝关节支具和辅助设备。对于部分患者，手术固定肩胛骨可以改善功能。需监测视网膜病变、听力损失和呼吸功能。

预后

FSHD 不会缩短寿命，但约 20% 的 50 岁以上患者需要使用轮椅。

先天性肌病

先天性肌病是通过肌肉活检表现（见图 19.1D）进行定义的，并且与大量的基因突变有关。它们通常在出生时即表现出肌张力低下和随后的运动发育迟缓。如果儿童能存活过围生期，大多数先天性肌病表现为相对非进展性，可能直到 10～20 岁或 20～30 岁才被诊断出来。先天性肌病常见的临床表现包括肌肉体积减少、身体瘦长、面部细长狭窄、骨骼异常（上腭高弓、漏斗胸、脊柱后侧弯、髋关节脱位和高弓足）以及肌肉牵张反射消失或减弱。

代谢性肌病

代谢性肌病是由于负责能量生产的酶（包括糖原、脂质及线粒体代谢的酶）突变引起的肌肉疾病。典型情况下，这些疾病在大龄儿童或成人中表现为运动不耐受、肌肉痉挛、肌痛以及与肌红蛋白尿相关的反复横纹肌溶解。新生儿和婴儿可能会出现严重的多系统障碍，这些往往是致命的。

糖和糖原代谢障碍

定义和流行病学

肌肉短期的无氧能量需求主要依赖于葡萄糖及其糖原储存。糖和糖原代谢障碍（称为糖原病）有两种不同的综合征：①无运动不耐受或肌红蛋白尿的静态固定性无力症状；②有运动不耐受、疼痛、痉挛和肌红蛋白尿的动态症状。酸性麦芽糖酶缺乏症（糖原贮积症Ⅱ型）是第一种情况的例子，可以用酶替代疗法治疗，这对儿童型有延长生命的作用。麦卡德尔病是第二种情况的例子。发病率因地区和种族群体而异。例如，酸性麦芽糖酶缺乏症在非裔美国人中的发病率高达 1∶14 000。麦卡德尔病的患病率约为 1∶100 000。

遗传学和病理学

所有这些疾病都是由负责葡萄糖或糖原代谢的酶突变引起的。肌肉活检通常显示肌膜下有糖原蓄积。

临床表现

酸性麦芽糖酶缺乏症通常有严重的婴儿型（有呼吸和心脏受累），以及缓慢进展的成人肌病（最初可表现为呼吸肌无力）。麦卡德尔病表现为与运动相关的严重肌肉痉挛和挛缩，以及后期出现的固定性肌病。许多患者会注意到"第二风"现象，即短暂休息后可以恢复更好的运动耐受。

诊断和鉴别诊断

诊断依据肌肉活检的特征性表现，结合对酶活性的进一步研究或特定基因突变的检测。鉴别诊断包括其他糖原贮积症、脂质代谢障碍或线粒体疾病。

治疗

FDA 批准的唯一一种糖原贮积症的治疗方法是对婴儿型或成人发病的酸性麦芽糖酶缺乏症进行酶替代疗法。针对酸性麦芽糖酶缺乏症遗传机制的治疗方法预计在不久的将来进入临床试验。

预后

疾病谱系广泛，包括从严重致命的婴儿型疾病到成人较轻的症状。

脂肪酸代谢障碍

脂质代谢障碍与葡萄糖和糖原代谢障碍不同，其代谢紊乱在于脂肪酸的酶促分解。许多患者在儿童期表现为禁食引发的低酮低血糖性脑病发作。血清脂肪酸谱常显示肉碱减少、长链部分增加，这取决于突变是发生在极长链、长链还是中链脂肪酸代谢中。成人通常表现为运动不耐受和肌红蛋白尿，可能发展为轻度肢带型肌病。最常见的脂肪酸代谢障碍是肉碱棕榈酰转移酶Ⅱ（CPT Ⅱ）缺乏症。该疾病范围从致命的新生儿型到成人型，表现为肌痛和反复肌红蛋白尿，常由运动、发热疾病或禁食引发。诊断通常通过检测骨骼肌中 CPT Ⅱ 活性降低并进行基因检测确诊。

线粒体肌病

定义和流行病学

线粒体肌病可以在任何年龄发病，严重程度或无力程度各异，影响多个器官系统，并具有任何遗传模

pattern of inheritance. Mutations affect enzymes necessary for normal mitochondrial function and can be mitochondrial or nuclear. The overall prevalence for mitochondrial disorders is thought to be approximately 1:8500; however, the prevalence of individual mitochondrial syndromes is much lower and ranges from just a handful of cases, to 1 to 6 per 100,000.

Genetics and Pathology

Mutations can occur in both mitochondrial DNA (in which case inheritance is maternal) and nuclear DNA (autosomal dominant, recessive, or X-linked). Mitochondrial disorders produce biochemical defects proximal to the respiratory chain (involving substrate transport and usage) or within the respiratory chain. On muscle biopsy, muscle fibers contain abnormal mitochondria. Pathologically, these fibers have a "ragged red" appearance on biopsy stains (trichrome) and fail to react for cytochrome C oxidase.

Clinical Presentation

Despite the diversity, certain patterns are characteristic for mitochondrial disorders, including slowly progressive myopathy and myalgias, which worsen with exertion or illness, and ptosis and/or ophthalmoplegia.

Diagnosis and Differential Diagnosis

The diagnosis is based on clinical history with recognition of multisystemic involvement, serum lactate levels, which can be elevated at rest, and characteristic findings on muscle biopsy. Diagnosis is confirmed by mitochondrial or nuclear genetic testing.

Treatment

Treatment is largely supportive and includes identification of other multisystem involvement, including diabetes, cardiac and ophthalmologic involvement, and hearing loss. Many agents have been tried in mitochondrial diseases, including coenzyme Q10, creatine, and carnitine. Aerobic exercise may reduce fatigue and improve muscle function, although there are no large trials of efficacy for either supplements or exercise.

Prognosis

The severity and prognosis depend partially on the load of abnormal mitochondrial DNA as well as the degree of multisystem involvement. Certain clinical syndromes with more predictable prognosis have been described.

MUSCLE CHANNELOPATHIES

The muscle channelopathies are a spectrum of disorders due to mutations in muscle ion channels commonly divided into the nondystrophic myotonias and periodic paralyses. Most are inherited in an autosomal dominant fashion, with episodic symptoms, often triggered by temperature or certain foods.

Nondystrophic Myotonias
Definition and Epidemiology

Nondystrophic myotonias are due to dysfunction of sodium or chloride channels resulting in hyperexcitable muscle and myotonia. The overall worldwide prevalence for nondystrophic myotonias is 1:100,000.

Genetics

Nondystrophic myotonias are caused by mutations in the muscle chloride (CLCN1) or sodium (SCN4A) channel genes causing alterations of depolarization and hyperpolarization of the muscle fiber membrane.

Clinical Presentation

As the name implies, patients have myotonia (see Table 19.2). Chloride channel mutations have a characteristic warm-up of myotonia with repetition. Sodium channel myotonias typically have more eye closure myotonia and can demonstrate a paradoxical worsening of myotonia with activity (paramyotonia). Symptoms usually start in the first decade, and patients can have a characteristic muscular build.

Diagnosis and Differential Diagnosis

Diagnosis is based on family history, clinical examination, and electrodiagnostic testing. It is confirmed by genetic testing. The differential diagnosis includes myotonic dystrophy and secondary causes of myotonia (other myopathies and drugs associated with myotonia—e.g., statins, fibric acid derivatives, and colchicine).

Treatment

Treatment for nondystrophic myotonias consists of non-mutation–specific sodium-channel blockade: mexiletine, a class IB antiarrhythmic, is the first-line therapy, but ranolazine, phenytoin, procainamide, and flecainide can be considered. Certain sodium-channel myotonias respond to the carbonic anhydrase inhibitor acetazolamide.

Periodic Paralyses
Definition and Epidemiology

The periodic paralyses are disorders that present with episodic weakness often triggered by exercise or food. Overall prevalence for the primary periodic paralyses varies between conditions from 1:100,000 to 1:1,000,000.

Genetics and Pathology

Periodic paralysis is caused by mutations in the calcium (CACN1AS), sodium (SCN4A), and potassium-channel (KCNJ2) genes that result in depolarized but inexcitable sarcolemma and episodes of paralysis. Hyperkalemic periodic paralysis is due to sodium-channel mutations that lead to persistent inward sodium current causing both myotonia and paralysis. Hypokalemic periodic paralysis can be caused by calcium-, sodium-, and potassium-channel mutations and is due to an anomalous gating pore current that, in low potassium conditions, produces a depolarizing current larger than hyperpolarizing potassium currents. Andersen-Tawil syndrome is due to loss of function in a potassium inward rectifier.

Clinical Presentation

Common to all are attacks of weakness first presenting in childhood or early adulthood, often brought on by rest after exercise, or in the mornings, and associated with changes in extracellular potassium. Hyperkalemic periodic paralysis is associated with either high or normal extracellular potassium, triggered by potassium-rich foods. In hypokalemic periodic paralysis attacks are associated with low extracellular potassium and are triggered by carbohydrates, stress, alcohol, or rest after exercise. Andersen-Tawil syndrome is characterized by the clinical triad of attacks of flaccid paralysis, dysmorphic features (wide-set eyes, narrow mandible, low-set ears, bent fifth finger, and common origin for the second and third toes), and polymorphic ventricular tachyarrhythmias.

Diagnosis and Differential Diagnosis

Diagnosis is based in family history and clinical history, supported by electrodiagnostic testing and confirmed by genetic testing.

Treatment

In all of the periodic paralyses disorders mild exercise at onset of weakness can abort attacks of paralysis. Treatment for acute attacks

式。突变影响维持线粒体正常功能所需的酶，可以是线粒体基因或核基因突变。总体上，线粒体疾病的患病率约为1∶8500；但单个线粒体综合征的患病率低得多，从仅有少数几例到每10万人中1～6例不等。

遗传学和病理学

突变可发生在线粒体DNA（此时遗传为母系遗传）和核DNA（常染色体显性、隐性或X连锁遗传）。线粒体疾病会产生呼吸链前的生化缺陷（涉及底物运输和利用）或呼吸链内的缺陷。在肌肉活检中，肌纤维含有异常线粒体。从病理学上看，这些纤维在三色染色法活检标本上呈现"破碎红纤维"外观，且对细胞色素C氧化酶无反应。

临床表现

尽管临床表现多样，但某些模式是线粒体疾病的特征性表现，包括缓慢进展的肌病和肌痛（在运动或疾病时加重），以及上睑下垂和（或）眼肌麻痹。

诊断和鉴别诊断

诊断依据临床病史识别的多系统受累、静息时升高的血清乳酸水平，以及肌肉活检的特征性改变。通过线粒体或核基因检测确诊。

治疗

治疗以支持性为主，包括识别其他多系统受累，如糖尿病、心脏和眼科受累以及听力损失。已经尝试了多种药物治疗线粒体疾病，如辅酶Q10、肌酸和肉碱，但疗效尚不确定。有氧运动可能减轻疲劳，改善肌肉功能，但尚无大规模的疗效试验。

预后

严重程度和预后部分取决于异常线粒体DNA的负荷以及多系统受累的程度。某些临床综合征具有更可预测的预后。

肌肉离子通道病

肌肉离子通道病是一组由肌肉离子通道突变引起的疾病谱，通常分为非营养不良性肌强直和周期性瘫痪。大多数以常染色体显性方式遗传，症状呈阵发性，常由温度或某些食物触发。

非营养不良性肌强直

定义和流行病学

非营养不良性肌强直是由于钠或氯通道功能障碍引起的肌肉过度兴奋和肌强直。全球非营养不良性肌强直的总体患病率为1∶100 000。

基因

非营养不良性肌强直由肌肉氯通道（CLCN1）或钠通道（SCN4A）基因突变引起，导致肌纤维膜去极化和超极化改变。

临床表现

顾名思义，患者有肌强直（见表19.2）。氯通道突变表现为重复活动后肌强直的特征性预热现象。钠通道肌强直通常有明显的眼睑闭合肌强直，并可表现为活动后肌强直反常加重（副肌强直）。症状通常在10岁前开始出现，患者可能有特征性的肌肉构造。

诊断和鉴别诊断

诊断依据家族史、临床检查和电生理检查，并通过基因检测确诊。鉴别诊断包括强直性肌营养不良和引起肌强直的继发原因（其他肌病和药物相关肌强直，如他汀类药物、纤维酸衍生物和秋水仙碱）。

治疗

非营养不良性肌强直的治疗包括非突变特异性的钠通道阻滞：美西律（ⅠB类抗心律失常药）是一线治疗，但雷诺嗪、苯妥英、普鲁卡因胺和氟卡尼也可考虑。某些钠通道肌强直可能对碳酸酐酶抑制剂乙酰唑胺有反应。

周期性瘫痪

定义和流行病学

周期性瘫痪是一类以阵发性无力为主要表现的疾病，常由运动或饮食诱发。原发性周期性瘫痪的总体患病率为1/100万至1/10万。

遗传学和病理学

周期性瘫痪是由钙（CACN1AS）、钠（SCN4A）和钾通道（KCNJ2）基因突变引起的，导致肌膜去极化但不可兴奋，从而出现瘫痪发作。高钾性周期性瘫痪是由钠通道突变引起，导致持续内向钠电流，引起肌强直和瘫痪。低钾性周期性瘫痪可由钙、钠和钾通道突变引起，是由于异常的门控孔电流，在低钾条件下产生大于超极化电流的去极化电流。Andersen-Tawil综合征是由于内向整流钾通道功能丧失引起的。

临床表现

所有类型的共同特点是无力发作首发于儿童期或成年早期，常由运动后休息引发或在早晨发作，并伴有细胞外钾浓度变化。高钾性周期性瘫痪与细胞外钾升高或正常有关，由富钾食物诱发。低钾性周期性瘫痪发作与细胞外钾降低有关，由碳水化合物、应激、酒精或运动后休息诱发。Andersen-Tawil综合征表现为临床三联征：弛缓性瘫痪发作、畸形特征（眼距宽、下颌窄、耳低位、小指弯曲、第二和第三足趾合并）和多形性室性心动过速。

诊断和鉴别诊断

诊断依据家族史和临床病史，辅以电生理诊断检查，并通过基因检测确诊。

治疗

在所有周期性瘫痪疾病中，在无力发作初期进行适度运动可以中止瘫痪发作。急性发作的治疗包括碳水

consists of carbohydrates (hyperkalemic periodic paralysis) or potassium supplementation (hypokalemic periodic paralysis). Prophylactic treatment for all the periodic paralyses consists of carbonic anhydrase inhibitors.

ACQUIRED MYOPATHIES

Unlike the inherited myopathies, the acquired myopathies are typically secondary to another process: toxic, autoimmune, inflammatory, or infectious. Pathologic changes can be distinctive and are not due to mutations in muscle-related proteins. Clinically, symptoms appear acutely or subacutely.

Inflammatory Myopathies

The idiopathic inflammatory myopathies can be divided into dermatomyositis/polymyositis and sporadic inclusion body myositis (Table 19.8).

Dermatomyositis/Polymyositis

Definition and epidemiology. Dermatomyositis/polymyositis (DM/PM) are acquired idiopathic diseases of muscle characterized by inflammation and variable symmetrical proximal muscle weakness, associated with elevated serum creatine kinase and irritable features on electromyography. The overall annual incidence is approximately 1 in 100,000.

Pathology. Dermatomyositis shows a pathognomonic pattern on muscle biopsy of perifascicular atrophy and perivascular inflammatory infiltrates and positive pericapillary membrane attack complex staining (see Fig. 19.1E). In contrast, polymyositis shows endomysial inflammatory infiltrates with invasion of non-necrotic fibers.

Clinical presentation. Dermatomyositis can occur at any age with an acute to insidiously progressive onset of symmetrical proximal muscle weakness with characteristic skin changes, which include heliotrope rash, shawl sign (maculopapular violaceous rash in V-shape around neck), Gottron nodules (erythematous papular rash on the extensor surfaces of the hands or fingers), and mechanic's hands (dry, cracked skin on the dorsal or ventral hands). In contrast, polymyositis is largely a diagnosis of exclusion, occurring in adults without associated skin changes. Myalgias are more common in polymyositis. Both DM/PM can be associated with respiratory weakness, interstitial lung disease, difficulty swallowing, or cardiomyopathy. Both DM/PM can be associated with underlying malignancy (dermatomyositis more frequently than polymyositis), so screening for malignancy is recommended especially in patients over age 40.

Diagnosis and differential diagnosis. Diagnosis is based on clinical history and examination findings in conjunction with irritable changes on electromyography (e.g., fibrillation potentials and positive sharp waves) and characteristic muscle biopsy. In about 30%, both DM/PM can be associated with myositis specific autoantibodies (see Table 19.2). Antibodies can help define a clinical syndrome and guide treatment. For example, patients with anti-Jo-1 antibodies can have interstitial lung disease and methotrexate may need to be avoided due to pulmonary toxicity. Patients may be at higher risk to develop malignancy with antibodies to transcription intermediary factor (TIF)-1gamma (anti-p155, anti-p155/140) and to nuclear matrix protein (NXP)-2 (anti-MJ or anti-p140). Muscle biopsy can help differentiate from other inflammatory myopathies associated with systemic disease (e.g., sarcoidosis).

Treatment. For both DM/PM the first line of treatment is prednisone. Steroid-sparing immunosuppressive therapies (e.g., methotrexate, azathioprine) are often added for those patients requiring long-term therapy in order to reduce the required dose of prednisone or to replace prednisone completely. In patients who do not respond to conventional therapy or have severe symptoms, intravenous immunoglobulin is used. Rituximab may also be effective.

Prognosis. Most patients respond to immunosuppressive therapies.

Sporadic Inclusion Body Myositis

Definition and epidemiology. Sporadic inclusion body myositis (s-IBM) is an idiopathic, slowly progressive muscle condition in older adults (occurring in more men than women), associated with inflammation and characteristic pathologic changes on muscle biopsy. It is the most common inflammatory muscle disease in patients over 50, affecting 3.5 per 100,000.

Pathology. Muscle biopsies resemble polymyositis with endomysial inflammatory infiltrates and invasion of non-necrotic fibers. Distinctive for IBM are vacuoles rimmed by mitochondria, secondary mitochondrial changes, and electron microscopy, which shows 15- to 18-nm tubulofilamentous inclusions.

Clinical presentation. S-IBM causes slowly progressive, often asymmetric weakness. It occurs usually after 50 years of age in an initially distinctive pattern, including distal forearm muscles (distal finger flexors) and quadriceps wasting and weakness. This can progress to involve almost any muscle and can affect swallowing in up to 70% of patients.

Diagnosis and differential diagnosis. Diagnosis is based on clinical history and examination and characteristic muscle pathology. In clinically challenging cases autoantibody levels directed against cytoplasmic 5′-nucleotidase 1A (anti-cN1A) can be helpful, with an estimated specificity around 90%. The main differential diagnosis is other idiopathic inflammatory myopathies or late-onset inherited

Myopathy	Sex	Typical Age at Onset	Pattern of Weakness	Creatine Kinase	Muscle Biopsy	Response to Immunosuppressive Therapy
Dermatomyositis	Women > men	Childhood and adult	Proximal > distal, respiratory weakness, dysphagia	Increased (up to 50× normal)	Perifascicular atrophy, inflammation, complement deposition on capillaries	Yes
Polymyositis	Women > men	Adult	Proximal > distal	Increased (up to 50× normal)	Endomysial inflammation; invasion of non-necrotic fibers	Yes
Sporadic inclusion body myositis	Men > women	Elderly (>50 yr)	Proximal and distal; predilection for finger and wrist flexors, knee extensors	Increased (<10× normal)	Endomysial inflammation, rimmed vacuoles; electron microscopy: 15- to 18-nm tubulofilaments	No

TABLE 19.8 Idiopathic Inflammatory Myopathies

化合物（高钾性周期性瘫痪）或补钾（低钾性周期性瘫痪）。所有周期性瘫痪的预防性治疗是碳酸酐酶抑制剂。

获得性肌病

与遗传性肌病不同，获得性肌病通常是继发于另一种疾病过程：毒性、自身免疫性、炎症性或感染性。病理变化可以具有特征性，并不是由于肌肉相关蛋白的突变导致。临床上，症状可呈急性或亚急性出现。

炎症性肌病

特发性炎症性肌病可以分为皮肌炎/多发性肌炎和散发性包涵体肌炎（表19.8）。

皮肌炎/多发性肌炎

定义和流行病学 皮肌炎/多发性肌炎（DM/PM）是获得性的特发性肌肉疾病，其特点是肌肉炎症和不同程度的对称性近端肌无力，伴有血清肌酸激酶（CK）升高和肌电图上的特征性改变。总体年发病率约为1/10万。

病理学 皮肌炎在肌肉活检上显示特征性表现，包括束周萎缩和血管周围炎性浸润，以及毛细血管周围膜攻击复合物染色阳性（见图19.1E）。相比之下，多发性肌炎表现为肌内膜炎性浸润，并累及未坏死的纤维。

临床表现 皮肌炎可在任何年龄发病，急性或渐进性出现对称性近端肌无力，并有特征性皮肤改变，包括向阳性皮疹、披肩征（颈部呈V形的紫红色丘疹性皮疹）、Gottron结节（手部或手指伸肌面的红斑性丘疹）和技工手（手背或掌侧的干裂皮肤）。相比之下，多发性肌炎主要是通过排除诊断，发生在成人且无相关皮疹。肌痛在多发性肌炎中更常见。DM/PM均可伴有呼吸肌无力、间质性肺病、吞咽困难或心肌病。DM/PM均可与潜在恶性肿瘤相关（皮肌炎较多发性肌炎更常见），因此建议40岁以上的患者筛查恶性肿瘤。

诊断和鉴别诊断 诊断依据临床病史和检查结果，结合肌电图上特征性改变（如纤颤电位和正锐波）和特征性的肌肉活检。约30%的DM/PM患者可检测到肌炎特异性自身抗体（见表19.2）。抗体检测可以帮助界定临床综合征并指导治疗。例如，有抗Jo-1抗体的患者可能伴有间质性肺病，需避免使用氨甲蝶呤（具有肺毒性）。携带转录中间因子（TIF）-1γ（抗p155、抗p155/140）和核基质蛋白（NXP）-2（抗MJ或抗p140）抗体的患者可能有较高的恶性肿瘤风险。肌肉活检可有助于鉴别其他与系统性疾病相关的炎症性肌病（如结节病）。

治疗 DM/PM的一线治疗是泼尼松。对于需要长期治疗的患者，常常加用免疫抑制剂（如氨甲蝶呤、硫唑嘌呤），以减少泼尼松的需求剂量或完全替代泼尼松。对于常规治疗无反应或症状严重的患者，可以使用静脉注射免疫球蛋白。利妥昔单抗也可能有效。

预后 大多数患者对免疫抑制治疗有效。

散发性包涵体肌炎

定义和流行病学 散发性包涵体肌炎（s-IBM）是一种特发性、缓慢进展的肌肉疾病，多见于老年人（男性多于女性），与炎症和肌肉活检中的特征性病理改变有关。它是50岁以上患者中最常见的炎症性肌病，发病率为3.5/10万。

病理学 肌肉活检表现类似多发性肌炎，有肌内膜炎性浸润和对未坏死肌纤维的累及。IBM的特点是有被线粒体包围的空泡、继发性的线粒体改变，以及在电子显微镜下可见15～18 nm的管状细丝包涵体。

临床表现 s-IBM导致缓慢进展的、常不对称性的无力。通常在50岁以后出现，最初表现为前臂远端肌肉（远端手指屈肌）和股四头肌的萎缩和无力。这种情况可能进展至累及几乎任何肌肉，并可影响多达70%患者的吞咽功能。

诊断和鉴别诊断 诊断依据临床病史和体格检查，以及特征性的肌肉病理改变。在临床诊断困难的情况下，检测针对胞质5′-核苷酸酶1A（抗cN1A）的自身抗体可能有帮助，其特异性估计为90%。主要鉴别诊断包括其他特发性炎症性肌病或晚发遗传性肌病。

表19.8 特发性炎症性肌病

肌病	性别	典型发病年龄	无力的模式	肌酸激酶	肌肉活检	对免疫抑制治疗的反应
皮肌炎	女性＞男性	儿童期和成人	近端＞远端，呼吸无力、吞咽困难	增加（高达正常值的50倍）	束周萎缩，炎症，毛细血管上补体沉积	有
多发性肌炎	女性＞男性	成人	近端＞远端	增加（高达正常值的50倍）	肌内膜炎症，非坏死纤维的浸润	有
散发性包涵体肌炎	男性＞女性	老年（＞50岁）	近端和远端；尤其是手指和手腕屈肌、膝关节伸肌	增加（＜正常值的10倍）	肌内膜炎症，镶边空泡；电子显微镜：15～18 nm的管状细丝	无

myopathies. The prominent hand weakness can be misinterpreted as neurogenic (e.g., amyotrophic lateral sclerosis) and electrodiagnostic studies can help differentiate the two.

Treatment. Unlike the other inflammatory myopathies, IBM does not respond to immunosuppression. Treatment is supportive.

Prognosis. Most patients with s-IBM progress to needing a wheelchair over 10 to 15 years. Swallowing difficulty can be life-threatening.

Myopathy With HMGCR Antibodies

Patients typically present with proximal greater than distal symmetric weakness and myalgia. Most patients, but not all, report concurrent or prior exposure to statins. The CK is usually high. EMG can show muscle fiber irritability with myotonic discharges. Laboratory testing is positive for autoantibodies against 3-hydroxy-3-methylglutaryl coenzyme A reductase (HMGCR). Muscle biopsy shows a necrotizing myopathy. Treatment includes discontinuation of statin therapy and corticosteroids or IVIG. With early recognition and treatment, patients can recover markedly.

Infectious Myositis

An acute viral myositis can occur in the setting of viral infections. Patients develop muscle pain, proximal weakness, and elevated CK levels. The disorder is self-limited but when severe can be associated with myoglobinuria and occasionally with renal failure.

An inflammatory myopathy can occur in the setting of human immunodeficiency virus infection, either in early or in later acquired immunodeficiency syndrome. The clinical presentation resembles polymyositis. The patient's condition may improve with corticosteroid therapy. The disorder must be distinguished from the toxic myopathy caused by zidovudine, which responds to dose reduction. Although rarely seen, tuberculosis can present with muscle abscess (pyomyositis) either in the setting of pulmonary or disseminated disease or in isolation.

Myopathies Caused by Endocrine and Systemic Disorders/Corticosteroid Myopathy

Thyroid studies should be part of the evaluation in any adult with muscle weakness. Patients with hyperthyroidism often have some degree of proximal weakness but this is rarely the presenting manifestation of thyrotoxicosis. Hypothyroid myopathy is associated with proximal weakness and myalgias, muscle enlargement, slow relaxation of the reflexes, and marked (up to 100-fold) increase of the serum CK level.

Excess corticosteroids can result from endogenous Cushing's syndrome; however, muscle weakness is rarely the presenting manifestation of Cushing's syndrome.

The most common endocrine myopathy is an iatrogenic **corticosteroid myopathy**, due to exogenous glucocorticoid administration. CK is typically low or normal and EMG normal. Muscle biopsy can show type 2 fiber atrophy. Therapy consists of reducing the corticosteroid dose to the lowest possible level, exercise, and adequate nutrition.

Toxic Myopathies

Many drugs, for example hydroxychloroquine, have been associated with muscle damage, proximal weakness, elevated CK levels, myopathic EMG readings, and abnormalities on muscle biopsy. Symptoms generally improve after stopping the medication.

Critical illness myopathy, also termed acute quadriplegic myopathy, develops in a patient in the intensive care setting and is often discovered when a patient is unable to be weaned off a ventilator. The cause of the diffuse weakness is the prolonged daily use of either high-dose intravenous glucocorticoids or nondepolarizing neuromuscular blocking agents, often both. Patients often have had sepsis and multiorgan failure. The diagnosis of critical illness myopathy is often clinical but can be confirmed by muscle biopsy, which shows the loss of myosin-thick filaments on electron microscopic examination. Treatment is discontinuation of the offending agents and early intensive physical therapy.

SUGGESTED READINGS

Amato AA, Griggs RC: Overview of the muscular dystrophies, Handb Clin Neurol 101:1–9, 2011.

Hamel J, Tawil R: Facioscapulohumeral muscular dystrophy: update on pathogenesis and future treatments, Neurotherapeutics 15(4):863–871, 2018.

Hehir MK, Logigian EC: Electrodiagnosis of myotonic disorders, Phys Med Rehabil Clin N Am 24:209–220, 2013.

Jackson CE, Barohn RJ: A pattern recognition approach to myopathy, Continuum (Minneap Minn) 19(6 Muscle Disease):1674–1697, 2013.

Lemmers RJ, Tawil R, Petek LM, et al: Digenic inheritance of an SMCHD1 mutation and an FSHD-permissive D4Z4 allele causes facioscapulohumeral muscular dystrophy type 2, Nat Genet 44(12):1370–1374, 2012.

Mammen AL: Statin-associated autoimmune myopathy, N Engl J Med 374:664–669, 2016.

Matthews E, Fialho D, Tan SV, et al: The non-dystrophic myotonias: molecular pathogenesis, diagnosis and treatment, Brain 133(Pt 1):9–22, 2010.

McGrath ER, Doughty CT, Amato AA: Autoimmune myopathies: updates on evaluation and treatment, Neurotherapeutics. 15(4):976–994, 2018.

Pfeffer G, Majamaa K, Turnbull DM, et al: Treatment for mitochondrial disorders, Cochrane Database Syst Rev (4):CD004426, 2012.

Statland JM, Bundy BN, et al: Mexiletine for symptoms and signs of myotonia in nondystrophic myotonia: a randomized controlled trial, J Am Med Assoc 308(13):1357–1365, 2012.

Statland JM, Tawil R: Facioscapulohumeral muscular dystrophy: molecular pathological advances and future directions, Curr Opin Neurol 24(5):423–428, 2011.

Thornton CA, Wang E, Carrell EM: Myotonic Dystrophy: approach to therapy, Curr Opin Genet Dev 44:135–140, 2017.

Wheeler TM, Leger AJ, Pander SK, et al: Targeting nuclear RNA for in vivo correction of myotonic dystrophy, Nature 488(7409):111–115, 2012.

显著的手部无力可能被误诊为神经源性（如肌萎缩侧索硬化），电生理检查有助于鉴别。

治疗　不像其他炎症性肌病，IBM 对免疫抑制治疗无反应。治疗主要是支持性治疗。

预后　大多数 s-IBM 患者在 10～15 年内需要使用轮椅。吞咽困难可能危及生命。

HMGCR 抗体相关肌病

患者通常表现为近端大于远端的对称性肌无力和肌痛。大多数但并非所有患者报告有同时或先前接触他汀类药物的经历。CK 通常升高。肌电图可显示肌纤维兴奋性伴有肌强直放电。实验室检查 3-羟基-3-甲基戊二酰辅酶 A 还原酶（HMGCR）的自身抗体呈阳性。肌肉活检显示坏死性肌病。治疗包括停用他汀类药物和糖皮质激素或静脉免疫球蛋白。及时识别并治疗后，患者可显著恢复。

感染性肌炎

在病毒感染的背景下可出现急性病毒性肌炎。患者出现肌痛、近端无力和 CK 升高。该病是自限性的，但严重时可伴有肌红蛋白尿，并偶有肾衰竭。

在人体免疫缺陷病毒感染的早期或后期获得性免疫缺陷综合征中也可出现炎症性肌病，临床表现类似多发性肌炎。患者的状况可能在糖皮质激素治疗下有所改善。需与由齐多夫定引起的中毒性肌病相鉴别，后者可通过减少剂量治疗。虽然很少见，但结核病也可以表现为肌肉脓肿（化脓性肌炎），可能发生在肺部或广泛性疾病的背景下，也可单独出现。

内分泌和系统性疾病引起的肌病/皮质类固醇肌病

在评估任何成人肌无力时，甲状腺功能检查应是必要的。甲状腺功能亢进患者通常有一定程度的近端无力，但这很少是甲状腺功能亢进的首发表现。甲状腺功能减退性肌病与近端肌无力和肌痛、肌肉肥大、反射松弛减慢以及血清 CK 水平显著升高（高达 100 倍）有关。

过量的皮质类固醇可能由内源性库欣综合征引起，但肌无力很少是库欣综合征的首发表现。

最常见的内分泌性肌病是医源性**皮质类固醇肌病**，由外源性糖皮质激素使用引起。CK 通常正常或偏低，肌电图正常。肌肉活检可见 2 型纤维萎缩。治疗包括尽可能减少糖皮质激素剂量、运动和营养支持。

中毒性肌病

许多药物，如羟氯喹等，都与肌肉损伤、近端无力、CK 升高、肌电图异常和肌肉活检异常有关。停药后症状通常会改善。

危重症肌病，也称为急性四肢瘫痪性肌病，发生在重症监护病房的患者中，通常在无法脱离呼吸机时被发现。弥漫性无力的原因是长期使用大剂量静脉糖皮质激素或非去极化神经肌肉阻滞剂，通常两者并用。患者通常有感染中毒症和多器官衰竭。危重症肌病的诊断通常是临床诊断，但可通过肌肉活检确诊，活检可见电子显微镜下肌球蛋白-粗肌丝丢失。治疗是停用致病药物，并进行早期积极的物理治疗。

推荐阅读

Amato AA, Griggs RC: Overview of the muscular dystrophies, Handb Clin Neurol 101:1–9, 2011.

Hamel J, Tawil R: Facioscapulohumeral muscular dystrophy: update on pathogenesis and future treatments, Neurotherapeutics 15(4):863–871, 2018.

Hehir MK, Logigian EC: Electrodiagnosis of myotonic disorders, Phys Med Rehabil Clin N Am 24:209–220, 2013.

Jackson CE, Barohn RJ: A pattern recognition approach to myopathy, Continuum (Minneap Minn) 19(6 Muscle Disease):1674–1697, 2013.

Lemmers RJ, Tawil R, Petek LM, et al: Digenic inheritance of an SMCHD1 mutation and an FSHD-permissive D4Z4 allele causes facioscapulohumeral muscular dystrophy type 2, Nat Genet 44(12):1370–1374, 2012.

Mammen AL: Statin-associated autoimmune myopathy, N Engl J Med 374:664–669, 2016.

Matthews E, Fialho D, Tan SV, et al: The non-dystrophic myotonias: molecular pathogenesis, diagnosis and treatment, Brain 133(Pt 1):9–22, 2010.

McGrath ER, Doughty CT, Amato AA: Autoimmune myopathies: updates on evaluation and treatment, Neurotherapeutics. 15(4):976–994, 2018.

Pfeffer G, Majamaa K, Turnbull DM, et al: Treatment for mitochondrial disorders, Cochrane Database Syst Rev (4):CD004426, 2012.

Statland JM, Bundy BN, et al: Mexiletine for symptoms and signs of myotonia in nondystrophic myotonia: a randomized controlled trial, J Am Med Assoc 308(13):1357–1365, 2012.

Statland JM, Tawil R: Facioscapulohumeral muscular dystrophy: molecular pathological advances and future directions, Curr Opin Neurol 24(5):423–428, 2011.

Thornton CA, Wang E, Carrell EM: Myotonic Dystrophy: approach to therapy, Curr Opin Genet Dev 44:135–140, 2017.

Wheeler TM, Leger AJ, Pander SK, et al: Targeting nuclear RNA for in vivo correction of myotonic dystrophy, Nature 488(7409):111–115, 2012.

Neuromuscular Junction Disease

Emma Ciafaloni

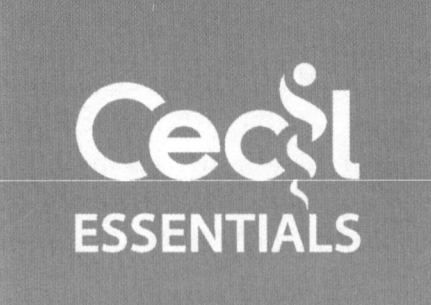

Neuromuscular junction diseases are caused by abnormal neuromuscular transmission of the action potential from the nerve terminal to the muscle, and they can be autoimmune (myasthenia gravis, Lambert-Eaton syndrome), hereditary (congenital myasthenic syndromes), or toxic (botulism, organophosphate intoxication).

MYASTHENIA GRAVIS

Definition/Epidemiology/Pathology

Myasthenia gravis (MG) is a rare autoimmune disease caused by antibodies against the postsynaptic acetylcholine receptors (AChR Ab) in the neuromuscular junction. All ages are affected but incidence is higher in women younger than 40 and in men older than 50. Prevalence is approximately 20 in 100,000. Transient neonatal MG occurs in about 12% of newborns of myasthenic mothers and is caused by transplacental passive transfer of antibodies from the mother to the fetus. Thymoma is found in 10% of patients with MG and thymic hyperplasia is present in 65%.

Clinical Presentation

MG is characterized by fluctuating, fatigable weakness either isolated to the ocular muscles (ocular MG) or involving ocular as well as limb, bulbar, and respiratory muscles (generalized MG). The majority of patients present first with ocular symptoms (blurred vision, double vision, droopy eyelids), but about 15% of cases present with bulbar symptoms first (dysarthria, dysphagia, shortness of breath) or limb weakness. Ptosis is usually asymmetric. Myasthenia crisis is a true neurologic emergency that occurs in 15% to 20% of patients and consists of severe dysphagia or respiratory failure requiring ventilator support and/or tube feeding in an ICU setting.

Diagnosis and Differential Diagnosis

The diagnosis of MG is based on a combination of clinical history, physical examination, and confirmatory tests. The ice pack test is a simple and relatively sensitive test to differentiate ptosis caused by MG from other causes of ptosis. In this test an ice pack is applied to the ptotic eye for 2 minutes and an improvement of 2 mm or more in ptosis supports MG.

Edrophonium chloride (Tensilon) is a short-acting acetylcholinesterase inhibitor administered intravenously to demonstrate symptom improvement in patients with MG. A positive Tensilon test is defined as an unequivocal improvement in strength in an affected muscle after 2 to 5 minutes from administration of 2 mg incremental doses up to 10 mg. Atropine should be available during a Tensilon test because bradycardia and hypotension are possible side effects. Edrophonium testing can be positive in other disorders.

Electrodiagnostic testing with 3 Hz repetitive nerve stimulation (RNS) demonstrates a compound muscle action potential (CMAP) decrement more than 10% in about 50% to 75% of patients with generalized MG but is abnormal in less than 50% of patients with purely ocular symptoms. Single fiber electromyography (SFEMG) is the most sensitive test in the diagnosis of MG and reveals increased jitter and blocking in 99% of patients with generalized MG and in 97% of those with purely ocular MG when a weak muscle is tested. SFEMG is usually available only in specialized EMG laboratories.

Serum antibody testing for AchR Ab (binding antibody) is positive in about 80% of patients with generalized MG and 50% of patients with purely ocular symptoms. Muscle specific tyrosine kinase (Anti MuSK) antibody is detected in a portion of seronegative patients, more frequently women.

Chest CT should be performed to rule out thymoma, found in approximately 10% of seropositive myasthenic patients. Thyroid function should be evaluated because thyroid disease is commonly associated with MG. Electrodiagnostic and serum antibody testing help with differentiating MG from motor neuron disease, Lambert-Eaton myasthenic syndrome (LEMS), and Guillain-Barré syndrome (GBS).

Treatment

Pyridostigmine 30 to 60 mg every 4 hours improves symptoms in most patients with MG; it is used alone to treat purely ocular and generalized cases with only minimal or mild weakness, or in combination with immunosuppressant drugs in patients with more severe manifestations. Prednisone is effective in improving muscle weakness in a short period of time, but long-term use is associated with side effects. Azathioprine and mycophenolate mofetil are used for long-term treatment and as steroids-sparing agents. Eculizumab is a complement inhibitor recently approved for patients with generalized MG with positive AChR antibody. Plasmapheresis and IVIG are used for cases with severe bulbar or generalized weakness, respiratory crisis, and in refractory patients who do not respond to oral immunomodulating medications. Thymoma resection is indicated in all patients with MG and thymoma. Thymectomy is also recommended in patients with nonthymomatous autoimmune MG to increase the probability of remission or improvement. Thymectomy is usually not recommended in patients over age 60. Some medications may exacerbate the symptoms of MG or precipitate the initial signs and symptoms of the disease (Table 20.1).

Prognosis

Most patients with MG who are optimally treated experience improvement or remission of their symptoms. About 10% of patients with MG experience refractory symptoms despite optimal treatment. Mortality is currently less than 5%.

神经肌肉接头疾病

李雨贤 译 杨沫 陈玮琪 审校 王伊龙 通审

神经肌肉接头疾病是由从神经末梢向肌肉传递的动作电位传导异常引起的，可分为自身免疫性（重症肌无力、兰伯特-伊顿综合征）、遗传性（先天性肌无力综合征）或中毒性（肉毒中毒、有机磷中毒）。

重症肌无力

定义、流行病学和病理学

重症肌无力（MG）是一种罕见的自身免疫性疾病，由神经肌肉接头突触后膜乙酰胆碱受体抗体（AChR Ab）引起。所有年龄段均可发病，但40岁以下女性和50岁以上男性发病率较高。患病率约为20/10万。患肌无力的母亲其新生儿中约有12%出现一过性新生儿MG，这是由于抗体经母体胎盘被动转运至胎儿体内所致。10% MG患者伴发胸腺瘤，65% MG患者存在胸腺增生。

临床表现

MG的特征是波动性、易疲劳的肌无力，可能只孤立累及眼外肌（眼肌型MG），也可能眼肌、四肢、延髓支配肌和呼吸肌均有受累（全身型MG）。多数患者首先出现眼部症状（视物模糊、复视、上睑下垂），但约15%的病例首先出现延髓症状（构音障碍、吞咽困难、气短）或肢体无力。上睑下垂通常为非对称性。肌无力危象是一种神经系统急症，在15%～20%的MG患者中会出现，表现为严重的吞咽困难或呼吸衰竭，需要在重症监护室应用呼吸机支持和（或）鼻饲营养。

诊断和鉴别诊断

MG的诊断需要结合临床病史、体格检查和确诊试验。冰敷试验是一种简单而相对敏感的测试方法，用以区分MG引起的上睑下垂和其他原因引起的上睑下垂。此试验中，用冰袋敷在上睑下垂的眼睛上2 min，如果上睑下垂改善2 mm或以上，则支持为MG。

依酚氯铵（腾喜龙）是一种短效乙酰胆碱酯酶抑制剂，MG患者静脉应用后可有症状改善。依酚氯铵试验阳性的定义是，给药剂量从2 mg递增至10 mg，2～5 min后受影响肌肉的力量明确改善。由于可能出现心动过缓和低血压的副作用，因此在进行依酚氯铵试验时应准备阿托品。其他疾病的依酚氯铵试验结果也可能呈阳性。

3 Hz重复神经刺激（RNS）的电生理检查结果显示，50%～75%的全身型MG患者的复合肌肉动作电位（CMAP）递减超过10%，但有不到50%的单纯眼部症状患者出现异常。单纤维肌电图（SFEMG）是诊断MG最敏感的检测方法，在检测力弱肌肉时，99%的全身型MG患者和97%的单纯眼肌型MG患者表现为颤抖（jitter）增宽和阻滞（blocking）。单纤维肌电图通常只能在专门的肌电图室进行。

约80%的全身型MG患者和50%的单纯眼部症状患者的血清AChR Ab（结合抗体）检测呈阳性。部分血清学阴性患者可检测到肌肉特异性酪氨酸激酶抗体（Anti MuSk），女性患者更常见。

应进行胸部CT检查以排除胸腺瘤。血清学阳性的肌无力患者中约10%发现胸腺瘤。应评估甲状腺功能，因为甲状腺疾病通常与MG相关。电生理和血清抗体检测有助于将MG与运动神经元病、兰伯特-伊顿肌无力综合征（LEMS）和吉兰-巴雷综合征（GBS）进行鉴别。

治疗

溴吡斯的明30～60 mg，每4 h一次，可改善大多数MG患者的症状；它可单独用于治疗仅有轻微或轻度肌无力的单纯眼肌型和全身型病例，也可与免疫抑制剂联合应用治疗表现较严重的患者。泼尼松能在短期内有效改善肌无力，但长期使用会产生副作用。硫唑嘌呤和吗替麦考酚酯可用于长期治疗，也可起到减少类固醇的作用。依库珠单抗是一种补体抑制剂，近期被批准用于AChR抗体阳性的全身型MG患者。血浆置换和静脉注射免疫球蛋白适用于严重延髓型肌无力或全身无力、呼吸危象的患者，以及口服免疫调节药物无效的难治性患者。胸腺瘤切除术适用于所有MG合并胸腺瘤的患者。非胸腺瘤自身免疫性MG患者也建议进行胸腺切除术，以提高病情缓解或好转的可能性。通常不建议对60岁以上的患者进行胸腺切除术。某些药物可能会加重MG的症状或诱发疾病初期症状和体征的进展（表20.1）。

预后

多数接受最佳治疗的MG患者的症状都会得到改善或缓解。约有10%的MG患者尽管接受了最佳治疗，但仍会出现难治性症状。目前MG死亡率低于5%。

TABLE 20.1 Drugs to Be Avoided or Used With Caution in Myasthenia Gravis

- D-penicillamine
- Penicillins
- Telithromycin
- Interferon-α
- Aminoglycoside antibiotics
- Fluoroquinolones
- Nitrofurantoin
- Tetracyclines
- Sulfonamides
- Botulinum toxin
- Magnesium, magnesium salts contained in some laxatives and antacids
- Neuromuscular blocking agents such as succinylcholine and vecuronium should only be used by an anesthesiologist familiar with MG
- Quinine, quinidine or procainamide
- β-blockers (propranolol; timolol maleate eyedrops)
- Calcium-channel blockers
- Iodinated contrast agents
- Checkpoint inhibitors: pembrolizumab
- Anesthetics: Methoxyflurane, succinylcholine

LAMBERT-EATON MYASTHENIC SYNDROME

Definition/Epidemiology/Pathology

LEMS is an acquired, presynaptic neuromuscular transmission disorder caused by antibodies against the P/Q type voltage-gated calcium channel (VGCC). P/Q VGCC antibodies cause reduced Ca$^+$ influx into the presynaptic nerve terminal, resulting in decreased acetylcholine release and neuromuscular transmission failure. LEMS is associated with cancer, usually small cell lung carcinoma, in 60% of cases. LEMS may predate tumor detection by up to 3 years. LEMS is very rare and more common in men (3:1).

Clinical Presentation

LEMS should be suspected whenever the triad of muscle weakness, dry mouth, and decreased or absent reflexes is present. Patients have fluctuating weakness and fatigability of proximal limb and trunk muscles, with the lower limbs more severely affected than the upper ones. Difficulty walking is a common symptom. Dysphagia, dysarthria, and ocular symptoms (ptosis, blurred vision, and diplopia) are less common than in MG. Tendon reflexes are hypoactive or absent and may increase following short exercise of the muscle. Autonomic manifestations (dry mouth, impotence, decreased sweating, orthostatic hypotension, and slow pupillary reflexes) occur in 75% of patients.

Diagnosis and Differential Diagnosis

Serum antibodies against P/Q VGCCs are found in nearly all cases of paraneoplastic LEMS and in about 90% of non-paraneoplastic cases. Electrodiagnostic testing can help confirm the diagnosis by demonstrating reduced CMAP amplitudes in distal hand muscles; CMAP facilitation of at least 100% after 10″ maximal voluntary contraction or high frequency RNS (post-tetanic facilitation); and CMAP decrement greater than 10% with low frequency RNS. Patients diagnosed with LEMS should be screened and monitored with chest CT for lung cancer, especially if they are smokers and over age 50. LEMS and MG can be differentiated with electrodiagnostic and antibody testing.

Treatment

Symptomatic treatment with 3,4 diaminopyridine (3,4-DAP) 5 to 10 mg every 3 to 4 hours and up to a maximum daily dose of 80 to 100 mg is most effective in improving muscle strength in patients with LEMS. Side effects at doses up to 60 mg per day are rare. Acral and perioral paresthesias occur within minutes from a dose and resolve in about 15 minutes. It is contraindicated in patients with seizures. Pyridostigmine 60 mg every 4 hours is also used to improve symptoms. In patients in whom symptoms are not adequately controlled with 3,4-DAP and pyridostigmine, immunomodulation with prednisone, azathioprine, or mycophenolate mofetil is used. Severe weakness is treated with plasmapheresis or IVIG. The underlying cancer should be treated.

Prognosis

In paraneoplastic LEMS the prognosis is determined by the underlying cancer. The presence of LEMS in patients with small cell lung cancer (SCLC) is associated with longer survival from the malignancy. Non-paraneoplastic LEMS, when optimally treated, has an excellent prognosis and normal life expectancy, although patients may continue to experience various degrees of muscle weakness.

BOTULISM

Definition/Epidemiology/Pathology

Botulism is a rare, potentially lethal, paralytic illness caused by the neurotoxin produced by the anaerobic, spore-forming bacterium *Clostridioides botulinum*. Botulinum toxin blocks voluntary and autonomic cholinergic neuromuscular junctions by binding irreversibly to the presynaptic nerve endings where it inhibits the release of acetylcholine. Human forms of the disease include food-borne botulism most commonly caused by home-canned food, wound botulism with most cases occurring among "black tar" heroin users, and infant botulism occurring usually in the second month of life due to intestinal colonization. Outbreaks of food-borne botulism occur in prison inmates due to ingestion of pruno, an alcoholic drink made illicitly in prison. About 145 botulism cases are reported each year in the United States; approximately 15% are food-borne, 65% are infant, and 20% are wound botulism.

Clinical Presentation

The disease is characterized by symmetric descending flaccid paralysis starting with blurred or double vision, ptosis, dysphagia, dry mouth, dysarthria, and muscle weakness. Symptoms usually start 18 to 36 hours after ingesting contaminated food.

Botulism should be suspected in any infant with poor feeding and sucking, constipation, dilated pupils, weak cry, poor tone, and respiratory distress. Sensory examination and mental status are normal.

Diagnosis and Differential Diagnosis

All suspected cases of botulism need to be reported to public health authorities immediately. Local health department and CDC laboratories can confirm the diagnosis by detecting the toxin in serum, stool, or gastric or wound aspirate specimens. Electrodiagnostic testing can also confirm the diagnosis by demonstrating persistent post-tetanic facilitation of CMAP of at least 20%, a decremental response greater than 10% with slow RNS, and increased jitter and blocking on SFEMG. Electrodiagnostic tests are also helpful in differentiating botulism from Guillain-Barré syndrome and myasthenia gravis.

Treatment

Prompt intensive care support with mechanical ventilation and parenteral feeding as needed are crucial in reducing mortality. Timely

表 20.1　重症肌无力患者应避免或谨慎使用的药物
• D-青霉胺 • 青霉素类 • 替利霉素 • 干扰素-α • 氨基糖苷类抗生素 • 氟喹诺酮类 • 呋喃妥因 • 四环素类 • 磺胺类 • 肉毒杆菌毒素 • 镁、某些缓泻药和抗酸药中含有的镁盐 • 琥珀胆碱和维库溴铵等神经肌肉阻滞剂应该只能由熟悉重症肌无力的麻醉医师使用 • 奎宁、奎尼丁或普鲁卡因胺 • β受体阻滞剂（普萘洛尔，马来酸噻吗洛尔滴眼液） • 钙通道阻滞剂 • 碘造影剂 • 检查点抑制剂：帕博利珠单抗 • 麻醉剂：甲氧氟烷、琥珀胆碱

兰伯特-伊顿肌无力综合征

定义、流行病学和病理学

兰伯特-伊顿肌无力综合征（LEMS）是一种获得性突触前膜神经肌肉传递障碍，由针对 P/Q 型电压门控钙离子通道（VGCC）的抗体引起。P/Q VGCC 抗体会导致神经末梢突触前膜的 Ca^+ 内流减少，从而导致乙酰胆碱释放减少和神经肌肉传递障碍。60% 的 LEMS 与癌症有关，通常是小细胞肺癌。LEMS 可能早于肿瘤 3 年出现。LEMS 非常罕见，男性相对常见（3∶1）。

临床表现

只要出现肌无力、口干、反射减弱或消失的三联征，就应怀疑 LEMS。患者的四肢近端肌肉和躯干肌会出现波动性无力和易疲劳，下肢比上肢受影响更严重。行走困难是一种常见症状。吞咽困难、构音障碍和眼部症状（上睑下垂、视物模糊和复视）较 MG 患者少见。腱反射减弱或消失，但在肌肉短时间运动后可能会增强。75% 的患者会出现自主神经受累表现（口干、阳痿、少汗、体位性低血压和瞳孔反射减慢）。

诊断和鉴别诊断

在几乎所有副肿瘤性 LEMS 病例和约 90% 的非副肿瘤性病例中，均可发现针对 P/Q VGCC 的血清抗体。电生理检查可帮助确诊：手部远端肌肉 CMAP 波幅降低；10 s 最大自主收缩或高频重复神经刺激后 CMAP 波幅增高至少 100%（强直后易化）；低频重复神经刺激 CMAP 波幅降低超过 10%。诊断 LEMS 的患者应通过胸部 CT 进行肺癌筛查和监测，尤其是吸烟者和 50 岁以上患者。LEMS 和 MG 可通过电生理诊断和抗体检测加以鉴别。

治疗

使用 3,4-二氨基吡啶（3,4-DAP）进行对症治疗，对改善 LEMS 患者的肌力最为有效，每 3～4 h 一次，每次 5～10 mg，每日最大剂量为 80～100 mg。每日最大剂量 60 mg 的副作用罕见。服药后几分钟内会出现指端和口周感觉异常，约 15 min 后症状可缓解。癫痫发作患者禁用。溴吡斯的明 60 mg 每 4 h 一次，也可用于改善症状。对于 3,4-DAP 和溴吡斯的明不能充分控制症状的患者，可使用泼尼松、硫唑嘌呤或吗替麦考酚酯进行免疫调节治疗。肌无力严重者可应用血浆置换或 IVIG 治疗。需对基础癌症进行治疗。

预后

副肿瘤性 LEMS 的预后取决于基础癌症。小细胞肺癌（SCLC）患者出现 LEMS 与较长的恶性肿瘤生存期有关。非副肿瘤性 LEMS 在接受最佳治疗后，预后良好，预期寿命正常，但患者可能会持续出现不同程度的肌无力。

肉毒中毒

定义、流行病学和病理学

肉毒中毒是一种罕见的由厌氧性芽孢杆菌——肉毒梭菌产生的神经毒素引起的潜在致死的麻痹性疾病。肉毒毒素通过不可逆地与神经末梢突触前膜结合，抑制乙酰胆碱的释放，从而阻断随意和自主胆碱能神经肌肉接头的信号传递。人类肉毒中毒的形式包括食源性肉毒中毒，最常见的是由家庭罐装食品引起的肉毒中毒；伤口肉毒中毒，大部分病例发生在"黑焦油"海洛因吸食者中；婴儿肉毒中毒，通常发生在出生后的第 2 个月，由肠道定植引起。食源性肉毒中毒曾在监狱囚犯中暴发，原因是囚犯摄入了监狱酒（pruno），即一种在监狱中非法制造的酒精饮料。美国每年报告的肉毒中毒病例约为 145 例，其中约 15% 是食源性肉毒中毒，65% 是婴儿肉毒中毒，20% 是伤口肉毒中毒。

临床表现

该病的特征是对称性下行性弛缓性瘫痪，开始时伴有视物模糊或复视、上睑下垂、吞咽困难、口干、构音障碍和肌无力。症状通常在摄入受污染食物 18～36 h 后开始出现。

如果婴儿出现喂养困难、吮乳不畅、便秘、瞳孔散大、哭声微弱、肌张力减低或呼吸窘迫，应怀疑是否发生肉毒中毒。患儿感觉检查和精神状态一般正常。

诊断和鉴别诊断

所有疑似肉毒中毒的病例都需要立即向公共卫生部门报告。当地卫生部门和疾病预防控制中心实验室可通过检测血清、粪便、胃或伤口抽吸物标本中的毒素来确诊。电生理检查也可通过以下方法确诊：CMAP 的持续强直后易化至少达到 20%，低频重复神经刺激递减反应超过 10%，单纤维肌电图显示颤抖增宽和阻滞。电生理检查也有助于肉毒中毒与吉兰-巴雷综合征和重症肌无力的互相鉴别。

治疗

及时提供重症监护支持、机械通气和必要的肠外营

administration of equine antitoxin within the first 24 hours may arrest the progression of paralysis and decrease the duration of illness. The antitoxin is provided by the CDC through the local health departments. Children younger than 12 months old should not be fed honey because it can contain *Clostridioides botulinum*.

Prognosis

The proportion of patients with botulism who die has fallen from 50% to between 3% and 5% in the past 50 years. Recovery of muscle strength may take several months. Mortality in untreated botulism is 60%.

ORGANOPHOSPHATE POISONING

Organophosphorus compounds (OPs) are used as pesticides and developed for chemical warfare. Exposure to even small amounts of an OP can be fatal and death is usually caused by respiratory failure. OPs cause inhibition of acetylcholinesterase (AChE) resulting in accumulation of acetylcholine at the cholinergic receptor sites, producing continuous stimulation of cholinergic fibers throughout the nervous system. A combination of an antimuscarinic agent (e.g., atropine), AChE reactivator, such as one of the pyridinium oximes (i.e., pralidoxime, trimedoxime, obidoxime, and HI-6), and diazepam are used for the treatment of OP poisoning in humans.

❖ For a deeper discussion on this topic, please see Chapter 394, "Disorders of Neuromuscular Transmission," in *Goldman-Cecil Medicine*, 26th Edition.

SUGGESTED READINGS

Palace J, Newsom-Davis J, Lecky B: A randomized double-blind trial of prednisolone alone or with azathioprine in myasthenia gravis, Neurology 50:1778–1783, 1998.

Pascuzzi RM, Coslett HB, Johns TR: Long-term corticosteroid treatment of myasthenia gravis: report of 116 patients, Ann Neurol 515:291–298, 1984.

Passaro DJ, Werner SB, McGee J: Wound botulism associated with black tar heroin among injecting drug users, J Am Med Assoc 279(11):859–863, 1998.

Sanders DB, Wolfe GI, Benatar M, et al: International consensus guidance for management of myasthenia gravis, Neurology 87(4):419–425, 2016.

Sobel J, Tucker N, Sulka A: Foodborne botulism in the United States, 1990-2000, Emerg Infect Dis 10:1606–1611, 2004.

Tim R, Massey J, Sanders D: Lambert-Eaton myasthenic syndrome: electrodiagnostic findings and response to treatment, Neurology 54:2176–2178, 2000.

Underwood K, Rubin S, Deakers T: Infant botulism: a 30 year experience spanning the introduction of botulism immune globulin intravenous in the intensive care unit at Children's Hospital Los Angeles, Pediatrics 120(6):1380–1385, 2007.

Vugia DJ, Mase SR, Cole B: Botulism from drinking pruno, Emerg Infect Dis 15:69–71, 2009.

Wirtz P, Lang B, Graus F: P/Q-type calcium channel antibodies, Lambert-Eaton myasthenic syndrome and survival in small cell lung cancer, J Neuroimmunol 164:161–165, 2005.

Wolfe GI, Kaminski HJ, Aban IB, et al: Randomized trial of thymectomy in myasthenia gravis, N Engl J Med 375:511–522, 2016.

养对降低死亡率至关重要。在最初的 24 h 内及时应用马抗毒素可阻止瘫痪的进展并缩短病程。抗毒素由疾病预防控制中心通过当地卫生部门提供。不要给 12 个月以下的儿童喂食蜂蜜，因为蜂蜜中可能含有肉毒梭菌。

预后

在过去的 50 年中，肉毒中毒患者的死亡比例已从 50% 下降到 3% ~ 5%。肌肉力量的恢复可能需要几个月的时间。未经治疗的肉毒中毒死亡率为 60%。

有机磷中毒

有机磷化合物（OP）被用作杀虫剂，并为化学战而开发。即使接触少量有机磷化合物也会致命，死亡通常由呼吸衰竭所致。有机磷化合物会抑制乙酰胆碱酯酶（AChE），导致乙酰胆碱在胆碱能受体部位的积聚，从而对整个神经系统的胆碱能纤维产生持续刺激。联合应用抗毒蕈碱药（如阿托品）、乙酰胆碱酯酶再激活剂［如吡啶肟类药物（解磷定、双解磷、双复磷和 HI-6）之一］和地西泮可用于治疗人有机磷化合物中毒。

❖ 有关此专题的深入讨论，请参阅 *Goldman-Cecil Medicine* 第 26 版第 394 章"神经肌肉传递障碍"。

推荐阅读

Palace J, Newsom-Davis J, Lecky B: A randomized double-blind trial of prednisolone alone or with azathioprine in myasthenia gravis, Neurology 50:1778–1783, 1998.

Pascuzzi RM, Coslett HB, Johns TR: Long-term corticosteroid treatment of myasthenia gravis: report of 116 patients, Ann Neurol 515:291–298, 1984.

Passaro DJ, Werner SB, McGee J: Wound botulism associated with black tar heroin among injecting drug users, J Am Med Assoc 279(11):859–863, 1998.

Sanders DB, Wolfe GI, Benatar M, et al: International consensus guidance for management of myasthenia gravis, Neurology 87(4):419–425, 2016.

Sobel J, Tucker N, Sulka A: Foodborne botulism in the United States, 1990-2000, Emerg Infect Dis 10:1606–1611, 2004.

Tim R, Massey J, Sanders D: Lambert-Eaton myasthenic syndrome: electrodiagnostic findings and response to treatment, Neurology 54:2176–2178, 2000.

Underwood K, Rubin S, Deakers T: Infant botulism: a 30 year experience spanning the introduction of botulism immune globulin intravenous in the intensive care unit at Children's Hospital Los Angeles, Pediatrics 120(6):1380–1385, 2007.

Vugia DJ, Mase SR, Cole B: Botulism from drinking pruno, Emerg Infect Dis 15:69–71, 2009.

Wirtz P, Lang B, Graus F: P/Q-type calcium channel antibodies, Lambert-Eaton myasthenic syndrome and survival in small cell lung cancer, J Neuroimmunol 164:161–165, 2005.

Wolfe GI, Kaminski HJ, Aban IB, et al: Randomized trial of thymectomy in myasthenia gravis, N Engl J Med 375:511–522, 2016.

SECTION II

Geriatrics

21　The Aging Patient, 294

第 2 篇

老年医学

21 老年患者，295

21

The Aging Patient

Laura A. Previll, Mitchell T. Heflin, Harvey Jay Cohen

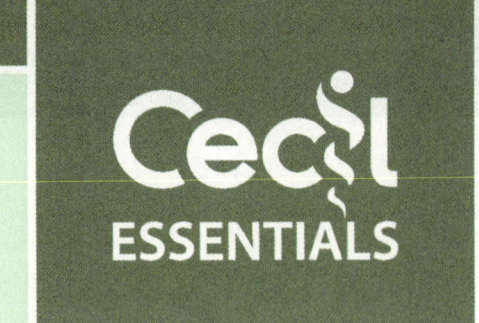

INTRODUCTION

The aging of the world's population compels all health care team members to gain competency in geriatrics, the clinical science of assessment, prevention, and treatment of illness in older adults. A basic grasp of geriatrics requires understanding at epidemiologic, biologic, and clinical levels. The provider must appreciate the impact of aging on presentation of and predisposition to certain conditions, must identify goals of care, and must select appropriate treatment strategies. Moreover, care of older adults demands a multifaceted approach, accounting for individual, family, and community resources. Finally, the practice of geriatrics requires an appreciation for systems of care that include interprofessional teams working in a variety of settings ranging from home to hospital to long-term care to community settings. This chapter will provide an introduction to geriatrics and the essentials of caring for older adults.

Over the last century, the number of Americans over the age of 65 years increased from 3 million to nearly 51 million in 2016, accounting for 16% of the population. During the same period the population over age 85 grew rapidly, expanding from 100,000 in 1900 to nearly 6.4 million in 2016. By 2030, the number of adults over age 65 will likely reach 74 million, or 21% of the total population. Ten million of those people will be over age 85 (Fig. 21.1). A report from the National Institute on Aging and the US State Department points out that this phenomenon is not isolated to the United States. Around the globe, the percentage of the population over 65 years of age will increase by 25% to 50% over the next 25 years and by 140% in developing nations.

EPIDEMIOLOGY OF AGING

Most experts believe that the rapid growth of the population of older adults reflects the many health care successes of the twentieth century. Fries, in his landmark paper, attributes the extension of the human lifespan to "the elimination of premature death, particularly neonatal mortality." Improvements in other aspects of public health, including adequate nutrition and housing, safe drinking water, immunizations, and antibiotics, have led to lower rates of mortality throughout childhood and early adulthood, affording an opportunity for more people to survive to late life. Examination of survival curves across the twentieth century demonstrates a marked change in the shape of the overall graph from nearly linear in 1900 to rectangular in the 1990s, with much of the mortality compressed into late life (Fig. 21.2). However, despite advances in public health, life expectancy at birth continues to vary by race and gender and social drivers of health affect the ability to achieve old age for many. As of 2016, the greatest average life expectancy at birth by ethnicity was in Hispanic females compared to non-Hispanic black males who average 10 years fewer. Although the overall average population life expectancy at birth rose dramatically in the 20th century from 47 years to nearly 77 years with up to 10% of the birth cohort surviving to age 95, the maximum lifespan defined as the age of the oldest surviving humans has remained remarkably stable at around 114 years.

THE BIOLOGY OF AGING

The relatively static nature of the maximum lifespan reflects the human body's limits at the cellular, tissue, and organ level in dealing with the stresses of aging. Across cell types and organ systems, certain consistent age-related alterations in physiologic function exist. Variability in tissue and organ function decreases, as evidenced by less fluctuation in heart rate or hormone secretion. Organ systems also exhibit predictable declines in function over time Table 21.1. These changes are most evident at times of stress, and ultimately these systems are slower to react and recover. The overall result is an impaired ability to deal with any demands within a narrow range. This progressive restriction in the capacity to maintain homeostasis can be depicted as a steady tapering in the reserve available in multiple organ systems as time progresses (Fig. 21.3). In this situation an individual may function within the normal range in the absence of crisis, but stress such as acute illness may exceed his or her capacity to restore function and recover health. The result at best may be a decline in health and ability, and at worst, death.

THEORIES OF AGING

Scientific research provides a number of plausible theories of aging, which can be grouped into two major categories. *Error* or *damage theories* propose that aging occurs because of persistent threats from damaging agents derived from environmental stressors and an ever-declining ability to respond to or repair this damage. *Program theories* postulate that genetic and developmental factors most significantly determine the biologic life course and the maximal age of the organism. In actuality, biologic aging may reflect a complex combination of many types of events. In a landmark paper outlining specific "Hallmarks of Aging," Lopez-Ortin suggests nine possible molecular or genetic mechanisms through which physiologic systems age. This section provides an introduction to some of these theories (Fig. 21.4). The end of the chapter also describes the emerging field of geroscience related to these criteria.

The free radical theory of aging proposes that oxidative metabolism results in an excess of highly reactive byproducts, called *oxygen free radicals,* which damage proteins, DNA, and lipids. Molecular injury eventually leads to cell dysfunction and ultimately to tissue and organ

老年患者

鲁晓春　付治卿　译　付治卿　鲁晓春　审校　李小鹰　通审

引言

在世界人口老龄化时代，医疗护理团队的每位成员都需要掌握老年医学的专业知识。老年医学作为一门专注于老年疾病评估、预防和治疗的临床学科，要求从流行病学、生物学和临床等多个层面深入理解老年疾病。医务人员必须了解衰老如何影响特定疾病的临床表现和发病倾向，明确照护目标，制订合适的治疗方案。此外，老年照护需要充分了解和综合考虑个体、家庭和社区等各方面资源后制订方案。最后，老年医学的实践还要求了解照护系统，他们是在家庭、医院、长期照护的社区等各种环境中工作的跨专业团队。本章将介绍老年医学的基础知识和老年照护的核心要点。

在过去一个世纪里，美国65岁以上人口从300万激增至2016年的近5100万，达到总人口的16%。同期，85岁以上人口也快速增长，从1900年的10万增至2016年的近640万。预计到2030年，65岁以上人口将达到7400万，占总人口的21%，其中约1000万人超过85岁（图21.1）。美国国家老龄化研究所和国务院的报告指出，这一现象并非美国独有。放眼全球，未来25年内65岁以上人口比例将增长25%～50%，发展中国家更是会激增140%。

衰老的流行病学

大多数专家认为，老年人口的迅速增长是20世纪医疗保健取得诸多成就的体现。Fries在其里程碑式论文中提出，人类寿命的延长归功于"消除早逝，特别是消除了新生儿夭折"。公共卫生的其他进步，包括充足的营养和住房、安全的饮用水、疫苗接种和抗生素的使用，降低了整个儿童期和成年早期的死亡率，让更多人有机会活到晚年。对整个20世纪的生存曲线的分析显示，人类生存曲线整体形状发生了明显的变化，从1900年的近乎直线变为1990年代的矩形，人类死亡主要集中在晚年（图21.2）。然而，尽管公共卫生取得了进步，出生时的预期寿命仍然因种族、性别和社会健康因素的不同而有所差异，这些因素影响着许多人能否存活到老年。截至2016年，按种族划分，西班牙裔女性的出生时预期寿命最长，而非西班牙裔黑人男性的平均寿命要短10年。尽管在20世纪，总体出生人口的平均预期寿命从47岁大幅提升至近77岁，有高达10%的出生队列能活到95岁，但定义为最长寿者的最大寿命却出奇地稳定在大约114岁左右。

衰老生物学

人类最大寿命相对稳定的特性反映了人体在细胞、组织和器官层面应对衰老压力的极限。在不同类型细胞和器官系统中，存在某些一致的与年龄相关的生理功能变化。组织和器官功能变化的波动范围降低，表现为心率或激素分泌的波动程度降低。器官系统的功能也会随着时间的推移出现可预知的衰退（表21.1）。这些变化在应激时最为明显，最终这些系统的反应速度和恢复能力将会越来越慢。总体结果是，在狭窄范围内应对任何需求的能力都会受损。随着时间的推移，机体保持和恢复体内稳态的能力进行性下降，这种现象可以理解为多器官系统可用的储备能力稳定地衰减（图21.3）。在这种情况下，个体可以在没有危机的情况下处于正常范围，但是像急性疾病这样的应激就可能超出其修复功能和恢复健康的能力。这种急性应激最好的康复结果可能是健康和能力出现下降，最坏的情况是死亡。

衰老理论

科学研究发现了多种关于衰老的理论，可分为两大类。错误或损伤理论认为，衰老是因为持续受到环境压力等损伤性因素作用，而机体对这些损伤的响应或修复能力不断下降。程序理论则假设，遗传和发育因素在很大程度上决定了生物的生命历程和有机体的最大寿命。实际上，生物学上的衰老可能反映了多种类型事件的复杂组合。在一篇名为"衰老的标志"的里程碑式论文中，Lopez-Ortin提出了九种可能的分子或遗传机制，这些机制与生理系统衰老紧密相关。本篇介绍了其中一些理论（图21.4）。本章末尾还将描述与这些准则相关的新兴老年科学领域。

衰老的自由基理论提出生物氧化代谢过程中会产生过量的高活性副产品，即氧自由基，它们会损伤蛋白质、DNA和脂质。分子损伤最终会引起细胞功能障

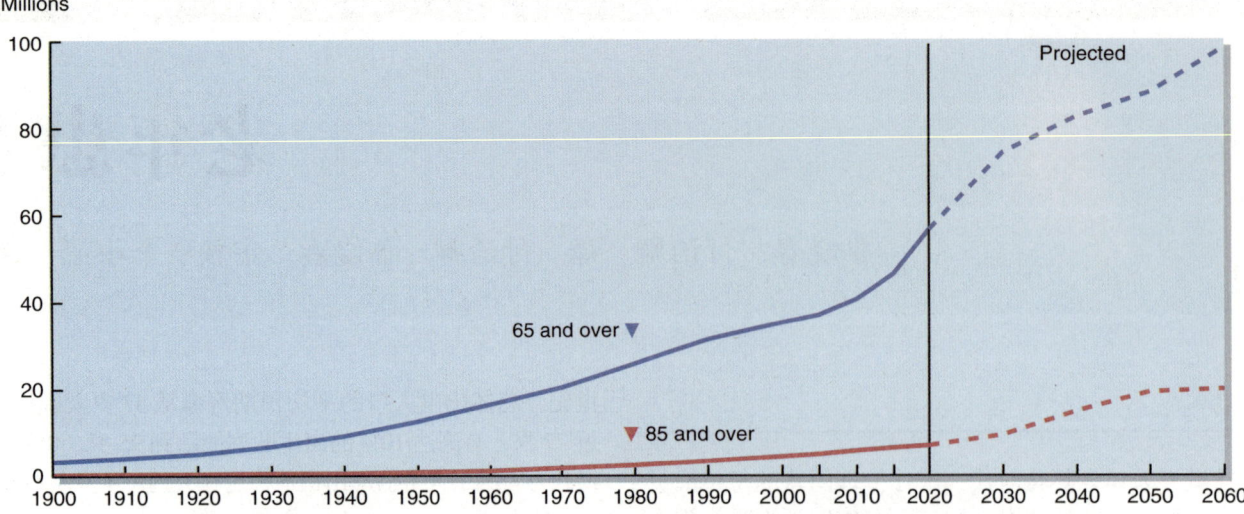

Fig. 21.1 Population age 65 and over and age 85 and over, selected years, 1900-2014, and projected years, 2020-2060. (From Federal Interagency Forum on Aging-Related Statistics: Older Americans 2016: key indicators of well-being. Federal Interagency Forum on Aging-Related Statistics, Washington, D.C., 2016, U.S. Government Printing Office.)

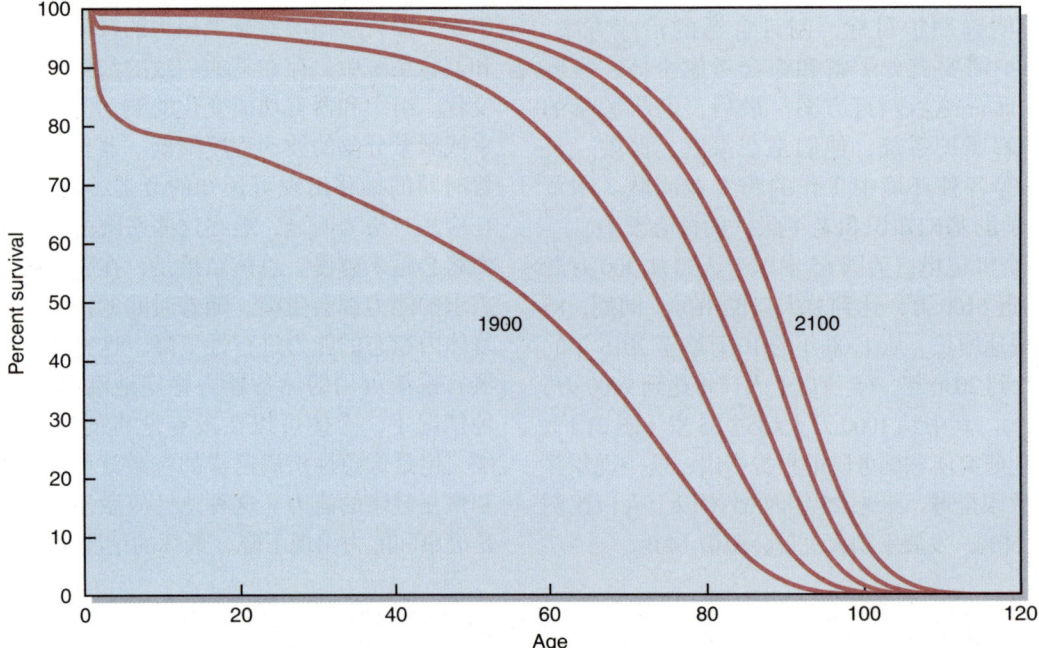

Fig. 21.2 Survival function for SSA population. Population survival curves based on period life tables for: 1900, 1950, 2000 and projected years 2050 and 2100. (From Bell, F.C. and Miller, M. L. Actuarial Study No. 120. Life Tables for the United States Social Security Area 1900-2100. [2005]. https://www.ssa.gov/oact/NOTES/as120/LifeTables_Body.html.)

disrepair. A second theory asserts that the accumulation of glucose-related molecules on proteins contributes to their dysfunction and degradation. These "glycosylated" molecules become more abundant over time and lead to impaired function at the tissue and organ level. Theory proponents point to the many chronic problems that routinely arise in patients with diabetes mellitus as proof of the significance of this phenomenon.

A different line of reasoning asserts that human lifespan and aging result from genetic-based timing mechanisms. Older theories suggest that evolutionary pressures are biased for traits that promote health and reproduction in early adulthood, possibly at the expense of health and function in late life. Furthermore, little selective pressure exists against negative traits that emerge in late life, leaving humans prone to the ill effects of aging. Geneticists have identified, among species of fruit flies and certain nematodes, specific genes that result in a significant prolongation in the organism's lifespan. Further exploration of specific modification to gene expression, also called epigenetics, has led to improved understanding of the influence of environmental factors

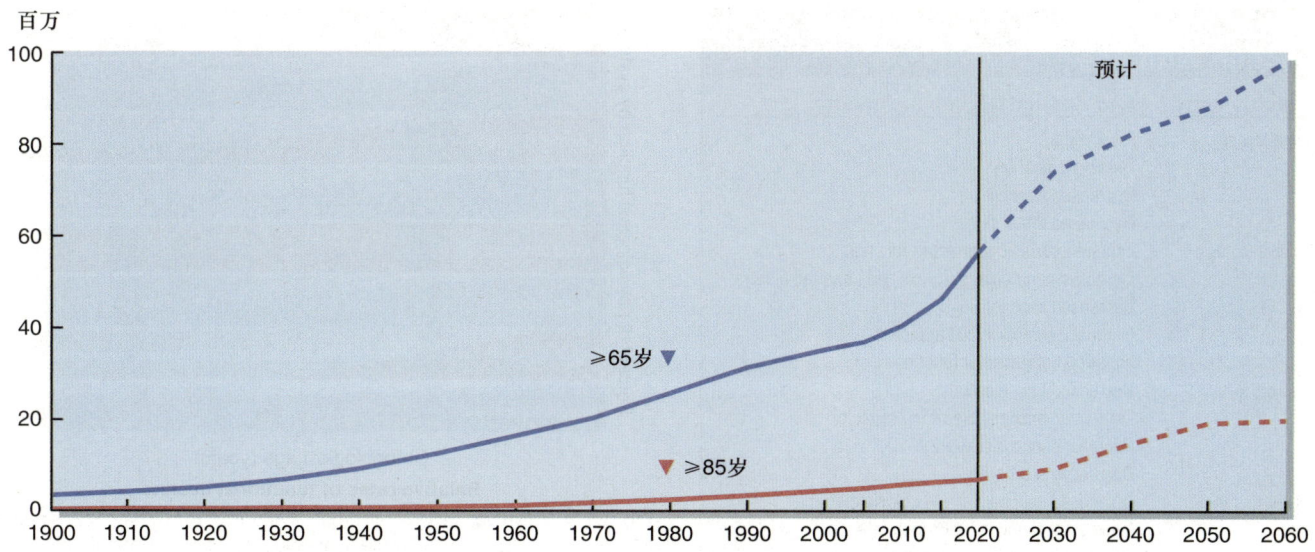

图 21.1　≥65 岁和 ≥85 岁人口数量增长趋势（1900—2014 年实际人口数和 2020—2060 年预期人口数）（引自 Federal Interagency Forum on Aging-Related Statistics：Older Americans 2016：key indicators of well-being. Federal Interagency Forum on Aging-Related Statistics，Washington，D.C.，2016，U.S. Government Printing Office.）

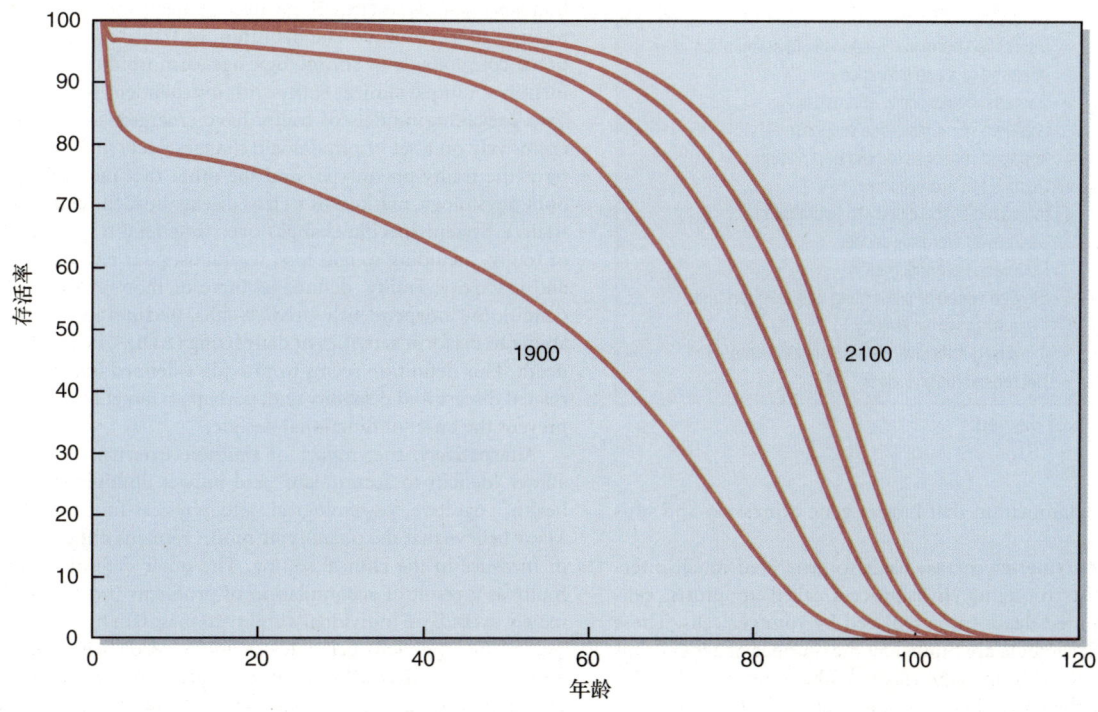

图 21.2　美国社会保障局（SSA）人口的生存函数。基于 1900 年、1950 年、2000 年以及预计的 2050 年和 2100 年寿命表的人口生存曲线（引自 Bell，F.C. and Miller，M. L. Actuarial Study No. 120. Life Tables for the United States Social Security Area 1900—2100.［2005］. https://www.ssa.gov/oact/NOTES/as120/LifeTables_Body.html.）

碍，导致组织和器官的损伤。另一种理论认为，蛋白质相关的糖基分子积累导致蛋白质功能障碍和降解。这些"糖基化"分子随时间变得更加丰富，并导致组织和器官层面的功能受损。该理论支持者指出，糖尿病患者经常出现的许多慢性问题都是这种现象的重要性的体现。

另一种不同的推定性理论认为，人类的寿命和衰老是由基因控制的时间机制所导致的。早期理论认为，进化压力偏向于在成年早期促进健康和繁殖的特征，可能会牺牲晚年的健康和功能。此外，晚年出现的负面特征几乎没有选择压力，因此人类容易受到衰老的不良影响。遗传学家在果蝇和某些线虫物种中发现了特定长寿基因，这些基因导致生物体寿命显著延长。对特定基因表达调节修饰的进一步研究，也称为

TABLE 21.1 Changes in Physiologic Function With Age

Organ System	Age-Related Decline in Function
Special senses	Presbyopia
	Lens opacification
	Decreased hearing
	Decreased taste, smell
Cardiovascular	Impaired intrinsic contractile function
	Increased ventricular stiffness and impaired filling
	Decreased conductivity
	Increased systolic blood pressure
	Impaired baroreceptor function
Respiratory	Decreased lung elasticity
	Decreased maximal breathing capacity
	Decreased mucus clearance
	Decreased arterial P_{O_2}
Gastrointestinal	Decreased esophageal and colonic motility
Renal	Decreased glomerular filtration rate
Immune	Decreased cell-mediated immunity
	Decreased T-cell number
	Increased T-suppressor cells
	Decreased T-helper cells
	Loss of memory cells
	Decline in antibody titers to known antigens
	Increased autoimmunity
Endocrine	Decreased hormonal responses to stimulation
	Impaired glucose tolerance
	Decreased androgens and estrogens
	Impaired norepinephrine responses
Autonomic nervous	Impaired response to fluid deprivation
	Decline in baroreceptor reflex
	Increased susceptibility to hypothermia
Peripheral nervous	Decreased vibratory sense
	Decreased proprioception
Central nervous	Slowed speed of processing and reaction time
	Decreased verbal fluency
	Increased difficulty learning new information
Musculoskeletal	Decreased muscle mass

P_{O_2}, Partial pressure of oxygen.

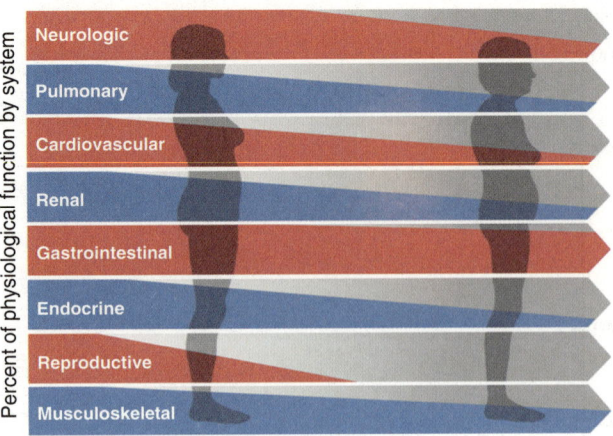

Fig. 21.3 Relative decline by organ system. (From Khan SS, Singer BD, Vaughan DE. [2017]. Molecular and physiological manifestations and measurement of aging in humans. Aging Cell, 16[4], 624-633.)

ASSESSMENT OF FRAILTY

Biologic changes of aging portend the increased vulnerability of humans to illness and functional decline in late life—a state commonly referred to as "frailty." The definition of frailty moves beyond traditional components of chronologic age, comorbidity, and disability to identify a unique clinical entity with independent predictive capacity. Two prevailing models of frailty have emerged—one focused more exclusively on a set of physiologic changes occurring in a cyclical pattern (the frailty phenotype) and the other that includes measures of both physiologic markers as well as disease burden (cumulative deficit frailty). System-specific changes over time lend a specific phenotype of frailty, including weight loss, weakness, poor endurance, slowness, and inactivity. Frailty, defined as three or more of these phenotypic conditions, independently predicts falls, declines in mobility, loss of ability to perform activities of daily living (ADLs), hospitalization, and death. This definition seems to provide a defined link between aging-related disease and disability and, perhaps, a target for interventions to prevent the onset of functional decline.

Alternatively, the impact of multiple external factors over time allows "deficits to accumulate" and impact multiple facets of overall health, cognitive, psychological, and physical function (Fig. 21.5). Many believe that the phenotypic model remains difficult to recognize or measure in the clinical setting. The other definition conceives of frailty as a result of accumulation of problems (or deficits) that ultimately exceeds an individual's ability to maintain function and health. This count of deficits generates an index predictive of disability and death. To some degree both models capture different aspects of complex and heterogeneous phenomena of vulnerability to declines in health and function with aging.

CLINICAL CARE OF OLDER ADULTS

Caring for older adults requires a strong foundation in the basics of internal medicine or family medicine integrated with an appreciation for the complexity and heterogeneity of the impact of aging on health and well-being. The clinician must possess strong diagnostic skills, given that older adults may have unique presentations or multiple comorbid conditions and functional decline. In addition, the clinician must monitor for a number of nonspecific conditions, such

such as chronic inflammation that impact gene expression and ultimately lifespan.

Study of the enzyme telomerase has also generated much interest among theorists on aging. In a process called apoptosis, cells undergo programmed death to be replaced by younger cells. These divisions and replacements are limited by the number of generations intrinsic to a specific cell line (the Hayflick phenomenon). As telomeres located on the ends of chromosomes are depleted, cell aging and demise eventually occur. The enzyme telomerase prevents telomere shortening and may increase a cell's number of allotted replications and thereby extend the lifespan of the organism. Of course, this advantage must be weighed against the price of "immortality," namely the increased risk of malignancy. Both apoptosis and cellular senescence are considered protective mechanisms against malignancy. The accumulation of senescent cells contributes to the biology of aging through secretion of various proteins that serve as inhibitory factors for halting cellular growth and division. In this way, regenerative capacities diminish when senescent cells shift the balance of cellular communication.

表 21.1	生理功能随年龄的变化
器官系统	与年龄相关的功能下降
特殊感官	老视
	晶状体混浊
	听力下降
	味觉、嗅觉减退
心血管	固有收缩功能受损
	心室僵硬度增加、充盈受损
	电传导性降低
	收缩压升高
	压力感受器功能受损
呼吸	肺顺应性降低
	最大呼吸能力下降（每分最大自主通气量）
	分泌物清除能力下降
	黏液清除率降低
	动脉氧分压下降
胃肠	食管和结肠蠕动能力下降
肾	肾小球滤过率降低
免疫	细胞介导的免疫力降低
	T 细胞数量减少
	T 抑制细胞增加
	T 辅助细胞减少
	记忆细胞丢失
	已知抗原的抗体滴度下降
	自身免疫增强
内分泌	应激引起的激素反应下降
	葡萄糖耐量受损
	雄激素和雌激素减少
	去甲肾上腺素反应受损
自主神经	对液体容量不足的反应减弱
	压力感受器反射减弱
	对低体温的敏感性增加
外周神经	振动感减弱
	本体感觉减弱
中枢神经	处理速度和反应时间减慢
	语言流畅性下降
	学习新信息更困难
肌肉骨骼	肌肉量减少

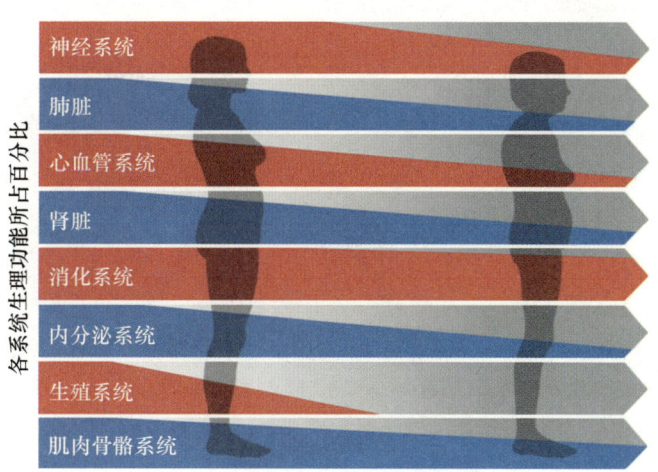

图 21.3 各器官系统的相对衰退情况（引自 Khan SS, Singer BD, Vaughan DE.［2017］. Molecular and physiological manifestations and measurement of aging in humans. Aging Cell, 16［4］, 624-633.）

衰弱的评估

随着年龄的增长，人体对疾病的易感性增加，同时生理功能减退，这种状态被称为衰弱。衰弱的定义超越了传统的时间年龄、共病状态和残疾等组分，是一个具有独立预测能力的独特临床概念。目前存在两种主要的衰弱模型：一种模型侧重于生理变化的周期性模式（表型衰弱）；另一种模型则包含了生理标志物和对疾病负担的估算（缺陷累积型衰弱）。随着时间推移，特定系统的变化产生特定的衰弱表型，如体重减轻、虚弱、耐力差、行动迟缓和缺乏活力。衰弱被定义为具备上述三个及以上表型特征，可独立预测跌倒、活动能力下降、日常生活活动能力（ADL）丧失、住院和死亡。这一定义似乎在衰老相关疾病和失能之间提供了一种明确的联系，或许也是预防功能衰退的干预目标。

另外，多种外部因素的长期影响可能导致"缺陷累积"，进而影响整体健康、认知、心理和身体功能的多个方面（图 21.5）。许多人认为表型模型在临床环境下仍然难以识别和评估。第二种模型（缺陷累积模型）是个体问题（或缺陷）累积的结果，严重超出了个体维持功能和健康的能力。根据这种缺陷计算获得的衰弱指数能预测失能和死亡。在某种程度上，这两种模型都捕捉到了随着年龄增长，易受健康和功能衰退影响的复杂和异质现象的不同方面。

老年人的临床照护

照顾老年人需要具备扎实的内科或家庭医学基础知识，并了解老龄化对健康和福祉影响的复杂性和异质性。鉴于老年人可能有独特的表现或多种并发症和功能衰退，临床医生必须具备很强的诊断技能。此

表观遗传学，使人们更深理解到环境因素（如慢性炎症）如何影响基因表达并最终影响寿命。

端粒酶的研究也引发了衰老理论学者的极大兴趣。在一种被称为凋亡的过程中，细胞经历程序性死亡，被更年轻的细胞所取代。这些分裂和替代受到特定细胞系固有的代数限制（Hayflick 现象）。随着位于染色体末端的端粒耗尽，细胞最终会衰老和死亡。端粒酶可以阻止端粒缩短，并可能增加细胞的固有复制次数，从而延长生物体的寿命。当然，这一优势必须与"长生不老"的代价（即恶性肿瘤的风险增加）进行权衡。凋亡和细胞衰老都被认为是对抗恶性肿瘤的保护性机制。衰老细胞通过分泌各种蛋白质作为抑制因子阻止细胞生长和分裂，从而促进衰老生物学的发展。这样，当衰老细胞改变了细胞交流的平衡时，再生能力就会减弱。

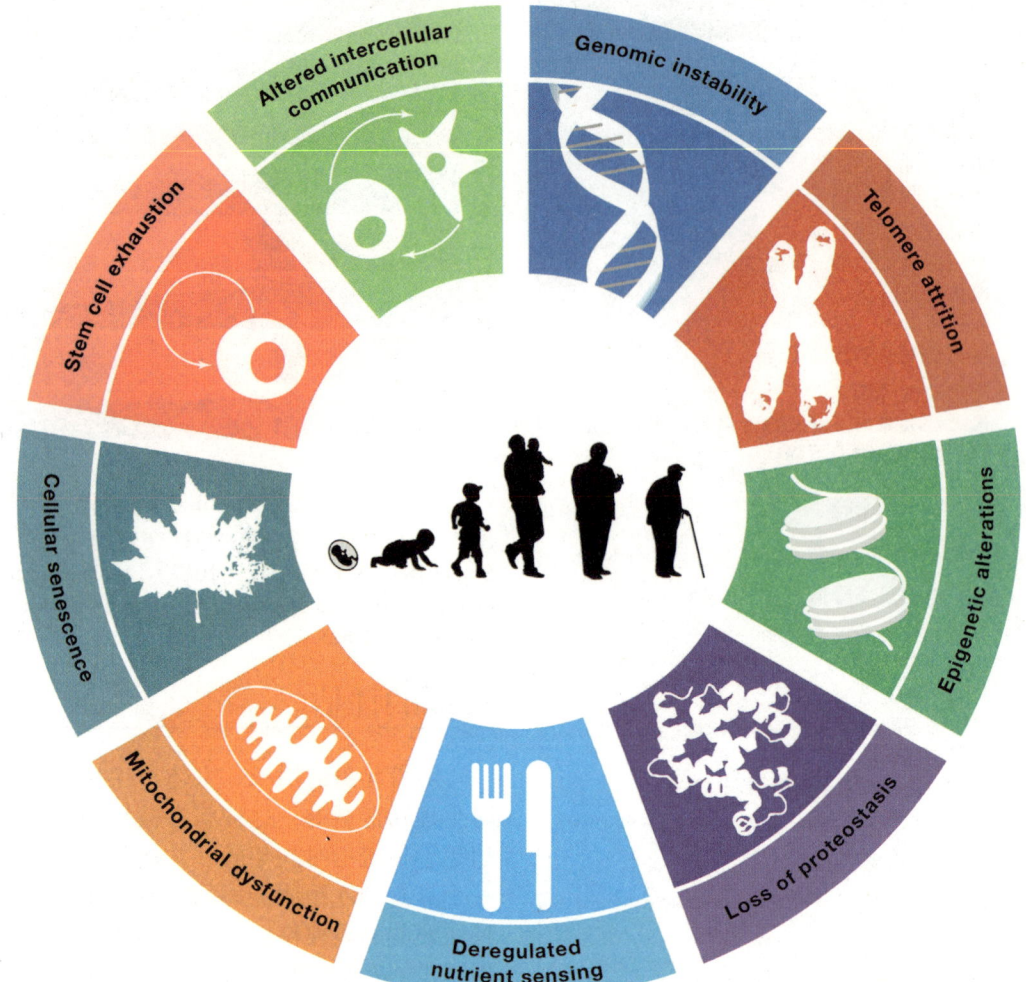

Fig. 21.4 The hallmarks of aging. (From López-Otín C, Blasco MA, Partridge L, et al [2013]. The Hallmarks of Aging. Cell, 153[6], 1194-1217.)

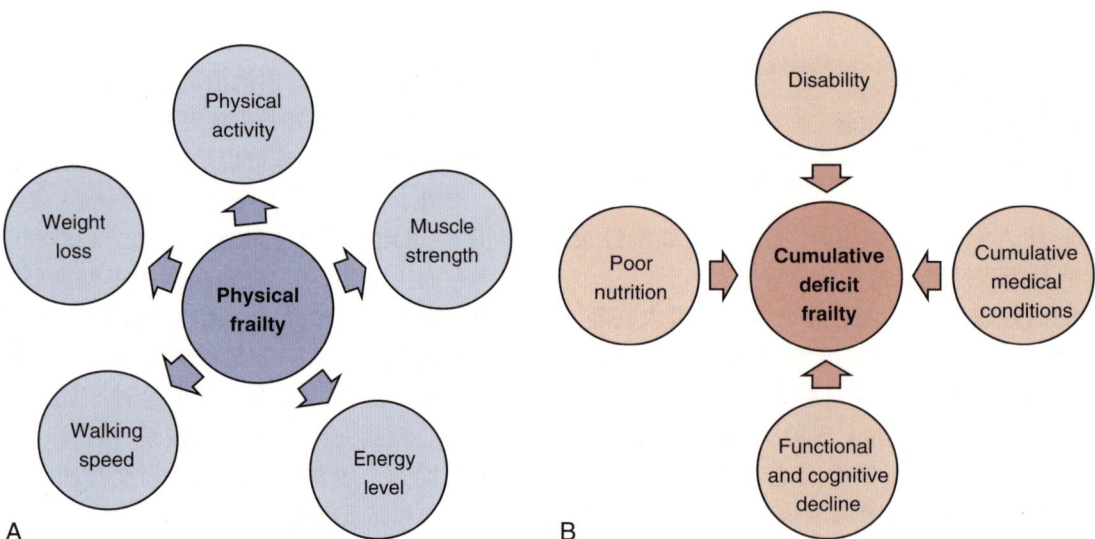

Fig. 21.5 Two major frailty theories. (A) Physical frailty or phenotypic frailty and (B) cumulative deficit frailty. (From Walston, J, Bandeen-Roche, K, Buta, B, et al. Moving frailty toward clinical practice: NIA Intramural Frailty Science Symposium Summary. J Am Geriatr Soc, 67: 1559-1564, 2019.)

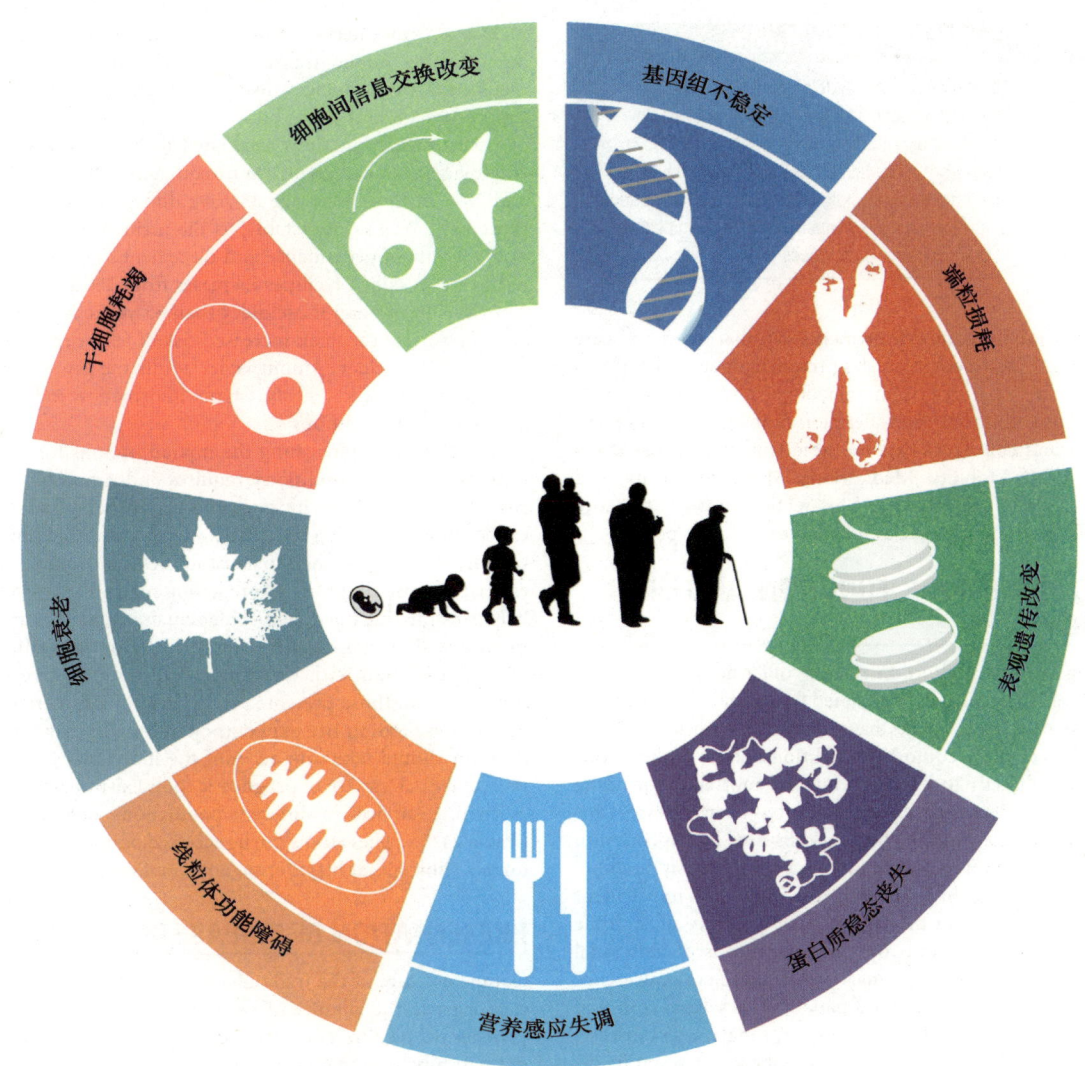

图 21.4 衰老的标志（引自 López-Otín C，Blasco MA，Partridge L，et al［2013］. The Hallmarks of Aging. Cell，153［6］，1194-1217.）

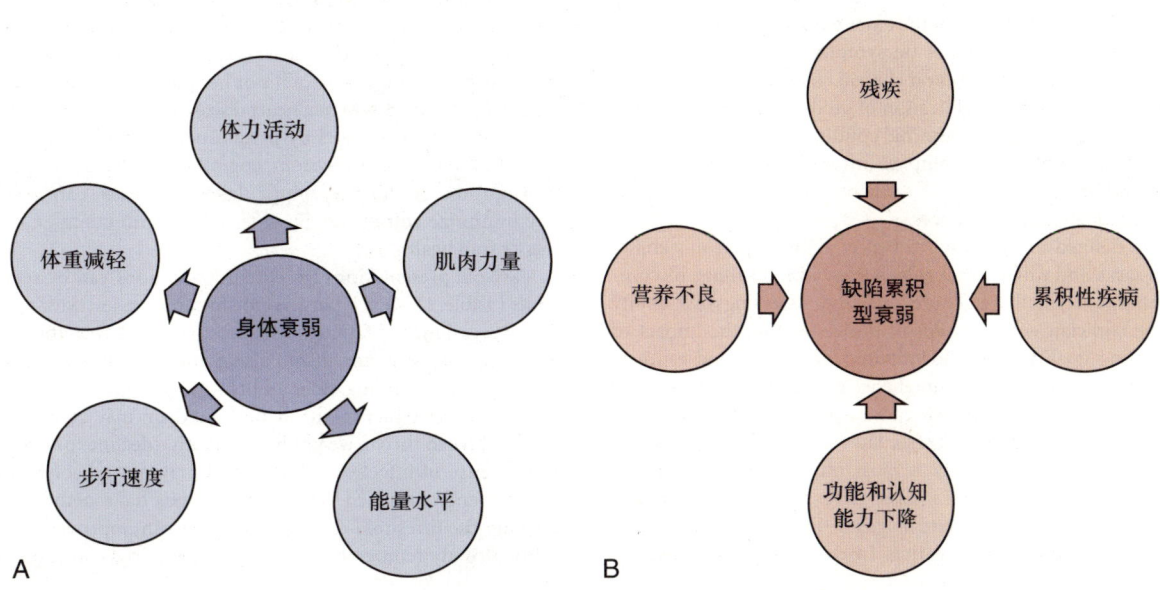

图 21.5 两种主要的衰弱理论。（A）身体衰弱或表型衰弱，（B）缺陷累积型衰弱（引自 Walston，J，Bandeen-Roche，K，Buta，B，et al. Moving frailty toward clinical practice：NIA Intramural Frailty Science Symposium Summary. J Am Geriatr Soc，67：1559-1564，2019.）

TABLE 21.2	The Geriatric 5-M's
Mind	Mentation, dementia, delirium, depression
Mobility	Impaired gait and balance, fall injury prevention
Medications	Polypharmacy, de-prescribing, optimal prescribing, adverse medication effects and medication burden
Multi-Complexity	Multi-morbidity, complex bio-psycho-social situations
Matters Most	Each individual's own meaningful health outcome goals and care preferences

as problems with mobility, mood, or mentation that affect self-care capacity and safety. Treatment strategies present unique challenges as well, often requiring a balance of pharmacologic and nonpharmacologic interventions with careful consideration of the individual's goals for care. Tinetti and colleagues capture these tenants of geriatrics as the five M's: "Mind, Mobility, Medications, Multi-complexity, and Matters Most to Me" (Table 21.2). This section presents the core components of the comprehensive assessment of the older patient.

COMORBID CONDITIONS, FUNCTION, AND LIFE EXPECTANCY

With advancing age and declines in reserve, older adults experience high rates of chronic illness and often related functional decline. Eighty percent of those over age 65 years have at least one chronic illness, and 50% have two or more comorbid conditions. Some of these conditions contribute directly to increased rates of mortality, including the leading causes of death among older adults—heart disease, cancer, stroke, lung disease, and Alzheimer's disease. Many common diseases, however, primarily threaten function and result in disability and institutionalization. Arthritis, hearing loss, and vision impairment are all important problems in this respect. The presence of multiple comorbid conditions compounds the disabling effects of individual diseases and further complicates management. In the era of evidence and guidelines, a clinician caring for a patient with several common chronic conditions, such as diabetes mellitus, coronary artery disease, and osteoporosis, may feel compelled to prescribe six or seven medications to remain in compliance with current recommendations. This practice can result in "polypharmacy" (described later), adding significant cost to the patient with limited accounting for risks, benefits, and individual preferences. In addition to considering the discrete management of individual diseases, care of the older adult requires assessment of the overall impact of treatment on symptoms, function, and life expectancy. To address this common clinical challenge, the American Geriatrics Society maintains publication of guiding principles on care of older persons with multiple comorbid conditions that highlights the importance of accounting for complex interactions between conditions, risks, and benefits of various treatment options, overall prognosis, and patient goals and preferences.

Function, defined formally by Reuben et al., is "a person's ability to perform tasks and fulfill social roles across a broad range of complexity"—more succinctly, self-care capacity. Assessing this ability provides the clinician with a means of understanding the impact of illness, assessing quality of life, identifying care needs, and estimating progress and prognosis. Comprehensive assessment of function should include questions about self-care capacity as well as objective measures of cognition and mobility (see later sections for details about the latter two). Self-care capacity is most often divided into basic, instrumental, and advanced ADLs. Basic ADLs include those actions that maintain personal health and hygiene, including transferring, bathing, toileting, dressing, and eating. Instrumental ADLs (IADLs) include activities necessary for living independently, specifically driving or using public transportation, cooking, shopping, managing medications and finances, using the telephone (or other communication device), and doing housework. Advanced ADLs include social or occupational functions associated with activities such as hobbies, employment, or caregiving. Approximately 30% of adults over age 65 and 78% of those over age 85 have difficulty with IADLs or one or more basic ADLs. Predictably, as the incidence of disability rises, so does the rate of dependence and placement in skilled facilities. Long-term care in skilled facilities increases from 2% among those aged 65 to 74 to 14% among those older than 85 years. Impairment in ADLs is also associated with an increased risk of falls, depression, and death in the affected elder. Among older adults the assessment of self-care capacity provides key health status information independent of age and comorbid conditions.

For clinicians, navigating the myriad options for management of multiple chronic conditions requires individualized assessment of risks, benefits, and specific goals of various therapies. Estimates of life expectancy, integrating the impact of age, comorbid illness, and function, have been generated to assist in medical decision making. These estimates assist clinicians in predicting median survival and thus can help in estimating the potential life remaining, which can impact treatment decision making. For example, the options offered to a frail 85-year-old man with less than 3 years left to live may be quite different from those presented to his healthy counterpart of the same age with a median life expectancy of 5 to 7 years. In addition, any decision should take into account the individual patient's goals and preferences. A variety of prognostic tools exist to assist clinicians with estimating survival in different populations and care circumstances (Table 21.3). These tools can be accessed online in an interactive fashion for clinicians at http://eprognosis.ucsf.edu/.

PRESENTATION OF DISEASE IN THE OLDER ADULT

Competent care of the frail older adult starts with recognition of disease, even in the absence of signs and symptoms typically present in younger people. Presentation of disease among older adults may differ dramatically from that expected in younger patients; manifestations of distress may be subtle or nonspecific, and improvement is less obvious and slower. These phenomena occur for a number of reasons. As noted previously, older adults experience high rates of comorbid illness, which may confound the clinician's ability to diagnose a problem accurately. For example, a patient with heart disease and chronic obstructive pulmonary disease who visits the office because of dyspnea may be experiencing a flare of his or her pulmonary disease or an atypical presentation of ischemic heart disease or both. Reporting of symptoms may also be affected by psychosocial factors, including limited access to the health care system, cognitive problems, or minimization of symptoms as "normal aging." Likewise, health care professionals may minimize complaints by older adults with complex medical illness or frail health.

Variable presentations for certain conditions can be seen in older adults (Table 21.4). Hyperthyroidism can manifest with apathy, malaise, depression, and fatigue, while lacking classic symptoms of tremor, tachycardia, or sweating. It can also manifest with heart failure and is highly prevalent among older adults with new-onset atrial fibrillation. Likewise, older patients with hypothyroidism may atypically demonstrate failure to thrive, weight loss, cognitive decline, or depression. In the presence of infection, older adults may not reliably mount fever or experience localized symptoms. Studies have demonstrated that lowering the threshold definition of fever can improve the diagnostic utility of body temperature as a sign of bacterial infection. Although

表21.2 老年医学5M原则	
心智（Mind）	精神，痴呆，谵妄，抑郁
行动能力（Mobility）	步态和平衡受损，预防跌倒损伤
药物（Medications）	多重用药，减少处方药，优化处方，药物不良反应和药物负担
多重复杂性（Multi-Complexity）	多病症，复杂的生物-心理-社会情况
我最关注的事情（Matters Most to Me）	对每个人自身而言有意义的健康结果目标和护理意愿

外，临床医生还必须监测一些非特异性情况，如影响自理能力和安全的行动、情绪或精神问题。治疗策略也提出了独特的挑战，通常需要平衡药物和非药物干预，并仔细考虑个人的护理目标。Tinetti及其同事将老年医学的这些原则概括为五个M："心智（Mind）、行动能力（Mobility）、药物（Medications）、多重复杂性（Multi-complexity）和我最关注的事情（Matters Most to Me）"（表21.2）。本篇将介绍老年患者综合评估的核心内容。

共病、功能和预期寿命

随着年龄的增长和生理储备的下降，老年人的慢性病发病率很高，而且往往与功能下降有关。80%的65岁以上老年人至少患有一种慢性疾病，50%的老年人处于两种或两种以上疾病的共病状态。其中一些疾病直接导致老年人死亡率增高，如心脏病、癌症、卒中、肺部疾病和阿尔茨海默病。然而，更多常见疾病主要影响老年人身体功能，导致失能和进入护理机构。关节炎、听力下降和视力障碍都是这方面的主要问题。多种疾病共存不仅加重了单一疾病的损害，也使老年疾病的管理更加复杂困难。在循证医学和指南时代，当临床医生诊治一个同时患几种常见慢性病（如糖尿病、冠状动脉疾病和骨质疏松症）的患者时，可能会觉得不得不开六、七种药才能符合当前的推荐规范。这种做法会导致"过多用药"（后文详述），在有限考虑风险、获益和个人意愿的情况下造成患者的治疗成本上升。对于老年患者的医疗管理，不仅需要考虑单个疾病的特殊处置，更需要评估治疗对于症状、功能、生存期的总体影响。为了应对这一常见的临床挑战，美国老年医学会持续发布针对多病共存老年人的照护指导原则，强调了考虑病情、各种治疗方案的风险和获益、总体预后以及患者的目标和意愿之间复杂相互影响的重要性。

Reuben等将"功能"正式定义为"一个人在多种复杂情况下执行任务和履行社会角色的能力"，简言之，就是自理能力。临床医生通过对患者功能的评估，能够了解疾病的影响、评估生活质量、识别护理需求、估计疾病进展和预后。功能的综合评估应包括患者自理能力的问询以及认知和活动能力的客观测量（关于后两者的详情，请参阅下文）。自理能力通常分为基本日常生活活动能力、工具性日常生活活动能力和高级日常生活活动能力。基本日常生活活动能力（ADL）包括维持个人健康和卫生的活动，包括移动、洗浴、如厕、穿衣和进食。工具性日常生活活动能力（IADL）包括独立生活所需的活动，特别是驾驶或使用公共交通工具、烹饪、购物、管理药物和财务、使用电话（或其他通信设备）以及做家务。高级日常生活活动能力则包括与爱好、就业或护理等活动相关的社会或职业能力。大约30%的65岁以上人群和78%的85岁以上人群在IADL、一项或多项ADL方面存在困难。可预见的是，随着失能发生率的上升，老年人照护依赖性和入住专业养老机构的比例也相应上升。65～74岁人群在专业机构接受长期护理的比例为2%，85岁以上人群则增长到14%。ADL受损与老年人跌倒、抑郁、死亡风险增加相关。在老年人中，自我照顾能力的评估可提供与年龄和共病无关的关键健康状况信息。

临床医生在制订管理多种慢性病的合理方案时，需要对各种治疗方法的风险、获益和具体目标进行个性化评估。一些研究整合年龄、共病和功能的影响，制订了预期寿命估算工具用以协助医疗决策。临床医生可以运用这些估算工具预测患者的中位生存期，估计可能影响治疗决策选择的潜在剩余生存时间。例如，向一位衰弱、预期寿命不足3年的85岁老年人提供的治疗方案，可能与向同龄、中位生存期为5～7年的健康老年人提供的治疗方案截然不同。另外，任何医疗决策都应考虑患者的个人目标和意愿。有多种预后评估工具可帮助临床医生估计不同人群和护理环境下的生存率（表21.3）。临床医生可通过 http://eprognosis.ucsf.edu/ 在线获取这些工具的互动快讯。

老年人的疾病表现

称职的衰弱老年照护，首先要在缺乏年轻人典型症状和体征的情况下识别出他们的疾病。老年人的疾病表现可能与年轻患者明显不同，痛苦表现可能很微弱或没有特异性，而疾病的好转也很缓慢而不明显。出现这些现象的原因有很多。如前所述，老年人存在共病的比例很高，这可能会影响临床医生准确诊断的能力。例如，一名患有心脏病和慢性阻塞性肺疾病的患者因呼吸困难就诊，可能是肺病复发或缺血性心脏病的不典型表现，或两者兼而有之。患者对症状的描述可能受到心理社会因素的影响，包括他们难以获得医疗保健系统的服务、存在认知问题，或是将某些症状认为是"正常衰老"的表现而忽略。同样，医护人员可能会在诊治那些有复杂共病或衰弱状况的老年人时，对其主诉未予重视。

某些疾病在老年人中会有不同的表现（表21.4）。甲状腺功能亢进症（甲亢）可表现为淡漠、乏力、抑郁和疲劳，而缺乏震颤、心动过速或出汗等典型症状。甲亢还可表现为心力衰竭，在新发心房颤动的老年人中发病率很高。同样，患有甲状腺功能减退症的老年患者可能表现出精神萎靡、体重减轻、认知能力下降或抑郁等非

TABLE 21.3 Clinical Decisions Influenced by Life Expectancy

Life Expectancy	Clinical Decision Examples
Short-term, <2 years	Minimize major, invasive surgical procedures
	Discuss goals of care and when to consider hospice care
	Discontinue statin therapy
Mid-term, 2–3 years	Aggressive blood pressure and lipid management in the setting of diabetes less likely to prevent microvascular complications
Long-term	Discontinue colon cancer screening if <7 years
	Limited benefit to A_{1C} target <8.0% if <5 years
	Discontinue prostate cancer screening if <10 years
	Limit breast cancer screening if <5 years

Adapted from Yourman LC, Lee SJ, Schonberg MA, et al. Prognostic indices for older adults: a systematic review. JAMA. 2012;307(2):182-192.

TABLE 21.4 Presentations of Disease in Older Adults[a]

Diagnosis	Potential Presenting Symptoms and Signs
Myocardial infarction	Altered mental status
	Fatigue
	Fever
	Functional decline
Infection	Altered mental status
	Functional decline
	Hypothermia
Hyperthyroidism	Altered mental status
	Anorexia
	Atrial fibrillation
	Chest pain
	Constipation
	Fatigue
	Weight gain
Depression	Cognitive impairment
	Failure to thrive
	Functional decline
Electrolyte disturbance	Altered mental status
	Falls
	Fatigue
	Personality changes
Malignancy	Altered mental status
	Fever
	Pathologic fracture
Pulmonary embolus	Altered mental status
	Fatigue
	Fever
	Syncope
Vitamin deficiency	Altered mental status
	Ataxia
	Dementia
	Fatigue
Fecal impaction	Altered mental status
	Chest pain
	Diarrhea
	Urinary incontinence
Aortic stenosis	Altered mental status
	Fatigue

[a]This table represents only a limited list of select disease processes and presentations; it is not meant to serve as an exhaustive reference for use during patient care activities.

chest pain remains the most common and important symptom of ischemic heart disease, dyspnea in the absence of chest pain is a commonly reported symptom, particularly in older adults and those with multiple comorbidities.

In truth, any medical illness may manifest nonspecifically among older adults, particularly those in frail health. Nonspecific symptoms related to an underlying illness include changes in mentation, difficulty with balance and falls, new urinary incontinence (UI), and a general change in functional ability. These presentations are often referred to as the "geriatric syndromes" and are detailed later. A lack of understanding of how disease presentation differs among older adults can lead to delays in diagnosis and treatment and result in worse outcomes. Research indicates that altered presentation predicts not only suboptimal care, but future functional decline and increased mortality.

MEDICATIONS

Medication-related problems are very common in older adults. In the United States, outpatients over age 65 take a median of four prescription medications daily, and nearly 40% are on five or more. Although medications may be indicated for specific medical conditions, use of multiple medications or polypharmacy increases the risk for drug-drug interactions and associated adverse drug events. Altered pharmacokinetics and pharmacodynamics contribute to adverse drug events, which are a common cause of hospitalization and morbidity in older persons. It is for this reason that certain medications can be considered "potentially inappropriate" in older adults. Common changes in pharmacokinetics include changes in body composition, with increased fat stores and decreased body water. Fat-soluble medications, such as benzodiazepines, have a prolonged duration of effect because of this phenomenon. Age-related declines in glomerular filtration rates result in decreased clearance of many medications, including such drugs as gabapentin, nitrofurantoin, and direct oral anticoagulants. Accurate calculations of creatinine clearance will inform drug choice and dosing and improve prescribing safety. Pharmacodynamic changes include decreased sensitivity to certain commonly prescribed drugs, such as β-blockers, and increased sensitivity to other agents, such as narcotics and warfarin.

Given the risks of medication use in older adults, health care professionals and systems must employ strategies to improve both the effectiveness and safety of prescribing as well as when to "de-prescribe" certain medications. Evidence-based recommendations include the following:

- Maintain an up-to-date medication list, including over-the-counter medications and herbal supplements.
- Comprehensively review medications at each visit with special attention at the time of transitions between care settings (e.g., after hospitalization). A clear indication for each medication, and documentation of response to therapy (particularly for chronic conditions) should be included.
- Assess for duplication and drug-drug or drug-disease interactions. Using a drug information database will help with this process.
- Assess adherence and affordability and inquire about the patient's system for administering medications (e.g., a pillbox).
- Assess for specific classes of medications commonly associated with adverse events: antiplatelet agents, anticoagulants, analgesics

表 21.3	受预期寿命影响的临床决策
预期寿命	临床决策示例
短期，<2 年	尽量减少重大创伤性外科手术 讨论护理目标以及何时考虑临终关怀 停止他汀类药物治疗
中期，2～3 年	在糖尿病患者中积极进行血压和血脂管理 不再考虑预防微血管并发症
长期	如果 < 7 年，停止结肠癌筛查 如果 < 5 年，HbA1c < 8.0% 的益处有限 如果 < 10 年，停止前列腺癌筛查 如果 < 5 年，减少乳腺癌筛查

改编自 Yourman LC，Lee SJ，Schonberg MA，et al. Prognostic indices for older adults：a systematic review. JAMA. 2012；307（2）：182-192.

表 21.4	老年人的疾病表现[a]
诊断	可能出现的症状和体征
心肌梗死	精神状态改变 疲劳 发热 功能下降
感染	精神状态改变 功能下降 低体温
甲亢	精神状态改变 厌食 心房颤动 胸痛 便秘 疲劳 体重增加
抑郁	认知障碍 精神萎靡 功能减退
电解质紊乱	精神状态改变 跌倒 疲劳 性格改变
恶性肿瘤	精神状态改变 发热 病理性骨折
肺栓塞	精神状态改变 疲劳 发热 晕厥
维生素缺乏症	精神状态改变 共济失调 痴呆 疲劳
粪便嵌塞	精神状态改变 胸痛 腹泻 尿失禁
主动脉瓣狭窄	精神状态改变 疲劳

[a] 本表仅列出了部分疾病过程和表现，不作为患者诊疗过程中的详尽参考。

典型症状。老年人感染时也可能不会明显发热或出现局部症状。研究表明，这种情况下，降低发热的阈值定义可以提高体温作为细菌感染征象的诊断效力。虽然胸痛仍是缺血性心脏病最常见和最重要的症状，但不伴胸痛的呼吸困难也是常见症状，尤其是在老年人和有共病的人群中。

事实上，在老年人，特别是衰弱状态的人群，任何疾病的临床表现都可以是非特异性的。与潜在疾病相关的非特异性症状包括精神状态改变、平衡困难和跌倒、新出现的尿失禁以及功能状态的总体变化。这些症状通常被称为"老年综合征"，下文将详细介绍。对老年人疾病的差异性表现缺乏了解会延误诊断和治疗，导致不良临床结局。研究表明，不典型的临床表现不仅预示患者可能无法得到最佳的治疗，而且预示着进一步功能下降和死亡率的增加。

药物

药物相关问题在老年人中非常普遍。美国 65 岁以上门诊患者每天服用的处方药物种类的中位数是 4 种，近 40% 的患者服用 5 种或更多。虽然药物可能适用于特定疾病，但使用多种药物会增加药物间相互作用和药物相关不良事件的风险。药代动力学和药效学的改变会导致药物不良事件，是老年人住院和发病的常见原因。因此，某些药物在老年人中可能需要慎用。机体的衰老性改变导致老年人药代动力学不同于年轻人，这些常见变化包括身体成分的变化，如脂肪储存增加，体内水分减少。由于这种改变，苯二氮䓬类等脂溶性药物的作用时间会延长。与年龄相关的肾小球滤过率下降会导致许多药物的清除率下降，包括加巴喷丁、硝基呋喃妥因和直接口服抗凝剂等药物。准确计算肌酐清除率将为药物选择和剂量确定提供依据，从而提高处方的安全性。老年人药效学也有变化，包括对某些常用处方药物（如 β 受体阻滞剂）的敏感性降低，而对其他一些药物（如麻醉剂和华法林）的敏感性增加。

鉴于老年人用药的风险，医疗保健专业人员和系统必须采取措施来提高处方的有效性和安全性，以及决定何时停用某些药物。基于证据的推荐包括以下内容：

- 及时更新药物清单，包括非处方药和草药。
- 每次就诊时进行全面药物核查，在护理机构间（如出院后）转运时需要特别关注。明确每种药物的应用指征并记录治疗反应。
- 检查重复用药，评估药物间或药物-疾病间的相互影响。使用药物信息数据库将对这一过程有所帮助。
- 评估服药依从性和可负担性，并询问患者确保服药的方法（如使用药盒）。
- 评估常见不良事件相关的特定药物类别：抗血小板药物、抗凝药物、镇痛药［特别是麻醉药和非甾体抗炎药（NSAID）］、降压药［特别是血管紧张素转换酶（ACE）抑制剂和利尿剂］、

(particularly narcotics and nonsteroidal anti-inflammatory drugs [NSAIDs]), antihypertensives (particularly angiotensin-converting enzyme [ACE] inhibitors and diuretics), insulin and hypoglycemic agents, and psychotropics.
- Be suspicious that new symptoms arise from adverse effects of current drugs, not new disease.
- Minimize or avoid use of anticholinergic medications, which present specific risks.

In addition to following these general principles, prescribing clinicians also benefit from consulting lists of potentially inappropriate medications. The Beers List of Potentially Inappropriate Medications (PIMs) provides an evidence-based guide to drugs that should be avoided if possible or used with caution in older adults. A clear and rational approach to prescribing and ongoing management of medications that accounts for indication, interactions, and adherence may reduce the risk of common adverse events.

COGNITION

Dementia

The prevalence of dementia increases with age, with estimates ranging from 20% to 50% after age 85. The most common forms of dementia include Alzheimer's disease, Lewy body dementia, and vascular dementia. The latter is commonly present in combination with Alzheimer's disease in a condition termed *mixed etiology dementia*. Dementia is characterized by impairment in one or more cognitive domains severe enough to disrupt function or occupation. Mild cognitive impairment (MCI) is present when an individual has discernible cognitive limitations without apparent deficits in IADLs. Patients with MCI develop dementia at a rate of approximately 15% per year. Dementia is associated with a higher risk of falls, functional impairment, institutionalization, and death. Caregivers of demented individuals also face increased rates of stress and health problems. Clinicians diagnose dementia through symptom and functional history (often including the input of caregivers), cognitive assessment, and physical examination. A number of instruments, including the MOCA (see Chapter 5), clock-drawing test, and the Mini-Cog, are validated screening tools. The time-tested Mini Mental State Examination (MMSE) offers an assessment of multiple cognitive domains but does not provide adequate measure of executive function. It is also prone to lack of sensitivity in individuals with high premorbid intelligence and lack of specificity in those with low levels of education. Validated assessments of executive function include the clock-drawing test, verbal fluency test, and the Trail Making test part B. Instruments also exist for collecting data regarding patient function from a relative or caregiver. In patients suspected of having dementia, personal safety with respect to firearms, driving, and the home environment should be assessed. A careful medication review and physical examination, including vital signs, complete neurologic assessment, including gait and balance, are, of course, essential in evaluating for dementia to reveal findings that point to a specific cause.

Delirium

The differential diagnosis for cognitive problems other than dementia is broad, and includes delirium, mood disturbance, and drug effects. The differentiation of dementia and delirium may present the most significant challenge, particularly in hospitalized elders (Table 21.5). Delirium is characterized as an abrupt change in global cognitive function, whereas dementia is chronic and affects specific cognitive domains over time. Differentiation often hinges on history, which may be lacking at presentation. Delirium, sometimes called "altered mental status," affects more than 2 million hospitalized persons each year. Its incidence is variably estimated at 25% to 60% among patients

TABLE 21.5 Features of Delirium Versus Dementia

Feature	Delirium	Dementia
Onset	Acute	Insidious
Course	Fluctuating, lucid at times	Generally stable
Duration	Hours to weeks	Months to years
Alertness	Abnormally low or high	Usually normal
Perception	Illusions and hallucinations common	Usually normal
Memory	Immediate and recent impaired	Recent and remote impaired
Thought	Disorganized	Impoverished
Speech	Incoherent, slow, or rapid	Word-finding difficulty
Physical illness or medication causative	Frequently	Usually absent

in acute care settings and results in extra hospital days and related expenditures. Delirium is also associated with prolonged hospital stay, increased costs, increased readmission rates to the hospital (12% to 65% at 6 months), higher in-hospital and 1-year mortality, and incident dementia. The Confusion Assessment Method (CAM) offers a validated framework for identifying delirium (https://consultgeri.org/try-this/general-assessment/issue-13.pdf). Per the CAM, delirium is likely present if the patient has both an acute onset of confusion with fluctuating course and inattention and either disorganized thinking or altered level of consciousness. According to Inouye and colleagues, key vulnerability factors for delirium include older age, cognitive impairment, comorbid illness, and impairments in vision and hearing. Precipitating factors related to acute illness include hypoxia, electrolyte abnormalities, dehydration, and malnutrition as well as medications and alcohol withdrawal. Delirium can also be a presenting sign for a number of serious medical conditions (see Table 21.2). Although treatment of delirium is difficult and revolves around the underlying medical issues, controlled trials have demonstrated that a multimodal intervention is effective in reducing rates of delirium in high-risk patients. There is evidence that the use of physical restraints in combative or confused older adults leads to increased morbidity and mortality. Nonpharmacologic management strategies include reorientation and preservation of sleep patterns, family or caregiver presence at the bedside, and early mobilization. "Chemical restraint" use, such as prescribing low dose antipsychotics, similarly has limited benefit. The use of pharmacologic agents, specifically neuroleptics, should be reserved for patients in whom nonpharmacologic strategies do not help and the patient presents a risk of harm to self or others.

MENTAL HEALTH

Older adults commonly experience depressive symptoms, with prevalence estimates as high as 15% to 19% among those over age 75, although in community-dwelling elders, major depressive disorder is actually less common than in younger adults. The presence of comorbid illness and grief often confound the presentation of depression. As a result, it can remain undetected despite its significant adverse impact on quality of life, morbidity, and mortality. Suicide rates are almost twice as high among older persons when compared with the general population, with the rate highest for white men over 85 years of age. Among older adults, depression can present with cognitive, functional, or sleep problems, as well as complaints of fatigue or low energy. Several instruments have been developed and validated for

胰岛素和降血糖药，以及抗精神病药物。
- 对患者新发症状应怀疑是否为药物的不良反应，而不一定是新发疾病。
- 尽量减少或避免使用有特殊风险的抗胆碱能药物。

除了遵循上述一般原则外，临床医生处方时还可以参考潜在不适当药物清单。Beers 潜在不适当药物清单（PIM）为老年人尽可能避免或谨慎使用的药物提供了循证指南。根据药物的适应证、相互作用和依从性，采用明确合理的方法开具处方并对药物进行持续管理，可降低常见不良事件的风险。

认知

痴呆

痴呆的患病率随年龄增长而增加，85 岁以上老年人的患病率估计高达 20%～50%。最常见的痴呆包括阿尔茨海默病、路易体痴呆和血管性痴呆。血管性痴呆常与阿尔茨海默病同时存在，称为混合性痴呆。痴呆以一个或多个认知域受损为特征，其严重程度足以影响日常生活或工作能力。轻度认知障碍（MCI）是指个体具有可察觉的认知受损，但没有明显影响 IADL。每年约有 15% 的 MCI 患者病情恶化发展为痴呆。痴呆与较高的跌倒、功能损害、住院以及死亡风险增高相关。痴呆患者的照护者也面临更高的压力和更多的健康问题。临床医生通过症状询问、功能史评估（常兼顾照护者的意见）、认知评估和体格检查来诊断痴呆。许多评价工具，包括 MOCA（见第 5 章）、画钟测验和简易认知评估量表（Mini-Cog）等，都是经过验证的筛选工具。广泛使用的简易精神状态量表（MMSE）可评估多个认知领域，但对执行功能的评估不够充分。对发病前智力水平较高的患者敏感性较低，对教育水平较低的人特异性较低。经过验证的执行功能测试包括画钟测验、言语流畅性测试和连线测验 B。此外，还有一些工具专门用于从亲属或照护者处收集患者功能的信息。对于怀疑有痴呆的患者，应评估涉及枪支、驾驶和家庭环境相关的人身安全问题。对痴呆患者进行仔细的药物审查和体格检查（包括生命体征），全面的神经系统评估（包括步态和平衡）是必不可少的，有助于揭示某些导致痴呆的特殊原因。

谵妄

除痴呆外，认知问题的鉴别诊断范围很广，包括谵妄、情绪障碍和药物作用。痴呆和谵妄的鉴别可能是最大的挑战，尤其是对住院老人而言（表 21.5）。谵妄的特点是整体认知功能的突发改变，而痴呆则是慢性的，会随着时间的推移影响特定的认知领域。鉴别通常取决于病史，而病史可能是患者发病时所缺乏的。谵妄有时被称为"精神状态改变"，每年影响 200 多万住院患者。在急症护理环境中，其发病率估计在 25%～60% 之间，会导致住院天数和相关支出增加。

表 21.5　谵妄和痴呆的特征比较

特征	谵妄	痴呆
发作形式	急性起病	隐袭起病
病程	波动性，间断清醒	一般较稳定
持续时间	数小时至数周	数月至数年
警觉力	异常减低或增高	通常正常
知觉	错觉和幻觉常见	通常正常
记忆	即刻和近期记忆下降	近期和远期记忆下降
思维	无条理的	贫乏的
语言	不合逻辑，缓慢或过快	找词困难
躯体疾病或药物因素	常有	一般没有

谵妄还与住院时间延长、费用增加、再入院率增加（6 个月时为 12%～65%）、院内死亡率和 1 年死亡率升高以及痴呆的发生有关。意识模糊评估法（CAM）为识别谵妄提供了一个有效的框架（https://consultgeri.org/try-this/general-assessment/issue-13.pdf）。根据 CAM，如果患者既有急性发作的精神状态改变和波动性病程，又有注意力障碍，还伴有思维紊乱或意识水平改变，则很可能患有谵妄。根据 Inouye 及其同事的研究，谵妄的主要易患因素包括老年、认知障碍、共病以及视听觉障碍。与急性病相关的诱发因素包括缺氧、电解质紊乱、脱水、营养不良、药物和酒精戒断。谵妄也可能是多种严重疾病的先兆（表 21.2）。虽然谵妄的治疗很困难，需要解决多方面潜在的医疗问题，但临床对照试验已经证明，多模态干预可以有效降低高危患者的谵妄发生率。有证据表明，在具有挑衅性或意识混乱的老年人中使用物理约束会增加谵妄的发病率和死亡率。非药物治疗策略包括重新调整和保持睡眠模式、家人或照顾者在床边陪伴以及尽早活动。使用"化学约束"（如处方小剂量抗精神病药物）同样效果有限。药物（尤其是抗精神病药物）治疗应仅限于非药物治疗无效且有可能伤害自身或他人的患者。

心理健康

抑郁症状在老年人中很常见，75 岁以上人群患病率高达 15%～19%，但重度抑郁症在社区老年人中实际上比年轻人更少见。共病和悲伤常常使抑郁症的表现变得复杂。因此，尽管抑郁对生活质量、发病率和死亡率有重大不良影响，但它仍难以被发现。老年人的自杀率几乎是普通人群的 2 倍，其中 85 岁以上白人男性的自杀率最高。老年人抑郁症往往不典型，表现为认知、功能或睡眠问题，有时以疲劳、精力不足为主诉。目前已开发并验证了几种用于筛查老年人抑郁症的工具。询问患者两个关于情绪和快感缺失的简单问题（"过去 2 周，您是否感到失望、抑郁或绝望"和"过去 2 周，您是否觉得做事缺乏兴趣或乐趣"），可能与使用长量表工具一样有效。长量表在门诊也是有用

screening for depression in elders. Asking two simple questions about mood and anhedonia ("Over the past 2 weeks have you felt down, depressed, or hopeless?" and "Over the past 2 weeks have you felt little interest or pleasure in doing things?") may be as effective as using longer instruments. Longer screening questionnaires, such as the Geriatric Depression Screen (GDS) or Patient Health Questionnaire (PHQ-9), are also useful tools in the ambulatory setting. Any positive screening test result should trigger a full diagnostic interview. When screening for depression in elders, it is particularly important to have systems in place to provide feedback of screening results, a readily accessible means of making an accurate diagnosis, and a mechanism for providing treatment and careful follow-up. Randomized trials indicate that the addition of counseling to pharmacologic therapy confers additional benefit for older, frail patients with depression. Anxiety is more common than depression among older adults and may similarly result in physical and cognitive symptoms, insomnia, agitation, psychosis, and isolation. Clinicians should consider a diagnosis of generalized anxiety, panic, or agoraphobia in older adult patients with any of these symptoms.

SLEEP

Sleep disorders are present in more than 50% of older adults and have a negative impact on health and quality of life. Sleep disorders or disturbance are associated with cognitive impairment, poor health status, functional decline, and increased mortality. This may stem in part from changes in sleep structure with aging such as decreased deep (stage N3) sleep, longer sleep latency, and decreased sleep efficiency. Moreover, a variety of comorbid factors present in later life have adverse effects on sleep quality, including medical conditions, medications, psychosocial factors, and disruptive or disabling symptoms such as pain or nocturia. This includes drug and alcohol use as well as use of prescription and over-the-counter sedative hypnotics, which can cause sleep fragmentation and rebound insomnia. Additionally, medications commonly prescribed for insomnia, such as benzodiazepines and non-benzodiazepine hypnotics, are linked with cognitive impairment and falls. The mainstay of treatment for insomnia among older adults is careful attention to addressing the variety of comorbid factors and behaviors that lead to sleep disruption. The following is a sleep hygiene resource: https://www.nhlbi.nih.gov/files/docs/public/sleep/healthy_sleep.pdf. Strong evidence supports cognitive-behavioral therapy for insomnia (CBT-I) and other nonpharmacologic approaches including stimulus control, sleep restriction, and relaxation techniques. Older adults also suffer higher rates of other primary sleep disorders, including sleep apnea, periodic leg movements of sleep, and REM sleep behavior disorder. Eliciting a history of daytime somnolence and/or sleep partner complaints characteristic of these disorders should lead to completion of a diagnostic polysomnogram, which then guides initiation of appropriate therapies.

MOBILITY

Problems with mobility are common among older persons. Among those over age 65, 20% of men and 32% of women report difficulty with one or more of five specific physical activities (stooping or kneeling, reaching overhead, writing, lifting 10 pounds, or walking two to three blocks). Among these, respondents cite problems with walking most commonly. Difficulties with balance and gait present significant risks for older adults. Approximately 30% of community-dwelling elders fall each year. The annual incidence of falls approaches 50% in patients over 80 years of age. Five percent of falls in older adults result in fracture or hospitalization. According to the CDC, the rate of deaths from falls among persons aged 65 years or older increased 31% from 2007 to 2016. Risk factors for falls include a history of falls, fear of falling, decreased vision, cognitive impairment, medications (particularly anticholinergic, psychotropic, and cardiovascular medications), peripheral neuropathy, diseases causing problems with strength and coordination, and environmental factors. Effective interventions for people with a history of falls or who are at risk for falling involve addressing multiple contributing factors. Clinicians and health care professionals should regularly inquire about recent falls or a fear of falling in older patients. For patients who report falling, the assessment should include review of circumstances of the fall(s), measure of orthostatic vital signs, visual acuity testing, cognitive evaluation, and gait and balance assessment. A brief physical examination maneuver called the "Timed get up and go" (TUG) has the patient arise from a sitting position, walk 10 feet, turn, and return to the chair to sit. A time of more than 12 seconds to complete the process, or observation of postural instability or gait impairment, suggests an increased risk of falling. Gait speed, an additional measure of mobility, predicts changes in ability and health status in older adults. Gait speed is measured over a 10-meter span with the patient walking at a comfortable pace. A speed of less than 1.0 m/sec is associated with increased mortality; 0.8 m/sec predicts difficulty navigating outside the home; and a speed of less than 0.6 m/sec predicts a high risk of falls and functional decline. For those found to be at risk for falls, providers should ask about possible causative agents and provide education about home safety. High-risk patients should be referred for evaluation by a physical therapist and consideration should be given to the utility of assistive devices and a supervised exercise program (Table 21.6).

VISION AND HEARING

Problems with vision and hearing are very common among older adults and frequently complicate the management of comorbid conditions and accelerate functional decline. Significant vision loss occurs in 16% to 18% of adults over age 65. Common causes include glaucoma, cataracts, age-related macular degeneration, and retinopathy from hypertension and diabetes. Decreased visual acuity increases fall risk and has been associated with all-cause mortality in older adults. Such problems may be detectable with regular testing via bedside tools such as the Snellen or Jaeger eye chart. Given the implications of vision loss for function and safety, a general ophthalmologic examination every 1 to 2 years is recommended for all older adults. Fortunately, many ophthalmologic centers recognize the multifaceted challenges faced by older adults with vision impairment. They offer specialized low vision clinics providing care from optometrists, occupational therapists, and social workers with a focus on improving quality of life and maintaining independence.

Hearing loss affects an estimated 40% to 66% of those over age 75. It is associated with depression, social isolation, poor self-esteem, cognitive decline, and functional disability. Pure tone audiometry is the reference standard for screening for hearing loss, but a simple whispered voice test is also highly sensitive and specific. Ideally, all older adults would undergo annual hearing screen by questionnaire and handheld audiometry. Unfortunately, the lack of reimbursement for hearings aids under most insurance plans, including Medicare, presents a major barrier for many older adults.

CONTINENCE

UI affects up to 30% of community-dwelling older adults and at least half of those residing in skilled nursing facilities. It occurs more frequently in women, but this gender disparity narrows as the rate of UI

的筛查工具，如老年抑郁量表（GDS）或患者健康问卷（PHQ-9）。任何阳性初筛结果都应进一步施行全面诊断性访谈。在对老年人进行抑郁症筛查时，尤其重要的是要有一套系统来提供筛查结果的反馈信息、一种易于使用的准确诊断方法，以及一种提供治疗和随访的机制。随机试验表明，在药物治疗的基础上增加心理咨询，可为老年衰弱抑郁症患者带来额外的获益。在老年人中焦虑比抑郁更常见，同样会导致躯体和认知症状、失眠、烦躁、精神病和孤独。对于有上述症状的老年患者，临床医生应考虑诊断为广泛性焦虑症、恐慌症或陌生环境恐惧症。

睡眠

超过50%的老年人存在睡眠障碍，这影响了老年人的健康和生活质量。睡眠障碍或紊乱与认知障碍、健康状况不佳、功能衰退和死亡率增加有关。部分原因可能是随着年龄的增长睡眠结构发生了变化，如深睡眠（N3阶段）减少、睡眠潜伏期延长和睡眠效率降低。此外，晚年生活中的各种合并因素也会对睡眠质量产生不利影响，如医疗条件、药物、社会心理因素以及疼痛、夜尿等干扰性或致残性症状。其中包括毒品、酒精的滥用以及处方和非处方的镇静催眠类药物的应用，它们可能引发睡眠片段化和反弹性失眠。常用于治疗失眠的药物（如苯二氮䓬类和非苯二氮䓬类镇静催眠药）与认知障碍和跌倒有关。治疗老年人失眠的主要方法是仔细观察并解决导致睡眠中断的各种共病因素和行为。以下是睡眠卫生资源：https://www.nhlbi.nih.gov/files/docs/public/sleep/healthy_sleep.pdf）。有充分的证据表明，认知行为疗法可用于治疗失眠（CBT-I），其他非药物性的方法，如刺激控制、睡眠限制以及放松技巧等也同样有效。老年人患其他原发性睡眠障碍的概率也更高，包括睡眠呼吸暂停、睡眠周期性腿动和快速眼动睡眠行为障碍。如果了解到日间嗜睡或睡眠伴侣抱怨这些疾病的特征性表现时，应进行诊断性多导睡眠图检查，然后开始指导进行适当治疗。

活动能力

活动能力问题在老年人中很常见。据报道，65岁以上人群中约20%的男性和32%的女性在五项特定身体活动中［弯腰或跪下，举手过头，书写，举10磅（4.54 kg）重物，或步行两至三个街区］会有一项或多项困难。其中，受访者最常提到的是行走问题。平衡力差和步态障碍给老年人带来了很大的风险。每年约有30%的社区老年人发生跌倒，80岁以上老年人跌倒的年发生率接近50%。约5%老年人跌倒会出现骨折或需要住院。跌倒的风险因素包括跌倒史、对跌倒的恐惧、视力下降、认知障碍、药物（特别是抗胆碱能药物、抗精神病药物和心血管药物）、周围神经病变、影响力量和协调性的疾病及环境因素。对有跌倒史老年人或跌倒高危人群的有效处置包括对多个因素的干预。医疗人员应定期询问老年患者最近跌倒或恐惧跌倒的情况。对于报告跌倒的患者，评估应包括回顾跌倒时的情况、测量直立位生命体征、视力测试、认知评估以及步态和平衡评估。"起立-行走"计时测试（TUG）是一种快速便捷的检查策略，要求患者从坐位站起，行走10ft（3.048 m），转身返回椅子并坐下（记录所需时间）。完成整个过程的时间如果超过12s或观察到姿势不稳或步态障碍，则提示跌倒的风险增加。步速是衡量运动能力的一项指标，能预测老年人的功能和健康状况的变化。步速的测量要求患者以舒适的步伐在10 m跨度上行走，测得步速小于1.0 m/s与死亡率增加相关；步速0.8 m/s提示患者难以外出旅行；步速低于0.6 m/s预示跌倒高风险和功能衰退。对于检查发现的有跌倒风险的患者，医疗人员需要检查其所有与跌倒可能相关的药物，并提供居家安全教育。高风险患者应转诊接受物理治疗师的评估，并考虑使用辅助器械和有监督的锻炼计划（表21.6）。

视觉和听觉

视力和听力问题在老年人中非常常见，常使共病控制更加复杂化并加速功能衰退。65岁以上人群中视力丧失的发生率为16%～18%，常见原因包括青光眼、白内障、年龄相关性黄斑变性，以及高血压和糖尿病引起的视网膜病变。视力下降增加了跌倒的风险，与全因死亡率相关。视力问题可以通过床边工具如Snellen或Jaeger视力表进行定期测试来发现。鉴于视力丧失对功能和安全性的影响，建议所有老年人每1～2年进行一次常规眼科检查。此外，眼科中心已经认识到具有视力障碍的老年人所面临的多方面的挑战。他们为此成立了专门的低视力诊所，由验光师、作业治疗师和社会工作者提供服务，目的是提高这些老年人的生活质量及保持其独立性。

估计有40%～66%的75岁以上老年人受到听力损失的影响。听力损失与抑郁、社交孤立、自尊心差、认知能力下降和功能障碍有关。纯音测听是用于筛查听力受损的标准测试。此外，简单的耳语测试也具有高度敏感性和特异性。理想的情况是每年所有老年人都可以通过问卷和手持式听力计进行听力筛查。然而，包括美国Medicare（美国政府向65岁以上的人提供医疗保险）在内的多数保险计划都没有将助听器纳入医保范围，这给许多老年人造成了很大的障碍。

失禁

多达30%的社区老年人和至少一半的专业护理机构老年人会受到尿失禁（UI）的影响。尿失禁在女性

TABLE 21.6 Recommended Components of Clinical Assessment and Management for Older Persons Living in the Community Who Are at Risk for Falling

Assessment and Risk Factor	Management
Circumstances of previous falls[a]	Change in environment and activity to reduce the likelihood of recurrent falls
Medication use • High-risk medications (e.g., benzodiazepines, other sleep medications, neuroleptics, antidepressants, anticonvulsives, or Class IA antiarrhythmics—including quinidine, procainamide, and disopyramide)[a,b,c] • Four or more medications[c]	Review and reduction of medications
Vision[a] • Acuity <20/60 • Decreased depth perception • Decreased contrast sensitivity • Cataracts	Ample lighting without glare; avoidance of multifocal glasses while walking; referral to an ophthalmologist
Postural blood pressure (after ≥5 min in a supine position, immediately after standing, and 2 min after standing)[c] • ≥20 mm Hg (or ≥20%) drop in systolic pressure, with or without symptoms, either immediately or after 2 min of standing	Diagnosis and treatment of underlying cause, if possible; review and reduction of medications; modification of salt restriction; adequate hydration; compensatory strategies (e.g., elevating head of bed, rising slowly, or performing dorsiflexion exercises); pressure stockings; pharmacologic therapy if the above strategies fail
Balance and gait[b,c] • Patient's report or observation of unsteadiness • Impairment on brief assessment (e.g., the "get up and go" test or performance-oriented assessment of mobility)	Diagnosis and treatment of underlying cause, if possible; reduction of medications that impair balance; environmental interventions; referral to physical therapist for assistive devices and for gait, balance, and strength training
Targeted neurologic examinations • Impaired proprioception[a] • Impaired cognition[a] • Decreased muscle strength[b,c]	Diagnosis and treatment of underlying cause, if possible; increase in proprioceptive input (with an assistive device or appropriate footwear that encases the foot and has a low heel and thin sole); reduction of medications that impair cognition; awareness on the part of caregivers of cognitive deficits; reduction of environmental risk factors; referral to physical therapist for gait, balance, and strength training
Targeted musculoskeletal examinations of legs (joints and range of motion) and examination of feet[a]	Diagnosis and treatment of underlying cause, if possible; referral to physical therapist for strength, range-of-motion, and gait and balance training, and for assistive devices; use of appropriate footwear; referral to podiatrist
Targeted cardiovascular examination[b] • Syncope • Arrhythmia (if there is known cardiac disease, abnormal electrocardiogram, and syncope)	Referral to cardiologist; carotid-sinus massage (in case of syncope)
Home-hazard evaluations after hospital discharge[b,c]	Removal of loose rugs and use of nightlights, nonslip bathmats, and stair rails; other interventions as necessary

Adapted from Tinetti ME: Clinical practice. Preventing falls in elderly persons, N Engl J Med 348(1):42-49, 2003.
[a]Recommendation of this assessment is based on observations that the finding is associated with an increased risk of falling.
[b]Recommendation of this assessment is based on one or more randomized controlled trials of a single intervention.
[c]Recommendation of this assessment is based on one or more randomized controlled trials of a multifactorial intervention strategy that included this component.

in men increases after age 85. The impact of UI on health ranges from increased risk of skin irritation, pressure wounds, and falls, to social isolation, functional decline, and depression. For caregivers of older adults, UI complicates physical care and can contribute to decisions for placement in skilled nursing facilities. Common comorbid conditions include diabetes mellitus, heart failure, arthritis, and dementia.

A systematic approach to the investigation of UI can often reveal a cause and potential solution. It is important to first determine if the incontinence is acute or chronic in nature. Acute causes of incontinence are often attributable to specific medical problems, including infection, metabolic disturbance, or medication effects. The pneumonic DIAPERS recalls the various potential acute causes of UI (D, delirium; I, infection; A, atrophic vaginitis; P, pharmaceuticals; E, excess urine output from congestive heart failure [CHF] or hyperglycemia; R, restricted mobility; and S, stool impaction). If the UI is chronic, then further history can characterize the nature of the symptoms from among four types. Urge incontinence from detrusor overactivity is the most common type. Patients with this problem will complain of urinary frequency, nocturia, and a sudden onset of urge to void. Stress incontinence occurs with incompetence of pelvic musculature or urethral sphincter and is characterized by small amounts of leakage with laughing, sneezing, coughing, or even standing. Overflow incontinence results from urinary retention, often related to prostatic hyperplasia in men or bladder atony in patients with diabetes or spinal cord injury. Patients often have constant dribbling or leakage without a true sense of needing to void. Finally, functional incontinence results from comorbid conditions that limit a patient's ability to act on or interpret the need to void, mobility problems such as arthritis, and weakness or cognitive problems. Table 21.7 describes the various types of incontinence and suggested approaches. Of course, older adults with multiple comorbid conditions often have incontinence that results from a combination of chronic and/or acute causes.

Continence problems are frequently treatable but are often not raised by patients as a concern. A targeted history and physical

表 21.6 对有跌倒风险的社区老年人进行临床评估和管理的推荐

评估和危险因素	管理措施
以前跌倒的情况[a]	改变环境和活动，减少再次跌倒的可能性
药物使用 • 高危药物（如苯二氮䓬类药物、其他睡眠药物、神经安定药、抗抑郁药、抗惊厥药或 IA 类抗心律失常药，包括奎尼丁、普鲁卡因胺和丙吡胺）[a,b,c] • 四种或更多药物[c]	审查并减少用药
视觉[a] • 敏锐度 < 20/60 • 深度感知下降 • 对比敏感度降低 • 白内障	照明充足，无眩光；行走时避免戴多焦点眼镜；转诊至眼科医生
体位性血压变化（仰卧位 ≥ 5 min 后、站立后立即和站立后 2 min）[c] • 收缩压下降 20 mmHg（或 20%），有或没有症状，站立后立即或 2 min 后	诊断和治疗潜在病因（如有可能）；审查和减少用药；调整限盐措施；充分补水；代偿策略（如抬高床头、缓慢站起或进行背伸运动）；穿弹力袜；如果上述策略失败则应用药物治疗
平衡和步态[b,c] • 患者报告或被观察到步态不稳 • 简要评估（如"起立-行走"计时测试或平衡与步态量表评估）中的受损	诊断和治疗潜在病因（如有可能）；减少损害平衡的药物；环境干预；转诊给物理治疗师进行辅助器具以及步态、平衡和力量训练
有针对性的神经系统检查 • 本体感觉受损[a] • 认知障碍[a] • 肌肉力量下降[b,c]	诊断和治疗潜在病因（如有可能）；增加本体感觉输入（使用辅助设备或适当的鞋袜包裹脚部并穿低跟薄底的鞋）；减少损害认知功能的药物；提高护理人员对认知障碍的认识；减少环境危险因素；转诊给物理治疗师进行步态、平衡和力量训练
有针对性的腿部肌肉骨骼（关节和活动范围）检查和足部检查[a]	诊断和治疗潜在病因（如有可能）；转诊至物理治疗师进行力量、运动范围、步态和平衡训练以及辅助器具训练；穿合适的鞋袜；转诊至足科医生
有针对性的心血管检查[b] • 晕厥 • 心律失常（如果已知有心脏病、心电图异常和晕厥）	转诊至心脏病专家；颈动脉窦按摩（以防晕厥）
出院后的家庭风险评估[b,c]	撤除松散的地毯，使用夜灯、防滑浴垫和楼梯扶手；其他必要的干预措施

改编自 Tinetti ME：Clinical practice. Preventing falls in elderly persons, N Engl J Med 348（1）：42-49, 2003.
[a] 本评估的建议是基于与跌倒风险增加相关的观察结果。
[b] 该评估的建议基于一项或多项针对单一干预措施的随机对照试验。
[c] 该评估的建议基于一项或多项包含该组成部分的多因素干预策略的随机对照试验。

当中发生更为常见，但是随着男性在 85 岁之后 UI 的增加，这种性别差异逐渐减小。尿失禁对健康的影响广泛，不仅增加了皮肤刺激、压疮和跌倒的风险，还导致社交孤立、功能衰退和抑郁。对于老年照护者而言，尿失禁使身体护理更加复杂，并可能最终促使照护者下决心将患者转入专业护理机构。常见的并存疾病包括糖尿病、心力衰竭、关节炎和痴呆。

对尿失禁的系统性调查通常可以揭示原因和潜在解决方案。首先确定尿失禁是急性还是慢性的非常重要。急性尿失禁通常归因于特定的医学问题，包括感染、代谢紊乱或药物影响。缩写词（译者注：原文 pneumonic 应为 mnemonic）DIAPERS 涵盖了尿失禁潜在的急性病因 [D，谵妄；I，感染；A，萎缩性阴道炎；P，药物；E，充血性心力衰竭（CHF）或高血糖引起的过多排尿；R，运动受限；S，便秘]。如果是慢性尿失禁，进一步的病史采集有助于提示症状的特征是以下四类型中的哪一种。急迫性尿失禁是最常见的类型，由逼尿肌过度活动导致。这类患者会主诉尿频、夜尿和尿急。压力性尿失禁是由于盆底肌或尿道括约肌功能障碍引起的，特征是在大笑、打喷嚏、咳嗽甚至是站立动作时有少量尿液溢出。充盈性尿失禁由尿潴留导致，通常与男性前列腺增生、糖尿病或脊髓损伤引起的膀胱失弛缓症相关。患者常有持续的滴尿或漏尿，但没有真正需要排尿的感觉。最后一种是功能性尿失禁，是由伴随疾病限制了患者进行排尿或解决排尿需求而引起的，如关节炎等运动问题及虚弱或认知问题。表 21.7 描述了各种类型的尿失禁和建议的处理方法。当然，有多种共病的老年人的尿失禁通常是由慢性和（或）急性的综合原因引起的。

排尿问题通常是可治疗的，但患者往往不会主动提及。有针对性的病史采集和体格检查有助于识别原因并给予适当的干预。应该每半年进行一次关于 UI 的

TABLE 21.7 Causes, Types, and Treatment of Urinary Incontinence

Type	Definition	Cause	Treatment
Stress	Leakage associated with increased intra-abdominal pressure (coughing, sneezing)	Hypermobility of the bladder base, frequently caused by lax perineal muscles	Pelvic muscle exercise, timed voiding, α-adrenergic drugs, estrogens, surgery
Urge	Leakage associated with a precipitous urge to void	Detrusor hyperactivity (outflow obstruction, bladder tumor, detrusor instability), idiopathic (poor bladder), compliance (radiation cystitis), hypersensitive bladder	Bladder training, pelvic muscle exercise, bladder-relaxant drugs (anticholinergics, oxybutynin, tolterodine, imipramine)
Overflow	Leakage from a mechanically distended bladder	Outflow obstruction, enlarged prostate, stricture, prolapsed cystocele, acontractile bladder (idiopathic, neurologic [spinal cord injury, stroke, diabetes])	Surgical correction of obstruction, intermittent catheter drainage
Functional	Inability or unwillingness to void	Cognitive impairment, physical impairment, environmental barriers (physical restraints, inaccessible toilets), psychological problems (depression, anger, hostility)	Prompted voiding, garment and padding, external collection devices

examination can often identify the cause of UI and lead to appropriate intervention. Asking about and documenting the presence or absence of UI should be done biannually, as well as determining whether the UI, if present, is bothersome to the patient or caregiver. In addition to a history of acute and chronic causes, a targeted physical examination should include an assessment for fluid overload, genital and rectal examination, and neurologic evaluation. Urine and blood tests are indicated to evaluate for infection, metabolic causes, and renal dysfunction. In addition, for patients suspected of having urinary retention, catheterization or ultrasound can help define the postvoid residual and determine any need for catheter placement and further urologic evaluation. Many institutions now offer more specialized evaluation and care through incontinence clinics, which offer a multidisciplinary approach to management, addressing both pharmacologic and nonpharmacologic options. Effective nonpharmacologic options include scheduled toileting, bladder training, and biofeedback. Use of these strategies may avoid the use of medications with frequent adverse effects, such as anticholinergic medications for detrusor overactivity.

Like UI, fecal incontinence (FI) is an underreported and undermanaged issue among older adults with multiple factors contributing to etiology. FI is present in 45% or more of nursing home residents and is much more common in those with impaired mobility, dementia, chronic constipation or diarrhea. Ensuring prevention of constipation and associated overflow diarrhea is essential in management. Issues with muscular weakness that commonly contribute to fecal incontinence have excellent potential for treatment with specific types of physical therapy targeting pelvic floor muscles.

NUTRITION

Older adults experience high rates of malnutrition related to multiple causes, including medical illness, dental problems, or access issues related to limited mobility, cost, or cognitive problems. Approximately 15% of older outpatients and half of hospitalized elders are malnourished and have associated increases in morbidity and mortality. The utility of general laboratory testing is limited, but a combination of serial weight measurements and inquiries about changing appetite can reveal nutritional problems in the older adults. Vulnerable elders with an involuntary weight loss of 10% or more in 1 year or less should undergo further evaluation for undernutrition. This includes assessment of medical or medication-related causes, dental status, problems with acquiring or preparing food, appetite and intake, swallowing ability, and previous directions for dietary restrictions. Obese older adults suffer from high rates of malnutrition, but it is often unrecognized. They should also be screened routinely for nutrition concerns.

SOCIAL AND LEGAL ISSUES

Evaluation of the social history for older persons includes assessment of resources for direct caregiving and financial support available. These issues become particularly important for frail older adults, given their physical and economic vulnerability.

Caregiving

The clinician should always inquire about who is providing care for the older patient, including both personal care with ADLs and help with IADLs, such as transportation, medications, food preparation, finances, and housekeeping. This list should include both formal caregivers, such as home health professionals or hired aides, and informal caregivers, such as family members, neighbors, or friends. The majority of elder care provided in the United States is delivered by informal caregivers. Over 34 million people in the United States provide informal care for older adults and, of these, 15.7 million are caring for persons suffering from dementia. Seventy-five percent of informal caregivers are women and 39% are over age 65. The stress of providing daily care can have serious deleterious effects on the caregiver's health. Studies have demonstrated adverse effects on blood pressure and immune function and increased rates of cardiovascular disease and death. In addition, caregivers have alarmingly high rates of psychological illness, with symptoms of depression reported in up to 50%. This problem is particularly prevalent in those providing care for patients with dementia. The presence of mental illness further raises the risk of verbal or physical abuse or neglect of the patient. The clinician must recognize caregiver problems early and consider referral to a social worker, patient resource manager, or, when available, a geriatric assessment team. Key risk factors for caregiver stress include a frail family caregiver; a patient with cognitive impairment, emotional disturbance, substance abuse, sleep disruption, or behavioral problems; low income or financial strain; and acute illness or hospitalization. Heath care professionals should recognize signs and symptoms of physical or mental strain and regularly inquire about caregiver burden with an offer to talk apart from the patient if need be.

A number of resources exist to support caregivers and provide strategies for problem solving and self-care. Community-based programs provide assistance with meals, transportation, and respite care options through volunteer organizations or subsidized programs. Counseling on both the physical and emotional aspects of care has been demonstrated to reduce health risks to the caregiver and delay institutionalization, including in-home or institutional respite stays to provide caregivers with precious time off. Studies consistently demonstrate that such services are underused by caregivers. One resource

表 21.7　尿失禁的分类、病因和治疗

分类	定义	原因	治疗
压力性	与腹内压升高相关的渗漏（咳嗽、打喷嚏）	膀胱底部过度活动，常由会阴肌肉松弛引起	盆底肌锻炼、定时排尿、α-肾上腺素能药物、雌激素、手术
急迫性	与急促排尿有关的渗漏	逼尿肌过度活动（流出道梗阻、膀胱肿瘤、逼尿肌不稳定）、特发性（膀胱功能低下）、顺应性降低（放射性膀胱炎）、过敏性膀胱	膀胱训练、盆底肌锻炼、膀胱松弛药物（抗胆碱能药、奥昔布宁、托特罗定、丙咪嗪）
充盈性	因膀胱机械性扩张引起渗漏	流出道梗阻、前列腺增生、膀胱狭窄、膀胱膨出脱垂、膀胱收缩［特发性、神经源性（脊髓损伤、卒中、糖尿病）］	手术矫正梗阻、间歇性导管引流
功能性	不能或不愿意排尿	认知障碍、身体障碍、环境障碍（身体限制、无法进入厕所）、心理问题（抑郁、愤怒、敌意）	提示性排尿、合适的服装和衬垫、外部收集装置

询问和记录，如果存在尿失禁，要评估其是否给患者和照护者带来困扰。除了询问急慢性病史外，有针对性的体格检查还应包括体液超负荷评估、生殖器和直肠检查以及神经系统评估。建议进行尿液和血液测试以评估感染、代谢原因和肾功能障碍。此外，如果怀疑患者有尿潴留，导尿或超声检查有助于确定排尿后残余尿量，确定是否需要留置尿管和进一步的泌尿系统评估。现在，许多机构通过尿失禁门诊提供更专业的评估和护理，并提供多学科的治疗策略，包括药物和非药物策略。有效的非药物方案包括定时如厕、膀胱训练和生物反馈。采用这些策略可以避免使用不良反应较多的药物，如治疗逼尿肌过度活动的抗胆碱能药物等。

与尿失禁类似，大便失禁（FI）在老年人中也是一个未被充分主诉和处理的问题，有多种病因与之相关。45%或更多的养老院老人会出现大便失禁，而在行动不便、痴呆、长期便秘或腹泻的老年人中更为常见。预防便秘和相关的溢出性腹泻是治疗的关键。导致大便失禁的肌无力问题很有可能通过针对盆底肌的特定物理疗法得到治疗。

营养

老年人营养不良的比例高，与多种原因相关，包括内科疾病、口腔问题，或行动不便、费用或认知障碍等导致营养获取不足的问题。大约15%的老年门诊患者和一半的住院老年人存在营养不良，并伴有发病率和死亡率的增加。虽然常规实验室检测发现营养不良的效用有限，但是通过连续测量体重和询问食欲改变相结合的方法可以发现老年人的营养问题。在一年或更短时间内，非主动的体重减轻10%及以上的脆弱老年人应进一步行营养不良评估，包括评估医疗或药物相关原因、牙齿状况、获得或准备食物的问题、食欲和摄入量、吞咽能力、以前的饮食限制情况。肥胖老年人也有较高的营养不良发生率，但往往不被识别，所以应定期对他们进行营养筛查。

社会和法律问题

老年人的社会史评估包括直接照护的资源和可获得的经济支持。鉴于衰弱老年人身体和经济的脆弱性，这些社会问题尤其重要。

照护

临床医生应经常询问谁在为老年患者提供日常起居（ADL）方面的个人护理和IADL方面的帮助（如交通、药物、食物准备、财务和家务）。提供照护的人员包括正式的照护者，如家庭保健专业人员或聘用的助手，也包括非正式照护者，如家庭成员、邻居或朋友。在美国，大部分老年人的照护工作都是由非正式护理人员提供的。美国有超过3400万人为老年人提供非正式照护，其中1570万人照护痴呆患者。75%的非正式照护者是女性，39%的年龄在65岁以上。日常照护的压力可能对照护者的健康有严重的危害，研究已经证明其对血压和免疫功能有不利影响，并且增加心血管疾病患病率和死亡率。此外，照护者的心理疾病发病率也高得惊人，抑郁症患病率高达50%。这个问题在痴呆患者的照护者当中尤为普遍。照护者有心理疾病会增加其对患者的言语或身体虐待或忽视的风险。临床医生必须及早发现照护者存在的问题，并考虑转诊给社会工作者、病例资源管理者，或在有条件情况下转给老年评估团队。照护人员压力的主要危险因素包括家庭照护者本身虚弱；照护的患者有认知障碍、情绪障碍、药物滥用、睡眠障碍或行为问题；低收入或经费紧张；急性疾病或住院。医务工作者应该注意识别照护者躯体或精神问题的体征和症状，并定期询问照护者负担，如果需要，应该避开患者进行询问。

有一些资源能给照护者提供支持，并提供解决问题和自我照顾的策略。社区项目通过志愿组织或补贴模式为照护者提供膳食、交通和临时看护的援助选择。已经证明对照护者提供躯体和情绪方面的咨询能够降低其健康风险；减少养老院制度化管理时间，包括在家中暂住或养老院暂歇期，为护理者提供宝贵的休息时间。但是研究表明，这些资料并没有得到充分利用。如下网站提供了有关护理的支持性讯信：https://eldercare.acl.gov/Public/Resources/Topic/Caregiver.aspx#UsefulLinks。

that provides resources and supportive information about caregiving is https://eldercare.acl.gov/Public/Resources/Topic/Caregiver.aspx#UsefulLinks.

Mistreatment

Older adults are particularly vulnerable to mistreatment due to poor health, functional dependence, and social isolation. Mistreatment is defined as either elder abuse (harm caused by others) or self-neglect. Self-neglect is thought to be the most common form of mistreatment, but true rates are difficult to estimate. Risk factors include cognitive impairment and recent functional decline. Elder abuse has been reported in 3% to 8% of the older adult population in the United States, although this is likely an underestimate due to underreporting by patients and lack of recognition by health care providers. Abuse assumes many forms including psychological, financial, physical, sexual, and neglect. Studies have demonstrated that neglect and abuse are associated with higher rates of nursing home placement and mortality among older adults. Signs of physical abuse include contusions, burns, bite marks, genital or rectal trauma, pressure ulcers, or unexplained weight loss. Other forms of abuse may be more difficult to discern on examination but can be improved with direct questions such as "Has anybody hurt you?"; "Are you afraid of anybody?"; or "Is anyone taking or using your money without your permission?" Any suspicion of abuse or neglect should be reported to Adult Protective Services. Of note, 44 states and the District of Columbia have laws mandating reporting of suspected elder abuse and the U.S. Department of Justice has a growing network of resources (https://www.justice.gov/elderjustice/about-eji).

Finances

The older adult population in the United States varies widely in measures of wealth. Although the overall rate of poverty among adults over age 65 has declined over the last 50 years, 9.3% of older adults still live at or below the poverty line, and the percentage is higher among African Americans (18.7%) and Hispanic individuals of any race (17.4%). Members of the health care team including providers should screen for financial problems because these issues have direct implications for health status and well-being. Older adults with limited means are more likely to have problems affording medications, meals, and basic amenities. Referrals to community resource networks can help identify options for help with basic needs, including housing options and congregate meals. Information on agencies and services in specific locales can be identified at https://eldercare.acl.gov/Public/Index.aspx.

Advance Care Planning

Advance directives come in a number of different forms and serve a variety of purposes. Ideally, these documents articulate a person's preferences for care in the event of serious illness or incapacitation. Often they will describe limits on care and circumstances in which life-sustaining or restoring measures may be withheld or even withdrawn. Traditionally, advance directives have included a living will and health care power of attorney. The living will often addresses situations in which the patient has a terminal illness, persistent vegetative state, or progressive neurologic condition and can include explicit directions for care management including withdrawal or withholding of specific measures, including artificial nutrition and hydration. Living wills are ideally paired with a companion document, the health care power of attorney, which designates the person's preferred decision maker, or proxy, in the event of an incapacitating illness. For patients who have not created a health care power of attorney, typically the spouse or other first-degree relative is the default decision maker. If no proxy is designated and no next of kin is available, guardianship may be obtained.

Guardianship is a legal proceeding whereby the court appoints a surrogate decision maker. The physician's responsibility includes determination of a person's capacity for independent decision making in the event of altered sensorium or progressive cognitive impairment. This involves an assessment of his or her ability to understand the situation, ask questions, weigh options and render an opinion and, in certain situations, may require a full geriatric or neuropsychological assessment. Traditional advance directives, particularly the living will, have been criticized as having limited utility in conveying specific preferences. Recently, more detailed forms have emerged to record very specific preferences and limits for measures such as hydration, nutrition, hospitalization, and resuscitation. Examples include the Medical Orders for Scope of Treatment (MOST) and Physician's Orders for Life Sustaining Treatment (POLST) forms https://polst.org/programs-in-your-state/. Of course, effective completion and application of any of these forms should include a goals of care conversation conducted with the primary care provider, ideally involving family caregivers. In addition, as preferences change over time depending on health status, health care providers should encourage older adults to revisit and renew their advance directives on an annual basis.

CONTEXTS OF CARE: SPECIAL CONSIDERATIONS

The Hospitalized Patient

Millions of older adults are hospitalized in the United States each year for a variety of acute illnesses and elective procedures. Fortunately, in the United States, Medicare Part A covers much of the cost associated with acute care, including hospitalization and short-term rehabilitation. While in the hospital, however, older adults can become vulnerable to myriad complications related to both their compromised health state and problems inherent to the acute care environment itself. As noted previously, delirium afflicts hospitalized elders at a very high rate and increases risk of prolonged hospital stays, nursing home admission, and death. Hospitalized older adults also experience the effects of immobilization, with loss of muscle strength and deconditioning. Acutely, these factors increase the risk of falls and impair function and ability to provide self-care. In addition, poor oral intake may result in malnutrition, and illness-related fluid losses may cause dehydration. As a result, hypotension and protein-calorie malnutrition are common problems. Immobility and malnutrition both predispose the acutely ill patient to the development of pressure wounds, which can develop in under 2 hours. All these problems worsen in the presence of delirium or depressed mood. Environmental factors also contribute to problems, including tethers such as catheters and intravenous lines (which increase risk of falls), noisy wards, and frequent tests and procedures that further disrupt diurnal rhythms and sleep. Up to one third of hospitalized older adults experience a decline in their ability to perform ADLs in the course of their hospitalization. Patients who experience declines in function during hospitalization have higher rates of rehospitalization, prolonged institutionalization, and mortality after discharge, and many (41%) never return to their preadmission level of function. To combat these problems, some hospitals have created specialized inpatient geriatric care units, often termed *acute care for elders (ACE) units*. These units incorporate adaptations in the physical environment and specially trained staff to provide safe, patient-centered care designed to maximize restoration of function and prevent common complications of hospitalization. In randomized trials, ACE units and their consultative counterpart, the mobile ACE (or MACE), have reduced lengths of stay, improved care transitions, and lowered readmissions. Likewise, geriatric evaluation and management (GEM) units (described later) offer specialized, team-based postacute care with an emphasis on rehabilitation and return to prior level of function.

虐待

老年人由于健康状况不佳、功能依赖和社会隔离而特别容易受到虐待。虐待被定义为受到虐待（由他人造成的伤害）或自我忽视。自我忽视被认为是最常见的虐待形式，但真实发生率很难估计。危险因素包括认知障碍和近期功能衰退。据报告，美国有3%～8%老年人受到过虐待。因为患者报告不足、医疗卫生人员缺乏认识，比例可能低估。虐待呈现多种形式，包括心理、经济、身体、性虐待和忽视。研究表明，忽视和虐待与老年人更高的养老院安置率和死亡率有关。身体虐待的迹象包括挫伤、烧伤、咬伤、生殖器或直肠创伤、压疮或不明原因的体重减轻。其他形式的虐待可能更难以在检查时辨别，但可以通过直接提问帮助识别，如"有人伤害你吗？""你害怕什么人吗？"或"是否有人未经您的许可而取走或使用您的钱款？"。任何怀疑虐待或忽视都应上报成人保护服务部门。美国44个州和哥伦比亚特区都有法律要求，报告可疑的老年人虐待。美国司法部拥有老年虐待资源网络，数据在不断增加（https://www.justice.gov/elderjustice/about-eji）。

财务

美国老年人的财富差异很大。虽然65岁以上老人的总体贫困率在过去50年有所减低，但9.3%的老年人仍然生活在贫困线以下，非裔（18.7%）和西班牙裔（17.4%）美国人处于贫困的比例更高。包括医务人员在内的医疗团队成员应筛查老年人的财务问题，因为这些问题对老年人健康状况和幸福感有直接影响。经济能力有限的老年人更容易出现药物供给、膳食和基本设施的问题。借助社区资源网络可以帮助老年人完成基本需求的选择，包括住房选择和膳食。有关特定地区代理和服务的信息请访问 www.eldercare.org。

预定医疗指示

预定医疗指示可以有多种不同的形式，并用于各种不同的目的。在理想情况下，预定医疗指示清楚表达了一个人在严重疾病或丧失能力的情况下的医疗选择。在预定医疗指示中通常会预先对医疗及场景做出限定，对何时保留或撤销生命维持及恢复措施做出预先指示。通常说来，预定医疗指示包括生前预嘱和医疗授权委托。生前预嘱主要解决当患者处于疾病终末期、持续植物状态或进行性神经疾病时，按照患者意愿对何时终止包括人工喂养和液体补充等特殊生命维持治疗做出明确指示。无行动能力患者的生前预嘱一般都有配套的医疗授权委托书，委托书中规定了其首选决策者或代理人。如果没有设定医疗授权委托人，通常默认患者的配偶或其他一级亲属为首选代理人。如果没有指定代理人也没有近亲，那么就可以（通过法律程序）指定监护者。

法定监护是由法院指定一名代理决策者的法律程序。医生有责任在患者感知能力改变或认知能力逐渐受损的情况下确定患者的独立决策能力。评估内容包括患者是否有能力了解自身所处情况、提出问题、权衡选择和发表意见。在某些情况下，可能需要进行全面的老年或神经心理评估。有人对传统的预定医疗指示，特别是生前预嘱提出批评，认为其传达患者的特殊选择权作用有限。最近，研究者开发出更详细的表格以记录对补液、营养、住院和复苏等措施的具体意向和限制，例如《治疗范围医嘱》（MOST）和《维持生命治疗医嘱》（POLST）表格（https://polst.org/programs-in-your-state/）。当然，有效填写和应用这些表格应与主要医疗服务提供者进行医疗目标对话，最好有家庭护理人员参与。此外，老年人的护理意向会随着健康状况的变化而改变，因此医疗服务提供者应鼓励老年人每年重新审视并更新其预定医疗指示。

照护环境：特殊考虑

住院患者

美国每年有数百万的老年人因各种急性疾病和择期手术住院治疗。美国国家医疗保险A部分涵盖了与急性护理相关的绝大部分花费，包括住院和短期康复治疗。然而，老年人在住院期间容易出现各种并发症，这可能与其健康状态受损有关，也与急诊环境本身固有的问题相关。如前所述，谵妄在住院老年人中的发病率非常高，并延长了住院时间，增加了转入养老院和死亡的风险。住院的老年人还会受活动受限的影响，肌肉力量下降，健康状况恶化。这些因素在短期内增加了跌倒的风险，损害了患者自理能力。此外，经口摄入不足可能导致营养不良，疾病相关的体液丢失，导致脱水。由此导致的低血压和蛋白质-热量营养不良是常见的问题。急性患者由于活动受限和营养不良容易发生压疮，甚至在2h内就可以出现。如果同时有谵妄和抑郁会使上述问题进一步恶化。环境因素同样影响病情转归，包括管路如导管和静脉输液管（增加跌倒的风险）、病房噪声，以及频繁的检查和操作，都会进一步扰乱患者的昼夜节律和睡眠。高达1/3老年人在住院期间出现日常生活活动能力下降，这部分患者住院时间长，再住院率和出院后死亡率都比较高，高达41%的患者再也无法恢复到其入院前的功能水平。为了解决上述问题，一些医院已经设立了专门的住院老年护理单元，即老年人急症照护（ACE）单元。这种护理单元对物理环境进行了适应性改造，并配备经过专业培训的工作人员，提供以患者为中心的安全护理，旨在最大限度地恢复患者的功能并预防住院期间的常见并发症。随机对照研究显示ACE单元及其配套的移动ACE（MACE）缩短了住院时间，改善了护理过渡并降低了再住院率。同样，老年评估管理（GEM）单元（稍后描述）提供了专业的、基于团队的急性期护理，重点是康复和帮助患者恢复到以前的功能水平。

Care Transitions

As noted previously, older adults experience high rates of complications during acute illness and require prolonged periods of time and sometimes admission for rehabilitation in various types of facilities in order to recover. For this reason, management in the postacute period represents a critical and complex time. Specifically, older adults with acute illness often find themselves transferred among different care settings and providers. Nearly one quarter of hospitalized older adults are discharged to skilled nursing facilities, and another 12% are discharged with home health care. Of those discharged to skilled facilities, about one fifth will return to the hospital within 30 days. Transitions in care represent high-risk episodes, and evidence shows that patients and caregivers frequently experience miscommunication, medication errors, and missed essential laboratory tests or appointments during this period. Recent trials have demonstrated a reduction in rehospitalization through a structured discharge and transition of care plan. This includes interdisciplinary team communication, medication reconciliation before and after discharge, careful planning for laboratory and appointment follow-up, communication with patients and caregivers about expectations and preferences, and specific coaching for patients and caregivers in symptom management. More information on care management in transitions is available at www.caretransitions.org.

SYSTEMS OF CARE

Ambulatory and Home Care

The majority of care for older adults occurs in the outpatient setting. Much of the cost of this care, including visit fees, laboratory tests, radiograph studies, and vaccinations, is covered under Medicare Part B, for which patients pay a monthly premium. Outpatient visits may occur with the physician, physician assistant, nurse practitioner, or clinical nurse specialists, depending on the nature of the problem and the structure of the setting. Other key members of the care team include social workers, pharmacists, psychologists, and physical and occupational therapists. Most assessments discussed in this chapter can be performed in outpatient settings, including functional assessments, cognitive and mood screening, gait and balance assessment, medication review, eye and ear examinations, and continence evaluations. Interview of a caregiver can augment the information collected. Care in this setting can be complicated, though, by problems with transportation and ineffective or inefficient communication among multiple providers, particularly for patients with multiple specialists.

Over the last several years, home care has reemerged as an effective means of providing health care for older adults. As with the outpatient setting, Medicare Part B will reimburse providers in part for services rendered in the home. In addition, if a rehabilitative or skilled service is needed (i.e., home nursing care or home physical therapy) Medicare Part A provides coverage. Patients receiving services in the home must be "homebound," implying that they are significantly functionally impaired and travel with assistance out of the home infrequently and usually only for medical purposes. Services rendered in the home include a full range of evaluations by teams of health care professionals depending on needs. Social workers often lead these visits and perform case management, assessing financial and other resource needs. Nurses, clinical nurse specialists, and/or nurse practitioners provide skilled services when necessary, including health education, symptom monitoring, or wound care. Physical and occupational therapy can assess mobility and home safety and greatly enhance function and independence. Furthermore, examination of a person's home environment can reveal much about his or her safety and nutrition and can facilitate education or intervention in these areas. Physicians may serve as medical directors of such programs but may also perform visits themselves to learn more about a given patient's health status. If significant concerns exist about a patient's safety, particularly in the setting of cognitive impairment, a home visit may provide information about the need for more urgent interventions, including referrals to Adult Protective Services. Research has demonstrated that coordinated home care programs can improve management of chronic disease, including dementia, diabetes mellitus, and congestive heart failure, as well as to reduce rehospitalization in patients with congestive heart failure. One home care model that began pushing the traditional boundaries of home care prior to 2001 is the hospital at home (HaH) program, which provides home-based acute care for older adults with specific illnesses identified in the ED. High quality care and patient satisfaction continue to aid in the spread of this model of care throughout the United States.

Long-Term Care

The phrase *long-term care* describes the array of services available to provide care for people with disability from chronic and acute conditions. This definition includes the services offered in the outpatient and home settings described previously. Most associate the term, however, with the system of nursing facilities providing personal and medical care for disabled adults of all ages. Skilled nursing facilities provide long-term care for those with permanent disabilities from chronic illness or short rehabilitative stays after acute illness (e.g., stroke) or procedures (e.g., joint replacement). The scope of services may also include end-of-life care in conjunction with a hospice care team. Facility staff includes licensed nurses who give 24-hour supervision, with much of the personal care provided by certified nursing assistants. Each facility also has a medical director overseeing various aspects of medical care. An attending physician, who may or may not be the medical director, performs scheduled patient visits every 30 to 60 days. Most SNFs also employ advanced practice providers (physician assistants or nurse practitioners), physical, occupational, and speech therapists for rehabilitation care, dietitians, social workers, and recreational therapists. Patients with moderate or severe dementia constitute approximately 60% of patients living in skilled nursing facilities. Although Medicare Part A provides payment for rehabilitative stays of 100 days or less (with a copayment for days 21 to 100), it does not finance long-term stays. Such patients pay out of pocket, through long-term care insurance, or through Medicaid, a joint federal and state assistance program. Medicaid constitutes between 45% and 65% of all payment sources for skilled nursing facility care in the United states.

For patients with less complex care needs, assisted living facilities or domiciliary care homes provide an alternative arrangement for long-term care. Although these facilities vary dramatically in their size and structure, most provide nonskilled care for patients who need some assistance with activities of daily living. Licensed nurses may be present during some specified periods of time, and other professions may visit the facility intermittently to provide services such as physical therapy. Assisted living facilities do not have medical directors, and patients normally continue to see a primary care provider in the outpatient setting. Unlicensed staff, including nursing aides, provide most of the personal care and assistance. Medicare does not cover the cost of assisted living. Medicaid provides some reimbursement for this type of care, but the majority of residents pay out of pocket or through other assistance programs, such as Social Security. For those with adequate means, a living option has emerged that combines independent living, assisted living, and skilled care in one location. Continuing care retirement communities allow residents to live within the same community while moving through or between levels of care. They offer residents convenient central resources, such as recreational and dining facilities, transportation, and onsite health care.

护理过渡

如前所述，老年人在急性疾病期间并发症发生率较高，需要更长的恢复时间，有时还需要入住各类康复机构以便康复。因此急性期后的治疗管理错综复杂，是他们康复的关键时间段。患有急性疾病的老年人常常需要在不同的医疗机构和照护者之间转移。近 1/4 的住院老年人被送往专业护理机构，另有 12% 的人出院后回归家庭护理。在出院到专业护理机构的患者中，约有 1/5 会在 30 天内重返医院。有证据表明，护理过渡是一种高危的过程，患者和护理人员在这段时间经常遇到错误沟通、用药错误及错过必要的实验室检测或预约检查。最近的试验表明，通过结构化（连贯安排）出院和护理过渡能减少再住院，具体措施包括跨学科团队沟通、出院前后的用药协调、化验和预约随访的周密计划、与患者和护理人员就期望和意向进行沟通，以及对患者和护理人员进行症状管理方面的具体指导。有关过渡期护理管理的更多信息，请访问 www.caretransitions.org。

照护系统

门诊和家庭照护

大多数老年人的照护要求多发生在门诊。主要医疗花费包括挂号、实验室检查、放射检查和疫苗接种等，都由国家医疗保险 B 部分支付，患者每月支付（国家医疗保险）保险费。根据问题的性质和门诊设置结构的不同，患者的门诊就诊可以由医生、医生助理、护士或临床护理专家进行。照护团队的其他主要成员包括社会工作者、药剂师、心理学家、物理和作业治疗师。本章讨论的大多数评估都可以在门诊进行，包括功能评估、认知和情绪筛查、步态和平衡评估、药物审查、眼耳检查和大小便失禁评估。和照护人员面谈可以增加收集的信息。然而，由于交通问题和多个医疗服务提供者之间沟通不畅或效率低下，尤其是一个患者同时需要多个专科医生时，照护工作可能会变得更加复杂。

在过去数年中，家庭照护已经重新成为为老年人提供医疗保健服务的有效手段。与门诊一样，国家医疗保险 B 部分将向照护提供者偿付部分家庭照护的费用，此外，如果需要康复或专业服务（如家庭护理或理疗），则需要医疗保险 A 计划提供保险。接受家庭照护的患者必须是"无法出门"的，这意味着他们的功能严重损害，除了在协助下就医外很少能够出门。家庭照护提供的服务主要是根据患者的需求，由来自多个专业的医疗团队对患者进行全面的评估。社会工作者通常组织这些探视评估、进行病例管理、财务评估和满足其他资源需求。必要时，护士、临床专科护士和（或）执业护士会提供专业服务，包括健康教育、症状监测或伤口护理。物理和作业治疗师可以评估患者活动能力和居家安全性，并大大提高患者功能和自理能力。此外，检查患者的家庭环境可以显示他（她）的安全性和营养状况，并有利于进行宣教和干预。医生既可以担任此类家庭照护计划的医疗主任，也可以亲自访问并了解特定患者的健康状况。如果患者的安全（特别是在认知障碍方面）存在重大问题，家访能提供所需要的紧急干预的信息，包括推荐其参加成人保护服务项目。研究表明，协作型家庭照护计划可以改进慢性疾病的管理，包括痴呆、糖尿病及充血性心力衰竭，并减少充血性心力衰竭患者的再住院。2001 年之前，一种名为"家庭医院"（HaH）的护理模式突破传统家庭护理的界限，为在急诊室确诊患有特殊疾病的老年人提供基于家庭的急症护理。高质量的护理和患者的满意度继续推动着这种护理模式在全美推广。

长期照护

长期照护一词指为因慢性和急性疾病而失能患者提供的一系列服务，包括前文描述的门诊和家庭照护。然而，大多数人将长期照护理解为对所有年龄的残疾成年人提供个人和医疗护理的照护机构系统。专业照护机构为因慢性疾病而导致的终生残疾患者提供长期护理，或是为急性疾病（如脑卒中）或手术（如关节置换）后的短期康复提供护理服务。长期照护的工作范围还包括与临终关怀护理团队合作进行的临终护理。该机构的工作人员包括提供 24 h 监护的执业护士，以及提供大部分个人护理的执业护理助理。每个机构还设有一名医务主任负责监督医疗的各个方面。主治医生（可以是或不是医疗主任）每 30～60 天需要对患者进行一次定期访视。大多数专业护理机构还聘请了高级医疗服务提供者（医生助理或主管护士），康复护理的物理治疗师、作业和语言治疗师，营养师，社会工作者和娱乐治疗师。中重度痴呆患者约占专业护理机构住院患者的 60%。国家医疗保险 A 部分赔付包括 100 天内的康复期付款（第 21～100 天有部分自费金额），但不会为超过 100 天的长期住院提供赔付。此时，患者需要自己付费、通过长期护理保险，或通过联邦和州参与的 Medicaid（美国医疗补助计划）支付。美国专业护理机构所有支付来源的 45%～65% 来自 Medicaid 医疗补助计划。

对于护理需求不太复杂的患者，生活辅助机构或家庭护理院为长期护理提供了另一种选择。这些机构规模大小和结构明显不同，但大多数能为日常生活需要协助的患者提供非技术护理。执业护士会在特定时间段值班，其他专业人员也会间断地到机构来为患者提供如物理治疗等服务。生活辅助机构不设医疗主任，患者仍照常去门诊与初级保健医生沟通。无执照的工作人员（包括护理辅助人员）则主要提供个人护理和帮助。Medicare（美国国家老年人医疗保险）不支付生活辅助机构的费用。Medicaid 可以为这种类型的护理提供部分报销，但大多数居民需要自己付费或通过其他如社会保障援助计划付费。对于经济富裕的人群，可以选择一种新出现的独立生活、生活辅助和专业护理相结合的生活方式。持续照护退休社区（CCRC）允许居民生活在同一社区内，同时又可以根据需要选择不同的护理级别，社区为居民提供便捷的中心资源，如娱乐和餐饮设施、交通及属地卫生保健。

Program of All-Inclusive Care for the Elderly

In the 1970s, a group providing care for older Chinese adults in San Francisco developed a model of long-term care centered in the community. Proponents of this model, entitled the Program of All-inclusive Care for the Elderly (PACE), believed that the community (rather than the institution) provided a better location to meet the chronic care needs of older adults. From its start as a community-based effort in California, the PACE model has grown with the support of private foundations and Medicare demonstration projects; now PACE is a benefit for older adults who qualify for both Medicare and Medicaid. Reimbursement is at 95% of the cost of nursing home care in the area where the patient lives. Participants must be over 55 and certified by the state to be eligible for nursing home care. The PACE program then uses combined Medicare and Medicaid funds otherwise slated to pay for the individual's long-term care to provide care in the community. Much of it is coordinated through senior centers offering an array of resources and services, including the following:

- Adult day care, offering nursing; physical, occupational, and recreational therapies; meals; nutritional counseling; social work; transportation; and personal care
- Medical care provided by a PACE physician familiar with the history, needs, and preferences of each participant
- Home health care and personal care
- All necessary prescription drugs
- Social services
- Medical specialists such as audiology, dentistry, optometry, podiatry, and speech therapy
- Respite care

When necessary, PACE participants are admitted to the hospital or nursing home. These services are provided under the auspices of the PACE program as part of the care package, and the program bears full financial risk. The benefits of care for older adults, particularly those of limited means, appear to be substantial.

See the National PACE Association website at www.npaonline.org for more information.

Geriatric Care

In caring for frail older adults with complex care needs, consultation with a geriatrician or geriatrics-focused interprofessional team can often provide highly useful information. The team can assist in the assessment and management of the specific conditions or situations described earlier. The geriatrician can advise on appropriate level or setting of care for an older adult as difficult decisions related to treatment options in the context of limited life expectancy occur. Geriatricians complete a minimum of 1 year of fellowship after residency training in internal medicine or family practice. After training they are eligible for board certification and qualified to work in a number of different settings, including the hospital, long-term care, home care, and outpatient clinics. Comprehensive assessment by a geriatrician or geriatrics team includes components detailed previously, including evaluation of the patient's medical condition, function, and social support. Normally the consultant will work with an interprofessional team that may include a nurse case manager, physician assistant and/or nurse practitioner, social worker, physical or occupation therapist, pharmacist, psychologist, and others. The outcome of the geriatric assessment is a comprehensive plan for safely restoring the patient to optimal function with mutually agreeable and realistic goals of care.

In the setting of acute illness, geriatricians also provide important services. As described earlier, ACE units can improve patient care and prevent iatrogenic complications. Similarly, once patients are medically stable, transfer to a specialized geriatrics care unit, often termed a geriatric evaluation and management unit, may be possible in some institutions, to provide a comprehensive medical assessment and plan for transition of care. Early consultation with a geriatrician and an interprofessional, transdisciplinary team in the acute care setting can help in the management of complex medical illness and with communication with patients and caregivers about post-hospitalization options. After hospitalization, locating facilities or services that offer comprehensive care by a geriatrician and interdisciplinary team is ideal, including a coordinated approach that uses specific strategies to manage transitions of care.

For a deeper discussion on this topic, please see Section IV, "Aging and Geriatric Medicine," in *Goldman-Cecil Medicine*, 26th Edition.

FUTURE DIRECTIONS: GEROSCIENCE, AN EMERGING FIELD

Frameworks of aging theory described previously provide a foundation for the emerging field of geroscience. The nine "hallmarks of aging" (see Fig. 21.4) introduced previously are considered a theoretical framework through which to study interventions that have the potential to influence the biology of aging and delay the emergence of most chronic diseases that appear to be driven by this mechanism. Through study of molecular mechanisms of aging, evidence is increasing to suggest ways humans can influence *healthspan*, which can be thought of as an overall delay of onset of chronic disease. Caloric restriction (CR), or the purposeful reduction of food intake, is the only intervention that has been shown to reproducibly extend maximal lifespan in certain laboratory animal models. In rats, lifespan increases an average of 20 months with a 40% reduction in calories. Rhesus monkeys enrolled in a trial of caloric restriction appear to have improvements in metabolic markers and a lower disease burden than controls after 15 years but have had no definitive extension in lifespan. The mechanism is not well understood but may be metabolically mediated. In observational studies in humans, those with lower average body temperature, lower insulin levels, and higher dehydroepiandrosterone sulfate (DHEAS) levels (all changes found in calorically restricted monkeys) appeared to survive longer. Current research is focused on similarly influencing the cellular biology of healthspan in human subjects and discovering chemical agents that mimic or mediate these metabolic effects.

Emergence of Geroscience Guided Therapies

Potential molecular targets that allow for the delayed onset of human disease are well described in animal models of cardiovascular, pulmonary, and musculoskeletal systems. Animal studies have shown delayed onset of aging with inhibition of mTOR pathway in multiple species. In recent years, translational clinical trials in humans evaluating geroscience guided therapies (GGTs) have begun to occur. The trials demonstrate promise toward impacting the trajectory of certain chronic diseases. The first human trial using senolytic therapy to ablate senescent cells showed potential for improvement in physical function in people with idiopathic pulmonary fibrosis. The emergence of translational geroscience as a multidisciplinary field has the potential to influence medical practice and outcomes in the coming years.

SUGGESTED READINGS

Boyd C, Smith CD, Masoudi FA, et al: Decision making for older adults with multiple chronic conditions: executive summary for the American geriatrics Society guiding principles on the care of older adults with Multimorbidity, J Am Geriatr Soc 67:665–673, 2019.

Campisi J: Aging, cellular senescence, and cancer, Annu Rev Physiol 75:685–705, 2013.

老年人全包式照护方案（PACE）

在20世纪70年代，旧金山的一个为华裔老年人群提供护理的团体开发了一种以社区为中心的长期照护模式，称为"老年人全包式照护方案"（PACE）。PACE的支持者们相信，社区（而不是某些机构）提供了一个更好的地点来满足老年人的慢性护理需求。从加利福尼亚州以社区为基础的初创开始，PACE模式在私人基金会和Medicaid示范项目的支持下逐渐发展；现在，对于那些同时享有医疗保险和医疗补助资金的老年人非常有益，报销费用占患者所在地区的护理院护理费用的95%。参加者必须年满55岁，并经国家证实有资格享有护理院护理。PACE计划将原本用于支付个人长期护理费用的医疗保险和医疗补助资金合并使用用于支付长期社区护理费用。其中大部分服务是通过提供系列资源和服务的老年人中心协调的，提供的一系列资源和服务如下：

- 成人日间照料提供：护理；物理、作业和娱乐治疗；膳食；营养咨询；社会工作；交通；个人护理。
- 由熟悉每位患者病史、需要和意愿的PACE医生提供医疗照护。
- 家庭保健和个人护理。
- 所有必需的处方药。
- 社会服务。
- 医学专家服务，如听力、口腔、验光、足部医疗和语言治疗等。
- 临时看护。

必要时，PACE参与者会被送入医院或护理院。这些服务是在PACE计划的支持下提供的，是"一揽子"护理服务的一部分。PACE计划承担全部财务风险。老年人，特别是生活拮据的老年人获益最大。

更多信息请访问（美国）国家PACE协会网站，网址为www.npaonline.org。

老年人照护

在照护复杂护理需求的衰弱老年人时，老年科医生或老年医学团队通常可以提供非常有用的信息。老年医学团队可以协助评估和管理前面所述的具体病症或特殊情况，老年科医生可以帮助那些有多种共病且预期寿命有限的老年人决定治疗策略，提供适当护理级别的建议。老年科医生需要在内科或全科住院医生培训结束后完成至少1年的专科培训，经过培训后才能有资格获得医学委员会认证，并有资格在以下不同的场所工作，包括医院、长期护理机构、家庭护理和门诊诊所。由老年科医生或老年医学团队进行的综合评估包括之前详述的内容，其中包括评估患者的医疗状况、功能和社会支持。通常，顾问会与跨专业团队合作，该团队包括一位病例管理护士、医生助理和（或）执业护士、社会工作者、物理或作业治疗师、药剂师、心理学家和其他人员。老年疾病评估最终是为了制订一个安全地帮助患者恢复最佳功能的全面计划，以及双方都同意的、切合实际的护理目标。

老年科医生在急性疾病诊治处理中也有重要作用。如前所述，老年人急症照护单元（ACE units）可以改善患者的照护，并预防医源性并发症。同样，一旦患者病情稳定，在一些机构就可以转到专门的老年病护理病房，通常称为老年评估管理单元，为护理过渡提供全面的医疗评估和计划。在急性疾病诊治处理过程中，及早向老年科医生和跨专业、跨学科团队咨询，有助于处理复杂的内科疾病，并能与患者和护理人员就出院后方案的制订进行沟通。入院后，理想的选择是由老年科医生和跨学科团队提供全面护理的机构或服务，包括协调使用特定策略来进行护理过渡。

有关此专题的深入讨论，请参阅 *Goldman-Cecil Medicine* 第26版第四篇"衰老与老年医学"。 ❖

未来方向：老年科学，一个新兴领域

前面介绍的老龄化理论框架为新兴的老年科学领域提供了基础。前文介绍的九个"衰老标志"（图21.4）被认为是理论框架，依靠这些理论，可以探索可能影响衰老生物学的干预措施，以延缓大多数由衰老机制驱动的慢性病的发生。通过对衰老分子机制的研究，越来越多的证据表明人类可以整体上推迟慢性疾病的发生，延长健康寿命。热量限制（CR）或有目的地减少食物摄入，是唯一一种在某些实验动物模型中延长最大寿命的可重复的干预措施。减少40%的卡路里摄入可使大鼠寿命平均延长20个月。参加热量限制试验的恒河猴在15年后代谢指标出现改善，疾病负担也低于对照组，但没有明确的整体寿命延长。热量限制具体机制尚不清楚，但可能是由代谢介导的。在人类观察性研究中，平均体温、胰岛素水平较低和硫酸脱氢表雄酮（DHEAS）水平较高的人似乎寿命更长，所有这些变化也都在热量受限的猴子身上发现。目前的研究重点是如何能在人类产生类似的细胞生物学作用以延长健康寿命，发现可模仿或调节这些代谢效应的化学药物。

老年科学引导疗法的兴起

在心血管、肺部和肌肉骨骼系统的动物模型中，可延缓人类疾病发生的潜在分子靶点已被充分描述。动物研究表明，在多个物种中抑制mTOR通路可延缓衰老的发生。近年来，评估老年科学引导疗法（GGT）的人体转化临床试验已开始进行。这些试验结果有望影响特定慢性病的发生、进展和预后。首例使用senolytic抗衰老疗法清除衰老细胞的人体试验显示，该疗法对于特发性肺纤维化患者可以改善其身体功能。作为一个多学科领域，老年转化医学的出现有可能在不远的将来影响医疗实践和改善衰老结局。

推荐阅读

Boyd C, Smith CD, Masoudi FA, et al: Decision making for older adults with multiple chronic conditions: executive summary for the American geriatrics Society guiding principles on the care of older adults with Multimorbidity, J Am Geriatr Soc 67:665–673, 2019.

Campisi J: Aging, cellular senescence, and cancer, Annu Rev Physiol 75:685–705, 2013.

Cesari M, Gambassi G, Abellan van Kan G, Vellas B: The frailty phenotype and the frailty index: different instruments for different purposes, Age Ageing 43:10–12, 2014.

Fries JF: Aging, natural death, and the compression of morbidity, N Engl J Med 303:130–135, 1980.

Goode PS, Burgio KL, Richter HE, et al: Incontinence in older women, J Am Med Assoc 303:2172–2181, 2010.

Gooneratne NS, Vitiello MV: Sleep in older adults: normative changes, sleep disorders, and treatment options, Clin Geriatr Med 30(3):591–627, 2014.

Khan SS, Singer BD, Vaughan DE: Molecular and physiological manifestations and measurement of aging in humans, Aging Cell 16(4):624–633, 2017.

Kim CS, Flanders SA: In the clinic: transitions of care, Ann Intern Med 158:ITC3-1, 2013.

Kirkland JL, Tchkonia T, Zhu Y, Niedernhofer LJ, Robbins PD: The clinical potential of senolytic drugs, J Am Geriatr Soc 65:2297–2301, 2017.

Li RM, Iadarola AC, Maisano CC, editors: Why population aging matters: a GlobaPerspective. A booklet prepared in follow-up to the 2007 Summit on global aging hosted by the U.S. State Department and the national Institute on aging, National Institute on Aging and the National Institutes of Health, March 2007.

López-Otín C, Blasco MA, Partridge L, Serrano M, Kroemer G: The hallmarks of aging, Cell 153(6):1194–1217, 2013.

Marcantonio ER: In the clinic. Delirium, Ann Intern Med 154, 2011:ITC6-1, 2011.

Mosqueda L, Dong X: Elder abuse and self-neglect: "I don't care anything about going to the doctor, to be honest…," J Am Med Assoc 306:532–540, 2011.

Reuben DB: Medical care for the final years of life: "When you're 83, it's not going to be 20 Years," J Am Med Assoc 302:2686–2694, 2009.

Reuben DB, Wieland DL, Rubenstein LZ: Functional status assessment of older persons: concepts and implications, Facts Res Gerontol 7:232, 1993.

Salzman B, Beldowski K, de la Paz A: Cancer screening in older adults, Am Fam Physician 96:659–667, 2016.

Steinman MA, Hanlon JT: Managing medications in clinically complex elders: "There's got to be a happy medium," J Am Med Assoc 304:1592–1601, 2010.

The 2019 American Geriatrics Society Beers Criteria® Update Expert Panel. American Geriatrics Society 2019 Updated AGS Beers Criteria® for Potentially Inappropriate Medication Use in Older Adults, J Am Geriatr Soc 67(4):674–694, 2019.

Tinetti M, Huang A, Molnar F: The geriatrics 5M's: a new way of communicating what we do, J Am Geriatr Soc 65(9):2115, 2017.

Wald HL, Ramaswamy R, Perskin MH, Roberts L, Bogaisky M, Suen W: The case for mobility assessment in hospitalized older adults: American geriatrics Society white paper executive summary, J Am Geriatr Soc 67:11–16, 2019.

Yourman LC, Lee SJ, Schonberg MA, Widera EW, Smith AK: Prognostic indices for older adults: a systematic review, J Am Med Assoc 307(2):182–192, 2012.

Cesari M, Gambassi G, Abellan van Kan G, Vellas B: The frailty phenotype and the frailty index: different instruments for different purposes, Age Ageing 43:10–12, 2014.

Fries JF: Aging, natural death, and the compression of morbidity, N Engl J Med 303:130–135, 1980.

Goode PS, Burgio KL, Richter HE, et al: Incontinence in older women, J Am Med Assoc 303:2172–2181, 2010.

Gooneratne NS, Vitiello MV: Sleep in older adults: normative changes, sleep disorders, and treatment options, Clin Geriatr Med 30(3):591–627, 2014.

Khan SS, Singer BD, Vaughan DE: Molecular and physiological manifestations and measurement of aging in humans, Aging Cell 16(4):624–633, 2017.

Kim CS, Flanders SA: In the clinic: transitions of care, Ann Intern Med 158:ITC3-1, 2013.

Kirkland JL, Tchkonia T, Zhu Y, Niedernhofer LJ, Robbins PD: The clinical potential of senolytic drugs, J Am Geriatr Soc 65:2297–2301, 2017.

Li RM, Iadarola AC, Maisano CC, editors: Why population aging matters: a GlobaPerspective. A booklet prepared in follow-up to the 2007 Summit on global aging hosted by the U.S. State Department and the national Institute on aging, National Institute on Aging and the National Institutes of Health, March 2007.

López-Otín C, Blasco MA, Partridge L, Serrano M, Kroemer G: The hallmarks of aging, Cell 153(6):1194–1217, 2013.

Marcantonio ER: In the clinic. Delirium, Ann Intern Med 154, 2011:ITC6-1, 2011.

Mosqueda L, Dong X: Elder abuse and self-neglect: "I don't care anything about going to the doctor, to be honest…," J Am Med Assoc 306:532–540, 2011.

Reuben DB: Medical care for the final years of life: "When you're 83, it's not going to be 20 Years," J Am Med Assoc 302:2686–2694, 2009.

Reuben DB, Wieland DL, Rubenstein LZ: Functional status assessment of older persons: concepts and implications, Facts Res Gerontol 7:232, 1993.

Salzman B, Beldowski K, de la Paz A: Cancer screening in older adults, Am Fam Physician 96:659–667, 2016.

Steinman MA, Hanlon JT: Managing medications in clinically complex elders: "There's got to be a happy medium," J Am Med Assoc 304:1592–1601, 2010.

The 2019 American Geriatrics Society Beers Criteria® Update Expert Panel. American Geriatrics Society 2019 Updated AGS Beers Criteria® for Potentially Inappropriate Medication Use in Older Adults, J Am Geriatr Soc 67(4):674–694, 2019.

Tinetti M, Huang A, Molnar F: The geriatrics 5M's: a new way of communicating what we do, J Am Geriatr Soc 65(9):2115, 2017.

Wald HL, Ramaswamy R, Perskin MH, Roberts L, Bogaisky M, Suen W: The case for mobility assessment in hospitalized older adults: American geriatrics Society white paper executive summary, J Am Geriatr Soc 67:11–16, 2019.

Yourman LC, Lee SJ, Schonberg MA, Widera EW, Smith AK: Prognostic indices for older adults: a systematic review, J Am Med Assoc 307(2):182–192, 2012.

SECTION III

Palliative Care

22 Palliative Care, 324

第 3 篇

缓和医疗

22　缓和医疗，325

22
Palliative Care

Brandon J. Wilcoxson, Erin M. Denney-Koelsch, Robert G. Holloway

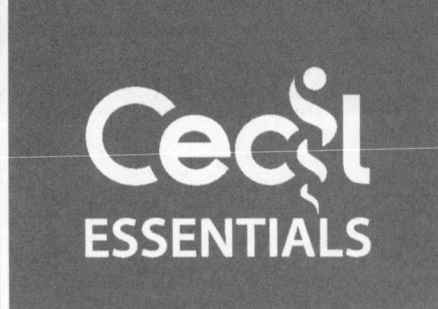

INTRODUCTION

Palliative care is both a philosophy of care and an area of specialization within several medical fields. The primary goal of palliative care is to minimize suffering and to support the best possible quality of life for patients and their families. Patients with serious and debilitating illness need and deserve excellent symptom control, assistance with difficult medical decisions, effective communication and collaboration among their providers, addressing of psychosocial problems, and an empathetic presence that fosters hope and healing relationships. Palliative care affirms life by supporting the patients' goals for the future in light of a full understanding of their medical condition, potentially including their hopes for cure, life-prolongation, relief from suffering, as well as preparation for death when time is short. This process includes exploring which life goals would be left undone if treatment does not go as hoped, who should make medical decisions for the patient if decision-making capacity is lost, and what limits might be set on aggressive therapy.

Palliative care provides an organized, structured system for delivering care by an interdisciplinary team, including physicians, nurses, social workers, chaplains, and counselors, as well as other health care professionals. Palliative care should be integrated within various health care settings including the hospital, emergency department, nursing home, home care, assisted living facilities, and outpatient settings. Palliative care remains very unevenly available, so many patients and families needlessly suffer, having either no, limited, or delayed access to appropriate palliative care. There is no evidence to suggest that early integration of palliative care shortens survival, yet many patients and health care professionals share an unspoken concern that it may hasten death. This common misconception, along with the misconception that palliative care is equivalent to end-of-life care, denies patients and families access to palliative care until late in the illness trajectory. Several prospective randomized controlled trials have compared early integration of specialty palliative care with standard care. These trials, primarily conducted in patients with advanced cancer, have shown improvements in important end points, including patient quality of life, rates of depression or anxiety, patient or caregiver satisfaction, and utilization of health services at the end of life. Two trials have also reported longer survival when palliative care is proactively integrated earlier than routine referral. Fig. 22.1 shows a visual concept of early integration of palliative care into a patient's disease course.

Basic palliative care should be part of the tool kit for all physicians who care for seriously ill patients. Specialty palliative care should be available for the more challenging symptom management, as well as the complex medical decision making that occurs in serious illness.

COMMON ILLNESS TRAJECTORIES AND PALLIATIVE CARE

There are four distinct trajectories of functional decline before dying. These trajectories have major implications for palliative care and health care delivery. Patients and families will also have different physical, psychological, social, and spiritual needs depending on the trajectory of their illness before they die. Being aware of these trajectories can help providers deliver appropriate care that integrates both disease-directed and palliative treatments.

Trajectory 1: Short Period of Evident Decline Before Death

Cancer typifies this trajectory. Function is preserved until rather late, followed by a predictable and precipitous decline over weeks to months. The onset of decline usually suggests metastatic tumor. A more predictable decline in function can assist in anticipating care needs, transitioning away from curative treatments toward a more exclusive emphasis on palliation, and eventually into hospice care. Not all malignancies follow this trajectory (e.g., prostate, breast) and some nonmalignant conditions (e.g., rapidly progressive dementias, amyotrophic lateral sclerosis) may follow this course.

Trajectory 2: Chronic Illness With Exacerbations and Sudden Dying

Congestive heart failure (CHF), chronic obstructive pulmonary disease (COPD), end-stage liver disease, and AIDS typify this trajectory. These organ system diseases represent chronic illnesses with occasional, acute exacerbations (e.g., physiologic stress that overwhelms the body's reserves), often requiring hospital admission. Patients can have a return of function after an exacerbation, but often not to the level of their baseline. They also may die suddenly during an exacerbation, but it is difficult to predict in advance. Prognosticating is very challenging in this trajectory. When patients choose to forego or stop aggressive life support, planning for aggressive symptom relief during a future exacerbation is essential.

Trajectory 3: Prolonged Dwindling

Dementia and frailty typify this trajectory. These patients have a prolonged course of physical and/or cognitive decline and become increasingly frail. Additional diagnoses include other neurodegenerative conditions (e.g., Parkinson's disease) and patients with multiple moderate to severe comorbidities (e.g., arthritis, visual impairment, past mild strokes, diabetes with neuropathy). Gradual decline in function, weight loss, fatigue, and low levels of activity are core features. Caregiver burden is usually immense. Prognosticating survival is

缓和医疗

阎格 译 张梦原 戴晓艳 审校 宁晓红 通审

引言

缓和医疗，既是一种照护理念，也是在多个医学领域均会涉及的一门专科。缓和医疗的主要目的是尽可能为患者与家属减少痛苦，并支持他们拥有尽可能好的生活质量。患有严重疾病及衰弱性疾病的患者需要并应当得到充分的症状控制、在困难医疗决策时得到帮助、在医疗服务提供者之间获得有效的沟通和协作、社会心理问题得以解决，以及得到帮助以建立希望和获得具有疗愈关系的同理性支持。缓和医疗通过充分理解患者的医疗状况，支持患者设定的未来目标从而支持到这个生命个体，这些目标可能包括他们对治愈、延长生命、缓解痛苦的期望，以及在生命时间有限时为死亡所做的准备。这个过程中会思考：如果治疗不如预期哪些人生目标将无法实现，在患者失去决策能力时将由谁为其做医疗决定，以及采取激进性治疗手段可能的局限性。

缓和医疗由跨学科团队提供有组织的、结构化的照护系统，这个团队包括医生、护士、社工、牧师、咨询师及其他医疗照护专业人员。缓和医疗应当整合到各种医疗照护环境中，包括医院、急诊、养老院、家庭照护、辅助型养老机构和门诊。缓和医疗的可及性非常不均衡，许多患者和家庭由于无法获得或只能有限地或不及时地获得适当的缓和医疗而遭受不必要的痛苦。没有证据表明早期将缓和医疗整合会缩短生存期，然而许多患者和医疗专业人员仍然担心其可能会加速死亡。这种普遍的误解，以及将缓和医疗误解等同于临终关怀，导致患者和家庭直至疾病发展的晚期才得以接触到缓和医疗。几项前瞻性随机对照试验将晚期癌症患者早期整合专业缓和医疗照护与标准照护进行比较，结果显示在重要的研究终点上有改善，包括患者生活质量、抑郁或焦虑的发生率、患者或照护者的满意度，以及生命末期医疗服务的使用情况等。有两项临床试验报告指出，与常规转诊相比，更早地积极整合缓和医疗可以使患者的生存期延长。图22.1显示了将缓和医疗早期整合到患者疾病进程的模式图。

基础缓和医疗应当成为所有照护重病患者的医生的基本技能的一部分。对更具挑战的症状管理以及在严重疾病中出现的复杂医疗决策应当交由专业缓和医疗团队处理。

常见疾病轨迹与缓和医疗

在生命结束前，有四种不同的功能衰退轨迹。这些疾病轨迹对缓和医疗和医疗照护服务的提供有重要影响。患者离世前，患者和家庭在不同的疾病轨迹中会有不同的身体、心理、社会和精神需求。了解这些疾病轨迹有助于医护人员将针对疾病的治疗和缓和治疗相结合。

轨迹1：离世前短期内明显衰退

癌症是这种疾病轨迹的典型代表。患者的功能一直保持到相对较晚的阶段，在随后在几周到几个月内出现可预测性的急剧下降。这种衰退的开始通常提示肿瘤已转移。功能的可预测性下降有助于提前预见照护需求，从治愈性治疗转向更专注于缓解症状的治疗，最终进入安宁疗护。值得注意的是，并非所有恶性肿瘤都遵循这一轨迹（如前列腺癌、乳腺癌就不符合这个轨迹），而一些非恶性疾病可能也符合这一轨迹（如快速进展的痴呆、肌萎缩侧索硬化症）。

轨迹2：慢性疾病加重和突然死亡

充血性心力衰竭（CHF）、慢性阻塞性肺疾病（COPD）、终末期肝病和艾滋病是这种疾病轨迹的典型代表。这些器官系统疾病表现为慢性病伴有偶发的急性加重（如生理应激超过身体储备），通常需要住院治疗。患者在病情加重后可能恢复部分功能，但通常无法回到基线水平。他们也可能在急性加重期间突然死亡，但很难提前预测。在这种疾病轨迹中预测生存期极具挑战性。当患者选择放弃或停止激进性生命支持时，提前为病情再次恶化时积极的症状管理进行准备至关重要。

轨迹3：长期缓慢衰退

痴呆和衰弱是这种疾病轨迹的典型代表。这些患者经历长期的身体和（或）认知下降，并且越来越衰弱。其他疾病还包括神经退行性疾病（如帕金森病），以及患有多种中重度合并症（如关节炎、视力障碍、轻度卒中史、伴有神经病变的糖尿病）的患者。功能逐渐下降、体重减轻、疲劳和活动能力下降是这个疾

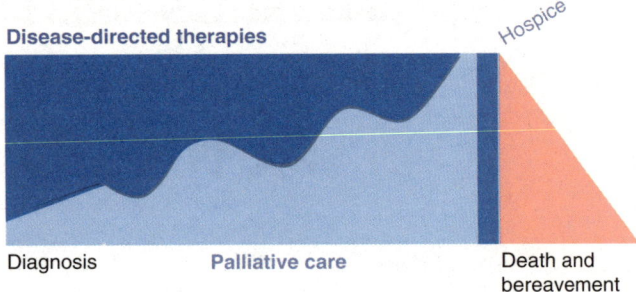

Fig. 22.1 Palliative care and hospice.

difficult and complications, such as pneumonia and fractures, may be terminal events. The benefits and burdens of artificial nutrition and hydration must be balanced in the late stages.

Trajectory 4: Severe Acute Brain Injury

Sudden impairment trajectories are those that stem from sudden neurologic injury that can lead to profound cognitive and functional impairment. These include the causes of severe acute brain injury: stroke, hypoxic ischemic encephalopathy, and traumatic brain injury. The vast majority of deaths occur either early after the event, when treatments are withheld or withdrawn, or in the chronic stage in survivors who have accumulating debility. The diagnoses in this trajectory represent the leading cause of adult disability. At the extremes of impairment are chronic disorders of consciousness (vegetative and minimally conscious states) and locked-in syndrome. But there is a vast spectrum of severe impairments short of these extremes that raise questions about how to manage potentially severe debility with little or uncertain chances of improvement. This trajectory requires a health care system responsive to negotiating goals of treatment with patients and surrogates who may consider these future health states to be "worse than death."

INTRODUCING PALLIATIVE CARE TO PATIENTS AND FAMILIES

Patients with serious, potentially life-threatening illnesses and their families are very vulnerable and initially may be frightened about the prospect of receiving palliative care. This fear develops from the association of palliative care with end-of-life care and some have even used the term "supportive care" to avoid this negative association. Such concerns, however, can be addressed by reinforcing that palliative care is intended to augment the usual treatment plan and that the integration of palliative care is designed to meet several objectives: (1) to ensure that pain and symptom control, psychosocial distress, spiritual issues, and practical needs are addressed throughout the continuum of care; (2) to make certain that patients and families obtain the information they need in an ongoing and comprehensible manner to understand their prognosis and treatment options. This process incorporates their values and preferences, and is sensitive to changes in the patient's condition over time; (3) palliative care seeks to provide seamless care coordination across settings with high-quality communication among providers; and (4) for those patients who are not going to recover, palliative care prepares patients and families, to the extent possible, for the dying process and for death, including options for hospice care, opportunities for personal growth and bereavement support.

SUFFERING AND SYMPTOM MANAGEMENT

Palliative care aims to relieve suffering, which is defined as severe distress related to events that threaten the stability of personhood or interconnectedness of the physical, psychological, spiritual, and social aspects of self. Beginning with simple, open-ended screening questions, such as "*In what ways are you suffering most?*" and following with more domain-related screening questions (e.g., physical, psychological, spiritual, social) may allow for more probing and multidimensional inquiries to better understand the various sources of and contributions to an individual's suffering.

One of the first steps in the care of any seriously ill patient is to control pain and other forms of physical suffering. There are striking similarities between the burden of symptoms experienced in patients dying of cancer and noncancer conditions. Although the profile of symptoms may differ, each disease carries with it troubling symptoms that can potentially be addressed and managed.

Physical Symptoms
Pain

Uncontrolled pain dominates all other experiences, and most pain can be relieved using basic pain management strategies. This includes a detailed history and physical examination, categorizing the likely type or types (i.e., somatic, visceral, neuropathic) and severity (rated on a 0-10 scale) of pain, knowledge about proper opioid dosing strategies, and judicious use of consultations and invasive interventions (e.g., nerve blocks, epidural analgesia). The overarching three-tiered approach is to use nonopioids (e.g., acetaminophen, nonsteroidal antiinflammatory drugs) for mild pain, weak opioids (e.g., hydrocodone or codeine) for mild-to-moderate pain, and strong opioids (e.g., morphine, hydromorphone, fentanyl, methadone) for moderate to severe pain.

Developing an opioid regimen. Most seriously ill patients with chronic moderate to severe pain should be initially started on around-the-clock dosing using a short-acting opioid. Table 22.1 shows the equianalgesic dosing, usual starting doses, half-lives, and durations for the commonly available opioid agents. Once the total daily dosing has been determined (sum of all scheduled and as-needed doses), the patient may be switched to a long-acting opioid to cover the baseline requirements. As-needed opioids for breakthrough pain should be approximately 10% of the total daily dose every 1 to 2 hours orally or every 30 to 60 minutes subcutaneously or intravenously. If a patient is requiring more than four to six breakthrough doses per day, he/she should be in contact with the prescribing clinician for reevaluation of dosing. Continuous intravenous or subcutaneous infusions of opioids may be needed for rapid control of severe pain.

There are additional opioid selection recommendations for patients with renal insufficiency (avoid morphine and codeine; use hydromorphone and oxycodone with caution; methadone and fentanyl are optimal) and hepatic insufficiency (cautiously use fentanyl, hydromorphone, oxycodone, or methadone; avoid or decrease dose of morphine). Methadone is useful in palliative care because of its excellent oral bioavailability, lack of active metabolites in renal impairment, low cost, flexible route of administration (PO, IV, SC), and possible effect on both neuropathic and somatic pain. However, it does have a dose-dependent, progressively long half-life and arrhythmogenic potential; therefore, an ECG should be considered prior to starting.

Opioid adverse effects. Adverse effects with opioids exist and can be serious. Constipation occurs with all opioids, and it should be anticipated and treated by starting the patient on an appropriate bowel regimen. In refractory cases, one may consider use of methylnaltrexone, if all other methods have been exhausted.

Respiratory depression with opioid use is rare, as long as the opioid is dosed appropriately and proportionately to the severity of symptoms. Therefore, respiratory diseases, such as congestive heart failure, chronic obstructive pulmonary disease, and lung cancer should not

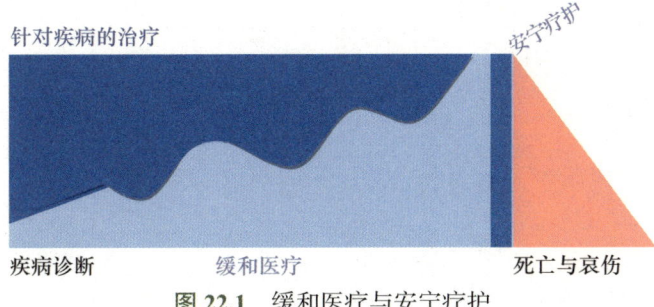

图 22.1 缓和医疗与安宁疗护

病轨迹的核心特征。照护者的负担通常非常沉重。预测生存期很困难，肺炎和骨折等并发症可能成为终末事件。在末期阶段必须权衡人工营养和水化的利弊。

轨迹 4：严重急性脑损伤

突发损伤轨迹是指由突发的神经损伤导致严重的认知和功能障碍。这些严重急性脑损伤的原因包括：卒中、缺氧缺血性脑病和创伤性脑损伤。绝大多数死亡发生在事件发生后、不采用或停止治疗的早期阶段，或是在衰弱逐渐积累的幸存者所进入的慢性阶段。这一轨迹中的诊断是成人残疾的主要原因。极端情况包括慢性意识障碍（植物状态和微意识状态）和闭锁综合征。但在这些极端情况之外，还有许多严重的情况。如何管理潜在的、改善机会微乎其微的严重失能状态仍值得探索。在这一疾病轨迹中，患者及其代理决策人可能认为未来的状况"比死亡更糟"，他们需要医疗系统能够回应其协商治疗目标的需求。

向患者及其家人介绍缓和医疗

患有严重、可能危及生命疾病的患者及其家人非常脆弱，最初可能会对接受缓和医疗感到恐惧。这种恐惧源于他们将缓和医疗与临终关怀联系在一起，有些人甚至使用"支持治疗"一词来避免这种负面关联。然而，这种担忧可通过强化以下认识来解决：强调缓和医疗旨在支持常规治疗计划，并指出整合缓和医疗旨在实现以下几个目标：①确保在整个连续照护过程中，解决疼痛和症状控制、心理与社会困扰、精神问题和实际需求。②确保患者和家庭能够持续地、以便于他们理解的方式获得其所需的信息，以帮助他们理解预后和治疗选择。这个过程需要融合患者与家庭的价值观和偏好，并对患者病情的变化保持敏感。③缓和医疗寻求在不同照护环境中进行无缝的照护协调，并在照护提供者之间保持高质量沟通。④对于那些无法康复的患者，缓和医疗尽可能地帮助患者及其家庭对离世过程和死亡进行准备，包括安宁疗护的选择、个人成长的机会和丧亲支持。

痛苦与症状管理

缓和医疗旨在缓解痛苦，这个痛苦指的是与威胁人格稳定或个体的身体、心理、精神和社会方面相互联结的相关事件引发的严重困扰。从简单、开放式的筛查问题开始，例如，"让您感到最痛苦的是哪些方面？"。随后是更多领域相关的筛查问题（例如身体、心理、精神、社会层面）来进行更深入和多维度的探询，以便更好地理解患者痛苦的具体来源。

在任何重病患者的照护中，首要步骤之一是控制疼痛和其他的身体痛苦症状。癌症和非癌症患者在临终阶段所经历的症状负荷有着惊人的相似之处。尽管症状表现可能不同，但每种疾病都伴随着可能需要解决和控制的痛苦症状。

躯体症状

疼痛

无法控制的疼痛会压倒所有其他的体验，而大多数疼痛可以通过基本的疼痛管理策略得到缓解。这包括详细的病史和体格检查，明确可能的疼痛类型（如躯体性、内脏性、神经性）并评估严重程度（以 0～10 级评分），正确的阿片类药物剂量调整，谨慎使用会诊和侵入性干预（如神经阻滞、硬膜外镇痛）。缓解疼痛的三阶梯干预方法为，使用非阿片类药物（如对乙酰氨基酚、非甾体抗炎药）治疗轻度疼痛，使用弱阿片类药物（如氢可酮或可待因）治疗轻度至中度疼痛，使用强阿片类药物（如吗啡、氢吗啡酮、芬太尼、美沙酮）治疗中度至重度疼痛。

制订阿片类药物使用方案 对于大多数患有中度至重度慢性疼痛的重病患者，最初应使用短效阿片类药物定时给药。表 22.1 显示了常见阿片类药物的等效镇痛剂量、常规起始剂量、半衰期和持续时间。一旦确定了每日总剂量（包括所有计划内和按需给药剂量的总和），患者可以转换为长效阿片类药物以覆盖基础需求。按需使用阿片类药物处理暴发痛，剂量约为每日总剂量的 10%，每 1～2 h 口服一次，或每 30～60 min 皮下或静脉注射一次。如果患者每天需要处理的暴发痛的次数超过 4～6 次，应联系处方医生重新评估给药方案。快速控制严重疼痛可能需要持续静脉或皮下注射阿片类药物。

对肾功能不全的患者，针对阿片类药物的选择的建议包括：避免使用吗啡和可待因，谨慎使用氢吗啡酮和羟考酮，美沙酮和芬太尼是最佳选择；针对肝功能不全的患者，则建议谨慎使用芬太尼、氢吗啡酮、羟考酮或美沙酮，避免使用或减少吗啡的剂量。美沙酮在缓和医疗中很有用，它具有很好的生物利用度，在肾功能不全时没有活性代谢产物，价格低、给药途径灵活（口服、静脉注射、皮下注射均可使用），对神经性和躯体性疼痛都有效。然而，它有剂量依赖性、半衰期会逐渐延长以及引发心律失常的潜在风险，在使用前应进行心电图检查。

阿片类药物不良反应 阿片类药物存在不良反应，并且可能会很严重。所有阿片类药物都会引起便秘，因此应提前预见并通过采取适当的通便方案来处理。在难治性病例中，若所有的通便方法都无效，可考虑使用甲基纳曲酮。

只要阿片类药物遵循了合适的剂量滴定并与症状的严重程度成比例，很少会发生呼吸抑制。因此，患有

TABLE 22.1 Equianalgesics for Adults

Pain	Medication	EQUIANALGESIC DOSE (FOR CHRONIC DOSING)			USUAL STARTING DOSES ADULT >50 KG; FOR OPIOID NAÏVE PATIENTS (◆ ½ DOSE FOR ELDERLY, OR SEVERE RENAL OR LIVER DISEASE)				Relative Generic Cost
		IM/IV Onset 15–30 min	PO Onset 30–60 min		Parenteral	PO	Half-Life	Duration	
Moderate to severe	Morphine	10 mg	30 mg		2.5–5 mg IV/SC q3–4h (◆1.25–2.5 mg)	5–15 mg q3–4h (IR or oral solution) (◆2.5–7.5 mg)	1.5–2 h (includes active metabolites)	3–7 h	$ (IR tablet) $$ (solution) $$ (ER generic) $$$$ (ER brand)
	Oxycodone	Not available	20 mg		Not available	5–10 mg q3–4h (◆2.5 mg)	3–4 h	4–6 h	$$ (comb. w/APAP) $$ (IR tablet) $$$ (solution) $$$ (ER brand)
	Hydromorphone	1.5 mg	7.5 mg		0.2–0.6 mg IV/SC q2–3h (◆0.2 mg)	1–2 mg q3–4h (◆0.5–1 mg)	2–3 h	4–5 h	$ (tablet) $$$ (solution) $$$$ (ER tablet)
	Methadone	Oral:IV 2:1	24 h oral morphine dose	Oral morphine:methadone ratio	1.25–2.5 mg q8h (◆1.25 mg)	2.5–5 mg q8h (◆1.25–2.5 mg)	15–190 h (N.B. large variation)	6–12 h	$ (tablet) $ (solution)
			<30 mg	2:1					
			31–99 mg	4:1					
			100–299 mg	8:1					
			300–499 mg	12:1					
			500–999 mg	15:1					
			1000–1200 mg	20:1					
			>1200 mg	Consider consult					
	Fentanyl (Duragesic Patch)	100 µg (single dose) (T1/2 life and duration of parenteral doses variable)	24 h oral morphine dose	Initial patch dose	25–50 µg IV q1–3h (◆12.5–25 µg)	12.5 µg/hr q72h (transdermal) (◆Not recommended for opioid naïve)	7 h (lozenge) 12–22 h (buccal) 13–22 h (transdermal)	60+ min (lozenge) 120+ min (buccal; not well studied) 48–72 h (transdermal)	$$$ (transdermal) $$$$ (buccal) $$$$ (buccal)
			30–59 mg	12.5 µg/hr					
			60–134 mg	25 µg/hr					
			135–224 mg	50 µg/hr					
			225–314 mg	75 µg/hr					
			315–404 mg	100 µg/hr					
Mild to moderate	Codeine	130 mg (IM only)	200 mg		15–30 mg IM/SC q4h (◆7.5–15 mg) IV contraindicated	30–60 mg q3–4h (◆15–30 mg)	3 h	4–6 h	$$ (combination with APAP) $$$ (tablet)
	Hydrocodone	Not available	30 mg		Not available	5 mg q3–4h (◆2.5 mg)	3 h	4–6 h	$$ (comb. with ibuprofen) $ (combination with APAP)

表 22.1 成人镇痛药物等剂量转换

疼痛程度	药物	等效镇痛剂量（肌注/静注 起效时间：15~30 min）	等效镇痛剂量（口服 起效时间：30~60 min）（适用于慢性疼痛）	常规起始剂量。适用于体重>50 kg，未使用过阿片类药物的成年患者，有严重肾、肝疾病患者剂量减半（◆老年患者）肠外	常规起始剂量 口服	半衰期	持续时间	相对费用
中度至重度	吗啡	10 mg	30 mg	2.5~5 mg 静脉/皮下注射 每 3~4 h 给药一次（◆1.25~2.5 mg）	5~15 mg 每 3~4 h 给药一次（即释或口服溶液）（◆2.5~7.5 mg）	1.5~2 h（包括活性代谢物）	3~7 h	$（即释片）$$（溶液）$$（仿制缓释片）$$$$（品牌缓释片）
	羟考酮	不可用	20 mg	不可用	5~10 mg 每 3~4 h 给药一次（◆2.5 mg）	3~4 h	4~6 h	$$（与对乙酰氨基酚的合剂）$$（即释片）$$$（溶液）$$$（品牌缓释片）
	氢吗啡酮	1.5 mg	7.5 mg	0.2~0.6 mg 静脉/皮下注射 每 2~3 h 给药一次（◆0.2 mg）	1~2 mg 每 3~4 h 给药一次（◆0.5~1 mg）	2~3 h	4~5 h	$（片剂）$$$（溶液）
	美沙酮	口服:静脉 2:1	口服吗啡:美沙酮的比例关系： 2:1 4:1 8:1 12:1 15:1 20:1 咨询专科医生 24 h 口服吗啡剂量： <30 mg 30~99 mg 100~299 mg 300~499 mg 500~999 mg 1000~1200 mg >1200 mg	1.25~2.5 mg 每 8 h 给药一次（◆1.25 mg）	2.5~5 mg 每 8 h 给药一次（◆1.25~2.5 mg）	15~190 h（注意：差异化巨大）	6~12 h	$（片剂）$（溶液）
	芬太尼（多瑞吉 芬太尼透皮贴剂）	100 μg（单次剂量）（肠外剂量的半衰期和持续时间可变）	24 h 口服吗啡剂量： 30~59 mg　　12.5 μg/h 60~134 mg　　25 μg/h 135~224 mg　　50 μg/h 225~314 mg　　75 μg/h 315~404 mg　　100 μg/h	25~50 μg/h 静脉每 1~3 h 给药一次（◆12.5~25 μg）	12.5 μg/h 每 72 h（透皮）贴（◆不推荐用于未使用过阿片类药物的患者）	7 h（含片）12~22 h（颊黏膜）13~22 h（透皮）	60+ min（含片）120+ min（颊黏膜；研究尚少）48~72 h（透皮）	$$$（透皮）$$$$（含片）$$$$（颊黏膜）
轻度至中度	可待因	130 mg（仅限肌内注射）	200 mg	15~30 mg 肌肉/皮下注射 每 4 h（禁用静脉注射）（◆7.5~15 mg）	30~60 mg 每 3~4 h（◆15~30 mg）	3 h	4~6 h	$$（与对乙酰氨基酚的合剂）$$$（片剂）
	氢可酮	不可用	30 mg	不可用	5 mg 每 3~4 h（◆2.5 mg）	3 h	4~6 h	$$（与布洛芬的合剂）$（与对乙酰氨基酚的合剂）

exclude opioid use in these patients. In fact, opioids can provide these patients with the additional benefit of relieving dyspnea. Furthermore, respiratory depression is almost always preceded by sedation. Therefore, if sedation develops, decreasing the dose of the opioid usually prevents respiratory depression.

Other predictable but less common side effects include nausea, myoclonus, urinary retention, pruritus, and delirium. Some of these side effects are time-limited with initiation and can be managed by dose reduction or opioid rotation.

If patients have had severe adverse effects from opioids in the past, the particular opioid associated with the adverse effects should be avoided, and other opioids should be used with caution (start with a very low dose). To avoid precipitating adverse effects in elderly and debilitated patients, recommended starting doses should be reduced by approximately 50%. Naloxone should be rarely used unless a clear overdose is suspected or if life-threatening complications occur.

Opioid crisis and abuse. The United States is currently facing a public health crisis related to opioid abuse/misuse. According to the National Institute on Drug Abuse, in 2017, more than 47,000 Americans died as a result of an opioid overdose, including prescription opioids, heroin, and illicitly manufactured fentanyl, a powerful synthetic opioid. That same year, an estimated 1.7 million people in the United States suffered from substance use disorders related to prescription opioid pain relievers, and 652,000 suffered from a heroin use disorder. Given this escalating problem, risk factors for potential opioid abuse or misuse should be screened for, including any lifetime personal or family history of substance abuse, as well as certain psychosocial characteristics (e.g., history of psychiatric illness or poor socioeconomic status) before initiating an opioid regimen. When patients with such risk factors develop painful, potentially life-limiting medical conditions, they deserve adequate pain treatment, but with extreme caution because of the risk of reactivating or aggravating abuse behavior. If risk factors are present, special precautions should be taken to minimize the risk of abuse, including clearly defined and adhered to prescribing contracts. These contracts outline an agreement with the patient, ensuring face-to-face encounters for all renewals, placing limits on opioid dosing (max daily amount) and requiring that dose adjustments can only be made after direct conversation with the prescriber. One single prescriber should be responsible for all opioid prescriptions and renewals, and one pharmacy should be used. If clinicians are inexperienced with such prescribing or there is difficulty with contract compliance, formal consultation with specialists in palliative care and/or addiction medicine should be considered.

Evidence abounds that pain is under-treated in many medical settings, including those patients who are severely and even terminally ill (especially women, the elderly, the cognitively impaired, and those from underrepresented groups). Some under-treatment stems from fears about addiction as well as concerns about the possibility of hastening death. When patients with prior addiction problems are excluded, the incidence of new addictive behavior when opioids are used to treat pain in those with a well-defined, serious illness is rare. Similarly, there are very little data to suggest that properly prescribed opioids hasten death. In fact, current evidence supports the idea that opioids may prolong life in these patients and enhance quality of life in those with advanced illness and major pain or dyspnea.

Adjuvant analgesia. Adjuvant analgesia includes both pharmacologic and nonpharmacologic therapies that may be effective in treating pain. The World Health Organization recommends that adjuvant medications be considered in all cases of pain management. Adjuvants should be tried before opioids in cases of chronic, nonmalignant pain. For malignant, moderate to severe pain, combination therapy with an opioid and an adjuvant has been shown to achieve better pain relief with less toxicity than continued escalation of the opioid alone. Adjuvants should be targeted to the particular type of pain (somatic, neuropathic, and visceral). For somatic pain, NSAIDS, acetaminophen, bisphosphonates, and corticosteroids have proven effective. For neuropathic pain, antidepressants (tricyclic and selective serotonin and norepinephrine reuptake inhibitors), anticonvulsants, and even topical analgesics (e.g., lidocaine patch) have provided relief. For visceral pain, anticholinergics have been used effectively. For a list of examples of commonly prescribed adjuvants, along with usual starting doses, please refer to Table 2.3 in Quill et al. *Primer of Palliative Care,* 7th edition. Prescribers who are unfamiliar with the use of these medications for pain management are encouraged to consult further with specialists in palliative care or pain management.

Other Symptoms

There are numerous non-pain physical symptoms that can dominate and overwhelm the clinical picture in any given patient. These include dyspnea, nausea and vomiting, constipation, anorexia-cachexia, fatigue, bleeding, agitation, apathy, myoclonus, pruritus, and specific functional deficits. Each symptom requires a structured approach to the history and physical examination with a full exploration of the potential etiologies and treatment options informed by the prognosis and preferences of the patient and family. A few of these are discussed in more detail here, but for practical information geared toward basic management of symptoms in palliative care refer to Quill et al., *Primer of Palliative Care,* 7th ed.

Dyspnea. Dyspnea is defined by the American Thoracic society as "a subjective experience of breathing discomfort." It is a common symptom at the end of life, experienced by patients suffering from diseases such as cancer, COPD, CHF, and pulmonary fibrosis. Dyspnea is very distressing, and when severe, requires urgent intervention.

The first step in management is identification of the underlying cause/disease, followed by treatment directed towards the particular etiology. After the underlying etiology is addressed, if dyspnea remains a prominent symptom, there are several general measures which can be done. These include reducing the need for exertion, repositioning the patient to a more upright position, keeping the compromised lung down in unilateral disease and improving air circulation by opening windows/doors or using a bedside fan.

Opioids are the preferred agents for symptomatically treating dyspnea because they effectively suppress awareness of the sensation of shortness of breath. Most routes of administration are effective except the use of nebulized opioids. There is emerging evidence that low-dose, sustained-release morphine may provide lasting relief of dyspnea, mainly in COPD patients. Some providers avoid the use of opioids for dyspnea out of fear of causing respiratory depression. However, in the absence of preexisting carbon dioxide (CO_2) retention, respiratory depression is uncommon in patients who are on carefully titrated dosages of opioids.

Anxiety and dyspnea frequently exacerbate one another. It is important to treat an anxious dyspneic patient with opioids first to reduce breathlessness and then follow with a benzodiazepine if anxiety persists.

Nausea and vomiting. Nausea and vomiting are some of the most distressing symptoms for patients. Studies have shown that these symptoms are experienced by up to 78% of patients with advanced cancer at some point during their disease course. They also occur in other advanced illnesses, including end-stage cardiac, renal, and liver disease. Persistent nausea and vomiting can affect appetite, pain management, and the quality of interactions with family members or friends.

CHF、COPD 和肺癌等呼吸系统疾病的患者不应排斥阿片类药物的使用。事实上，阿片类药物可以给这些患者带来缓解呼吸困难的作用。此外，在出现呼吸抑制之前几乎都是先出现镇静的效果。因此，一旦患者出现镇静即减少阿片类药物剂量通常可以预防呼吸抑制的发生。

其他可预见但不太常见的副作用包括恶心、肌阵挛、尿潴留、瘙痒和谵妄。这些副作用通常是自限性的，可以通过降低剂量或阿片类药物的轮替来解决。

如果患者过去使用阿片类药物曾经出现严重的不良反应，应避免使用与不良反应相关的特定阿片类药物，并谨慎使用其他阿片类药物（从非常低的剂量开始）。为了避免在老年和虚弱患者中引发可预见的不良反应，推荐起始剂量应减少约 50%。除非怀疑有明确的药物过量或危及生命的并发症发生，否认很少使用纳洛酮。

阿片类药物危机和滥用 美国正面临与阿片类药物滥用 / 误用相关的公共卫生危机。根据美国国家药物滥用研究所的数据，2017 年，超过 4.7 万美国人死于阿片类药物使用过量，包括处方阿片类药物、海洛因和非法制造的强效合成阿片类药物芬太尼。同年，美国约 170 万人存在与处方阿片类镇痛药物相关的毒品滥用，65.2 万人存在海洛因滥用。鉴于这一日益严重的问题，在开始阿片类药物治疗之前，应筛查潜在的阿片类药物滥用或误用的危险因素，包括个人或家族物质滥用史，以及某些社会心理特征（如精神疾病史或社会经济地位差）。当有这些危险因素的患者出现疼痛、可能危及生命的医疗状况时，他们应得到充分的疼痛治疗，但由于有重新激活或加重滥用行为的风险，治疗必须极为谨慎。若存在危险因素，应采取特别的预防措施以最大限度减少滥用风险，包括明确定义并严格遵守的处方规定：处方规定应包含与患者的协议，确保所有续药都面对面进行，限定阿片类药物的剂量（每日最大剂量），并要求只有在与处方医生直接面谈后才能调整剂量。所有阿片类药物的处方和续药应由单一处方医生负责，并在同一家药房进行。如果临床医生在此类处方方面缺乏经验或存在难以确保规定执行的情况，应考虑向缓和医疗和（或）药物成瘾专家正式咨询。

有大量证据表明，在许多医疗环境中患者的疼痛治疗不足，包括那些重病甚至末期患者（尤其是女性、老年人、认知障碍患者和弱势群体）。部分治疗不足的状况源于对成瘾的恐惧以及对可能加速死亡的担忧。在排除了患者从前存在成瘾问题的情况下，使用阿片类药物治疗由明确严重疾病引发的疼痛时，成瘾的发生率很低。同样，几乎没有数据显示处方合理的阿片类药物会加速死亡。实际上，现有证据支持阿片类药物可能延长这些患者的生命，并提高那些患有晚期疾病以及严重疼痛或呼吸困难的患者的生活质量。

辅助镇痛 辅助镇痛包括对疼痛有效的药物和非药物方法。世界卫生组织建议在所有疼痛案例中都应考虑辅助镇痛药物。对慢性非恶性疼痛的病例，应在使用阿片类药物之前尝试辅助镇痛药物。对于恶性疾病引发的中度至重度疼痛，与单纯使用阿片类药物持续增加剂量相比，阿片类药物联合辅助药物治疗已被证明能更好地缓解疼痛且毒性更低。应针对特定类型的疼痛（如躯体性、神经性和内脏性）给予不同的辅助镇痛药物。对于躯体性疼痛，非甾体抗炎药、对乙酰氨基酚、双膦酸盐和皮质类固醇已被证明有效。对于神经性疼痛，抗抑郁药（三环类、选择性 5-羟色胺和去甲肾上腺素再摄取抑制剂）、抗惊厥药，甚至局部镇痛药（如利多卡因贴片）可帮助缓解疼痛。对于内脏性疼痛，可使用抗胆碱类药物。关于常用辅助镇痛药物的示例及其常规起始剂量，请参阅 Quill 等人所著 *Primer of Palliative Care* 第 7 版中的表 2.3。对不熟悉这些疼痛管理药物使用方法的医生，应多咨询缓和医疗或疼痛管理专科医生。

其他症状

任何患者都可能出现许多疼痛以外的身体症状，这些症状可能占据主导地位并使病情复杂化。这些症状包括呼吸困难、恶心和呕吐、便秘、厌食-恶病质、疲乏、出血、烦躁不安、淡漠、肌阵挛、瘙痒和特定功能缺陷。每种症状都需要用结构化的方法进行病史采集和体格检查，并充分探讨潜在的病因和治疗选择，最终应根据预后和患者及其家庭的偏好来做出最终临床决策。下面将详细讨论其中的一些症状，但有关缓和医疗中症状基本管理的更实用的信息请参阅 Quill 等人所著 *Primer of Palliative Care* 第 7 版。

呼吸困难 美国胸科协会将呼吸困难定义为"一种主观的呼吸不适的体验"。它是生命末期的常见症状，常见于癌症、COPD、CHF 和肺纤维化的患者。呼吸困难令人十分痛苦，当症状严重时需要紧急干预。

症状管理的第一步是识别潜在的原因 / 疾病，然后针对特定病因进行治疗。在解决潜在病因后，如果呼吸困难仍然是突出症状，可以采取一些综合措施。这些措施包括：减少运动引发的耗氧需求，将患者调整到更直立的位置，在单肺疾病的情况下让受损的肺在下方，以及打开门窗或使用床边风扇来改善空气流通。

阿片类药物是治疗呼吸困难的首选药物，这类药物能有效抑制患者气短的感觉。除了雾化外，阿片类药物在大多数给药途径下都有效。有越来越多证据表明，低剂量、缓释吗啡能为 COPD 患者持久缓解呼吸困难。一些医生出于对药物引起呼吸抑制的担忧而不敢使用阿片类药物治疗呼吸困难。实际上，在没有二氧化碳（CO_2）潴留的情况下，于严格滴定的情况下使用阿片类药物，患者发生呼吸抑制的情况很罕见。

焦虑和呼吸困难经常相互影响加剧症状。对于合并焦虑的呼吸困难患者，首先使用阿片类药物来减少呼吸急促是非常重要的，如果焦虑持续存在，则随后加用苯二氮䓬类药物。

恶心和呕吐 恶心和呕吐是患者最痛苦的症状之一。研究表明，高达 78% 的晚期癌症患者会在其疾病过程中某个阶段经历这个症状。恶心和呕吐也会发生在其他晚期疾病中，包括终末期心脏病、肾病和肝病。持续的恶心和呕吐会影响食欲、疼痛管理以及与家人或朋友之间的互动质量。

When evaluating patients with nausea and vomiting, it is important to first consider whether the symptoms are a result of intra-abdominal factors (e.g., gastroparesis, ileus, gastric outlet obstruction, bowel obstruction) or extra-abdominal factors (drugs, electrolyte abnormalities, central nervous system metastases). The goal is to identify and treat underlying reversible causes first.

In most cases, empiric pharmacologic treatment is necessary to immediately control symptoms. There are a number of pharmacologic agents that have been shown to be useful for nausea/vomiting, depending on the etiology. One of the most useful is haloperidol. When nausea and vomiting are due to increased intracranial pressure, a steroid such as dexamethasone is useful. Metoclopramide may be useful in situations of delayed gastric emptying or early satiety. When nausea and vomiting are due to inner-ear pathology or motion sickness, antihistamines can help manage vertigo.

In addition, high dosages of a combination of agents may be required for adequate control of symptoms. Treating patients with a scheduled dose of antiemetics can often prevent recurrent nausea. If the patient is too nauseated to tolerate oral medications, consider SC, IV, or PR routes.

Constipation. Palliative care patients are at particularly high risk for developing constipation due to a combination of factors, including decreased PO intake, impaired mobility and use of opioid analgesics.

Pharmacologic options for management of constipation include stool softeners (docusate sodium), stimulants (Senokot and bisacodyl), and osmotic agents (polyethylene glycol, lactulose, magnesium hydroxide, magnesium citrate). The key to adequate management of constipation in the palliative care setting is prevention, which involves initiation of a maintenance bowel regimen. If the patient has a history of constipation, the preferred maintenance regimen should be the patient's regular home regimen. If constipation has never been a problem in the past, starting with senna can be a good option. Docusate may also be used initially; however, the efficacy of docusate alone is limited, and most patients will require addition of a bowel stimulant, like senna or bisacodyl. Osmotic agents, such as polyethylene glycol or lactulose, are effective additions to most bowel regimens but may also bring about adverse effects such as bloating and flatulence. Rectal suppositories and enemas may be necessary when constipation is severe. Avoid bulk-forming agents (psyllium, methylcellulose) in palliative care patients, as these agents can lead to impactions with inadequate fluid intake.

All of the above medications may be used in combination when managing constipation. However, maximizing the dose/frequency of current bowel medications will typically provide desired effects and should be done prior to addition of other medications.

Medical Marijuana

Cannabis has several beneficial health effects although clinical data are limited because of restrictions on research.

The body contains an endogenous network known as the endocannabinoid system, which involves two receptors, CB1 and CB2. As endocannabinoids interact with these receptors, they impact many physiologic processes, including gastrointestinal (GI) function, appetite, metabolism, pain, memory, movement, immunity, and inflammation. Cannabis contains phytocannabinoids, Δ-tetrahydrocannabinol (THC) and cannabidiol (CBD), which interact with these receptors much the same way that endocannabinoids do, thereby providing the various medicinal effects that are observed with cannabis use.

THC is the primary psychoactive constituent of cannabis. Observed effects include impairments of learning, memory, spatial orientation, and attention. However, patients also report benefits including antiemetic, analgesic, and anti-inflammatory properties. CBD lacks the THC-induced intoxicating properties, and the presence of CBD in a cannabis product is actually believed to counteract the psychosis-inducing effects of THC. CBD has reported benefits of anticonvulsant, anxiolytic, anti-inflammatory, and neuroprotective properties; however, none of these have been verified. Synthetic cannabinoids currently marketed are dronabinol, a biochemically identical form of THC, and nabilone, a THC analogue. Both can be prescribed clinically for nausea and/or vomiting, appetite stimulation, pain, and spasticity.

The National Academies of Sciences, Engineering, and Medicine (NASEM) published a comprehensive literature review on the health effects of cannabis and concluded that there is substantial evidence that cannabis is effective (1) for the treatment of chronic pain, (2) as an antiemetic in chemotherapy-induced nausea and vomiting, and (3) for muscle spasticity syndromes in MS. As far as adverse effects, the NASEM concluded that there is substantial evidence for an association between cannabis smoking and respiratory disease, motor vehicle collisions (MVCs), lower birthweight offspring, and schizophrenia or other psychoses.

Medicolegal realities surrounding medical cannabis are rapidly evolving in the United States. As of publication of this book, 33 US states and the District of Columbia have programs authorizing cannabis use for specific medical conditions. Because cannabis is illegal under federal law, clinicians cannot prescribe it and pharmacies cannot dispense it as they would with other pharmaceuticals. States require health care professionals to be registered in order to certify patients for cannabis use. Cannabis is then supplied to patients through state-licensed medical cannabis dispensaries, in various forms, including vaporized oils or plant material, sublingual tinctures, and oral capsules.

Psychological Distress

Depression, anxiety, and delirium are all common in the palliative care setting. They are frequently under-recognized and under-treated, although appropriate diagnosis and treatment can have significant improvement in a patient's quality of life.

Depression and Anxiety

Almost all patients in palliative care and their families experience normal sadness/grief as illness advances. Depression, however, is more enduring, persistent, intense, and may be associated with hopelessness, helplessness, worthlessness, and guilt. Two questions, found to have high sensitivity for depression screening, include: "*Are you depressed?*" and "*Do you have much interest and pleasure in doing things?*" A more formal exploration is indicated if the patient gives a positive answer to either of these questions. One should be cautious about overusing somatic symptoms to diagnose depression (e.g., fatigue, anorexia, sleep disturbance) because they frequently overlap with physiological changes associated with advanced disease. Terminally ill patients with depression are at higher risk of suicide and suicidal ideation, and they may have increased desires and requests for hastened death.

Anxiety symptoms may be triggered by a range of medical transitions, such as the initial diagnosis of serious illness, a recurrence of illness, treatment side effects/failure, or discussion of hospice. The patient may also have underlying fears related to their disease and end-of-life, including uncontrolled pain, isolation, abandonment, loss of control, worry about family members or even the idea of death/dying.

Regarding treatment of depression and anxiety, first recognize and address contributions from physical symptoms (e.g., uncontrolled pain), medical causes (e.g., hypothyroidism, hyperthyroidism), and medications. Effective pharmacologic and nonpharmacologic treatments exist for both depression and anxiety, though treatment selection depends on symptom intensity, patient prognosis, and treatment benefits and burdens. Other members of the interdisciplinary team

在评估恶心和呕吐的患者时，首先要考虑这些症状是由腹腔内因素（如胃轻瘫、麻痹性肠梗阻、胃出口梗阻、肠道梗阻）还是腹腔外因素（药物、电解质异常、中枢神经系统转移）引起的。目标是首先识别并治疗潜在的可逆性病因。

在大多数情况下，需要经验性药物治疗来迅速控制症状。针对不同的病因，许多药物已被证明对恶心和呕吐有效。其中最有效的是氟哌啶醇。当恶心和呕吐是由于颅内压升高引起时，可使用类固醇类药物如地塞米松。甲氧氯普胺可用于胃排空延迟或早饱的情况。当恶心和呕吐是由内耳病变或晕动病引起时，抗组胺药可以帮助控制眩晕。

此外，可能需要多种药物高剂量联合应用来充分控制症状。计划性地给予患者止吐药通常可以预防恶心症状的再发。如果患者无法耐受口服药物，可考虑皮下、静脉或直肠给药。

便秘 由于多种因素的共同作用，缓和医疗的患者特别容易发生便秘，这些因素包括口服摄入减少、活动受限和使用阿片类镇痛药。

治疗便秘的药物选择包括大便软化剂（多库酯钠）、刺激性泻药（番泻苷类药物和比沙可啶）和渗透性泻药（聚乙二醇、乳果糖、氢氧化镁、柠檬酸镁）。在缓和医疗中有效管理便秘的关键是预防，这就需要有一个持续性的肠道管理方案。如果患者有便秘史，首选的维持方案应是患者在家中使用的常规治疗方案。如果患者既往从未有过便秘的困扰，初始选择可以考虑番泻叶。多库酯也可以作为初始选择，但单独使用多库酯效果有限，大多数患者需要加用肠道刺激剂，如番泻叶或比沙可啶。渗透性药物，如聚乙二醇或乳果糖，是大多数肠道管理方案的有效补充，但也可能带来腹胀和胀气等不良反应。当便秘严重时，可能需要使用直肠栓剂和灌肠剂。应避免对缓和医疗患者使用容积性泻药（洋车前子、甲基纤维素），因为这些药物在液体摄入不足的情况下可能导致嵌塞。

在治疗便秘时，上述所有药物均可联合使用。当然，在增加其他药物之前，通常应先将当前肠道药物的剂量和频率最大化以达到预期效果。

医用大麻

大麻有一些有益的健康效果。但由于研究受限，临床数据有限。人体包含一个称为内源性大麻素系统的网络，它涉及两种受体，CB1和CB2。内源性大麻素与这些受体相互作用，影响许多生理过程，包括胃肠功能、食欲、代谢、疼痛、记忆、运动、免疫和炎症。大麻含有植物大麻素、Δ-四氢大麻酚（THC）和大麻二酚（CBD），它们与这些受体的相互作用方式与内源性大麻素类似，从而产生了使用大麻时观察到的各种药用效果。

THC是大麻的主要精神活性成分，观察到的效果包括对学习、记忆、空间定向和注意力的损害。此外，患者也报告了包括止吐、镇痛和抗炎特性在内的益处。CBD不具有THC引起的致幻特性，被认为可以抵消THC诱发的精神症状。CBD已被报道具有抗惊厥、抗焦虑、抗炎和神经保护特性，然而这些都未被验证。目前上市的合成大麻素包括生化上与THC相同的屈大麻酚（dronabinol）和THC类似物大麻隆（nabilone）。两者都可以在临床上用于治疗恶心和（或）呕吐、刺激食欲、治疗疼痛和痉挛。

美国国家科学院、工程院和医学院（NASEM）发表了一份关于大麻对健康影响的综合文献综述，并得出如下结论：有大量证据表明大麻在以下方面是有效的：①治疗慢性疼痛，②作为止吐药用于化疗引起的恶心和呕吐，③用于多发性硬化症的肌肉痉挛综合征。就不良反应而言，NASEM指出，有大量证据表明吸食大麻与呼吸系统疾病、机动车事故、后代低出生体重和精神分裂症或其他精神疾病之间存在关联。

在美国关于医用大麻的法律正在迅速演变。截至本书出版时，美国33个州和哥伦比亚特区已授权大麻用于特定的医疗项目。由于大麻在联邦法律下是非法的，临床医生不能开具处方，药房也不能像其他药品一样发放大麻。各州要求医疗专业人员注册，从而为患者使用大麻提供认证。可通过州政府许可的有医用大麻分发权限药房向患者供应多种剂型的大麻，包括挥发性油剂或植物药材、舌下酊剂和口服胶囊。

心理困扰

抑郁、焦虑和谵妄在缓和医疗环境中都很常见。尽管适当的诊断和治疗可以显著改善患者的生活质量，但它们经常被忽视且得不到充分的治疗。

抑郁与焦虑

几乎所有缓和医疗的患者及家庭在疾病进展时都会经历正常的悲伤/哀伤。然而，抑郁更为持久、持续和强烈，并可能与绝望、无助、无价值和内疚感有关。两个敏感性较高的用于筛查抑郁的问题是："你感到抑郁吗？"和"你做事情有兴趣和愉悦感吗？"。如果患者对其中任何一个问题给出阳性回答，则需要进行更正式的评估。应注意不要过度使用躯体症状（如疲劳、厌食、睡眠障碍）来诊断抑郁，这些症状经常与晚期疾病相关的生理变化相重叠。患有抑郁症的终末期患者自杀和有自杀意念的风险更高，他们可能会有更强烈的加速死亡的愿望和要求。

焦虑症状可能由一系列医疗上的变化触发，例如严重疾病的初次诊断、疾病复发、治疗副作用或治疗失败或讨论到安宁疗护。患者可能还有对疾病和生命终结相关的潜在恐惧，包括无法控制的疼痛、孤独、被抛弃、失控感、对家人的担忧，或是对死亡/濒死的想法。

关于抑郁和焦虑的治疗，首先要识别和处理身体症状（如无法控制的疼痛）、疾病原因（如甲状腺功能减退症、甲状腺功能亢进症）和药物的影响。对于抑郁和焦虑，尽管治疗选择取决于症状强度、患者预后以及治疗的获益和负担，药物和非药物方面均有有效的方法。跨学科团队中的其他成员（社工、牧师和心理学专家）在抑郁及焦虑评估和持续管理中经常发挥关键性作用。

(social worker, chaplain, and psychologist) often play a critical role in assessment and ongoing management.

Delirium

Delirium, an acquired and fluctuating disorder of consciousness and cognition, occurs commonly in the palliative care setting. The level of psychomotor activity can vary from hyperactive ("agitated" delirium) to hypoactive ("quiet" delirium). Nearly 80% of the delirium in the palliative care setting is the hypoactive variant. As a result, it is often under-diagnosed or misdiagnosed as depression and fatigue. The most common causes of delirium in palliative care include medications (e.g., opioids), metabolic disorders due to progressive organ failure, and infection. Meticulous attention to the history from collateral sources (e.g., nurses, caregiver) and a detailed medication history are essential for an accurate diagnosis. While delirium may reverse if an obvious cause is identified and removed, frequently it represents an important marker of progressive illness; therefore, cognitive improvements may be transient and incomplete. In addition to etiology-specific treatment (e.g., change or stop medications, treat infection, oxygen, hydration, bisphosphonates), environmental interventions are recommended for all patients (e.g., quiet reassurance, gentle reorientation, optimize sensory input, minimize night disruptions). Pharmacologic management should be used sparingly and cautiously and may include antipsychotic medications, benzodiazepines, and psychostimulants (for the hypoactive variant). Keep in mind that benzodiazepines can sometimes have a paradoxical effect, worsening confusion and agitation in delirium.

Spiritual and Existential Suffering

Spiritual and existential distress is prevalent in patients and families with serious illness, especially at the end of life. Spirituality is about one's relationship with and responses to transcendent questions that confront one as a human being (e.g., search for meaning and purpose in life). Religion is a set of texts, practices, and beliefs about the transcendence shared by a community. Spirituality is broader than religion. The spiritual issues of seriously ill and dying patients often center on questions of meaning, value, and relationships. Dying patients want to be assured of their value in the face of actual or perceived threats to their intactness as a human being (e.g., physical and cognitive declines, altered appearances). Spirituality can help people find hope in despair and can help restore purpose.

One of the goals of palliative care is to relieve spiritual and existential distress. Patients and families often welcome such discussions. Examples of open-ended questions to facilitate this dialogue include: "*Are you at peace with all of this?*" and "*Is faith (religion, spirituality) important to you?*" Acknowledgement and empathetic listening are the most important responses for most clinicians, as opposed to trying to provide "correct answers."

Other strategies for fostering hope and meaning include developing caring relationships, setting attainable goals, involving the patient in the decision-making process, affirming the patient's worth, using lighthearted humor (when appropriate), and reminiscing with life review. It is important, however, to know one's professional boundaries and refer to chaplains or clergy from the patient's faith traditions if questions move beyond the realm of general exploration (e.g., "*It sounds like it would be good to explore this with someone with more experience than I have. Would it be okay for me to send our chaplain in to discuss this with you?*").

COMMUNICATION AND CARE COORDINATION

Excellent communication skills are central to palliative care, including communication with patients, family members, other physicians, nurses, and other members of the health care team. The overarching aim is to assist the patient and family in establishing the goals of current and future treatment in a shared decision-making process.

Negotiating Goals of Care

When negotiating goals of treatment in palliative care, the focus is often to assist with the following decisions: to help decide types and aggressiveness of disease-directed therapies; to ensure optimum palliation of symptoms; to assist in hospice determinations; to discuss initiating, withholding or withdrawing therapies; to facilitate advance care planning; and to initiate surrogate decision making if the patient lacks capacity. These discussions occur at various time points in the course of advancing illness when new and important information is learned and needs to be communicated to the patient and family. The need to renegotiate goals should also be anticipated when triggers of advancing disease suggest limited life expectancy or excessive suffering. These discussions are almost always variants of "bad news" discussions.

The overall approach to communication and negotiating goals of care is standard among all patients, illnesses, and situations (Table 22.2). This includes running an effective family meeting, with or without the patient present. Initial elements include establishing the proper setting, identifying key stakeholders, and "doing your homework" (i.e., discussing potential plans with all relevant subspecialties who may have communicated with the patient and family). When the meeting begins, find out what the patient and family understand about the medical condition and ask what additional information they want to know. Keep an open mind and try to hold back on a fixed agenda (e.g., to "get the DNR" or to "stop futile care"). This allows patients and family members sufficient time to "tell their stories" and provides the context within which effective decision making can occur. In general, the more patients and families speak in the early parts of such meetings, the better.

The provider then needs to share prognostic information and discuss the benefits and burdens of the available treatment options. Alerting the patient or family of impending bad news with a warning shot (e.g., "*I am afraid I have some difficult news to share with you*") is a useful initial communication strategy. The amount of information should be paced with frequent pauses to allow time for emotional responses. Comprehension should be frequently checked, and questions should be encouraged using an "ask-tell-ask" strategy. The skilled clinician can flexibly assess, probe, and pace the content and depth of the discussion in an emotionally responsive (acknowledge, explore, empathize, and legitimize) and culturally competent manner. This includes the ability to understand and respect diverse religious practices and differing preferences about degree of truth telling. When appropriate, the clinician should make recommendations based on scientific knowledge as well as awareness of a patient's values and preferences and be prepared to help resolve conflicts among the patient, family members, and providers. Finally, providers need to develop strategies to preserve and potentially reframe hope, including ways to "*hope for the best*" and simultaneously "*prepare for the worst.*" Commitments to minimize suffering and to not abandon the patient and family are essential. At the end of the discussions, the provider should summarize key aspects of what was reviewed and establish a follow-up plan for future communications and treatments.

Estimating and Communicating Prognosis

A core component of information shared in the palliative care setting is prognosis. Understanding prognosis is central to making decisions (e.g., treatment, comfort measures, hospice). Prognosis is a prediction of possible future outcomes of a disease (e.g., survival, symptoms, function, quality of life, family and financial impact) with or without treatment. Most patients and families want to know prognosis. Since

谵妄

谵妄是一种获得性和波动性的意识和认知障碍，在缓和医疗场景中十分常见。患者精神运动活动的水平可从激越（"躁动型"谵妄）到淡漠（"安静型"谵妄）。缓和医疗中，近80%的谵妄是淡漠型。因此，谵妄经常被漏诊或误诊为抑郁和疲劳。缓和医疗中谵妄最常见原因包括药物（如阿片类药物）、由于器官衰竭进展引起的代谢紊乱和感染。仔细收集来自其他信息来源（如护士、照护者）的病史信息以及详细的用药史对谵妄的准确诊断至关重要。尽管在识别和去除明显原因后，谵妄有可能逆转，但它通常是疾病进展的重要标志；因此，认知的改善可能只是暂时和不完全的。除了针对特定病因的治疗（如更换或停用药物、治疗感染、吸氧、水化、使用双膦酸盐），还需要关注所有谵妄患者的环境因素（如安抚、温和的定位引导、优化感官感受、减少夜间干扰等）。药物治疗应谨慎使用，包括抗精神病药物、苯二氮䓬类药物和精神兴奋剂（用于淡漠型谵妄）。需要注意的是，苯二氮䓬类药物有时会产生相反的效果，导致谵妄的意识混乱和躁动症状加重。

精神痛苦和存在性痛苦

精神和存在性困扰在重病患者及其家属中普遍存在，尤其在临近生命尽头的阶段。精神（译者注：Spirituality译法有争议，此处译为精神）是关于个人作为人类与所面临的超越性问题的关系和反应（如寻找生命的意义和目的）。宗教则是一套由一个社交群体所共享的、关于超越性的文本、实践和信仰。精神相关的概念比宗教更广泛。重病和终末期患者的精神相关问题通常集中在意义、价值和关系的层面上。临终患者希望在面对人的完整性受到实际的或感知上的威胁（如身体和认知的下降，外貌的改变）时，其价值能够被肯定。精神，可以帮助人们在绝望中找到希望，并助力其恢复目标。

缓和医疗的目标之一是缓解精神层面和存在层面的困扰，患者和家属通常也愿意展开这类讨论。促进这类谈话的开放式问题可以是："你对发生的这一切感到内心平静吗"和"信仰（宗教，精神层面）对你来说重要吗"。对于大多数临床医生来说，认同患者表述的内容以及富有同理心的倾听是最重要的回应方式，而不是试图提供所谓的"正确答案"。

另外，有助于找到希望和意义的其他方法包括建立关怀关系，设定可实现的目标，让患者参与到决策过程中来，肯定其价值，在适当时候带入轻快的幽默感，以及进行生命回顾。同时，医护人员了解自己的职业界限很重要，在问题超出常规的范畴时需要转介至患者信仰体系中的牧师或神职人员（如"听起来，跟比我更有经验的人来探讨这件事会更好一些，我可以请牧师来和您讨论这个问题吗？"）。

沟通与照护协调

出色的沟通技巧是缓和医疗的核心，包括与患者、家属、其他医护人员及医疗团队其他成员的沟通。沟通的主要目标是在共同决策过程中，协助患者和家属确立当前和未来的治疗目标。

协商照护目标

缓和医疗在协商治疗目标时，重点通常在于协助进行以下决策：帮助决定针对疾病治疗的类型和积极程度；确保症状得到最佳缓解；协助确定进入安宁疗护；讨论启动、不进行或撤除治疗；促进预立照护计划；在患者缺乏决策能力时启动代理决策机制。在疾病进展过程中的多个时间点，当出现新的重要信息并需要传达给患者和家属时，就会进行这类讨论。也应预见到，在疾病进展提示预期寿命有限或过度痛苦时，都需要重新协商照护目标。这些讨论几乎都是不同形式的关于"坏消息"的讨论。

与不同的患者、不同疾病和不同情境下的患者沟通和协商照护目标的总体方法是标准化的（表22.2）。需要召开一场患者在场或者不在场的、有效的家庭会议。家庭会议的基本元素包括设置好适当的环境，确定关键利益相关者，以及"做好准备工作"（即，和所有可能已经与患者和家属沟通过的相关专业医疗人员讨论潜在可行的计划）。会议开始时，了解患者和家属对病情的理解，并询问他们还希望了解哪些信息。医护人员需保持开放的心态，尽量不要试图完成某个固定的目标（如"获取拒绝心肺复苏同意书"或"停止无效治疗"），这样可以让患者和家属有充分的时间"讲述他们的故事"，从而为有效决策提供出背景信息。一般来说，在这类家庭会议的早期，患者和家属说得越多，会议效果越好。

医护人员需要告知患者及家属预后相关信息并讨论治疗选项的利弊。在初始沟通环节，使用预警语（如"恐怕我有一些不好的消息要告诉你"）来提醒患者或家属即将到来的坏消息是一种有效的策略。向患者及家属传递的信息量应该适度，并经常停顿，以便为其留出情绪反应的时间。应经常核实患者及家属的理解程度，并鼓励使用"问-说-问"的策略来提问。沟通技能熟练的临床医生可以通过采用呼应患方情感（承认、探索、共情和合理化）及适合本地文化的方式来灵活地评估、探究和调整讨论的内容和深度。这需要医生理解和尊重不同的宗教习俗以及患方对真相告知程度的想法。在适当的时候，临床医生应根据科学知识以及患者的价值观和偏好提出建议，并随时准备为解决患者、家属和照护者之间的冲突提供帮助。最后，医护人员需要找到保护和重建希望的方法，包括让患者"期待最好的结果"，同时"为最坏的情况做准备"。向患者及家属承诺会尽可能减轻他们的痛苦并且不会放弃他们是至关重要的。在讨论结束时，医护人员应总结所讨论的关键点，并制订出未来沟通和治疗的随诊计划。

评估和沟通预后

在缓和医疗中，共享信息的核心是预后。理解预后对于做出医疗决策（如治疗、舒适措施、安宁疗护）至关重要。预后指的是对疾病（在治疗或不治疗的情况下）未来发展结果的预测（如生存期、症状、功能、生

TABLE 22.2	General Strategy for Communicating and Negotiating Goals of Care in Common Palliative Care Settings
Step 1	Prepare and establish setting
	Do not have a rigid preset agenda
Step 2	Ask patient and family what they know and understand
	Provide sufficient time for patients and families to "tell their story"
	Active listening skills
Step 3	Find out how much patient and family want to know
	Acknowledge and explore emotions
Step 4	Give information in small amounts, and frequently check understanding
	Discuss prognosis and benefits and burdens of treatment options
	Be mindful of overly optimistic and pessimistic predictions
	Be prepared to make recommendations
Step 5	Respond to emotions and empathetic response
	Convey honesty and reframe hope
	Use "I wish" statements
Step 6	Summarize, establish and implement plan, follow-up
	Possible time-limited trial

there are some patients and families that may not want to know prognosis or may want it communicated in a particular way, it is essential to begin by finding out what the patient and family knows and wants to know.

Inaccurate predictions may lead to poor decision making. Physicians tend to overestimate survival in patients with advanced cancer by about 30%, and the bias is more pronounced the longer the physician-patient relationship. Overly optimistic predictions can lead to overuse of ineffective or unwanted disease-directed treatment, delay in hospice referrals, false expectations, unnecessary tests and procedures, and poor symptom control. Therefore, accurately estimating and communicating prognosis is central to optimal decision making in advanced illness and at the end of life.

In advanced illnesses, common factors found to be predictive of short-term survival (i.e., less than 6 months) include performance status, anorexia-cachexia syndrome, delirium, and dyspnea. The Palliative Performance Scale can be used to measure and track a patient's functional status. It is available in a variety of websites and books. In addition to a physician's subjective predictions of survival, there exist models to assist with prognostic estimates, including generic models for particular populations (e.g., hospice enrollees) as well as disease-specific models (e.g., cancers, heart failure, liver disease, stroke, AIDS, spinal cord compression). Hospice eligibility criteria also differ for specific diseases. While not uniformly reliable, these criteria can be useful in formulating estimates where prognosis might be 6 months or less if the disease is allowed to run its natural course (a prognostic criterion). One example of this is the Functional Assessment Staging (FAST) scale used to determine hospice eligibility for Alzheimer's/dementia patients.

For an individual patient, however, prognostic uncertainty remains the rule. Therefore, it is important to integrate both evidence and experience-based medicine and present the information in formats tailored to the particular patient (verbal descriptions, numeric, frequencies, or graphics). Prognostic estimates should be bounded with ranges to convey realistic uncertainty, being sure to allow for exceptions in both directions. For example, "*in my experience, patients with your condition live on average a few weeks to a few months. It could be longer, but it could also be shorter.*" For survival-oriented prognoses (e.g., "*How long do I have?*"), be mindful of overly optimistic prognoses, remembering to think of and convey the lower bound (e.g., "*some may live longer, but others may, unfortunately, live shorter*"). For quality of life-oriented prognoses (e.g., "*What will life be like?*"), be mindful of overly pessimistic predictions, remembering the power of adaptation and engendering hope by helping patients and families find new meaning.

END-OF-LIFE CARE

The Role of Diagnostic Tests and Invasive Procedures

Several questions should be considered in determining the appropriateness of aggressive medical or palliative interventions near the end of life: What is the goal or expected outcome of the proposed intervention? What is the probable efficacy of the intervention? What is the patient's baseline level of function and life expectancy? What are the potential side effects and burdens of the intervention? What are the patient's and family's wishes, values, and preferences?

The range of medical and palliative options available is huge, so the challenge is to determine what makes sense to enhance the well-being of each patient at their particular stage of illness. Palliative interventions range from pure symptom management and support to invasive options, such as chemotherapy, radiotherapy, surgical/endoscopic interventions, stenting procedures, thoracentesis, paracentesis, pericardiocentesis, home inotropic therapy, noninvasive ventilation, antibiotics, or transfusions. The challenge is to individualize discussions, so that patients can take full advantage of treatments that will help them meet their goals without having their experience dominated by near futile invasive treatments.

Role of Hospice

Hospice care is a specialized form of palliative care aimed at those patients and families in the terminal stages of illness. The National Hospice and Palliative Care Organization defines hospice as follows: *Considered to be the model for quality, compassionate care for people facing a life-limiting illness or injury, hospice and palliative care involve a team-oriented approach to expert medical care, pain management, and emotional and spiritual support expressly tailored to the person's needs and wishes. Support is provided to the person's loved ones as well. The focus of hospice relies on the belief that each of us has the right to die pain free and with dignity, and that our loved ones will receive the necessary support to allow us to do so.*

Since the establishment of the Medicare Hospice Benefit in 1982, use of hospice for end-of-life care has grown steadily. In 2015, more than 1.6 million patients were served by hospice programs in the United States. Cancer used to be the most common diagnosis for patients dying in hospice programs. However, in 2017, Alzheimer's disease was reported as the top principal diagnosis for hospice patients. COPD, heart failure and cancer were listed among the top five. In 2015, the median length of stay for patients in hospice was 23 days.

In most cases, hospice care is provided in the person's home. Hospice care can also be provided in freestanding hospice centers, hospitals, and nursing homes or other long-term care facilities. In order to qualify for the Medicare Hospice Benefit, two physicians must sign a statement certifying that the patient's prognosis for survival, if the disease runs its natural course, is likely to be 6 months or less. Hospice criteria exist to assist in making these determinations for common medical conditions (see section, Estimating and Communicating Prognosis). The Medicare Hospice Benefit covers most costs related to terminal care without a deductible, which includes palliative medications, nursing oversight, supplies, and bereavement care. Hospice also covers up to 2 to 4 hours of custodial caregiver services per day;

表 22.2	缓和医疗中沟通与协商照护目标的通用策略
第一步	环境准备 不要有固定的预设议程
第二步	询问患者及家属他们知道和理解的病情信息 给予患者及家属充分的时间讲述他们的故事 运用积极倾听的技巧
第三步	了解患者及家属想要了解多少信息 认可并探索情感
第四步	少量并逐步地提供信息,并经常确认患者及家属的理解程度 讨论预后及治疗方案的利弊 注意要避免过于乐观或悲观的预估 做好提出建议的准备
第五步	对情感给予同理性回应 传达诚实的情感并帮助患者及家属重塑希望 使用"我希望……"的句式
第六步	总结、制订及实施计划,随访 给予可能的限时试验治疗的建议

活质量、对家庭和经济条件的影响)。大多数情况下,患者和家属希望知道预后。有些患者和家属可能不想知道预后,或希望以某个特定的方式获知,因此非常重要的是首先厘清患者和家属已知和他们想知道的信息。

预估不准确可能导致低质量的决策。医生倾向于将晚期癌症患者的生存期高估约30%,而且医生与患者相处时间越长,这种偏差越明显。过于乐观的预测可导致过度使用无效的或患者不想要的、以控制疾病为目的的治疗,延误向安宁疗护的转诊,使患者产生虚假的期望,进行不必要的检查和操作,以及症状控制不佳。因此,准确预估和沟通预后对于在晚期疾病和终末期阶段做出最佳决策至关重要。

在晚期疾病中,生存期短(如不足6个月)的常见预测因素包括功能状态、厌食-恶病质综合征、谵妄和呼吸困难。缓和医疗功能量表可用于测量和跟踪患者的功能状态。该量表可在各种网站和书籍中找到。除了医生对生存期的主观预测外,一些模型可以协助进行预后估算,包括特定人群的通用模型(如安宁疗护准入筛查)以及特定疾病(如癌症、心力衰竭、肝病、卒中、艾滋病、脊髓压迫)模型。不同疾病的安宁疗护准入标准不同。虽然这些标准并非始终可靠,但在疾病自然发展情况下预后可能是6个月或更短时,这些标准仍有参考价值。其中一个例子是功能评估分期(FAST)量表,它是筛查阿尔茨海默病/痴呆患者安宁疗护准入资格的量表。

然而,对单个患者来说,预后的不确定性仍是常态,因此,将证据和医学经验整合,并以适合特定患者的形式(口头描述、数字、概率或图表)呈现这个信息十分重要。预后的估算应该以范围来界定,以显示出现实中的不确定性,并考虑到比预估时间更长或更短的情况。例如,"根据我的经验,处于您这种状况的患者平均生存时间为几周到几个月。可能会更长,但也可能会更短"。对于生存期相关的问题(如"我还能活多久?"),要注意避免过于乐观的估计,并考虑和传达较低的预期(如"有些人可能会活得更长,但不幸的是,另一些人可能会活得更短")。对于生活质量相关问题(如"以后的生活会是什么样?"),则需要注意避免过于悲观的预测,要重视患者适应变化的能力,并通过帮助患者和家属找到新的人生意义来激发希望。

生命末期照护

诊断性检查和侵入性措施的作用

在临近生命终点时是否适合启动激进性医疗措施还是缓和医疗干预措施,应考虑以下几个问题:干预的目标或预期结果是什么?干预的可能效果有哪些?患者的基线功能水平和预期寿命如何?干预的潜在副作用和负担是什么?患者和家属的愿望、价值观和偏好是什么?

医疗干预和缓和照护的选择范围是非常广泛的,因此挑战在于如何在疾病的不同阶段确定合理的、提升患者生活状况的干预方法。缓和医疗的干预措施囊括了从纯粹的症状管理和支持到侵入性干预措施,如化疗、放疗、手术/内镜干预、支架置入、胸腔穿刺、腹腔穿刺、心包穿刺、家庭正性肌力疗法、无创通气、抗生素或输血。因此,挑战主要在于开启个性化讨论,从而让患者能够充分利用有助于他们实现照护目标的干预,且不会被无效的侵入性治疗所主导。

安宁疗护的作用

安宁疗护是一种针对处于疾病终末期的患者和家属的特殊的缓和医疗模式。美国国家安宁疗护和缓和医疗组织将安宁疗护定义如下:安宁疗护和缓和医疗被认为是为面临生命有限的疾病或创伤的患者提供优质、富有同理的照护模式,这个过程需要通过团队完成专业的医疗照护、疼痛管理以及根据个人需求和愿望量身定制的情感和精神支持。这种照护同样为患者的亲人提供支持。安宁疗护的重点在于相信每个人都有权利在无痛苦和有尊严的情况下离世,他们的亲人也应获得必要的支持,从而助力我们帮助到患者。

自1982年设立《联邦医疗保险安宁疗护福利》以来,安宁疗护在生命终末期照护中的使用稳步增长。2015年,美国有超过160万患者接受了安宁疗护服务。癌症曾是安宁疗护项目中死亡患者最常见的诊断。然而,在2017年,阿尔茨海默病成为安宁疗护患者主诊断的首位。COPD、心力衰竭和癌症都位居前五。2015年,安宁疗护患者的中位住院时间为23天。

多数情况下,安宁疗护是在患者的家中提供的,也可以在独立的安宁疗护中心、医院、养老院或其他长期照护机构中提供。为了符合《联邦医疗保险安宁疗护福利》的资格审查,须有两名医生共同签署一份声明,证明如果疾病按自然过程发展,患者的预期寿命可能为6个月或更短。为安宁疗护设定标准是为了协助根据常见医疗状况做出决策(见"评估和沟通预后"部分)。《联邦医疗保险安宁疗护福利》涵盖了与终末期照护相关的大部分费用,无需自付,费用包括缓和性治疗相关药物、护理照护服务、医疗用品和丧亲关怀。安宁疗护还涵盖每天2~4h的看护服务;当然,如果患者选择在

however, family and/or friends must provide the remaining care if the patient is to stay at home. Hospice can supplement care in a skilled nursing facility, but patients themselves or their insurance would be responsible for the nursing home room and board charges. The hospice benefit includes bereavement care for the family after the patient's death.

Discussing hospice with patients and families can be challenging. First, some may view the transition to hospice as a way of "giving up" or "giving in to death." It is often initially viewed as a "bad news" discussion given that patients and families need to confront the fact that disease-directed treatment is no longer effective and that prognosis is likely to be 6 months or less. Second, given the reimbursement restrictions, patients may also need to forgo particular types of treatment that are important to them (e.g., acute hospital or ICU-level care, dialysis, chemotherapy, milrinone for heart failure).

Last Hours and Days of Living

An integral aspect of palliative care is preparing and guiding the patient and caregivers through the dying process. When prognosis is measured in hours to days there are typical signs and symptoms that usually occur. Patients become weak and fatigued and gradually lose mobility. There is also a gradual and predictable decrease in food and fluid intake. Most patients do not experience hunger and thirst, and the associated mouth dryness that occurs is easily palliated with small sips or sponges of cold water. Caregivers will frequently ask about intravenous hydration. In rare instances, intravenous or subcutaneous fluids may temporarily improve mental status and energy in the final days of life. Most of the time, however, the benefits are difficult to discern and the excessive fluids may contribute to end-of-life physiologic conditions (edema, ascites, effusions, and pulmonary secretions) that do not improve longevity and may worsen comfort.

As patients become weaker, there is a predictable decrease in the level of consciousness with increasing periods of somnolence, eventually giving way to a comatose state. Education about this process should include associated changes in respiratory patterns, including prolonging periods of apnea, interspersed with episodes of hyperpnea and deep breathing (Cheyne-Stokes respirations). During this process caregivers often feel they are on a "roller-coaster ride," and gentle guidance on what to expect can allay concerns. As consciousness wanes, swallowing slows and the cough reflex weakens. As a result, saliva pools in the oropharynx and can result in noisy respiration ("death rattle"), which can usually be palliated to some degree with scopolamine (transdermal), glycopyrrolate (PO, IV, SC) or hyoscyamine (PO disintegrating tablets or sublingual solution). Families should be reminded that these symptoms are a natural part of the dying process and that persistent shortness of breath is relatively uncommon but can be treated with opiates and benzodiazepines, if needed.

As death approaches, reduced perfusion causes cooling and cyanosis of the extremities, as well as a reduced volume and darkening of the urine. Most deaths are relatively peaceful, but a few can be preceded by periods of intense agitation and restlessness (hyperactive terminal delirium). Antipsychotic medications and conventional doses of benzodiazepines can usually treat terminal delirium. Prior to and when death occurs, families should be encouraged to carry out cultural or religious rituals that are important to them. Providers should express condolences, be available for questions and responsive to intense emotional reactions that sometimes occur. A short condolence card or letter is almost always appreciated. If possible, efforts should be made to follow up with family members and caregivers deemed at risk for complicated bereavement and grief.

COMMON ETHICAL CHALLENGES IN PALLIATIVE CARE

Patient Capacity and Surrogate Decision Making

When discussing goals of care, it is essential to determine if a patient has capacity to make medical decisions. Adults are presumed to have capacity, unless determined by the court. However, many medical conditions can alter a patient's ability to make decisions for themselves (e.g., delirium, dementia, sedation). As many as 25% of adult inpatients are found to lack capacity. In order to be found to have capacity, a patient must (1) be able to comprehend the factual information about their medical condition and treatment options, (2) understand the risks and benefits of the treatment options and the consequences of that decision, (3) be able to accept or reject the proposed treatment voluntarily, and (4) provide reliable choice over time. A physician, psychiatrist, or ethics consultant may determine a patient's capacity to make a medical decision. Only a court can determine legal competence. In the event that the patient lacks capacity, a surrogate decision-maker must be consulted. This could be a health care proxy (legally designated by the patient when he/she did have capacity), a legal next-of-kin, or a court-appointed guardian. When there is question about a patient's capacity, which surrogate decision-maker is legally appropriate, or if the surrogate appears to be making decisions contrary to the patient's best interests, an ethics consultation should be obtained.

When Patients and Families Want Near Futile Treatment

The patient autonomy movement in medicine has led to patients and families taking an active role in their own medical decision making. This is generally a positive development except in two circumstances: (1) when physicians stop taking an active role using their expertise to guide patients in their decision making, thereby abdicating their professional responsibility of advocating for the best possible treatment based on the patient's medical condition and personal values, and (2) when patients or their families want and even demand near futile treatment toward the end of their lives despite physician's advice that treatment has much more burden than benefit. Physicians might try to respond to patients who want "everything" by suggesting that they want to try everything that is "more likely to help than harm," but avoid any treatment that is most likely to "do more harm than good." However, some patients and families will accept no limits on treatment no matter what the burden and the improbability of success. Of course, truly futile treatment should not be offered or provided upon request, but absolute futility has been difficult to define in many cases.

Feeding Tube Questions

Many patients gradually stop eating and drinking as a natural part of the dying process, but this can be very hard for patients and families to accept in light of fears about "starving to death" and in view of seemingly simple technologies that can potentially combat and even reverse the problem. In fact, with few exceptions, feeding tubes have not been shown to prolong life in most advanced illnesses such as metastatic cancer or advanced Alzheimer's disease. It is important to know about the exceptions (e.g., esophageal and oropharyngeal cancers, amyotrophic lateral sclerosis, acute stroke) but also to have an open discussion about the natural progression of diminished eating and drinking as many illnesses advance. If there is uncertainty about whether a particular patient might benefit from a feeding tube, and patient and family are clear about wanting to give it a try, the clinician can frame the decision as a "time-limited trial" to see how the patient tolerates tube feeding psychologically as well as physiologically in a specified timeframe. A potential framework for such a trial is that a nasogastric tube has a built-in time limit of about a month before a PEG tube needs to be inserted. Explaining to patients and families about the positive

家中接受安宁疗护，家人和（或）朋友必须负责其余时间的照护。安宁疗护可作为在专业护理机构中的补充照护，但患者本人及其保险需要支付护理机构食宿费用。安宁疗护福利包括了患者去世后对家属的丧亲关怀。

与患者和家属讨论安宁疗护是具有挑战性的。首先，有些人可能将转诊安宁疗护视为"放弃"或"向死亡妥协"。由于患者和家属需要面对针对疾病的治疗不再有效、并且预后可能只有6个月或更短的事实，因此讨论安宁疗护通常被视为讨论"坏消息"。其次，由于报销的限制，患者可能还需要放弃一些对他们来说重要的治疗（如急救医院或ICU治疗、透析、化疗、心力衰竭的米力农治疗等）。

临终前最后数小时及数天

缓和医疗的一个重要方面是为患者和照护者在经历临终过程时提供准备和指导。当生存时间以小时或以天计算时，通常会出现一些典型的症状和体征。患者会变得虚弱、疲劳，并逐渐失去活动能力。食物和液体摄入也会逐渐减少。大多数患者不会感到饥饿和口渴，口干的症状可以通过少量饮水或用海绵蘸冷水擦拭口腔来缓解。照护者经常会询问是否需要静脉输液。在极少数情况下，静脉或皮下输液可帮助患者在生命最后几天暂时改善精神状态，但大多数情况下，静脉补液的益处难以评估，过量液体会导致生命终末期身体状况恶化（如水肿、腹水、积液和肺部分泌物），并不会延长寿命，反而可能会降低舒适度。

随着患者愈加虚弱，意识水平会出现可预测的下降，嗜睡的时间会不断延长，最终进入昏迷状态。对这个过程认知教育需要包含患者呼吸模式的变化：呼吸暂停期延长，期间有过度呼吸和深呼吸的片段（称为潮式呼吸）。在此过程中，照护者的心情常常像"坐过山车"，因此帮助他们了解可预期的情况可以减轻他们的担忧。随着意识逐渐减退，吞咽会变得更慢，咳嗽反射也会减弱，这会导致唾液积聚在口咽部，可能导致呼吸时发出声响（即"临终喉鸣"），通常可通过使用东莨菪碱贴片，格隆溴铵（口服、静脉或皮下）或莨菪碱（口服崩解片或舌下溶液）达到一定程度的缓解。应提醒家属，这些症状是临终过程的自然部分。持续的呼吸困难相对少见，但如果需要，可以用阿片类药物和苯二氮䓬类药物进行处理。

随着死亡临近，灌注减少会导致四肢冰冷、发绀，以及尿量减少、尿色变深。大多数死亡过程相对平静，但少数人可能出现剧烈的躁动和不安（激越型终末期谵妄）。抗精神病类药物和常规剂量的苯二氮䓬类药物通常可以缓解终末期谵妄。在死亡前和死亡发生时，应鼓励家属进行重要且有意义的文化或宗教仪式。医护人员应表达哀悼之情，随时准备回答问题，并对家属可能出现的强烈情绪反应做出回应。简短的慰问卡片或哀悼信很受家人们的欢迎。如果可能，应对具有复杂性哀伤风险的家属和照护者进行随访。

缓和医疗中常见的伦理挑战

患者决策能力和代理决策

在讨论照护目标时，确定患者是否有能力进行相关医疗决策至关重要。除非法院另有裁定，否则成年人被默认具有决策能力。然而，许多医疗状况可能会改变患者的决策能力（如谵妄、痴呆、镇静）。多达25%的成年住院患者缺乏决策能力。判断患者拥有决策能力，必须满足以下几点：①能够理解其医疗状况和不同治疗选择的信息；②理解不同治疗选择的风险和收益以及该决策的后果；③能够自愿接受或拒绝被建议的治疗；④可以做出可靠的选择。医生、精神科医生或伦理顾问都可以参与判断患者是否有能力做出医疗决策，但只有法院才能确定法律层面的决策能力。如患者缺乏决策能力，则必须咨询其代理决策者。代理决策者可以是患者在有能力时指定的合法医疗代理人、法定近亲或法院指定的监护人。当已经存在合法的代理决策人但患者的决策能力存疑或代理决策人疑似做出违背患者最佳利益的决定时，应进行伦理咨询。

面对患者和家属对无效治疗的需求

医学中的患者自主权运动使得患者和家属在自己的医疗决策中发挥了积极的作用。一般来说这会是正向作用，以下两种情况除外：①医生停止使用专业知识引导患者进行决策，从而放弃了基于患者医疗状况和个人价值观来促进患者得到最佳治疗的职业责任；②尽管医生已经告知治疗带来的负担远大于益处，患者或其家属仍希望甚至要求在生命末期接受接近无效的治疗。医生可能会通过建议他们尝试"利大于弊"的治疗方式来回应想要"一切治疗"的患者，并避免可能"弊大于利"的治疗。然而，无论治疗的负担多重，成功的可能性多低，一些患者和家属仍会要求所有治疗。医生不应提供或应患方要求提供无效的治疗，但在许多情况下很难界定什么是完全无效的治疗。

喂食管路相关问题

许多患者在临终过程中会逐渐停止进食和饮水，但患者和家属可能很难接受，他们害怕患者被"饿死"，希望存在可以对抗甚至逆转这一问题的简单技术。事实上，除了少数情况如食管癌、口咽癌、肌萎缩侧索硬化症、急性卒中等，在大多数晚期疾病（如转移性癌症或晚期阿尔茨海默病），喂食管路并不能延长生命。了解上述少数情况很重要，但也需要对疾病进展而自然出现的进食和饮水减少的情况随时进行开放式讨论。如果不确定患者是否能从喂食管路中受益，并且患者和家属明确表示希望尝试，临床医生可以通过"限时尝试"的方法来观察患者在指定时间段内在心理和身体上对管饲的耐受情况来做出决定。鼻胃管是一种潜在的限时试验，当需要放置经皮内窥镜胃造口管（PEG）时，会先尝试放置鼻胃管约1个月。尽量向患者和家属解释自然进食的好处（如气味、味道和享受，而且即使只是少量进食也有这样

aspects (smell, taste, and enjoyment) of natural feeding of real food, even in small amounts, may help focus the decision on important quality of life issues, rather than more technical, physiological issues.

Proportionate Palliative Sedation

Proportionate palliative sedation is the use of gradually escalating levels of sedation to help relieve intractable and distressing physical symptoms at the end of a patient's life. The goal is to achieve the lowest level of sedation that adequately relieves the patient's uncontrolled suffering, not to intentionally end a patient's life or hasten a patient's death. Although unconsciousness may eventually be the outcome of proportionate palliative sedation, this is not the intended aim.

Terminally ill patients receiving proportionate palliative sedation should have do-not-resuscitate (DNR) and do-not-intubate (DNI) orders before the treatment is initiated. Patients with capacity should provide verbal or written consent prior to initiating the process because capacity usually will be compromised once it is started. If the patient lacks capacity, the decision to initiate proportionate palliative sedation would be made by the patient's surrogate decision maker.

Medications used to achieve adequate symptom control include sedatives (lorazepam, midazolam, and phenobarbital) in the form of continuous IV infusions. Careful monitoring of the patient's level of sedation/agitation is very important in order to determine need for additional bolus doses or titration of infusion rate. A formal palliative care consult is strongly recommended to help guide this process.

Examples of conditions when proportionate palliative sedation might be initiated include agitated terminal delirium, unrelenting nausea and vomiting, intractable pain, and unrelenting dyspnea in actively dying patients who do not respond to the usual palliative treatments.

Request for Hastened Death

The prevalence of suicidal ideation and suicide attempts is higher in patients with advanced life-limiting illness compared to those without serious disease. In Oregon, where physician-assisted suicide is legally permitted (subject to safeguards), the prevalence of a patient wanting to explore a health care professional's willingness to help hasten death is about 1/50, whereas only about 1/500 die using physician-assisted suicide. The motivation behind such initial explorations may relate to relentless physical suffering, disfigurement, hopelessness, loss of dignity, fear of being a burden, or a "cry for help." Most enduring requests from patients with progressive medical illnesses, however, arise not from inadequate symptom control, but from a patient's belief about dignity, meaning, and control over the circumstances of death. Although some providers might be uncomfortable exploring such requests, before responding, a systematic approach should be used to evaluate and understand the root causes of these requests. A careful evaluation includes a precise clarification and exploration as to exactly what the patient is asking and why. Is the request based on transient thoughts about ending life (common) or a serious appeal for assistance (relatively rare)? Does the request occur in the context of intense physical suffering, psychological despair, an existential crisis, or a combination of factors? Does the patient have full decision-making capacity? Is the request proportionate to the level of suffering? Evaluating such requests can be emotionally fatiguing and conflicting, and clinicians need self-awareness in distinguishing their emotions from the patient's, including tending to one's own support by sharing the burden of such requests with trusted colleagues.

Responding to such a request should first include evaluation for potentially reversible contributions to suffering. This will often include treating physical and psychological symptoms, aggressive attempts to foster hope, consulting psychiatrists or spiritual counselors, and creative brainstorming with trusted colleagues and team members. Some requests for hastened death persist, despite optimal palliative care. In such circumstances, the clinician should seek out a second opinion and confront the possibilities. These possibilities include withdrawal of life-sustaining interventions, palliative sedation, voluntary cessation of oral intake, and assisted suicide. As of publication, it is legal in nine jurisdictions: California, Colorado, District of Columbia, Hawaii, Montana, Maine [starting January 1, 2020], New Jersey, Oregon, Vermont, and Washington. While it is important to support the patient, the clinician must balance integrity and non-abandonment. This may include drawing specific boundaries of what the clinician can and cannot do, while still searching in earnest for a mutually acceptable solution.

PROSPECTUS FOR THE FUTURE

Palliative care became an officially recognized subspecialty within the United States in 2006. Physicians from 10 specialties can be board certified in hospice and palliative medicine, following completion of a fellowship. These specialties include: family medicine, internal medicine, emergency medicine, pediatrics, physical medicine and rehabilitation, anesthesiology, psychiatry, neurology, radiology, and surgery. As patients live longer with chronic illness, there will be an increasing need to fully integrate palliative care providers and programs within hospitals, nursing homes, and the outpatient setting; and to ensure that all primary care providers and non-palliative specialists develop the skill sets needed to provide basic palliative care. There is a compelling need for continued education and research to improve the overall palliative approach to care for everyone and to better define the optimal timing, setting, and delivery of palliative care to improve the quality of life and lessen the suffering of patients and families with advanced illness.

SUGGESTED READINGS

Ben Amar M: Cannabinoids in medicine: a review of their therapeutic potential, J Ethnopharmacol (Review) 105(1-2):1–25, 2006.

Buss MK, Rock LK, McCarthy EP: Understanding palliative care and hospice: a review for primary care providers, Mayo Clin Proc 92(2):280–286, 2017.

Ebbert JO, Scharf EL, Hurt RT: Medical Cannabis, Mayo Clinic Proc 93(12):1842–1847, 2018.

Ferrell B, Twaddle M, Melnick A, Meier DE: National consensus project clinical practice guidelines for quality palliative care guidelines, 4th edition, J Palliat Med 21(12):1684–1689, 2018.

Goldstein NE, Morrison RS, editors: Evidence-Based Practice of Palliative Medicine, Philadelphia, 2013, Elsevier.

Harris PS, Stalam T, Ache KA, et al: Can hospices predict which patients will die within six months? J Palliat Med 17:894–898, 2014.

Moryl N, Coyle N, Foley KM: Managing an acute pain crisis in a patient with advanced cancer: "This is as much of a crisis as a code", JAMA 299:1457–1467, 2008.

Mouhamed Y, Vishnyakov A, Qorri B, et al: Therapeutic potential of medicinal marijuana: an educational primer for health care professionals, Drug Healthc Patient Saf 10:45–66, 2018.

National Institute on Drug Abuse, National Institute of Health: Opioid Overdose Crisis, 2019, Retrieved from https://www.drugabuse.gov/drugs-abuse/opioids/opioid-overdose-crisis.

Quill TE, Abernethy AP: Generalist plus specialist palliative care–creating a more sustainable model, N Engl J Med 368:1173–1175, 2013.

Quill TE, Periyakoil V, Denney-Koelsch E, et al: Primer of palliative care, ed 7, Illinois, 2019, American Academy of Hospice and Palliative Medicine.

Temel JS, Greer JA, El-Jawahri A, et al: Effects of early integrated palliative care in patients with lung and GI cancer: a randomized clinical trial, J Clin Oncol 35(8):834–841, 2017.

Trecki J. A perspective regarding the current state of the opioid epidemic. JAMA Netw Open. Published online January 18, 20192(1):e187104.

的好处）可能有助于将决策聚焦在更重要的生活质量问题上，而不是更多地将焦点放在技术性、生理性问题上。

适度缓和镇静

适度缓和镇静是指用逐渐加深的镇静程度来帮助缓解患者生命末期的顽固性痛苦症状。其目标是通过最低的镇静程度来达到充分缓解患者难以控制的痛苦的目的，而非故意结束患者的生命或加速其死亡。尽管适度缓和镇静会导致患者失去意识，但这并不是缓和镇静预期的目标。

接受适度缓和镇静的终末期患者在开始治疗前应有"不进行心肺复苏"（DNR）和"不进行插管"（DNI）的医疗指示。具有决策能力的患者在启动缓和镇静前应提供口头或书面同意，因为一旦开始，其决策能力通常会受到影响。如果患者没有决策能力，应由其代理决策者决定是否启动适度缓和镇静。

实现充分症状控制的药物包括持续静脉输注的镇静剂（如劳拉西泮、咪达唑仑和苯巴比妥）。仔细监测患者的镇静/躁动水平非常重要，以确定是否需要额外的注射剂量或调整输注速度。强烈推荐通过正式的缓和医疗会诊来指导这一过程。

在常规缓和医疗无效的濒死患者中，可能需要启动适度缓和镇静的情况包括：激越型终末期谵妄、持续性恶心呕吐、顽固性疼痛以及持续性呼吸困难。

面对加速死亡的请求

与没有严重疾病的患者相比，患有危及生命疾病的终末期患者有更高的自杀意念和企图。在允许医生协助自杀（在有相关程序的保障下进行）的俄勒冈州，希望医护人员帮助加速死亡的患者比例约为1/50，而真正使用医生协助自杀死亡的患者比例大约只有1/500。这些探索医助自杀背后的动机可能与持续的身体痛苦、容貌改变、绝望、尊严丧失、害怕成为负担或"求救心态"有关。然而，大多数患有进展性疾病的患者持续请求医助自杀并非因为症状控制不充分，而是源于患者对死亡过程中尊严、意义和控制的信念。尽管一些医护人员对进一步探寻这类请求感到不适，但在回应之前，应全面评估和理解这些请求的根本原因。仔细的评估包括精确地澄清和探索患者究竟在问什么以及为什么问这些，该请求是暂时的结束生命的想法（常见）还是严肃的协助自杀的请求（相对罕见）？该请求是否发生在强烈的身体痛苦、心理绝望、存在性危机或多种因素的背景下？患者是否具有完全的决策能力？该请求是否与其痛苦程度相匹配？评估此类请求可能会导致情感疲惫和矛盾，临床医生需要拥有自我意识，从而将自己的情绪和患者的情绪区分开，也可以通过与可信赖的同事分享这类请求给自己带来的负担来获得支持。

回应此类请求应首先评估潜在的、可逆的导致痛苦的因素，通常包括治疗身体和心理症状，积极尝试重建患者的希望，咨询精神科医生或精神顾问，以及与可信赖的同事和团队成员进行创造性的头脑风暴。即使在拥有最佳的缓和医疗的情况下，一些加速死亡的请求仍然持续存在。在这种情况下，临床医生应寻求第二意见，并面对各种可能性。这些可能性包括撤回维持生命的干预措施、缓和镇静、自愿停止口服摄入和协助自杀。截至出版时，协助自杀在美国以下九个地区是合法的：加利福尼亚、科罗拉多、哥伦比亚特区、夏威夷、蒙大拿、缅因（自2020年1月1日起）、新泽西、俄勒冈、佛蒙特和华盛顿。虽然支持患者很重要，但临床医生必须平衡诚信和不放弃的原则，这需要明确界定医生可以和不可以做什么，同时真诚地寻找双方都能接受的解决方案。

未来展望

2006年缓和医疗在美国成为官方认可的亚专科。来自10个专业的医生在完成专科培训后可以获得安宁疗护和缓和医疗委员会的认证。这些专业包括：家庭医学、内科、急诊医学、儿科、物理康复科、麻醉科、精神病科、神经科、放射科和外科。随着慢病患者带病生存时间的延长，将缓和医疗全面整合到医院、养老院和门诊环境中的需求将会不断增加；同时需要确保所有初级医疗提供者和非缓和医疗专家补充所需的技能以提供基本的缓和医疗服务。迫切需要持续的教育和研究来改善缓和医疗理念，从而为每个人提供更好的照护，优化缓和医疗的最佳介入时机、照护环境和提供方式，以提高晚期疾病患者和家庭的生活质量并减轻他们痛苦。

推荐阅读

Ben Amar M: Cannabinoids in medicine: a review of their therapeutic potential, J Ethnopharmacol (Review) 105(1-2):1–25, 2006.

Buss MK, Rock LK, McCarthy EP: Understanding palliative care and hospice: a review for primary care providers, Mayo Clin Proc 92(2):280–286, 2017.

Ebbert JO, Scharf EL, Hurt RT: Medical Cannabis, Mayo Clinic Proc 93(12):1842–1847, 2018.

Ferrell B, Twaddle M, Melnick A, Meier DE: National consensus project clinical practice guidelines for quality palliative care guidelines, 4th edition, J Palliat Med 21(12):1684–1689, 2018.

Goldstein NE, Morrison RS, editors: Evidence-Based Practice of Palliative Medicine, Philadelphia, 2013, Elsevier.

Harris PS, Stalam T, Ache KA, et al: Can hospices predict which patients will die within six months? J Palliat Med 17:894–898, 2014.

Moryl N, Coyle N, Foley KM: Managing an acute pain crisis in a patient with advanced cancer: "This is as much of a crisis as a code", JAMA 299:1457–1467, 2008.

Mouhamed Y, Vishnyakov A, Qorri B, et al: Therapeutic potential of medicinal marijuana: an educational primer for health care professionals, Drug Healthc Patient Saf 10:45–66, 2018.

National Institute on Drug Abuse, National Institute of Health: Opioid Overdose Crisis, 2019, Retrieved from https://www.drugabuse.gov/drugs-abuse/opioids/opioid-overdose-crisis.

Quill TE, Abernethy AP: Generalist plus specialist palliative care–creating a more sustainable model, N Engl J Med 368:1173–1175, 2013.

Quill TE, Periyakoil V, Denney-Koelsch E, et al: Primer of palliative care, ed 7, Illinois, 2019, American Academy of Hospice and Palliative Medicine.

Temel JS, Greer JA, El-Jawahri A, et al: Effects of early integrated palliative care in patients with lung and GI cancer: a randomized clinical trial, J Clin Oncol 35(8):834–841, 2017.

Trecki J. A perspective regarding the current state of the opioid epidemic. JAMA Netw Open. Published online January 18, 20192(1):e187104.

SECTION IV

Alcohol and Substance Use

23 Alcohol and Substance Use, 344

第 4 篇

酒精和物质使用

23 酒精和物质使用，345

23

Alcohol and Substance Use

Richard A. Lange, Joaquin E. Cigarroa

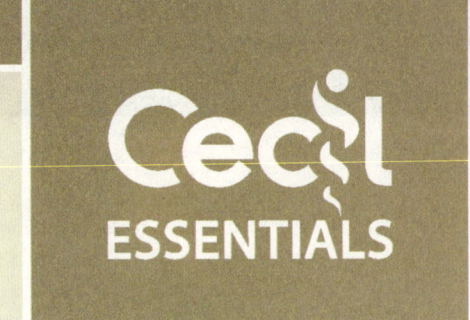

ALCOHOL USE

Alcohol use is a major public health problem worldwide, accounting for 3 million deaths (5.3% of all deaths) annually. One in six US adults binge drinks (i.e., a pattern of drinking that brings a person's blood alcohol concentration to 0.08 g percent [80 mg/dL] or above, which typically happens when men consume five or more drinks or women consume four or more drinks in about 2 hours) about four times a month, consuming about seven drinks per binge. Alcohol use is the third leading preventable cause of death in the United States (exceeded only by cigarette smoking and hypertension) and claims over 88,000 lives annually, or 9.8% of all US deaths. Alcohol use accounts for 28% of all traffic-related deaths in the United States, or approximately 10,500 vehicular deaths annually, and is a major contributor to risky sexual behavior, domestic violence, homicide, and suicide. In 2010, the estimated alcohol-related costs in the United States were $249 billion, 77% of which was attributable to binge drinking. These costs resulted from losses in workplace productivity, health care expenditures, criminal justice costs, and other expenses.

DEFINITION AND EPIDEMIOLOGY

The American Psychiatric Association has specific criteria for the diagnosis of *alcohol use disorder*; these 11 criteria are described in the *Diagnostic and Statistical Manual of Mental Disorders,* Fifth Edition, and are listed in Table 23.1. Alcohol use disorder is further characterized as mild, moderate, or severe, based on the number of criteria the individual meets; two to three criteria indicate a mild disorder, four to five criteria a moderate disorder, and six or more a severe disorder. The so-called *binge drinker* is defined as a man who typically consumes five or more drinks or a women who consumes four or more drinks on a single occasion. Nearly 50% of alcohol use disorder risk is heritable (i.e., transmissible from parent to offspring), with the other 50% attributable to environmental factors.

In 2016, 136.7 million Americans aged 12 or older reported current use of alcohol and 65.3 million reported binge alcohol use in the past month (Fig. 23.1). This number of people who were current binge drinkers corresponds to about 1 in 4 people aged 12 or older (Fig. 23.2) and nearly half of current alcohol users. Additionally, 16.3 million reported heavy alcohol use in the past month (see Fig. 23.1), which means that 1 in 8 (12%) current alcohol users or 1 in 4 (25%) binge drinkers reported heavy alcohol use. Although the prevalence of ethanol use is highest in individuals younger than 30 years of age, survey data suggest that about two thirds of persons over age 30 consume it.

In 2016, 73% of men and 66% of women aged 18 years or older reported drinking in the past year, and 7.8% of men and 4.2% of women were diagnosed with an alcohol use disorder. Native American individuals had the highest prevalence of alcohol use disorder (9.2%), followed by non-Hispanic white (5.9%), black (5.6%), Hispanic (5.1%), Pacific Islander (3.5%), and Asian (3.0%) individuals. Alcohol use peaks in younger adults, with those aged 21 through 25 years having the highest prevalence of past-year drinking (83%) and those aged 18 through 25 years having the highest prevalence of alcohol use disorder (11%).

PHARMACOLOGIC AND METABOLIC FACTORS

After oral ingestion, alcohol is absorbed predominantly in the small intestine, and its rate of intestinal absorption is accelerated by the simultaneous ingestion of carbohydrates and carbonated beverages. Prolonged retention of alcohol in the stomach, as occurs when food is consumed before drinking, delays alcohol absorption because absorption in the stomach is considerably slower than in the duodenum. Once in the blood, alcohol equilibrates rapidly across all membranes, including the blood-brain barrier, thereby accounting for the prompt onset of its euphoric effects. Maximal blood alcohol concentrations are reached 45 to 75 minutes after alcohol is ingested.

The liver metabolizes approximately 90% of ethanol to acetaldehyde via the alcohol dehydrogenase pathway; subsequently, acetaldehyde is converted by aldehyde dehydrogenase to acetate, which enters the Krebs cycle. At low or moderate serum concentrations of ethanol, the alcohol dehydrogenase pathway functions almost exclusively in metabolizing ethanol. At high concentrations, the microsomal ethanol oxidizing system (CYP2E1) contributes to metabolism. Less than 10% of ethanol is excreted unchanged through the skin, kidneys, and lungs. Elimination of alcohol from the body is affected by obesity, food intake, previous exposure to alcohol, and variability among individuals in the efficiency of the alcohol and aldehyde dehydrogenase systems. These enzymatic variations also influence a person's risk of developing an alcohol use disorder. The mechanism is thought to involve elevated acetaldehyde levels resulting from a more rapid conversion of ethanol (in cases of alcohol dehydrogenase variants with higher enzymatic activity) or slower elimination of acetaldehyde oxidation (in cases of aldehyde dehydrogenase variants with reduced enzymatic activity). Acetaldehyde causes facial flushing, nausea, and tachycardia, which make individuals reduce their intake of alcohol.

MECHANISMS OF ALCOHOL-INDUCED ORGAN DAMAGE

The major organs that are susceptible to damage by alcohol are the liver, pancreas, heart, brain, and bone (Table 23.2). Several alcohol-related

酒精和物质使用

向小军　龙江　译　郝伟　审校

酒精使用

酒精使用是全球主要的公共卫生问题,每年导致300万人死亡(占所有死亡人数的5.3%)。1/6的美国成人每个月约狂饮4次[狂饮是一种饮酒模式,指个体的酒精浓度达到每100 ml 血液中含 0.08 g 酒精(80 mg/dl)或更高,通常见于在约2 h 内饮酒≥5个标准杯的男性或饮酒≥4个标准杯的女性],每次狂饮消耗约7个标准杯。酒精使用是美国第三大可预防的死亡原因(仅次于吸烟和高血压),每年导致88 000人死亡,占美国总死亡人数的9.8%。酒精使用导致的交通事故死亡人数占美国所有交通相关死亡的28%,即每年约10 500人死于车祸,并且是导致危险性行为、家庭暴力、谋杀和自杀的主要因素。据估计,2010年美国与酒精相关的经济损失为2490亿美元,其中77%归因于狂饮。这些经济损失来自于工作生产力的损失、医疗保健支出、刑事司法成本和其他费用。

定义与流行病学

美国精神病学协会对酒精使用障碍有具体的诊断标准;《精神疾病诊断与统计手册》第5版(DSM-5)中描述了11项诊断标准(表23.1)。根据个体符合的诊断标准数量,酒精使用障碍被进一步划分为轻度、中度或重度:符合2~3项标准为轻度酒精使用障碍;符合4~5项标准为中度酒精使用障碍;符合≥6项标准为重度酒精使用障碍。其中,狂饮者被定义为通常在单次饮酒中饮酒≥5个标准杯的男性,或≥4个标准杯的女性。酒精使用障碍的遗传风险(即从父母传给子代)约为50%,其余50%归因于环境因素。

2016年,1.367亿12岁及以上的美国人报告当前使用酒精,其中6530万人报告在过去1个月内狂饮(图23.1)。当前狂饮者的人数相当于12岁及以上的人中每4人就有约1人酗酒(图23.2),几乎占当前酒精使用者的1/2。此外,1630万人报告在过去1个月内重度酒精使用(图23.1),这意味着每8个当前酒精使用者中就有1人(12%)或每4个狂饮者中就有1人(25%)报告重度酒精使用。尽管酒精使用的患病率在30岁以下人群中最高,但调查数据表明,约2/3的30岁以上个体饮酒。

2016年,在18岁及以上人群中,73%的男性和66%的女性报告在过去1年中曾饮酒,其中7.8%的男性和4.2%的女性被诊断为酒精使用障碍。美国原住民的酒精使用障碍患病率最高(9.2%),其次是非西班牙裔白人(5.9%)、黑人(5.6%)、西班牙裔人(5.1%)、太平洋岛民(3.5%)和亚洲人(3.0%)。酒精使用在成年早期达到顶峰,21~25岁年龄组过去1年酒精使用的患病率最高(83%),18~25岁年龄组酒精使用障碍的患病率最高(11%)。

药理学和代谢因素

饮酒后,酒精主要在小肠被吸收,同时摄入碳水化合物和碳酸饮料会加速这一过程。如果饮酒前先进食,酒精在胃中的停留时间会延长,从而减缓吸收,因为胃的吸收能力远低于十二指肠。一旦进入血液,酒精会迅速在全身各组织间达到平衡,包括穿透血脑屏障,因此能快速产生欣快感。血中酒精浓度通常在饮酒后45~75 min达到峰值。

肝通过乙醇脱氢酶途径将约90%的乙醇代谢为乙醛。随后,乙醛被乙醛脱氢酶转化为乙酸,进入克雷布斯循环(Krebs cycle,即三羧酸循环)。在乙醇血清浓度低或中等时,乙醇脱氢酶途径几乎专门用于代谢乙醇。在高浓度时,微粒体乙醇氧化系统(CYP2E1)参与代谢。不足10%的乙醇由皮肤、肾和肺以原型排出。酒精的体内清除过程受肥胖、食物摄取、酒精暴露史,以及乙醇和乙醛脱氢酶系统活性个体差异的影响。这些酶活性的差异也会影响个体罹患酒精使用障碍的风险。所涉及的机制包括由于乙醇转化太快(在乙醇脱氢酶活性增高的情况下)导致乙醛水平升高或由于乙醛的氧化清除变慢(在乙醛脱氢酶的活性降低的情况下)导致乙醛水平升高。乙醛会导致面部潮红、恶心和心动过速,这些症状会使个体减少酒精摄入。

酒精导致器官损害的机制

容易被酒精损害的主要器官包括肝、胰腺、心脏、脑和骨骼(表23.2)。多种与酒精相关的疾病是由各种

TABLE 23.1 Criteria for the Diagnosis of Alcohol Use Disorder

Two or More of the Following in the Previous 12 Months

1. Recurrent alcohol use resulting in a **failure to fulfill major** obligations at work, school, or home
2. Recurrent alcohol use in situations in which it is physically **hazardous**
3. Continued alcohol use despite having persistent or **recurrent social or interpersonal problems** caused or exacerbated by the effects of alcohol
4. **Tolerance**, as defined by:
   - need for markedly increased amounts of alcohol to achieve intoxication or desired effect; and/or
   - markedly diminished effect with continued use of the same amount of alcohol
5. **Withdrawal**, as manifested by:
   - characteristic alcohol withdrawal syndrome; and/or
   - alcohol is taken to relieve or avoid withdrawal symptoms
6. Alcohol is often taken in **larger amounts** or over a longer period than was intended
7. Persistent desire or **unsuccessful efforts to diminish** or to control alcohol use
8. A great deal of **time** is spent in activities necessary to obtain, use, or recover from the effects of alcohol
9. Important social, occupational, or recreational **activities are relinquished or reduced** because of alcohol use
10. Alcohol use is **continued despite knowledge** of having a persistent or recurrent physical or psychological problem that is likely to have been caused or exacerbated by alcohol use
11. **Craving** or a strong desire or urge to use a specific type of alcohol

Modified from the American Psychiatric Association: Diagnostic and statistical manual of mental disorders, ed 5, Washington, D.C., 2013, American Psychiatric Press.

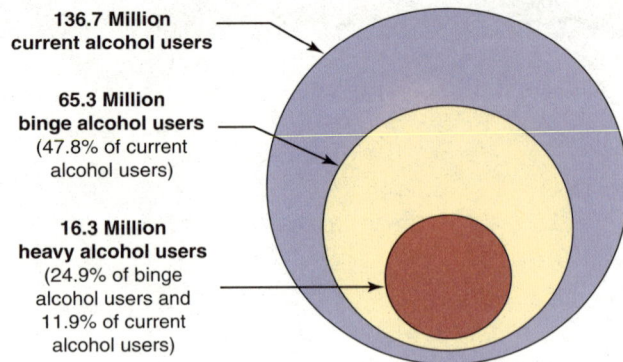

Fig. 23.1 Current, binge, and heavy alcohol use among persons aged 12 years or older according to the National Survey on Drug Use and Health (2016). Binge drinking is defined as males consuming five or more drinks on an occasion and for females consuming four or more drinks on an occasion. Heavy alcohol use is defined as binge drinking on 5 or more days in the past 30 days. (Substance Abuse and Mental Health Services Administration. [2017]. Key substance use and mental health indicators in the United States: Results from the 2016 National Survey on Drug Use and Health [HHS Publication No. SMA 17-5044, NSDUH Series H-52]. Rockville, MD: Center for Behavioral Health Statistics and Quality, Substance Abuse and Mental Health Services Administration.)

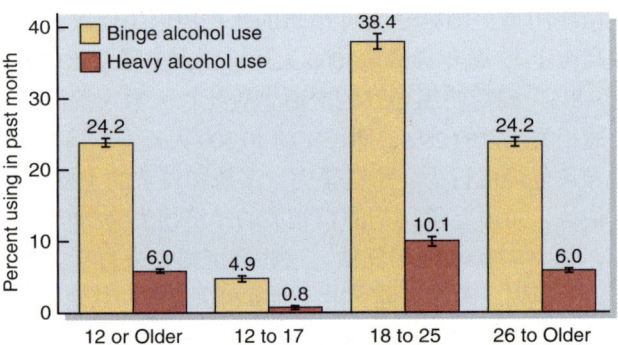

Fig. 23.2 Past month binge and heavy alcohol use among persons aged 12 years or older, by age group, according to the National Survey on Drug Use and Health (2016). Binge drinking is defined as males consuming five or more drinks on an occasion and for females consuming four or more drinks on an occasion. Heavy alcohol use is defined as having had five or more drinks on the same occasion on each of 5 or more days in the previous 30 days. (Substance Abuse and Mental Health Services Administration. [2017]. Key substance use and mental health indicators in the United States: Results from the 2016 National Survey on Drug Use and Health [HHS Publication No. SMA 17-5044, NSDUH Series H-52]. Rockville, MD: Center for Behavioral Health Statistics and Quality, Substance Abuse and Mental Health Services Administration. Retrieved from https://www.samhsa.gov/data.)

medical disorders are caused by various nutritional deficiencies; ethanol is deficient in proteins, minerals, and vitamins. Therefore, the initial management of the alcoholic patient must attend to suggested dietary deficiencies (e.g., thiamine) and electrolyte deficiencies, including potassium, magnesium, calcium, and zinc.

Alcohol-related liver disease is the leading preventable cause of hepatic failure in the industrialized world. Genetic factors are thought to play a role in susceptibility to this disorder, since alcoholic liver disease is more prevalent in white individuals than in other ethnic groups (despite a similar magnitude of ethanol consumption). The histopathologic features of alcoholic liver disease include fatty infiltration, hepatitis, fibrosis, and end-stage cirrhosis.

CLINICAL PRESENTATION

Acute Alcohol Intoxication

Mild ethanol intoxication produces slurred speech, ataxia, irregular eye movements, and poor coordination. Signs of central nervous system (CNS) depression and associated cerebellar or vestibular dysfunction include dysarthria, ataxia, and nystagmus. Although blood alcohol concentrations are not precisely correlated with the degree of intoxication and the clinical effect of ethanol widely varies among individuals, stupor and coma usually develop at blood concentrations approaching 400 mg/dL. Blood levels of 500 mg/dL often are fatal; however, it is important to understand that death may occur even when the blood alcohol concentration is as low as 300 mg/dL.

Withdrawal Syndrome (Convulsions)

Alcohol withdrawal occurs in three stages. The signs of minor withdrawal usually appear 6 to 12 hours after the discontinuation of ethanol and are caused by central adrenergic hyperexcitability; they consist of anxiety, tremors, sweating, tachycardia, diarrhea, and insomnia. Additional evidence of autonomic nervous system hyperactivity often appears within 12 to 24 hours and includes increased startle response, nightmares, and visual hallucinations. Alcohol withdrawal seizures (so-called *rum fits*) are generalized clonic-tonic convulsions that occur

表 23.1　酒精使用障碍的诊断标准

在过去 12 个月中，出现以下 2 种及以上情况：
1. 反复使用酒精导致无法履行工作、学校或家庭中的重要义务
2. 在对身体有害的情况下仍反复使用酒精
3. 尽管酒精使用引起或加剧持续或反复的社会或人际问题，但仍然继续使用酒精
4. 耐受性，定义如下：
   - 需要显著增加饮酒量以达到陶醉或期望的效果；和（或）
   - 继续使用等量的酒精时，效果明显减弱
5. 戒断症状，表现如下：
   - 特征性的酒精戒断综合征；和（或）
   - 为了缓解或避免戒断症状而饮酒
6. 酒精的摄入量和持续时间通常超过预期
7. 持续希望或努力减少或控制酒精使用，但未成功
8. 花费大量时间在获取酒精、使用酒精或从酒精影响中恢复的必要活动中
9. 由于酒精使用而放弃或减少重要的社交、职业或娱乐活动
10. 尽管知道已存在可能由酒精使用引起或加剧的持续或反复的躯体或心理问题，但仍然继续使用酒精
11. 对特定类型的酒精有强烈的渴求或冲动

改编自 the American Psychiatric Association: Diagnostic and statistical manual of mental disorders, ed 5, Washington, D.C., 2013, American Psychiatric Press.

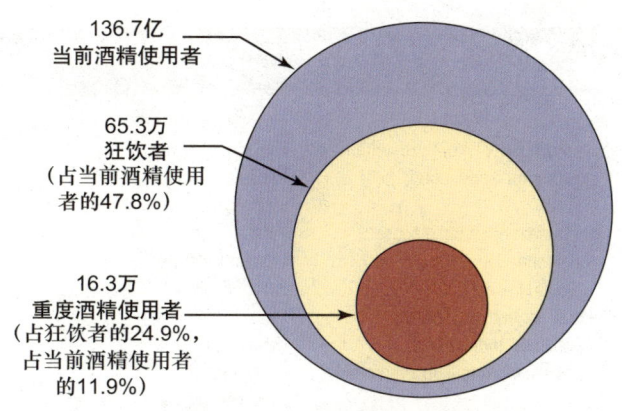

图 23.1　根据 2016 年美国国家药物使用和健康调查，12 岁及以上人群中当前酒精使用、狂饮和重度酒精使用的情况。狂饮者的定义为男性单次饮酒 ≥ 5 个标准杯或女性饮酒 ≥ 4 个标准杯。重度酒精使用者的定义为在过去 30 天中有 ≥ 5 天存在狂饮行为［Substance Abuse and Mental Health Services Administration.（2017）. Key substance use and mental health indicators in the United States: Results from the 2016 National Survey on Drug Use and Health（HHS Publication No. SMA 17-5044，NSDUH Series H-52）. Rockville, MD: Center for Behavioral Health Statistics and Quality, Substance Abuse and Mental Health Services Administration. Retrieved from https://www.samhsa.gov/data.］

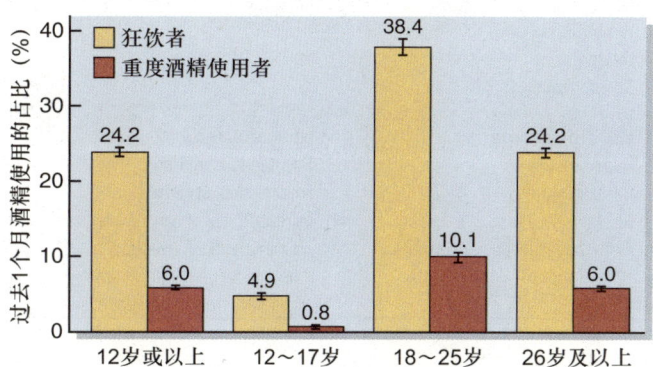

图 23.2　根据 2016 年美国国家药物使用和健康调查，12 岁及以上人群中过去 1 个月狂饮和重度酒精使用的情况。狂饮的定义为在单次饮酒中男性饮酒 ≥ 5 个标准杯或女性饮酒 ≥ 4 个标准杯。重度酒精使用的定义为在过去 30 天内有 ≥ 5 天存在狂饮行为［Substance Abuse and Mental Health Services Administration.（2017）. Key substance use and mental health indicators in the United States: Results from the 2016 National Survey on Drug Use and Health（HHS Publication No. SMA 17-5044，NSDUH Series H-52）. Rockville, MD: Center for Behavioral Health Statistics and Quality, Substance Abuse and Mental Health Services Administration. Retrieved from https://www.samhsa.gov/data］

营养缺乏引起的；乙醇中缺乏蛋白质、矿物质和维生素。因此，对患者的初步治疗必须注意可能的营养缺乏（如维生素 B_1）和电解质缺乏（包括钾、镁、钙和锌）。

在工业化国家，酒精性肝病是肝衰竭的主要可预防原因。遗传因素被认为在该病的易感性方面发挥作用，因为酒精性肝病在白人中比其他种族群体中更为普遍（即使饮酒量相似）。酒精性肝病的组织病理学特征包括脂肪浸润、肝炎、纤维化和晚期肝硬化。

临床表现

急性酒精中毒

轻度乙醇中毒会导致口齿不清、共济失调、眼球运动不规律和协调能力下降。中枢神经系统（CNS）抑制及相关的小脑或前庭功能障碍的体征包括构音障碍、共济失调和眼球震颤。尽管血液酒精浓度与中毒程度无明确的相关性，且乙醇的临床效应在不同个体间差异很大，但血液酒精浓度接近 400 mg/dl 时通常会出现昏睡和昏迷。血液酒精浓度达到 500 mg/dl 时往往是致命的；然而，即使血液酒精浓度为 300 mg/dl 也可能导致死亡，了解这一点至关重要。

戒断综合征（抽搐）

酒精戒断分为 3 个阶段。轻微戒断的体征通常在停止饮酒后 6～12 h 出现，由中枢肾上腺素能过度兴奋引起；这些症状包括焦虑、震颤、出汗、心动过速、腹泻和失眠。自主神经系统功能亢进的其他表现通常在 12～24 h 出现，包括惊跳反应增加、噩梦和幻视。酒精戒断性癫痫发作（即朗姆酒发作）是指全身性强

TABLE 23.2 Medical Complications of Alcohol Use

Neurologic	Electrolyte or Nutritional
Encephalopathy (Wernicke, with oculomotor dysfunction; gait ataxia)	Thiamine deficiency
	Niacin deficiency
	Folate deficiency
Marchiafava-Bignami disease (demyelination of corpus callosum)	Vitamin B_{12} deficiency
	Vitamin D deficiency
	Zinc deficiency
Central pontine myelinosis	Hypokalemia
Cognitive dysfunction	Hypomagnesaemia
Amnesia (i.e., Korsakoff syndrome)	Hypocalcaemia
Dementia	Ketoacidosis
Cerebellar degeneration	Hypoglycemia
Peripheral neuropathy	Hypertriglyceridemia
Seizures	Malnutrition
Hematologic	**Endocrine**
Anemia (often with macrocytosis)	Diabetes mellitus
Leukopenia	Gynecomastia
Thrombocytopenia	
Gastrointestinal	**Musculoskeletal**
Esophagitis	Myopathy
Esophageal varices	Osteoporosis
Gastritis	Testicular atrophy
Gastrointestinal bleeding	Amenorrhea
Pancreatitis	Infertility
Hepatitis	
Cirrhosis	
Splenomegaly	
Cardiovascular	**Miscellaneous**
Hypertension	Spontaneous abortion
Cardiomyopathy	Fetal alcohol syndrome
Stroke	Increased risk of cancer (breast, oropharyngeal, esophageal, hepatocellular, colorectal)
Arrhythmias (especially atrial fibrillation)	
	Accidents, trauma, violence, suicide

TABLE 23.3 CAGE: An Alcoholism Screening Test

1. Have you ever felt you should *cut down* on your drinking?
2. Have people *annoyed* you by criticizing your drinking?
3. Have you felt *guilty* about your drinking?
4. Have you ever had a drink first thing in the morning to steady your nerves or to get rid of a hangover (i.e., as an *eye-opener*)?

12 to 48 hours after the discontinuation of ethanol and are estimated to occur in 2% to 5% of alcoholics.

Delirium Tremens

Delirium tremens (DTs) is characterized by delirium (a confused state with varying levels of consciousness), hallucinations, disorientation, agitation, tremor (caused by marked autonomic nervous system over activity), tachycardia, hypertension, fever, and diaphoresis. It occurs in approximately 5% of alcoholics who discontinue or decrease their alcohol use, most often in chronic heavy users with underlying neurologic damage. If unrecognized and untreated, the in-hospital mortality rate of DTs approaches 25%; with early recognition and treatment the mortality is only 1% to 4%.

TREATMENT

Intervention strategies in alcohol users are designed to modify the individual's attitudes, knowledge, and skills to prevent alcohol misuse. In the outpatient setting, increased frequency of contact between the primary care physician and the patient increases the likelihood of detection, intervention, and prevention of heavy alcohol consumption. All scheduled office visits should include alcohol screening, assessment, and brief attempts at intervention (one or more discussions lasting 10 to 15 minutes), if indicated, as studies show that this approach decreases alcohol intake and its consequences. Behavioral or pharmacologic treatment should be considered because two thirds of treated patients have a reduction in the amount of consumption (by more than 50%) as well as the consequences of consumption (e.g., alcohol-related injury or job loss). A year after treatment, one third of patients are either abstinent or drink moderately without consequences.

Screening and Intervention Strategies

The National Institute on Alcohol Abuse and Alcoholism (NIAAA) provides several web-based guidelines for alcohol screening during the routine health examination (www.niaaa.nih.gov). A four-step plan exists with which physicians can (1) screen patients for alcohol use, (2) assess for the presence of alcohol-related problems, (3) provide advice concerning appropriate action, and (4) monitor the patient's progress. For the current drinker, the physician should inquire about the number of drinks consumed per day, number of days per week on which ethanol is consumed, and total number of drinks consumed per month. Alcohol consumption that exceeds 14 drinks per week or three drinks per day should trigger an in-depth assessment of alcohol-related problems. The physician should ascertain if the individual is at risk for alcohol-related problems, has an existing problem, or may be alcohol-dependent. Difficulties with work-related, interpersonal, or family relationships and/or evidence of high-risk behavior despite self-reported low-risk consumption indicate that the individual is at risk for alcohol use disorder.

The CAGE questionnaire (each of the letters in the acronym refers to one of the questions) (Table 23.3) is a useful screening tool for identifying *alcohol-dependent individuals*. A positive response to two or more of the four questions is indicative of a potential alcohol problem and should prompt questions regarding the quantity and frequency of consumption.

The 2013 US Preventive Services Task Force (USPSTF) recommendation identified one-item screeners such as the Single Item Alcohol Screening Questionnaire (SASQ) and the Alcohol Use Disorders Identification Test (AUDIT) as having the best accuracy to screen for any level of *unhealthy alcohol use* among adults. The SASQ asks, "How many times in the past year have you had 5 [for men]/4 [for women] or more drinks in a day?", where one or more occasions in the previous year constitutes a positive screen. AUDIT (Table 23.4) is the most widely validated instrument for use in primary care settings. Utilizing 10 items and taking 2 to 3 minutes to complete, it is better suited to settings where visit times are longer or when it can be completed and scored before a clinician visit. Evidence supports the use of brief (1-item) instruments as initial screeners, where high sensitivity and lower specificity would be desirable, followed by a longer instrument, such as AUDIT, with greater specificity.

表 23.2	酒精使用的躯体并发症
神经系统	电解质或营养
脑病（韦尼克脑病伴眼球运动功能失调；步态不稳、共济失调）	维生素 B_1 缺乏症
	烟酸缺乏症
马-比二氏病（胼胝体脱髓鞘）	叶酸缺乏症
脑桥中枢髓鞘病	维生素 B_{12} 缺乏症
认知功能障碍	维生素 D 缺乏症
遗忘（如科萨科夫综合征）	锌缺乏症
痴呆	低钾血症
小脑变性	高镁血症
周围神经病	低钙血症
癫痫发作	酮症酸中毒
	低血糖
血液系统	高甘油三酯血症
贫血（通常伴有大红细胞症）	营养不良
白细胞减少症	
血小板减少症	内分泌系统
消化系统	糖尿病
食管炎	男性乳房发育
食管静脉曲张	肌肉骨骼系统
胃炎	肌病
消化道出血	骨质疏松症
胰腺炎	睾丸萎缩
肝炎	闭经
肝硬化	不孕不育
脾大	
	其他
心血管系统	自然流产
高血压	胎儿酒精综合征
心肌病	癌症风险增加（乳腺癌、口咽癌、食管癌、肝细胞癌、结直肠癌）
卒中	
心律失常（特别是心房颤动）	
	意外事故、创伤、暴力、自杀

表 23.3	CAGE：酒精中毒筛查测试
1. 你是否曾觉得应该减少饮酒？	
2. 是否曾有人批评你饮酒而激怒了你？	
3. 你是否因为饮酒而觉得内疚？	
4. 你是否曾有过早上起来第一件事就是饮酒来稳住自己的神经或去掉宿醉感（如作为醒脑剂）？	

直-阵挛性发作，发生于停止饮酒后 12～48 h 内，据估计 2%～5% 的酒瘾者会出现这种情况。

震颤性谵妄

震颤性谵妄（DT）的特征是谵妄（一种意识水平不同的意识模糊状态）、幻觉、定向障碍、激越、震颤（由自主神经系统功能亢进引起）、心动过速、高血压、发热和出汗。这种情况见于约 5% 的酒瘾者中，在停止或减少饮酒后发生，最常见于有潜在神经损伤的慢性重度酒精使用者。如果未被识别和治疗，DT 的住院死亡率接近 25%；如果早期被识别和治疗，死亡率仅为 1%～4%。

治疗

酒精使用者的干预策略旨在改变个体的态度、知识和技能，以防止酒精滥用。在门诊环境中，增加初级保健医生与患者的接触频率可提高识别、干预和预防重度酒精使用的可能性。所有门诊预约患者均应进行酒精筛查、评估，以及简短干预（单次或多次讨论，持续 10～15 min），因为研究表明这种方法可以减少酒精摄入及其不良后果。应考虑行为治疗或药物治疗，因为 2/3 接受治疗的患者饮酒量减少（超过 50%），饮酒的不良后果减少（如与酒精相关的损伤或失业）。治疗 1 年后，1/3 的患者可以实现完全戒酒或适量饮酒而没有不良后果。

筛查和干预策略

美国国立酒精滥用与酒精中毒研究所（NIAAA）的官方网站（www.niaaa.nih.gov）提供了多个可在常规健康体检中使用的在线酒精筛查指南。医生可以采取以下四步法：①对患者进行酒精使用的筛查；②对存在的酒精相关问题进行评估；③提供针对酒精使用可采取的适当行动的建议；④监测患者的进展。对于当前酒精使用者，医生应询问每天饮酒的标准杯数量、每周饮酒的天数，以及每月饮酒的总标准杯数量。如果每周饮酒超过 14 个标准杯或每天饮酒超过 3 个标准杯，则应进行对酒精相关问题的深度评估。医生应确定个体是否有酒精相关问题的风险、已存在酒精相关问题或可能存在酒精依赖。如果自我报告的饮酒风险低，但存在工作、人际关系或家庭关系相关问题和（或）存在高风险行为的证据，则表明个体存在酒精使用障碍的风险。

CAGE 问卷（缩写的每个字母代表问卷中的一个问题）（表 23.3）是用于识别酒精依赖的有效筛查工具。对 4 个问题中的 2 个及以上问题做出肯定回答，表明可能存在酒精使用问题，应进一步询问有关饮酒量和频率的问题。

2013 年美国预防服务工作组（USPSTF）的建议认为，单项筛查工具［如单项酒精筛查问卷（SASQ）和酒精使用障碍筛查量表（AUDIT）］在筛查成人不健康饮酒行为方面的准确性最高。SASQ 中的问题是："在过去 1 年中，你有多少次在 1 天内饮酒超过 5 个标准杯（男性）/4 个标准杯（女性）？"其中，过去 1 年中有 ≥1 次即为筛查阳性。AUDIT（表 23.4）是在初级保健机构中使用最广泛的筛查工具。它共包含 10 个项目，完成问卷需要 2～3 min，其更适合于随诊次数多或在医生就诊前能完成量表评估和评分的机构。目前的证据支持使用简短的（单项）工具（敏感性高和特异性较低是可取的）进行初步筛查，随后使用 AUDIT 等特异性更高的较长的问卷。

TABLE 23.4 Alcohol Use Disorders Identification Test (AUDIT)

Questions	No. Items/Time to Administer	Scoring Notes
1. How often do you have a drink containing alcohol? 　0. Never 　1. Monthly or less 　2. Two to four times a month 　3. Two so three times a week 　4. Four or more times a week	10 items 2–5 min	Scoring: ≥8 considered a positive screen for hazardous or harmful drinking. In general: Scores between 8 and 15 are most appropriate for simple advice focused on the reduction of hazardous drinking Scores between 16 and 19 suggest brief counseling and continued monitoring Scores of 20 and above clearly warrant further diagnostic evaluation for alcohol dependence
2. How many drinks containing alcohol do you have on a typical day when you are drinking? 　0. 1 or 2 　1. 3 or 4 　2. 5 or 6 　3. 7 to 9 　4. 10 or more		
3. How often do you have six[a] or more drinks on one occasion? 　0. Never 　1. Less than monthly 　2. Monthly 　3. Weekly 　4. Daily or almost daily		
4. How often during the last year have you found that you were not able to stop drinking once you had started? *(same options as #3)*		
5. How often during the last year have you failed to do what was normally expected from you because of drinking? *(same options as #3)*		
6. How often during the last year have you needed a first drink in the morning to get yourself going after a heavy drinking session? *(same options as #3)*		
7. How often during the last year have you had a feeling of guilt or remorse after drinking? *(same options as #3)*		
8. How often during the last year have you been unable to remember what happened the night before because you have been drinking? *(same options as #3)*		
9. Have you or someone else been injured as a result of your drinking? 　0. No 　1. Yes, but not in the last year 　2. Yes, during the last year		
10. Has a relative or friend or a doctor or other health worker been concerned about your drinking or suggested you cut down? *(same options as #9)*		

[a]The US version asks about five or more drinks, reflecting standard drink sizes in the United States.

On physical examination, evidence of alcoholic liver disease may be exhibited as jaundice, hepatomegaly, palmar erythema, male gynecomastia, spider angiomata, and ascites. The serum γ-glutamyltransferase concentration typically is elevated in individuals who drink excessively.

Low-Risk Drinking

A standard drink contains 12 g of alcohol, an amount similar to that found in one 12-oz bottle of beer or wine cooler, one 5-oz glass of wine, or 1.5 oz. of distilled (e.g., 80 proof) spirits. In men older than age 64 years and in women older than 21 years, the limit for moderate drinking is one drink per day. For younger men, moderate drinking is defined as no more than two drinks per day. For the same amount of ingested ethanol, women and older adult men achieve a higher blood concentration of ethanol than younger men owing to their smaller volume of body water. A reasonable blood alcohol level should not exceed 50 mg/dL.

A blood-alcohol level as low as 80 mg/dL may exceed the legal definition for driving under the influence (DUI) or driving while intoxicated (DWI). In national surveys, the strategy of the *designated driver* appears to be effective at preventing unsafe driving by drinkers at risk for DWI. Complete abstinence is recommended for people with a history of alcohol use disorder, other serious medical conditions (e.g., liver disease), and pregnancy.

Nonpharmacologic Therapies

Psychosocial interventions efficacious in treating heavy alcohol use or alcohol use disorder include brief interventions, motivational enhancement therapy, cognitive-behavioral therapy, behavioral approaches, family therapies, and 12-step programs (the recovering alcoholic moves through 12 specific steps aided by his or her attendance at regular meetings within a self-help peer group). Although these therapies provide similar efficacy, brief interventions—which are commonly 15 to 20 minutes long—are most practical in outpatient medical settings. When more intensive psychosocial therapy is needed, it may be most feasible for a therapist trained in the specific method to provide it in concert with a medical practitioner who can prescribe an alcohol treatment medication.

表 23.4　酒精使用障碍筛查量表（AUDIT）		
问题	条目数量/所需时间	评分说明
1. 你多久喝一次含酒精饮料？ 　0. 从不 　1. 每月≤1次 　2. 每月2～4次 　3. 每周2～3次 　4. 每周≥4次	10个条目 2～5 min	得分≥8分被认为是危险或有害性饮酒筛查阳性 一般情况下： 8～15分者最适合向其提供简单的建议，重点是减少危险饮酒 16～19分者建议进行简短咨询和持续监测 ≥20分者需要进一步的诊断评估，以确定是否为酒精依赖
2. 当你饮酒时，通常一天喝多少个标准杯？ 　0. 1～2个 　1. 3～4个 　2. 5～6个 　3. 7～9个 　4. ≥10个		
3. 你多久一次性饮酒≥6个标准杯[a]？ 　0. 从不 　1. 每月≤1次 　2. 每月1次 　3. 每周1次 　4. 每天或几乎每天1次		
4. 过去1年中，你有多少次一开始喝酒就停不下来？（选项与第3题相同）		
5. 过去1年中，你有多少次因为喝酒而未能完成分内的事情？（选项与第3题相同）		
6. 过去1年中，你有多少次在大量饮酒后需要在早晨喝一杯酒来让自己振作起来？（选项与第3题相同）		
7. 过去1年中，你有多少次在喝酒后感到内疚或懊悔？（选项与第3题相同）		
8. 过去1年中，你有多少次因为喝酒而记不得前一晚发生的事情？（选项与第3题相同）		
9. 你或他人是否因你的饮酒而受伤？ 　0. 没有 　1. 是的，但不是在过去1年 　2. 是的，在过去1年内		
10. 是否有亲戚、朋友、医生或其他医疗工作者对你的饮酒表示过担忧或建议你减少饮酒？（选项与第9题相同）		

[a] 美国版问卷中此处为"≥5个标准杯"，反映了美国标准杯的大小。

在体格检查中，酒精性肝病可能表现为黄疸、肝大、肝掌、男性乳房发育、蜘蛛痣和腹腔积液。血清γ-谷氨酰转移酶水平升高通常见于过度饮酒的个体。

低风险饮酒

1个标准杯含有12 g酒精，这相当于1瓶12盎司（≈350 ml）的啤酒或冰镇果酒饮料、1杯5盎司（≈148 ml）的葡萄酒或1.5盎司（≈44 ml）的蒸馏酒（如40°酒）。对于64岁以上的男性和21岁以上的女性，适量饮酒的上限是每天1个标准杯。对于年轻男性，适量饮酒的定义为每天≤2个标准杯。由于体内水分含量较少，摄入相同量的酒精后，女性和老年男性的血液酒精浓度高于年轻男性。合理的血液酒精水平应≤50 mg/dl。

即使血液酒精水平低至80 mg/100 ml，也可能超出酒后驾驶（DUI）或醉酒驾驶（DWI）的法定定义［译者注：在中国，酒后驾驶（酒驾）是指车辆驾驶人员血液中的酒精含量≥20 mg/100 ml但<80 mg/100 ml的驾驶行为，而醉酒驾驶（醉驾）是指车辆驾驶人员血液中的酒精含量≥80 mg/100 ml的驾驶行为］。在美国全国性调查中，代驾策略似乎能有效防止有DWI风险的饮酒者进行不安全驾驶。对于有酒精使用障碍史者、有其他严重医疗状况（如肝病）者及孕妇，建议完全戒酒。

非药物治疗

心理社会干预可有效治疗重度酒精使用或酒精使用障碍，包括简短干预、动机增强治疗、认知行为疗法、行为治疗、家庭治疗和12步法（正在康复的酒瘾者通过参加自助同伴组织的定期会议完成12个具体步骤）。尽管这些治疗的疗效类似，但简短干预（通常为15～20 min）在门诊环境中最为实用。当需要更深入的社会心理治疗时，最可行的方法是由接受过特定方法培训的治疗师与能开具酒精治疗药物处方的医生共同提供治疗。

Considerations for Drug Interventions

Three medications are approved by the US Food and Drug Administration (FDA) to treat alcohol use disorders: disulfiram, naltrexone (oral and long-acting injectable formulations), and acamprosate. Medications are prescribed to less than 9% of patients who are likely to benefit from them, despite their inclusion in clinical practice guidelines as first-line treatments for moderate to severe alcohol use disorder. Medications should be administered in conjunction with psychosocial interventions to enhance treatment adherence.

Disulfiram (Antabuse) inhibits aldehyde dehydrogenase (i.e., the enzyme that converts acetaldehyde to acetate), resulting in a 5- to 10-fold increase in serum acetaldehyde concentrations when alcohol is consumed. This produces uncomfortable symptoms (e.g., facial flushing, tachycardia, nausea, vomiting, and headache), which act to deter alcohol consumption. Because of low medication compliance and limited efficacy, disulfiram is rarely prescribed.

Naltrexone is an opioid receptor antagonist. In clinical trials, a combination of naltrexone and psychosocial intervention reduced the number of drinking days, induced a longer period of abstinence from ethanol, and decreased the relapse rate in heavy drinkers when compared with psychosocial intervention alone: it reduced the likelihood of a return to any drinking by 5% and binge-drinking risk by 10%. Naltrexone is administered orally in a dose of 50 mg daily for 12 weeks, although larger doses (i.e., 100 to 150 mg daily) and a longer duration of administration may improve its success in preventing relapse. In 2006, the FDA approved a once-a-month injectable form of naltrexone (380 mg intramuscular) for the treatment of alcohol use disorders; this form appears to be more effective than the pill form at maintaining abstinence, since it eliminates the problem of medication compliance.

Naltrexone can be initiated while the individual is still drinking, thereby permitting treatment to be provided in a community-based setting without the need for enforced abstinence or detoxification. Some recovering alcoholics develop somnolence, nausea or vomiting when naltrexone is initiated. Because hepatic toxicity may occur at high doses ($\geq$300 mg), periodic testing of liver function is recommended. Naltrexone is contraindicated in subjects receiving opioids, given that opiate withdrawal is an unintended adverse effect of the drug.

Acamprosate (Campral), a structural analog of γ-amino butyric acid (GABA), decreases excitatory glutamatergic neurotransmission during alcohol withdrawal. The recommended dosage is 666 to 1000 mg 3 times daily, and its most common side effects are diarrhea and intestinal cramping. In placebo-controlled trials, acamprosate reduced relapse rates and increased abstinence from ethanol. In comparative trials, it did not appear to be as efficacious as naltrexone. Acamprosate should be used once abstinence is achieved; since it is not metabolized by the liver, it can be given safely to individuals with alcoholic liver disease.

The use of several other pharmacologic agents has been associated with a reduction in alcohol consumption, including ondansetron (a selective serotonin reuptake inhibitor), topiramate (an anticonvulsant), baclofen (a GABA agonist), sodium oxybate (the sodium salt of gamma-hydroxybutyrate), nalmefene (an opioid antagonist), and varenicline (a nicotinic acetylcholine-receptor and dopamine partial agonist), but none of these agents has been approved by the FDA for treatment of alcohol dependence.

Fetal Alcohol Spectrum Disorders

Alcohol freely crosses the placenta and is teratogenic. It is a leading preventable cause of birth defects with mental deficiency, with up to 1 in 100 children in the United States being born with fetal alcohol spectrum disorders (FASDs). The scope of disabilities and malformations varies and depends on the amount of alcohol consumed, the frequency of exposure, the stage of fetal development when alcohol is present, maternal parity, nutrition, genetic susceptibility, and individual variation in maternal and fetal alcohol metabolism.

The term FASD is used to characterize the full range of prenatal alcohol damage, varying from mild to severe and encompassing a broad array of physical defects and cognitive, behavioral, and emotional deficits. It includes conditions such as fetal alcohol syndrome (FAS), alcohol-related neurodevelopmental disorder (ARND), and alcohol-related birth defects (ARBDs).

FAS, the most severe form of FASD, is characterized by (a) growth retardation (i.e., height or weight $\geq$10th percentile); (b) neurodevelopmental abnormalities (i.e., microcephaly, hyperactivity, irritability, altered motor skills, learning disabilities, seizure disorders, and mental retardation); and (c) dysmorphic facial features (i.e., short palpebral fissures, smooth philtrum, and a thin upper lip). Children with typical dysmorphic facial features who lack the other features have partial FAS. Children with ARBDs have typical facies associated with FAS as well as anomalies in other organs (i.e., cardiac, renal, skeletal, auditory) but no growth retardation or neurodevelopmental abnormalities. Children with ARND exhibit behavioral or cognitive abnormalities in the absence of dysmorphic facial features.

Although the damage from prenatal exposure to alcohol cannot be reversed, children with FASDs benefit from early diagnosis and aggressive intervention with physical, occupational, speech and language, and educational therapies. Early recognition can also benefit the impaired mother, resulting in access to alcohol treatment and a better social situation for the entire family.

Although the recognition of FASD is important, its prevention is essential. Given that no safely established level of alcohol consumption in pregnancy exists, recommendations suggest that pregnant women maintain abstinence. In addition, women who are considering pregnancy or are already pregnant must be counseled about the effects of alcohol on the fetus.

Medical Management of Alcohol Withdrawal and Delirium Tremens

Patients admitted to a general medical hospital who have a history of heavy alcohol use have an approximately 2% to 7% chance of developing severe alcohol withdrawal syndrome (SAWS). Appropriate identification, prophylaxis, and treatment of withdrawal are essential in reducing morbidity and mortality associated with this disorder. Unfortunately, individual symptoms or signs do not effectively predict or exclude SAWS. The most effective method for predicting SAWS in acute care settings is use of a risk assessment tool that combines findings from a patient's history and clinical examination. The Prediction of Alcohol Withdrawal Severity Scale (Table 23.5) performs best for predicting the development of SAWS and requires an interview, examination (heart rate), and testing (blood alcohol).

For the patient with probable alcohol withdrawal, comorbid conditions that may coexist or mimic the symptoms of withdrawal (e.g., infection, trauma, hepatic encephalopathy, drug overdose, gastrointestinal bleeding, and metabolic derangements) should be excluded. Once this has been accomplished, the patient should be placed in a quiet and protective environment and should receive parenteral thiamine and multivitamins to decrease the risk of Wernicke encephalopathy or Korsakoff amnestic syndrome.

The Revised Clinical Institute for Withdrawal Assessment for Alcohol (CIWA-Ar) scale (available at https://umem.org/files/uploads/1104212257_CIWA-Ar.pdf), a measure of withdrawal severity, is useful in guiding symptom-triggered therapy in medically stable (i.e., non-ICU or postoperative) patients. Benzodiazepines are the only medications proved to ameliorate symptoms and to decrease the risk of

药物干预的注意事项

FDA批准了3种用于治疗酒精使用障碍的药物：双硫仑（戒酒硫）、纳曲酮（包括口服剂型和长效注射剂型）和阿坎酸（坎普拉尔）。尽管这些药物已被纳入临床实践指南作为中重度酒精使用障碍的一线治疗药物，但在可能受益于这些药物的患者中，不足9%的患者被开具了这些药物的处方。药物治疗应与心理社会干预联合使用，以增强治疗依从性。

双硫仑能抑制乙醛脱氢酶（将乙醛转化为乙酸的酶），饮酒后会导致血清中乙醛浓度增加5～10倍。这会产生不适症状（如面部潮红、心动过速、恶心、呕吐和头痛），从而抑制饮酒。由于用药依从性低和效果有限，医生很少开具双硫仑的处方。

纳曲酮是一种阿片受体拮抗剂。在临床试验中，相比于单纯心理社会干预，纳曲酮联合心理社会干预可减少饮酒天数，延长戒断期，并降低重度饮酒者的复发率。它可将重新开始饮酒的可能性降低5%，狂饮的风险降低10%。纳曲酮口服剂量为50 mg/d，持续12周，虽然更大剂量（即100～150 mg/d）和更长时间的给药可能提高其预防复饮的成功率。2006年，FDA批准了每月1次的纳曲酮注射剂型（380 mg肌内注射）用于治疗酒精使用障碍。在维持戒断状态方面，这种剂型可能比片剂更有效，因为它消除了药物依从性的问题。

纳曲酮可以在个体仍在饮酒时开始使用，从而允许在社区环境中提供治疗，而不需要强制戒断或脱毒。一些正在康复的酒瘾者在开始使用纳曲酮时可能会出现嗜睡、恶心或呕吐。由于高剂量（≥300 mg）可能导致肝毒性，建议定期检测肝功能。正在接受阿片类药物治疗的患者禁用纳曲酮，因为该药可导致阿片戒断。

阿坎酸是γ-氨基丁酸（GABA）的结构类似物，可在酒精戒断期间减少兴奋性谷氨酸能神经传递。推荐剂量为666～1000 mg，3次/日，其最常见的副作用是腹泻和肠绞痛。在安慰剂对照试验中，阿坎酸可降低复饮率并提升戒断率。在比较试验中，其疗效似乎不如纳曲酮。一旦成功戒酒，应使用阿坎酸，因为它不经过肝代谢，酒精性肝病患者可以安全使用。

多种其他药物可减少酒精消耗，包括昂丹司琼（选择性5-羟色胺再摄取抑制剂）、托吡酯（抗癫痫药）、巴氯芬（GABA激动剂）、羟丁酸钠（γ-羟基丁酸钠）、纳美芬（阿片受体拮抗剂）和伐尼克兰（尼古丁乙酰胆碱受体和多巴胺部分激动剂），但这些药物均未被FDA批准用于治疗酒精依赖。

胎儿酒精谱系障碍

酒精可以自由透过胎盘，并具有致畸作用。它是导致先天性智力缺陷的首要可预防原因。在美国，每100个儿童中有1个儿童在出生时患有胎儿酒精谱系障碍（FASD）。患者残疾和畸形的范围不同，并取决于饮酒量、饮酒频率、酒精摄入时的胎儿发育阶段、母体生育次数、营养状况、遗传易感性及母体和胎儿酒精代谢的个体差异。

FASD是指程度从轻微到严重的一系列产前酒精损伤，包括各种身体缺陷和认知、行为及情感缺陷。FASD包括胎儿酒精综合征（FAS）、酒精相关的神经发育障碍（ARND）和酒精相关的出生缺陷（ARBD）等。

FAS是FASD最严重的形式，其特征包括：①生长迟缓（即身高或体重≤第10百分位数）；②神经发育异常（即小头畸形、多动、易怒、运动技能改变、学习障碍、癫痫发作和智力低下）；③面部畸形特征（即睑裂短、人中平滑和上唇薄）。具有典型面部畸形特征但缺乏其他特征的儿童可被诊断为部分FAS。ARBD儿童具有与FAS相关的典型面容及其他器官（即心脏、肾、骨骼、听觉）异常，但没有生长迟缓或神经发育异常。ARND儿童表现为行为或认知异常，但没有面部畸形特征。

虽然产前暴露于酒精所造成的损害无法逆转，但FASD儿童可以从早期诊断和积极干预中受益，包括身体、职业、言语-语言治疗及教育治疗。早期识别还可使母体受益，从而接受酒精治疗，并为整个家庭提供更好的社会环境。

尽管识别FASD很重要，但其预防也至关重要。鉴于妊娠期没有确定的安全饮酒水平，建议孕妇不要饮酒。此外，必须告知考虑妊娠或已经怀孕的女性有关酒精对胎儿的影响。

酒精戒断和震颤性谵妄的医疗管理

在综合医院就诊的有重度酒精使用史的患者中，2%～7%可能发展为严重酒精戒断综合征（SAWS）。适当地识别、预防和治疗戒断症状对于降低SAWS相关发病率和死亡率至关重要。不幸的是，个体症状或体征并不能有效预测或排除SAWS。在急性治疗环境中，预测SAWS的最有效方法是使用风险评估工具，其结合了患者病史和临床检查结果。酒精戒断严重程度预测量表（表23.5）在预测SAWS发生方面的表现最佳，它需要进行访谈、检查（心率）和检测（血液酒精浓度）。

对于可能存在酒精戒断的患者，应排除可能共存或类似戒断症状的合并症（如感染、创伤、肝性脑病、药物过量、消化道出血和代谢紊乱）。排除上述问题后，患者应在安静且安全的环境中接受肠外维生素B_1和多种维生素治疗，以减小韦尼克脑病或科萨科夫遗忘综合征的风险。

修订版临床机构酒精戒断状态评定（CIWA-Ar）量表（https://umem.org/files/uploads/1104212257_CIWA-Ar.pdf）可衡量戒断的严重程度，并在病情稳定的（即非重症监护病房或术后）患者中指导根据症状严重程度进行治疗。苯二氮䓬类药物是唯一被证明可以改善症状

TABLE 23.5 The Prediction of Alcohol Withdrawal Severity (AW) Scale

Part A: Threshold Criteria (yes or no; no point):
Have you consumed any amount of alcohol (i.e., been drinking) within the last 30 days? OR did the patient have a "+" BAL upon admission? IF the answer to either is YES, proceed with test:

Part B: Based on Patient Interview (1 point each):
1. Have you been intoxicated or drunk within the last 30 days?
2. Have you ever undergone alcohol use disorder rehabilitation treatment or treatment for alcoholism (i.e., inpatient or outpatient treatment programs or AA attendance)?
3. Have you ever experienced previous episodes of alcohol withdrawal, regardless of severity?
4. Have you ever experienced blackouts?
5. Have you ever experienced alcohol withdrawal seizures?
6. Have you ever experienced delirium tremens or DTs?
7. Have you combined alcohol with other "downers" like benzodiazepines or barbiturates during the last 90 days?
8. Have you combined alcohol with any other substance of abuse during the last 90 days?

Part C: Based on Clinical Evidence (1 point each):
1. Was the patient's BAL on presentation ≥200 mg/dL?
2. Is there evidence of increased autonomic activity (i.e., HR >120/min, tremor, sweating, agitation, nausea)?

Maximum score = 10 points.
This instrument is intended as a **SCREENING TOOL**. The greater the number of positive findings, the higher the risk for the development of AWS.
A score of **>4 suggests HIGH RISK** for moderate to severe (complicated) AWS; prophylaxis and/or treatment may be indicated.

AA, Alcoholics Anonymous; *AWS*, alcohol withdrawal syndrome; *BAL*, blood alcohol level; *DT*, delirium tremens

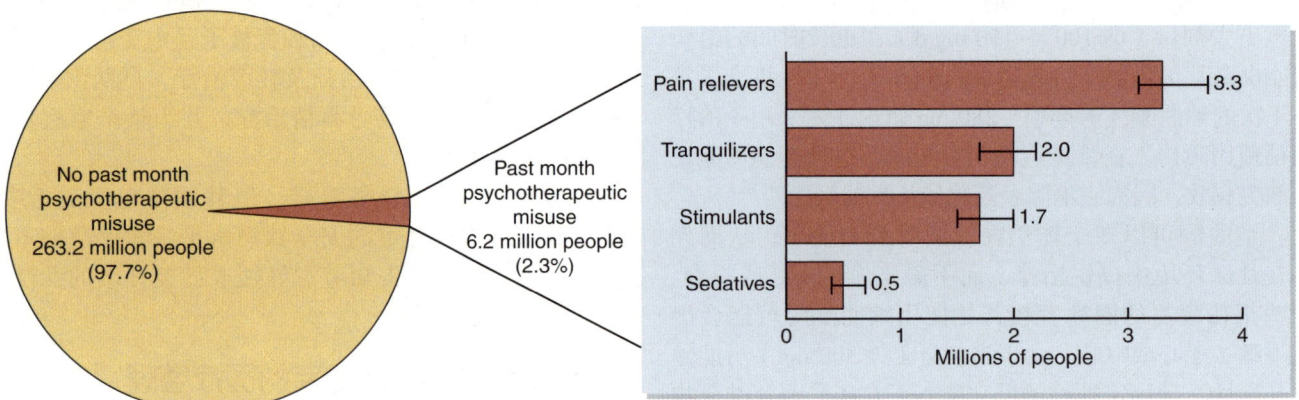

Fig. 23.3 Numbers of past month prescription psychotherapeutic misusers among persons aged 12 years or older according to the National Survey on Drug Use and Health (2016). (Substance Abuse and Mental Health Services Administration. [2017]. Key substance use and mental health indicators in the United States: Results from the 2016 National Survey on Drug Use and Health [HHS Publication No. SMA 17-5044, NSDUH Series H-52]. Rockville, MD: Center for Behavioral Health Statistics and Quality, Substance Abuse and Mental Health Services Administration. Retrieved from https://www.samhsa.gov/data.)

seizures and DTs in patients with alcohol withdrawal. Typically, diazepam (5 to 20 mg), chlordiazepoxide (50 to 100 mg), or lorazepam (1 to 4 mg) is administered intravenously every 5 to 10 minutes until symptoms subside, with the last of these medications preferred in patients with advanced cirrhosis, considering that the liver minimally metabolizes it. All benzodiazepines appear to be similarly efficacious in treating alcohol withdrawal, but long-acting agents may be more effective in preventing withdrawal seizures and are associated with fewer rebound symptoms. Conversely, short-acting agents may offer a lower risk of oversedation. For the patient who is resistant to benzodiazepines, intravenous phenobarbital (130 to 260 mg administered intravenously every 15 minutes until symptoms are controlled) may be given. If the agitation is not controlled by phenobarbital, propofol (0.3 to 1.25 mcg/kg/hr for maximum 48-hour infusion) can be tried, with intubation strongly recommended.

PRESCRIPTION DRUG ABUSE

According to the 2016 National Survey on Drug Use and Health, an estimated 6.2 million Americans aged 12 years or older used prescription-type psychotherapeutic drugs nonmedically in the past month (Fig. 23.3). This estimate represents 2.3% of the population aged 12 years or older. More people in the United States now die of prescription drug overdose (i.e., the nonmedical use of prescription-type pain relievers, tranquilizers, stimulants, and sedatives) than accidental vehicular trauma.

Sedatives and Hypnotics

Benzodiazepines and barbiturates are the major sedative-hypnotic drugs among the commonly abused agents that are listed in Table 23.6. The patient with sedative-hypnotic intoxication may have slurred speech,

表 23.5　酒精戒断严重程度预测量表

A 部分：阈值标准（"是"或"否"；不计分）：
您在过去 30 天内是否有过饮酒？或患者入院时 BAL 是否为"＋"？如果任一问题的答案为"是"，则继续进行测试：

B 部分：基于患者访谈（每个问题 1 分）：
1. 您在过去 30 天内是否有过酒精中毒或醉酒？
2. 您是否曾接受过酒精使用障碍的康复治疗或酒精中毒的治疗（如住院或门诊治疗项目或参加 AA 会议）？
3. 无论戒断的严重程度如何，您是否经历过酒精戒断发作？
4. 您是否经历过"断片"？
5. 您是否经历过酒精戒断性癫痫发作？
6. 您是否经历过 DT？
7. 您在过去 90 天内是否曾将酒精与其他"镇静剂"（如苯二氮䓬类药物或巴比妥类药物）合用？
8. 您在过去 90 天内是否曾将酒精与其他滥用物质合用？

C 部分：基于临床证据（每个问题 1 分）：
1. 患者是否在入院时 BAL ≥ 200 mg/dl？
2. 是否有自主神经系统功能亢进的证据（如心率＞ 120 次 / 分、震颤、出汗、焦虑、恶心）？

最高分为 10 分
此工具为筛查工具。阳性发现的数量越多，发展为 AWS 的风险越高
得分＞ 4 分表明发展为中重度（复杂性）AWS 的风险高；可能需要预防和（或）治疗

AA，匿名戒酒者协会；AWS，酒精戒断综合征；BAL，血液酒精水平；DT，震颤性谵妄。

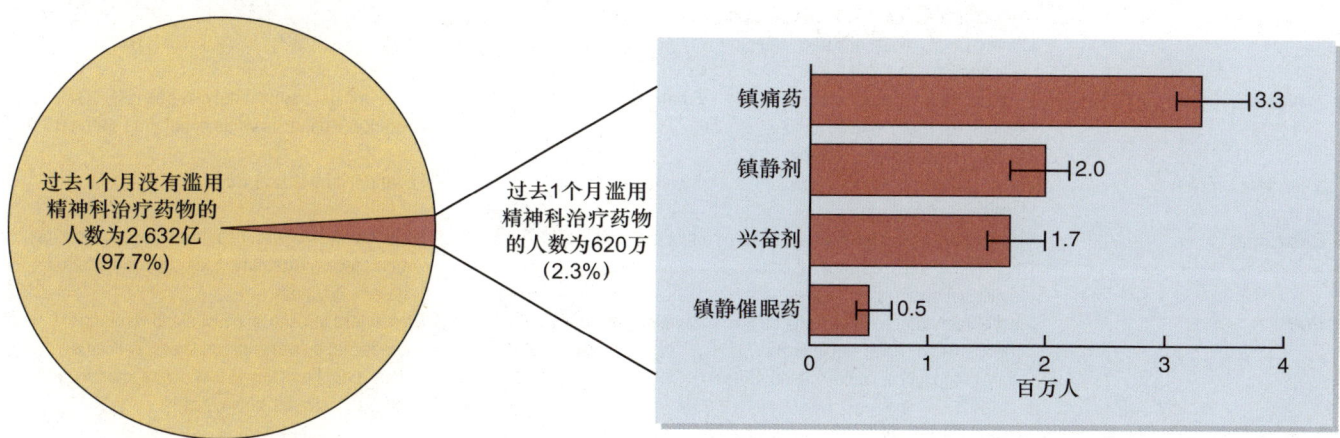

图 23.3　根据 2016 年美国国家药物使用和健康调查，12 岁及以上人群中过去 1 个月滥用精神科治疗药物的情况 [Substance Abuse and Mental Health Services Administration.（2017）. Key substance use and mental health indicators in the United States：Results from the 2016 National Survey on Drug Use and Health（HHS Publication No. SMA 17-5044，NSDUH Series H-52）. Rockville, MD：Center for Behavioral Health Statistics and Quality, Substance Abuse and Mental Health Services Administration. Retrieved from https：//www.samhsa.gov/data]

并降低酒精戒断患者癫痫发作和 DT 风险的药物。通常情况下，地西泮（5～20 mg）、氯氮卓（50～100 mg）或劳拉西泮（1～4 mg）每 5～10 min 静脉注射 1 次，直到症状消退，晚期肝硬化患者首选劳拉西泮，因其不经过肝代谢。所有苯二氮䓬类药物在治疗酒精戒断方面的疗效相似，但长效药物可能在预防戒断性癫痫发作方面更有效，且反弹症状较少。相反，短效药物过度镇静的风险较低。对苯二氮䓬类药物有耐药性的患者可静脉使用苯巴比妥（每 15 min 静脉注射 130～260 mg，直到症状控制）。如果苯巴比妥不能控制激越，可尝试使用丙泊酚 [0.3～1.25 μg/（kg·h），最多输注 48 h]，强烈建议气管插管。

处方药物滥用

根据 2016 年美国国家药物使用和健康调查，在 12 岁及以上的美国人中，估计有 620 万人在过去 1 个月内非医疗使用处方类精神科药物（图 23.3）。这一估计数字占美国 12 岁及以上人口的 2.3%。目前，美国因处方药过量而死亡的人数 [即非医疗使用处方类镇痛药（译者注：指强效阿片类镇痛药）、镇静剂、兴奋剂和镇静催眠药] 多于意外车祸死亡的人数。

镇静催眠药

苯二氮䓬类药物和巴比妥类药物是常被滥用的主要镇静催眠药，常见的滥用药物如表 23.6 所示。镇静催眠药中毒的患者可能出现口齿不清、运动不协调、

TABLE 23.6 Commonly Abused Drugs

Substance: Category and Name	Examples of Commercial and Street Names	How Administered[a]	Intoxication Effects and Potential Health Consequences
Cannabinoids			Euphoria, slowed thinking and reaction time, drowsiness, inattention, confusion, impaired balance and coordination, enhanced perception, cough, frequent respiratory infections, impaired memory and learning, increased heart rate, anxiety, panic attacks, tolerance, addiction
Hashish	Boom, gangster, hash, hash oil, hemp	Smoked, swallowed	
Marijuana	Blunt, dope, ganja, grass, herb, joint, bud, Mary Jane, pot, reefer, green trees, smoke, sinsemilla, skunk, weed	Smoked, swallowed	
K2/Synthetic Marijuana	Spice, K2, fake weed, Yucatan fire, skunk, moon rocks	Smoked, swallowed	Vomiting, agitation, hallucinations, hypertension, myocardial infarction, death, withdrawal and addiction symptoms
Sedative-Hypnotics (CNS Depressants)			Reduced pain and anxiety, feeling of well-being, lowered inhibitions, labile mood, impaired judgment, poor concentration, fatigue, confusion, impaired coordination and memory, respiratory depression and arrest, addiction
Benzodiazepines (Other Than Flunitrazepam)	Ativan, Halcion, Klonopin, Librium, ProSom, Restoril, Serax, Tranxene, Valium, Xanax, Doral; candy, downers, sleeping pills, tranks	Swallowed	Sedation, drowsiness, dizziness
Flunitrazepam[b]	Rohypnol; forget-me pill, Mexican Valium, R2, roach, Roche, roofies, roofinol, rope, rophies, woolfies	Swallowed, snorted	Visual and gastrointestinal disturbances, urinary retention, amnesia while under drug's effects
Sleep Medications	Ambien (zolpidem), Sonata (zaleplon), Lunesta (eszopiclone)	Swallowed	Sedation, drowsiness, dizziness
Barbiturates	Amytal, Nembutal, phenobarbital, Seconal; barbs, reds, red birds, phennies, tooies, yellows, yellow jackets	Injected, swallowed	Sedation, drowsiness, depression, unusual excitement, fever, irritability, poor judgment, slurred speech, dizziness
GHB[b]	γ-hydroxybutyrate; G, Georgia home boy, grievous bodily harm, liquid ecstasy, soap, scoop, goop, liquid X, geeb, Gina	Swallowed	Drowsiness, dizziness, nausea and vomiting, headache, loss of consciousness, hallucinations, peripheral vision loss, nystagmus, loss of reflexes, seizures, coma, death
Dissociative Drugs			Increased heart rate and blood pressure, impaired function, memory motor loss, numbness, nausea and vomiting
PCP and Analogues	Phencyclidine; angel dust, boat, hog, love boat, peace pill	Injected, smoked, swallowed	Possible decrease in blood pressure and heart rate, panic, aggression, violence, suicidal ideation; loss of appetite, depression
Ketamine[a]	Ketalar SV; cat Valiums, K, Special K, vitamin K	Injected, smoked, snorted	At high doses: delirium, depression, respiratory depression and arrest, amnesia while under drug's effects
Salvia Divinorum	Salvia, shepherdess's herb, maria pastora, magic mint, sally-d	Chewed, smoked swallowed	
Dextromethorphan (DXM)	Found in some cough and cold medications: Robo, Robotripping, Triple C	Swallowed	Euphoria, slurred speech, confusion, dizziness, distorted visual perceptions
Hallucinogens			Altered states of perception and feeling, nausea, chronic mental disorders, persisting perception disorder (flashbacks)
LSD	Lysergic acid diethylamide; acid, blotter, cubes, microdot, yellow sunshines, blue heaven	Swallowed, absorbed through mouth tissues	LSD: flashbacks, hallucinogen persisting perception disorder LSD and mescaline: increased body temperature, heart rate, blood pressure, loss of appetite, sleeplessness, numbness, weakness, tremors, impulsive behavior, rapid shift in emotion
Mescaline	Buttons, cactus, mesc, peyote	Smoked, swallowed	

Continued

表 23.6　常见滥用药物

物质：类别和名称	商品名和街头名称举例	摄入方式[a]	中毒效应及潜在的健康影响
大麻素			欣快、思维和反应减慢、嗜睡、注意力不集中、意识模糊、平衡和协调能力受损、感觉增强、咳嗽、频繁呼吸道感染、学习记忆功能受损、心率加快、焦虑、惊恐发作、耐受、成瘾
大麻脂（哈希什）	Boom、gangster、hash、hash oil、hemp	吸食、口服	
大麻烟（大麻植物顶端的花蕊和叶子）	Blunt、dope、ganja、grass、herb、joint、bud、Mary Jane、pot、reefer、green trees、smoke、sinsemilla、skunk、weed	吸食、口服	
K2/合成大麻	Spice、K2、fake weed、Yucatan fire、skunk、moon rocks		呕吐、激越、幻觉、高血压、心肌梗死、死亡、戒断和成瘾症状
镇静催眠药（CNS抑制剂）			疼痛和焦虑减轻、幸福感、抑制力下降、情绪波动、判断力受损、注意力不集中、疲劳、意识模糊、协调能力和记忆功能受损、呼吸抑制和暂停、成瘾
苯二氮䓬类药物（氟硝西泮除外）	劳拉西泮（Ativan）、三唑仑（Halcion）、氯硝西泮（Klonopin）、氯氮卓（利眠宁）、艾司唑仑（ProSom）、替马西泮（Restoril）、奥沙西泮（Serax）、氯拉卓酸（Tranxene）、地西泮（Valium）、阿普唑仑（赞安诺）、夸西泮（Doral）；candy、安眠药、睡眠药丸、镇静药	口服	镇静、嗜睡、头晕
氟硝西泮[b]	氟硝西泮（Rohypnol）；忘我药丸、墨西哥安定、R2、roach、Roche、roofies、roofinol、rope、rophies、woolfies	口服、鼻吸	视觉和胃肠道功能紊乱、尿潴留、用药后失忆
催眠药	唑吡坦（Ambien）、扎来普隆（Sonata）、艾司佐匹克隆（Lunesta）	口服	镇静、嗜睡、头晕
巴比妥类药物	异戊巴比妥（阿米他）、戊巴比妥（耐波他/宁眠泰尔/必妥）、苯巴比妥、司可巴比妥（速可）；barbs、reds、red birds、phennies、tooies、yellows、yellow jackets	注射、口服	镇静、嗜睡、抑郁、异常兴奋、发热、易激惹、判断力差、口齿不清、头晕
GHB[b]	γ-羟基丁酸；G、Georgia home boy、grievous bodily harm、liquid ecstasy、soap、scoop、goop、liquid X、geeb、Gina	口服	嗜睡、头晕、恶心和呕吐、头痛、意识丧失、幻觉、周边视觉丧失、眼球震颤、反射消失、癫痫发作、昏迷、死亡
分离性药物			心率加快、血压升高、功能受损、记忆动力丧失、麻木、恶心和呕吐
PCP及其类似物	苯环利定；天使粉、boat、hog、love boat、安宁丸	注射、吸食、口服	可能出现血压下降和心率减慢、惊恐、攻击行为、暴力、自杀意念；食欲减退、抑郁
氯胺酮[a]	Ketalar SV；cat Valiums、K、Special K、维生素K	注射、吸食、鼻吸	大剂量时：谵妄、抑郁、呼吸抑制和暂停、用药物后失忆
墨西哥鼠尾草	Salvia、shepherdess's herb、maria pastora、magic mint、sally-d	咀嚼、吸食、口服	
右美沙芬（DXM）	一些镇咳药和感冒药中含有：Robo、Robotripping、Triple C	口服	欣快、口齿不清、意识模糊、头晕、视觉失真
致幻剂			感知和感觉状态改变、恶心、慢性精神障碍、持续感知障碍（闪回）
LSD	麦角酸二乙胺；acid、blotter、cubes、microdot、yellow sunshines、blue heaven	口服、经口腔组织吸收	LSD：闪回、致幻剂持续感知障碍 LSD和麦司卡林：体温升高、心率加快、血压升高、食欲减退、失眠、麻木、虚弱、震颤、冲动行为、情绪急剧变化
麦司卡林	Buttons、cactus、mesc、peyote	吸食、口服	

TABLE 23.6 Commonly Abused Drugs—cont'd

Substance: Category and Name	Examples of Commercial and Street Names	How Administered[a]	Intoxication Effects and Potential Health Consequences
Psilocybin	Magic mushrooms, purple passion, shrooms, little smoke	Swallowed	Nervousness, paranoia, panic
Opioids and Morphine Derivatives			Pain relief, euphoria, drowsiness, respiratory depression and arrest, pinpoint pupils, nausea, confusion, constipation, sedation, unconsciousness, seizures, coma, tolerance, addiction
Codeine	Empirin with Codeine, Fiorinal with Codeine, Robitussin A-C, Tylenol with Codeine, OxyContin, Roxicodone, Vicodin; Captain Cody, Cody, schoolboy (with glutethimide: doors and fours, loads, pancakes and syrup)	Injected, swallowed	Less analgesia, sedation, and respiratory depression than morphine
Other Opioid Pain Relievers Oxycodone, hydrocodone bitartrate hydromorphone, oxymorphone, meperidine, propoxyphene	Tylox, OxyContin, Percodan, Percocet; Oxy, O.C., oxycotton, oxycet, hillbilly, heroin, percs Vicodin, Lortab, Lorcet; vike, Watson-387 Dilaudid; juice, smack, D, footballs, dillies Opana, Numorphan, Numorphone; biscuits, blue heaven, blues, Mrs. O, octagons, stop signs, O bomb Demerol, meperidine hydrochloride; demmies, pain killer Darvon, Darvocet	Chewed, injected, snorted, suppositories, swallowed	For oxycodone—muscle relaxation/twice as potent an analgesic as morphine; high abuse potential
Fentanyl	Actiq, Duragesic, Sublimaze; apache, China girl, China white, dance fever, friend, goodfella, jackpot, murder 8, TNT, Tango and Cash	Injected, smoked, snorted	80–100 times more potent an analgesic than morphine
Heroin	Diacetylmorphine; brown sugar, dope, H, horse, junk, skag, skunk, smack, white horse, China white, cheese (with OTC cold medicine and antihistamine)	Injected, smoked, snorted	Staggering gait
Morphine	Roxanol, Duramorph, M, Miss Emma, monkey, white stuff	Injected, smoked, swallowed	
Opium	Laudanum, paregoric; big O, black stuff, block, gum, hop	Smoked, swallowed	
Stimulants			Increased heart rate, blood pressure, body temperature; feelings of exhilaration, increased energy and mental alertness, tremors, rapid or irregular heart beat; reduced appetite, irritability, anxiety, panic, paranoia, violent behavior, psychosis, weight loss, insomnia, heart failure, seizures, coma
Amphetamine	Adderall, Biphetamine, Dexedrine; bennies, black beauties, crosses, hearts, LA turnaround, speed, truck drivers, uppers	Injected, smoked, snorted, swallowed	Rapid breathing, hallucinations, loss of coordination, restlessness, delirium, panic, impulsive behavior, Parkinson's disease, tolerance, addiction
Methamphetamine	Desoxyn; chalk, christina, cookies, cotton candy, crank, crystal, dunk, fire, gat, garbage, glass, go fast, go-go, ice, meth, no doze, no stop, pookie, rocket fuel, scooby snacks, speed, tina, trash, tweak, uppers, wash, white cross, yaba, yellow barn	Injected, smoked, snorted, swallowed	Memory loss, cardiac and neurologic damage, impaired memory and learning, tolerance, addiction, severe dental problems
Methylphenidate	Ritalin, Concerta; JIF, MPH, R-ball, Skippy, the smart drug, vitamin R	Injected, snorted swallowed	Increase or decrease in blood pressure, psychotic episodes, digestive problems,

表 23.6 常见滥用药物（续表）

物质：类别和名称	商品名和街头名称举例	摄入方式 a	中毒效应及潜在的健康影响
赛洛西宾	神奇蘑菇、紫色激情、shrooms、little smoke	口服	紧张、偏执、惊恐
阿片类物质和吗啡衍生物			缓解疼痛、欣快、嗜睡、呼吸抑制和暂停、针尖样瞳孔、恶心、意识模糊、便秘、镇静、意识丧失、癫痫发作、昏迷、耐受、成瘾
可待因	阿司匹林-可待因合剂、头痛粉-可待因合剂、感冒合剂（Robitussin A-C）、酚麻美敏混悬液（泰诺）-可待因合剂、盐酸羟考酮控释片（奥施康定）、盐酸羟考酮制剂、维柯丁；Captain Cody、Cody、schoolboy（同时服用格鲁米特：doors and fours、loads、pancakes and syrup）	注射、口服	镇痛、镇静和呼吸抑制的作用小于吗啡
其他阿片类镇痛药			
羟考酮、氢可酮、酒石酸氢吗啡酮、羟吗啡酮、哌替啶、右丙氧芬	泰勒宁、奥施康定、羟考酮（Percodan）、Percocet；Oxy、O.C.、oxycotton、oxycet、hillbilly、heroin、percs 维柯丁、洛塔布、洛赛特；vike、Watson-387、氢吗啡酮（Dilaudid）；juice、smack、D、footballs、dillies、欧帕纳、纽莫芬、纽莫酮；biscuits、blue heaven、blues、Mrs. O、octagons、stop signs、O bomb 杜冷丁、盐酸哌替啶；demmies、painkiller 达尔丰、达福赛	咀嚼、注射、鼻吸、栓剂、口服	羟考酮：肌肉松弛/镇痛效果是吗啡的两倍；滥用可能性大
芬太尼	Actiq、Duragesic、Sublimaze；apache、China girl、China white、dance fever、friend、goodfella、jackpot、murder 8、TNT、Tango、Cash	注射、吸食、鼻吸	镇痛效果是吗啡的 80~100 倍
海洛因	二乙酰吗啡；brown sugar、dope、H、horse、junk、skag、skunk、smack、white horse、China white、cheese（与 OTC 感冒药和抗组胺药一起使用）	注射、吸食、鼻吸	蹒跚步态
吗啡	Roxanol、Duramorph、M、Miss Emma、monkey、white stuff	注射、吸食、口服	
鸦片	鸦片酊、帕利高特；big O、black stuff、block、gum、hop	吸食、口服	
兴奋剂			心率加快、血压升高、体温升高；兴奋、精力和精神警觉性增强、震颤、心搏加快或不规则；食欲减退、易激惹、焦虑、惊恐、偏执、暴力行为、精神病、体重减轻、失眠、心力衰竭、癫痫发作、昏迷
苯丙胺	阿德拉、必飞腾、Dexedrine；bennies、black beauties、crosses、hearts、LA turnaround、speed、truck drivers、uppers	注射、吸食、鼻吸、口服	呼吸急促、幻觉、协调能力缺失、烦躁不安、谵妄、惊恐、冲动行为、帕金森病、耐受、成瘾
甲基苯丙胺	Desoxyn；chalk、christina、cookies、cotton candy、crank、crystal、dunk、fire、gat、garbage、glass、go fast、go-go、ice、meth、no doze、no stop、pookie、rocket fuel、scooby snacks、speed、tina、trash、tweak、uppers、wash、white cross、yaba、yellow barn	注射、吸食、鼻吸、口服	记忆丧失、心脏和神经系统损伤、学习记忆功能受损、耐受、成瘾、严重口腔问题
哌甲酯	利他林、专注达；JIF、MPH、R-ball、Skippy、聪明药、维生素 R	注射、鼻吸、口服	血压升高或降低、精神疾病发作、消化系统问题

TABLE 23.6 Commonly Abused Drugs—cont'd

Substance: Category and Name	Examples of Commercial and Street Names	How Administered[a]	Intoxication Effects and Potential Health Consequences
Cocaine	Cocaine hydrochloride; blow, bump, C, candy, Charlie, coke, crack, flake, rock, snow, toot	Injected, smoked, snorted	Chest pain, respiratory failure, nausea, abdominal pain, stroke, malnutrition, nasal damage from snorting
MDMA[b] (Methylenedioxymethamphetamine)	Adam, clarity, ecstasy, Eve, lover's speed, peace, uppers, Molly	Injected, snorted, swallowed	Mild hallucinogenic effects, increased tactile sensitivity, empathic feelings, chills, sweating, nystagmus, ataxia, teeth clenching, muscle cramping, impaired memory and learning, lowered inhibition
Synthetic Cathinone (Methylenedioxypyrovalerone (MDPV), Mephedrone ("Drone," "Meph," or "Meow Meow"), and Methylone)	Bath salts, drone, meph, meow meow, ivory wave, bloom, cloud nine, lunar wave, vanilla sky, white lightning, scarface	Injected, smoked, swallowed	Chest pain, paranoia, hallucinations, panic attacks, excited delirium, rhabdomyolysis, renal failure, high abuse and addiction potential
Other Compounds			
Inhalants	Solvents (paint thinners, gasoline), glues, gases (butane, propane, aerosol propellants, nitrous oxide), nitrites (isoamyl, isobutyl, cyclohexyl); laughing gas, poppers, snappers, whippets	Inhaled through nose or mouth	Stimulation, loss of inhibition, headache, nausea or vomiting, slurred speech, loss of motor coordination, wheezing, unconsciousness, cramps, weight loss, muscle weakness, depression, memory impairment, damage to cardiovascular and nervous systems, sudden death
Anabolic Steroids	Anadrol, Oxandrin, Durabolin, Depo-Testosterone, Equipoise; roids, juice, gym candy, pumpers	Injected, swallowed, topical	No intoxication effects. Hypertension, blood clotting and cholesterol changes, hostility and aggression, acne, prostate cancer, reduced sperm production, shrunken testicles, breast enlargement. In females: menstrual irregularities, beard development, and other masculine characteristics.

CNS, Central nervous system.
[a]Taking drugs by injection can increase the risk of infection through needle contamination with staphylococci, human immunodeficiency virus, hepatitis, and other organisms.
[b]Associated with sexual assaults (e.g., date rape).

incoordination, unsteady gait, impaired attention or memory, stupor, and coma. The psychiatric manifestations of intoxication include inappropriate behavior, labile mood, and impaired judgment and social functioning. On physical examination, the person may have respiratory depression or even arrest, nystagmus, and hyperreflexia. Although benzodiazepines rarely depress respiration to the extent that barbiturates do (and, as a result, have a much wider margin of safety), the effects of these drugs are additive with those of other CNS depressants, such as ethanol. Chronic use may produce physical and psychological dependence and a potentially dangerous withdrawal syndrome.

Benzodiazepines potentiate the effects of GABA, which inhibits neurotransmission. They are available as short-acting agents (temazepam [Restoril] and triazolam [Halcion]), intermediate-acting agents (alprazolam [Xanax], chlordiazepoxide [Librium], estazolam [ProSom], lorazepam [Ativan], and oxazepam [Serax]), and long-acting agents (clorazepate [Tranxene], clonazepam [Klonopin], diazepam [Valium], flurazepam [Dalmane], halazepam [Paxipam], Prazepam [Centrax], and quazepam [Doral]). Flunitrazepam (Rohypnol, also known as *roach, rophies, circles, Mexican valium, forget me pill, wolfies,* or *rope*) is a popularly abused benzodiazepine that is not legally available in the United States but is often smuggled here from other countries. It has been implicated in cases of date rape and is known as a club drug because adolescents and young adults often use it at nightclubs and bars or during all-night dance parties called raves.

In persons with an acute benzodiazepine overdose, respiratory depression is the major danger. Flumazenil (Romazicon), a competitive antagonist of benzodiazepines, can be given intravenously for acute overdose. Although it reverses the sedative effects of benzodiazepines, flumazenil may not completely reverse respiratory depression, and it may cause seizures in patients with physical dependence or concurrent tricyclic antidepressant poisoning.

Benzodiazepine cessation may precipitate withdrawal symptoms, depending on the half-life of the specific agent, the duration of use, and the dose. Such withdrawal is characterized by intense anxiety, insomnia, irritability, perceptual changes, hypersensitivity to light and sound, psychosis, hallucinations, palpitations, hyperthermia, tachypnea, diarrhea, muscle spasms, tremors, and seizures. Withdrawal symptoms usually peak 2 to 3 days after the discontinuation of a short-acting agent and 5 to 10 days after discontinuation of a longer-acting one; however, panic attacks and nightmares may recur for months. In general, agents with shorter half-lives produce more intense withdrawal symptoms compared with agents with longer half-lives. Benzodiazepines should be discontinued gradually over a period of several weeks (e.g., 4 to 8 weeks) to prevent seizures and avoid severe withdrawal symptoms. Whether switching to a long-acting agent such as diazepam improves detoxification is unclear. Few evidence-based treatment recommendations for pharmacotherapy of benzodiazepine withdrawal are available but include antidepressant agents for depression and sleep problems,

表 23.6 常见滥用药物（续表）

物质：类别和名称	商品名和街头名称举例	摄入方式 [a]	中毒效应及潜在的健康影响
可卡因	盐酸可卡因；blow、bump、C、candy、Charlie、coke、crack、flake、rock、snow、toot	注射、吸食、鼻吸	胸痛、呼吸衰竭、恶心、腹痛、卒中、营养不良、鼻吸引起的鼻腔损伤
MDMA [b]（亚甲基二氧甲基苯丙胺）	摇头丸、Adam、clarity、ecstasy、Eve、lover's speed、peace、uppers、Molly	注射、鼻吸、口服	轻度致幻作用、触觉敏感性增强、共鸣感、寒战、出汗、眼球震颤、共济失调、牙关紧闭、肌肉痉挛、学习记忆功能受损、抑制力下降
合成卡西酮［亚甲基二氧吡咯戊酮（MDPV）、甲氧麻黄酮或3,4-亚甲基二氧甲卡西酮］	"浴盐"；drone、meph、"喵喵"、ivory wave、bloom、cloud nine、lunar wave、vanilla sky、white lightning、scarface	注射、吸食、口服	胸痛、妄想、幻觉、惊恐发作、兴奋性谵妄、横纹肌溶解综合征、肾衰竭、滥用和成瘾的可能性大
其他化合物			
吸入剂	溶剂（油漆稀释剂、汽油），胶水，气体（丁烷、丙烷气溶胶推进剂、一氧化二氮），亚硝酸盐（异戊基、异丁基、环己基）；笑气、poppers、snappers、whippets	经鼻或经口吸入	兴奋、抑制力丧失、头痛、恶心或呕吐、口齿不清、运动协调能力丧失、喘息、意识丧失、痉挛、体重减轻、肌无力、抑郁、记忆力减退、心血管和神经系统受损、猝死
合成代谢类固醇	康复龙、氧雄龙、苯丙酸诺龙、环戊丙酸睾酮、宝丹酮；roids、juice、gym candy、pumpers	注射、口服、局部使用	无中毒效应。高血压、凝血和胆固醇变化、敌意和攻击性、痤疮、前列腺癌、精子生成减少、睾丸萎缩、乳房增大。女性：月经不调、胡须生长和其他男性特征

CNS，中枢神经系统。
[a] 注射吸毒会增加因针头污染而感染葡萄球菌、HIV、肝炎病毒和其他微生物的风险。
[b] 与性侵犯（如约会强奸）有关。

步态不稳、注意力或记忆力损伤、木僵和昏迷。中毒的精神表现包括行为失常、情绪不稳定、判断力和社会功能受损。体格检查时，患者可能会出现呼吸抑制甚至暂停、眼球震颤和反射亢进。虽然苯二氮䓬类药物很少会像巴比妥类药物那样抑制呼吸（因此安全范围更广），但这类药物与其他中枢神经系统抑制剂（如乙醇）的作用可以叠加。因此，长期使用可能导致躯体和心理依赖及潜在的戒断综合征。

苯二氮䓬类药物可增强 GABA 的作用，而 GABA 可抑制神经传递。该类药物分为短效药物（替马西泮和三唑仑），中效药物（阿普唑仑、氯氮卓、艾司唑仑、劳拉西泮和奥沙西泮）和长效药物（氯拉卓酸、氯硝西泮、地西泮、氟西泮、哈拉西泮、普拉西泮和夸西泮）。氟硝西泮（又称 roach、rophies、circles、墨西哥安定、忘我药丸、wolfies 或 rope）是一种常被滥用的苯二氮䓬类药物，虽在美国无法合法购买，但经常从其他国家走私到美国。由于青少年和年轻人经常在夜总会和酒吧或被称为"狂欢"的通宵舞会上使用氟硝西泮，因此其常与约会强奸案关联，并被称为俱乐部毒品。

对于苯二氮䓬类药物急性过量使用的患者，呼吸抑制是主要的危险。氟马西尼是一种苯二氮䓬类药物的竞争性拮抗剂，可静脉注射用于治疗急性药物过量。虽然氟马西尼可逆转苯二氮䓬类药物的镇静作用，但它可能无法完全逆转呼吸抑制，并可能导致苯二氮䓬类躯体依赖或同时服用三环类抗抑郁药中毒的患者出现癫痫发作。

停用苯二氮䓬类药物可导致戒断症状，这取决于特定药物的半衰期、使用时间和剂量。这类戒断症状的特点是强烈焦虑、失眠、易激惹、知觉改变、对光和声音过度敏感、精神病、幻觉、心悸、高热、呼吸急促、腹泻、肌肉痉挛、震颤和癫痫发作。戒断症状通常在停用短效制剂 2~3 天后达到高峰，在停用长效制剂 5~10 天后达到高峰。然而，惊恐发作和噩梦可能在数月内反复出现。一般来说，与半衰期较长的药物相比，半衰期较短的药物会产生更强烈的戒断症状。苯二氮䓬类药物应在数周内（如 4~8 周）逐渐停用，以防止癫痫发作并避免出现严重的戒断症状。尚不清楚改用地西泮等长效药物是否有助于脱毒治疗。关于苯二氮䓬类药物戒断的药物治疗，循证治疗建议很少，但可使用抗抑郁药（治疗戒断时的抑郁和睡眠问题）和心境稳定剂［尤其是卡

as well as mood stabilizers, especially carbamazepine (200 mg twice per day), although empirical evidence for these approaches is limited. Propranolol can be given to decrease tachycardia, hypertension, and anxiety.

Barbiturates may be short acting (pentobarbital and secobarbital), intermediate acting (amobarbital, aprobarbital, and butabarbital), or long acting (mephobarbital and phenobarbital). The symptoms of acute intoxication with the withdrawal from barbiturates are similar to those of benzodiazepines. For acute barbiturate overdose, oral charcoal and alkalinization of the urine (to a pH >7.5) with forced diuresis are effective in lowering the blood concentration. For patients with hemodynamic compromise refractory to aggressive supportive therapy, barbiturate elimination can be increased by hemodialysis or charcoal hemoperfusion. The effective treatment of withdrawal symptoms requires estimating the daily dose of the abused drug and substituting an equivalent phenobarbital dose to stabilize the patient, after which the dose of phenobarbital is tapered over 4 to 14 days, depending on the half-life of the abused drug. Benzodiazepines may also be used for detoxification, and propranolol and clonidine may help reduce symptoms.

Abuse of γ-hydroxybutyrate (GHB) has increased substantially over the last decade in the United States. This drug is abused for its sedative, euphoric, and bodybuilding effects. GHB is a metabolite of the neurotransmitter GABA, and it also influences the dopaminergic system. It potentiates the effects of endogenous or exogenous opiates. The ingestion of GHB results in immediate drowsiness and dizziness, with the feeling of a *high*. These effects can be potentiated by the concomitant use of alcohol or benzodiazepines. Similar to flunitrazepam and ketamine, GHB is a popular club drug, and it has been implicated in cases of date rape. Its street names include *G, liquid E, liquid X, fantasy, geeb, Georgia home boy, scoop,* and *grievous bodily harm*. Adverse effects that may occur within 15 to 60 minutes of its ingestion include headache, nausea, vomiting, hallucinations, loss of peripheral vision, nystagmus, hypoventilation, cardiac dysrhythmias, seizures, and coma. In rare instances, these adverse effects have led to death. The withdrawal from GHB becomes clinically apparent within 12 hours and may last up to 12 days.

Opioids

Opioids include the natural and semisynthetic alkaloid derivatives of opium as well as the purely synthetic drugs that mimic heroin. They bind to opioid receptors in the brain, spinal cord, and gastrointestinal tract; in addition, they act on several other CNS neurotransmitter systems, including dopamine, GABA, and glutamate, to produce analgesia, CNS depression, and euphoria. With continued opioid use, tolerance and physical dependence develop. As a result, the user must use larger amounts of the drug to obtain the desired effect, and withdrawal symptoms may occur if use is discontinued. Opioid misuse includes the misuse of prescription opioid pain relievers or the use of heroin. The commonly abused opioids include heroin, morphine, codeine, oxycodone (OxyContin, OxyIR, Oxecta, Roxicodone, or combination products, such as Percocet, Percodan, Tylox, Combunox), meperidine (Demerol), propoxyphene (Darvon), hydrocodone (Vicodin, Lortab, Lorcet), hydromorphone (Dilaudid), buprenorphine (Temgesic), and fentanyl (Sublimaze).

In 2016, there were 11.8 million past-year opioid misusers aged 12 or older in the United States, the vast majority of whom (97%) misused prescription pain relievers. The 2016 National Survey on Drug Use and Health reported that 53% of subjects who abused prescription pain relievers obtained them from friends or relatives (40% were given, 9% bought, and 4% stolen), and about one third (35%) indicated that they obtained pain relievers through prescription(s); only 6% were bought from a drug dealer.

Deaths from opioid overdoses have increased dramatically over the last decade. Opioids were involved in 47,600 overdose deaths in 2017 (68% of all drug overdose deaths), with synthetic opioids (other than methadone) the main driver of drug overdose deaths. Deaths involving synthetic opioids in the United States increased from roughly 3000 in 2013 to more than 30,000 in 2018. Synthetic opioids like fentanyl—which is 50 times more potent than heroin and 100 times more potent than morphine—are now involved in twice as many deaths as heroin.

Acute opioid overdose produces pulmonary congestion, with resultant cyanosis and respiratory distress, and changes in mental status that may progress to coma. Other manifestations include fever, pinpoint pupils, and seizures. Unsterile intravenous practices can lead to skin abscesses, cellulitis, thrombophlebitis, wound botulism, meningitis, rhabdomyolysis, endocarditis, hepatitis, or human immunodeficiency virus (HIV) infection. Neurologic complications from intravenous heroin use include transverse myelitis, inflammatory polyneuropathy, and peripheral nerve lesions.

For acute opioid overdose, the patient's respiratory status must be assessed and supported. Naloxone should be administered intravenously and repeated at 2- to 3-minute intervals, often in escalating doses; the patient should respond within minutes with increases in pupil size, respiratory rate, and level of alertness. If no response occurs, opioid overdose is excluded, and other causes of somnolence and respiratory depression must be considered. Naloxone should be titrated carefully, since it may precipitate acute withdrawal symptoms in opioid-dependent patients.

Withdrawal symptoms may appear as early as 6 to 10 hours after the last injection of heroin. Initially the individual often has feelings of drug craving, anxiety, restlessness, irritability, rhinorrhea, lacrimation, diaphoresis, and yawning; these signs are followed by dilated pupils, piloerection, anorexia, nausea, vomiting, diarrhea, abdominal cramps, bone pain, myalgia, tremors, muscle spasms, and, in rare cases, seizures. These symptoms and signs peak at 36 to 48 hours and then subside over 5 to 10 days, if untreated. A protracted abstinence syndrome characterized by bradycardia, hypotension, mild anxiety, sleep disturbance, and decreased responsiveness may occur for up to 5 months.

Treatment for opioid use disorder combines medication with behavioral health services, which is associated with a reduction in deaths from overdose, less opioid use and relapse, and prevention of infectious diseases. Several drugs that target the μ-opioid receptor can be used to manage opioid withdrawal: the full agonist methadone, the partial agonist buprenorphine, and the antagonist naltrexone.

Withdrawal from opioids can be managed with methadone, a long-acting synthetic agonist drug, as withdrawal symptoms of methadone develop more slowly and are less severe than those caused by heroin. Methadone is more highly regulated than the other opioid treatment drugs (i.e., classified as a schedule II substance in the United States) and is usually administered to patients via observed dosing in specialized clinics since it may be abused, diverted, or misused. Methadone can be given twice daily and tapered over 7 to 10 days. Methadone use, in both therapeutic doses and overdoses, has been associated with QTc interval prolongation and torsade de pointes, which, in some cases, has been fatal.

Buprenorphine can alleviate opioid withdrawal signs and symptoms, reduce craving, and block the subjective effects (e.g., so-called drug-liking) of other opioids. Accordingly, treatment with buprenorphine can be titrated to patients' withdrawal symptoms, yielding a well-tolerated transition to treatment. It is available in a daily mucosal formulation (which is also subject to diversion and misuse), as a subdermal implant administered every 6 months, or a monthly subcutaneously injected, extended-release formulation. It is also combined with naloxone in a formulation (Suboxone) developed to decrease the potential for abuse. This combination is available for use in two

马西平（200 mg，2次/日）]，尽管这些方法的经验证据有限。普萘洛尔可以减轻心动过速、高血压和焦虑。

巴比妥类药物可分为短效制剂（戊巴比妥和司可巴比妥）、中效制剂（异戊巴比妥、阿普比妥和布他比妥）或长效制剂（甲苯比妥和苯巴比妥）。巴比妥类药物的急性中毒症状和戒断症状与苯二氮䓬类药物相似。对于急性巴比妥类药物过量，口服活性炭和强制利尿碱化尿液（使尿液pH值>7.5）可有效降低血药浓度。对于积极支持治疗无效的血流动力学受损患者，可通过血液透析或活性炭血液灌流增加巴比妥酸盐的排出。有效治疗戒断症状需要估算滥用药物的每日剂量，并用同等剂量的苯巴比妥替代，以稳定患者病情，然后根据滥用药物的半衰期，在4~14天内逐渐减少苯巴比妥的剂量。苯二氮䓬类药物也可用于脱毒治疗，普萘洛尔和可乐定有助于减轻症状。

在过去十年中，γ-羟丁酸（GHB）的滥用在美国大幅增加。该药因其镇静作用、欣快作用和健美效果而被滥用。GHB是神经递质GABA的代谢产物，也会影响多巴胺能系统。它能增强内源性或外源性阿片类物质的作用。摄入GHB后会立即出现嗜睡、头晕和兴奋感。同时服用酒精或苯二氮䓬类药物会增强这些效果。与氟硝西泮和氯胺酮类似，GHB也是一种流行的俱乐部毒品，并与约会强奸案相关。其街头名称包括G、liquid E、liquid X、fantasy、geeb、Georgia、homeboy、scoop和grievous bodily harm。摄入GHB后15~60 min可能出现的不良反应包括头痛、恶心、呕吐、幻觉、周边视觉丧失、眼球震颤、通气不足、心律失常、癫痫发作和昏迷。在极少数情况下，这些不良反应会导致死亡。从临床上看，服用GHB后的戒断症状在12 h内变得明显，并可能持续长达12天。

阿片类药物

阿片类药物包括天然阿片类药物、半合成阿片生物碱衍生物，以及作用与海洛因类似的纯合成药物。它们可与脑、脊髓和胃肠道中的阿片受体结合。此外，它们还可作用于多种中枢神经递质系统，包括多巴胺、GABA和谷氨酸，从而产生镇痛作用、中枢抑制作用和欣快感。持续使用阿片类药物会产生耐受性和躯体依赖性。因此，使用者必须使用更大剂量的药物才能获得所需的效果，如果停止使用，可能出现戒断症状。阿片类药物滥用包括处方阿片类镇痛药滥用或海洛因滥用。常被滥用的阿片类药物包括海洛因、吗啡、可待因、羟考酮[奥施康定、OxyIR、Oxecta、Roxicodone或复方制剂（如羟考酮/对乙酰氨基酚、阿司匹林/羟考酮、Tylox、布洛芬/羟考酮）]、哌替啶、右丙氧芬、二氢可待因酮、氢吗啡酮、丁丙诺啡和芬太尼。

2016年，在美国12岁及以上人群中，有1180万人在过去1年中滥用阿片类药物，其中绝大多数（97%）为滥用处方阿片类镇痛药。2016年美国国家药物使用和健康调查报告显示，53%的处方镇痛药滥用者是从朋友或亲戚那里获得药物（40%为赠与，9%为购买，4%为偷窃），约1/3（35%）通过处方获得药物，只有6%是从毒贩那里购买的。

在过去十年中，死于阿片类药物过量的人数急剧增加。2017年，有4.76万例药物过量死亡与阿片类药物有关（占所有药物过量死亡的68%），其中合成阿片类药物（美沙酮除外）是导致过量死亡的主要药物。美国涉及合成阿片类药物的死亡人数从2013年的约3000人增加到2018年的3万多人（译者注：根据美国疾病预防控制中心发布的数据，2022年1月—2023年1月有超过10.9万美国人死于药物过量。其中，66%以上的死亡病例与芬太尼有关）。合成阿片类药物（如芬太尼）的药效是海洛因的50倍，是吗啡的100倍，目前导致的死亡人数是海洛因的2倍。

阿片类药物急性过量会造成肺充血，导致发绀和呼吸窘迫、精神状态改变，并可能发展为昏迷。其他表现还包括发热、针尖样瞳孔和癫痫发作。静脉吸毒使用未经消毒的针头可导致皮肤脓肿、蜂窝织炎、血栓性静脉炎、伤口肉毒中毒、脑膜炎、横纹肌溶解综合征、心内膜炎、肝炎或HIV感染。静脉注射海洛因引起的神经系统并发症包括横贯性脊髓炎、炎症性多发性神经病和周围神经病变。

对于阿片类药物急性过量患者，必须对其呼吸状况进行评估和支持治疗。应静脉注射纳洛酮，每隔2~3 min可重复注射，剂量通常会递增；患者应在数分钟内出现瞳孔扩大、呼吸频率加快、警觉性提高。如果没有反应，则可排除阿片类药物过量的可能性，必须考虑导致嗜睡和呼吸抑制的其他原因。由于纳洛酮可能诱发阿片类药物依赖者的急性戒断症状，因此应谨慎滴定纳洛酮的剂量。

戒断症状最早可能在最后一次注射海洛因后6~10 h出现。患者最初通常表现为对药物的渴求、焦虑、烦躁不安、易激惹、流涕、流泪、出汗和打呵欠；随后会出现瞳孔扩大、立毛肌竖起、厌食、恶心、呕吐、腹泻、腹部绞痛、骨痛、肌痛、震颤、肌肉痉挛等症状，少数情况下还会出现癫痫发作。如果不加以治疗，这些症状和体征会在36~48 h出现，然后5~10天消退。以心动过缓、低血压、轻度焦虑、睡眠障碍和反应迟钝为特征的稽延戒断综合征可能会持续长达5个月。

阿片类药物使用障碍的治疗应结合药物治疗和行为健康服务，以减少药物过量导致的死亡，减少阿片类药物的使用和复吸，以及预防传染病。多种针对μ-阿片受体的药物可用于控制阿片类药物的戒断症状，包括完全激动剂美沙酮、部分激动剂丁丙诺啡和拮抗剂纳曲酮。

美沙酮（一种长效合成阿片受体激动剂）可治疗阿片类药物的戒断症状，因为美沙酮的戒断症状比海洛因的戒断症状出现更晚，且严重程度更低。与其他阿片类药物相比，美沙酮受到更严格的监管（在美国被列为二类管控物质），由于其可能被滥用、流弊或误用，因此通常在专门诊所根据患者的实际用药情况调整美沙酮剂量。美沙酮每天给药2次，7~10天逐渐减量。无论是正常治疗剂量还是过量使用美沙酮，患者都可能出现QTc间期延长和尖端扭转型室性心动过速，甚至导致死亡。

丁丙诺啡可减轻阿片类药物的戒断症状和体征，减少渴求，并阻断其他阿片类药物的主观效应（即药物喜好）。因此，可根据患者的戒断症状来调整丁丙诺啡的

different forms—under the tongue or in the cheek—and decreases withdrawal symptoms for about 24 hours.

Naltrexone, a long-acting opioid antagonist that blocks impulsive opioid use, is an option for maintenance treatment to prevent relapse. It can be given orally daily or via injectable depot and implantable formulations every 60 to 90 days. It should only be administered after the patient is thoroughly detoxified because it may precipitate withdrawal. Pharmacotherapy must be combined with psychotherapy and structured rehabilitation to achieve an optimal outcome.

Finally, clonidine reduces autonomic hyperactivity and is particularly effective if combined with a benzodiazepine.

Amphetamines

Amphetamines have been used therapeutically for weight reduction and treatment of attention-deficit disorder and narcolepsy. Similar to cocaine, they cause a release of monoamine neurotransmitters (dopamine, norepinephrine, and serotonin) from presynaptic neurons. In addition, however, they have neurotoxic effects on dopaminergic and serotonergic neurons. Their euphoric and reinforcing effects are mediated through dopamine and the mesolimbic system, whereas their cardiovascular effects are caused by the release of norepinephrine. Chronic use leads to neuronal degeneration in dopamine-rich areas of the brain, which may increase the risk for the eventual development of Parkinson's disease.

Amphetamines can be abused orally, intranasally, intravenously, or by smoking. The most frequently used drugs are dextroamphetamine (Dexedrine), methamphetamine (Desoxyn), and methylphenidate (Ritalin). Illicit use of amphetamines has increased substantially, in part because (a) they are easily and quickly synthesized from ephedrine or pseudoephedrine and (b) their psychotropic effects may persist for up to 24 hours. The anorexiants, phenmetrazine and phentermine, which are structurally and pharmacologically similar to amphetamine, also have been used illicitly.

Tolerance to the stimulant effects of amphetamines develops rapidly, and toxic effects can occur with higher doses. Acute amphetamine toxicity is characterized by excessive sympathomimetic effects, including tachycardia, hypertension, hyperthermia, cardiac tachyarrhythmia, tremors, seizures, and coma. The patient may experience irritability, hypervigilance, paranoia, stereotyped compulsive behavior, and tactile, visual, or auditory hallucinations. The clinical picture may simulate an acute schizophrenic psychosis. The symptoms of withdrawal are similar to those seen with cocaine (see discussion of cocaine), but the acute psychosis and paranoia are often pronounced.

The treatment of amphetamine abuse centers on a quiet environment, benzodiazepines for anxiety, and sodium nitroprusside for severe hypertension. Antipsychotics, such as haloperidol, can reduce the agitation and psychosis by blocking the effect of dopamine on the CNS receptor. Urine acidification with ammonium chloride accelerates amphetamine excretion.

ILLICIT DRUG ABUSE

Cocaine

Among individuals 12 years old or older in 2016, 1.9 million had used cocaine within the previous month, including 432,00 users of crack. Cocaine can be taken orally or intravenously; alternatively, because it is well absorbed through all mucous membranes, abusers may achieve a high blood concentration after intranasal, sublingual, vaginal, or rectal administration. Its freebase form (called *crack* because of the popping sound it makes when heated) is heat stable, and it can be smoked. Crack cocaine is considered to be the most potent and addictive form of the drug. Euphoria occurs within seconds after crack cocaine is smoked, and is short lived. Compared with smoking crack cocaine or intravenous injection of the drug, mucosal administration results in a slower onset of action, a later peak effect, and a longer duration of action. The blood half-life is approximately 1 hour. The drug's major metabolite is benzoylecgonine, which can be detected in the urine for 2 to 3 days after a single dose.

An intense, pleasurable reaction lasting 20 to 30 minutes occurs after cocaine use, after which rebound depression, agitation, insomnia, and anorexia occur, which are then followed by fatigue, hypersomnolence, and hyperphagia (the *crash*). This crash usually lasts 9 to 12 hours but occasionally may last up to 4 days. Users often ingest the drug repetitively at relatively short intervals to recapture the euphoric state and to avoid the crash. On occasion, sedatives or alcohol are ingested concomitantly to reduce the intensity of anxiety and irritability associated with the crash. The combination of cocaine and intravenously administered heroin (so-called *speedball, snowball, blanco, boy-girl, Bombita, Belushi,* or *dynamite*) is often used so that the abuser can experience the cocaine-induced euphoria and then *float* down on the opiate. Unfortunately, this combination has been reported to cause sudden death. People who use cocaine in temporal proximity to the ingestion of ethanol produce the metabolite cocaethylene, which has also been implicated in cocaine-related deaths.

Cocaine blocks the presynaptic reuptake of norepinephrine and dopamine, producing an excess of these neurotransmitters at the site of the postsynaptic receptor. Thus, cocaine acts as a powerful sympathomimetic agent, resulting in tachycardia, hypertension, tachypnea, hyperthermia, agitation, pupillary dilation, peripheral vasoconstriction, and seizures. Cocaine causes potent vasoconstriction of cerebral arteries and, therefore, may result in a stroke. It is associated with myocardial ischemia and arrhythmias and, in rare cases, with myocardial infarction in young persons with normal or only minimally diseased coronary arteries. The principal mechanisms of ischemia and infarction are coronary arterial vasoconstriction, thrombosis, platelet aggregation, tissue plasminogen activator inhibition, increased myocardial oxygen demand, and accelerated atherosclerosis (Fig. 23.4).

For patients with cocaine-induced hypertension or tachycardia, labetalol and benzodiazepines are usually effective in lowering systemic arterial pressure and heart rate. Patients with acute cocaine-related myocardial infarction should receive aspirin, heparin, nitroglycerin, and, if indicated, reperfusion therapy (with a thrombolytic agent or primary coronary intervention). The use of β-adrenergic blockers should be avoided when possible, since ischemia may be worsened by unopposed α-adrenergically mediated coronary arterial vasoconstriction. Patients with a normal electrocardiogram or nonspecific changes can be managed safely with observation.

The immediate treatment of acute cocaine intoxication includes obtaining vascular and airway access, if needed, and careful electrocardiographic monitoring. Benzodiazepines can be given to control CNS agitation; haloperidol or risperidone can be used in the severely agitated patient. A supportive environment is needed, but detoxification is not required, given that few physical signs of true dependence are present.

Most chronic cocaine abusers have psychological dependence and an intense craving for cocaine. Personal and group therapies are important adjuncts to pharmacologic treatment, but relapse is common and is difficult to manage. Although no medication is FDA approved for treatment of cocaine addiction, disulfiram, modafinil, anticonvulsants (e.g., topiramate and tiagabine), serotonin reuptake inhibitors (e.g., citalopram), serotonin receptor antagonists (e.g., ondansetron), and GABA receptor agonists (e.g., baclofen) have shown some promise in promoting cocaine abstinence.

治疗剂量，使患者在治疗过渡期耐受良好。丁丙诺啡有日用黏膜剂型（也可能被流弊和滥用）、每6个月使用1次的皮下植入剂型（译者注：指Titan Pharmaceuticals生产的Probuphine，已于2020年退市）或每月使用1次的皮下注射缓释剂。丁丙诺啡和纳洛酮的复方制剂（赛宝松）可减少滥用的可能性。这种复方制剂有舌下含片和颊黏膜贴剂，可在24 h内减轻戒断症状。

纳曲酮是一种阿片受体拮抗剂，可阻止阿片类药物的冲动性使用，是预防复吸的维持治疗选择。纳曲酮可每日口服，也可每60～90天注射或植入1次（译者注：目前国外上市的仅有30天注射1次的长效针剂，我国刚上市了持续约150天的纳曲酮植入剂）。由于纳曲酮可能诱发戒断症状，因此只有在患者彻底脱毒后才能使用。药物治疗必须与心理治疗和康复治疗相结合才能取得最佳疗效。

可乐定能降低自主神经系统功能亢进，与苯二氮䓬类药物联用的效果尤佳。

苯丙胺类药物

苯丙胺类药物已被用于减重、治疗注意力缺陷障碍和发作性睡病。与可卡因类似，苯丙胺类药物也会导致突触前神经元释放单胺类神经递质（多巴胺、去甲肾上腺素和5-羟色胺）。此外，它们还会对多巴胺能神经元和5-羟色胺能神经元产生神经毒性作用。苯丙胺类药物的欣快和强化效应通过中脑边缘多巴胺系统介导，而其对心血管的影响则是由去甲肾上腺素的释放引起。长期服用会导致大脑中富含多巴胺区域的神经元变性，这可能会增加最终罹患帕金森病的风险。

苯丙胺类药物的滥用方式包括口服、鼻吸、静脉注射或吸食。最常用的药物是右苯丙胺、甲基苯丙胺和哌甲酯。苯丙胺类药物的非法使用大幅增加，部分原因包括：①易于通过麻黄碱或伪麻黄碱快速合成；②精神作用可持续长达24 h。抑制食欲药物（芬美曲秦和芬特明）的化学结构和药理作用与苯丙胺相似，也可能被非法使用。

对苯丙胺类药物兴奋作用的耐受性发展迅速，剂量越大越容易产生毒性反应。急性苯丙胺中毒的特征是过度拟交感效应，包括心动过速、高血压、高热、快速型心律失常、震颤、癫痫发作和昏迷。患者可能出现易激惹、过度警觉、偏执、刻板的强迫行为，以及幻触、幻视或幻听。临床表现可与急性精神分裂样精神病相似。苯丙胺类药物的戒断症状与可卡因类似，但急性精神病和偏执通常很明显。

苯丙胺类药物滥用的主要治疗包括将患者置于安静的环境、使用苯二氮䓬类药物（抗焦虑）和硝普钠（治疗严重高血压）。抗精神病药（如氟哌啶醇）可通过阻断多巴胺对中枢神经系统受体的作用来减轻激越和精神病症状。用氯化铵酸化尿液可加速苯丙胺的排泄。

非法药物滥用

可卡因

2016年，在美国12岁及以上人群中，有190万人在近1个月内使用过可卡因，其中包括4.32万名快克可卡因（crack）使用者。可卡因可通过口服或静脉注射滥用；此外，由于可卡因能被所有黏膜吸收，滥用者可通过鼻内、舌下、阴道或直肠给药而达到较高的血药浓度。它的游离基形态（因加热时发出"啪啪"的声音而被称为"crack"）具有热稳定性，因此可以吸食。快克可卡因被认为是药效最强、最容易上瘾的毒品。吸食快克可卡因后数秒内即可产生欣快感，且持续时间很短。与吸食或静脉注射快克可卡因相比，黏膜给药起效较慢，药效峰值出现较晚，作用持续时间较长。快克可卡因在血液中的半衰期约为1 h。该药物的主要代谢产物是苯甲酰基可卡因，一次服药后2～3天内可在尿液中检测到。

吸食可卡因后会出现持续20～30 min的强烈愉悦反应，之后会出现反跳性抑郁、激越、失眠和厌食，接着出现疲劳、嗜睡和暴食（"崩溃"）。这种"崩溃"通常会持续9～12 h，但偶尔也会持续4天。吸毒者通常会在相对较短的间隔时间内反复吸食毒品，以重获欣快状态，避免"崩溃"。吸毒者有时会同时摄入镇静剂或酒精，以减轻"崩溃"带来的焦虑和易激惹。滥用者经常会使用可卡因和静脉注射海洛因的组合（即所谓的speedball、snowball、blanco、boy-girl、Bombita、Belushi或dynamite），从而先体验到可卡因引起的欣快感，然后在阿片类制剂的作用下飘飘欲仙。不幸的是，据报道这种组合可能会导致猝死。在摄入乙醇的同时使用可卡因会产生代谢产物古柯乙烯，这种物质也与可卡因导致的猝死有关。

可卡因可阻断突触前对去甲肾上腺素和多巴胺的再摄取，从而在突触后受体部位产生过量的去甲肾上腺素和多巴胺。因此，可卡因是一种强效拟交感神经药，可导致心动过速、高血压、呼吸急促、高热、激越、瞳孔扩大、外周血管收缩和癫痫发作。可卡因能使脑动脉剧烈收缩，因此可能导致卒中。可卡因与心肌缺血和心律失常有关，在极少数情况下，冠状动脉正常或仅有轻微病变的年轻人也会发生心肌梗死。缺血和梗死的主要机制是冠状动脉血管收缩、血栓形成、血小板聚集、抑制组织纤溶酶原激活物、心肌需氧量增加和动脉粥样硬化加速（图23.4）。

对于可卡因诱发的高血压或心动过速患者，拉贝洛尔和苯二氮䓬类药物通常能有效降低全身动脉压和减慢心率。可卡因相关急性心肌梗死患者应接受阿司匹林、肝素、硝酸甘油治疗，并在必要时接受再灌注治疗（使用溶栓药物或直接冠状动脉介入治疗）。应尽可能避免使用β受体阻滞剂，因为缺血可能会因α肾上腺素能介导的冠状动脉血管收缩而恶化。心电图正常或有非特异性改变的患者可观察病情变化，随时处理。

急性可卡因中毒的紧急治疗包括在必要时开放静脉通道和气道，并进行严密的心电图监测。可使用苯二氮䓬类药物控制中枢神经系统激越；对于严重激越的患者，可使用氟哌啶醇或利培酮。患者需要一个支持性的环境，但由于很少出现依赖的体征，因此不需要脱毒治疗。

大多数慢性可卡因滥用者都有心理依赖和对可卡因的强烈渴求。个体和团体心理治疗是药物治疗的重要辅助手段，但复吸现象仍然很常见，且难以控制。虽然

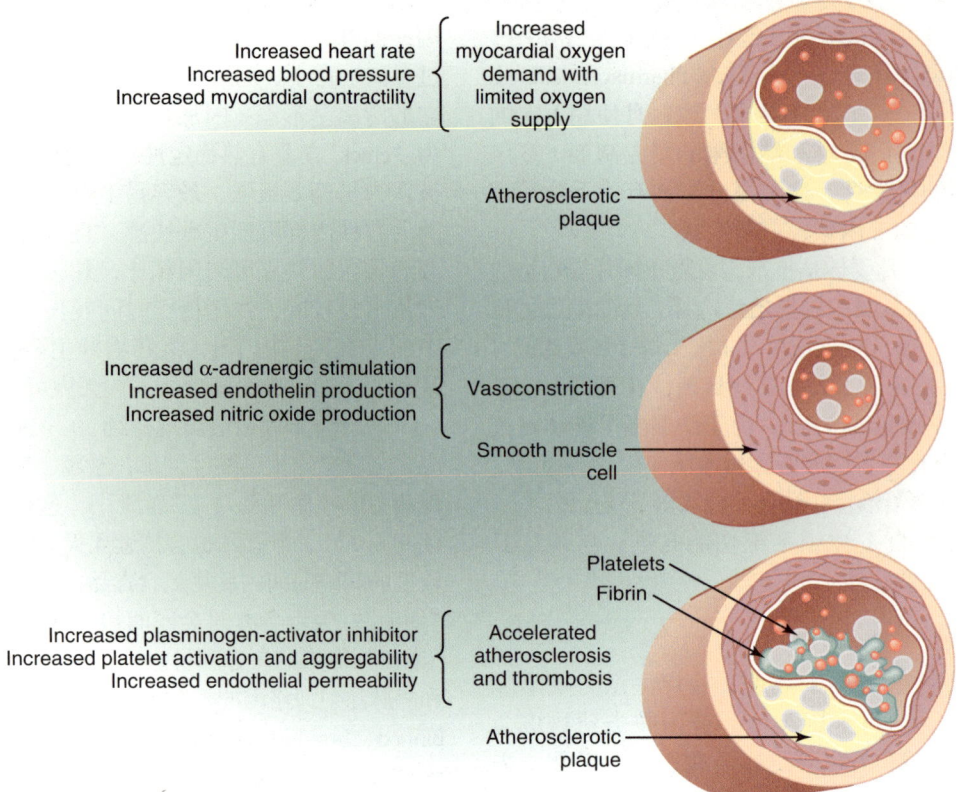

Fig. 23.4 The mechanisms by which cocaine may induce myocardial ischemia or infarction. Cocaine may cause increases in the determinants of myocardial oxygen demand when oxygen supply is limited *(top)*, when intense vasoconstriction of the coronary arteries occurs *(middle)*, or when accelerated atherosclerosis and thrombosis are present *(bottom)*.

Cannabis

The cannabinoid drugs include marijuana (the dried flowering tops and stems of the hemp plant) and hashish (a resinous extract of the hemp plant). Marijuana is the most commonly used "illicit" drug in the United States, recognizing that it is now legalized for recreational use in many states and for medical indications in most states. In 2016, an estimated 24 million Americans had used it in the past month. Between 2007 and 2016, the rate of use increased from 5.8% to 8.9% of the U.S. population, and the number of users increased from 14.5 million to 24 million. This increase reflects the increase in marijuana use by adults aged 26 years or older and, to a lesser extent, the increase in marijuana use among young adults aged 18 to 25 years (Fig. 23.5). In 2018 about 1 in every 13 young adults (8%) aged 19 to 28 was a daily or near daily marijuana user.

Marijuana use disorder occurs when someone experiences clinically significant impairment caused by the recurrent use of marijuana, including health problems, persistent or increasing use, and failure to meet major responsibilities at work, school, or home. Approximately 4.0 million people aged 12 or older in 2016 had a marijuana use disorder in the past year, which represents 1.5% of persons aged 12 years or older.

Marijuana and hashish are among the drugs most commonly used by adolescents, with approximately one third (36%) of 12th graders admitting use at least once and 5.8% reporting that they are daily or nearly daily users. Most of their pharmacologic effects come from metabolites of δ-9-tetrahydrocannabinol, which bind to specific cannabinoid receptors located in the CNS, spinal cord, and peripheral nervous system. The primary mode of use is smoking, with mood-altering and intoxicating effects noted within 3 minutes and peak effects in approximately 1 hour. However, vaping cannabis extracts and synthetic cannabinoids ("fake marijuana") in electronic cigarette devices has become increasingly popular. The acute physiologic effects are dose-related and often include increased heart rate, conjunctival congestion, dry mouth, fine tremor, muscle weakness, and ataxia. Psychoactive effects include euphoria, enhanced perception of colors and sounds, drowsiness, inattentiveness, and inability to learn new facts. Tolerance and physical dependence occur, and chronic users may experience mild withdrawal symptoms of irritability, restlessness, anorexia, insomnia, or mild hyperthermia. Rarely, acute psychosis with panic reactions occurs. The treatment of withdrawal is supportive and includes reassurance; benzodiazepines may be used in severely agitated patients. Cannabinoids have been used as antiemetic agents in patients with cancer receiving chemotherapy, for weight stimulation (in patients with cancer or HIV infection), and in the treatment of glaucoma.

Severe pulmonary illnesses have been reported in hundreds of otherwise healthy young persons who have "vaped" cannabis extracts (i.e., tetrahydrocannabinol products) in e-cigarettes, with one third requiring mechanical ventilation and some experiencing death. Initial symptoms include shortness of breath, cough, chest pain fever, gastrointestinal issues (i.e., nausea, vomiting, diarrhea, and abdominal pain), and weight loss, which occurs days or weeks after vaping. Bilateral infiltrates are present on chest imaging. Although most patients (>80%) reported having used tetrahydrocannabinol products in e-cigarette

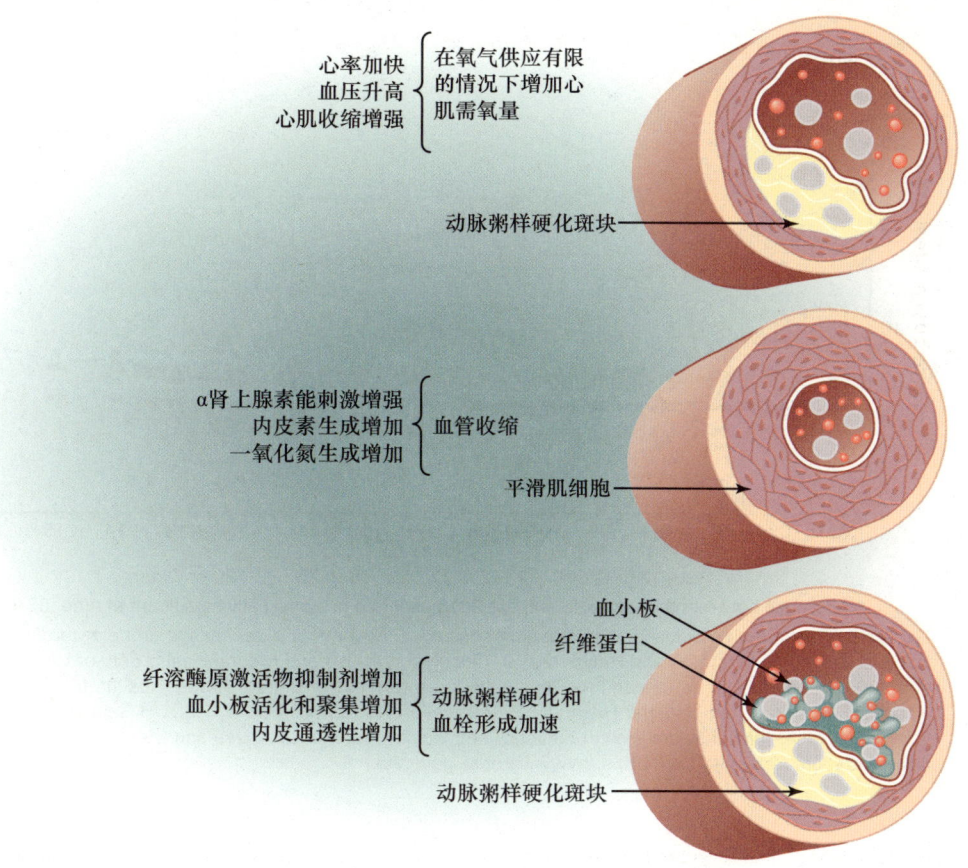

图 23.4 可卡因诱发心肌缺血或梗死的机制。当氧气供应受限（上图）、冠状动脉血管强烈收缩（中图）、动脉粥样硬化和血栓形成加速（下图）时，可卡因可能导致心肌需氧量增加

FDA 尚未批准任何药物用于治疗可卡因成瘾，但双硫仑、莫达非尼、抗惊厥药（如托吡酯和加巴喷丁）、5-羟色胺再摄取抑制剂（如西酞普兰）、5-羟色胺受体拮抗剂（如昂丹司琼）和 GABA 受体激动剂（如巴氯芬）在促进可卡因戒断方面已显示出一定的应用前景。

大麻

大麻类物质包括大麻烟（大麻植物的干花顶端和茎）和大麻脂（哈希什；大麻植物的树脂提取物）。大麻烟是美国最常使用的"非法"药物。目前在美国大多数州，大麻的医疗用途已合法化，而在许多州，大麻的娱乐用途也已经合法化。2016 年，估计有 2400 万美国人在最近 1 个月内使用过大麻。2007—2016 年，美国人口的大麻使用率从 5.8% 增至 8.9%，使用者人数从 1450 万增至 2400 万。这一增长反映了 26 岁及以上人群使用大麻的增加，其次是 18～25 岁年轻人（图 23.5）。2018 年，19～28 岁的年轻人中每 13 人约有 1 人（8%）每天或几乎每天吸食大麻。

大麻使用障碍是指个体因目前使用大麻而出现临床上的严重损害，包括健康问题、持续或逐渐增加大麻使用量，以及无法履行工作、学校或家庭中的主要责任。2016 年，12 岁及以上人群中约有 400 万人在过去 1 年中存在大麻使用障碍，占该人群的 1.5%。

大麻烟和大麻脂是青少年最常吸食的毒品之一，约 1/3（36%）的十二年级学生承认至少吸食过 1 次，

5.8% 的学生表示每天或几乎每天吸食。大麻的药理作用主要来源于其代谢产物 δ-9-四氢大麻酚，其可与位于中枢神经系统、脊髓和外周神经系统的特异性大麻素受体结合。大麻的主要使用方式是吸食，3 min 内即可改变情绪和产生令人陶醉的效果，约 1 h 后效果达到峰值。然而，在电子烟设备中吸食大麻提取物和合成大麻素（"假大麻"）也越来越流行。大麻的急性生理效应与剂量有关，通常包括心率加快、结膜充血、口干、细微震颤、肌无力和共济失调。精神兴奋作用包括欣快感、对颜色和声音的感知增强、嗜睡、注意力不集中及无法学习新知识。大麻会产生耐受性和躯体依赖性，长期吸食者可能出现易激惹、不安、厌食、失眠或轻度发热等轻微戒断症状。极少数情况下会出现伴有惊恐反应的急性精神病。戒断治疗是支持性的，包括安抚；严重激越患者可使用苯二氮䓬类药物。大麻素已被用作接受化疗的癌症患者的止吐药、刺激食欲（癌症患者或 HIV 感染者）及治疗青光眼的药物。

据报道，数百名既往健康的年轻人"吸食"电子烟中的大麻提取物（即四氢大麻酚产品）后出现了严重的肺部疾病，其中 1/3 需要机械通气，部分吸食者死亡。最初的症状包括呼吸急促、咳嗽、胸痛、发热、胃肠道症状（即恶心、呕吐、腹泻和腹痛）及体重减轻，这些症状在吸食后数天或数周出现。胸部影像学检查可见双肺浸润。尽管大多数患者（＞ 80%）报告在出现严重肺部症状之前曾使用过电子烟设备中的四氢大麻酚产品，

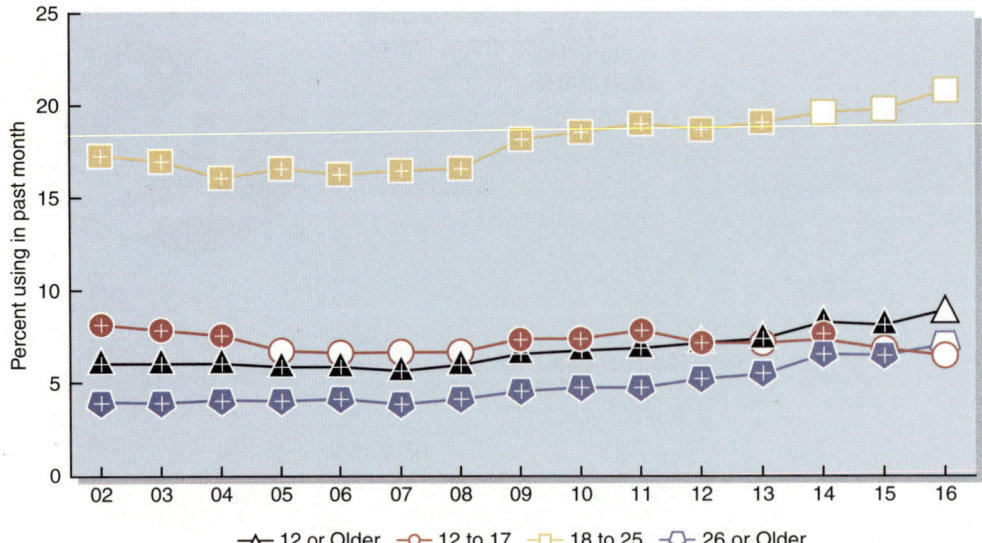

Fig. 23.5 Past-month marijuana use among persons aged 12 years or older, by age group according to the National Survey on Drug Use and Health (2016). (Substance Abuse and Mental Health Services Administration. [2017]. Key substance use and mental health indicators in the United States: Results from the 2016 National Survey on Drug Use and Health [HHS Publication No. SMA 17-5044, NSDUH Series H-52]. Rockville, MD: Center for Behavioral Health Statistics and Quality, Substance Abuse and Mental Health Services Administration. Retrieved from https://www.samhsa.gov/data.)

devices prior to the development of their severe pulmonary symptoms, a wide variety of products and devices have been reported. E-cigarette liquids and aerosols contain a variety of chemical constituents that may have adverse health effects, including propylene glycol, glycerin, hydrocarbons, nitrosamines, volatile organic chemicals, and toxic metals, flavoring compounds (i.e., diacetyl and 2,3-pentanedione), and THC-based oils and vitamin E acetate.

Synthetic marijuana is a psychoactive designer drug composed of a mixture of herbs, spices, or shredded plant material that is sprayed with synthetic chemicals that mimic the effects of cannabis when smoked or prepared as a tea. They have been sold widely in "head shops" as well as through the internet and are best known by the brand names K2 and Spice. Spice products are popular among young people; of the illicit drugs most used by high school seniors, they are second only to marijuana. Synthetic cannabis can precipitate acute psychosis or a worsening of previously stable psychotic disorders; they also may trigger a chronic (long-term) psychotic disorder among vulnerable individuals, such as those with a family history of mental illness. K2 ingestion has been associated with myocardial infarction and death. Regular users may experience withdrawal and addiction symptoms.

Hallucinogens and Dissociative Drugs

Hallucinogens (drugs that cause hallucinations) include lysergic acid diethylamide (LSD), mescaline, psilocybin, and ibogaine. *Dissociative drugs* distort perceptions of sight and sound and produce feelings of detachment (dissociation) without causing hallucinations. They include phencyclidine (PCP), ketamine, salvia, and dextromethorphan (a widely available cough suppressant).

LSD is the most potent of the hallucinogenic drugs. Although it is known to interact with serotonin receptors in the cerebral cortex and *locus ceruleus*, its precise psychoactive mechanism is unknown. Within 30 minutes of its oral ingestion, sympathomimetic effects appear, including mydriasis, hyperthermia, tachycardia, elevated blood pressure, diaphoresis, dry mouth, increased alertness, tremors, and nausea. Within 2 hours, the psychoactive effects become apparent, with heightened perceptions (highly intensified colors, smells, sounds, and other sensations), body distortions, mood variations, and visual hallucinations. An acute panic reaction may occur, sometimes leading to self-injury or suicide. After approximately 12 hours, the syndrome begins to subside, but fatigue and tension may persist for another day. Flashbacks (brief recurrences of the hallucinations) may occur days or even weeks after the last dose but tend to disappear without treatment. Acute panic reactions are best treated in a supportive environment; benzodiazepines can be given to severely agitated patients.

PCP is a potent, addictive hallucinogen that produces a prompt stimulant effect similar to that of amphetamines, with feelings of euphoria, power, and invincibility. Patients may have hypertension, tachycardia, hyperthermia, bidirectional nystagmus, slurred speech, ataxia, hallucinations, extreme agitation, and rhabdomyolysis. With more severe reactions, patients may be brought to medical attention in a coma-like state, with open eyes and pupils that are partially dilated, a decreased pain response, brief periods of excitation, and muscle rigidity. On occasion, PCP users may have hypertensive urgency, seizures, and bizarre (often violent) behavior, which lead to suicide or extreme violence toward others. Tolerance and mild withdrawal symptoms have been seen in daily users, but the major problem is drug craving. Treatment entails a quiet environment, sedation with benzodiazepines, hydration, haloperidol for terrifying hallucinations, and suicide precautions. Continuous gastric suction and acidification of the urine with intravenous ammonium chloride or ascorbic acid may aid in the drug's excretion, but acidification may increase the risk of renal failure if rhabdomyolysis is present.

Ketamine is a rapidly acting general anesthetic; unlike most anesthetics, it produces only mild respiratory depression and appears to stimulate the cardiovascular system. Adverse effects, including delirium

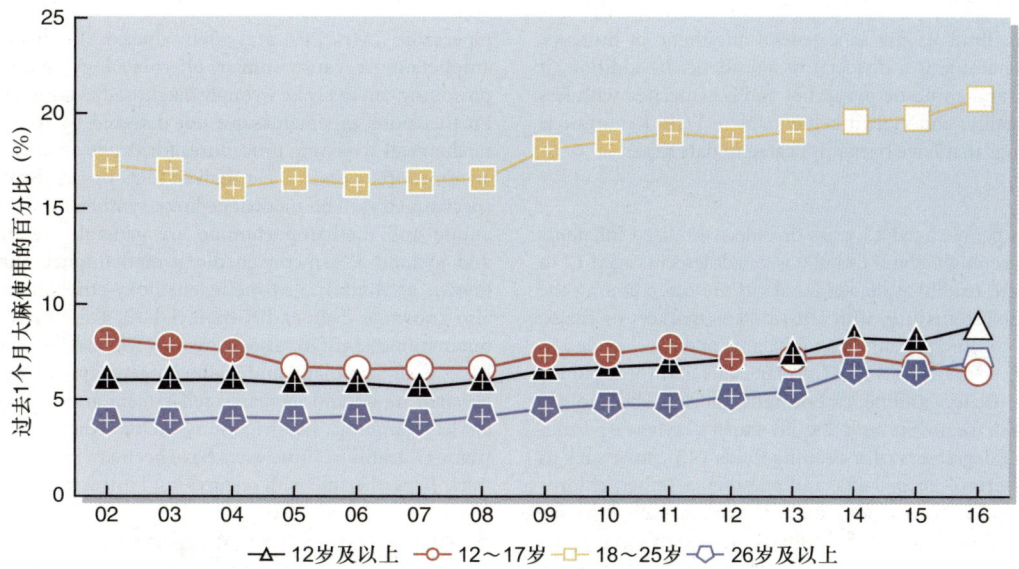

图 23.5 根据美国全国毒品使用和健康调查（2016 年），按年龄组划分的 12 岁或 12 岁以上人群过去 1 个月大麻使用的情况 [Substance Abuse and Mental Health Services Administration.（2017）. Key substance use and mental health indicators in the United States：Results from the 2016 National Survey on Drug Use and Health（HHS Publication No. SMA 17-5044，NSDUH Series H-52）. Rockville，MD：Center for Behavioral Health Statistics and Quality，Substance Abuse and Mental Health Services Administration. Retrieved from https://www.samhsa.gov/data.]

但报告的产品和设备种类繁多。电子烟液体和气溶胶中含有多种可能对健康产生不良影响的化学成分，包括丙二醇、甘油、碳氢化合物、亚硝胺、挥发性有机化学物质和有毒金属、调味化合物（即双乙酰和 2,3-戊二酮），以及以四氢大麻酚为基础的精油和醋酸维生素 E。

合成大麻烟是一种具有精神活性的策划药，由草药、香料或切碎的植物材料混合物组成，喷洒合成化学物质后，在吸食或泡茶时能模拟大麻的效果。它们在"头店"和互联网上广泛销售，最著名的品牌名称是 K2 和 Spice。Spice 在年轻人中很流行，是美国高中生使用最多的非法药物，仅次于大麻烟。合成大麻可诱发急性精神病或使已稳定的精神病性障碍恶化；它们还可能在易感人群（如有精神病家族史者）中诱发慢性（长期）精神病性障碍。吸食 K2 与心肌梗死和死亡有关。经常服用者可能出现戒断和成瘾症状。

致幻剂和分离性药物

致幻剂（可产生幻觉的药物）包括麦角酰二乙胺（LSD）、麦司卡林、赛洛西宾和伊博格碱。分离性药物可扭曲视觉和听觉感知，产生分离（解离）感，但不会导致幻觉（译者注：分离性药物能产生幻觉，如幻视、幻听等），包括苯环己哌啶（PCP）、氯胺酮、墨西哥鼠尾草和右美沙芬（一种广泛使用的止咳药）。

LSD 是致幻剂中药效最强的一种。虽然它能与大脑皮质和蓝斑核中的 5-羟色胺受体相互作用，但其确切的精神活性机制尚不清楚。在口服 LSD 后 30 min 内即可出现拟交感神经作用，包括瞳孔扩大、高热、心动过速、血压升高、出汗、口干、警觉性增高、震颤和恶心。在 2 h 内，精神活性作用开始显现，表现为知觉增强（颜色、气味、声音和其他感觉高度强化），身体扭曲，情绪变化和幻视。患者可能会出现急性惊恐反应，有时会导致自伤或自杀。约 12 h 后，各种症状开始消退，但疲劳和紧张可能会持续 1 天。在最后一次服药后数天甚至数周，可能出现闪回（幻觉的短暂重现），但通常无须治疗即可消失。急性惊恐反应最好在支持性环境中进行治疗；严重激越患者可服用苯二氮䓬类药物。

PCP 是一种强效的成瘾性致幻剂，可产生类似苯丙胺类药物的快速兴奋剂效果，使人感到欣快、充满力量和不可战胜。患者可能出现高血压、心动过速、高热、双向眼球震颤、口齿不清、共济失调、幻觉、极度激越和横纹肌溶解综合征。对于更严重的反应，患者可能会被送往医疗机构，处于类似昏迷的状态，表现为双眼睁开、瞳孔部分扩大、对疼痛的反应降低、短暂兴奋期和肌强直。PCP 使用者有时会出现高血压急症、癫痫发作和怪异（通常是暴力）行为，导致自杀或对他人使用极端暴力。每日使用者会出现耐受性和轻微的戒断症状，但核心问题是药物渴求。治疗措施包括提供安静的环境、使用苯二氮䓬类药物镇静、补充水分、使用氟哌啶醇治疗幻觉、预防自杀。持续抽吸胃液和酸化尿液（静脉注射氯化铵或抗坏血酸）可帮助药物排泄，但如果出现横纹肌溶解综合征，酸化尿液可能会增加肾衰竭的风险。

氯胺酮是一种快速起效的全身麻醉剂；与大多数麻醉剂不同，氯胺酮仅产生轻微的呼吸抑制，可能还会刺激心血管系统。谵妄和幻觉等不良反应限制了氯胺酮作为全身麻醉剂的临床使用。与 PCP 类似，氯胺酮也是一种分离性麻醉剂。此外，氯胺酮还具有镇痛和催眠作

and hallucinations, limit its use as a general anesthetic in humans. Similar to PCP, ketamine is a dissociative anesthetic. In addition, it has both analgesic and amnestic properties and is associated with less confusion, irrationality, and violent behavior than PCP. Ketamine is one of the club drugs that have been implicated in date rape.

Inhalants

Of the 1.8 million people aged 12 years or older who used inhalants in the past year to get high, about 684,000 were adolescents aged 12 to 17. Because they are readily available, inhalants are often among the first drugs that adolescents use, with felt-tip pens/markers or magic markers the most common agents. The inhalants may be classified as (1) *organic solvents*, including toluene (airplane glue and spray paint), paint thinners, kerosene, gasoline, carbon tetrachloride, shoe polish, acetone (nail polish removers and Liquid Paper), xylene (permanent markers), and degreasers (dry cleaning fluids); (2) *gases*, such as butane, propane, aerosol propellants, and anesthetics (ether, chloroform, halothane, and nitrous oxide); and (3) *nitrites*, such as cyclohexyl nitrite, amyl nitrite, and butyl nitrite (room deodorizer). These substances are most often inhaled by children or young adolescents, after which they produce dizziness and intoxication within minutes. Prolonged exposure or daily use may lead to hearing loss, bone marrow depression, cardiac arrhythmias, cerebral degeneration, peripheral neuropathies, and damage to the liver, kidneys, or lungs. A characteristic "glue sniffer's rash" around the nose and mouth is sometimes seen after prolonged use. In rare instances, death may occur, most likely from hypoxemia, cardiac arrhythmias, pneumonia, or aspiration of vomit while unconscious. Detoxification is rarely required for the patient who has abused these substances, but psychiatric treatment may be needed to prevent relapse.

Designer Drugs

The term *designer drug* refers to illicit synthetic drugs, many of which have increased potency in comparison with their parent compounds. The most common designer drugs include analogs of fentanyl, meperidine, piperazine, and methamphetamines. Several fentanyl derivatives, initially sufentanil, alfentanil, remifentanil, carfentanil and, more recently, acetylfentanyl, 6-butyrfentanyl, 4-MeO-butyrfentanyl, isobutyrylfentanyl, furanylfentanyl, α-methylfentanyl (China white), 3-methylfentanyl or TMF, p-methylfentanyl, methylacetylfentanyl, acrylfentanyl, 2-fluorofentanyl, fluoroacetylfentanyl, ocfentantanyl are illegally manufactured. These derivatives do not have recognized medical uses, are often not detected by routine drug testing, and have worsened the opioid crisis and number of drug-related deaths. Because these drugs are approximately 1000 times as potent as heroin, it is not surprising that fatal overdoses from respiratory depression have been reported.

The major meperidine derivatives are 1-methyl-4-phenyl-4-propionoxypiperidene (MPPP) and 1-methyl-4-phenyl-1, 2, 3, 6-tetrahydropyridine (MPTP), each of which produces euphoria similar to that caused by heroin. In some users, MPTP causes neuronal degeneration in the substantia nigra, which produces an irreversible form of Parkinson's disease.

Piperazines, a new class of designer drugs of abuse, are commonly sold as party pills in the form of tablets, capsules, or powders on the drug black market and in so-called head shops or over the internet under the names of Frenzy, Bliss, Charge, Herbal ecstasy, A2, Legal X, and Legal E. 1-Benzylpiperazine (BZP) is the most prevalent of these compounds. Aside from BZP and 1-(3,4-methylenedioxybenzyl) piperazine (MDBP), the phenylpiperazine derivatives 1-(3-trifluoromethylphenyl) piperazine (TFMPP), 1-(3-chloro phenyl) piperazine (mCPP), and 1-(4-methoxyphenyl) piperazine (MeOPP) are often abused. Because piperazines and amphetamines cause similar pharmacologic symptoms, piperazine poisoning can easily be wrongly diagnosed as amphetamine poisoning. Furthermore, piperazines are not detected by routinely used immunochemical screening procedures for drugs of abuse, but they require an appropriate toxicologic analysis (e.g., by gas chromatography-mass spectrometry). The methylenedioxy synthetic derivatives of amphetamine and methamphetamine are generally referred to as *ecstasy* and include 3, 4-methylenedioxy methamphetamine (MDMA, also known as *Adam*); 3, 4-methylenedioxy-ethylamphetamine (MDEA, also known as *Eve*); and N-methyl-1-(3, 4-methylenedioxyphenyl)-2-butanamine (MBDB, also known as *Methyl-J* or *Eden*). These drugs have CNS stimulant and hallucinogenic properties. They produce elevated mood and increased self-esteem and may cause acute panic, anxiety, paranoia, hallucinations, tachycardia, nystagmus, ataxia, and tremor. Deaths in some users have been attributed to cardiac arrhythmias, hyperthermia with seizures, and intracranial hemorrhage.

PROSPECTUS FOR THE FUTURE

Immunotherapy (i.e., vaccine development) has emerged as a promising approach to treat abuse of drugs like methamphetamine, heroin, and cocaine. By sequestering the drugs in the periphery without allowing the drug to cross the blood-brain barrier, the toxic and rewarding effects of the drugs are reduced. A novel pharmacokinetic approach to the treatment of drug toxicity involves the development of compounds that can be administered safely to humans and that accelerate the metabolism of the drug to inactive components. For example, catalytic antibodies have been developed to accelerate cocaine metabolism and are administered parentally. In experimental animals, mutations of human butyrylcholinesterase (one of the enzymes responsible for the metabolism of cocaine) accelerate cocaine metabolism and antagonize cocaine's behavioral and toxic effects.

SUGGESTED READINGS

Edenberg HJ, McClintick JN: Alcohol dehydrogenases, aldehyde dehydrogenases, and alcohol use disorders: a critical review, Alcohol Clin Exp Re 42:2281–2297, 2018.

Haight BR, Learned SM, Laffont CM, et al: For the RB-US-13-0001 Study Investigators. Efficacy and safety of a monthly buprenorphine depot injection for opioid use disorder: a multicentre, randomised, double-blind, placebo-controlled, phase 3 trial, Lancet 393:778–790, 2019.

Jonas DE, Amick HR, Feltner C, et al: Pharmacotherapy for adults with alcohol use disorders in outpatient settings: a systematic review and meta-analysis, J Am Med Assoc 311:889–1900, 2014.

Kaner EFS, Beyer FR, Muirhead C, et al: Effectiveness of brief alcohol interventions in primary care populations, Cochrane Database Syst Rev 2, 2018, Art.No.: CD004148, 2018.

Kranzler HR, Soyka: Diagnosis and pharmacotherapy of alcohol use disorder: a review, J Am Med Assoc 320:815–824, 2018.

O'Connor EA, Perdue LA, Senger CA, et al. Screening and behavioral counseling interventions to reduce unhealthy alcohol use in adolescents and adults: an updated systematic review for the U.S. Preventive Services Task Force. Evidence Synthesis No. 171. AHRQ Publication No. 18-05242-EF-1. Rockville, MD: Agency for Healthcare Research and Quality, 2018.

Peacock A, Leung J, Larney S, et al: Global statistics on alcohol, tobacco and illicit drug use: 2017 status report, Addiction 113:1905–1926, 2018.

Schulenberg JE, Johnston LD, O'Malley PM, Bachman JG, Miech RA, Patrick ME: Monitoring the Future national survey results on drug use, 1975–2018: volume II, College students and adults ages 19–60, Ann Arbor, 2019, Institute for Social Research, The University of Michigan, Available at http://monitoringthefuture.org/pubs.html#monographs. Accessed September 2019.

用。与 PCP 相比，它较少引起意识模糊、失去理智和暴力行为。氯胺酮是与约会强奸相关的俱乐部毒品。

吸入剂

在美国 12 岁及以上人群中，180 万人在过去 1 年为获得快感而使用过吸入剂，其中约 68.4 万人是 12～17 岁的青少年。由于很容易买到，吸入剂通常是青少年最初使用的毒品，其中最常见的是圆珠笔 / 标记笔或魔术标记笔中的化学物质。吸入剂可分为：①有机溶剂，包括甲苯（航模粘合胶和喷漆）、油漆稀释剂、煤油、汽油、四氯化碳、鞋油、丙酮（指甲油去除剂和修正液）、二甲苯（永久性标记笔）和脱脂剂（干洗液）；②气体，如丁烷、丙烷、气溶胶推进剂和麻醉剂（乙醚、氯仿、氟烷和一氧化二氮）；③亚硝酸盐，如亚硝酸环己基酯、亚硝酸戊酯和亚硝酸丁酯（室内除臭剂）。这些物质最常被儿童或青少年吸入，吸入后数分钟内即可产生头晕和中毒症状。长期接触或每天使用可能会导致听力下降、骨髓抑制、心律失常、大脑退化、周围神经病，以及肝、肾或肺部损害。长期使用后，口鼻周围有时会出现特征性的"嗅胶疹"。在极少数情况下，吸入剂可能导致死亡，可能的原因主要包括低氧血症、心律失常、肺炎或在昏迷时吸入呕吐物。滥用吸入剂的患者很少需要脱毒治疗，但可能需要接受精神科治疗，以防止复吸。

策划药

策划药一词是指非法合成毒品，其中许多药物的药效比其母体化合物更强。最常见的策划药包括芬太尼、哌替啶、哌嗪和甲基苯丙胺的类似物。目前已非法生产出多种芬太尼衍生物，包括最初的舒芬太尼、阿芬太尼、瑞芬太尼、卡芬太尼，还有相对近期的乙酰芬太尼、6-丁酰基芬太尼、4-甲基丁酰基芬太尼、异丁酰基芬太尼、呋喃芬太尼、α-甲基芬太尼（China white）、3-甲基芬太尼或 TMF、对甲基芬太尼、甲基乙酰基芬太尼、丙烯酰芬太尼、2-氟芬太尼、氟乙酰基芬太尼、邻芬太尼。这些衍生物没有公认的医疗用途，常规毒品检测通常无法测出，这加剧了阿片类药物危机，增加了与毒品相关的死亡人数。由于这类药物的效价约为海洛因的 1000 倍（译者注：芬太尼的药效是海洛因的 30～50 倍，卡芬太尼的药效是海洛因的约 10 000 倍），因此有因呼吸抑制而过量致死的报道。

主要的哌替啶衍生物包括 1-甲基-4-苯基-4-丙氧基哌啶（MPPP）和 1-甲基-4-苯基-1,2,3,6-四氢吡啶（MPTP），这两种物质产生的欣快感与海洛因相似。在一些使用者中，MPTP 可导致黑质神经元变性，从而导致不可逆的帕金森病。

哌嗪类药物是一类新的策划药，通常以片剂、胶囊或粉末的形式作为派对用药在毒品黑市、头店（head shops）或互联网上出售，其名称包括 Frenzy、Bliss、Charge、Herbal ecstasy、A2、Legal X 和 Legal E。1-苄基哌嗪（BZP）是这些化合物中最常见的一种。除了 BZP 和 1-（3,4-亚甲基二氧苯基）哌嗪（MDBP）外，苯基哌嗪衍生物 1-（3-三氟甲基苯基）哌嗪（TFMPP）、1-（3-氯苯基）哌嗪（mCPP）和 1-（4-甲氧基苯基）哌嗪（MeOPP）也经常被滥用。由于哌嗪类药物和苯丙胺类药物会引起相似的药理症状，因此哌嗪中毒很容易被误诊为苯丙胺中毒。然而，滥用药物的常规免疫化学检测无法检测到哌嗪类药物，需要进行适当的毒理学分析（如气相色谱-质谱法）。苯丙胺和甲基苯丙胺的亚甲二氧基合成衍生物通常被称为摇头丸，包括 3,4-亚甲基二氧甲基苯丙胺（MDMA；又称 Adam）、3,4-亚甲基二氧乙基苯丙胺（MDEA；又称 Eve）和 N-甲基-1-（3,4-亚甲基二氧苯基）-2-丁胺（MBDB；又称 Methyl-J 或 Eden）。这些药物具有中枢神经兴奋作用和致幻作用，可使人情绪高涨、自信心增强，并可能导致急性惊恐、焦虑、偏执、幻觉、心动过速、眼球震颤、共济失调和震颤。部分使用者因心律失常、高热惊厥和颅内出血而死亡。

未来展望

免疫治疗（即疫苗开发）已成为治疗甲基苯丙胺、海洛因和可卡因等药物滥用的一种前景广阔的方法［译者注：目前针对成瘾的免疫治疗（特别是疫苗）仍处于研究和试验阶段，尚未正式上市用于治疗药物成瘾］。通过将药物封闭在外周组织而不让其穿过血脑屏障，可以减少药物毒性，降低其奖赏效应。治疗药物中毒的一种新型药代动力学方法是开发可安全给药的化合物，其可加速药物代谢为非活性成分。例如，已经开发出催化抗体来加速可卡因的代谢，并可通过注射的方式给药（译者注：尚未应用于临床）。在实验动物中，人类丁酰胆碱酯酶（可卡因代谢酶之一）突变可加速可卡因的代谢，并拮抗可卡因的作用和毒性效应。

推荐阅读

Edenberg HJ, McClintick JN: Alcohol dehydrogenases, aldehyde dehydrogenases, and alcohol use disorders: a critical review, Alcohol Clin Exp Re 42:2281–2297, 2018.

Haight BR, Learned SM, Laffont CM, et al: For the RB-US-13-0001 Study Investigators. Efficacy and safety of a monthly buprenorphine depot injection for opioid use disorder: a multicentre, randomised, double-blind, placebo-controlled, phase 3 trial, Lancet 393:778–790, 2019.

Jonas DE, Amick HR, Feltner C, et al: Pharmacotherapy for adults with alcohol use disorders in outpatient settings: a systematic review and meta-analysis, J Am Med Assoc 311:889–1900, 2014.

Kaner EFS, Beyer FR, Muirhead C, et al: Effectiveness of brief alcohol interventions in primary care populations, Cochrane Database Syst Rev 2, 2018, Art.No.: CD004148, 2018.

Kranzler HR, Soyka: Diagnosis and pharmacotherapy of alcohol use disorder: a review, J Am Med Assoc 320:815–824, 2018.

O'Connor EA, Perdue LA, Senger CA, et al. Screening and behavioral counseling interventions to reduce unhealthy alcohol use in adolescents and adults: an updated systematic review for the U.S. Preventive Services Task Force. Evidence Synthesis No. 171. AHRQ Publication No. 18-05242-EF-1. Rockville, MD: Agency for Healthcare Research and Quality, 2018.

Peacock A, Leung J, Larney S, et al: Global statistics on alcohol, tobacco and illicit drug use: 2017 status report, Addiction 113:1905–1926, 2018.

Schulenberg JE, Johnston LD, O'Malley PM, Bachman JG, Miech RA, Patrick ME: Monitoring the Future national survey results on drug use, 1975–2018: volume II, College students and adults ages 19–60, Ann Arbor, 2019, Institute for Social Research, The University of Michigan, Available at http://monitoringthefuture.org/pubs.html#monographs. Accessed September 2019.

Soyka M: Treatment of benzodiazepine dependence, N Engl J Med 376:1147–1157, 2017.

Substance Abuse and Mental Health Services Administration. (2017). Key substance use and mental health indicators in the United States: Results from the 2016 National Survey on Drug Use and Health (HHS Publication No. SMA 17-5044, NSDUH Series H-52). Rockville, MD: Center for Behavioral Health Statistics and Quality, Substance Abuse and Mental Health Services Administration. Available at https://www.samhsa.gov/data/sites/default/files/NSDUH-FFR1-2016/NSDUH-FFR1-2016.pdf. Accessed September 2019.

Wood E, Albarqouni L, Tkachuk S, et al: Will this hospitalized patient develop severe alcohol withdrawal syndrome? The rational clinical examination systematic review, J Am Med Assoc 320:825–833, 2018.

Wozniak JR, Riley EP, Charness ME: Clinical presentation, diagnosis, and management of fetal alcohol spectrum disorder, Lancet Neurol 18:760–770, 2019.

Soyka M: Treatment of benzodiazepine dependence, N Engl J Med 376:1147–1157, 2017.

Substance Abuse and Mental Health Services Administration. (2017). Key substance use and mental health indicators in the United States: Results from the 2016 National Survey on Drug Use and Health (HHS Publication No. SMA 17-5044, NSDUH Series H-52). Rockville, MD: Center for Behavioral Health Statistics and Quality, Substance Abuse and Mental Health Services Administration. Available at https://www.samhsa.gov/data/sites/default/files/NSDUH-FFR1-2016/NSDUH-FFR1-2016.pdf. Accessed September 2019.

Wood E, Albarqouni L, Tkachuk S, et al: Will this hospitalized patient develop severe alcohol withdrawal syndrome? The rational clinical examination systematic review, J Am Med Assoc 320:825–833, 2018.

Wozniak JR, Riley EP, Charness ME: Clinical presentation, diagnosis, and management of fetal alcohol spectrum disorder, Lancet Neurol 18:760–770, 2019.

索引 Index

A

Absence epilepsy
   childhood, 198, 204
   juvenile, 198
Absence seizures, atypical, 194
Acamprosate (Campral), for alcoholism, 352
Acetylcholine
   botulism and, 288
   Lambert-Easton myasthenic syndrome and, 288
   myasthenia gravis and, 286
Acid maltase deficiency (Pompe disease), 278
Acquired immunodeficiency syndrome (AIDS)
   dementia and, 52
Acquired myopathies, 282-284
Action tremor, 122
Activities of daily living (ADL), 298
Acute alcohol intoxication, 346
Acute autoimmune brachial neuritis, 250
Acute brain injury, severe, palliative care and, 326
Acute disseminatedencephalomyelitis (ADEM), 240
Acute inflammatory demyelinating polyneuropathy, 258-260
Acute low back pain, 90
Acute quadriplegic myopathy, 284
Acute stress disorder, 60-62
Acute transient monocular blindness, 100
Acute viral myositis, 284
Adie pupils, 96
Adjustment insomnia, 32
Adjuvant analgesia, 330
Advance directives, in older adults, 314
Afferent pupillary defect, 94, 98
Aging, 292-320, 296f
   biology of, 294, 298f, 298t
   epidemiology of, 294, 296f
   frailty phenotype and, 298, 300f
   memory and, 52
   population, 296f
   theories of, 294-298, 298t, 300f
Agnosia, 40-42
Agoraphobia, 60
Akinesia, 116
Alcohol consumption, low-risk drinking and, 352
Alcohol-dependent individuals, 348
Alcohol intoxication, acute, 346
Alcohol-related liver disease, 346
Alcohol use, 344
   clinical presentation of, 346-348
   commonly abused drugs, 356t-360t
   considerations for drug interventions in, 352
   definition of, 344
   delirium tremens in, 348
   epidemiology of, 344, 346f
   liver disease caused by, 346
   medical complications of, 348t
   nonpharmacologic therapies for, 350
   organ damage in, 344-346, 348t
   pharmacologic and metabolic factors in, 344
   in pregnancy, 352
   prospectus for future, 370
   screening and intervention strategies for, 348-350, 348t-350t
   treatment of, 348-354

Page numbers followed by "f" indicate figures, "t" indicate tables, and "b" indicate boxes.

A

失神癫痫
   儿童，199，205
   青少年，199
非典型失神发作，195
阿坎酸（坎普拉尔），治疗酒精中毒，353
乙酰胆碱
   肉毒中毒，289
   兰伯特-伊顿肌无力综合征，289
   重症肌无力，287
酸性麦芽糖酶缺乏症（糖原贮积症Ⅱ型），279
获得性免疫缺陷综合征（AIDS）
   痴呆，53
获得性肌病，283-285
动作性震颤，123
日常生活活动能力（ADL），299
急性酒精中毒，347
急性自身免疫性臂丛神经炎，251
严重急性脑损伤，缓和医疗，327
急性播散性脑脊髓炎（ADEM），241
急性炎症性脱髓鞘性多发性神经病，259-261
急性腰痛，91
急性四肢瘫痪性肌病，285
急性应激障碍，61-63
急性短暂性单眼失明，101
急性病毒性肌炎，285
阿迪瞳孔，97
适应性失眠，33
辅助镇痛，331
预定医疗指示，老年人，315
传入性瞳孔障碍，95，99
衰老，293-321，297f
   生物学，295，299f，299t
   流行病学，295，297f
   衰弱表型，299，301f
   记忆，53
   人口，297f
   理论，295-299，299t，301f
失认症，41-43
广场恐惧症，61
运动不能，117
酒精消耗，低风险饮酒，353
酒精依赖，349
急性酒精中毒，347
酒精性肝病，347
酒精使用，345
   临床表现，347-349
   常见滥用药物，357t-361t
   药物干预的注意事项，353
   定义，345
   震颤性谵妄，349
   流行病学，345，347f
   酒精性肝病，347
   并发症，349t
   非药物治疗，351
   器官损害，345-347，349t
   药理学和代谢因素，345
   妊娠期，353
   未来展望，371
   筛查和干预策略，349-351，349t-351t
   治疗，349-355

页码数字中，"f"代表"图"，"t"代表"表格"，"b"代表"框"。

withdrawal syndrome (convulsions) in, 346-348
    medical management of, 352-354
Alcohol use disorder
    criteria for diagnosis of, 346t
    definition of, 344
Alcohol Use Disorders Identification Test (AUDIT), 348, 350t
Alcohol Withdrawal Severity (AW) Scale, prediction of, 354t
Alemtuzumab, for multiple sclerosis, 236
Alexia without agraphia, 40
"Altered mental status", 306
Alzheimer disease, 44-50
    diagnostic criteria for, 48t
    familial *vs.* sporadic, 48t
Amaurosis fugax, 100, 156-158
Ambulatory care, for older adults, 316
Amnesia, 52
Amphetamine, 356t-360t, 364
    for ADHD, 146
    piperazines and, 370
    treatment of abuse with, 364
β-Amyloid (Ab), in Alzheimer disease, 44
Amyloid angiopathy, 160
Amyloid autonomic neuropathy, 72
Amyotrophic lateral sclerosis (ALS), 244-248
    clinical presentation of, 244-246
    definition of, 244
    diagnosis and differential diagnosis of, 246
    epidemiology of, 244
    pathology of, 244
    symptoms and signs associated with, 246t
    treatment for, 246
Anabolic steroids, 356t-360t
Anhidrosis, 68
Anisocoria, 92, 96f
Anomia, 36-40
Anosognosia, 42
Anterior cerebral artery (ACA), stroke associated with, 158, 164t
Anterograde amnesia, 52
Anticoagulation
    for spinal cord injury, 184
    in stroke patients, 174
    for stroke prevention, secondary, 174
Anticonvulsants, for neuropathic pain, 258t
Antidepressant medications
    for bipolar disorders, 62
    for depression, 62t
Antiepileptic drugs, discontinuing of, 214
Anti-myelin oligodendrocyte glycoprotein disorder, 240
Antiplatelet therapy
    for stroke prevention, 170
Antipsychotic medications, for bipolar disorders, 64
Anton syndrome, 100
Anxiety, 60-62, 60t
    in older adults, 306-308
    palliative care and, 332-334
    somatic symptoms of, 64t
Aortic stenosis
    in older adults, 304t
Aphasia, 36-40
    types of, 40t
    in writing, 40, 40f
Apnea, 26
Apnea-hypopnea index (AHI), 26
Apoptosis, 298
Apraxia, 40-42, 42f
Argyll-Robertson pupils, 94-96
Aspirin
    for stroke prevention
        primary, 170

戒断综合征（抽搐），347-349
    医疗管理，353-355
酒精使用障碍
    诊断标准，347t
    定义，345
酒精使用障碍筛查量表（AUDIT），349，351t
酒精戒断严重程度预测量表，355t
阿仑单抗，治疗多发性硬化，237
不伴有失写症的失读症，41
"精神状态改变"，307
阿尔茨海默病，45-51
    诊断标准，49t
    家族性 *vs.* 散发性，49t
一过性黑矇，101，157-159
门诊照护，老年人，317
遗忘症，53
苯丙胺，357t-361t，365
    ADHD，147
    哌嗪类药物，371
    药物滥用，365
β 淀粉样蛋白（Aβ），见于阿尔茨海默病，45
淀粉样血管病，161
淀粉样变性自主神经病变，73
肌萎缩侧索硬化（ALS），245-249
    临床表现，245-247
    定义，245
    诊断和鉴别诊断，247
    流行病学，245
    病理学，245
    症状和体征，247t
    治疗，247
合成代谢类固醇，357t-361t
无汗症，69
瞳孔不等，93，97f
命名性失语，37-41
病感失认症，43
大脑前动脉（ACA），与卒中相关，159，165t
顺行性遗忘，53
抗凝治疗
    脊髓损伤，185
    卒中患者，175
    卒中的二级预防，175
抗惊厥药，治疗神经病理性疼痛，259t
抗抑郁药
    双相障碍，63
    抑郁，63t
抗癫痫药，停药，215
抗髓鞘少突胶质细胞糖蛋白抗体病，241
抗血小板治疗
    卒中预防，171
抗精神病药，治疗双相障碍，65
安东综合征，101
焦虑，61-63，61t
    老年患者，307-309
    缓和医疗，333-335
    躯体症状，65t
主动脉瓣狭窄
    老年患者，305t
失语症，37-41
    类型，41t
    书写失语症，41，41f
呼吸暂停，27
呼吸暂停-低通气指数（AHI），27
凋亡，299
失用症，41-43，43f
阿-罗瞳孔，95-97
阿司匹林
    卒中预防
        一级，171

secondary, 174
    for Sturge-Weber syndrome, 152
Assisted suicide, 340
Astrocytomas, 216, 222
    anaplastic, 222
Ataluren, for Duchenne muscular dystrophy, 272
Atherosclerosis
    stroke caused by, 160, 162f
Atonic seizure, 196
Atrial fibrillation
    stroke prevention in, 170, 174
Atrophy, multiple system, 70
Attention-deficit/hyperactivity disorder (ADHD), 146
Aura
    of migraine, 76, 204
    of seizures, 192, 204
Autism spectrum disorder, 144-146
Automatisms, 196-198
Autonomic nervous system
    disorders of, 68-74
        clinical presentation of, 68-70
        definition and epidemiology of, 68
        diagnosis and differential diagnosis of, 70-72, 70f
        pathology of, 68
        prognosis of, 72
        treatment for, 72
Axonalpolyneuropathies, symmetrical, 250
Azathioprine, for myasthenia gravis, 286

B

Babinski sign, 244-246
Baclofen, for alcoholism, 352
Barbiturates
    abuse of, 354-360, 356t-360t
    to induced coma, 182
Basilar artery, 158f, 160
    migraine associated with, 204
Behavior, major disorders of, 56-66, 60t
Benign intracranial hypertension, 86
Benign paroxysmal positional vertigo (BPPV), 110, 112f
Benzodiazepines
    abuse of, 356t-360t, 360
    for alcohol withdrawal, 360-362
    for bipolar disorders, 64
    for epilepsy, 204
Beta-interferons (BIFN), for multiple sclerosis, 232
Binge drinker, 344
Binswanger disease, 50
Bipolar disorders, 56-60
Blindness
    acute transient monocular, 100
    cortical, 100
Blood flow
    cerebral, 160-162, 162f
Blood pressure
    orthostatic, 70-72, 70f
Botulinum toxin, for headache, 82
Botulism, 288-290
Brachial plexopathy, 248
Brachial plexus, 248
    disorders of, 248-250
Bradykinesia, 116
Brain
    biopsy of, 220
    function of, criteria for cessation of, 24t
    herniation of, 14, 222
    mass lesion, in coma, 14
Brain death, 22, 24t
Brain injury, traumatic, 180-186

二级, 175
    Sturge-Weber综合征, 153
协助自杀, 341
星形细胞瘤, 217, 223
    间变性, 223
阿塔鲁伦, 治疗进行性假肥大性肌营养不良, 273
动脉粥样硬化
    导致卒中, 161, 163f
失张力发作, 197
心房颤动
    卒中预防, 171, 175
萎缩, 多系统, 71
注意缺陷多动障碍（ADHD）, 147
先兆
    偏头痛, 77, 205
    癫痫发作, 193, 205
孤独症谱系障碍, 145-147
自动症, 197-199
自主神经系统
    疾病, 69-75
        临床表现, 69-71
        定义和流行病学, 69
        诊断和鉴别诊断, 71-73, 71f
        病理学, 69
        预后, 73
        治疗, 73
轴索性多发性神经病, 对称性, 251
硫唑嘌呤, 治疗重症肌无力, 287

B

巴宾斯基征, 245-247
巴氯芬, 治疗酒精中毒, 353
巴比妥类药物
    滥用, 355-361, 357t-361t
    诱发昏迷, 183
基底动脉, 159f, 161
    偏头痛, 205
主要行为障碍, 57-67, 61t
良性颅内高压, 87
良性阵发性位置性眩晕（BPPV）, 111, 113f
苯二氮䓬类药物
    滥用, 357t-361t, 361
    酒精戒断, 361-363
    双相障碍, 65
    癫痫, 205
β-干扰素（BIFN）, 治疗多发性硬化, 233
狂饮者, 345
Binswanger病, 51
双相障碍, 57-61
盲
    急性短暂性单眼盲, 101
    皮质盲, 101
血流量
    脑, 161-163, 163f
血压
    直立位血压, 71-73, 71f
肉毒毒素, 治疗头痛, 83
肉毒中毒, 289-291
臂丛神经病, 249
臂丛, 249
    疾病, 249-251
运动迟缓, 117
脑
    活检, 221
    功能丧失的标准, 25t
    脑疝, 15, 223
    占位性病变, 昏迷, 15
脑死亡, 23, 25t
颅脑损伤, 181-187

future of, 186
management, 180-182
prognosis of, 186
second impact syndrome in, 180
Brain tissue, injury to, 162-164
Brain tumors, 216
headaches caused by, 84-86, 84t, 216-218
metastatic, 216
visual loss caused by, 100
Brainstem
infarcts of, 164
locked-in syndrome and, 22
mass lesion, in coma, 14
Breathing, sleep-disordered, 26-28
Broca aphasia, 40
Brown-Sequard syndrome, 184
Brudzinski reflex, 16, 18f
Bulbospinal muscular atrophy (BSMA), 248
Buprenorphine, for opioid abuse, 362-364

C

CAGE questionnaire, 348, 348t
Calcitonin gene-related peptide (CGRP), for migraine, 78
Caloric restriction (CR), lifespan and, 318
Caloric testing, 20
Campylobacter jejuni
Guillain-Barré syndrome associated with, 258
Cannabidiol (CBD), 332
Cannabinoids, 356t-360t
Cannabis, 366-368, 368f
Carbamazepine, 206, 206t
Cardiac arrest, coma after, prognosis in, 20-22
Cardioembolism, stroke caused by, 154
Caregiving, in older adults, 312-314
Carotid artery
blood supply from, 158
internal, stroke associated with, 158, 164t
plaque in, visual loss caused by, 100
Carotid endarterectomy, 170
Carpal tunnel syndrome, 256-258
Catamenial epilepsy, 188
Cataplexy, narcolepsy with, 28
Cataract, 92
Catatonic stupor, 22
Cauda equina syndrome, 90
Central nervous system (CNS) tumors, 216-224
clinical presentation of, 216-218
definition/epidemiology of, 216
diagnosis/differential, 218-220, 218f-220f
pathology of, 216
prognosis of, 222
treatment of, 220-222
Central sleep apnea, 28
Cerebellar ataxias, 132-134, 134t
Cerebellum, 116, 118f
Cerebral edema, after traumatic brain injury, 182
Cerebral infarction, 164
Cerebral perfusion pressure (CPP), 160-162
in traumatic brain injury, 182
Cerebral venous sinus thrombosis, 100
Cerebrospinal fluid (CSF)
in demyelinating neuropathy, 256
hypocretin level in, in narcolepsy, 28
IgG in, multiple sclerosis, 228
investigation of, 6
in multiple sclerosis, 228, 230f
seizures and, 202
Cerebrovascular disease, 154-178
clinical presentation of, 164-166

未来展望，187
管理，181-183
预后，187
二次撞击综合征，181
脑组织，损伤，163-165
脑肿瘤，217
头痛，85-87，85t，217-219
转移性，217
视力丧失，101
脑干
梗死，165
闭锁综合征，23
占位性病变，昏迷，15
呼吸，睡眠障碍，27-29
Broca失语症（运动性失语症），41
布朗-塞卡综合征，185
布鲁津斯基反射，17，19f
延髓脊肌萎缩（BSMA），249
丁丙诺啡，治疗阿片类药物滥用，363-365

C

CAGE问卷，349，349t
降钙素基因相关肽（CGRP），治疗偏头痛，79
热量限制（CR），延长寿命，319
冷热水试验，21
空肠弯曲菌
吉兰-巴雷综合征，259
大麻二酚（CBD），333
大麻素，357t-361t
大麻，367-369，369f
卡马西平，207，207t
心脏停搏后昏迷，预后，21-23
心源性栓塞，导致卒中，155
照护，老年人，313-315
颈动脉
血液供应，159
颈内动脉，与卒中相关，159，165t
斑块，引起视力丧失，101
颈动脉内膜切除术，171
腕管综合征，257-259
月经性癫痫，189
发作性睡病，猝倒，29
白内障，93
紧张性木僵，23
马尾综合征，91
中枢神经系统（CNS）肿瘤，217-225
临床表现，217-219
定义/流行病学，217
诊断/鉴别诊断，219-221，219f-221f
病理学，217
预后，223
治疗，221-223
中枢性睡眠呼吸暂停，29
小脑性共济失调，133-135，135t
小脑，117，119f
脑水肿，颅脑损伤后，183
脑梗死，165
脑灌注压（CPP），161-163
颅脑损伤，183
脑静脉窦血栓形成，101
脑脊液（CSF）
脱髓鞘性神经病，257
下丘脑分泌素水平，发作性睡病，29
IgG，多发性硬化，229
检查，7
多发性硬化，229，231f
癫痫发作，203
脑血管疾病，155-179
临床表现，165-167

common forms of, 156t
definitions of, 154
diagnosis and differential diagnosis of, 166-168
epidemiology of, 154
modifiable risk factors of, 154-158, 156t
Parkinsonism and, 122
pathology of, 158-164
prognosis of, 176
vascular anatomy of, 158-160, 158f
vascular pathogenesis of, 160-162
Ceruloplasmin, in Wilson's disease, 128
Cervical radiculopathy, 88-90
Cervical spinal myelopathy, cervical spondylitis and, 88-90
Cervical spondylosis, 88-90, 90t
Channelopathies
    epilepsy in, 190
    muscle, cardiomyopathies associated with, 280-282
Charcot-Marie-Tooth disease (CMT), 260
Chemotherapy, for brain tumors, 220
Chiari malformation, type 1 (CMI), 138-140
Cholinesterase inhibitors, for Alzheimer disease, 48-50
Chorea, 124-126, 126t
Chronic inflammatory demyelinating polyneuropathy (CIDP), 260
Chronic paroxysmal hemicrania, 82
Chronic relapsing inflammatory optic neuropathy (CRION), 242
Circle of Willis, 158
Cladribine, oral, for multiple sclerosis, 238
Clonidine, for opioid withdrawal, 364
Clopidogrel, for stroke prevention, 174-176
Clostridioides botulinum, 288
Cluster headache, 82
Cocaine, 356t-360t, 364
    heroin with, 364
    myocardial ischemia or infarction caused by, 364, 366f
Codeine, 326, 328t, 356t-360t
Cognitive-behavioral therapy, for alcoholism, 350
Coital headache, 84
Coma, 14
    differential diagnosis of, 16
    emergency management in, 18t
    history in, 14
    neurologic signs in, 16f
    normal computed tomography scan, 18t
    pharmacologic, in traumatic brain injury, 182
    prognosis in, 20-22, 20f
    separation of structural from metabolic causes of
        motor response in, 16-18
        pupillary reactivity, 18
        reflex eye movements, 20
Coma-like states, 22
Complex partial seizure (CPS), 192, 192t
Computed tomography (CT)
    in coma, 14, 18t
    in neurologic disease, 8-10, 12t
    in stroke, 166, 166f
Concussion
    grading of, 182
    post-concussive syndrome, 182
Conduction aphasia, 40
Confusion, 14
Confusion Assessment Method (CAM), 306
Congenital malformations, 138-144, 140t
Congenital muscular dystrophies, 276t
Congenital myopathies, 278
Consciousness
    diagnostic approach of, 14-20
    disorders of, 14-24
    pathophysiologic factors of, 14
    seizures and, 192

常见形式，157t
定义，155
诊断和鉴别诊断，167-169
流行病学，155
可控的危险因素，155-159，157t
帕金森综合征，123
病理学，159-165
预后，177
血管解剖学，159-161，159f
血管发病机制，161-163
铜蓝蛋白，见于肝豆状核变性，129
颈神经根病，89-91
脊髓型颈椎病，颈椎病，89-91
颈椎病，89-91，91t
离子通道病
    癫痫，191
    肌肉，心肌病相关，281-283
夏科-马里-图思病（CMT），261
化疗，脑肿瘤，221
Chiari 畸形，1 型（CM1），139-141
胆碱酯酶抑制剂，治疗阿尔茨海默病，49-51
舞蹈症，125-127，127t
慢性炎症性脱髓鞘性多发性神经病（CIDP），261
慢性阵发性偏侧头痛，83
慢性复发性炎症性视神经病变（CRION），243
Willis 环，159
克拉屈滨，口服，治疗多发性硬化，239
可乐定，治疗阿片类物质戒断，365
氯吡格雷，卒中预防，175-177
肉毒梭菌，289
丛集性头痛，83
可卡因，357t-361t，365
    海洛因，365
    引起心肌缺血或心肌梗死，365，367f
可待因，327，329t，357t-361t
认知行为疗法，治疗酒精中毒，351
性交头痛，85
昏迷，15
    鉴别诊断，17
    急诊管理，19t
    病史，15
    神经系统体征，17f
    正常计算机断层成像，19t
    药源性，见于颅脑损伤，183
    预后，21-23，21f
    鉴别结构性病因和代谢性病因
        运动反应，17-19
        瞳孔对光反射，19
        反射性眼球运动，21
类昏迷状态，23
复杂部分性发作（CPS），193，193t
计算机断层成像（CT）
    昏迷，15，19t
    神经系统疾病，9-11，13t
    卒中，167，167f
脑震荡
    分级，183
    脑震荡后综合征，183
传导性失语症，41
意识模糊，15
意识模糊评估法（CAM），307
先天性畸形，139-145，141t
先天性肌营养不良，277t
先天性肌病，279
意识
    诊断方法，15-21
    意识障碍，15-25
    病理生理因素，15
    癫痫发作，193

Constipation
    with opioid use, 326
    in palliative care, 332
Conventional angiography, 10-12
Convulsions, 192
    in alcohol withdrawal, 346-348
Corneal reflection test, 96
Corpus callosum, 36
    agenesis of, 140
Cortical blindness, 100
Cortical dementia, 46t
Cortical development, malformations of, 144
Cortical spreading depression, 78
Cortical syndromes, 36-42
    anatomy in, 36, 36f-38f
    clinical assessment of, 36
    and localization, 38t
    prospectus for future, 42
    regional, 36-42
Corticobasal syndrome, 122
Corticosteroid myopathy, 284
Crack cocaine, 364
Cranial neuralgias, 78t, 88
Creutzfeldt-Jakob disease (CJD)
    dementia in, 52
Critical illness myopathy, 284
Critical illness polyneuropathy (CIP), 260

D

Damage theories, 294
Decerebrate posturing, 16-18
Declarative memory, 52
Decorticate posturing, 16-18
Delirium, 14, 306, 306t
    hyperactive terminal, 338
    palliative care and, 334
Delirium tremens (DTs), 348
    medical management of, 352-354
Delusional disorder, 64-66
Dementia, 44-54, 306
    acquired immunodeficiency syndrome and, 52
    causes of, 46t
    from chronic meningitis, 52
    cortical vs. subcortical, 46t
    delirium vs., 306
    diffuse Lewy body disease and, 50
    etiologic diagnosis of, 46t
    frontotemporal, 50
    with Lewy bodies, 122
    major syndromes of, 44-52
    Montreal Cognitive Assessment for, 44, 48t
    in normal-pressure hydrocephalus, 50-52
    palliative care and, 324-326
    Parkinson's disease and, 50
    from prion infection, 52
Demyelinating disorder, 98-100, 226-242
    neuromyelitis optica, 98-100
    optic neuritis, 98
Dentatorubropallidoluysianatrophy (DRPLA), 126
Depression, 56
    in epilepsy, 188
    in older adults, 304t
    in palliative care, 332-334
Depressive disorders, 56-60
    psychotherapies and antidepressant medications for, 62t
Dermatomyositis/polymyositis, 282
Designer drugs, 370
Developmental disorders, 144-148
Devic disease, 98-100, 238-240

便秘
    使用阿片类药物，327
    缓和医疗，333
传统血管造影，11-13
惊厥，193
    酒精戒断，347-349
角膜映光测试，97
胼胝体，37
    发育不全，141
皮质盲，101
皮质性痴呆，47t
皮质发育，畸形，145
皮质扩散性抑制，79
皮质综合征，37-43
    解剖学，37，37f-39f
    临床评估，37
    定位，39t
    未来展望，43
    局灶，37-43
皮质基底节综合征，123
皮质类固醇肌病，285
快克可卡因，365
脑神经痛，79t，89
克-雅病（CJD）
    痴呆，53
危重症肌病，285
危重症多发性神经病（CIP），261

D

损伤理论，295
去大脑强直，17-19
陈述性记忆，53
去皮质强直，17-19
谵妄，15，307，307t
    激越型终末期，339
    缓和医疗，335
震颤性谵妄（DT），349
    医疗管理，353-355
妄想性障碍，65-67
痴呆，45-55，307
    获得性免疫缺陷综合征，53
    病因，47t
    继发于慢性脑膜炎，53
    皮质性 vs. 皮质下，47t
    谵妄 vs. 痴呆，307
    弥漫性路易体病，51
    病因诊断，47t
    额颞叶，51
    路易体，123
    主要综合征，45-53
    蒙特利尔认知评估量表，45，49t
    正常压力脑积水，51-53
    缓和医疗，325-327
    帕金森病，51
    朊病毒感染，53
脱髓鞘疾病，99-101，227-243
    视神经脊髓炎，99-101
    视神经炎，99
齿状核-红核-苍白球-路易体萎缩症（DRPLA），127
抑郁，57
    癫痫，189
    老年患者，305t
    缓和医疗，333-335
抑郁障碍，57-61
    心理治疗和抗抑郁药，63t
皮肌炎／多发性肌炎，283
策划药，371
发育障碍，145-149
Devic 病，99-101，239-241

Dexamethasone, for vasogenic edema, with brain tumor, 222
Dextromethorphan (DXM), 356t-360t
Diabetes mellitus
　　autonomic neuropathy and, 68
　　lumbosacral polyradiculoplexopathy in, 260
Diabetic lumbosacral polyradiculoplexopathy, 260
Diabetic neuropathy, 260
Dietary therapy, for epilepsy, 208
Diffuse Lewy body disease, 50
Dimethyl fumarate, for multiple sclerosis, 236
Diplopia, monocular, 96
Dipyridamole, aspirin with, for stroke prevention, 174-176
Diroximel fumarate, for multiple sclerosis, 236
Dissociative drugs, 356t-360t, 368-370
Disulfiram (Antabuse), 352
Dizziness, 108-114
　　clinical presentation of, 108-110
　　definition, 108
　　differential diagnosis for, 110-112, 110t
　　differentiating central from peripheral, 108, 110t
　　epidemiology, 108
　　treatment for, 112-114
Doll's eyes maneuver, 20, 96
Dorsal induction, disorders of, 138-140
Double vision, 96
Dravet syndrome, 190
Dronabinol, 332
Drop seizures, 196
Drug abuse
　　illicit drugs in, 364-370
　　prescription drugs in, 354-364, 354f
Drug-induced movement disorders, 128
Drugs
　　hearing loss caused by, 106
　　Parkinsonism induced by, 122
Duchenne muscular dystrophy, 270
Dying process, 338-340
Dysautonomias
　　benign, 68
　　in traumatic spinal cord injury, 184
Dyspnea
　　in palliative care, 330
Dystonia, 128-130
Dystrophin, 268-270
Dystrophin-glycoprotein complex (DGC), 264, 268f
Dystrophinopathies, 268-272

E

Ecstasy, 370
Edaravone, for amyotrophic lateral sclerosis, 246
Edrophonium chloride (Tensilon), for myasthenia gravis, 286
Electroencephalography, 8
　　of absence seizures, 200-202
　　inpatient video long-term monitoring in, 202
　　for seizure diagnosis, 200-202
　　　　of juvenile myoclonic epilepsy, 198
　　　　of Lennox-Gastaut syndrome, 198
　　for seizure evaluation, 202
Electrolyte disturbance, in older adults, 304t
Electromyography, 8
　　in peripheral neuropathies, 244
Electrophysiologic studies, neurologic, 8
Empty sella syndrome, 86
Encephalopathy
　　metabolic, 14
　　Wernicke, 352
Endocrine disorders
　　myopathies caused by, 284
Endolymphatic hydrops, 106

地塞米松，治疗脑肿瘤引起的血管源性水肿，223
右美沙芬（DXM），357t-361t
糖尿病
　　自主神经病，69
　　腰骶多发性神经根神经丛病，261
糖尿病腰骶多发性神经根神经丛病，261
糖尿病神经病变，261
饮食治疗，治疗癫痫，209
弥漫性路易体病，51
二甲基富马酸，治疗多发性硬化，237
复视，单眼，97
双嘧达莫，与阿司匹林联用，预防卒中，175-177
富马酸地洛西美，治疗多发性硬化，237
分离性药物，357t-361t，369-371
双硫仑（戒酒硫），353
头晕，109-115
　　临床表现，109-111
　　定义，109
　　鉴别诊断，111-113，111t
　　鉴别中枢性和周围性，109，111t
　　流行病学，109
　　治疗，113-115
玩偶眼试验，21，97
背侧诱导，障碍，139-141
复视，97
Dravet综合征，191
屈大麻酚，333
跌倒发作，197
药物滥用
　　非法药物，365-371
　　处方药物，355-365，355f
药物诱发的运动障碍，129
药物
　　导致听力损失，107
　　诱发帕金森综合征，123
进行性假肥大性肌营养不良，271
临终过程，339-341
自主神经功能障碍
　　良性，69
　　外伤性脊髓损伤，185
呼吸困难
　　缓和医疗，331
肌张力障碍，129-131
抗肌萎缩蛋白，269-271
抗肌萎缩蛋白-糖蛋白复合物（DGC），265，269f
抗肌萎缩蛋白病，269-273

E

摇头丸，371
依达拉奉，治疗肌萎缩侧索硬化，247
依酚氯铵（腾喜龙），治疗重症肌无力，287
脑电图，9
　　失神发作，201-203
　　住院患者视频长程监测，203
　　癫痫发作诊断，201-203
　　　　青少年肌阵挛性癫痫，199
　　　　Lennox-Gastaut综合征，199
　　癫痫发作评估，203
电解质紊乱，老年人，305t
肌电图，9
　　周围神经病，245
电生理检查，神经电生理，9
空蝶鞍综合征，87
脑病
　　代谢性，15
　　韦尼克脑病，353
内分泌紊乱
　　引起肌病，285
内淋巴积液，107

Endomysium, 264
Ependymomas, 218
Epigenetics, 296-298
Epilepsy, 188-214
    activity restrictions in, 188
    benign Rolandic, 196
    classification of, 188, 196
    clinical manifestations of, 190-200
    definitions of, 188
    diagnosis of, 200-202
    differential diagnosis of, 202-204, 204t
    epidemiology of, 188
    etiology of, 190f
    genetic counseling and pregnancy in, 210-212
    genetics of, 190
    history and examination of, 200
    idiopathic/genetic, 198, 204
    nocturnal, 188
    pathology of, 188-190
    prognosis of, 212-214
    psychosocial concerns in, 212
    seizure threshold in, 188
    surgery of, 206-208
    symptomatic seizures and, 190t
    treatment of, 204-210
Epileptic spasms, 196
Epimysium, 264
Epworth Sleepiness Scale (ESS), 26, 28t
Error theories, 294
Essential tremor, 122-124, 124t
Ethanol intoxication, mild, 346
Ethosuximide, 204, 206t
Evoked potentials (EPs), 8
    in multiple sclerosis, 228
Excessive daytime sleepiness (EDS), disorders of, 26
Existential suffering, 334
External beam radiation, for brain tumors, 220
Eye movement
    evaluation of, 96, 98f, 98t
    ophthalmoplegia, 96
        causes of, 98t
    reflex, in coma, 20

F

Facioscapulohumeral muscular dystrophy, 276-278
Familial Alzheimer disease, 48t
Familial amyloid neuropathies, 260-262
Familial prion disease, 126
Fascicles, 264
Fasciculation, 244
Fat-soluble medications, 304
Fatty acids, metabolic disorders of, 278-280
Febrile seizures, 200
Fecal impaction, in older adults, 304t
Fentanyl, 328t
    abuse of, 356t-360t
Fetal alcohol spectrum disorders (FASDs), 352
Fever
    headache with, 84
    in traumatic brain injury, 182
Fibrillation, 244
Figure-4 sign, 192-194
Finances, in older adults, 314
Fingolimod, for multiple sclerosis, 234-236
Fluids, palliative care and, 338
Flunitrazepam, 356t-360t, 360
Focal epilepsy, 196-198, 204-206
    combined generalized and, 198-200
Focal post-traumatic epilepsy, 198

肌内膜，265
室管膜瘤，219
表观遗传学，297-299
癫痫，189-215
    限制活动，189
    良性运动性，197
    分类，189，197
    临床表现，191-201
    定义，189
    诊断，201-203
    鉴别诊断，203-205，205t
    流行病学，189
    病因，191f
    遗传咨询和妊娠，211-213
    遗传，191
    病史和体格检查，201
    特发性/遗传性，199，205
    夜间发作，189
    病理学，189-191
    预后，213-215
    社会心理问题，213
    癫痫发作阈值，189
    手术，207-209
    症状性癫痫发作，191t
    治疗，205-211
癫痫性痉挛，197
肌外膜，265
Epworth 嗜睡量表（ESS），27，29t
错误理论，295
特发性震颤，123-125，125t
轻度乙醇中毒，347
乙琥胺，205，207t
诱发电位（EP），9
    多发性硬化，229
白天过度嗜睡（EDS）障碍，27
存在性痛苦，335
外线束辐射，治疗脑肿瘤，221
眼球运动
    评估，97，99f，99t
    眼肌麻痹，97
        病因，99t
    反射性，昏迷时，21

F

面肩肱型肌营养不良，277-279
家族性阿尔茨海默病，49t
家族性淀粉样神经病，261-263
家族性朊病毒病，127
肌束，265
肌束震颤，245
脂溶性药物，305
脂肪酸，代谢障碍，279-281
热性惊厥，201
粪便嵌塞，老年人，305t
芬太尼，329t
    滥用，357t-361t
胎儿酒精谱系障碍（FASD），353
发热
    头痛，85
    颅脑损伤，183
肌纤维震颤，245
4字征，193-195
财务，老年人，315
芬戈莫德，治疗多发性硬化，235-237
液体，缓和医疗，339
氟硝西泮，357t-361t，361
局灶性癫痫，197-199，205-207
    合并全面性癫痫，199-201
局灶性外伤后癫痫，199

Foramen ovale, patent, paradoxical embolism and, 160
Fragile X syndrome, 146-148
Frailty
    aging and, 298, 300f
    palliative care and, 324-326
Free radical theory of aging, 294-296
Frontal absence seizures, 198
Frontal lobe epilepsy (FLE), 198
Frontal lobe seizure, 192t
Frontal sinusitis, 84
Frontotemporal dementias, 50
Function, definition of, 302
Functional movement disorders, 134
Funduscopy, 96-98, 98f

G

Gabapentin, 206, 206t
Generalized seizures, 194
    focal and, 198-200
Generalized tonic-clonic (GTC) seizure, 192-194
    in idiopathic epilepsy, 198
Genetic testing
    for Huntington's disease, 124
    in neurologic diseases, 12, 12t
Geriatric 5-M's, 302, 302t
Geriatric care, 318
"Geriatric syndromes", 304
Geroscience guided therapies, emergence of, 318
Giant cellarteritis (GCA), 86
Glasgow Coma Score, 180-182, 182t, 186
Glatiramer acetate, for multiple sclerosis, 232
Glaucoma, 100
Glioma, low-grade, 220
Global aphasia, 40
Glossopharyngeal neuralgia, 88
Glucose metabolism disorders, 278
Glycogen metabolism disorders, 278
Glycogenosis, 278
Guardianship, 314
Guillain-Barré syndrome, 68, 258-260

H

"Hallmarks of Aging", 294
Hallucinations, visual, 100
    in diffuse Lewy body disease, 50
Hallucinogens, 356t-360t, 368-370
Hamartin, 150
Hashish, 356t-360t
Hastened death, request for, 340
Hayflick phenomenon, 298
Head injuries, retrograde amnesia and, 52
Headache, 76-90
    assessment of, questions in, 78t
    brain tumors and, 216-218
    cervicogenic, 88
    classification of, 76-86, 78t
    cluster, 82
    cranial neuralgias, 78t, 88
    daily
        chronic, 84
        new persistent, 84
    definition and epidemiology of, 76
    differential diagnosis for, 84t
    evaluation of, 86-88
    in giant cellarteritis, 86
    in idiopathic intracranial hypertension, 86
    in idiopathic intracranial hypotension, 86
    muscle-contraction, 82-84

卵圆孔未闭，反常栓塞，161
脆性X染色体综合征，147-149
衰弱
    衰老，299，301f
    缓和医疗，325-327
衰老的自由基理论，295-297
额叶失神发作，199
额叶癫痫（FLE），199
额叶癫痫发作，193t
额窦炎，85
额颞叶痴呆，51
功能，定义，303
功能性运动障碍，135
眼底镜检查，97-99，99f

G

加巴喷丁，207，207t
全面性癫痫发作，195
    局灶性癫痫发作，199-201
全面性强直-阵挛（GTC）发作，193-195
    特发性癫痫，199
基因测定
    亨廷顿病，125
    神经系统疾病，13，13t
老年医学5M原则，303，303t
老年人照护，319
"老年综合征"，305
老年科学引导疗法，兴起，319
巨细胞动脉炎（GCA），87
格拉斯哥昏迷评分，181-183，183t，187
醋酸格拉默，治疗多发性硬化，233
青光眼，101
胶质瘤，低级别，221
全面性失语症，41
舌咽神经痛，89
糖代谢障碍，279
糖原代谢障碍，279
糖原病，279
监护，315
吉兰-巴雷综合征，69，259-261

H

"衰老的标志"，295
幻视，101
    弥漫性路易体病，51
致幻剂，357t-361t，369-371
Hamartin蛋白，151
大麻脂（哈希什），357t-361t
加速死亡，请求，341
Hayflick现象，299
头部损伤，逆行性遗忘，53
头痛，77-91
    评估，79t
    脑肿瘤，217-219
    颈源性，89
    分类，77-87，79t
    丛集性，83
    脑神经痛，79t，89
    每日头痛
        慢性，85
        新发持续性，85
    定义和流行病学，77
    鉴别诊断，85t
    评估，87-89
    巨细胞动脉炎，87
    特发性颅内高压，87
    特发性颅内低压，87
    肌收缩性，83-85

post-traumatic, 86
short-lasting unilateral neuralgiform headache with conjunctival tearing, 84
in sinusitis, 84
structural brain lesions in, clinical features suggesting, 84t
tension-type, 82-84
Hearing impairments, 100-106
auditory dysfunction, symptoms of, 100-102, 102f
auditory system, examination of, 102
Hearing loss
causes of, 102-106, 104t
treatment of, 106
Hematoma
intracerebral, 172
Hemianopia, 92
Hemicrania, paroxysmal, 82
Hemispheric mass lesions, 14
Hemorrhage
intracerebral, 160, 172-174
Heparin
stroke and, 172
in traumatic spinal cord injury, 186
Heroin, 356t-360t
with cocaine, 364
Hippocampal sclerosis, 188-190
Hippus, 96
HMGCR antibodies, myopathies with, 284
Holoprosencephaly (HPE), 140, 142f
Homonymous field defects, 92, 94f
Horner syndrome, 94
cluster headache with, 82
Hospice, 336-338
Human immunodeficiency virus (HIV) infection
primary CNS lymphoma and, 216
Huntington's disease, 124-126
phenocopies of, 126
Hydrocephalus
intracerebral hemorrhage with, 172-174
noncommunicating, 14
normal-pressure, dementia in, 50-52
Hydrocodone, 326, 328t
Hydromorphone, 326, 328t
γ-Hydroxybutyrate (GHB), 362
Hyperhidrosis, 68
Hypermotor seizures, 198
Hypertension
cerebral blood flow and, 160-162, 162f
Hyperthyroidism
in older adult, 302-304, 304t
Hyperventilation, 204
for elevated intracranial pressure, 182
Hypnagogic hallucinations, narcolepsy with, 28
Hypnic headache, 84
Hypnotics, abuse of, 354-362
Hypomania, in bipolar disorder, 60
Hypopneas, 26
Hypothyroidism
in older adult, 302-304

I

Ice pack test, for myasthenia gravis, 286
Ictal phase, 192
Ictus, 192
Idiopathic acute optic neuritis, 242
Idiopathic anxiety disorders, 60
Idiopathic hypersomnia, 28-30
Idiopathic inflammatory myopathies, 282t
Idiopathic intracranial hypertension, 86
visual loss in, 100

外伤后，87
短暂性单侧神经痛样头痛伴结膜充血和流泪，85
鼻窦炎，85
结构性脑损伤，临床特征，85t
紧张型，83-85
听力障碍，101-107
听觉功能障碍，症状，101-103，103f
听觉系统，检查，103
听力损失
病因，103-107，105t
治疗，107
血肿
颅内，173
偏盲，93
偏侧头痛，阵发性，83
幕上占位性病变，15
出血
脑，161，173-175
肝素
卒中，173
外伤性脊髓损伤，187
海洛因，357t-361t
可卡因，365
海马硬化，189-191
虹膜震颤，97
HMGCR抗体，肌病，285
前脑无裂畸形（HPE），141，143f
同向视野缺损，93，95f
霍纳综合征，95
丛集性头痛，83
安宁疗护，337-339
人类免疫缺陷病毒（HIV）感染
原发性中枢神经系统淋巴瘤，217
亨廷顿病，125-127
拟表型，127
脑积水
脑出血，173-175
非交通性，15
正常压力，痴呆，51-53
氢可酮，327，329t
氢吗啡酮，327，329t
γ-羟基丁酸（GHB），363
多汗症，69
过度运动性癫痫发作，199
高血压
脑血流量，161-163，163f
甲状腺功能亢进症
老年患者，303-305，305t
过度换气，205
颅内压升高，183
睡前幻觉，发作性睡病，29
睡眠性头痛，85
催眠药，滥用，355-363
轻躁狂，见于双相障碍，61
低通气，27
甲状腺功能减退症
老年患者，303-305

I

冰敷试验，重症肌无力，287
癫痫发作期，193
发作，193
特发性急性视神经炎，243
特发性焦虑障碍，61
特发性嗜睡症，29-31
特发性炎症性肌病，283t
特发性颅内高压，87
视力丧失，101

Idiopathic intracranial hypotension, 86
Imaging
    neurologic, 8-12
Indomethacin, for cluster headache, 82
Infantile spasms, 200
Infectious myositis, 284
Inflammatory disorders, 226-242
Inflammatory myopathies, 282-284, 282t
    idiopathic, 282t
Inhalants, abuse of, 356t-360t, 370
Inherited/genetic ataxias, 132-134
Injury, types of, 180
Insomnia, 30-32
Intensive care unit (ICU)
    traumatic spinal cord injury, 184
Intention tremor, 122
Interictal phase, 192
Internuclear ophthalmoplegia, 96
Intracerebral hemorrhage (ICH), 160, 172-174. See also Subarachnoid hemorrhage
Intracranial hypertension, idiopathic
    cerebral venous sinus thrombosis, 100
    headache caused by, 86
Intracranial hypotension, headache caused by, 86
Intracranial pressure (ICP)
    in traumatic brain injury, 182
Intravenous gammaglobulin, for Guillain-Barré syndrome, 258-260
Intubation
    in traumatic brain injury, 182
    nasotracheal, in traumatic spinal cord injury, 182
Ischemic optic neuropathy, 100
"Ischemic penumbra", 164
Ishihara color plates, 92

J

Jacksonian march, 198
Juvenile myoclonic epilepsy (JME), 198

K

Kayser-Fleischer corneal rings, in Wilson's disease, 128
Kennedy disease, 248
Ketamine, 356t-360t, 368-370
Ketogenic diet, 208
Korsakoff amnestic syndrome, 352
Korsakoff syndrome, 52

L

Lacosamide, 206t
Lambert-Eaton myasthenic syndrome (LEMS), 68, 288
Lamotrigine, 206t
    for bipolar disorders, 58-60
Lateral frontal seizures, 198
Leber hereditary optic neuropathy, 100
Lennox-Gastaut syndrome (LGS), 198
Lewy bodies, 50, 116
Light-near dissociation, 92-94
Limb-girdle muscular dystrophies, 268
Limbic system, seizures associated with, 196-198
Locked-in syndrome, 22, 22t
Low pressure headache, 86
Lumbar puncture, See also Cerebrospinal fluid
    in comatose patient, 16
    complications of, 6
    contraindications to, 6
    in demyelinating neuropathy, 256
    indications for, 12t
Lumbosacral plexopathy, 250
Lumbosacral plexus, disorders of, 248-250

特发性颅内低压，87
成像
    神经系统，9-13
吲哚美辛，治疗丛集性头痛，83
婴儿痉挛症，201
感染性肌炎，285
炎症性疾病，227-243
炎症性肌病，283-285，283t
    特发性，283t
吸入剂，滥用，357t-361t，371
遗传性共济失调，133-135
损伤，类型，181
失眠，31-33
重症监护病房（ICU）
    外伤性脊髓损伤，185
意向性震颤，123
发作间期，193
核间性眼肌麻痹，97
脑出血（ICH），161，173-175；参见蛛网膜下腔出血

特发性颅内高压
    脑静脉窦血栓形成，101
    引起头痛，87
颅内低压，引起头痛，87
颅内压（ICP）
    颅脑损伤，183
静脉注射丙种球蛋白，治疗吉兰-巴雷综合征，259-261
插管
    颅脑损伤，183
    经鼻气管插管，见于外伤性脊髓损伤，183
缺血性视神经病变，101
"缺血半暗带"，165
石原色盲板，93

J

贾克森扩布，199
青少年肌阵挛性癫痫（JME），199

K

Kayser-Fleischer角膜环（K-F环），见于肝豆状核变性，129
肯尼迪病，249
氯胺酮，357t-361t，369-371
生酮饮食，209
科萨科夫遗忘综合征，353
科萨科夫综合征，53

L

拉考沙胺，207t
兰伯特-伊顿肌无力综合征（LEMS），69，289
拉莫三嗪，207t
    双相障碍，59-61
额叶外侧癫痫发作，199
莱伯遗传性视神经病，101
Lennox-Gastaut综合征（LGS），199
路易体，51，117
光-近分离，93-95
肢带型肌营养不良，269
边缘系统，癫痫发作，197-199
闭锁综合征，23，23t
低颅压头痛，87
腰椎穿刺，参见脑脊液
    昏迷患者，17
    并发症，7
    禁忌证，7
    脱髓鞘性神经病，257
    适应证，13t
腰骶丛神经病，251
腰骶丛疾病，249-251

Lysergic acid diethylamide (LSD), 356t-360t, 368

M

Magnesium, for migraine prevention, 80-82
Magnetic resonance imaging (MRI)
    vs. computed tomography, 12t
    for acute lower back pain, 90
    of brain tumors, 218
    in multiple sclerosis, 228, 230f
    in neurologic disease, 8-10
Maintenance of wakefulness test (MWT), 26
Malignancy, in older adult, 304t
Malingering, 66
Mammalian target of rapamycin (mTOR), 150
Mannitol, for elevated intracranial pressure, 182
Marijuana, 332, 356t-360t, 368
Maxillary sinusitis, 84
McArdle disease, 278
Mechanical ventilation
    in traumatic spinal cord injury, 184
Medications, for epilepsy, 204-206
Melatonin, for insomnia, 32
Memory
    disturbances to, 44-54
    function of, isolated disorders of, 52-54
    structure of, 52
Ménière disease, 110
Meniere's syndrome, 106
Meningeal irritation, in coma, 14
Meningioma, 222
Meningismus, 84
Meningitis
    chronic, dementia and, 52
    identification of, 14-16
Mental disorders, classification of, 56
Mental health, of older adults, 306-308
Meperidine
    abuse of, 356t-360t
    derivatives of, 370
Mephedrone, 356t-360t
Mescaline, 356t-360t
Mesial temporal sclerosis, 188-190
Metabolic coma, multifocal disorders indicating, 16t
Metabolic myopathies, 278
Methadone, 326, 328t
Methamphetamine, 356t-360t. *See also* Amphetamine
1-methyl-4-phenyl-1, 2, 3, 6-tetrahydropyridine (MPTP), 370
3, 4-methylenedioxy methamphetamine (MDMA), 370
Methylenedioxymethamphetamine (MDMA), 356t-360t
Methylenedioxypyrovalerone (MDPV), 356t-360t
Methylone, 356t-360t
Methylphenidate, 356t-360t
    for ADHD, 146
Methylprednisolone, for multiple sclerosis, 232
Metoclopramide, Parkinsonism and, 122
Middle cerebral artery (MCA), stroke associated with, 158, 164t, 172
Migraine, 76-82, 168
    acute attack, 80
    auras of, 76, 204
    with basilar aura, 76
    in children, 76
    classification of, 78t
    complications of, 76
    definition of, 76
    familial hemiplegic, 76
    pathophysiology of, 78
    prevention of, 80-82, 82t
    treatment of, 78-80, 80f
        in emergency room, 80

麦角酸二乙胺（LSD），357t-361t，369

M

镁，预防偏头痛，81-83
磁共振成像（MRI）
    vs. 计算机断层成像，13t
    急性腰痛，91
    脑肿瘤，219
    多发性硬化，229，231f
    神经系统疾病，9-11
清醒维持测验（MWT），27
恶性肿瘤，老年人，305t
诈病，67
哺乳动物雷帕霉素靶蛋白（mTOR），151
甘露醇，颅内压升高，183
大麻，333，357t-361t，369
上颌窦炎，85
麦卡德尔病，279
机械通气
    外伤性脊髓损伤，185
药物，治疗癫痫，205-207
褪黑素，治疗失眠症，33
记忆
    记忆障碍，45-55
    功能，孤立性记忆障碍，53-55
    结构，53
梅尼埃病，111
梅尼埃综合征，107
脑膜刺激征，见于昏迷，15
脑膜瘤，223
脑膜刺激征，85
脑膜炎
    慢性，痴呆，53
    诊断，15-17
精神障碍，分类，57
心理健康，老年人，307-309
哌替啶
    滥用，357t-361t
    衍生物，371
甲氧麻黄酮，357t-361t
麦司卡林，357t-361t
内侧颞叶硬化，189-191
代谢性昏迷，由多灶性病变提示，17t
代谢性肌病，279
美沙酮，327，329t
甲基苯丙胺，357t-361t；参见苯丙胺
1-甲基-4-苯基-1,2,3,6-四氢吡啶（MPTP），371
3,4-亚甲基二氧甲基苯丙胺（MDMA），371
亚甲基二氧甲基苯丙胺（MDMA），357t-361t
亚甲基二氧吡咯戊酮（MDPV），357t-361t
3,4-亚甲基二氧甲卡西酮，357t-361t
哌甲酯，357t-361t
    ADHD，147
甲泼尼龙，治疗多发性硬化，233
甲氧氯普胺，帕金森综合征，123
大脑中动脉（MCA），与卒中相关，159，165t，173
偏头痛，77-83，169
    急性发作，81
    先兆，77，205
    基底先兆性，77
    儿童，77
    分类，79t
    并发症，77
    定义，77
    家族性偏瘫型，77
    病理生理学，79
    预防，81-83，83t
    治疗，79-81，81f
        急诊治疗，81

Migrainous infarction, 76
Migralepsy, 76
Mild cognitive impairment (MCI), 306
    Alzheimer disease and, 48-50
Mild ethanol intoxication, 346
Mini Mental State Examination (MMSE), 306
Mistreatment, in older adults, 314
Mitochondrial myopathies, 278-280
Mitoxantrone, for multiple sclerosis, 234
Mixed etiology dementia, 306
Modified Medical Research Council Motor Strength Testing Scale, 272t
Monomethyl fumarate, for multiple sclerosis, 236
Montreal Cognitive Assessment (MoCA), for dementia, 44, 48t
Mood
    major disorders of, 56-66, 60t
        prospectus for future of, 66
Morphine, 326, 328t, 356t-360t
Motor neuron diseases, 244-248
    acquired, 248
    clinical spectrum of, 248t
    prognosis of, 248
    spinal muscular atrophy, 248
    symptom management for, 248t
Motor system disorders, 116-136
Motor unit, symptom localization in, 8t
Movement disorders, 116-134, 120t
    hyperkinetic, 116
    hypokinetic, 116
Multifocal disorders, indicating metabolic coma, 16t
Multiple sclerosis (MS), 226-238
    clinical presentation of, 226-228
    clinically isolated syndrome in, 226
    definition of, 226
    diagnosis of, 228
        criteria for, 228, 228t
        evoked potentials in, 228
        magnetic resonance imaging in, 228, 230f
        optical coherence tomography, 228
        spinal fluid analysis in, 228
    differential diagnosis of, 228-230, 232t
    disease modifying medications for, 234t
    epidemiology of, 226
    pathology of, 226
    prognosis of, 230-232
    progressive, 226
    relapsing remitting, 226-228, 234
    symptoms and management of, 232t
    treatment of, 232-238
Multiple sleep latency test (MSLT), 26
Multiple system atrophy (MSA), 70, 120-122
Muscle, organization and structure of, 264, 266f-268f
Muscle biopsy, in peripheral neuropathy, 256
Muscle channelopathies, 280-282
Muscle cramping, 264
Muscle diseases, 264-284
Muscle fibers, skeletal, 264
Muscle-contraction headache, 82-84
Muscular dystrophies, 268
Myasthenia gravis, 286, 288t
Myasthenic syndrome, Lambert-Easton, 288
Myelomeningocele (MMC), 138
Myocardial infarction, in older adult, 304t
Myocardial ischemia, cocaine-induced, 364, 366f
Myoclonic seizures, 194
Myoclonus dystonia syndrome, 130
Myopathy(ies)
    acquired, 282-284
    acute quadriplegic, 284

偏头痛性梗死, 77
偏头痛癫痫, 77
轻度认知障碍（MCI）, 307
    阿尔茨海默病, 49-51
轻度乙醇中毒, 347
简易精神状态量表（MMSE）, 307
虐待, 老年人, 315
线粒体肌病, 279-281
米托蒽醌, 治疗多发性硬化, 235
混合性痴呆, 307
改良医学研究会运动力量测试量表, 273t

富马酸单甲酯, 治疗多发性硬化, 237
蒙特利尔认知评估量表（MoCA）, 评估痴呆, 45, 49t
心境
    主要障碍, 57-67, 61t
        未来展望, 67
吗啡, 327, 329t, 357t-361t
运动神经元病, 245-249
    获得性, 249
    临床谱系, 249t
    预后, 249
    脊髓性肌萎缩, 249
    症状管理, 249t
运动系统疾病, 117-137
运动单位, 症状定位, 9t
运动障碍, 117-135, 121t
    多动性, 117
    少动性, 117
多灶性病变, 提示代谢性昏迷, 17t
多发性硬化（MS）, 227-239
    临床表现, 227-229
    临床孤立综合征, 227
    定义, 227
    诊断, 229
        诊断标准, 229, 229t
        诱发电位, 229
        磁共振成像, 229, 231f
        光学相干断层成像, 229
        脑脊液分析, 229
    鉴别诊断, 229-231, 233t
    疾病修饰药物, 235t
    流行病学, 227
    病理学, 227
    预后, 231-233
    进展型, 227
    复发-缓解型, 227-229, 235
    症状和管理, 233t
    治疗, 233-239
多次小睡睡眠潜伏时间试验（MSLT）, 27
多系统萎缩（MSA）, 71, 121-123
肌肉, 组成和结构, 265, 267f-269f
肌肉活检, 周围神经病, 257
肌肉离子通道病, 281-283
肌肉痉挛, 265
肌肉疾病, 265-285
骨骼肌纤维, 265
肌收缩性头痛, 83-85
肌营养不良, 269
重症肌无力, 287, 289t
兰伯特-伊顿肌无力综合征, 289
脊髓脊膜膨出（MMC）, 139
心肌梗死, 老年人, 305t
心肌缺血, 可卡因诱发, 365, 367f
肌阵挛发作, 195
肌阵挛-肌张力障碍综合征, 131
肌病
    获得性, 283-285
    急性四肢瘫痪性, 285

assessment of, 264, 266f
congenital, 278
corticosteroid, 284
critical illness, 284
diagnostic testing of, 268
electromyographyin, 244
in endocrine and systemic disorders, 284
examination of, 264-266, 270t
with HMGCR antibodies, 284
inflammatory, 282-284, 282t
inherited, 268-278
metabolic, 278
mitochondrial, 278-280
muscle channelopathies and, 280-282
muscle weakness and, characteristic patterns of, 272t
overview of, 266t
toxic, 284
Myositis
    acute viral, 284
    infectious, 284
    sporadic inclusion body, 282-284
Myotonias
    electromyographyin, 244
    nondystrophic, 280
Myotonic dystrophy, 274-276

N

Nabilone, 332
Nalmefene, for alcoholism, 352
Naloxone, 362
Naltrexone
    for alcoholism, 352
    to block opioid abuse, 364
Narcolepsy, 28
Natalizumab, for multiple sclerosis, 234
Nausea
    in palliative care, 330-332
Neck stiffness
    cervical spondylosis with, 88-90
    giant cellarteritis with, 86
Neglect, hemispatial, 40-42
Nerve biopsy, 256
Nerve conduction studies, 8
    in peripheral neuropathies, 244
Nervous system, 12f
Neural tube defects (NTD), 138
Neurocutaneous disorders, 148-152
Neurodegeneration, dementia and, 44
Neurofibromatosis 1, 148, 148f, 150t
Neurofibromatosis 2, 148-150, 150t
Neurofibromin, 148
Neurogenic claudication, 90
Neurogenic shock, 182
Neuroimaging
    of epilepsy, 202
    for ventral induction disorders, 140
Neurologic disease
    categories of, 8t
Neurologic evaluation, 4-12
    examination in, 4-6, 10t
        final common pathway and, 4
    history of, 4
    hypotheses of, 4
    localization in, 4
    prospectus for future, 12
Neurologic symptoms, potential localizing value of, 6t
Neuromuscular diseases, 244-254
    classification of, 246t
    clinical features of, 246t

评估，265，267f
先天性，279
皮质类固醇肌病，285
危重症，285
诊断性检查，269
肌电图，245
内分泌和系统性疾病，285
检查，265-267，271t
HMGCR 抗体，285
炎症性，283-285，283t
遗传性，269-279
代谢性，279
线粒体肌病，279-281
肌肉离子通道病，281-283
肌无力，特征模式，273t
概述，267t
中毒性，285
肌炎
    急性病毒性，285
    感染性，285
    散发性包涵体，283-285
肌强直
    肌电图，245
    非营养不良性，281
强直性肌营养不良，275-277

N

大麻隆，333
纳美芬，治疗酒精中毒，353
纳洛酮，363
纳曲酮
    酒精中毒，353
    阻断阿片类物质滥用，365
发作性睡病，29
那他珠单抗，治疗多发性硬化，235
恶心
    缓和医疗，331-333
颈强直
    颈椎病，89-91
    巨细胞动脉炎，87
偏侧忽视，41-43
神经活检，257
神经传导检查，9
    周围神经病，245
神经系统，13f
神经管缺陷（NTD），139
神经皮肤疾病，149-153
神经退行性变，痴呆，45
神经纤维瘤病 1 型，149，149f，151t
神经纤维瘤病 2 型，149-151，151t
神经纤维瘤蛋白，149
神经源性跛行，91
神经源性休克，183
神经影像学
    癫痫，203
    腹侧诱导障碍，141
神经系统疾病
    分类，9t
神经系统评估，5-13
    检查，5-7，11t
        最终共同通路，5
    病史，5
    假设，5
    定位，5
    未来展望，13
神经系统症状，潜在定位价值，7t
神经肌肉疾病，245-255
    分类，247t
    临床特征，247t

Neuromuscular junction disease, 286-290
    botulism, 288-290
    Lambert-Easton myasthenic syndrome, 288
    myasthenia gravis, 286
    organophosphate poisoning, 290
Neuromyelitis optica (NMO), 98-100, 238-240, 238f
Neuronal migration and organization, disorders of, 144
Neuropathic disorders
    based on symptoms, differential diagnosis of, 254t
    hereditary, 254t
Neuropathic pain, 256, 258t
Neuropathy
    associated with pain, 254t
    peripheral, 258
        classification and causes of, 250t
        diabetic, 260
        laboratory studies of, 256t
        mononeuropathies, 252t, 256-258
        symptomatic treatment for, 258t
    toxic-induced, 260
    vasculitic, 250
Neurostimulators, 208
New daily persistent headache, 84
Nondeclarative memory, 52
Nondystrophic myotonias, 280
NREM parasomnias, 32
Nutrition, in older adults, 312
Nystagmus, 92-94, 108, 110t

O

Obsessive-compulsive disorder, 60
Occipital lobe epilepsy, 196
Occipital neuralgia, 88
Ocrelizumab, for multiple sclerosis, 236
Ofatumumab, for multiple sclerosis, 236-238
Older adults
    care transitions, 316
    clinical care of, 298-302, 302t
        cognition in, 306
        comorbid conditions in, 302
        continence in, 308-312, 312t
        function and, 302
        hearing in, 308
        life expectancy and, 302, 304t
        medications in, 304-306
        mobility in, 308, 310t
        mental health in, 306-308
        nutrition in, 312
        sleep in, 308
        vision in, 308
    geriatric care for, 318
    hospitalized patient and, 314
    presentation of disease in, 302-304, 304t
    social and legal issues of, 312-314
        advance directives, 314
        caregiving, 312-314
        finances, 314
        mistreatment, 314
    systems of care for, 316-318
Oligodendrogliomas, 222
Olivopontocerebellar degeneration, with prominent cerebellar dysfunction, 120-122
Ondansetron, for alcoholism, 352
Ophthalmology, for ventral induction disorders, 140-142
Ophthalmoscopy, 96
Opioid abuse, 330
Opioid crisis, 330
Opioids
    abuse of, 356t-360t

神经肌肉接头疾病，287-291
    肉毒中毒，289-291
    兰伯特-伊顿肌无力综合征，289
    重症肌无力，287
    有机磷中毒，291
视神经脊髓炎（NMO），99-101，239-241，239f
神经元迁移和组织异常，145
神经疾病
    基于症状的鉴别诊断，255t
    遗传，255t
神经病理性疼痛，257，259t
神经病
    疼痛，255t
    周围神经病，259
        分类和病因，251t
        糖尿病神经病变，261
        实验室检查，257t
        单神经病，253t，257-259
        对症治疗，259t
    中毒性，261
    血管炎性，251
神经刺激器，209
新发每日持续性头痛，85
非陈述性记忆，53
非营养不良性肌强直，281
NREM 异态睡眠，33
营养，老年人，313
眼球震颤，93-95，109，111t

O

强迫症，61
枕叶癫痫，197
枕神经痛，89
奥瑞珠单抗，治疗多发性硬化，237
奥法木单抗，治疗多发性硬化，237-239
老年人
    护理过渡，317
    临床照护，299-303，303t
        认知，307
        共病，303
        失禁，309-313，313t
        功能，303
        听觉，309
        期望寿命，303，305t
        药物，305-307
        活动能力，309，311t
        心理健康，307-309
        营养，313
        睡眠，309
        视觉，309
    照护，319
    住院患者，315
    疾病表现，303-305，305t
    社会和法律问题，313-315
        预定医疗指示，315
        照护，313-315
        财务，315
        虐待，315
    照护系统，317-319
少突胶质细胞瘤，223
橄榄脑桥小脑变性，严重小脑功能障碍，121-123

昂丹司琼，治疗酒精中毒，353
眼科，腹侧诱导障碍，141-143
眼底镜检查，97
阿片类药物滥用，331
阿片类药物危机，331
阿片类药物
    滥用，357t-361t

equianalgesic table for, 328t
palliative care in, 330
in renal or hepatic insufficiency, 326
in traumatic brain injury, 182
Opium, 356t-360t
Optic nerve, compression of, 100
Optic neuritis, 98-100
Optic neuropathy, 98-100
ischemic, 100
Optical coherence tomography, in multiple sclerosis, 228
Organophosphate poisoning, 290
Organophosphorus compounds (OPs), 290
Orthostatic blood pressure, 70-72, 70f
Orthostatic hypotension, 68, 72
treatment of, 72t
Orthostatic intolerance, 70
Otosclerosis, 104
Oxcarbazepine, 206t
Oxycodone, 326, 328t
Oxygen free radicals, aging and, 294-296
Ozanimod, for multiple sclerosis, 236

P

Pain, 326-330
intensity of, in headache, 86-88
neuropathic, 256, 258t
Palliative care, 322-340, 326f
common illness trajectories and, 324-326
chronic illness with exacerbations and sudden dying, 324
prolonged dwindling, 324-326
severe acute brain injury, 326
short period of evident decline before death, 324
communication and care coordination in, 334-336
diagnostic tests and invasive procedures in, role and use of, 336
estimating and communicating prognosis, 334-336
ethical challenges in, 338-340
feeding tube questions, 338-340
futile treatment in, 338
last hours and days of living and, 338
negotiating goals of care, 334, 336t
patient capacity and surrogate decision making in, 338
to patients and families, 326
physical symptoms in, 326-332
prospectus for future, 340
request for hastened death in, 340
role of hospice in, 336-338
suffering and symptom management in, 326-334
Palsy, ulnar, 258
Panic attacks, 60, 204
Paradoxical embolism, stroke caused by, 160
Paradoxical insomnia, 32
Paralyses, periodic, 280-282
Paraneoplastic cerebellar degeneration, 134
Parasomnias, 32-34
Parenteral nutrition
in traumatic spinal cord injury, 186
Parinaud syndrome, 92-94
Parkinsonism, 116-122, 120t-122t
atypical, 120-122
diagnosis of, red flags in, 122t
differential diagnosis for, 120t
idiopathic Parkinson's disease, 116-120
medications for, 124t
secondary, 122
Parkinson's disease, 50
Paroxysmal dyskinesias, 132
Pentobarbital, to induce coma, 182
Perimysium, 264
Periodic limb movement disorder (PLMD), 30

等效镇痛剂量表，329t
缓和医疗，331
肾功能不全或者肝功能不全，327
颅脑损伤，183
鸦片，357t-361t
视神经受压，101
视神经炎，99-101
视神经病，99-101
缺血性，101
光学相干断层成像，多发性硬化，229
有机磷中毒，291
有机磷化合物（OP），291
直立位血压，71-73，71f
体位性低血压，69，73
治疗，73t
直立不耐受，71
耳硬化症，105
奥卡西平，207t
羟考酮，327，329t
氧自由基，老化，295-297
奥扎莫德，治疗多发性硬化，237

P

疼痛，327-331
强度，头痛，87-89
神经病理性，257，259t
缓和医疗，323-341，327f
常见疾病轨迹，325-327
慢性疾病加重和突然死亡，325
长期缓慢衰退，325-327
严重急性脑损伤，327
离世前短期内明显衰退，325
沟通与照护协调，335-337
诊断性检查和侵入性措施，作用和使用，337
评估和沟通预后，335-337
伦理挑战，339-341
喂食管路相关问题，339-341
无效治疗，339
临终前最后数小时及数天，339
协商照护目标，335，337t
患者能力和替代决策，339
患者和家人，327
躯体症状，327-333
未来展望，341
加速死亡的请求，341
安宁疗护的作用，337-339
痛苦与症状管理，327-335
麻痹，尺神经，259
惊恐发作，61，205
反常栓塞，引起卒中，161
矛盾性失眠，33
周期性瘫痪，281-283
副肿瘤性小脑变性，135
异态睡眠，33-35
肠外营养
外伤性脊髓损伤，187
帕里诺综合征，93-95
帕金森综合征，117-123，121t-123t
非典型，121-123
诊断，"红旗征"，123t
鉴别诊断，121t
特发性帕金森病，117-121
药物，125t
继发性，123
帕金森病，51
发作性运动障碍，133
戊巴比妥，诱导昏迷，183
肌束膜，265
周期性肢体运动障碍（PLMD），31

Periodic limb movements in sleep, 30
Periodic paralyses, 280-282
Peripheral nerves, disorders of, 250-256
Peripheral neuropathy, 258
    classification and causes of, 250t
    diabetic, 260
    laboratory studies of, 256t
    mononeuropathies, 252t, 256-258
    polyneuropathies
        acquired, specific, 258-260
        hereditary, 260
    symptomatic treatment for, 258t
Persistent depressive disorder, 56
Persistent vegetative states (PVS), 22
Personality, definition of, 66
Personality disorders, 60t, 66
Petit mal, 194, 194f
Petit mal epilepsy, 198
Phencyclidine (PCP), 368
Phenobarbital, 206t
Phenothiazine, for migraine, 80
Phenytoin, 206t
    in traumatic brain injury, 182
Phobia, 60
Phosphenes, 100
Photopsias, 100
Physiologic anisocoria, 92-94
Plasma membrane, 264
Plasmapheresis
    for Guillain-Barré syndrome, 258-260
    for myasthenia gravis, 286
Plexopathy
    brachial, 248
    lumbosacral, 250
Poisoning
    organophosphate, 290
Polymyalgia rheumatica (PMR)
    with giant cellarteritis, 86
Polyneuropathies, 258-260
    acquired, specific, 258-260
    hereditary, 260
    symmetrical axonal, 250
Polyradiculoplexopathy, lumbosacral, diabetic, 260
Polysomnography (PSG), 26
Population aging, 294
Port-wine birthmark, in Sturge-Weber syndrome, 152
Positron emission tomography (PET)
    for epilepsy, 202
    functional imaging, 12
Post-concussive syndrome (PCS), 182
Posterior cerebral artery (PCA), stroke associated with, 158, 164t
Postherpetic neuralgia, 88
Postictal phase, 192
Postictal state, 14
Post-traumatic headache, 86
Post-traumatic stress disorder, 60-62
Prechiasmal pathway, 92
Prednisone
    for myasthenia gravis, 286
    for temporal arteritis, 86
Pregabalin, 206t
Pregnancy
    alcohol consumption in, 352
    management during and after, 212
Presbycusis, 102-104
Prevalent muscular dystrophies, 274t
Primary exertional headache, 84
Primary lateral sclerosis, 248
Primary stabbing headache, 84

睡眠周期性肢体运动, 31
周期性瘫痪, 281-283
周围神经疾病, 251-257
周围神经病, 259
    分类和病因, 251t
    糖尿病性, 261
    实验室检查, 257t
    单神经病, 253t, 257-259
    多发性神经病
        特殊获得性, 259-261
        遗传性, 261
    对症治疗, 259t
持续性抑郁障碍, 57
持续植物状态（PVS）, 23
人格, 定义, 67
人格障碍, 61t, 67
小发作, 195, 195f
癫痫小发作, 199
苯环己哌啶（PCP）, 369
苯巴比妥, 207t
吩噻嗪类, 治疗偏头痛, 81
苯妥英, 207t
    颅脑损伤, 183
恐惧症, 61
光幻视, 101
闪光感, 101
生理性瞳孔不等, 93-95
质膜, 265
血浆置换
    吉兰-巴雷综合征, 259-261
    重症肌无力, 287
神经丛病
    臂丛神经病, 249
    腰骶丛神经病, 251
中毒
    有机磷, 291
风湿性多肌痛（PMR）
    巨细胞动脉炎, 87
多发性神经病, 259-261
    特殊获得性, 259-261
    遗传性, 261
    对称性轴索性, 251
糖尿病腰骶多发性神经根神经丛病, 261
多导睡眠监测（PSG）, 27
人口老龄化, 295
葡萄酒色胎记, 见于 Sturge-Weber 综合征, 153
正电子发射断层成像（PET）
    癫痫, 203
    功能成像, 13
脑振荡后综合征（PCS）, 183
大脑后动脉（PCA）, 与卒中相关, 159, 165t
带状疱疹后神经痛, 89
发作后期, 193
发作后状态, 15
外伤后头痛, 87
创伤后应激障碍, 61-63
视交叉前通路, 93
泼尼松
    重症肌无力, 287
    颞动脉炎, 87
普瑞巴林, 207t
妊娠
    饮酒, 353
    孕期和产后管理, 213
老年性耳聋, 103-105
常见的肌营养不良, 275t
原发性劳力性头痛, 85
原发性侧索硬化, 249
原发性针刺样头痛, 85

Prion infection, dementia and, 52
Program of All-inclusive Care for the Elderly (PACE), 318
Program theories, 294
Progressive multifocal leukoencephalopathy (PML)
    natalizumab associated with, 234
Progressive muscular atrophy, 248
Progressive supranuclear palsy (PSP), 122
Propofol, to induce coma, 182
Proportionate palliative sedation, 340
Pseudotumor cerebri, 100
Psilocybin, 356t-360t
Psychiatric syndromes, 56, 58t
    causes of, 58t
Psychogenic amnesia, 52-54
Psychogenic unresponsiveness, 22
Psychological distress, 332-334
Psychophysiologic insomnia, 32
Psychosis, 64
Psychotic disorders, 64-66, 64t
Ptosis, 94
    myasthenia gravis and, 286
Pulmonary embolism
    in older adult, 304t
Pupillary reactivity, in coma, 18
Pupils, examination of, 92-96, 96f
Pursuit eye movements, 96
Pyridostigmine
    for Lambert-Easton myasthenic syndrome, 288
    for myasthenia gravis, 286

Q
Quadrantanopsias, 92

R
Radiculopathy, cervical, 88-90
Ramelteon, for insomnia, 32
Rapid eye movement behavior disorder, 32-34
Rapid-onset dystonia, 130
Reflex epilepsies, 198
Respiratory depression, with opioid use, 326-330
Restraints, in confused older adults, 306
Retrograde amnesia, 52
Rett syndrome, 146
Rinne test, 102
Rum fits, 346-348

S
Saccadic eye movements, 96
Salicylates, hearing loss caused by, 106
Salvia divinorum, 356t-360t
Schizencephaly, 144
Schizoaffective disorder, 64
Schizophrenia, 64
Schwannomas
    in neurofibromatosis, 150
    vestibular, 104, 104f
Scotomas, 92
    scintillating, 92
Secondarily generalized tonic-clonic seizures, 192-194
Sedative-hypnotics, abuse of, 356t-360t
Sedatives, abuse of, 354-362
Seizures, 188. *See also* Epilepsy
    brain tumor causing, 216-218
    classification of, 190-192
    electrographic, 192
    febrile, 200
    focal, 192-194
    generalized, 190-192

朊病毒感染，痴呆，53
老年人全包式照护方案（PACE），319
程序理论，295
进行性多灶性白质脑病（PML）
    那他珠单抗，235
进行性肌萎缩，249
进行性核上性麻痹（PSP），123
丙泊酚，诱导昏迷，183
适度缓和镇静，341
假性脑瘤，101
赛洛西宾，357t-361t
精神病综合征，57，59t
    病因，59t
心因性遗忘症，53-55
心因性反应迟钝，23
心理困扰，333-335
心理生理性失眠，33
精神病，65
精神病性障碍，65-67，65t
上睑下垂，95
    重症肌无力，287
肺栓塞
    老年人，305t
瞳孔对光反射，昏迷时，19
瞳孔，检查，93-97，97f
追踪眼球运动，97
溴吡斯的明
    兰伯特-伊顿肌无力综合征，289
    重症肌无力，287

Q
象限偏盲，93

R
颈神经根病，89-91
雷美替安，治疗失眠症，33
快速眼动行为障碍，33-35
快速发作的肌张力障碍，131
反射性癫痫，199
呼吸抑制，阿片类药物使用，327-331
约束，意识障碍老年人，307
逆行性遗忘，53
Rett 综合征，147
林纳试验，103
朗姆酒发作，347-349

S
眼扫视运动，97
水杨酸盐，引起听力损失，107
墨西哥鼠尾草，357t-361t
脑裂畸形，145
分裂情感障碍，65
精神分裂症，65
神经鞘瘤
    神经纤维瘤病，151
    前庭神经鞘瘤，105，105f
暗点，93
    闪光暗点，93
继发性全面性强直-阵挛发作，193-195
镇静催眠药，滥用，357t-361t
镇静药，滥用，355-363
癫痫发作，189；参见癫痫
    脑肿瘤导致，217-219
    分类，191-193
    电图性，193
    热性惊厥，201
    局灶性，193-195
    全面性，191-193

nonconvulsive, 20
partial, 192
in stroke, acute, 168
subclinical, 192
symptomatic causes of, 188, 190t
in traumatic brain injury, early onset, 182
Self-care capacity, 302
Semiology, of seizure, 192
Septo-optic dysplasia, 140
Serotonin agonists, for migraine, 80
Serum creatinekinase, elevated causes for, 268, 274t
Short-lasting unilateral neuralgiform headache with conjunctival tearing, 84
Short-term memory, 52
Shy-Drager syndrome, 120-122
Simple partial seizure (SPS), 192
Single Item Alcohol Screening Questionnaire (SASQ), 348
Single-photon emission computed tomography (SPECT), for epilepsy, 202
Siponimod, for multiple sclerosis, 236
Skeletal muscle fibers, 264
Sleep, disorders of, 26-34
    agents promoting wakefulness for, 28t
    excessive daytime sleepiness in, 26
    idiopathic hypersomnia in, 28-30
    insomnia in, 30-32
    Kleine-Levin syndrome in, 30
    narcolepsy in, 28
    in older adults, 308
    parasomnias in, 32-34
    periodic limb movement disorder in, 30
    sleep-disordered breathing in, 26-28
Sleep hygiene, 32, 32t
Sleep medications, 356t-360t
Sleep paralysis, narcolepsy with, 28
Sleep terrors, 32
Sleepwalking, 32
Sleep-disordered breathing, 26-28
Sleep-state misperception, 32
Small cell lung carcinoma (SCLC)
    Lambert-Easton myasthenic syndrome with, 288
Small-fiber neuropathies, 254
Snellen chart, 92, 94f
Social phobia, 60
Sodium oxybate, in narcolepsy, 28
Somatic symptom disorders, 60, 60t, 66
Sphenoidal sinusitis, 84
Spina bifida, 138
Spinal cord compression
    cervical spondylosis with, 88-90
Spinal cord injury, traumatic, 180-186
    future of, 186
    management of, 182-184
    prognosis of, 186, 186t
Spinal cord syndromes, 184
Spinal fluid analysis, in multiple sclerosis, 228
Spinal muscular atrophy (SMA), 248
Spinal shock, 184
Spinocerebellarataxia, 132
Spiritual suffering, 334
Sporadic Alzheimer disease, 48t
Sporadic inclusion body myositis, 282-284
Sporadic/acquired ataxias, 134
Stapedectomy, 104
Statins, for stroke prevention, 176
Status epilepticus, 208-210, 210t
    nonconvulsive, 20
Status migrainosus, 76
Stenting
    for cardiac complications, 174
Stimulants, 356t-360t

非惊厥性发作，21
部分性发作，193
急性卒中，169
亚临床，193
症状性发作的病因，189，191t
颅脑损伤，早期发作，183
自理能力，303
症状学，癫痫发作，193
透明隔-视神经发育不良，141
5-羟色胺激动剂，治疗偏头痛，81
血清肌酸激酶，升高的原因，269，275t
伴结膜充血和流泪的短暂性单侧神经痛样头痛，85
短期记忆，53
Shy-Drager 综合征，121-123
简单部分性发作（SPS），193
单项酒精筛查问卷（SASQ），349
单光子发射计算机断层成像（SPECT），用于癫痫，203
西尼莫德，治疗多发性硬化，237
骨骼肌纤维，265
睡眠障碍，27-35
    促觉醒药物，29t
    白天过度嗜睡，27
    特发性嗜睡症，29-31
    失眠，31-33
    克莱恩-莱文综合征，31
    发作性睡病，29
    老年人，309
    异态睡眠，33-35
    周期性肢体运动障碍，31
    睡眠呼吸障碍，27-29
睡眠卫生，33，33t
催眠药，357t-361t
睡眠麻痹，发作性睡病，29
睡惊症，33
睡行症，33
睡眠呼吸障碍，27-29
失眠状态错觉，33
小细胞肺癌（SCLC）
    兰伯特-伊顿肌无力综合征，289
小纤维神经病，255
斯内伦视力表，93，95f
社交恐惧症，61
羟丁酸钠，治疗发作性睡病，29
躯体症状障碍，61，61t，67
蝶窦炎，85
脊柱裂，139
脊髓压迫症
    颈椎病，89-91
脊髓损伤，外伤性，181-187
    未来展望，187
    管理，183-185
    预后，187，187t
脊髓综合征，185
脑脊液分析，多发性硬化，229
脊髓性肌萎缩（SMA），249
脊髓休克，185
脊髓小脑性共济失调，133
精神痛苦，335
散发性阿尔茨海默病，49t
散发性包涵体肌炎，283-285
散发性/获得性共济失调，135
镫骨足板切除术，105
他汀类药物，卒中预防，177
癫痫持续状态，209-211，211t
    非惊厥性，21
偏头痛持续状态，77
支架置入
    心脏并发症，175
兴奋剂，357t-361t

Stroke
    definition of, 154
    epidemiology of, 154
    ischemic, 154, 164
        acute treatment of, 170-172, 172t
        clinical manifestations of, 164t
        evidence-based primary prevention of, 170t
    mimics and differential diagnosis of, 168t
    prevention of
        primary, 170
        secondary, 174-176
    rehabilitation and recovery of, 174
    risk factors for, 156t
    treatment of, 168-176
Sturge-Weber syndrome, 152
Subarachnoid hemorrhage, 164
    coma associated with, 14
Subcortical dementia, 46t
Subependymal giant cell astrocytomas (SEGA), for tuberous sclerosis complex, 150
Sudomotor failure, 70
Sumatriptan, 80
Supplementary motor seizures, 198
Swinging light test, 92
Sydenham chorea, 126t, 128
Symmetrical axonalpolyneuropathies, 250
Symptomatic generalized epilepsies, 198
Syncope
    convulsive, 204
Syringomyelia, 140
Systemic disorders, myopathies caused by, 284

T

Tardive dyskinesia, medications and, 128
Telomerase
    aging and, 298
Temozolomide, for glioblastoma, 220
Temporal lobe epilepsy (TLE), 196-198
Temporal lobe seizures, 192t
Tensilon test, 286
Tension-type headache, 82-84
Teratogenicity, 212
Teriflunomide, for multiple sclerosis, 236
Δ-Tetrahydrocannabinol (THC), 332
Thiamine
    deficiency of, in Korsakoff syndrome, 52
Third cranial nerve palsy, 94
Thoughts, major disorders of, 56, 60t
Thrombolytic therapy
    for stroke, ischemic, 170-172
Thunderclap headache, 84
Thymectomy, for myasthenia gravis, 286
Thymoma
    myasthenia gravis and, 286
Tics, 130-132
"Timed get up and go" (TUG), 308
Tinnitus, 100, 102f
    subjective, 100-102
Tissue biopsies, neurologic, 6-8
Todd paralysis, 168, 194
Tonic pupils, 96
Tonic seizure, 196
Topiramate, 206t
    for alcoholism, 352
Tourette syndrome, 130-132
Toxic myopathies, 284
Toxic-induced neuropathies, 260
Transient global amnesia, 52
Transient ischemic attack (TIA), 158

卒中
    定义，155
    流行病学，155
    缺血性，155，165
        急性期治疗，171-173，173t
        临床表现，165t
        循证一级预防，171t
    卒中模拟病和鉴别诊断，169t
    预防
        一级，171
        二级，175-177
    康复治疗，175
    危险因素，157t
    治疗，169-177
Sturge-Weber综合征，153
蛛网膜下腔出血，165
    昏迷，15
皮质下痴呆，47t
室管膜下巨细胞星形细胞瘤（SEGA），结节性硬化症，151
汗腺功能衰竭，71
舒马普坦，81
辅助运动区癫痫，199
摆动光测试，93
Sydenham舞蹈症（小舞蹈症），127t，129
对称性轴索性多发性神经病，251
症状性全面性癫痫，199
晕厥
    惊厥性，205
脊髓空洞症，141
系统性疾病，导致肌病，285

T

迟发性运动障碍，药物，129
端粒酶
    老化，299
替莫唑胺，治疗胶质母细胞瘤，221
颞叶癫痫（TLE），197-199
颞叶癫痫发作，193t
依酚氯铵试验，287
紧张型头痛，83-85
致畸性，213
特立氟胺，治疗多发性硬化，237
Δ-四氢大麻酚（THC），333
维生素B₁
    缺乏，见于科萨科夫综合征，53
第Ⅲ脑神经麻痹，95
思维，主要思维障碍，57，61t
溶栓治疗
    缺血性卒中，171-173
霹雳性头痛，85
胸腺切除术，治疗重症肌无力，287
胸腺瘤
    重症肌无力，287
抽动症，131-133
"起立-行走"计时测试（TUG），309
耳鸣，101，103f
    主观性，101-103
组织活检，神经系统，7-9
Todd瘫痪，169，195
强直性瞳孔，97
强直发作，197
托吡酯，207t
    酒精中毒，353
抽动秽语综合征，131-133
中毒性肌病，285
中毒性神经病变，261
短暂性全面性遗忘，53
短暂性脑缺血发作（TIA），159

Transverse myelitis (TM), 98-100
    acute, 240-242
Tremor, 122-124, 124t
    action, 122
    essential, 122-124, 124t
    intention, 122
Tricyclic antidepressants
    for neuropathic pain, 258t
    tension-type headache and, 84
Trigeminal autonomic cephalgia, 82
Trigeminal neuralgia, 88
Triptans, for migraine, 80
Tube feeding
    palliative care and, 338-340
Tuberin, 150
Tuberous sclerosis complex (TSC), 150-152
    clinical presentation of, 150
    definition/epidemiology, 150
    diagnosis/differential, 150
    pathology of, 150
    prognosis for, 150-152
    treatment for, 150

U

Ulnar palsy, 258
Ultrasonography
    of carotid arteries, 12
    vertebral arteries, 12
Uncinate seizures, 196-198
Urinary incontinence, causes, type, and treatment of, 312t

V

Vagal failure, 70
Valproate, 206t
Varenicline, for alcoholism, 352
Vascular dementia, 50
Vascular malformations, epilepsy associated with, 202
Vasculitic neuropathies, 250
Vasogenic edema, brain tumor causing, 222
Vegetative states, persistent, 22
Vena cava filter
    inpatients with traumatic spinal cord injury, 184
Ventral induction, disorders of, 140-144
    clinical presentation of, 142
    definition/epidemiology, 140
    diagnosis/differential, 142
    pathology/embryology, 140-142, 142f
    prognosis for, 144
    treatment of, 144, 144t
Ventriculoperitoneal shunt, 86
Vertebral arteries, 158
Vertigo, 76, 108-114
    benign paroxysmal positional, 110, 112f
    clinical presentation of, 108-110
    definition, 108
    differential diagnosis for, 110-112, 110t
    differentiating central from peripheral, 108, 110t
    epidemiology, 108
    treatment for, 112-114
    vestibular schwannoma with, 104
Vestibular schwannomas, hearing loss and, 104, 104f
Vestibular system, basic concepts of, 108
Vestibulo-ocular reflex, 108
Viral myositis, acute, 284
Vision, eye movement and, disorders of, 92-100
    binocular visual loss, 100
    visual system, examination of, 92-98, 94f
        acuity in, 92

横贯性脊髓炎（TM），99-101
    急性，241-243
震颤，123-125，125t
    动作性，123
    特发性，123-125，125t
    意向性，123
三环类抗抑郁药
    神经病理性疼痛，259t
    紧张型头痛，85
三叉神经自主神经性头痛，83
三叉神经痛，89
曲普坦类，治疗偏头痛，81
管饲
    缓和医疗，339-341
Tuberin 蛋白，151
结节性硬化症（TSC），151-153
    临床表现，151
    定义和流行病学，151
    诊断与鉴别诊断，151
    病理学，151
    预后，151-153
    治疗，151

U

尺神经麻痹，259
超声检查
    颈动脉，13
    椎动脉，13
钩回发作，197-199
尿失禁的分类、病因和治疗，313t

V

迷走神经功能衰竭，71
丙戊酸，207t
伐尼克兰，治疗酒精中毒，353
血管性痴呆，51
血管畸形，癫痫，203
血管炎性神经病，251
血管源性水肿，脑肿瘤引起，223
持续植物状态，23
腔静脉滤器
    外伤性脊髓损伤住院患者，185
腹侧诱导，障碍，141-145
    临床表现，143
    定义和流行病学，141
    诊断与鉴别诊断，143
    病理学与胚胎学，141-143，143f
    预后，145
    治疗，145，145t
脑室腹腔分流术，87
椎动脉，159
眩晕，77，109-115
    良性阵发性位置性，111，113f
    临床表现，109-111
    定义，109
    鉴别诊断，111-113，111t
    中枢性与周围性的鉴别，109，111t
    流行病学，109
    治疗，113-115
    前庭神经鞘瘤，105
前庭神经鞘瘤，听力损失，105，105f
前庭系统，基本概念，109
前庭-眼反射，109
急性病毒性肌炎，285
视觉与眼动疾病，93-101
    双眼视力丧失，101
    视觉系统，检查，93-99，95f
        视力，93

eye movements in, 96, 98f, 98t
funduscopy in, 96-98, 98f
monocular visual loss, 98-100
oculomotor function, components of, 96
pupils in, 92-96, 96f
visual fields in, 92, 94f
Visual fields, 92, 94f
Visual hallucinations, 100
　in diffuse Lewy body disease, 50
Visual illusions, 100
Visual loss
　binocular, 100
　giant cellarteritis with, 86
　monocular, 98-100
Visual-evoked potential studies, 8
Vitamin B_2, for migraine prevention, 80-82
Vitamin B_{12} (cobalamin)
　deficiency, ataxia and, 134
Vitamin deficiency, in older adult, 304t
Vitamin E
　deficiency of, ataxia and, 134
Vomiting
　headache with, 84
　in palliative care, 330-332

W

Wallenberg syndrome, 158
Warfarin
　for stroke prevention
　　primary, 170
　　secondary, 174
Weber test, 102
Wernicke aphasia, 40
Wernicke encephalopathy, 352
West syndrome, 200
Wilson's disease, 128, 130f
Withdrawal syndrome, 346-348

Z

Zonisamide, 206t

眼球运动, 97, 99f, 99t
眼底镜检查, 97-99, 99f
单眼视力丧失, 99-101
眼球运动功能, 组成成分, 97
瞳孔, 93-97, 97f
视野, 93, 95f
视野, 93, 95f
幻视, 101
　弥漫性路易体病, 51
视错觉, 101
视力丧失
　双眼, 101
　巨细胞动脉炎, 87
　单眼, 99-101
视觉诱发电位检查, 9
维生素 B_2, 预防偏头痛, 81-83
维生素 B_{12}（钴胺素）
　缺乏, 共济失调, 135
维生素缺乏症, 老年人, 305t
维生素 E
　缺乏, 共济失调, 135
呕吐
　头痛, 85
　缓和医疗, 331-333

W

Wallenberg 综合征, 159
华法林
　卒中预防
　　一级, 171
　　二级, 175
韦伯试验, 103
Wernicke 失语症（感觉性失语症）, 41
韦尼克脑病, 353
West 综合征, 201
肝豆状核变性, 129, 131f
戒断综合征, 347-349

Z

唑尼沙胺, 207t